GRIEVE'S MODERN MUSCULOSKELETAL PHYSIOTHERAPY

For Elsevier:
Senior Content Strategist: Rita Demetriou-Swanwick
Content Development Specialist: Nicola Lally
Project Manager: Umarani Natarajan
Designer/Design Direction: Miles Hitchen
Illustration Manager: Lesley Frazier
Illustrator: Graphic World Illustration Studio

GRIEVE'S MODERN MUSCULOSKELETAL PHYSIOTHERAPY

FOURTH EDITION

Edited by

Gwendolen Jull Dip Phty, Grad Dip Manip Ther, MPhty, PhD, FACP
Emeritus Professor, Physiotherapy, School of Health and Rehabilitation Sciences, University of Queensland, Brisbane, Australia

Ann Moore PhD, FCSP, FMACP, Dip TP, Cert Ed
Professor of Physiotherapy and Head of the Centre for Health Research, School of Health Sciences, University of Brighton, UK

Deborah Falla BPhty (Hons), PhD
Professor, Pain Clinic, Center for Anesthesiology, Emergency and Intensive Care Medicine
Professor, Department of Neurorehabilitation Engineering
Universitätsmedizin Göttingen, Georg-August-Universität, Germany

Jeremy Lewis BApSci (Physio), PhD, FCSP
Consultant Physiotherapist, London Shoulder Clinic, Centre for Health and Human Performance, London, UK
Consultant Physiotherapist, Central London Community Healthcare NHS Trust, UK
Professor (Adjunct) of Musculoskeletal Research, Clinical Therapies, University of Limerick, Ireland
Reader in Physiotherapy, School of Health and Social Work, University of Hertfordshire, UK

Christopher McCarthy PhD, FCSP, FMACP
Consultant Physiotherapist, St Mary's Hospital, Imperial College Healthcare, UK

Michele Sterling PhD, MPhty, BPhty, Grad Dip Manip Physio, FACP
Director, CRE in Road Traffic Injury
Associate Director, Centre of National Research on Disability and Rehabilitation (CONROD)
Professor, School of Allied Health, Menzies Health Institute Queensland, Griffith University, Australia

Foreword by
Karim Khan MD, PhD, FASCM
Editor of the British Journal of Sports Medicine
Director, Department of Research & Education, Aspetar Orthopaedic and Sports Medicine Hospital, Qatar
Professor, Faculty of Medicine, University of British Columbia, Canada

ELSEVIER

Edinburgh   London   New York   Oxford   Philadelphia   St Louis   Sydney   Toronto 2015

ELSEVIER

First edition 1986
Second edition 1994
Third edition 2005

Chapter 44.b: Model B: Linda-Joy Lee. LJ Lee Physiotherapist Corp retains copyright to illustrations.

Chapter 46.b: The Pelvic Girdle: A Look at How Time, Experience And Evidence Change Paradigms: Diane Lee retains copyright to her own illustrations.

ISBN 978-0-7020-5152-4

Notices

Knowledge and best practice in this field are constantly changing. As new research and experience broaden our understanding, changes in research methods, professional practices, or medical treatment may become necessary.

Practitioners and researchers must always rely on their own experience and knowledge in evaluating and using any information, methods, compounds, or experiments described herein. In using such information or methods they should be mindful of their own safety and the safety of others, including parties for whom they have a professional responsibility.

With respect to any drug or pharmaceutical products identified, readers are advised to check the most current information provided (i) on procedures featured or (ii) by the manufacturer of each product to be administered, to verify the recommended dose or formula, the method and duration of administration, and contraindications. It is the responsibility of practitioners, relying on their own experience and knowledge of their patients, to make diagnoses, to determine dosages and the best treatment for each individual patient, and to take all appropriate safety precautions.

To the fullest extent of the law, neither the Publisher nor the authors, contributors, or editors, assume any liability for any injury and/or damage to persons or property as a matter of products liability, negligence or otherwise, or from any use or operation of any methods, products, instructions, or ideas contained in the material herein.

your source for books, journals and multimedia in the health sciences
www.elsevierhealth.com

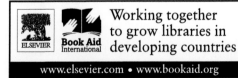
Working together to grow libraries in developing countries
www.elsevier.com • www.bookaid.org

The publisher's policy is to use paper manufactured from sustainable forests

Printed and bound in the United Kingdom

Last digit is the print number: 9 8 7 6 5 4 3 2

Contents

■ PART V
FUTURE DIRECTIONS

PREFACE TO THE FOURTH EDITION

The first edition of *Grieve's Modern Manual Therapy: The Vertebral Column* was published in 1986 and its editor was the late Gregory Grieve. The convention of a roughly 10 year period between editions has been preserved for the fourth edition of this seminal text. Time is needed to allow for the furtherance of research and the knowledge base and for its translation to clinical practice. A review of the content of the four editions of this text is not unexpectedly, witness to the major changes in knowledge, evidence base, practice and its delivery over the past 30 years.

There has been a change in title of the text, from *Grieve's Modern Manual Therapy* to *Grieve's Modern Musculoskeletal Physiotherapy*. This change has been made to reflect historical development. Physiotherapists have been practising manipulative therapy from the early part of the 20th century under successive medical mentors such as Edgar Cyriax and James Mennell and subsequently under James Cyriax, John Mennell and the leading osteopath, Alan Stoddard. It was in the 1950s and 1960s that leading physiotherapists developed concepts or methods of manipulative therapy practice that were eagerly sought by the physiotherapy world internationally. These early concepts placed a major focus on articular dysfunction. Manipulative therapy and/or manual therapy became a method of management, as reflected in the title of the earlier editions of this text. The last 20 years in particular have seen quite significant shifts in models of musculoskeletal pain and care which have spurred and directed contemporary practice and research. Musculoskeletal disorders are now well embedded within a biopsychosocial context which provides a wider understanding and appreciation of the associated pain, functional impairments and activity limitations. Advances in the neurosciences (e.g. the pain sciences, sensorimotor sciences) as well as the behavioural sciences have changed practice. The earlier concepts and practices of manipulative therapy have grown and developed and transitioned into more comprehensive methods of management. It was therefore time to make the title of this fourth edition reflective of contemporary practice. Hence the name change to *Grieve's Modern Musculoskeletal Physiotherapy*.

Since the third edition of this text was published, the physiotherapy world has been saddened by the passing of some of the original leaders in the field, namely Geoffrey Maitland, Robin McKenzie and Robert (Bob) Elvey. All had a passion for the discipline and for enhanced patient care. We are sure that they along with Gregory Grieve would be pleased with the way the clinical art and evidence base of manipulative and musculoskeletal physiotherapy has and will continue to develop. This text with contributions from contemporary researchers and clinicians is built upon their legacy.

GJ
AM
DF
JL
CM
MS

Australia, United Kingdom, Germany 2015

ACKNOWLEDGEMENTS

There are approximately 140 international researchers and clinicians who have contributed to this multi-authored text and the editors thank them sincerely for not only their chapters, but for the years of work and experience behind their words. They are all to be congratulated on outstanding work. They are often forging new territory that translates into new or better quality assessment and management practices to the benefit of both the patients and practitioners. You are all making a significant contribution to musculoskeletal physiotherapy internationally.

Thanks are also given to the publishers Elsevier, Oxford and in particular to Rita Demetriou-Swanwick and Veronika Watkins who started the ball rolling and to Nicola Lally who rolled the ball to the finish line. Thanks are given to all Elsevier staff 'behind the scenes' for their work in collating and copy-editing all chapters to bring this complex text to fruition.

Finally, the editors would like to acknowledge the work of Jeffrey Boyling who was the lead editor of the second and third editions of *Grieve's Modern Manual Therapy*. We as editors of this fourth edition are very well aware of your vision for these previous and acclaimed editions. On behalf of the readership, we thank you for your contribution and the massive amount of work and time you devoted to this important international text. Fly high in your (semi) retirement!

GJ
AM
DF
JL
CM
MS

Australia, United Kingdom, Germany 2015

FOREWORD

If you are a physiotherapist and you see patients of any age with musculoskeletal problems then this book is your best value investment. Investment in the broad sense – a valuable way to use your time and cognitive effort. If you teach at any level of a physiotherapy programme, this book will broaden your appreciation for your profession no matter how well trained you are. If you are a student, by definition passionate about health with a spirited love of life, you will find this book both a crutch and a ladder.

Grieve's Modern Musculoskeletal Physiotherapy captures the wisdom of over 100 of the world's leading physiotherapists and scientists in related fields. It was created in 11 countries. You are holding 500,000 hours of expertise in your hands. That would take you 250 years to acquire solo.

One of the joys of life is being on a steep learning curve. It is not marketed the way travel companies promote lounging poolside with a drink. But think of schussing through an alpine forest or conversing fluently in a new language. Think of any occasion when you have gained mastery and you know the buzz of negotiating a steep learning curve successfully.

This revamped edition of *Grieve's* guides you to professional pleasures. For me, the wisdom and clarity of illustration in Chapter 7 (Neuromuscular adaptations to exercise) is just one an example. Chapter 31 (Therapeutic exercise) provided a remarkably novel approach for this old dog. High quality science mashes up with practical relevance. See Chapter 1 for a concise overview of the chapters and the innovations.

In the 3rd edition foreword, Lance Twomey wrote 'This is a bold book.' A decade later, *Grieve's* 4th edition is not an evolution – it is a revolution. It is a complete synthesis of the different clinically successful physiotherapy approaches that satisfy patients the world over. It outlines patient-based approaches that are far greater than a sum of techniques. It captures how physiotherapy science and practice have advanced dramatically decade over decade since Gregory Grieve launched his almost 900-page tome in 1986.

Today's 53 chapters codify musculoskeletal physiotherapy that has the power to make a difference in every patient encounter. It provides an incontrovertible storyline that physiotherapy benefits from practice-based evidence and is a solidly evidence-based practice. The comprehensive nature of *Grieve's* adds to credibility by demonstrating a body of knowledge that distinguishes the musculoskeletal physiotherapy specialisation. As *Modern Musculoskeletal Physiotherapy*, this 'extended scope' 4th edition of *Grieve's* adds substantial value to an even broader group of the physiotherapy profession than did its vertebral column serving predecessors.

On behalf of all those who will benefit from this opus, I congratulate and thank the leadership team – Professors Gwen Jull, Ann Moore, Deborah Falla, Jeremy Lewis, Christopher McCarthy and Michele Sterling – together with each contributor to this book, for extending and very strongly reinforcing the field of modern musculoskeletal physiotherapy. The multi-year international commitment to *Grieve's* reflects the respect the editors have earned; they inspired, cajoled, and I suspect occasionally begged, to assemble a physiotherapy dream team. And judging by the team balance, the 5th and 6th editions are in good hands.

Karim Khan, MBBS, PhD, MBA
Director, Department of Research & Education
Aspetar Orthopaedic and Sports Medicine
Hospital, Qatar
Professor, Faculty of Medicine, University of British
Columbia, Canada

CONTRIBUTORS

Michael Adams BSc, PhD
Professor of Biomechanics, Centre for Comparative
  and Clinical Anatomy, University of Bristol, UK
Visiting Professor, Sir Run Run Shaw Hospital,
  Zheijang University, China

Caroline Alexander PhD, MSc, Grad Dip Phys
NIHR Senior Clinical Lecturer, Physiotherapy,
  Imperial College Healthcare NHS Trust
NIHR Senior Clinical Lecturer, Surgery and Cancer,
  Imperial College London, UK

Panos Barlas BSc, DPhil, LicAc
School of Health and Rehabilitation,
  Keele University, UK

Harsimran Singh Baweja BPT, PhD
Assistant Professor, Exercise and Nutritional Sciences,
  Physical Therapy, San Diego State University, USA

**Darren Beales BSc (Physiotherapy), M Manip
Ther, PhD**
Research Fellow, School of Physiotherapy and Exercise
  Science, Curtin University, Perth, Australia

David Beckwée MSc
Postdoctoral Researcher at the Vrije Universiteit
  Brussel (Brussels, Belgium) and Teacher at the
  Stichting Opleiding Musculoskeletale Therapie
  (SOMT) (Amersfoort, The Netherlands)
Department of Physiotherapy, Vrije University,
  Belgium

Kim Bennell BAppSci (Physio), PhD
Professor, Department of Physiotherapy, University of
  Melbourne, Melbourne, Australia

Joel E Bialosky PhD, PT
Clinical Assistant Professor, Physical Therapy,
  University of Florida, Gainesville, USA

**Leanne Bisset PhD, MPhty (Manipulative), MPhty
(Sports), BPhty**
Senior Lecturer, School of Rehabilitation Sciences,
  Griffith University, Gold Coast, Australia

John D Borstad PT, PhD
Associate Professor, Physical Therapy, Ohio State
  University, Columbus, USA

**Kathy Briffa BAppSc(Physiotherapy), Grad Dip Sports
Physiotherapy, MAppSc (Health Sc), PhD**
School of Physiotherapy and Exercise Science, Curtin
  University, Perth, Australia

**Rachelle Buchbinder MBBS (Hons), MSc,
PhD, FRACP**
Director, Monash Department of Clinical
  Epidemiology, Cabrini Institute
Professor, Department of Epidemiology and Preventive
  Medicine, School of Public Health and Preventive
  Medicine, Monash University, Melbourne, Australia

Barbara Cagnie PT, PhD
Assistant Professor, Rehabilitation Sciences and
  Physiotherapy, Ghent University, Ghent, Belgium

Lynne Caladine EdD, MSc
Head of School, School of Health Professions,
  University of Brighton, UK

Valentina Camomilla PhD
Doctor, Department of Movement, Human and Health
  Sciences, University of Rome 'Foro Italico', Italy

Aurelio Cappozzo PhD
Professor of Movement, Human and Health Sciences,
  University of Rome 'Foro Italico', Italy

Marco Cardinale PhD, MSc, BSc
Head of Sports Physiology, Sports Science, Aspire
  Academy, Doha, Qatar
Honorary Reader, Computer Science, University
  College London, London
Honorary Senior Lecturer, Medical Sciences,
  University of Aberdeen, Aberdeen, UK

Andrea Cereatti PhD
Assistant Professor, Information Engineering Unit,
  POLCOMING Department, University of Sassari,
  Sassari, Italy

**Helen Clare PhD, MAppSc, GradDipManipTher,
DipPhty**
Director of Education, McKenzie Institute
  International, Wellington, New Zealand
Director, Helen Clare Physiotherapy, Sydney, Australia

Nicholas Clark PhD, MSc, MCSP, MMACP, CSCS
Senior Lecturer in Sport Rehabilitation, School of
Sport, Health and Applied Science, St Mary's
University, Twickenham, London, UK

Gray Cook MSPT, OCS, CSCS
Co-Founder, Functional Movement Systems, Chatham,
UK

Jill Cook PhD, BAppSci
Professor, School of Primary Health Care, Monash
University, Virginia, Australia

Brooke Coombes BPhty, MPhty, Phd
Post-doctorate Research Fellow, Physiotherapy
Division, University of Queensland, Brisbane,
Australia

Michel W Coppieters PhD, PT
Professor, Move Research Institute, VU University
Amsterdam, Amsterdam, The Netherlands

**Sallie Cowan BAppSc (Physio), Grad Dip Manip
Physio, PhD**
Senior Research Fellow, Department of Physiotherapy,
University of Melbourne
Senior Research Fellow, Physiotherapy, St Vincents
Hospital, Melbourne
Director, Clifton Hill Physiotherapy, Melbourne,
Australia

Kay Crossley PhD, BAppSc (Physio)
School Health Rehab Sciences, University of
Queensland, Brisbane, Australia

Wim Dankaerts PT, MT, PhD
Musculoskeletal Rehabilitation Research Unit,
Department of Rehabilitation Sciences, Faculty of
Kinesiology and Rehabilitation Sciences, University
of Leuven, Leuven, Belgium

Lieven Danneels PT, PhD
Professor, Department of Physical Therapy and Motor
Rehabilitation, Ghent University, Ghent, Belgium

Elizabeth Dean PhD, MS, DipPT, BA
Professor, Physical Therapy, University of British
Columbia, Vancouver, Canada

Margot De Kooning MSc
Departments of Human Physiology and Physiotherapy,
Vrije University
Faculty of Medicine and Health Sciences, Antwerp
University, Antwerp, Belgium

Mark de Zee PhD
Associate Professor, Department of Health Science and
Technology, Aalborg University, Aalborg, Denmark

Patricia Dolan BSc, PhD
Reader in Biomechanics, Centre for Comparative and
Clinical Anatomy, University of Bristol, Bristol, UK
Visiting Professor, Sir Run Run Shaw Hospital,
Zheijang University, Zheijang, China

Jaap van Dieën PhD
Professor, Faculty of Human Movement Sciences,
University of Amsterdam, Amsterdam,
The Netherlands

Linda van Dillen PhD, PT
Associate Director of Musculoskeletal Research,
Professor of Physical Therapy, Professor of
Orthopaedic Surgery, Washington University School
of Medicine in St Louis, St Louis, USA

James Elliott PT, PhD
Assistant Professor, Physical Therapy and Human
Movement Sciences, Feinberg School of Medicine,
Northwestern University, Chicago and St Lucia,
USA
Honorary Senior Fellow, School of Health and
Rehabilitation Sciences, University of Queensland,
Brisbane, Chicago and St Lucia, Australia

Deborah Falla BPhty (Hons), PhD
Professor, Pain Clinic, Center for Anesthesiology,
Emergency and Intensive Care Medicine
Professor, Department of Neurorehabilitation
Engineering, Universitätsmedizin Göttingen, Georg-
August-Universität, Germany

Dario Farina PhD
Professor and Chair, Director of the Department,
Bernstein Center for Computational Neuroscience,
Bernstein Focus Neurotechnology Goettingen,
Department of Neurorehabilitation Engineering,
University Medical Center Goettingen, Georg-
August University, Germany

Michael Farrell BAppSc (Phty), MSc, PhD
Senior Research Fellow, Imaging, Florey Institute of
Neuroscience and Mental Health
Honorary Senior Research Fellow, Anatomy and
Neuroscience, University of Melbourne, Melbourne,
Australia

Kjartan Fersum PhD, MSc, Bsc
Researcher, Department of Global Public Health
and Primary Care, University of Bergen, Bergen,
Norway

**Gail Forrester-Gale MSc (Manual Therapy),
BSc Hons (Physiotherapy), PgCertificate Education,
MMACP; MCSP**
Senior Lecturer in Physiotherapy, Physiotherapy
Subject Group, Exercise, Sport and Rehabilitation,
Department of Applied Science and Health,
Coventry University, Coventry, UK

Simon French PhD, MPH, BAppSc
Assistant Professor, School of Rehabilitation Therapy,
Faculty of Health Sciences, Queen's University,
Kingston, Canada

Julie Fritz PT, PhD
Professor, Physical Therapy, University of Utah, Salt
Lake City, USA

**Graham Galloway BSc (H),
Grad Cert Comp Sci, PhD**
Professor, Centre for Advanced Imaging, University of
Queensland, Brisbane, Australia

Jill Gamlin MSc, Grad Dip Phys
Consultant Physiotherapist, Cambridgeshire,
Cambridge, UK

Sabata Gervasio PhD, MSc EE
Research Assistant, Health Science and Technology,
Aalborg University, Aalborg, Denmark

Karen Ginn PhD, MHPEd, GDManipTher, GDPhty
Associate Professor, Discipline of Biomedical Science,
Sydney Medical School, University of Sydney,
Sydney, Australia

Charlie Goldsmith BSc, MSc, PhD
Maureen and Milan Ilich/Merck Chair in Statistics for
Arthritis and Musculoskeletal Diseases, Arthritis
Research Centre of Canada
Professor of Biostatistics, Faculty of Health Sciences,
Simon Fraser University, Richmond, Burnaby and
Hamilton
Emeritus Professor of Biostatistics, Clinical
Epidemiology and Biostatistics, McMaster University,
Canada

**Sally Green PhD, BAppSci (Physiotherapy), Grad Dip
(Manipulative Physiotherapy)**
Professorial Fellow, School of Public Health and
Preventive Medicine, Monash University, Melbourne,
Australia

Susan Greenhalgh PhD, MA, GDPhys, (FCSP)
Doctor, Elective Orthopaedics, Bolton NHS
Foundation Trust, Bolton, UK

Alison Grimaldi BPhty, MPhty (Sports), PhD
Director, Physiotec Physiotherapy, Brisbane, Australia

Hubert van Griensven PhD, MSc (Pain), BSc, DipAc
Research Fellow, Centre for Health Research, School
of Health Sciences, University of Brighton,
Brighton, UK
Consultant Physiotherapist, Department of
Rehabilitation, Southend University Hospital NHS
Foundation Trust, Southend, UK

Jeremy Grimshaw MB ChB, PhD
Senior Scientist, Clinical Epidemiology Program,
Ottawa Hospital Research Institute
Professor, Department of Medicine, University of
Ottawa, Ottawa, Canada

Anita Gross BEcPT, MSc, Grad Dip MT
Associate Clinical Professor, Rehabilitation Science,
McMaster University
Clinical Lecturer, Physical Therapy, Western
University, Hamilton, London, Canada

Toby Hall MSc, PhD
Adjunct Associate Professor, School of Physiotherapy,
Curtin University of Technology
Senior Teaching Fellow, University of Western
Australia, Perth, Australia,

Stephen Harridge PhD
Professor, Centre of Human and Aerospace
Physiological Sciences, King's College London,
London, UK

Jan Hartvigsen PhD
Professor, Department of Sports Science and Clinical
Biomechanics, University of Southern Denmark
Senior Researcher, Nordic Institute of Chiropractic and
Clinical Biomechanics, Odense, Denmark

Eric Hegedus BSBA, MHSc, DPT
Professor and Chair, Physical Therapy, High Point
University, High Point, USA

Nicola Heneghan PhD, MSc
Birmingham, School of Sport, Exercise and
Rehabilitation Sciences, University of Birmingham,
Birmingham, UK

Lee Herrington PhD, MSc, BSc (Hons)
Senior Lecturer in Sports Rehabilitation, School of
Health Sciences, University of Salford
Technical Lead Physiotherapist, Physiotherapy, English
Institute of Sport, Manchester, UK

Jonathan Hill PhD, MSc, BSc
Lecturer in Physiotherapy, Arthritis Research UK
Primary Care Centre, Keele University, Keele, UK

Claire Hiller PhD, MAppSc, BAppSc
Research Fellow, Faculty of Health Sciences, University
of Sydney, Sydney, Australia

Rana Hinman BPhysio, PhD
Department of Physiotherapy, School of Health
Sciences, University of Melbourne, Melbourne,
Australia

Paul Hodges PhD, MedDr, DSc, BPhty (Hons)
Director, CCRE Spine, School of Health and
Rehabilitation Sciences, University of Queensland,
Brisbane, Australia

Melanie Holden PhD, BSc (Hons)
Doctor, Arthritis Research UK Primary Care Centre, Keele University, Keele, UK

Alan Hough PhD, BA (Hons), Grad Dip Phys
Honorary Associate Professor, School of Health Professions (NC), Faculty of Health & Human Sciences (NC), Plymouth University, Plymouth, UK

Venerina Johnston PhD, BPhty (Hons), Grad Cert OHS, (Cert Work Disability Prevention)
Academic, Division of Physiotherapy, University of Queensland, Brisbane, Australia

Gwendolen Jull Dip Phty, Grad Dip Manip Ther, MPhty, PhD, FACP
Emeritus Professor, Department of Physiotherapy, School of Health and Rehabilitation Sciences, University of Queensland, Brisbane, Australia

Joanne Kemp MSportsPhysio, BAppSc (Physio)
PhD Candidate, School of Health and Rehabilitation Sciences, University of Queensland, Brisbane
Research Associate, Australian Centre of Research into Injury in Sport and its Prevention (ACRISP), Federation University, Ballarat
Principal Physiotherapist, Bodysystem, Hobart, Australia

Justin Kenardy PhD
CONROD, University of Queensland, Brisbane, Australia

Peter Kent BAppSc (Physio), BAppSc (Chiro), Grad Dip (Manipulative Physiotherapy), PhD
Associate Professor, Institute of Sports Science and Clinical Biomechanics, University of Southern Denmark
Clinical Associate Professor, Institute of Regional Health Research, University of Southern Denmark, Odense, Denmark

Roger Kerry MSc
Associate Professor, Faculty of Medicine and Health Science, University of Nottingham, Nottingham, UK

Henri Kiers MSc
Human Movement Scientist, Physiotherapist, Research Group Lifestyle and Health, University of Applied Sciences Utrecht, Utrecht, The Netherlands

Kyle Kiesel PT, PhD
Professor, Physical Therapy, University of Evansville, Evansville, USA

Idsart Kingma PhD
Associate Professor, Human Movement Scientist, Research Institute MOVE, Faculty of Human Movement Sciences, VU University Amsterdam, Amsterdam, The Netherlands

Diane Lee BSR FCAMT
Director, Diane Lee & Associates, South Surrey, Canada

Linda-Joy Lee PhD, BSc(PT), BSc
Director of Curriculum & Mentorship, Dr Linda-Joy Lee Physiotherapist Corporation, North Vancouver
Founder & Director, Synergy Physiotherapy, North Vancouver, Canada
Honorary Senior Fellow, Physiotherapy, University of Melbourne, Australia
Associate Member, Centre for Hip Health & Mobility, Vancouver, Canada

Scott Lephart PhD
Dean and Professor, College of Health Sciences, Endowed Chair of Orthopaedic Research, University of Kentucky
Lexington, USA

Jeremy Lewis PhD, FCSP
Consultant Physiotherapist, London Shoulder Clinic, Centre for Health and Human Performance
Consultant Physiotherapist, Central London Community Healthcare NHS Trust, UK
Professor (Adjunct) of Musculoskeletal Research, Clinical Therapies, University of Limerick, Limerick, Ireland
Reader in Physiotherapy, School of Health and Social Work, University of Hertfordshire, London, UK

Ian Loram MA, PhD
Professor of Neuromuscular Control of Human Movement, Cognitive Motor Function Research Group, School of Healthcare Science, Manchester Metropolitan University, Manchester, UK

James Henry McAuley PhD
Senior Lecturer (Conjoint), Neuroscience Research Australia, School of Medical Sciences, University of New South Wales, Sydney, Australia

Christopher McCarthy PhD, FCSP, FMACP
Lead Orthopaedic Practitioner, St Mary's Hospital, Imperial College Healthcare, London, UK

Jenny McConnell BAppSci (Phty), Grad Dip Man Ther, M Biomed Eng
Visiting Senior Fellow, Melbourne University, Australia

Joy MacDermid PhD
Professor, Rehabilitation Sciences, McMaster University, Hamilton, Canada

Martin Mackey PhD, MSafetySc, GradDipEducStud(HigherEduc), BAppSc(Physio), BEc
Doctor, Senior Lecturer, Physiotherapy, University of Sydney, Sydney, Australia

Katie McMahon PhD, Hons, BSc
Doctor, Centre for Advanced Imaging, University of Queensland, Brisbane, Brisbane
Honorary Fellow, Wesley Research Institute, Australia

Stephen May MA, FCSP, Dip MDT, MSc, PhD
Doctor, Faculty of Health and Wellbeing, Sheffield Hallam University, Sheffield, UK

Claudia Mazzà PhD
Lecturer, Mechanical Engineering, University of Sheffield, Sheffield, UK

Niamh A Moloney BPhysio, MManipulative Therapy, PhD
Lecturer, Physiotherapy, University of Sydney, Sydney, Australia

Ann Moore PhD, FCSP, FMACP, Dip TP, Cert Ed
Professor of Physiotherapy and Head of the Centre for Health Research, School of Health Sciences, University of Brighton, Brighton, UK

Jane Morris Ed D, MA, GradDipPhys, MCSP, PG Cert HE, FHEA
Deputy Head of School, School of Health Sciences University of Brighton, Brighton, UK

Natalie Mrachacz-Kersting BSc, MEd, PhD
Associate Professor, Health Science and Technology, Aalborg University, Aalborg, Denmark

Robert J Nee PT, PhD, MAppSc
Associate Professor, Physical Therapy, Pacific University, Hillsboro, USA

Jo Nijs PhD, PT, MT
Associate Professor, Pain in Motion Research Group, Departments of Human Physiology and Rehabilitation Sciences, Faculty of Physical Education and Physiotherapy, Vrije Universiteit Brussel, Brussel, Belgium

Tze Siong Ng BSc (Hons) Physiotherapy, MA (Manual Therapy)
Senior Principal Physiotherapist, Ms, Rehabilitation, National University Hospital, Singapore

Shaun O'Leary BPhty(Hons), MPhty(Msk), PhD
Principal Research Fellow, CCRE (Spinal Pain Injury and Health), University of Queensland, Brisbane, Australia

Peter Osmotherly BSc, Grad Dip Phty, M Med Sci
Senior Lecturer in Physiotherapy, School of Health Sciences, University of Newcastle, Newcastle, Australia

Kieran O'Sullivan PhD, M Manip Ther, B Physio
Lecturer, Department of Clinical Therapies, University of Limerick, Limerick, Ireland

Peter O'Sullivan PhD
Professor, Physiotherapy, Curtin University, Perth, Australia

Ioannis Paneris BSc (Hons), MSc, MCSP, MMACP
Extended Scope Practitioner, Community and Medicine, Central Manchester University Hospitals – NHS Foundation Trust, Manchester, UK

Ruth Parry MCSP, MMedSci, PhD
Principal Research Fellow, Supportive, Palliative and End of Life Care Research Group, University of Nottingham, UK

George Peat PhD
Professor of Clinical Epidemiology, Arthritis Research UK Primary Care Centre, Keele University, Keele, UK

Nicola Petty DPT, MSc
Principal Lecturer, Centre for Health Research, School of Health Sciences, University of Brighton, Brighton, UK

Harry von Piekartz PhD, MSc PT
Professor, Department of Movement Science, University of Applied Science, Osnabrück Germany

Tania Pizzari PhD, BPhysio (Hons)
Doctor, Physiotherapy, La Trobe University, Melbourne, Australia

Ross Pollock BSc, MSc, PhD
Doctor, Centre of Human and Aerospace Physiological Sciences, King's College London, London, UK

Annelies Pool-Goudzwaard PhD, PT, MT
Senior Researcher, Neuroscience, Faculty of Medicine and Health Sciences, Erasmus MC University, Rotterdam, The Netherlands

John Rasmussen MSc, PhD
Professor, Mechanical and Manufacturing Engineering, Aalborg University, Aalborg, Denmark

Maree Raymer B Phty (Hons), MPhty St (Msk), Masters Health Management
Assistant Program Manager, Statewide Neurosurgical and Orthopaedic Physiotherapy Screening Clinics and Multidisciplinary Service, Physiotherapy, Royal Brisbane and Women's Hospital, Brisbane, Australia

Kathryn M Refshauge PhD, MBiomedE, GradDipManipTher, DipTher
Professor, Faculty of Health Sciences, University of Sydney, Sydney, Australia

Ebonie Rio BAppSci, BA Phys (Hons), Masters Sports Phys, PhD candidate
PhD Researcher, Physiotherapy Department, Monash University, Frankston, Australia

Darren A Rivett BAppSc(Phty), GradDipManipTher, MAppSc(ManipPhty), PhD
Professor of Physiotherapy, School of Health Sciences, University of Newcastle, Newcastle, Australia

Ulrik Röijezon PhD, PT
Assistant Professor, Department of Health Sciences, Luleå University of Technology, Luleå, Sweden

Shirley Sahrmann PT, PhD
Professor Emeritus, Physical Therapy, Washington University School of Medicine, St Louis, USA

Siobhan Schabrun PhD, BPhysio (Hons)
NHMRC Clinical Research Fellow, School of Science and Health, University of Western Sydney
Honorary Senior Fellow, School of Health and Rehabilitation Science, University of Queensland, Brisbane, Australia

Axel Meender Schäfer PhD
Verw Prof, Faculty of Social Work and Health, University of Applied Science and Art, Hildesheim, Germany

Annina Schmid PhD, MManipTher, PT OMT svomp
Post Doctoral Research Fellow, Nuffield Department of Clinical Neurosciences, Oxford University, Oxford, UK
School of Health and Rehabilitation Sciences, University of Queensland, Brisbane, Australia

Quentin Scott BPHTY, Post Grad Dip Manip Ther, FACP
Specialist Musculoskeletal Physiotherapist, Milton Physiotherapy, Brisbane, Australia

Hazel Screen BEng, MRes, PhD
Reader in Biomedical Engineering and Deputy Director of Taught Programmes, School of Engineering and Materials Science, Queen Mary University of London, London, UK

James Selfe PhD, MA, GDPhys, FCSP
Professor of Physiotherapy, School of Sport, Tourism and The Outdoors, University of Central Lancashire, Preston, UK

Jane Simmonds PD, MA, PGDIP, PGCHE, BAPP(SC), BPE
Professional Lead Physiotherapy, Allied Health and Midwifery, University of Hertfordshire
Clinical Specialist, Hypermobility Unit, Hospital of St John and St Elizabeth, London, UK

Kevin P Singer PhD, PT
Winthrop Professor, Surgery, University of Western Australia, Perth, Australia

Kathleen Sluka PT, PhD
Professor, Neurobiology of Pain Laboratory, University of Iowa, Iowa, USA

Ashley Smith PT, PhD(c)
PhD Student, University of Queensland Director, Evidence Sport and Spinal Therapy, Calgary, Canada, Division of Physiotherapy, NHMRC Centre of Clinical Excellence Spinal Pain, Injury and Health, University of Queensland, Brisbane, Australia

Anne Söderlund PhD, RPT
Professor, Physiotherapy, School of Health, Care and Social Welfare, Malardalen University, Västerås, Sweden

Michele Sterling PhD, MPhty, BPhty, Grad Dip Manip Physio, FACP
Associate Director of the Centre of National Research on Disability and Rehabilitation Medicine (CONROD)
Professor in the Centre of Musculoskeletal Research and the School of Allied Health, Griffith University, Brisbane, Australia

Maria Stokes PhD FCSP
Professor of Musculoskeletal Rehabilitation, Faculty of Health Sciences, University of Southampton, Southampton, UK

Leon Straker PhD, MSc, BAppSc
Professor of Physiotherapy, School of Physiotherapy and Exercise Science, Curtin University, Perth Australia

Peter William Stubbs BSc, MPhty, PhD
Research Officer, Neuroscience Research Australia, Australia
Post Doctoral Fellow, Research Department, Hammel Neurorehabilitation and Research Center, Aarhus University, Aarhus, Denmark

Brigitte Tampin Physio, Grad Dip Manip Ther, MSc, PhD
Adjunct Research Fellow, School of Physiotherapy and Exercise Science, Curtin University
Department of Physiotherapy, Sir Charles Gairdner Hospital, Perth Australia

Alan Taylor MCSP, MSc
Lecturer, Physiotherapy and Rehabilitation Sciences, University of Nottingham, Nottingham, UK

Carolyn Taylor BAppSc (Exercise & Sports Science), BAppSc (Physiotherapy)
Lecturer in Physiotherapy, La Trobe Rural Health School, La Trobe University, Melbourne, Australia

Julia Treleaven BPhty, PhD
Lecturer, CCRE Spine, Division of Physiotherapy, University of Queensland, Brisbane, Australia

Peter Vaes PhD
Head of Department, Rehabilitation Sciences and Physiotherapy, Vrije University of Brussels, Brussels, Belgium

Giuseppe Vannozzi PhD
University Researcher, Motor, Human and Health Sciences, University of Rome 'Foro Italico', Rome, Italy

Bill Vicenzino PhD, MSc, BPhty, GradDipSportsPhty
Professor, Division of Physiotherapy, School of Health and Rehabilitation Sciences, University of Queensland, Brisbane, Australia

Anne Wajon BAppSc (Phty), MAppSc (Phty), PhD
Director, Macquarie Hand Therapy, Macquarie University, Sydney, Australia

David Walton BScPT, MSc, PhD
Assistant Professor, School of Physical Therapy, Western University, London, Canada

Lyn Watson BAppSc Physio
Clinical Shoulder Physiotherapy Specialist, LifeCare, Prahran Sports Medicine Centre and Melbourne Orthopaedic Group, Prahran, Australia

Tim Watson PhD, BSc, FCSP
Professor of Physiotherapy, Department of Allied Health Professions and Midwifery, University of Hertfordshire, Hatfield, UK

Rod Whiteley PhD
Research & Education Physiotherapist, Rehabilitation Department, Aspetar Sports Medicine Hospital, Doha, Qatar

Nienke Willigenburg PhD
Post-Doctoral Student, Human Movement Scientist, Division of Sports Medicine, Sports Health and Performance Institute, Ohio State University, Ohio USA

PLATE 1

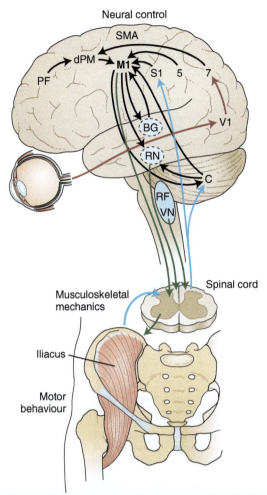

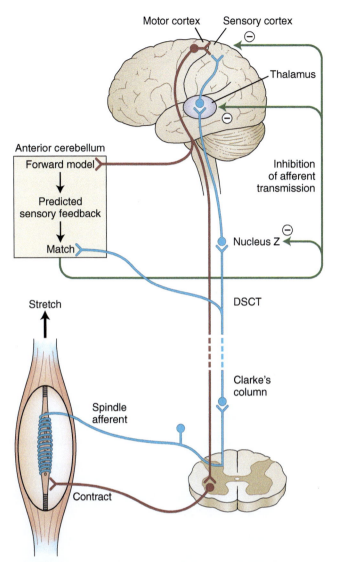

FIGURE 4-2 ■ Sensorimotor pathways through the central nervous system. The central nervous system is conventionally viewed as having a hierarchical organization with three levels: the spinal cord, brainstem and cortex. The spinal cord is the lowest level, including motor neurons, the final common pathway for all motor output, and interneurons that integrate sensory feedback from the skin, muscle and joints with descending commands from higher centres. The motor repertoire at this level includes stereotypical multijoint and even multilimb reflex patterns, and basic locomotor patterns. At the second level, brainstem regions such as the reticular formation (*RF*) and vestibular nuclei (*VN*) select and enhance the spinal repertoire by improving postural control, and can vary the speed and quality of oscillatory patterns for locomotion. The highest level of control, which supports a large and adaptable motor repertoire, is provided by the cerebral cortex in combination with subcortical loops through the basal ganglia and cerebellum.[36] Motor planning and visual feedback are provided through several parietal and premotor regions. The primary motor cortex (*M1*) contributes the largest number of axons to the corticospinal tract and receives input from other cortical regions that are predominantly involved in motor planning. Somatosensory information is provided through the primary somatosensory cortex (*S1*), parietal cortex area 5 (*5*) and cerebellar pathways. The basal ganglia (*BG*) and cerebellum (*C*) are also important for motor function through their connections with M1 and other brain regions. *RN,* Red nucleus; *V1,* Primary visual cortex; *7,* Region of posterior parietal cortex; *dPM,* Dorsal premotor cortex; *SMA,* Supplementary motor area; *PF,* Prefrontal cortex. (Reproduced with modification from Scott.[38])

FIGURE 4-3 ■ Neural pathways estimating position from sensory and motor information. Integration of muscle spindle afferents with expectations generated from motor output. When the muscle is stretched, spindle impulses travel to sensory areas of the cerebral cortex via Clarke's column, the dorsal spinocerebellar tract (*DSCT*), Nucleus Z, and the thalamus (shown in red). Collaterals of DSCT cells project to the anterior cerebellum. When a motor command is generated, it leads to co-activation of skeletomotor and fusimotor neurons (shown in blue). A copy of the motor command is sent to the anterior cerebellum where a comparison takes place between the expected spindle response based on that command and the actual signal provided by the DSCT collaterals. The outcome of the match is used to inhibit reafferent activity, preventing it from reaching the cerebral cortex. Sites of inhibition could be at Nucleus Z, the thalamus, or the parietal cortex itself. (Reproduced from Proske and Gandevia.[41])

PLATE 2

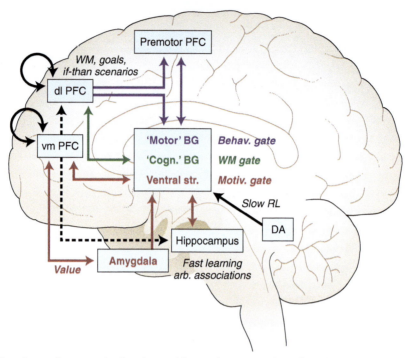

FIGURE 4-4 ■ Access of basal ganglia to motivational, cognitive and motor regions for selection and reinforcement learning. The basal ganglia are a group of interconnected subcortical nuclei that represent one of the brain's fundamental processing units. Interacting corticostriatal circuits contribute to action selection at various levels of analysis. Coloured projections reflect subsystems associated with value/motivation (red), working memory and cognitive control (green), procedural and habit learning (blue), and contextual influences of episodic memory (orange). Sub-regions within the basal ganglia (*BG*) act as gates to facilitate or suppress actions represented in frontal cortex. These include parallel circuits linking the BG with motivational, cognitive, and motor regions within the prefrontal cortex (*PFC*). Recurrent connections within the PFC support active maintenance of working memory (*WM*). Cognitive states in dorsolateral PFC (*dlPFC*) can influence action selection via projections to the circuit linking BG with the motor cortex. Dopamine (*DA*) drives incremental reinforcement learning in all BG regions, supporting adaptive behaviours as a function of experience. (Reproduced from Frank.[22])

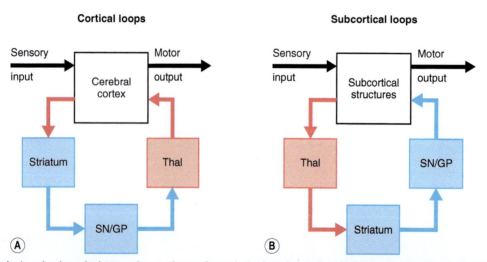

FIGURE 4-5 ■ Cortical and subcortical sensorimotor loops through the basal ganglia. (**A**) For corticobasal ganglia loops the position of the thalamic relay is on the return arm of the loop. (**B**) In the case of all subcortical loops the position of the thalamic relay is on the input side of the loop. Predominantly excitatory regions and connections are shown in red while inhibitory regions and connections are blue. *Thal*, Thalamus; *SN/GP*, Substantia nigra/globus pallidus. (Reproduced from Redgrave.[109])

PLATE 3

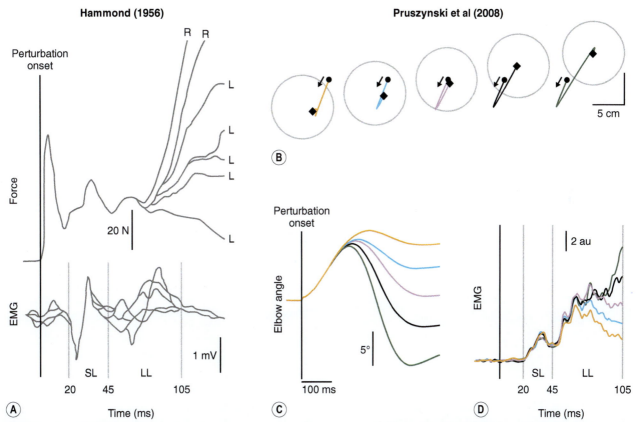

Hammond (1956)

Pruszynski et al (2008)

FIGURE 4-9 ■ Modulation of fast motor response by prior subject intent. **(A)** Example of how subjects can categorically modulate the long-latency (transcortical) stretch response according to verbal instruction. Subjects were verbally instructed to respond to a mechanical perturbation with one of two verbal instructions ('resist'/'let go'). The upper panel depicts force traces from individual trials aligned on perturbation onset and labelled according to the instruction. The bottom panel is the corresponding muscle activity, which shows modulation in the long-latency stretch response (*LL*) but not the short-latency (spinal) stretch response (*SL*). **(B)** Example of how subjects can continuously modulate their long-latency stretch response in accordance with spatial target position. Subjects were instructed to respond to an unpredictable mechanical perturbation by placing their hand inside one of the five presented spatial targets. Each plot represents exemplar hand kinematics as a function of target position. Subjects began each trial at the filled black circle, and the black diamond indicated final hand position. The small arrows indicate the approximate direction of motion caused by the perturbation. **(C)** Temporal kinematics for the elbow joint aligned on perturbation onset. **(D)** Pooled EMG aligned on perturbation onset and normalised to pre-perturbation muscle activity. Note that the long-latency stretch response exhibits graded modulation as a function of target position. (Reproduced from Pruszynski and Scott.[27])

PLATE 4

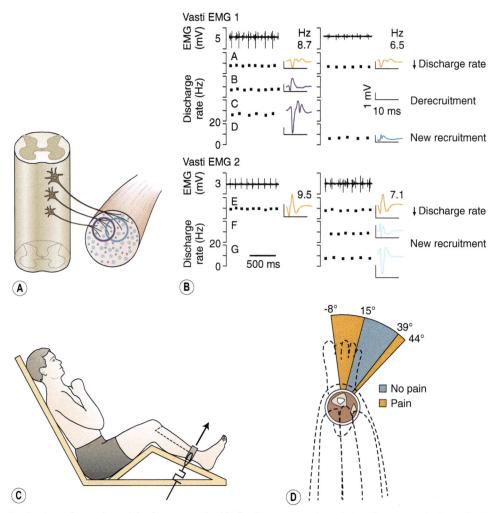

FIGURE 6-3 ■ Redistribution of muscle activity in acute pain. **(A)** During acute pain activity of motor units is redistributed within and between muscles. **(B)** Fine-wire electromyography (EMG) recordings are shown during contractions performed at identical force before (left) and during (right) pain for two recording sites in the vasti muscles. The time of discharge of individual motor units is displayed below the raw EMG recordings. The template for each unit is shown. Pain led to redistribution of activity of the motor units. Units A and E discharged at a slower rate during pain. Units B and C stopped discharging during pain and units F and G, which were not active prior to pain, began to discharge only during pain. These changes indicate that the participant maintained the force output of the muscle, by using a different population of motor units (i.e. redistribution of activity within a muscle). **(C)** Knee extension task. **(D)** The direction of force used by the participants to match the force during contractions with and without pain differed between trials. During pain, participants generated force more medially or laterally than in the pain-free trials. (A, B Redrawn from data from Tucker et al.;[26] C, D redrawn from data from Tucker et al.[64])

PLATE 5

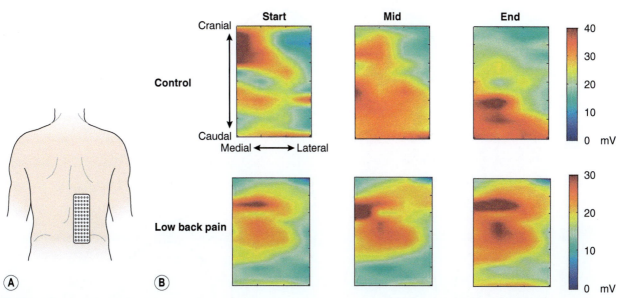

FIGURE 6-4 ■ Reduced redistribution of muscle activation in low back pain. Although healthy individuals redistribute muscle activity to maintain the motor output in the presence of fatigue, this is not observed in people with low back pain. **(A)** A 13 × 5 grid of electromyography electrodes was placed over the lumbar erector spinae in a group of healthy controls and people with chronic low back pain to assess the spatial distribution of erector spinae activity and change in the distribution during performance of a repetitive lifting task for ~200 second. **(B)** Representative topographical maps of the root mean square EMG amplitude from the right lumbar erector spinae muscle for a person with low back pain and a control. EMG maps are shown for the start, mid and end of a repetitive lifting task. Areas of blue correspond to low EMG amplitude and dark red to high EMG amplitude. Note the shift (redistribution) of activity in the caudal direction as the task progresses but for the control subject only. (Reprinted with permission from Falla et al.[17])

PLATE 6

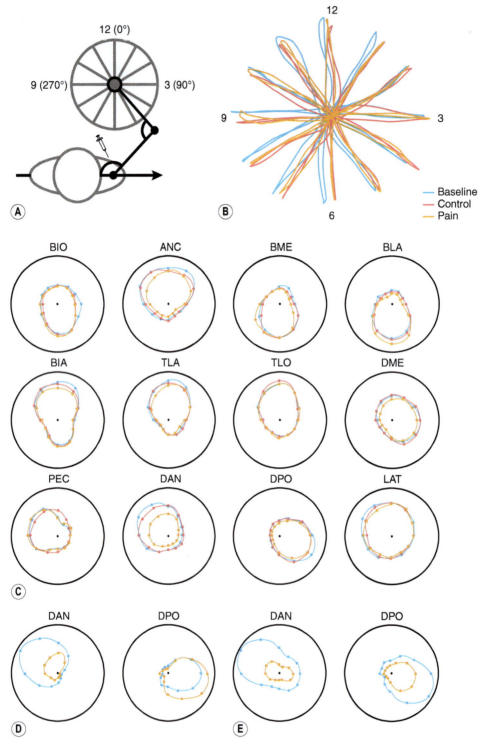

FIGURE 6-5 ■ Changes in muscle activity vary between individuals when challenged by pain, with no few consistent changes across participants. (**A**) Pain-free volunteers (*n*=8) performed multijoint reaching in the horizontal plane using a manipulandum, with the starting point at the centre of the circle. The subject had to reach the 12 targets depicted in A with each reaching movement lasting 1 second followed by a 5 second rest period at the target position before returning to the centre point over 1 second. Subjects performed the task at baseline, and following the injection of isotonic (control) and hypertonic (painful) saline. Saline was injected into the right anterior deltoid (*DAN*) muscle. (**B**) Representative example of endpoint trajectories recorded from one subject during the baseline (blue), control (magenta), and painful (red) conditions. Note that pain did not affect the kinematics of this controlled task. (**C**) Directional tuning of the EMG envelope peak value recorded from 12 muscles during the baseline (blue), the control (magenta), and pain (red) conditions. The 'shrinking' of the pain curves of the DAN muscle was due to a consistent decrease of the EMG activity of this muscle across subjects. Other muscles also change their activity, however the direction of change was different across subjects, demonstrating the variability in subject response. For example, the activity of the posterior deltoid (*DPO*), increased during pain in three subjects while it decreased in five subjects, so that on average it was unchanged. (**D**) Representative data from a single subject showing a decrease in DAN activity with a simultaneous increase in DPO activity during pain. (**E**) In contrast, representative data from another subject shows that decreased DAN activity occurred together with a decrease in DPO activity during pain. *ANC*, Anconeus; *BIA*, Brachialis; *BIO*, Brachioradialis; *BLA*, Lateral head of the biceps brachii; *BME*, Medial head of the biceps brachii; *DME*, Medial deltoid; *LAT*, Latissimus dorsi; *PEC*, Pectoralis major; *TLA*, Lateral head of the triceps brachii; *TLO*, Long head of the triceps brachii. (Reprinted with permission from Muceli et al.[3])

PLATE 7

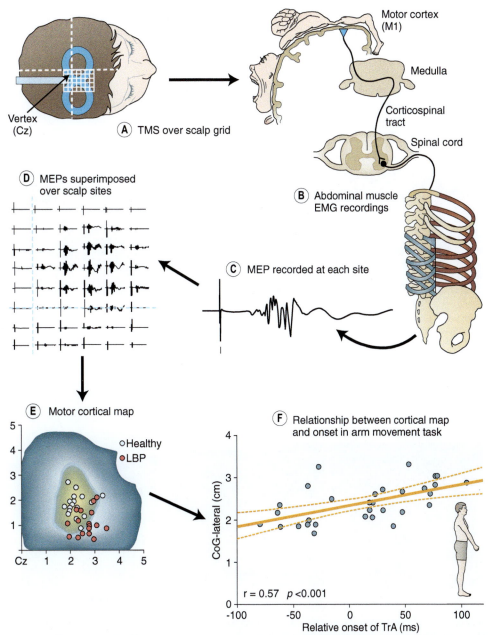

FIGURE 6-7 ■ Changes in motor cortex organization in low back pain. **(A)** Transcranial magnetic stimulation (*TMS*) was applied according to a grid over the motor cortex to stimulate the corticospinal pathway. **(B)** Electromyography was recorded from the transversus abdominis (*TrA*) muscle. **(C)** Motor evoked potentials (*MEP*) were recorded from stimuli applied at each point on the grid. **(D)** The amplitude of MEPs is larger when stimulation is applied to the cortical region with neural input to the muscle. **(E)** The gradient from low (blue) to high (light green) MEP amplitude is shown relative to the vertex (*Cz*). White/blue dots indicate the centre of the region with input to TrA in healthy participants, and the grey/orange indicates that for people with a history of LBP. The centre is positioned further posterior and lateral in the LBP group, providing evidence of reorganization of the motor cortex. **(F)** The degree of reorganization was correlated with the delay of the onset of activation of TrA EMG during an arm movement task.

PLATE 8

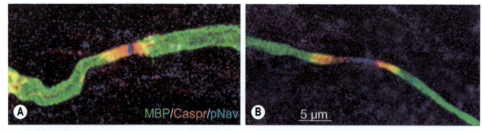

FIGURE 8-4 ■ Patients with CTS have elongated nodes of Ranvier. (**A**) Normal nodal architecture of a dermal myelinated fibre shown by a distinct band of voltage-gated sodium channels (*pNav*, blue) located in the middle of the gap between the myelin sheaths (green, myelin basic protein [*MBP*]). Paranodes are stained with contactin associated protein (*Caspr*, red). (**B**) A dermal myelinated fibre of a patient with carpal tunnel syndrome demonstrating an elongated node with an increased gap between the myelin sheaths. Voltage-gated sodium channels are dispersed within the elongated node.

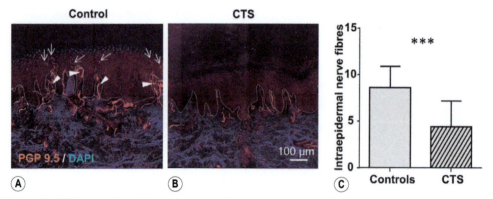

FIGURE 8-5 ■ Patients with CTS have a loss of small fibres. (**A**) Cross-section through a healthy skin taken on the lateropalmar aspect of the second digit. The dermal–epidermal junction is marked with a faint line with the epidermis located on top. Axons are stained with protein gene product 9.5 (a panaxonal marker, red) and cell nuclei are stained with DAPI (blue). There is an abundancy of nerve fibres in the subepidermal plexus as well as inside papillae (arrowheads). Many small fibres pierce the dermal–epidermal junction (arrows). (**B**) Skin of an age- and gender-matched patient with carpal tunnel syndrome (CTS) demonstrates a clear loss of intraepidermal nerve fibres and a less dense subepidermal plexus. (**C**) Graph confirms a substantial loss of intraepidermal nerve fibres (per mm epidermis) in patients with CTS ($p < 0.0001$, mean and standard deviations).

PLATE 9

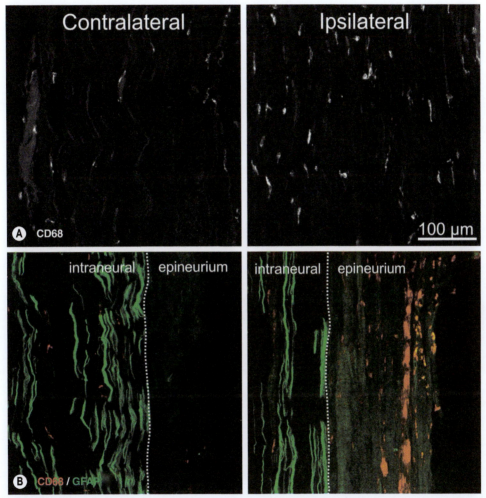

FIGURE 8-6 ■ Experimental mild nerve compression induces a local immune-inflammatory reaction intraneurally as well as in connective tissue. Longitudinal sections through non-operated (left) and mildly compressed (right) sciatic nerves of rats. (**A**) Top panel shows the presence of resident CD68+ macrophages in a non-operated nerve (left) and an intraneural activation and recruitment of macrophages beneath a mild nerve compression (right). (**B**) The activation and recruitment of CD68+ macrophages (red) within the epineurium following mild nerve compression (right) compared to a healthy nerve (left). Schwann cells are stained in green with glial fibrillary acid protein (GFAP).

PLATE 10

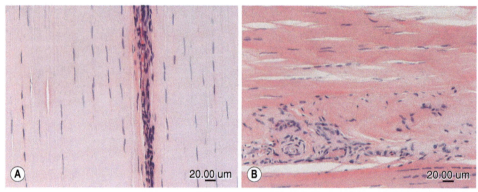

FIGURE 10-5 ■ Histological sections, viewed with a Nikon Eclipse 80i, from the energy-storing equine superior digital extensor tendon. Images compare (**A**) a healthy tendon and (**B**) a tendinopathic tendon. Note the aligned and ordered matrix in the healthy tendon, and clearly differentiated interfascicular matrix. By contrast, the tendinopathic sample shows the disordered matrix, rounded cells and increased cellularity. (Photographs taken in Professor Peter Clegg's laboratory, University of Liverpool.[33])

PLATE 11

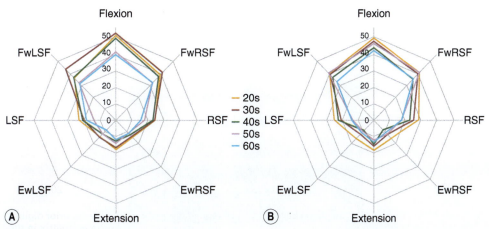

FIGURE 12-3 ■ The decline in range of motion in all planes, observed when using the combined movement examination of the lumbar spine. F, flexion; FwRSF, flexion with right side flexion; RSF, right side flexion; EwRSF, extension with right side flexion; E, extension; EwLSF, extension with left side flexion; LSF, left side flexion; FwLSF, flexion with left side flexion.

PLATE 12

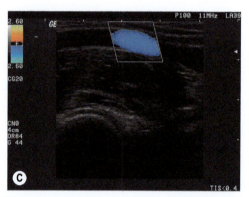

FIGURE 14-1 ■ Types of image display. **(C)** Colour Doppler.

PLATE 13

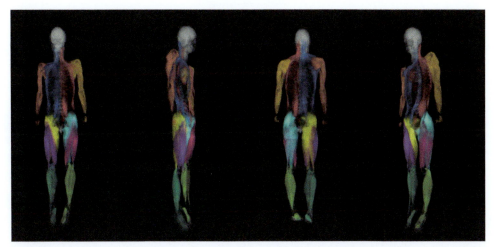

FIGURE 15-3 ■ An example of whole body magnetic resonance imaging using a three-dimensional semi-automated segmentation algorithm where the quantification of specific muscle volume and fat infiltration can be realized. (Images are courtesy of Dr Olof Dahlqvist-Leinhard, Linköping University, Sweden; Advanced MR Analytics http://amraab.se/).

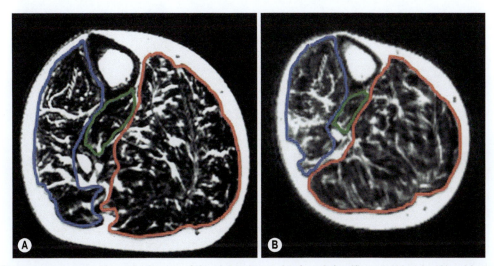

FIGURE 15-4 ■ Magnetic resonance (fat only) image of the right plantar (*red*) and dorsiflexors (*blue*) in (**A**) subject with incomplete spinal cord injury and (**B**) subject with chronic whiplash-associated disorder. Note the increased signal throughout the plantar/dorsiflexors in both subjects, suggestive of fatty infiltrates. Note: The posterior tibialis is highlighted in green.

PLATE 14

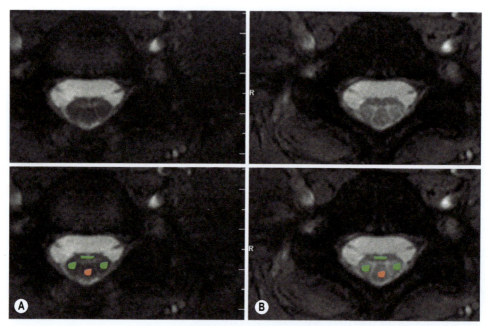

FIGURE 15-5 ■ Anatomically defined regions of interest (ROIs) on the **(A)** magnetization transfer (MT) and **(B)** non-MT-weighted image over the ventromedial and dorsolateral (green in colour plate, arrows in this figure) primarily descending motor pathways and the dorsal column (red in colour plate, circled in this figure) ascending sensory pathways of the cervical spinal cord. The non-magnetization transfer (non-MT) scan (B) is identical except that the MT saturation pulse is turned off and run as a separate co-registered acquisition. The MTR is calculated on a voxel-by-voxel basis using the formula of: MTR = 100*(non-MT − MT)/non-MT.

PLATE 15

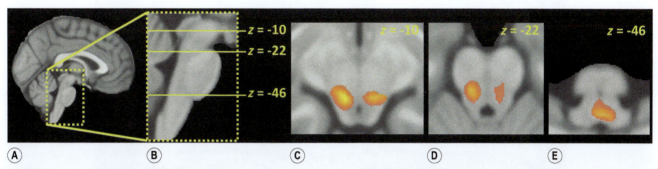

FIGURE 16-1 ■ **(A)** A midline sagittal view of the brain is provided to show the location of the brainstem, which is enclosed within the dashed box. **(B)** The brainstem outlined in panel A is enlarged and transverse lines indicate the axial level of images displayed in the remaining panels. The z-value refers to the distance in mm inferior to the anterior commissure. **(C)** An axial slice through the midbrain shows pain activations encompassing the ventrolateral regions of the periaqueductal grey. The aqueduct is visible on the image as a dark oval region at the midline between the symmetrical activations. **(D)** The parabrachial regions are incorporated within the pain activations on this axial slice at the upper level of the pons. **(E)** An axial slice through the upper (rostral) part of the medulla also cuts through the lowest portion of the pons (grey tissue highest in the panel). The pain activation overlays the midline nucleus raphe magnus, which is the human homologue of the rostroventral medulla in animals.

PLATE 16

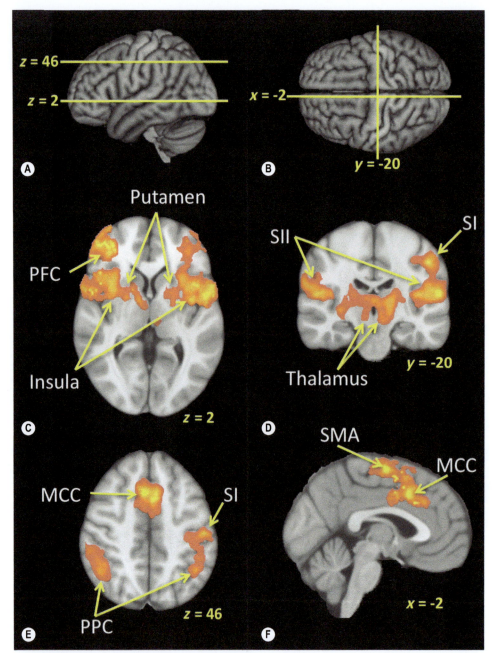

FIGURE 16-2 ■ **(A)** A three-dimensional rendering of the left hemisphere of human brain is traversed by two yellow lines that indicate the positions of axial slices shown in panels C and E. The *z*-values are the distances in mm of the lines above the anterior commissure. **(B)** The hemispheres are viewed from above to show the position of a sagittal slice 2 mm into the left hemisphere (*x* = –2) and a coronal slice 20 mm posterior to the anterior commissure (*y* = –20). The slices appear in panels D and F. **(C)** Pain activation commonly occurs in the insula and prefrontal cortex (*PFC*). Regions within the basal ganglia, such as the putamen can also show pain activation. **(D)** The thalamus is the projection site of inputs from the spinothalamic tract. The ventroposterior lateral nuclei of the thalamus project to the primary (*SI*) and secondary (*SII*) somatosensory cortices. **(E)** The midcingulate cortex (*MCC*) almost invariably activates in association with pain. The primary somatosensory cortex (*SI*) is less consistently activated during noxious stimulation. Pain activation in the posterior parietal cortex (*PPC*) predominates in the right hemisphere for stimuli on either side of the body, although the left PPC can also activate during pain. **(F)** The midcingulate cortex (*MCC*) is a midline structure that is proximal to, and has connections with, the supplementary motor area (*SMA*).

PLATE 17

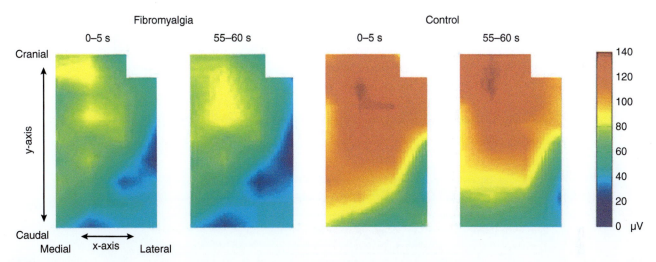

FIGURE 17-6 ■ Topographical mapping of muscle activity. Representative topographical maps (interpolation by a factor 8) of the EMG root mean square value from the right upper trapezius muscle for a person with fibromyalgia and a control subject. Maps are shown for the first and last 5 seconds of a 60-degree sustained shoulder abduction contraction. Areas of blue correspond to low EMG amplitude and dark red to high EMG amplitude. Note the shift of activity in the cranial direction as the task progresses but for the control subject only. (Reprinted with permission from Falla et al.[111])

PLATE 18

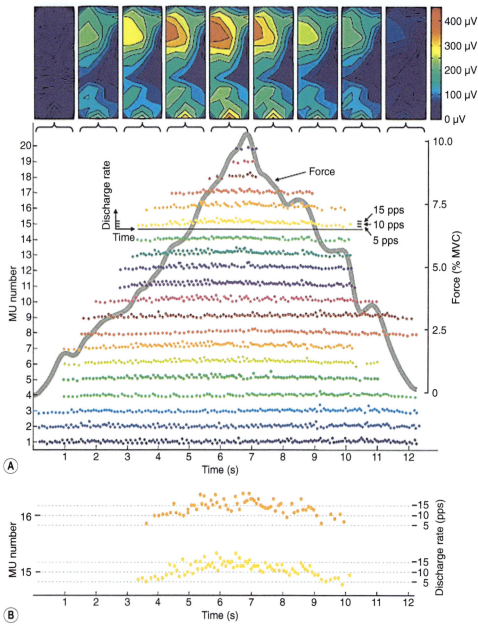

FIGURE 17-7 ■ Extraction of single motor unit discharge patterns from high-density surface EMG. **(A)** Motor unit discharge patterns during an increasing (6 seconds) and decreasing (6 seconds) force isometric contraction (to 10% of the maximum) of the abductor pollicis brevis muscle, as estimated from surface EMG recordings obtained with a 13 × 5 electrode grid. Each dot indicates a motor unit discharge at a time instant. The grey thick line represents the exerted muscle force. The upper panel depicts the root mean square EMG map under the electrode grid during the same muscle contraction. RMS values were calculated from signal epochs of 1-s duration. **(B)** The discharge times of two motor units from **(A)** are shown on a larger vertical scale to illustrate the discharge rate modulation during the contraction. MU: motor unit. (Reprinted with permission from Merletti et al.[119])

PLATE 19

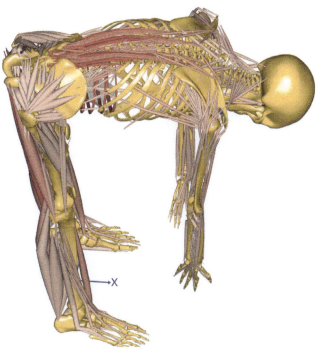

FIGURE 19-3 ■ Model of human lifting a load with spine and hip flexion. The model is developed in the AnyBody Modelling System™ and comprises more than 1000 individually activated muscles. The colour shading of the muscles indicates the level of activity. X indicates the x-direction of the global coordinate system.

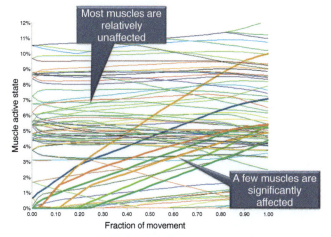

FIGURE 19-5 ■ The effect of a gradual 15° pelvic lateral tilt on muscle activation in the lumbar spine.

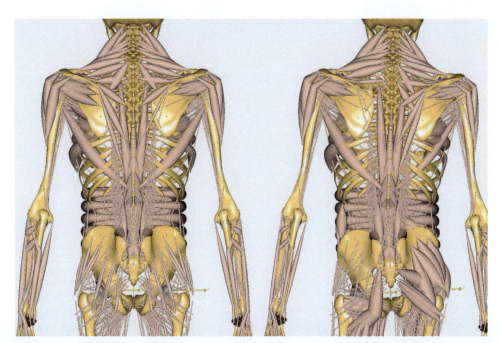

FIGURE 19-6 ■ Alteration of muscle forces (illustrated by the thickness of each fascicle) from symmetrical standing (left) to 10° pelvic lateral tilt (right).

PLATE 20

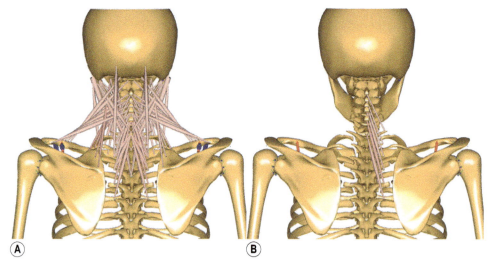

FIGURE 19-7 ■ Model of the cervical spine with (**A**) all the muscle and (**B**) the six fascicles of the semispinalis cervicis on the right side.

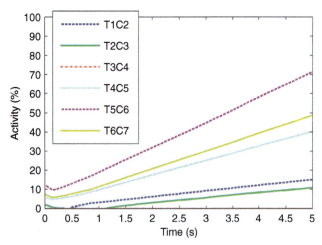

FIGURE 19-8 ■ The predicted activity of the six fascicles of the semispinalis cervicis during ramped extension.

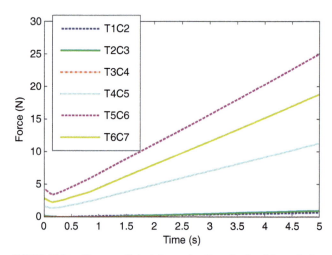

FIGURE 19-9 ■ The predicted force in the six fascicles of the semispinalis cervicis during ramped extension.

PLATE 21

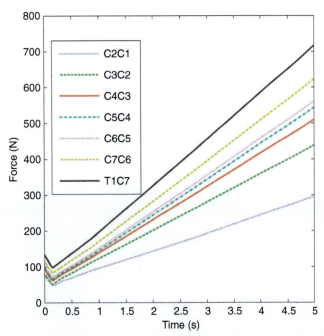

FIGURE 19-10 ■ The predicted reaction forces between the vertebrae in the cervical spine during ramped extension.

PLATE 22

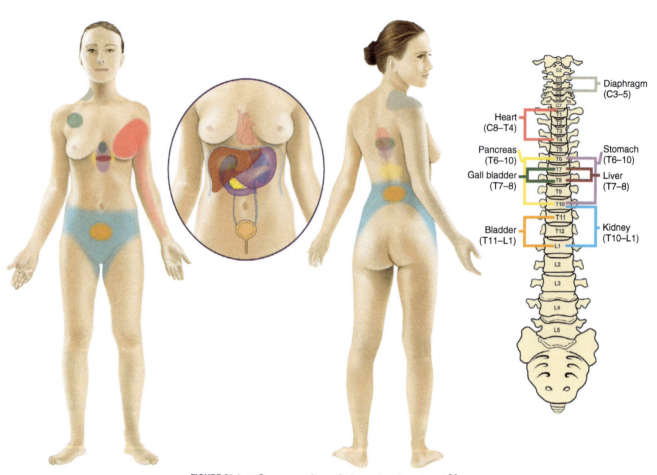

FIGURE 35-1 ■ Common sites of visceral pain referral.[5,6]

Diaphragm
(C3–5)

Heart
(C8–T4)

Pancreas
(T6–10)

Gall bladder
(T7–8)

Stomach
(T6–10)

Liver
(T7–8)

Bladder
(T11–L1)

Kidney
(T10–L1)

PLATE 23

HEALTH IMPROVEMENT CARD

Male (   ) Female (   )

Age 20-34 (   ) 35-39 (   ) 40-44 (   ) 50-54 (   ) 55-59 (   ) 60-64 (   ) 65-69 (   ) 70-74 (   )

Height (   ) metres or feet   Weight (   ) kilograms or pounds

Waist circumference (   ) centimetres or inches

Body mass index =
(SI [metric] units)
$$\frac{\text{weight (kg)}}{\text{height (m) x height(m)}}$$
(   ) kg/m²

OR

Body mass index =
(Imperial/US customary units)
$$\frac{\text{weight (lb)}}{\text{height (in) x height(in)}} \times 703$$
(   ) lb/in²

Biometrics scorecard

- helps you track measurable risk indicators which could over time damage your health, potentially leading to cancers, diabetes, respiratory diseases, heart disease, mental health problems and oral diseases.
- allows your health professional to help support you with information, advice, treatments (when indicated) and care
- enables you to improve your health through your own personalised action plan

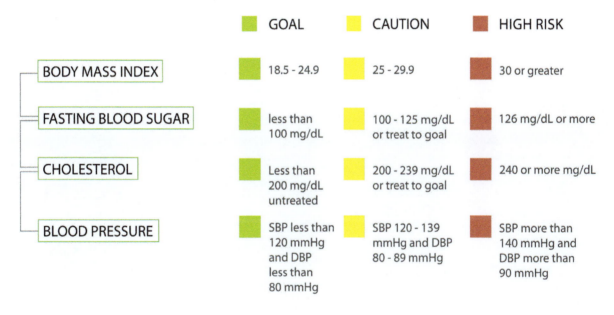

	GOAL	CAUTION	HIGH RISK
BODY MASS INDEX	18.5 - 24.9	25 - 29.9	30 or greater
FASTING BLOOD SUGAR	less than 100 mg/dL	100 - 125 mg/dL or treat to goal	126 mg/dL or more
CHOLESTEROL	Less than 200 mg/dL untreated	200 - 239 mg/dL or treat to goal	240 or more mg/dL
BLOOD PRESSURE	SBP less than 120 mmHg and DBP less than 80 mmHg	SBP 120 - 139 mmHg and DBP 80 - 89 mmHg	SBP more than 140 mmHg and DBP more than 90 mmHg

HEALTH IMPROVEMENT ACTION PLAN

my commitment		my goal:
my action		
health professional action		target date:

For details, visit www.whpa.org

With the support of IFPMA

FIGURE 37-4 ■ **Health Improvement Card.** (Source: Health Improvement Card. World Health Professions Alliance. Reprinted with permission. <http://www.ifpma.org/fileadmin/content/Publication/2011/ncd_Health-Improvement-Card_web-1.pdf>.[22])

PLATE 24

Lifestyle scorecard

- helps you understand how you can improve your health by changing your lifestyle
- allows your health professional to help you improve your health and well-being
- enables you to own and personalise your health improvement action plan

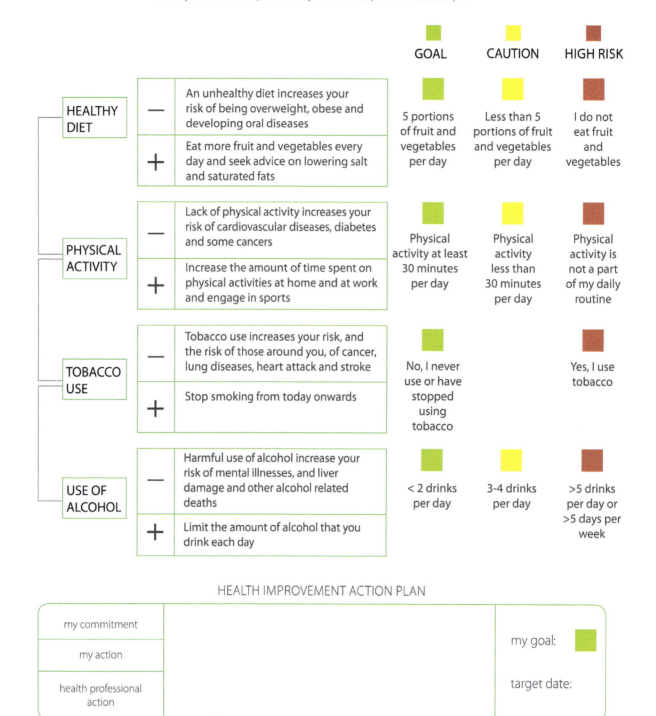

	GOAL	CAUTION	HIGH RISK
HEALTHY DIET — An unhealthy diet increases your risk of being overweight, obese and developing oral diseases	5 portions of fruit and vegetables per day	Less than 5 portions of fruit and vegetables per day	I do not eat fruit and vegetables
+ Eat more fruit and vegetables every day and seek advice on lowering salt and saturated fats			
PHYSICAL ACTIVITY — Lack of physical activity increases your risk of cardiovascular diseases, diabetes and some cancers	Physical activity at least 30 minutes per day	Physical activity less than 30 minutes per day	Physical activity is not a part of my daily routine
+ Increase the amount of time spent on physical activities at home and at work and engage in sports			
TOBACCO USE — Tobacco use increases your risk, and the risk of those around you, of cancer, lung diseases, heart attack and stroke	No, I never use or have stopped using tobacco		Yes, I use tobacco
+ Stop smoking from today onwards			
USE OF ALCOHOL — Harmful use of alcohol increase your risk of mental illnesses, and liver damage and other alcohol related deaths	< 2 drinks per day	3-4 drinks per day	>5 drinks per day or >5 days per week
+ Limit the amount of alcohol that you drink each day			

HEALTH IMPROVEMENT ACTION PLAN

my commitment		my goal:
my action		
health professional action		target date:

For details, visit www.whpa.org

With the support of IFPMA

Figure 37-4. Cont'd

PART I

INTRODUCTION TO THE TEXT

Gwendolen Jull • Ann Moore • Deborah Falla •
Jeremy Lewis • Christopher McCarthy • Michele Sterling

The theory and practice of musculoskeletal physiotherapy have grown and changed quite markedly in the decade following the publication of the third edition of this seminal text. This fourth edition aims to reflect this change and present some of the advances that have occurred in both the science and evidence base pertaining to the diagnosis and management of musculoskeletal disorders. The text also explores issues that will face clinicians and researchers over the next decade.

Several changes have been made in presenting this fourth edition. Firstly, there has been a name change from 'Grieve's Modern Manual Therapy: The Vertebral Column' to 'Grieve's Modern Musculoskeletal Physiotherapy'. This is to reflect the evolution in knowledge, models of diagnosis and contemporary practice. The original manipulative therapy concepts developed in the 1950s and 1960s by physiotherapists such as Geoffrey Maitland and Freddy Kaltenborn were presented essentially, as complete systems of assessment and management of musculoskeletal disorders. Painful musculoskeletal disorders were regarded broadly as manifestations of abnormal movement and articular dysfunction. Such concepts set physiotherapists on a path of detailed analysis of the 'symptoms and signs' of a patient's musculoskeletal disorder, which were interpreted on predominantly kinesiological, biomechanical and neurophysiological bases, taking the individual patient into account. It was recognized even then that the patho-anatomical model was not very helpful in designing manipulative therapy management programmes. Health professionals were first challenged about the inadequacy and limitations of regarding illness only on a biological basis by Engel in 1977,[1] who introduced the concept of a biopsychosocial model. A decade later, Waddell[2] presented for consideration a new clinical model for the treatment of low back pain which embraced the biopsychosocial principles. It spurred a massive volume of research internationally to understand psychological and social moderators and mediators not only of back pain, but of all chronic musculoskeletal disorders. There has also been a surge of research into the neurosciences pertaining to, for example, pain, movement and sensorimotor function in musculoskeletal disorders. The knowledge gained through this research has had and is having a profound influence on physiotherapists' approaches to the diagnosis and management of musculoskeletal disorders. The original concepts of manipulative therapy have grown to embrace new research-generated knowledge. There have been expansions in practice to embrace the evidence for, for example, the superiority of multimodal management approaches which include consideration of and attention to psychological or social moderators. The original manual therapy or manipulative therapy approaches have metamorphosed into musculoskeletal physiotherapy and this is recognized by the change in title of this text.

A second change is the expansion of the focus of the text from the vertebral column to the entire musculoskeletal system. In this edition, both the spine and extremities are considered for the first time. This was a logical progression of the scope of the text as the relevance of much of the basic, behavioural and clinical sciences and indeed the principles of practice are not confined to one body region. There can certainly be peculiarities in the nature of the disorders and their management in the various regions of the body and this has been respected, particularly in the section which overviews contemporary issues in practice (Part IV).

The third change is in the nature of the content of the text. The aims in assembling this multi-authored text were to capture some of the advances in the science and practices made in the last decade relevant to musculoskeletal physiotherapy, to look futuristically at emerging areas as well as presenting some of the current issues in practice. Initially, emphasis is placed on the advances in the sciences underpinning musculoskeletal physiotherapy practice, where there is commentary on topics such as pain, movement, motor control, the interaction between pain and motor control as well as neuromuscular adaptations to exercise. There is also consideration of applied anatomical structure as well as the current and future field of genetics in musculoskeletal pain. A new section of the text highlights the important area of measurement and presents the scope of current and emerging measurements for investigating central and peripheral aspects relating to pain, function and morphological change. It is important for clinicians to be intelligent and discriminating consumers of research. A section of the text has therefore been devoted to discussing some contemporary research approaches including quantitative and qualitative methods to gather, test and examine treatment effects in their broadest interpretation. Importantly, translational research is discussed, the process which ensures that evidence-based practices which are developed in the research environment genuinely make change in clinical practice and policy/procedures.

A sizeable portion of this text is devoted to the principles and broader aspects of management that are applicable to musculoskeletal disorders of both the spine and periphery. A range of topics have been chosen for this section to reflect the scope of musculoskeletal physiotherapy practice. Topics presented include models for management prescription, communication and pain management, as well as contemporary principles of management for the articular, nervous and sensorimotor systems. Recognizing the patient-centred and inclusive nature of contemporary musculoskeletal practice, there is discussion about how physiotherapists may include cognitive behavioural therapies in the management of people with chronic musculoskeletal disorders. In this broader context, self-management, occupational health, lifestyle and health promotion and musculoskeletal screening are presented as is the place of adjuvant physical modalities in pain management. A chapter is also devoted to cautions in musculoskeletal practice of which all clinicians must be aware. Over the last decade, there has been development of advanced practice roles for some musculoskeletal physiotherapists and these different models of practice are discussed.

Part IV of the text concentrates on contemporary issues in clinical practice. All regions of the spine are presented and, as mentioned, novel to this edition is presentation of discussion of topics pertaining to the upper and lower extremities. It is not possible to provide the full scope of management for any region and this was not the intention of this text. Rather, this section presents selected issues in current practice for a particular region or condition or the most topical approaches to the diagnosis and management of a region. A critical review of the evidence or developing evidence for approaches is provided and areas for future work are highlighted. It is recognized that some topics or fields of practice are not discussed, even in a text of this size. It is hoped nevertheless, that the reader gains a good understanding and appreciation of contemporary musculoskeletal physiotherapy.

REFERENCES

1. Engel GL. The need for a new medical model: a challenge for biomedicine. Science 1977;196:129–36.
2. Waddell G. A new clinical model for the treatment of low-back pain. Spine 1987;12:632–44.

PART **II**

ADVANCES IN THEORY AND PRACTICE

ADVANCES IN BASIC SCIENCE

Basic science is essential science and provides the foundation for the development of evidence-based therapeutic strategies. Over the past two decades in particular, there has been a surge in basic science in the field of musculoskeletal physiotherapy which has led to developments and advances in this discipline. Contemporary interventions for musculoskeletal disorders are no longer arbitrarily applied but rather are grounded on scientific discoveries in the field of musculoskeletal health and injury.

This Section brings together the views of some eminent experts in this field and presents 11 chapters which review research into basic mechanisms related to musculoskeletal health, pain and movement that are fundamental to musculoskeletal physiotherapy practice. First is a vital update on pain physiology where knowledge has increased enormously over the past decade. Modern pain neuroscience is used by the clinician for diagnostic and therapeutic purposes. The next collection of chapters covers the basic sciences that are essential to understand when assessing movement and muscle dysfunction and prescribing exercise. It presents the important areas of muscle neurophysiology, the sensorimotor mechanisms underlying postural control and recent research relating to motor control and motor learning. The interaction between pain and sensorimotor function is explored, and a contemporary theory for the effect of pain on sensorimotor function and potential mechanisms underlying sensorimotor disturbances in musculoskeletal pain is offered. It is valuable for clinicians to understand treatment effects, and a chapter presents exercise-induced neuromuscular adaptations with a focus on the muscle structural and neural adaptations to both strength and endurance training. Then follows a collection of chapters where other aspects of the musculoskeletal system vital to clinical practice are presented, including contemporary research into the peripheral nervous system in function and dysfunction, functional anatomy, and the area that continues to attract considerable interest, namely tendon health and pathology. The Section concludes with chapters dealing with important contemporary issues in musculoskeletal health and pain, namely, the role that genetics and lifestyle play in the development of chronic pain and the effects of ageing on the musculoskeletal system.

There have been tremendous advances in our understanding of musculoskeletal health and injury in recent years and the current state of knowledge is provided within this Section. An ongoing aim is to translate the benefits of advances in the basic sciences to the treatment of musculoskeletal disorders. Much knowledge is already being implemented in the contemporary management of musculoskeletal disorders as seen in Section 4 of this text.

CHAPTER 2

THE NEUROPHYSIOLOGY OF PAIN AND PAIN MODULATION: MODERN PAIN NEUROSCIENCE FOR MUSCULOSKELETAL PHYSIOTHERAPISTS

Jo Nijs • Margot De Kooning • David Beckwée • Peter Vaes

INTRODUCTION

Anatomy, arthrokinematics and neurophysiology are traditionally viewed as the key basic sciences for musculoskeletal physiotherapy. Neurophysiology is important for understanding how the brain controls body movements and how neuromuscular control can become a potential part of the treatment in patients with musculoskeletal pain. In addition, the neurophysiology of pain is important for musculoskeletal physiotherapy.

Modern pain neuroscience has evolved spectacularly over the past decades. Here we explain the basic principles of modern pain neuroscience, from the musculoskeletal tissues to the brain, and from the brain down the spinal cord back to the tissues. It will be explained that not all pain arises from damage in the musculoskeletal system, that all pain is in the brain, and that musculoskeletal physiotherapists can apply modern pain neuroscience for diagnostic, communicational and therapeutic purposes. In addition, specific information for better understanding (the underlying mechanisms of) musculoskeletal diagnosis and therapy is provided.

The chapter begins with a very brief overview of acute pain neurophysiology, followed by various key mechanisms involved in neuroplasticity (i.e. wind-up, long-term potentiation, central sensitization) and pain modulation (descending nociceptive inhibition and facilitation). An important part of the chapter is dedicated to the pain (neuro)matrix, and several 'boxes' throughout the chapter highlight the translation of modern pain neuroscience to clinical practice.

THE NEUROPHYSIOLOGY OF MUSCULOSKELETAL PAIN: FROM TISSUE NOCICEPTION TO THE PAIN NEUROMATRIX

Many tissues hold the capacity to alert the central nervous system of (potential) danger, and hence to produce action potentials that can be interpreted by the brain as pain. These include the skin, muscles, tendons, muscle fascia,[1] part of the menisci, ligaments, joint capsules, (osteochondral) bone and the nervous system itself. Besides low-threshold sensory receptors, important for touch (including texture and shape) and proprioception, high-threshold sensory receptors are available and respond to strong heat, cold and mechanical or chemical stimuli. Given their high threshold they respond preferentially, but certainly not exclusively, to noxious stimuli and are therefore called nociceptors. Many such nociceptors respond to multiple stimulus modalities (i.e. heat, cold, mechanical or chemical stimuli), making them polymodal nociceptors.

Each of the nociceptors is connected to an ion channel that opens once the nociceptor is activated by a stimulus (e.g. chemicals released from cell rupture). This allows for the stimulus (often tissue damage or one that holds the capacity to cause tissue damage such as a pin prick) to be converted into an electrical current: first a gradual potential, followed by an action potential. For instance, in patients where the neck muscles become highly tensed due to physical (over)use, mechanical pressure builds up inside the neck muscles, which causes the polymodal nociceptors to open their connecting ion channels, which results in an influx of positive charges in the neurons, generating an action potential (physiological response due to usual use). Following overuse and in cases of local inflammation, chemicals like potassium ions, histamine, serotonin, prostaglandins, pro-inflammatory cytokines and substance P are released from damaged tissue or produced by immune cells or sensory neurons. These chemicals lower the stimulus thresholds of the nociceptors significantly, which increases the chance of generating action potentials. This results in increased sensitivity to pain (recall you cannot even touch the skin of an acutely injured joint without triggering more pain).

Regardless of whether or not the sensitivity of the nociceptor is altered, the action potential arising from nociceptors can be transported by two types of nerve fibres: Aδ and C fibres. Fast pain is transmitted from the tissue to the central nervous system via Aδ fibres, which are small, myelinated nerve fibres with a high conduction speed. Fast pain is typically described by patients as sharp and localized, while slow (C-fibre) pain is duller and more diffuse, but lasts much longer. C fibres are small, unmyelinated nerve fibres with a low conduction speed.

Both Aδ and C fibres are primary sensory nerve fibres. Sensory information enters the central nervous system in the spinal cord, where these nerve fibres synapse on secondary afferent nerve fibres. These synapses are highly modulated by local (interneurons) and top-down (descending or brain-orchestrated) neurons, implying that not all action potentials entering the spinal cord will enter the brain (and hence not all action potentials arising from nociceptors trigger pain). This modulation of incoming danger messages is further detailed below (under the heading 'Brain-orchestrated pain modulation'). If the action potential from the primary afferent neuron is transferred to the secondary afferent neuron in the dorsal horn, then the incoming message will cross the body's midline in the spinal cord and can ascend to the brain, more precisely the thalamus, which spreads the message to several other brain regions involved in the pain (neuro)matrix (see below and Fig. 2-2). Even when the action potential makes it to the brain, it still remains unconscious until the brain has processed it. This implies that the various brain areas involved in processing the incoming messages, together referred to as the pain matrix, will decide whether or not the signals should be interpreted as threatening to the body's homeostasis or not (pain or no pain).

TEMPORAL SUMMATION AND WIND-UP

It is important to understand that not all nociceptive signals are perceived as pain, and not every pain sensation originates from nociception. Nevertheless, acute pain almost always originates from nociceptors in somatic or visceral tissue. However, when the nociceptors keep on 'firing' nociceptive impulses, the dorsal horn neurons may become hypersensitive.[5,6] This increased neuronal responsiveness is accomplished by neurotransmitters (e.g. glutamate, aspartate and substance P) that modulate the postsynaptic electric discharges with further transmission to supraspinal sites (thalamus, anterior cingulate cortex, insular cortex and somatosensory cortex) via ascending pathways.[5] The neurotransmitters initiate increased postsynaptic responses by triggering hyperexcitability of N-methyl-D-aspartate (NMDA) receptor sites of second-order neurons in the dorsal horn (Fig. 2-1). This mechanism is related to temporal summation of second pain or wind-up. Wind-up refers to the progressive increase of electrical discharges from the second-order neuron in the spinal cord in response to repetitive C-fibre stimulation, and is experienced in humans as increased pain.[7,8] Wind-up is part of the process known as central sensitization.[9]

BRAIN-ORCHESTRATED PAIN MODULATION

The brain orchestrates top-down pain-modulatory systems that are able to facilitate or inhibit nociceptive

---

BOX 2-1	The Nervous System as Source of Nociception and Pain: Neuropathic Pain Highlights for Clinicians

It is not only the musculoskeletal system that can generate nociception: the nervous system itself can be a source of nociception. Neuropathic pain is defined as '*pain arising as a direct consequence of a lesion or disease affecting the somatosensory system*'.[2] Neuropathic pain can be both peripheral (i.e. located in a nerve, dorsal root ganglion or plexus) and central (i.e. located in the brain or spinal cord). In the neuropathic pain definition, the term *lesion* points to the often available evidence from diagnostic investigations (e.g. imaging, neurophysiology, biopsies, laboratory tests) to reveal an abnormality (such as scar tissue) of the nervous system. Alternatively, lesion may refer to posttraumatic or postsurgical damage to the nervous system. For example, about 27% of patients develop chronic postsurgical pain following total hip or knee arthroplasty, but neuropathic pain is rare, accounting for 5.7% of all chronic pain patients.[3] This implies that following total hip or knee arthroplasty, damage to a peripheral nerve is rarely identified. Further addressing the neuropathic pain definition, the term *disease* refers to the underlying cause of the lesion, which is often clear: postherpetic neuralgia, cancer, stroke, vasculitis, diabetes mellitus, genetic abnormality, neurodegenerative disease, etc. Finally, *somatosensory* refers to information about the body per se including visceral organs, rather than information about the external world (e.g. vision, hearing, or olfaction).

Addressing the clinical signs of neuropathic pain, the location of neuropathic pain is neuroanatomically logical, implying that all neuropathic pains are perceived within the innervation territory of the damaged nerve, root, or pathway due to the somatotopic organization of the primary somatosensory cortex.[4] Patients with neuropathic pain often describe pain as burning, shooting, or pricking. Finally, sensory testing is of prime importance for the diagnosis of neuropathic pain.[2] This includes testing of the function of sensory fibres with simple tools (e.g. a tuning fork for vibration, a soft brush for touch and cold/warm objects for temperature), which typically assess the relation between the stimulus and the perceived sensation.[4] Several options arise here, all suggestive of neuropathic pain: hyperaesthesia, hypoaesthesia, hyperalgesia, hypoalgesia, allodynia, paraesthesia, dysaesthesia, aftersensations, etc. Again, the location of the sensory dysfunction should be neuroanatomically logical. The presence of neuropathic pain does not exclude the possibility of central sensitization pain (i.e. hyperexcitability of the central nervous system as often seen in chronic musculoskeletal pain – this concept is further detailed below) or vice versa. In fact, some patients evolve from neuropathic pain with severe but local signs and symptoms, to a widespread pain condition that cannot be explained by neuropathic pain solely. In such cases, central sensitization might account for the evolution to a widespread pain condition.

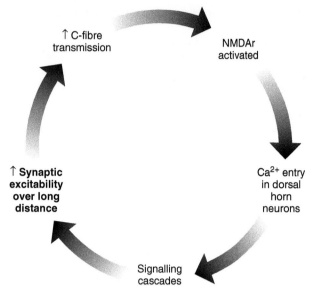

FIGURE 2-1 ■ The neurophysiology of temporal summation and wind-up. NMDAr, N-methyl D-aspartate receptors; ca²⁺, calcium ions.

input from the periphery.[15] This implies that all nociceptive stimuli arising from muscles, joints, skin or viscera are modulated in the spinal cord, more specifically the dorsal horn. Incoming messages (nociceptive stimuli) from the periphery enter the spinal cord in the dorsal horn where they synapse with secondary afferent neurons that have the capacity to send the messages to the brain. 'Have the capacity' implies that they do not always do that. These synapses are modulated by top-down (descending) neurons, which can either result in inhibition (descending inhibition) or augmentation (descending facilitation) of the incoming messages. In the case of the former, nociceptive stimuli may 'die' in the dorsal horn, implying that nociceptive stimuli will not result in pain. In such cases the person will never become aware of the nociception that has occurred. Descending facilitation implies that incoming messages are amplified and that the threshold in the dorsal horn for sending incoming messages to the brain is lower than normal.

In summary, the brain controls a brake (descending inhibition) and an accelerator (descending facilitation). Both modulatory mechanisms are further explained below, starting with descending facilitation.

Descending Nociceptive Facilitation

Output from the brainstem (i.e. nuclei in the mesencephalic pontine reticular formation) activates descending pathways from the rostral ventromedial medulla that enhances nociceptive processing at the level of the spinal dorsal horn.[16] Descending facilitatory pathways are not demonstrably involved during nociceptive processing in the normal state.

Catastrophizing, avoidance behaviour and somatization are factors that have been shown to prevent effective descending inhibition, and at the same time they activate descending facilitation.[17] Together, this may result in

How can we translate these findings to clinical practice? Is it required to translate these findings to clinical practice? This question relates to how wind-up is possibly created/facilitated by musculoskeletal treatment. Here we provide a viewpoint. When musculoskeletal physiotherapists apply hands-on techniques, and by doing so eliciting compression and hereby deliver identical nociceptive stimuli to the skin, muscles or joint capsules more often than once every 3 seconds, they are likely to trigger this mechanism of pain amplification.[10] In line with this reasoning, musculoskeletal physiotherapists should be aware that the vicinity of myofascial trigger points differs from normal muscle tissue by its lower pH levels (i.e. more acid), increased levels of substance P, calcitonin gene-related peptide and pro-inflammatory cytokines (i.e. tumour necrosis factor alpha and interleukine-1β), each of which has its role in increasing pain sensitivity.[11–13] Sensitized muscle nociceptors are more easily activated and may respond to normally innocuous and weak stimuli such as light pressure and muscle movement.[11,12] All this becomes even more important when one realizes how crucial it is to limit the time course of afferent stimulation of peripheral nociceptors. Indeed, tissue injury healing and focal pain recovery should occur within a period of approximately 3 months to prevent development of chronic widespread pain.[14] Progression towards chronic widespread pain is associated with injuries to deep tissues which do not heal within several months.[14]

sensitization of dorsal horn spinal cord secondary neurons.[17] Sustained arousal is likely to maintain sensitization of the brain circuitry involved in central sensitization pain.[18] It is important for clinicians to realize that pain cognitions like fear of movement and catastrophizing are not only of importance in patients with chronic pain, but may even be crucial at the stage of acute/subacute musculoskeletal disorders.[19]

Descending Nociceptive Inhibition

Stimulation of certain regions of the midbrain facilitates extremely powerful descending pain-modulating pathways that project, via the medulla, to neurons in the dorsal horn that control the ascending information in the nociceptive system.[20] These pain-inhibitory pathways arise mainly from the periaquaductal grey matter and the rostral ventral medulla in the brainstem.[20] The descending inhibitory pathways apply neurotransmitters such as serotonin[16] and noradrenaline. The main descending inhibitory action to the spinal dorsal horn is noradrenergic. In the dorsal horn, norepinephrine, through its action on alpha-2A-adrenoceptors, suppresses the release of excitatory transmitters from central terminals of primary afferent nociceptors.[21] In addition it may suppress postsynaptic responses of spinal pain-relay neurons.[21] One function of the descending inhibitory pathway is to 'focus/target' the excitatory state of the dorsal horn neurons by suppressing surrounding neuronal activity,[22] a role attributed to the 'diffuse noxious inhibitory controls' phenomenon.[23] In case of central sensitization and chronic widespread pain these descending pain-inhibitory pathways are malfunctioning.[24–27]

Exercise is a physical stressor that activates descending nociceptive inhibition, a mechanism often referred to as exercise-induced endogenous analgesia.[28] In some patients with chronic musculoskeletal pain (including chronic whiplash-associated disorders[29] and fibromyalgia[30]), exercise does not activate endogenous analgesia. Other populations such as people with chronic low back pain, do have a normal endogenous analgesic response to exercise.[31]

Likewise, manual joint mobilizations have been shown to activate descending nociceptive inhibition. For instance, animal research indicates that joint mobilization reduces postoperative pain by activation of the peripheral opioid pathway[32] and the involvement of the adenosinergic system.[33] Likewise, unilateral joint mobilization reduces bilateral hyperalgesia induced by chronic muscle or joint inflammation in animal models.[34] In humans, there is level A evidence for a significant effect of spinal manipulative therapy on increasing pressure pain thresholds at the remote sites of stimulus application supporting a potential central nervous system mechanism (i.e. activation of descending nociceptive inhibition).[35]

Until now we have learned how the brain tries to control what information comes in and what stays out. Next, let us have a look at what happens when nociceptive messages enter the brain. For a proper understanding of modern pain neuroscience, it is important to understand that incoming nociceptive messages, when they first enter the brain, are still not perceived consciously. At this point, we are not even aware of them. The brain will now start processing the nociception. For the processing of incoming nociceptive messages, the brain uses several brain regions that co-work to decide whether or not the nociceptive messages will be interpreted as dangerous or not (i.e. painful or not). When the brain decides that the messages are dangerous, then it will produce pain and it will let the same brain regions decide *how much* pain (pain severity) is produced. Although a specific role is attributed to each of these brain regions (see below), they do not function independently from one another; they co-work and communicate closely. Together this brain circuitry is called the pain matrix or pain neuromatrix (first proposed by Melzack to explain phantom pain[36]).

THE PAIN NEUROMATRIX

All pain is in the brain. The brain can produce pain without nociception and vice versa, which holds tremendous potential for musculoskeletal clinicians working with patients in pain. The brain produces pain by activating a circuitry: a number of brain regions that become active all together when a person is in pain (Fig. 2-2). These brain regions differ between individuals and possibly even for one individual in different circumstances, but they differ the most when comparing acute versus chronic pain. Nevertheless, the following brain regions are generally accepted as being involved in pain sensations:

- The primary and secondary **somatosensory cortex**, which is the primary area responsible for identifying the location of the pain in the body (i.e. the sensory-discriminative aspect of pain). The more attention one pays to the painful stimulus/painful region, the more activity is observed in the primary somatosensory cortex.[37] The amount of activity in the somatosensory cortex correlates with pain intensity in those with central sensitization pain.[38]
- One key brain area involved in the pain (neuro) matrix is the **amygdala** (the upper part of Fig. 2-2 illustrates its deep location in the brain), often referred to as the fear-memory centre of the brain:
  - The amygdala has a key role in negative emotions and pain-related memories.[39] In addition to the amygdala, the anterior cingulate cortex takes part of the central fear network in the brain.[40,41]
  - Recent research supports the cardinal role of the amygdala as a facilitator of chronic pain development, including sensitization of central nervous system pain pathways.[39,40,42–45]
  - In line with this is the finding that the amygdala, as well as the somatosensory cortex and insula, shows less activity during pain delivery in case of positive treatment expectations.[46] This is an important message for clinicians: it is advocated to question the patient's treatment expectations.

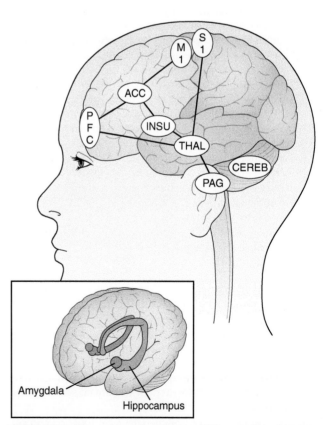

FIGURE 2-2 ■ The pain neuromatrix. *ACC*, anterior cingulate cortex; *CEREB*, cerebellum; *INSU*, insula; *M1*, primary motor cortex; *PAG*, periaqueductal grey; *PFC*, prefrontal cortex; *S1*, primary somatosensory cortex; *THAL*, thalamus.

Positive treatment expectations not only increase the likelihood of a positive treatment outcome, it also implies less activity in key areas involved in the pain neuromatrix. This should motivate clinicians to address negative treatment expectations, for instance by increasing treatment expectations during therapeutic pain neuroscience education.

- Movement therapy in musculoskeletal pain: Of major relevance for providing exercise therapy to patients with chronic musculoskeletal pain is the amygdala's role in pain memories and, more precisely, in memories of painful movements. Therefore the amygdala closely collaborates with the hippocampus and the anterior cingulate cortex (Fig. 2-2). Even though nociceptive pathology has often long subsided, the brains of patients with chronic musculoskeletal pain have typically acquired a protective pain memory,[47] which can be defined as a memory of movements that once elicited pain and prevents people from performing that 'dangerous' movement. For movements that once provoked pain, this implies protective behaviours like antalgic postures, antalgic movement patterns (including altered motor control), or even avoidance of such movements (fear of movement).

- The **thalamus** is important for sending the incoming (nociceptive) messages to other brain regions, including those listed above. In addition, the (sensory) thalamus, together with the periaqueductal grey (see below) is used as a target for deep brain stimulation in patients with neuropathic pain,[55] illustrating its role in descending analgesia. More precisely, the thalamus and the periaqueductal grey closely interact (i.e. activity in the periaqueductal grey inhibits the sensory thalamus and activation of the sensory thalamus activates the periaqueductal grey).[56] The thalamus activity differs in those with chronic pain: it shows less activity on the contralateral side.[37] A functional magnetic resonance imaging study showed increased anterior thalamic activity in those with central sensitization compared to the normal state.[38]

- The **brain stem**, which includes several key regions for orchestrating top-down pain inhibition (or endogenous analgesia). The brainstem has been identified as one of the key regions for the maintenance of central sensitization pain in humans, with increased brainstem activity in those with central sensitization compared to the normal state.[38] Within the brainstem the mesencephalic pontine reticular formation has been identified as a particularly important region showing increased activity in central sensitization.[38] The increased brainstem activity, and more specifically the mesencephalic pontine reticular formation, in central sensitization pain may reflect increased descending facilitation. Another (mid)brain stem area of importance is the periaqueductal grey, which – together with the dorsolateral prefrontal cortex – is another key centre for activating top-down endogenous analgesia.[55,56]

BOX 2-3   Long-Term Pain Memories are often Apparent in Patients with Chronic Musculoskeletal Pain

Kinesiophobia or fear of movement is seldom applicable to all kinds of physical activity, but rather applies to certain movements (e.g. neck extension in patients postwhiplash, overhead smashes in patients with shoulder impingement syndrome, or forward bending in patients with low back pain). Even though these movements provoked pain in the (sub)acute phase, or even initiated the musculoskeletal pain disorder (e.g. the pain initiated following an overhead smash), they are often perfectly safe to perform in a chronic stage. The problem is that the brain has acquired a long-term pain memory, associating such movements with danger/threat. Even preparing for such 'dangerous' movements is enough for the brain to activate its fear-memory centre and hence to produce pain (without nociception) and employ an altered (protective) motor control strategy.[48] Exercise therapy can address this by applying the 'exposure without danger' principle.[47] This implies addressing patients' perceptions about exercises, before and following performance of exercises and daily activities. This way, therapists try to decrease the anticipated danger (threat level) of the exercises by challenging the nature of and reasoning behind their fears, assuring the safety of the exercises, and increasing confidence in a successful accomplishment of the exercise. Such treatment principles are in line with those applied by psychologists during graded exposure in vivo,[49] a cognitive behaviour treatment that has yielded good outcomes in patients with chronic low back pain,[50,51] complex regional pain syndrome type I,[52] whiplash pain,[53] and work-related upper limb pain[54] (level B evidence). Studies examining whether musculoskeletal physiotherapists are capable of applying such treatment principles are warranted.

Recent experimental (basic) pain research reveals that extinction training during reconsolidation of threat memory is more effective than classical extinction training (i.e. exposure in vivo).[41] Extinction training results in increased connectivity between the prefrontal cortex and the amygdala, which implies that the prefrontal cortex inhibits the expression of pain memories by the amygdala. Precise timing of such extinction training (exposure in vivo principles) to coincide with pain memory reconsolidation (e.g. imagery of the movement that injured the shoulder or lower back) results in a disconnection between the prefrontal cortex and the amygdala.[41] This altered brain connectivity may be important for enabling extinction training to more permanently 'rewrite' the original pain memory. In clinical practice, this would imply that immediately before performing the threatening exercise or activity, we ask our patients to think back to the movement that once injured the painful body part (or to the accident that triggered the musculoskeletal pain disorder). However, before translating these basic pain research findings into clinical practice, more studies using pain memory reconsolidation are required, including studies showing that extinction training during reconsolidation of threat memory is more effective than classical extinction training also applies to clinical pain (i.e. studies in patients with musculoskeletal pain), and not only to experimental pain in healthy subjects.

Finally, different classes of neurons important for top-down pain inhibition have been identified in the rostral ventromedial medulla; ON-cells are known to promote nociception, and OFF-cells to suppress nociception.[57]

- The **anterior cingulate cortex**, an area important for the affective-motivational aspects of pain, including empathy and social exclusion.
  - The anterior cingulate cortex does not seem to be involved in coding stimulus intensity or location, but participates in both the affective and attentional concomitants of pain sensation.[37]
  - Studies have shown that social exclusion evokes social pain in excluded individuals, and neuroimaging studies suggest that this social pain is associated with activation of the dorsal anterior cingulate cortex, with further regulation of social pain being reflected in activation of the right ventrolateral prefrontal cortex.[58,59] Thus, the brain areas that are activated during the distress caused by social exclusion are also those activated during physical pain.[60] The pain of a broken heart is now an evidence-based metaphor for explaining to patients that all pain is in the brain, and that pain does not rely on tissue damage (cf. therapeutic pain neuroscience education).
  - With respect to empathy for pain, a core network consisting of bilateral anterior insular cortex and medial/anterior cingulate cortex has been identified.[61] For obtaining a modern understanding of pain, it is important to realize that activation in these areas overlaps with activation during directly experienced pain.
- The **prefrontal cortex**, an area responsible for the cognitive-evaluative dimension of pain:
  - The prefrontal cortex is important for anticipation and attention (vigilance) to pain and pain-provoking situations, which brings us to pain memories/previous painful experiences. For the latter, the prefrontal cortex closely communicates with the amygdala and the hippocampus. All together these brain areas can be viewed as the 'pain memories circuitry'.
  - The dorsolateral part of the prefrontal cortex has been identified as a key region involved in descending nociceptive inhibition/endogenous analgesia mediated by opioids.[62] Therefore, the dorsolateral prefrontal cortex has become a popular target for transcranial magnetic brain stimulation,[62] a non-invasive electrotherapy treatment for chronic (neuropathic) pain and depression. In case of more intense pain levels, pain catastrophizing is associated with decreased activity in several brain regions involved in top-down pain inhibition like the dorsolateral prefrontal cortex and the medial prefrontal cortex.[63]
  - Pain anticipation, or pain expectancies, can contribute to determining the intensity of pain. Indeed, expectancies have pain-modulatory effects and they closely relate to placebo effects. This is a powerful tool in clinical practice: clinicians can increase or decrease the patient's expectations for subsequent pain experiences (e.g. in response to treatments or daily activities). This is not soft science, but neuroscience: expectancies shape pain-intensity processing in the central nervous system, with strong effects on nociceptive portions of insula, cingulate and thalamus.[64] Expectancy effects on subjective experience are also driven by responses in other regions like the dorsolateral prefrontal cortex and the orbitofrontal cortex.[64] Naturally, these brain regions largely overlap with brain regions identified as playing a pivotal role in placebo analgesia, such as the anterior cingulate cortex, anterior insula, prefrontal cortex and periaqueductal grey.[65]
- The **insula**, a brain region that has a role in the emotional component of every pain sensation, but also contributes to the sensory-discriminative aspect of pain.[37]

CENTRAL SENSITIZATION

Central sensitization is defined as 'an augmentation of responsiveness of central pain-signalling neurons to input from low-threshold mechanoreceptors'.[67] While peripheral sensitization is a local phenomenon that is important for protecting damaged tissue during the early phases post injury, central sensitization means that central pain-processing pathways localized in the spinal cord and the brain become sensitized. Indeed, the process of central sensitization is neither limited to the dorsal horn, nor to pain amplification of afferent impulses. Central sensitization encompasses altered sensory processing in the brain and malfunctioning of pain-inhibitory mechanisms. Coding of the mechanism of wind-up involves multiple brain sites, including somatosensory (thalamus, anterior insula, posterior insula, primary somatic sensory cortex, secondary somatic sensory cortex), cognitive-evaluative/affective (anterior cingulate cortex and prefrontal cortex) and pain-modulating regions (rostral anterior cingulate cortex).[68] The elevated central nervous system reactivity inhibits functioning of regulatory pathways for the autonomic, endocrine and the immune systems.[69]

BOX 2-4	The Overlap between the Pain Neuromatrix and the Brain Regions Involved in Movement Control

For musculoskeletal physiotherapists it is important to realize that frequent activation in **motor-related areas** such as the striatum, cerebellum and supplementary motor area has been observed during (experimental) pain.[37] These areas are increasingly accepted as parts of the pain (neuro) matrix. In line with this is the finding that healthy subjects display a relation between pain catastrophizing and brain activity in regions involved in motor response and motor planning (i.e. thalamus, putamen and premotor cortex).[63] This implies that the pain neuromatrix partly overlaps with brain regions involved in movement control,[66] partly explaining why people who are in pain present with movement dysfunctions.

In those with central sensitization pain, the pain neuromatrix is likely to be overactive: increased activity is present in brain areas known to be involved in acute pain sensations and emotional representations like the insula, anterior cingulate cortex and the prefrontal cortex.[70] An overactive pain neuromatrix also entails brain activity in regions not involved in acute pain sensations, including various brain stem nuclei, dorsolateral frontal cortex and the parietal associated cortex.[70] Research findings also suggest a specific role of the brainstem for the maintenance of central sensitization in humans.[38]

Furthermore, *long-term potentiation of neuronal synapses* in the anterior cingulate cortex,[71] nucleus accumbens, insula and the sensorimotor cortex, as well as decreased gamma-aminobutyric acid-neurotransmission[72] represent two mechanisms contributing to the overactive pain neuromatrix. Long-term potentiation implies that synapses become much more efficient: a single action potential will lead to more presynaptic release of neurotransmitters, combined with more postsynaptic binding of neurotransmitters. This results in more efficient communication between neurons and even brain regions. This mechanism of long-term potentiation makes it possible for us to understand that the circuitry of different brain regions will be more easily (and longer) activated in those with chronic compared to acute pain. Long-term potentiation is one of the key mechanisms contributing to central sensitization.

The decreased availability of neurotransmitters like gamma-aminobutyric acid[72] (GABA) is a second mechanism contributing to the overactive pain neuromatrix. GABA is an important inhibitory neurotransmitter. Less available GABA neurotransmission, which can be the result of long-term stress, implies increased excitability of central nervous system pathways.

In acute musculoskeletal pain, the main focus for treatment is to reduce the nociceptive trigger. For that we have several non-pharmacological treatment options, including hands-on manual therapy and exercise therapy. Such a focus on peripheral pain generators is often effective for treatment of (sub)acute musculoskeletal pain.[73-76] In patients with chronic musculoskeletal pain, ongoing nociception rarely dominates the clinical picture. Chronic musculoskeletal pain conditions like osteoarthritis,[77] rheumatoid arthritis,[78] whiplash,[26,79,80] fibromyalgia,[9,81] low back pain,[82] pelvic pain,[83] and lateral epicondylitis,[84] are often characterized by brain plasticity that leads to hyperexcitability of the central nervous system (central sensitization) or vice versa. Cumulating evidence supports the clinical importance of central sensitization in patients with chronic musculoskeletal pain.[85-88] Still, not all patients with one of the above-mentioned diagnoses have central sensitization pain. Box 2-5 provides a brief overview on how to recognize central sensitization pain in clinical practice.

In such cases, musculoskeletal physiotherapists need to think and treat beyond muscles and joints.[91] Within the context of the management of chronic pain, it is crucial to consider the concept of central pain mechanisms like central sensitization.[92] Hence, in patients with chronic musculoskeletal pain and central sensitization it

---

BOX 2-5 | **Recognition of Central Sensitization Pain in Musculoskeletal Pain Patients**

For recognizing central sensitization pain in musculoskeletal pain patients with conditions like osteoarthritis, low back pain, or lateral epicondylalgia, the following clinical signs and symptoms can be of use. Central sensitization pain is typically characterized by disproportionate pain, implying that the severity of pain and related reported or perceived disability (e.g. restriction and intolerance to daily life activities, to stress, etc.) are disproportionate to the nature and extent of injury or pathology (i.e. tissue damage or structural impairments). In addition, patient self-reported pain distribution, as identified from the clinical history and/or a body chart, often reveals a large pain area with a non-segmental distribution (i.e. neuroanatomically illogical), or pain varying in (anatomical) location/travelling pain, including to anatomical locations unrelated to the presumed source of nociception. Finally, a score of 40 or higher on part A of the Central Sensitization Inventory,[89] which assesses symptoms common to central sensitization, provides a clinically relevant guide to alert healthcare professionals to the possibility that a patient's symptom presentation may indicate the presence of central sensitization.[90]

---

seems rational to target therapies at the central nervous system rather than muscles and joints. More precisely, modern pain neuroscience calls for treatment strategies aimed at decreasing the sensitivity of the central nervous system (i.e. desensitizing therapies). Therapeutic pain neuroscience education (Box 2-6) might be part of such a desensitizing approach to musculoskeletal pain, but further study is required to support this viewpoint.

DOES THE AUTONOMIC NERVOUS SYSTEM INFLUENCE PAIN?

The autonomic nervous system, together with the hypothalamus–pituitary–adrenal axis, accounts for the body's stress response systems. Pain is a stressor that activates the stress response systems, but at the same time the stress response systems can influence pain through several neurophysiologic mechanisms. It goes like this: once pain becomes apparent, the body activates its stress response systems, including the autonomic nervous system and the hypothalamus–pituitary–adrenal axis. Given the threatening nature of pain, it seems logical to understand that the body responds to pain with its 'fight or flight' system. This leads to increases in stress hormones like (nor)adrenaline and cortisol, which exert analgesic effects at the level of the brain (e.g. noradrenaline is an important neurotransmitter for enabling descending nociceptive inhibition[15]) and spinal cord (e.g. cortisol in the dorsal horn). The dorsal horn neurons contain glucocorticoid receptors, having pain-inhibitory capacity.[102] Thus, a normal response to stress is pain inhibition. Stress is a natural pain killer.

However, many of our patients with musculoskeletal pain experience the reverse: stress aggravates pain rather

| BOX 2-6 | Translating Modern Pain Neuroscience to Practice: Therapeutic Pain Neuroscience Education in Musculoskeletal Physiotherapy Practice |

The presence of central sensitization implies that the brain produces pain, fatigue and other 'warning signs' even when there is no real tissue damage or nociception. How can musculoskeletal physiotherapists translate our current understanding of pain neuroscience to clinical practice in patients with (chronic) musculoskeletal pain? The first thing to do is to explain to patients what pain is, and that all pain is in the brain. Therapeutic pain neuroscience education enables patients to understand the controversy surrounding their pain, including the lack of objective biomarkers or imaging findings. One of the main goals of therapeutic pain neuroscience education is changing pain beliefs through the reconceptualization of pain. The focus is convincing patients that pain does not per se result from tissue damage. Pain neuroscience education is generally welcomed very positively by patients.[93,94] We and other groups have shown that face-to-face sessions of therapeutic pain neuroscience education, in conjunction with written educational material, are effective for changing pain beliefs and improving health status in patients with various chronic pain disorders (level A evidence),[93,94] including those with chronic spinal pain.[95–100] More specifically, therapeutic pain neuroscience education is effective for improving maladaptive pain beliefs, and decreasing pain and disability in patients with chronic pain.[95–99] However, the effects are small and education is insufficient as a sole treatment.[94] Practice guidelines for therapeutic pain neuroscience education are available.[93,94]

Interestingly, one study revealed that therapeutic pain neuroscience education improves descending pain inhibition (i.e. conditioned pain modulation) in patients with fibromyalgia.[101] Larger studies should confirm these early findings, but if confirmed they point towards a remarkable mind–body interaction, and moreover one that can be influenced by physiotherapists.

than inhibiting pain. Indeed, stress triggers a switch in second messenger signalling for pronociceptive immune mediators in primary afferent nociceptors, possibly explaining pain and stress-induced symptom flares/exacerbations as typically seen in those with chronic musculoskeletal pain.[103] In addition, stress activates the dorsomedial nucleus of the hypothalamus and subsequent activation of ON-cells plus suppression of OFF-cells[104] (recall that ON- and OFF-cells are different types of neurons in the ventromedial medulla; ON-cells are known to promote nociception and OFF-cells to suppress nociception[57]). Together these central nervous system changes can result in stress-induced hyperalgesia (augmented nociceptive facilitation and suppressed nociceptive inhibition) instead of analgesia.[104] Likewise, chronic exercise stress has detrimental effects on GABA neurotransmission both at the spinal and supraspinal level, resulting in generalized hyperalgesia and disinhibition of the hypothalamic–pituitary–adrenal axis.[72]

Focussing on the role of the sympathetic branch of the autonomic nervous system, sympathetic activation may lead to lowered sensory and pain thresholds.[105] Enhanced sympathetic activation affects muscle spindle function, muscle microcirculation and muscle contractile properties, and consequently might even contribute to the development of central sensitization and chronic pain.[106]

The theoretical framework provided above underscores the importance of addressing stress management in patients with chronic musculoskeletal pain. Stress management programs target the cognitive emotional component of central sensitization pain.

The involvement of dysfunction in the autonomic nervous system (e.g. enhanced activity of the sympathetic nervous system) has been found in chronic widespread pain syndromes characterized by central sensitization (e.g. fibromyalgia[107–109]), but not in all patients with chronic widespread pain or central sensitization. Studying the relation between the autonomic nervous system and chronic widespread pain in a large sample ($n = 1574$), a dysregulation of the autonomic nervous system, including the balance between sympathetic and parasympathetic nervous system activity, was found to be unrelated to the presence of chronic widespread pain.[110] Also, no relation between a dysregulated sympathetic tone and pain intensity was present. But in persons experiencing chronic widespread pain, lower parasympathetic activity was associated with higher pain intensity suggesting that intense pain is a chronic stressor interfering with the parasympathetic activity.[110]

In more localized pain conditions (e.g. lower back pain[111]) there is no clear evidence of the involvement of dysfunctions in the autonomic nervous system. In chronic low back pain, not pain but the perceived disability was related to parasympathetic activity. Cardiac sympathetic activation and parasympathetic withdrawal are caused by psychological stressors,[112] suggesting that it is not the perceived pain as such, but how the patient reacts (i.e. what interpretations they give to painful stimuli) to the pain that may be the key link between the physical and mental aspects experienced.[111] Such observations indicate that interactions between the autonomic nervous system and pain are modulated by the pain neuromatrix.

Similar conclusions can be drawn in patients with chronic whiplash-associated disorders. In the acute stage diminished vasoconstrictive response as an indication of sympathetic nervous system activation has a predictive value for the transition from acute to chronic whiplash-associated disorders.[113] It has been hypothesized that increased acute autonomic activity and variations in hypothalamus–pituitary–adrenal axis activity after a (car) accident would predict an increased likelihood of subsequently developing whiplash-associated disorders.[102] However, the autonomic response to painful stimuli did not differ in chronic whiplash-associated disorders compared to healthy controls.[114] The autonomic nervous system activity or reactivity to pain appeared unrelated to either pain thresholds or endogenous analgesia.[114] However a subgroup of patients with chronic whiplash-associated disorders suffering from moderate post-traumatic stress demonstrated a reduced sympathetic reactivity to pain. This suggests that disturbances in the autonomic nervous system are not a general feature in chronic whiplash, but instead might be a trait of a subgroup experiencing a prolonged state of stress after the impact event.[114] With respect to the hypothalamus–pituitary–adrenal axis, cortisol (one of the major stress hormones and output product of the axis) did not differ either at baseline, nor following cognitive tests in patients with chronic whiplash-associated disorders versus healthy controls.[115]

CONCLUSION

Pain neuroscience has evolved spectacularly over the past 20 years. It is becoming increasingly recognized that musculoskeletal physiotherapy can benefit from pain neuroscience. With respect to diagnosis, musculoskeletal physiotherapists rely on pain neuroscience for the classification of nociceptive versus neuropathic versus central sensitization pain.[116,117] At the communicational level, musculoskeletal therapists can explain pain neuroscience to patients with (chronic) musculoskeletal pain. This strategy is known as therapeutic pain neuroscience education and aims at 'retraining' the patient's pain neuromatrix.[66] More importantly, it prepares the patient for a modern neuroscience approach to musculoskeletal physiotherapy, including hands-on treatment,[10] exercise therapy,[28,118] and behavioural interventions[49] that are inspired by advances in pain neuroscience.

REFERENCES

1. Taguchi T, Yasui M, Kubo A, et al. Nociception originating from the crural fascia in rats. Pain 2013;154(7):1103–14.
2. Treede RD, Jensen TS, Campbell JN, et al. Neuropathic pain: redefinition and a grading system for clinical and research purposes. Neurology 2008;70(18):1630–5.
3. Haroutiunian S, Nikolajsen L, Finnerup NB, et al. The neuropathic component in persistent postsurgical pain: a systematic literature review. Pain 2013;154(1):95–102.
4. Haanpää MTR. Diagnosis and classification of neuropathic pain. Pain Clinical Updates 2010;XVII(7).
5. Staud R, Smitherman ML. Peripheral and central sensitization in fibromyalgia: pathogenetic role. Curr Pain Headache Rep 2002;6(4):259–66.
6. Baranauskas G, Nistri A. Sensitization of pain pathways in the spinal cord: cellular mechanisms. Prog Neurobiol 1998;54(3):349–65.
7. Mendell LM, Wall PD. Responses of single dorsal cord cells to peripheral cutaneous unmyelinated fibres. Nature 1965;206:97–9.
8. Staud R, Robinson ME, Price DD. Temporal summation of second pain and its maintenance are useful for characterizing widespread central sensitization of fibromyalgia patients. J Pain 2007;8(11):893–901.
9. Meeus M, Nijs J. Central sensitization: a biopsychosocial explanation for chronic widespread pain in patients with fibromyalgia and chronic fatigue syndrome. Clin Rheumatol 2007;26(4):465–73.
10. Nijs J, Van Houdenhove B. From acute musculoskeletal pain to chronic widespread pain and fibromyalgia: application of pain neurophysiology in manual therapy practice. Man Ther 2009;14(1):3–12.
11. Shah JP, Phillips TM, Danoff JV, et al. An in vivo microanalytical technique for measuring the local biochemical milieu of human skeletal muscle. J Appl Physiol 1985;99(5):1977–84.
12. Shah JP, Gilliams EA. Uncovering the biochemical milieu of myofascial trigger points using in vivo microdialysis: an application of muscle pain concepts to myofascial pain syndrome. J Bodyw Mov Ther 2008;12(4):371–84.
13. Shah JP, Danoff JV, Desai MJ, et al. Biochemicals associated with pain and inflammation are elevated in sites near to and remote from active myofascial trigger points. Arch Phys Med Rehabil 2008;89(1):16–23.
14. Vierck CJ Jr. Mechanisms underlying development of spatially distributed chronic pain (fibromyalgia). Pain 2006;124(3):242–63.
15. Millan MJ. Descending control of pain. Prog Neurobiol 2002;66(6):355–474.
16. Suzuki R, Morcuende S, Webber M, et al. Superficial NK1-expressing neurons control spinal excitability through activation of descending pathways. Nat Neurosci 2002;5(12):1319–26.
17. Zusman M. Forebrain-mediated sensitization of central pain pathways: 'non-specific' pain and a new image for MT. Man Ther 2002;7(2):80–8.
18. Ursin H, Eriksen HR. Sensitization, subjective health complaints, and sustained arousal. Ann N Y Acad Sci 2001;933:119–29.
19. Swinkels-Meewisse IE, Roelofs J, Schouten EG, et al. Fear of movement/(re)injury predicting chronic disabling low back pain: a prospective inception cohort study. Spine 1976;31(6):658–64.
20. Purves D, Augustine GJ, Fitzpatrick D, et al., editors. Neuroscience. Sunderland: Sinauer Associations; 1997.
21. Pertovaara A. Noradrenergic pain modulation. Prog Neurobiol 2006;80(2):53–83.
22. Woolf CJ, Salter MW. Neuronal plasticity: increasing the gain in pain. Science 2000;288(5472):1765–9.
23. Le Bars D, Villanueva L. Electrophysiological evidence for the activation of descending inhibitory controls by nociceptive afferent pathways. Prog Brain Res 1988;77:275–99.
24. Staud R, Robinson ME, Price DD. Isometric exercise has opposite effects on central pain mechanisms in fibromyalgia patients compared to normal controls. Pain 2005;118(1–2):176–84.
25. Price DD, Staud R, Robinson ME, et al. Enhanced temporal summation of second pain and its central modulation in fibromyalgia patients. Pain 2002;99(1–2):49–59.
26. Banic B, Petersen-Felix S, Andersen OK, et al. Evidence for spinal cord hypersensitivity in chronic pain after whiplash injury and in fibromyalgia. Pain 2004;107(1–2):7–15.
27. Daenen L, Nijs J, Roussel N, et al. Dysfunctional pain inhibition in patients with chronic whiplash-associated disorders: an experimental study. Clin Rheumatol 2012;32(1):23–31.
28. Nijs J, Kosek E, Van Oosterwijck J, et al. Dysfunctional endogenous analgesia during exercise in patients with chronic pain: to exercise or not to exercise? Pain Physician 2012;15(Suppl. 3):ES205–13.
29. Van Oosterwijck J, Nijs J, Meeus M, et al. Lack of endogenous pain inhibition during exercise in people with chronic whiplash associated disorders: an experimental study. J Pain 2012;13(3):242–54.
30. Kosek E, Ekholm J, Hansson P. Modulation of pressure pain thresholds during and following isometric contraction in patients with fibromyalgia and in healthy controls. Pain 1996;64(3):415–23.
31. Meeus M, Roussel NA, Truijen S, et al. Reduced pressure pain thresholds in response to exercise in chronic fatigue syndrome but not in chronic low back pain: an experimental study. J Rehabil Med 2010;42(9):884–90.
32. Martins DF, Bobinski F, Mazzardo-Martins L, et al. Ankle joint mobilization decreases hypersensitivity by activation of peripheral opioid receptors in a mouse model of postoperative pain. Pain Med 2012;13(8):1049–58.
33. Martins DF, Mazzardo-Martins L, Cidral-Filho FJ, et al. Ankle joint mobilization affects postoperative pain through peripheral and central adenosine A1 receptors. Phys Ther 2013;93(3):401–12.
34. Sluka KA, Skyba DA, Radhakrishnan R, et al. Joint mobilization reduces hyperalgesia associated with chronic muscle and joint inflammation in rats. J Pain 2006;7(8):602–7.
35. Coronado RA, Gay CW, Bialosky JE, et al. Changes in pain sensitivity following spinal manipulation: a systematic review and meta-analysis. J Electromyogr Kinesiol 2012;22(5):752–67.
36. Wall B, Melzack R, editors. Textbook of Pain. 3rd ed. London: Churchill-Livingstone; 1994.
37. Peyron R, Laurent B, Garcia-Larrea L. Functional imaging of brain responses to pain. A review and meta-analysis. Neurophysiol Clin 2000;30(5):263–88.
38. Lee MC, Zambreanu L, Menon DK, et al. Identifying brain activity specifically related to the maintenance and perceptual

consequence of central sensitization in humans. J Neurosci 2008; 28(45):11642–9.

39. Li Z, Wang J, Chen L, et al. Basolateral amygdala lesion inhibits the development of pain chronicity in neuropathic pain rats. PLoS ONE 2013;8(8):e70921.

40. Kattoor J, Gizewski ER, Kotsis V, et al. Fear conditioning in an abdominal pain model: neural responses during associative learning and extinction in healthy subjects. PLoS ONE 2013; 8(2):26.

41. Schiller D, Kanen JW, Ledoux JE, et al. Extinction during reconsolidation of threat memory diminishes prefrontal cortex involvement. Proc Natl Acad Sci U S A 2013;110(50):20040–5.

42. Hadjikhani N, Ward N, Boshyan J, et al. The missing link: enhanced functional connectivity between amygdala and visceroceptive cortex in migraine. Cephalalgia 2013;29:29.

43. Kim JY, Kim SH, Seo J, et al. Increased power spectral density in resting-state pain-related brain networks in fibromyalgia. Pain 2013;154(9):1792–7.

44. Schwedt TJ, Schlaggar BL, Mar S, et al. Atypical resting-state functional connectivity of affective pain regions in chronic migraine. Headache 2013;53(5):737–51.

45. Simons LE, Moulton EA, Linnman C, et al. The human amygdala and pain: evidence from neuroimaging. Hum Brain Mapp 2014;35(2):527–38.

46. Schmid J, Theysohn N, Gass F, et al. Neural mechanisms mediating positive and negative treatment expectations in visceral pain: a functional magnetic resonance imaging study on placebo and nocebo effects in healthy volunteers. Pain 2013;16(13):381–3.

47. Zusman M. Mechanisms of musculoskeletal physiotherapy. Phys Ther Rev 2004;9:39–49.

48. Tucker K, Larsson AK, Oknelid S, et al. Similar alteration of motor unit recruitment strategies during the anticipation and experience of pain. Pain 2012;153(3):636–43.

49. Vlaeyen JWSMS, Linton SJ, Boersma K, et al. Pain-related fear. In: Exposure-Based Treatment of Chronic Pain. USA: IASP Press Seattle; 2012. p. 196.

50. Leeuw M, Goossens ME, van Breukelen GJ, et al. Exposure in vivo versus operant graded activity in chronic low back pain patients: results of a randomized controlled trial. Pain 2008;138(1):192–207.

51. Vlaeyen JW, de Jong J, Geilen M, et al. The treatment of fear of movement/(re)injury in chronic low back pain: further evidence on the effectiveness of exposure in vivo. Clin J Pain 2002; 18(4):251–61.

52. de Jong JR, Vlaeyen JW, Onghena P, et al. Reduction of pain-related fear in complex regional pain syndrome type I: the application of graded exposure in vivo. Pain 2005;116(3):264–75.

53. de Jong JR, Vangronsveld K, Peters ML, et al. Reduction of pain-related fear and disability in post-traumatic neck pain: a replicated single-case experimental study of exposure in vivo. J Pain 2008;9(12):1123–34.

54. de Jong JR, Vlaeyen JW, van Eijsden M, et al. Reduction of pain-related fear and increased function and participation in work-related upper extremity pain (WRUEP): effects of exposure in vivo. Pain 2012;153(10):2109–18.

55. Gray AM, Pounds-Cornish E, Eccles FJ, et al. Deep brain stimulation as a treatment for neuropathic pain: a longitudinal study addressing neuropsychological outcomes. J Pain 2013;15(3): 283–92.

56. Wu D, Wang S, Stein JF, et al. Reciprocal interactions between the human thalamus and periaqueductal gray may be important for pain perception. Exp Brain Res 2013;232(2):527–34.

57. Carlson JD, Maire JJ, Martenson ME, et al. Sensitization of pain-modulating neurons in the rostral ventromedial medulla after peripheral nerve injury. J Neurosci 2007;27(48):13222–31.

58. Yanagisawa K, Masui K, Furutani K, et al. Does higher general trust serve as a psychosocial buffer against social pain? An NIRS study of social exclusion. Soc Neurosci 2011;6(2):190–7.

59. Eisenberger NI, Lieberman MD, Williams KD. Does rejection hurt? An FMRI study of social exclusion. Science 2003; 302(5643):290–2.

60. Panksepp J. Neuroscience. Feeling the pain of social loss. Science 2003;302(5643):237–9.

61. Lamm C, Decety J, Singer T. Meta-analytic evidence for common and distinct neural networks associated with directly experienced pain and empathy for pain. Neuroimage 2011;54(3):2492–502.

62. Taylor JJ, Borckardt JJ, George MS. Endogenous opioids mediate left dorsolateral prefrontal cortex rTMS-induced analgesia. Pain 2012;153(6):1219–25.

63. Seminowicz DA, Davis KD. Cortical responses to pain in healthy individuals depends on pain catastrophizing. Pain 2006;120(3): 297–306.

64. Atlas LY, Wager TD. How expectations shape pain. Neurosci Lett 2012;520(2):140–8.

65. Kong J, Kaptchuk TJ, Polich G, et al. Placebo analgesia: findings from brain imaging studies and emerging hypotheses. Rev Neurosci 2007;18(3–4):173–90.

66. Puentedura EJ, Louw A. A neuroscience approach to managing athletes with low back pain. Phys Ther Sport 2012;13(3): 123–33.

67. Meyer RA, Campbell IT, Raja SN. Peripheral neural mechanisms of nociception. In: Wall PD, Melzack R, editors. Textbook of Pain. 3rd ed. Edinburgh: Churchill Livingstone; 1995. p. 13–44.

68. Staud R, Craggs JG, Robinson ME, et al. Brain activity related to temporal summation of C-fiber evoked pain. Pain 2007;129(1–2): 130–42.

69. Bell IR, Baldwin CM, Schwartz GE. Illness from low levels of environmental chemicals: relevance to chronic fatigue syndrome and fibromyalgia. Am J Med 1998;105(3A):S74–82.

70. Seifert F, Maihofner C. Central mechanisms of experimental and chronic neuropathic pain: findings from functional imaging studies. Cell Mol Life Sci: CMLS 2009;66(3):375–90.

71. Zhuo M. A synaptic model for pain: long-term potentiation in the anterior cingulate cortex. Mol Cells 2007;23(3):259–71.

72. Suarez-Roca H, Leal L, Silva JA, et al. Reduced GABA neurotransmission underlies hyperalgesia induced by repeated forced swimming stress. Behav Brain Res 2008;189(1):159–69.

73. Grunnesjo MI, Bogefeldt JP, Blomberg SI, et al. A randomized controlled trial of the effects of muscle stretching, manual therapy and steroid injections in addition to 'stay active' care on health-related quality of life in acute or subacute low back pain. Clin Rehabil 2011;25(11):999–1010.

74. Surenkok O, Aytar A, Baltaci G. Acute effects of scapular mobilization in shoulder dysfunction: a double-blind randomized placebo-controlled trial. J Sport Rehabil 2009;18(4):493–501.

75. Brantingham JW, Cassa TK, Bonnefin D, et al. Manipulative and multimodal therapy for upper extremity and temporomandibular disorders: a systematic review. J Manipulative Physiol Ther 2013;36(3):143–201.

76. Struyf F, Nijs J, Mollekens S, et al. Scapular-focused treatment in patients with shoulder impingement syndrome: a randomized clinical trial. Clin Rheumatol 2013;32(1):73–85.

77. Lluch Girbes E, Nijs J, Torres-Cueco R, et al. Pain treatment for patients with osteoarthritis and central sensitization. Phys Ther 2013;93(6):842–51.

78. Meeus M, Vervisch S, De Clerck LS, et al. Central sensitization in patients with rheumatoid arthritis: a systematic literature review. Semin Arthritis Rheum 2012;41(4):556–67.

79. Sterling M. Differential development of sensory hypersensitivity and a measure of spinal cord hyperexcitability following whiplash injury. Pain 2010;150(3):501–6.

80. Curatolo M, Petersen-Felix S, Arendt-Nielsen L, et al. Central hypersensitivity in chronic pain after whiplash injury. Clin J Pain 2001;17(4):306–15.

81. Staud R. Evidence of involvement of central neural mechanisms in generating fibromyalgia pain. Curr Rheumatol Rep 2002;4(4): 299–305.

82. Roussel NA, Nijs J, Meeus M, et al. Central sensitization and altered central pain processing in chronic low back pain: fact or myth? Clin J Pain 2013;29(7):625–38.

83. Kaya S, Hermans L, Willems T, et al. Central sensitization in urogynecological chronic pelvic pain: a systematic literature review. Pain Physician 2013;16(4):291–308.

84. Fernandez-Carnero J, Fernandez-de-Las-Penas C, de la Llave-Rincon AI, et al. Widespread mechanical pain hypersensitivity as sign of central sensitization in unilateral epicondylalgia: a blinded, controlled study. Clin J Pain 2009;25(7):555–61.

85. Smart KM, Blake C, Staines A, et al. Self-reported pain severity, quality of life, disability, anxiety and depression in patients classified with 'nociceptive', 'peripheral neuropathic' and 'central sensitisation' pain. The discriminant validity of mechanisms-based

classifications of low back (+/–leg) pain. Man Ther 2012;17(2): 119–25.

86. Sterling M, Jull G, Vicenzino B, et al. Sensory hypersensitivity occurs soon after whiplash injury and is associated with poor recovery. Pain 2003;104(3):509–17.

87. Jull G, Sterling M, Kenardy J, et al. Does the presence of sensory hypersensitivity influence outcomes of physical rehabilitation for chronic whiplash? – A preliminary RCT. Pain 2007;129(1–2): 28–34.

88. Coombes BK, Bisset L, Vicenzino B. Thermal hyperalgesia distinguishes those with severe pain and disability in unilateral lateral epicondylalgia. Clin J Pain 2012;28(7):595–601.

89. Mayer TG, Neblett R, Cohen H, et al. The development and psychometric validation of the central sensitization inventory. Pain Pract 2012;12(4):276–85.

90. Neblett R, Cohen H, Choi Y, et al. The Central Sensitization Inventory (CSI): establishing clinically significant values for identifying central sensitivity syndromes in an outpatient chronic pain sample. J Pain 2013;14(5):438–45.

91. Nijs J, Roussel N, Paul van Wilgen C, et al. Thinking beyond muscles and joints: therapists' and patients' attitudes and beliefs regarding chronic musculoskeletal pain are key to applying effective treatment. Man Ther 2012;18(2):96–102.

92. Gifford L, Butler D. The integration of pain sciences into clinical practice. J Hand Ther 1997;10:86–95.

93. Louw A, Diener I, Butler DS, et al. The effect of neuroscience education on pain, disability, anxiety, and stress in chronic musculoskeletal pain. Arch Phys Med Rehabil 2011;92(12):2041–56.

94. Nijs J, Paul van Wilgen C, Van Oosterwijck J, et al. How to explain central sensitization to patients with 'unexplained' chronic musculoskeletal pain: practice guidelines. Man Ther 2011;16(5): 413–18.

95. Van Oosterwijck J, Nijs J, Meeus M, et al. Pain neurophysiology education improves cognitions, pain thresholds, and movement performance in people with chronic whiplash: a pilot study. J Rehabil Res Dev 2011;48(1):43–58.

96. Moseley GL. Evidence for a direct relationship between cognitive and physical change during an education intervention in people with chronic low back pain. Eur J Pain 2004;8(1):39–45.

97. Moseley GL. Widespread brain activity during an abdominal task markedly reduced after pain physiology education: fMRI evaluation of a single patient with chronic low back pain. Aust J Physiother 2005;51(1):49–52.

98. Moseley GL. Joining forces – combining cognition-targeted motor control training with group or individual pain physiology education: a successful treatment for chronic low back pain. J Man Manip Ther 2003;11:88–94.

99. Moseley GL, Nicholas MK, Hodges PW. A randomized controlled trial of intensive neurophysiology education in chronic low back pain. Clin J Pain 2004;20(5):324–30.

100. Moseley GL. Combined physiotherapy and education is efficacious for chronic low back pain. Aust J Physiother 2002;48(4): 297–302.

101. Van Oosterwijck J, Meeus M, Paul L, et al. Pain physiology education improves health status and endogenous pain inhibition in fibromyalgia: a double-blind randomized controlled trial. Clin J Pain 2013;29(10):873–82.

102. McLean SA, Clauw DJ, Abelson JL, et al. The development of persistent pain and psychological morbidity after motor vehicle collision: integrating the potential role of stress response systems into a biopsychosocial model. Psychosom Med 2005;67(5): 783–90.

103. Khasar SG, Burkham J, Dina OA, et al. Stress induces a switch of intracellular signaling in sensory neurons in a model of generalized pain. J Neurosci 2008;28(22):5721–30.

104. Martenson ME, Cetas JS, Heinricher MM. A possible neural basis for stress-induced hyperalgesia. Pain 2009;142(3):236–44.

105. Caceres C, Burns JW. Cardiovascular reactivity to psychological stress may enhance subsequent pain sensitivity. Pain 1997; 69(3):237–44.

106. Passatore M, Roatta S. Influence of sympathetic nervous system on sensorimotor function: whiplash associated disorders (WAD) as a model. Eur J Appl Physiol 2006;98(5):423–49.

107. Martinez-Lavin M, Hermosillo AG, Mendoza C, et al. Orthostatic sympathetic derangement in subjects with fibromyalgia. J Rheumatol 1997;24(4):714–18.

108. Raj SR, Brouillard D, Simpson CS, et al. Dysautonomia among patients with fibromyalgia: a noninvasive assessment. J Rheumatol 2000;27(11):2660–5.

109. Furlan R, Colombo S, Perego F, et al. Abnormalities of cardiovascular neural control and reduced orthostatic tolerance in patients with primary fibromyalgia. J Rheumatol 2005;32(9):1787–93.

110. Barakat A, Vogelzangs N, Licht CM, et al. Dysregulation of the autonomic nervous system and its association with the presence and intensity of chronic widespread pain. Arthritis Care Res 2012;64(8):1209–16.

111. Gockel M, Lindholm H, Niemisto L, et al. Perceived disability but not pain is connected with autonomic nervous function among patients with chronic low back pain. J Rehabil Med 2008; 40(5):355–8.

112. Cacioppo JT, Malarkey WB, Kiecolt-Glaser JK, et al. Heterogeneity in neuroendocrine and immune responses to brief psychological stressors as a function of autonomic cardiac activation. Psychosom Med 1995;57(2):154–64.

113. Sterling M, Jull G, Vicenzino B, et al. Physical and psychological factors predict outcome following whiplash injury. Pain 2005; 114(1–2):141–8.

114. De Kooning M, Daenen L, Cras P, et al. Autonomic response to pain in patients with chronic whiplash associated disorders. Pain Physician 2013;16(3):E277–85.

115. Meeus M, Van Oosterwijck J, Ickmans K, et al. Interrelationships between pain processing, cortisol and cognitive performance in chronic whiplash-associated disorders. Clin Rheumatol 2014; [Epub ahead of print].

116. Nijs J, Van Houdenhove B, Oostendorp RA. Recognition of central sensitization in patients with musculoskeletal pain: application of pain neurophysiology in manual therapy practice. Man Ther 2010;15(2):135–41.

117. Smart KM, Blake C, Staines A, et al. The Discriminative validity of 'nociceptive,' 'peripheral neuropathic,' and 'central sensitization' as mechanisms-based classifications of musculoskeletal pain. Clin J Pain 2011;27(8):655–63.

118. Nijs J, Meeus M, Cagnie B, et al. A modern neuroscience approach to chronic spinal pain: combining pain neuroscience education with cognition-targeted motor control training. Phys Ther 2014;94(5):730–8.

CHAPTER 3

NEURO-ELECTROCHEMISTRY OF MOVEMENT

Harsimran Baweja

EDITOR'S INTRODUCTION

In this chapter the author, a neuro physiologist and physical therapist, has provided the reader with a detailed description of the complex neuro-electrochemistry underpinning movement. Descriptions of the neural pathways or 'circuitry' involved in movement are detailed elsewhere in this book; however, it is easy to forget the sophisticated neural physiology that is involved in the propagation, direction and conveyance of signals within these circuits. The neuro-electrochemical interactions within the nerve and those of synaptic transmission are described in detail. It is hoped that this chapter will remind us that our understanding of the neurophysiology of movement must start at an electrochemical level.

Multiple levels of the nervous system collaborate for the neurophysiological control of movement – how the nervous system controls the actions of muscles to produce human motion is akin to biomechanical principles. Several processes occur concurrently and in synchrony for activation signals to be generated by the neural tissues, leading to muscle contraction and production of forces for movement to be executed. At the most fundamental functional level of all, this is the motor unit. A motor unit consists of the anterior horn cell in the spinal cord, its motor neuron and all the muscle fibers it supplies.[1] The motor unit and its properties are discussed in greater depth later in this book. The objective of this chapter is to provide insight into the neuronal electrochemical physiology underlying the operation of excitable membranes on nerves, motor units and thereafter muscles in a global sense. This chapter includes the physiological properties of excitable membranes, resting membrane potential, action potentials and their propagation and transmission across the synapses.

Information is transmitted across nerve cells because of the electrical signals produced within them. One would then assume that neurons are good conductors of electricity, but they are not. Rather, the system has mechanisms set in place for producing these signals simply on the movement of ions across the nerve cell membranes. Typically, excitable membranes generate a negative potential, called the resting membrane potential. This is measured by recording the potential difference between the cytoplasmic and extracellular fluid. In the presence of a stimulus, an action potential momentarily eliminates the negative resting membrane potential and creates a positive potential. Action potentials are the signals that relay information along the axons from one structure to another within the nervous system. These information-packed neural signals arise due to ionic fluctuations, the selective permeability of the membranes to different species of ions and the uneven circulation of these ions across excitable membranes.

In order to comprehend muscle activation by the nervous system, it is important to review a few basic physical principles underlying 'neuro-electrochemistry'. These principles deal with the presence and flow of electric charge through electrical conductors[2,3] within the nervous system. These help one appreciate the flow of current along the excitable membranes, which enable the interaction of contractile proteins in muscles on a grander scale.

FUNDAMENTAL PRINCIPLES UNDERLYING NEURO-ELECTROCHEMISTRY

Electrical Potential and Current

Electrical potential is the difference between charged particles at any two points on a current-carrying conductor and is the cause of current flow. Very often it is interchangeably referred to as voltage, electromotive force or simply 'potential difference'. Electrical potential is measured in volts (V or ΔV for potential difference), which is defined as the amount of work (Joules; J) required to move one coulomb (C) of charge (Q) between any two points in a circuit (equation 1):

$$V = J/C \qquad [1]$$

Current is the rate at which the charged particles move between two points on an electrical conductor with a potential difference. Opposing charges move towards each other. That is charges with a negative polarity move towards areas of positive polarity and vice versa. Current (I) is measured in amperes (A) and is defined as the amount of charge (Q) crossing a given point on a conductor in one second (time; t) (equation 2):

$$I = Q/t \qquad [2]$$

We can compute the electrical potential of a 'neuronal' battery if we know the ionic concentrations on either side of the membrane. This forms the electrochemical basis for the resting membrane potential, which is discussed in greater depth, in the next section.

Conductance

The electrical conductance (G) of an electrical conductor is the ease at which an electric current passes through it. Electrical conductance is measured in Siemens (S). Simply put, conductance is dependent upon the length (L) and the cross-sectional area (A) of the conductor and the conductivity (proportionality constant; σ) of the material. This relation is described as equation 3:

$$G = \sigma \frac{A}{L} \qquad [3]$$

Resistance

The inverse of conductance is resistance. The electrical resistance (R) is the opposition to the passage of an electric current through an electric conductor. Electrical resistance shares some theoretical equivalents with the mechanical notion of friction. The SI unit of electrical resistance is the ohm (Ω). Resistance is the inverse of conductance and is dependent upon the same factors as conductance. These are length of the conductor, its cross-sectional area and the proportionality constant called resistivity (ρ). This relation is described in equation 4:

$$R = \rho \frac{L}{A} \qquad [4]$$

Ohm's law asserts an essential relation between the resistance, electrical potential and the current in an electrical conductor. Ohm's law states that the current through a conductor between two points is directly proportional to the potential difference across the two points.[4] In this relation resistance is the constant of proportionality, giving us the following (equation 5):

$$I = V/R \qquad [5]$$

where I is the current through a conductor. The SI unit for current is ampere (A), and R is the resistance of the conductor, measured in units of ohms.[5]

Taken together, these are some of the fundamental constructs[6] underlying the electrophysiological properties of excitable membranes and neurons. For example, neurons can be classified as fast-conducting and slow-conducting depending on their length, cross-sectional area and degree of myelination. The following sections discuss the electrochemical processes underlying some of these principles.

RESTING MEMBRANE POTENTIAL

The relatively inert membrane potential of electrically silent cells is known as the resting membrane potential.

In the nervous system, neurons act as batteries storing potential energy (E) because of charged particles across their membranes. The difference in polarity and concentration gradient of the ions present on either side of the membrane leads to an electrical potential difference. The Nernst equation describes this electrical potential within a neuronal 'battery' as (equation 6):

$$\begin{aligned} E &= \frac{RT}{zF} \ln \frac{[\text{concentration of ions}]_{outside}}{[\text{concentration of ions}]_{inside}} \\ &= 2.303 \frac{RT}{zF} \log_{10} \frac{[\text{concentration of ions}]_{outside}}{[\text{concentration of ions}]_{inside}} \end{aligned} \qquad [6]$$

where, R = gas constant, T = absolute temperature (Kelvins), z = valence (electrical charge) of the ions and F = Faraday constant (i.e., the amount of electric charge contained in one mole of a univalent ion). Given that at room temperature and normal atmospheric pressure (at sea level):[7]

$$RT/zF \cong 26\,mV/z \qquad [7]$$

one can work out the electric potential difference across a membrane if the ionic concentrations inside and outside the cell are known. Let us consider that the concentration gradient of K^+ outside the cell is ten times lesser than its concentration inside the cell. Inputting this together with equation 6 into equation 7 for K^+:

$$E_K = 2.303 * \frac{26\,mV}{z_K} \log_{10} \frac{[1]_{outside}}{[10]_{inside}} \qquad [8]$$

The valance of z for K^+ is +1 and log 1/10 equals −1. Solving for the equilibrium potential (E_K) and rewriting the equation 8 above:

$$E_K \cong 60 * -1 \cong -60\,mV \qquad [9]$$

The fundamental characteristic of voltage is that negatively charged ions move towards a higher voltage and positively charged ions move towards lower voltages. Consequently, the current in an electrical conductor always flows from higher voltage to lower voltage. In some cases, current can flow from a lower voltage to a higher voltage, but only at the expense of energy to push the positively charged ions against a higher potential gradient. From a biophysical point of view, this flow occurs due to the difference in ionic gradient across the membranes. These occur as a result of specific membrane permeability for potassium, sodium, calcium, chloride and bicarbonate ions, which result from changes in functional activity of various ion channels and ion transporters.

In summary, the membrane permeability for potassium is high, causing potassium ions to flow from the intracellular cytoplasm into the extracellular fluid carrying out a positive charge. Once the movement of potassium ions is balanced by the build-up of a negative charge on the inner surface of the membrane, resting membrane potential is established.[8-17]

Experimentally Measuring the Membrane Potential

The most popular electrophysiological method used to measure membrane potential is the voltage clamp method (Fig. 3-1).[18] Its name is derived from the ability to measure potential difference across voltage-gated ionic channels. Essentially, a voltage clamp allows the experimenter to control the membrane voltage and measure the transmembrane current required to maintain that voltage.[19-23]

In the early 1940s, Kenneth Cole[24] came up with the notion of voltage clamping. He tested the hypothesis that a cell's membrane potential could be experimentally maintained by using pair of electrodes and a feedback circuit, and discovered that it was feasible to do so. It was with the help of this technique that Hodgkin and Huxley conducted a series of seminal experiments[13,17,25-38] contributing to our basic understanding of the resting membrane potential and action potential. Together, their work led to Hodgkin and Huxley being conferred the Nobel Prize in Physiology and Medicine in 1963.[39,40]

In its simplest form, a voltage clamp consists of a two-electrode pair apparatus. A pair of electrodes is connected to a current generator and a pair is connected to a voltmeter. A stimulating electrode from the current generator and a recording electrode from the voltmeter are placed inside the cell. The second electrode from the current generator is placed outside the cell and acts as the ground electrode, while the second electrode from the voltmeter records the voltage from outside the membrane. The generator is used to deliver a current pulse through the membrane and the corresponding change in the transmembrane potential is recorded by the voltmeter. The advantages of performing voltage clamping include: (a) it eliminates the capacitive current (e.g. synaptic potentials); (b) the current flow is proportional to the number of open channels (i.e. membrane conductance); and (c) it offers control over the opening and closing of transmembrane ionic channels.[19-23]

The experimentally derived values of physiologically important ionic equilibrium potentials across the squid nerve cell membranes for K^+, Na^+, and Cl^- are −75, +55 and −60 mV, respectively.[41] The resting membrane potential of nerve cells is approximately −65 mV. Over a series of seminal experiments, Hodgkin and Katz[42,43] suggested that the membrane potential at rest is negative because: (a) the excitable membranes at rest are more permeable to K^+ than other physiologically important ion species; and (b) the ionic concentration of K^+ inside the neuron is greater than outside. Therefore, at rest the net ionic polarity inside a cell membrane is negative. The transmembrane ionic gradients equilibrium and transport is maintained by the Na^+/K^+ pump (commonly known as the sodium–potassium pump). This is discussed in greater detail in the next section.

Sodium–Potassium Pump

The resting membrane potential across excitable membranes and nerve cells is established by the Na^+/K^+

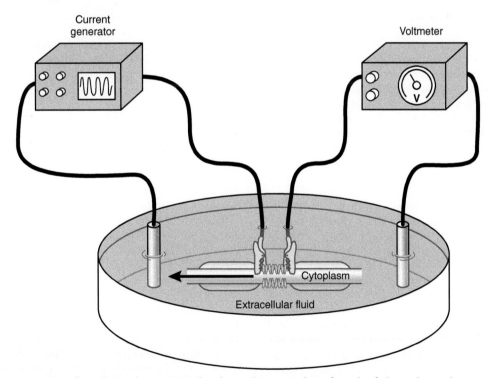

FIGURE 3-1 ■ Representation of a voltage clamp setup. A voltage clamp consists of a pair of electrodes each connected to a current generator and a voltmeter. A stimulating electrode from the current generator and a recording electrode from the voltmeter are placed inside the cell. The other electrode from the current generator is placed outside the cell and acts as the ground electrode, while the one from the voltmeter records the voltage from outside the membrane. The generator is used to deliver a current pulse through the membrane and the corresponding change in the membrane potential is recorded by the voltmeter. (Adapted from Adrian RH, Chandler WK, Hodgkin AL. Voltage clamp experiments in skeletal muscle fibres. J Physiol 1966;186(2):51P–2P.)

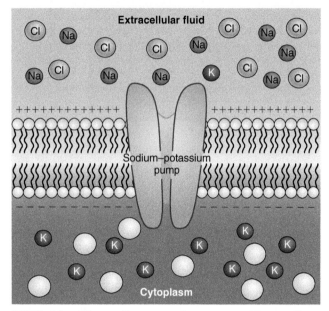

FIGURE 3-2 ■ The sodium–potassium pump. The sodium–potassium pump is a transmembrane antiporter molecule present on the phospholipid bilayer membrane. It helps the bidirectional transport of K⁺ and Na⁺ ions across the membrane. (Adapted from Hall JE, Guyton AC. Textbook of Medical Physiology. St. Louis, Mo: Elsevier Saunders; 2006.)

(sodium–potassium pump; Fig. 3-2). The separation and transport of potassium (K⁺) and relatively immobile bicarbonate (HCO₃⁻) ions from the intracellular cytoplasm, and the sodium (Na⁺) and chloride (Cl⁻) ions in the extracellular fluid causes a concentration gradient across the membranes. Because of concentration gradients, a cell cannot maintain the passive diffusion of sodium and potassium ions in and out of the membrane indefinitely. This is where the Na⁺/K⁺ pump comes in to play. It is a transmembrane antiporter molecule present on the phospholipid bilayer membrane. The primary mechanistic function of the Na⁺/K⁺ pump as a protein embedded in the membrane is that it can return Na⁺ and K⁺ ions to their regions of higher concentrations. The protein has binding sites for Na⁺ and ATP inside the cell and K⁺ on the outside of the cell. The Na⁺/K⁺ pump actively transports different ions across excitable membranes in opposite directions by expending one molecule of energy (ATP). The Na⁺/K⁺–ATPase enzyme promotes the transport of K⁺ out of the cell and Na⁺ into the cell.

The equilibrium potential for K⁺ is around −78 mV and is the primary driver for the resting membrane potential. But the resting membrane potential is typically around −65 mV. This suggests that the other ions such as Cl⁻, Na⁺ and HCO₃⁻ also contribute towards the resting membrane potentials, but to a proportionally smaller extent than K⁺. Because of the greater concentration gradient of Na⁺ in the extracellular fluid, the net ionic movement of Na⁺ is inwards. This deposit of Na⁺ within the intracellular cytoplasm generates a lesser negative charge inside the cell than the equilibrium potential of K⁺. Consequently, the resting membrane potential is sustained due to a relatively constant influx of Na⁺ and efflux of K⁺ across the nerve cell membrane. This would also imply that the Nernst equation is simplistic as it only considers

one permeant species of ions crossing the membrane at any given instance. Therefore, in 1943, David Goldman developed what is now known as the Goldman equation.[44] This equation accounts for not only the concentration gradients of multiple permeant ionic species, but also the relative permeability of the membrane to these ions. A simple version of the Goldman equation for Na⁺, K⁺, HCO₃⁻ and Cl⁻ can be written as (equation 10):

$$V = 60\log_{10}\frac{\begin{array}{c}P_{Na}[Na]_{outside} + P_K[K]_{outside} \\ + P_{HCO}[HCO]_{inside} + P_{Cl}[Cl]_{inside}\end{array}}{\begin{array}{c}P_{Na}[Na]_{inside} + P_K[K]_{inside} \\ + P_{HCO}[HCO]_{outside} + P_{Cl}[Cl]_{outside}\end{array}} \quad [10]$$

Where, V is the transmembrane voltage and P is the relative permeability of the membrane to these ions. It looks similar to the Nernst equation and is an extension of it to account for all the ionic species and their membrane permeability. It is important to note that the valence (z) has been eliminated, consequently inverting the concentrations of the anions (HCO₃⁻ and Cl⁻) relative to the cations (Na⁺ and K⁺).

So far, it has been assumed that neurons maintain steady ionic concentration gradients across their excitable membrane surfaces. But ions are never in a state of electrochemical homeostasis; rather resting membrane potential is a bit noisy in vivo. Unless nerve cells can restore the ions displaced during current flow during neural signalling and the constant ionic escape that occurs at rest, there will be a steady dissipation of the concentration gradients creating an imbalance. A group of plasma membrane proteins known as active transporters maintain the ionic concentration and gradient. Active transporters do this by forming complex molecules which they translocate and slowly supply energy in the form of ion concentration gradients across the membranes. In the case of a stimulus, the opening of ionic channels rapidly disintegrates this stored energy to being the cascade of processes involved in generating and transmitting the action potential.

ACTION POTENTIAL AND ITS PROPAGATION

We have established that bidirectional exchange of ions is the ionic basis for the production and occurrence of the membrane potential. This exchange occurs as a function of the membrane's permeability to various ions on either side. For the generation of an action potential within a neuronal cell, it is the interplay of these processes that underlies neuronal signalling. The reversal of polarity inside the cell (due to an influx of excessive Na⁺ by the Na⁺/K⁺ pump) relative to outside of the cell is referred to as depolarization. This typically requires an activation signal to trigger the influx of Na⁺ via the Na⁺/K⁺ pump. The return to resting membrane polarity due to an increase in the K⁺ efflux is known as repolarization.

An action potential is an all-or-none event. This means that the voltage threshold has to be breached

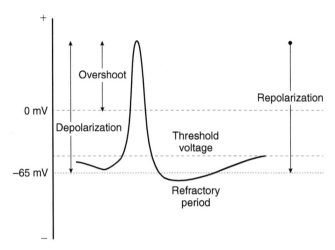

FIGURE 3-3 ■ A representative action potential and its phases. The initial depolarization, overshoot, repolarization and hyperpolarization (refractory period). The grey-dotted line indicates an arbitrary threshold potential. If the ionic imbalance leads to a potential generation greater than this voltage an action potential will be generated. This is the all-or-none principle. (Adapted from Hodgkin AL, Huxley AF. A quantitative description of membrane current and its application to conduction and excitation in nerve. J Physiol 1952;117(4):500–44.)

by an activation signal to cause the cascade of events that lead to an action potential. This can then be repeated once every few milliseconds until there is an activation signal (stimulus) providing the drive to alter the resting state.

An action potential arises from the temporary reversal of the membrane potential due to an increase in the permeability to Na^+.[30] The concurrent activation of many synapses leads to the activation of the ionic channels necessary to cause the reversal of the membrane polarity – depolarization. So the resting membrane potential that is originally negative now starts to become positive. This continues until the Na^+ channels are open, creating an influx of Na^+. Once the ionic channels transporting Na^+ into the cell close, the membrane permeability to K^+ is restored – repolarization and the ionic balance returns the potential to resting membrane potential. These are the sequence of events that occur within a neuronal cell during the generation of an action potential. This action potential is then quickly transmitted along the axon.[10,13,17,24-38,42,43,45-57]

Decomposing an Action Potential

Action potentials have a characteristic waveform that can be divided into phases. Each phase marks a particular ionic event leading to a change in the voltage across the membrane, rendering a characteristic waveform to the action potential. Figure 3-3 describes the typical waveform of an action potential. There are four basic parts to an action potential – the initial depolarization, overshoot, repolarization and hyperpolarization (refractory period). A stimulus triggers the action potential by causing a rapid and transient reversal of the permeability to Na^+ into the cytoplasm. This causes a rise in the membrane potential and is known as the initial

depolarization (change in polarity). During the rising phase, the depolarizing membrane potential momentarily becomes positive with respect to the extracellular fluid, causing greater positive potential to be recorded and is called an overshoot. The peak of the overshoot corresponds with the closure of the sodium channels, thus causing a fall in the potential (seen as the downward limb of the action potential in Fig. 3-3). This rapid decline in the membrane potential back to negative polarity is known as repolarization. Repolarization reflects the rapid intake of K^+ ions back into the cytoplasm. Similar to the overshoot, during repolarization excessive K^+ intake leads to an undershoot (below the resting membrane potential). This undershoot is known as the after hyperpolarization or refractory period. The beauty of the refractory period is that it is difficult to elicit another action potential during this phase. This is because as an action potential moves along the nerve axon, it leaves behind it the Na^+ channels inactivated and K^+ channels activated for a brief time. Hence, the period is defined by the time necessary to reactivate the Na^+ channels to open up and the K^+ channels to close down. This limits the number of action potentials that can be generated per unit time by a given cell. This is also the physiological phenomenon accounting for the unidirectional flow of current in nerve cells.

An intriguing concept of action potential generation is its all-or-none nature. This means the action potential will not initiate below a certain membrane potential, known as the threshold potential. The initial triggering stimulus could be a synaptic input or an external electric current that facilitates the spread of an action potential down the axon. The ionic channels mediating the rapid reversal of the membrane permeability are voltage-gated channels. These channels do not activate and open up completely unless a criterion voltage has been achieved on the outside of the membrane. There is a range of sub-critical depolarization, where the rate of Na^+ influx is less than the rate of K^+ efflux from within the cell (recall the resting membrane is favourably permeable to K^+ and requires the efflux of K^+ for depolarization). So there would be a certain level – the threshold – at which the efflux matches the influx leading to an unstable equilibrium above the resting membrane potential. Theoretically, an action potential would occur if at this point there was a net increase of Na^+ inwards; on the contrary, repolarization would occur if there was a net gain of K^+ inside the membrane. Therefore a threshold is defined as the depolarizing membrane potential at which the ionic potential of Na^+ entering is equal to that of K^+ exiting the cell.[58]

Action Potential Propagation

The voltage-dependent mechanisms underlying the generation of action potentials are also responsible for their transmission (Fig. 3-4). This means an action potential will propagate if there is a directional displacement of the transient membrane potential reversal across the nerve axon.

A depolarizing trigger such as a postsynaptic potential or an experimentally induced current injected into the

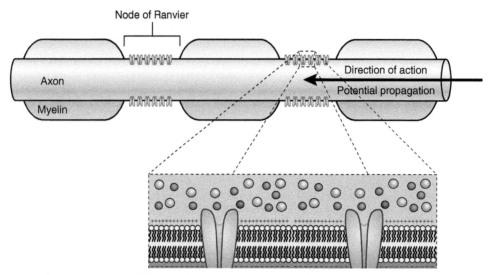

FIGURE 3-4 ■ Representation of action potential transmission along a myelinated neuronal axon. The transmission of action potentials along the axons of nerve fibers is facilitated by passive conductance due to the potential difference between the electrically active sites of the action potential and the inactive sites in the direction of propagation on the axon. (Adapted from Dodge FA, Frankenhaeuser B. Membrane currents in isolated frog nerve fibre under voltage clamp conditions. J Physiol 1958;143(1):76–90.)

membrane causes the local depolarization of the excitable membrane. This leads to the opening of voltage-gated Na^+ channels in that area (e.g. node of Ranvier on an axon). The opening of these channels leads to a transient increase on the influx of Na^+, depolarizing the membrane potential enough to breach the threshold initiating an action potential in that area. A small quantity of the current generated by the action potential flows passively along the axon by electronic conductance. This means that Na^+ does not move along the axon, but transfers its charge to neighbouring particles passively. This passive current flow causes the depolarization of membrane potential in the adjacent node of Ranvier (on an axon). Thus, the local depolarization initiates an action potential in this node, repeating the cascade of events in an ongoing cycle until the length of the axon is traversed. Consequently, the transmission of action potentials entails the organized current flow in two ways: active currents flowing through voltage-gated ion channels and passive flow of current through conductance.

The electrochemical mechanisms explained above render the following principal properties to the propagation of action potentials: (a) the propagation to action potentials is also an all-or-none event. This means that the magnitude of the action potentials measured across the length of its transmission remains constant; (b) due to the refractory nature of the involved ion channels, action potential propagation is unidirectional; and (c) action potentials have a measurable conduction velocity. The conduction velocity is dependent on the thickness of the axon, number of ionic channels lining the nodes of Ranvier, the state of neuronal myelination and the length of the axon. The rate of transmission is measureable by placing recording electrodes at varying distances on the axon. The mechanism of action potential propagation is comprehensible if one understands the generation of action potentials, the passive flow of current in conductors and axons and the functioning of voltage-gated ionic channels.

A NOTE ON SYNAPTIC TRANSMISSION

An activation signal is necessary for an action potential to develop and propagate through the axon of a nerve cell. This activation signal needs to possess the charge necessary to depolarize the cell membrane and cause the cascade of events leading to the generation and propagation of the action potential mentioned in the previous sections of this chapter. These activation signals are generated at and propagated via synapses: the functional connections between nerve cells which allow the flow of information across the length of the nervous system. Based on the specialized modus operandi, synapses are fundamentally classified into electrical and chemical synapses. While electrical synapses allow for the direct flow of current via gap junctions, chemical synapses cause the flow of current through neurotransmitter secretion across the synaptic junction.

In the case of an electrical synapse, the presynaptic and postsynaptic membranes are lined with pairs of communicating ion channels that are separated by a microscopic gap of 2–3 nanometers. The term gap junction is used to describe this space in an electrical synapse (Fig. 3-5). For the postsynaptic membrane to depolarize there needs to be an action potential traversing the presynaptic neuron and ample pairs of ionic channels and gap junctions to cause a sufficient transfer of the current to change the postsynaptic membrane threshold.[59] The advantages of having electrical synapses are that they allow for two-way communication within neurons. They work by high passive conductance of ionic current from one neuron to another along the series. The flow of current is very rapid compared with chemical synapses. One of the most important functions of electrical synapses is their role in emergency situations. Because of the speed of transmission across an electrical synapse, onset of the elicited motor response is very rapid, as needed in life-saving circumstances.[60]

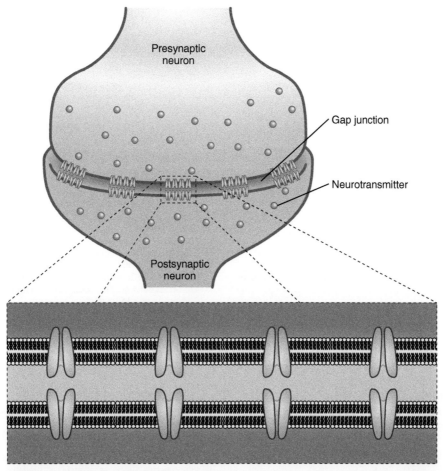

FIGURE 3-5 ■ Representations of an electric synapse. The presynaptic and postsynaptic membranes are lined with pairs of communicating ion channels that are separated by gap junctions. (Adapted from Hall JE, Guyton AC. Textbook of Medical Physiology. St. Louis, Mo: Elsevier Saunders; 2006.)

Chemical synapses use neurotransmitters to convey information from one neuron to another.[61-63] The 'gaps' in chemical synapses are considerably larger (~20–40 nanometers) than in electrical synapses and are known as synaptic clefts. Characteristic of these synapses are synaptic vesicles that store the chemical neurotransmitters. The release of the neurotransmitter from a synaptic vesicle occurs on the arrival of the action potential at the presynaptic end of the synapse.[64] The incoming action potential causes the opening of the Ca^{2+} voltage-gated channels at the presynaptic end.[65] Consequently, the increase of Ca^{2+} concentration in the presynaptic terminal mobilizes the vesicles towards the presynaptic membrane, where they fuse and release neurotransmitter into the cleft.[66-68] This release process is known as exocytosis.[69] Upon reaching the postsynaptic membrane the neurotransmitter binds with specific binding sites on the membrane. This causes the change in the conductance (increase or decrease) of the membrane potential in the postsynaptic neuron – causing excitation or inhibition based on the nature of the signal. Due to the cascade of events that occur for transmission to complete across a chemical synapse, the speed of transmission is relatively slower than across electrical synapses. Furthermore, synaptic vesicles release neurotransmitters in fixed quantities, also known as quanta.[70] This produces membrane potentials proportional to the quantum of received neurotransmitter in the postsynaptic neuron. In brief, this is the mechanism of interneuronal transfer of information.

SUMMARY

Excitable membranes on neural tissue generate electricity to transport signals across the nervous system and other cells. These signals are generated due to changes in the transmembrane resting potential. The resting membrane potential arises due to membrane permeability to physiologically important ion species which cause a transmembrane ionic gradient. Specifically, the resting membrane potential results from predominant membrane permeability to K^+. Action potentials are voltage-gated events that occur due to a transient reversal of the membrane permeability to Na^+. Upon the closure of these Na^+ channels the membrane potential reverts to its K^+ permeability, causing repolarization. As this is a voltage-gated event, momentarily during repolarization, another action potential cannot be elicited from the same site on the membrane.

Action potentials and their properties have been studied for years via a technique called voltage clamping developed in the 1940s. It allows for the control and regulation of the transmembrane potentials in a laboratory setting. Significant scientific work using this technique has established that the ionic gradients and their transmembrane potentials are the basis of the all-or-none nature of action potentials. The transmission of action potentials along the axons of nerve fibres is facilitated by passive conductance due to the potential difference between the electrically active sites of the action potential and the inactive sites in the direction of propagation on the axon.

Interneuronal communication and transmission of action potential occurs via specialized junctions between neurons. These junctions are called synapses. Based on their specialized mechanism of information transfer within the neural circuit, they are broadly categorized into electrical and chemical synapses. In electrical synapses, the passive yet direct flow of current across the gap junctions is the mechanism of transmission. Transmission across these synapses is a very rapid event and plays a functional role in evoking a quick motor response during life-threatening situations. In the case of chemical synapses, there is a cascade of events leading up to the release of neurotransmitters into the synaptic cleft. Neurotransmitters are released in fixed amounts – quanta. Upon their binding with sites in the postsynaptic membrane, information is transmitted to the next neuron. This process is relatively slower when compared with electrical synapses. This is the fundamental basis of how information is generated and transferred across the whole nervous system.

SUGGESTED READING

Cole KS. Membranes, Ions and Impulses: A Chapter of Classical Biophysics. Berkeley, CA: University of California Press; 1968.

Hodgkin AL. The Conduction of the Nervous Impulse. Springfield, IL: Charles C. Thomas; 1967.

Hodgkin AL. Chance and Design. Cambridge: Cambridge University Press; 1992.

Junge D. Nerve and Muscle Excitation. 3rd ed. Sunderland, MA: Sinauer Associates; 1992.

Katz B. Nerve, Muscle, and Synapse. New York: McGraw-Hill; 1966.

REFERENCES

1. Buchthal F, Schmalbruch H. Motor unit of mammalian muscle. Physiol Rev 1980;60(1):90–142.
2. Esty W, Millikan RA, McDougal WL. American Technical Society. Elements of Electricity. Chicago: American Technical Society; 1937.
3. Esty W, Millikan RA, McDougal WL. American Technical Society. Elements of Electricity: A Practical Discussion of the Fundamental Laws and Phenomena of Electricity and Their Practical Applications in the Business and Industrial World. Chicago: American Technical Society; 1944.
4. Ohm GS. Die GalvanischeKette, Mathematisch. Berlin: T. H. Riemann; 1827.
5. Millikan RA, Bishop ES. American Technical Society. Elements of electricity. Chicago: American Technical Society; 1917.
6. American Technical Society. Cyclopedia of Applied Electricity; A General Reference Work on Direct-Current Generators and Motors, Storage Batteries, Electrochemistry, Welding, Electric Wiring, Meters, Electric Light Transmission, Alternating-Current Machinery, Telegraphy, etc. Chicago: American Technical Society; 1914.
7. McNaught AD, Wilkinson A. International Union of Pure and Applied Chemistry. Compendium of Chemical Terminology: IUPAC recommendations. 2nd ed. Oxford [England]; Malden, MA, USA: Blackwell Science; 1997.
8. Baker PF, Hodgkin AL, Shaw TI. The effects of changes in internal ionic concentrations on the electrical properties of perfused giant axons. J Physiol 1962;164:355–74.
9. Frankenhaeuser B, Hodgkin AL. The effect of calcium on the sodium permeability of a giant nerve fibre. J Physiol 1955;128(2):40–1P.
10. Frankenhaeuser B, Hodgkin AL. The after-effects of impulses in the giant nerve fibres of Loligo. J Physiol 1956;131(2):341–76.
11. Frankenhaeuser B, Hodgkin AL. The action of calcium on the electrical properties of squid axons. J Physiol 1957;137(2):218–44.
12. Hawkins RD, Abrams TW, Carew TJ, et al. A cellular mechanism of classical conditioning in Aplysia: activity-dependent amplification of presynaptic facilitation. Science 1983;219(4583):400–5.
13. Hodgkin AL. The membrane resistance of a non-medullated nerve fibre. J Physiol 1947;106(3):305–18.
14. Hodgkin AL. Ionic movements and electrical activity in giant nerve fibres. Proc R Soc Lond B Biol Sci 1958;148(930):1–37.
15. Hodgkin AL, Horowicz P. The influence of potassium and chloride ions on the membrane potential of single muscle fibres. J Physiol 1959;148:127–60.
16. Hodgkin AL, Horowicz P. The effect of sudden changes in ionic concentrations on the membrane potential of single muscle fibres. J Physiol 1960;153:370–85.
17. Hodgkin AL, Huxley AF. Resting and action potentials in single nerve fibres. J Physiol 1945;104(2):176–95.
18. Dodge FA, Frankenhaeuser B. Membrane currents in isolated frog nerve fibre under voltage clamp conditions. J Physiol 1958;143(1):76–90.
19. Adrian RH, Chandler WK, Hodgkin AL. Voltage clamp experiments in skeletal muscle fibres. J Physiol 1966;186(2):51P–2P.
20. Adrian RH, Chandler WK, Hodgkin AL. Voltage clamp experiments in striated muscle fibers. J Gen Physiol 1968;51(5):188–92.
21. Adrian RH, Chandler WK, Hodgkin AL. Voltage clamp experiments in striated muscle fibers. J Gen Physiol 1968;51(Suppl. 5):188S+.
22. Adrian RH, Chandler WK, Hodgkin AL. Slow changes in potassium permeability in skeletal muscle. J Physiol 1970;208(3):645–68.
23. Adrian RH, Chandler WK, Hodgkin AL. Voltage clamp experiments in striated muscle fibres. J Physiol 1970;208(3):607–44.
24. Cole KS. Mostly membranes (Kenneth S. Cole). Annu Rev Physiol 1979;41:1–24.
25. Hodgkin AL, Huxley AF. Potassium leakage from an active nerve fibre. Nature 1946;158:376.
26. Hodgkin AL. The effect of potassium on the surface membrane of an isolated axon. J Physiol 1947;106(3):319–40.
27. Hodgkin AL. The local electric changes associated with repetitive action in a non-medullated axon. J Physiol 1948;107(2):165–81.
28. Hodgkin AL, Katz B. The effect of calcium on the axoplasm of giant nerve fibers. J Exp Biol 1949;26(3):292–4, pl.
29. Hodgkin AL, Katz B. The effect of temperature on the electrical activity of the giant axon of the squid. J Physiol 1949;109(1–2):240–9.
30. Hodgkin AL, Katz B. The effect of sodium ions on the electrical activity of giant axon of the squid. J Physiol 1949;108(1):37–77.
31. Hodgkin AL, Nastuk WL. Membrane potentials in single fibres of the frog's sartorius muscle. J Physiol 1949;108(3):Proc, 42.
32. Hodgkin AL. Conduction of the nervous impulse: some recent experiments. Br Med Bull 1950;6(4):322–5.
33. Hodgkin AL, Huxley AF. Propagation of electrical signals along giant nerve fibers. Proc R Soc Lond B Biol Sci 1952;140(899):177–83.
34. Hodgkin AL, Huxley AF. A quantitative description of membrane current and its application to conduction and excitation in nerve. J Physiol 1952;117(4):500–44.
35. Hodgkin AL, Huxley AF. The dual effect of membrane potential on sodium conductance in the giant axon of Loligo. J Physiol 1952;116(4):497–506.
36. Hodgkin AL, Huxley AF. The components of membrane conductance in the giant axon of Loligo. J Physiol 1952;116(4):473–96.
37. Hodgkin AL, Huxley AF. Currents carried by sodium and potassium ions through the membrane of the giant axon of Loligo. J Physiol 1952;116(4):449–72.

38. Hodgkin AL, Huxley AF. Movement of sodium and potassium ions during nervous activity. Cold Spring Harb Symp Quant Biol 1952;17:43–52.
39. Hodgkin, Huxley and Eccles. Medical Nobelists for 1963. Med Serv J Can 1964;20:191–5.
40. [Winners of the 1963 Nobel Prize in Medicine)]. Orv Hetil 1963;104:2477–8.
41. Hodgkin AL. The relation between conduction velocity and the electrical resistance outside a nerve fibre. J Physiol 1939;94(4): 560–70.
42. Hodgkin AL, Huxley AF, Katz B. Measurement of current-voltage relations in the membrane of the giant axon of Loligo. J Physiol 1952;116(4):424–48.
43. Hodgkin AL. A note on conduction velocity. J Physiol 1954;125(1): 221–4.
44. Goldman DE. Potential, impedance, and rectification in membranes. J Gen Physiol 1943;27(1):37–60.
45. Hodgkin AL. Evidence for electrical transmission in nerve: Part I. J Physiol 1937;90(2):183–210.
46. Cole KS, Hodgkin AL. Membrane and protoplasm resistance in the squid giant axon. J Gen Physiol 1939;22(5):671–87.
47. Hodgkin AL, Rushton WA. The electrical constants of a crustacean nerve fibre. Proc R Soc Med 1946;134(873):444–79.
48. Hodgkin AL, Huxley AF. Potassium leakage from an active nerve fibre. J Physiol 1947;106(3):341–67.
49. Hodgkin AL, Keynes RD. Sodium extrusion and potassium absorption in Sepia axons. J Physiol 1953;120(4):46P–7P.
50. Hodgkin AL, Keynes RD. The mobility and diffusion coefficient of potassium in giant axons from Sepia. J Physiol 1953;119(4): 513–28.
51. Hodgkin AL, Keynes RD. The potassium permeability of a giant nerve fibre. J Physiol 1955;128(1):61–88.
52. Hodgkin AL, Keynes RD. Active transport of cations in giant axons from Sepia and Loligo. J Physiol 1955;128(1):28–60.
53. Hodgkin AL, Horowicz P. Movements of Na and K in single muscle fibres. J Physiol 1959;145(2):405–32.
54. Caldwell PC, Hodgkin AL, Keynes RD, et al. The effects of injecting 'energy-rich' phosphate compounds on the active transport of ions in the giant axons of Loligo. J Physiol 1960;152:561–90.
55. Hodgkin AL. Chance and design in electrophysiology: an informal account of certain experiments on nerve carried out between 1934 and 1952. J Physiol 1976;263(1):1–21.
56. Kandel ER. Small systems of neurons. Sci Am 1979;241(3):66–76.
57. Kandel ER. Cellular insights into behavior and learning. Harvey Lect 1979;73:19–92.
58. Huxley AF. Hodgkin and the action potential 1935–1952. J Physiol 2002;538(Pt 1):2.
59. Galarreta M, Hestrin S. Electrical synapses between GABA-releasing interneurons. Nat Rev Neurosci 2001;2(6):425–33.
60. Bennett MV. Electrical synapses, a personal perspective (or history). Brain Res Brain Res Rev 2000;32(1):16–28.
61. Curtis DR, Phillis JW, Watkins JC. The chemical excitation of spinal neurones by certain acidic amino acids. J Physiol 1960; 150:656–82.
62. Curtis DR, Phillis JW, Watkins JC. Chemical excitation of spinal neurones. Nature 1959;183(4661):611–12.
63. Changeux JP. Chemical signaling in the brain. Sci Am 1993;269(5): 58–62.
64. Murthy VN, De Camilli P. Cell biology of the presynaptic terminal. Annu Rev Neurosci 2003;26:701–28.
65. Adler EM, Augustine GJ, Duffy SN, et al. Alien intracellular calcium chelators attenuate neurotransmitter release at the squid giant synapse. J Neurosci 1991;11(6):1496–507.
66. Miledi R. Transmitter release induced by injection of calcium ions into nerve terminals. Proc R Soc Lond B Biol Sci 1973;183(73): 421–5.
67. Schweizer FE, Ryan TA. The synaptic vesicle: cycle of exocytosis and endocytosis. Curr Opin Neurobiol 2006;16(3):298–304.
68. Sudhof TC. The synaptic vesicle cycle: a cascade of protein-protein interactions. Nature 1995;375(6533):645–53.
69. Heuser JE, Reese TS, Dennis MJ, et al. Synaptic vesicle exocytosis captured by quick freezing and correlated with quantal transmitter release. J Cell Biol 1979;81(2):275–300.
70. Del Castillo J, Katz B. Quantal components of the end-plate potential. J Physiol 1954;124(3):560–73.

CHAPTER 4

Postural Control and Sensorimotor Integration

Ian Loram

SUMMARY

Sensorimotor integration is central to sustained control of configuration (postural control). This chapter considers postural sensorimotor integration at the level of the whole system, which includes concurrent perceptual, executive and motor processes. These mechanisms provide a basis for physiotherapeutic practice. Multiple sensory modalities are combined with prior personal experience and converged to a set of movement possibilities. From these possibilities, control priorities are selected and passed to the motor system which generates coordinated inhibition and excitation of the entire muscular system. Within a main perception–selection–motor feedback loop, two levels of mechanism work together. The slow intentional system acting through central selection and optimization pathways (e.g. basal ganglia, premotor and prefrontal cortex, cerebellum) allows sequential optimization, selection and temporal inhibition of alternative possibilities up to a maximum rate of two to four selections per second. The fast habitual-reflexive system acting through previously facilitated transcortical, brain stem and spinal pathways implements coordinated responses to environmental stimuli with a latency as low as 50–100 ms. The main perception–selection–motor loop provides a mechanism for amplifying or diminishing maladaptive perceptions and selections. Restoration of maladapted function requires re-education of the central processes of perception and selection.

POSTURAL CONTROL

Posture simply means configuration of the body. The human body comprises multiple segments along a kinematic chain which includes feet, shanks, thighs, pelvis, spine, thorax, arms, neck and head. There are many possible configurations. Some configurations require little muscular energy to maintain whereas others require a great deal. In choosing a configuration one is constrained to provide the effort required to balance that configuration. The postural task is to maintain these segments in a desired configuration or choose some other control priority which allows configuration to adjust as required.

Passive structures, including joint surface, ligaments and inactive muscle, provide some degree of postural control.[1-3] For example, muscle naturally becomes stiffer when it is still and that stiffness dispels during movement,[2,4] thus assisting maintenance of configuration without impeding movement. It is possible to align the shanks, thighs, pelvis, spine, thorax, neck and head such that standing is temporarily possible with no muscle activity.[3,5,6] Passive stabilization through alignment, or through contact with external surfaces (e.g. floor, wall, table or chair), reduces the control and attentional demands of maintaining configuration. However, even allowing for passive stabilization, the free-standing upright aligned body is mechanically unstable. In the absence of sensory feedback even small departures from alignment will cause the body to fall.[2,7-13] During accurate alignment, the active muscular forces required to balance gravity are minimal. The time taken to fall from the aligned configuration increases exponentially with the accuracy of the initial alignment.[2,14-16] Hence, upright configuration is achieved most economically and most stably when alignment is controlled accurately.

Neural regulation is essential for postural control. Mechanical instability alone means sensorimotor feedback is required. Furthermore, daily life requires sensory and mechanical engagement with external objects and social engagement with other people: the required configurations are many and difficult to predict beyond a short time scale. Pre-computing motor solutions and storing them in a retrievable fashion is appropriate when the controlled 'system' and necessary constraints do not change.[17] Pre-computed building blocks of motor control known as motor primitives are stored within the motor cortex, brain stem and spinal cord. The sensorimotor system retrieves and combines these primitive components in the construction of posture and movement.[18-20] However, through fatigue, development and ageing the human system changes. Local pain, injury and irritation cause people to limit the ranges of desired configurations. These altered limits may be required swiftly and may also evolve gradually. Constraints on configuration and control strategy change with the need to catch, pick up and hold objects, look at computer monitors, communicate with other people, evade dangerous objects and generally negotiate the mechanical environment. Pre-computed solutions alone are insufficient. This kind of control, to handle changing constraints, requires flexibility for computing new motor solutions in the moment of activity.[21] Constructing new motor solutions in the moment of activity requires selection, recombination of existing possibilities and temporal inhibition of non-selected alternatives.[22] Thus within a main feedback loop retaining executive control of posture, the human postural system requires two kinds of feedback: a fast loop for implementing pre-computed control, and a slow loop for implementing control which is reconstructed during activity. The human nervous system has sensorimotor pathways corresponding to both loops.[23] In this chapter these loops are named as habitual-reflexive (fast) and intentional (slow). In control theory, the general paradigm which provides time for selection and optimization within the main feedback loop is known as intermittent control.[17,23,24] The continuous paradigm (e.g. servo control, continuous optimal control) has been the mainstay of postural and motor control since early physiological investigation into postural reflexes,[25,26] and since the 1960s from investigation of sensorimotor integration.[27] The more recently developed intermittent control paradigm includes and extends the explanatory power of the better known continuous paradigm.[23,24]

To summarize, postural mechanisms provide sustained control of an unstable multisegmental structure in known and unpredicted circumstances. This control requires neural integration of multiple sensory modalities with multiple possible goals and constraints.

SENSORIMOTOR INTEGRATION

Sensorimotor integration is central to postural control. Postural control can be understood as a main feedback loop combining concurrent elements of perception, selection and motor control[23,28] (Fig. 4-1) implemented through a range of neural pathways (Fig. 4-2).

Perception

The person receives multiple channels of information through their eyes, ears, skin, muscles, joints and other internal sources. Perception is the interpretive process of sensory analysis. Sensory information is uncertain and potentially ambiguous. Sensory accuracy and confidence are improved by integrating information between sensory modalities, and by combining sensory information with prior experience in a process described mathematically as Bayesian state estimation.[29-34] Prior personal experience influences the earliest stages of neural sensory representation through to later stages of perceptual decision making.[29] Through integrative analysis all sensory channels are converged to a smaller number of possibilities for movement stored as action representations in the frontal cortex.[23,35]

Selection

From the current possibilities, priorities are selected for postural and motor action. This response selection

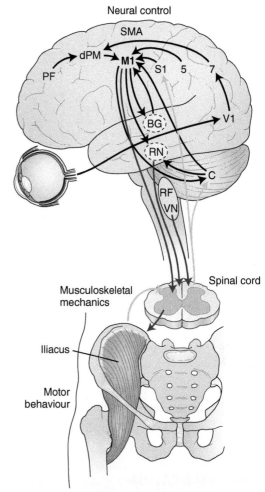

FIGURE 4-2 ■ Sensorimotor pathways through the central nervous system. The central nervous system is conventionally viewed as having a hierarchical organization with three levels: the spinal cord, brainstem and cortex. The spinal cord is the lowest level, including motor neurons, the final common pathway for all motor output, and interneurons that integrate sensory feedback from the skin, muscle and joints with descending commands from higher centres. The motor repertoire at this level includes stereotypical multijoint and even multilimb reflex patterns, and basic locomotor patterns. At the second level, brainstem regions such as the reticular formation (*RF*) and vestibular nuclei (*VN*) select and enhance the spinal repertoire by improving postural control, and can vary the speed and quality of oscillatory patterns for locomotion. The highest level of control, which supports a large and adaptable motor repertoire, is provided by the cerebral cortex in combination with subcortical loops through the basal ganglia and cerebellum.[36] Motor planning and visual feedback are provided through several parietal and premotor regions. The primary motor cortex (*M1*) contributes the largest number of axons to the corticospinal tract and receives input from other cortical regions that are predominantly involved in motor planning. Somatosensory information is provided through the primary somatosensory cortex (*S1*), parietal cortex area 5 (*5*) and cerebellar pathways. The basal ganglia (*BG*) and cerebellum (*C*) are also important for motor function through their connections with M1 and other brain regions. *RN*, Red nucleus; *V1*, Primary visual cortex; *7*, Region of posterior parietal cortex; *dPM*, Dorsal premotor cortex; *SMA*, Supplementary motor area; *PF*, Prefrontal cortex. For colour version see Plate 1. (Reproduced with modification from Scott.[38])

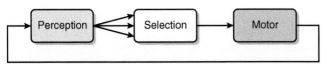

FIGURE 4-1 ■ Perception–selection–motor feedback loop. Sensorimotor integration forms a feedback loop in which selected motor control influences sensory analysis, perception and future selection. This feedback loop provides a mechanism for amplifying or diminishing the consequences of maladaptive selections.

process acts through central selection and optimization pathways such as those within the basal ganglia and cerebellum[22,36] and allows sequential optimization, selection and temporal inhibition of alternative possibilities up to a maximum low rate of two to four selections per second.[23,28,37]

Motor Control

Using parameters passed from the selection process, the motor system produces coordinated inhibition and excitation of the entire set of muscles, joints and implements control of configuration. These selections are executed through the slow and fast pathways working together within the main perception–selection–motor feedback loop. The slow intentional pathway provides control which is reformulated and executed sequentially within the main feedback loop with a variable latency of 180–500 ms.[28,37] Using preselected parameters, the fast loop acting through transcortical, brain stem and spinal pathways implements coordinated habitual-reflexive responses to environmental stimuli with a latency as low as 50–100 ms.[5]

The results of motor control generate sensory input which is interpreted, thus completing the feedback loop. The feedback loop is a dynamic system. Thus all maladapted features of postural control (symptoms) evolve through time, either constructively or destructively depending on whether feedback is mathematically negative or positive.

SENSORY INTEGRATION

Combination of sensory signals with prior expectation occurs centrally in areas including the mid-brain and cerebral cortex.[30,39,40] For example, the posterior parietal cortex receives input from the three sensory systems that enable localization of the body and external objects in space: the visual system, the auditory system and the somatosensory system. The posterior parietal cortex also receives input from the cerebellum which is increasingly thought to generate expected sensory signals from known motor commands[20] (Fig. 4-3). Much of the output of the posterior parietal cortex goes to areas of the frontal motor cortex.[20]

For postural control, the visual, vestibular, proprioceptive and cutaneous modalities work together to estimate where parts of the body are in relation to one another and the external world. These senses are commonly stated to be redundant, since postural control is possible with one or more modalities missing. However estimation is more accurate and more robust when different senses are combined.[40,42] A weighted combination of signals from all sensory modalities is combined with copies of motor signals passing through central neural networks trained by prior experience to produce equivalent expected sensory signals (Fig. 4-3).[20,41,43-45] This integration enables the nervous system to use all its available information and knowledge to resolve potential conflicts of interpretation.[43,44] For example, when you move your eyes causing the image of the world to move across your

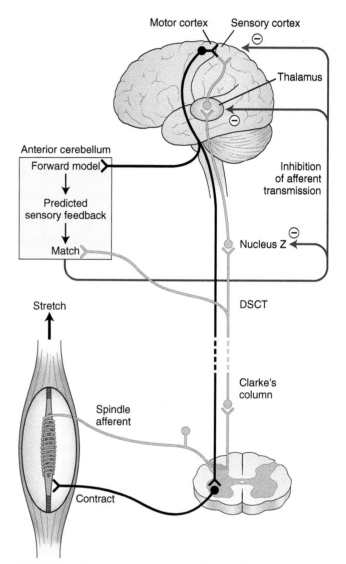

FIGURE 4-3 ■ Neural pathways estimating position from sensory and motor information. Integration of muscle spindle afferents with expectations generated from motor output. When the muscle is stretched, spindle impulses travel to sensory areas of the cerebral cortex via Clarke's column, the dorsal spinocerebellar tract (*DSCT*), Nucleus Z, and the thalamus (shown in red). Collaterals of DSCT cells project to the anterior cerebellum. When a motor command is generated, it leads to co-activation of skeletomotor and fusimotor neurons (shown in blue). A copy of the motor command is sent to the anterior cerebellum where a comparison takes place between the expected spindle response based on that command and the actual signal provided by the DSCT collaterals. The outcome of the match is used to inhibit reafferent activity, preventing it from reaching the cerebral cortex. Sites of inhibition could be at Nucleus Z, the thalamus, or the parietal cortex itself. For colour version see Plate 1. (Reproduced from Proske and Gandevia.[41])

retina, the world appears stationary because your nervous system knows that you are stationary relative to the ground and knows that you have moved your eyes rather than believe the external world has moved.[46]

Vision provides powerful sensory input to posture and balance,[47-49] illustrated by its famous ability in 'moving room' experiments to make young children fall over.[50,51] Vision signals movement of the external world relative to the eye via optic flow of the visual field across the whole retina.[52,53] Estimation of body movement from retinal information requires knowledge of eye-in-head movement, knowledge of head-on-neck movement and other joint movement down the kinematic chain.[54,55] For example, when fixing the fovea on stationary targets, together rotation of eye-in-head and head-on-neck signal movement of the head and trunk relative to the external target. Visual sensitivity to postural sway is high, allowing detection of sway about the ankle joint of only ~0.1 degree,[52,56] but this sensitivity decreases as distance to the visual target increases.[52,53] Closing one's eyes illustrates both an immediate reduction in stability and also that normally postural control without vision is possible.

Vestibular organs including the semicircular canals and otoliths register rapid rotation and translation of the head, respectively.[57-59] While commonly thought to sense acceleration, these organs contain substantial internal viscous damping, which means they measure damped acceleration that more closely resembles velocity.[46] Vestibular sensitivity to postural sway is an order of magnitude lower than vision and requires postural rotations about the ankle joint of approximately ~1 degree. Similar to vision, extraction of body motion from sensed head movement requires knowledge of head orientation with respect to the trunk.[57-60] Similar to vision, postural control is possible with vestibular loss, but balance is less robust and falls are more likely.[61-64] However, vestibular organs provide compelling sensory input of larger, faster head movements relevant to falls and balance. Most importantly, whereas vision alone cannot distinguish motion relative to the ground (self-motion) from motion of external objects relative to the eye (world motion), vestibular sensation alone provides an absolute measure of self-motion albeit motion of the head in space. Vestibular sensation is important for resolving ambiguity resulting from visual and proprioceptive sensation.[44]

Proprioception provides the sense of relative position and movement between neighbouring parts of the body. The sensory information derives mainly from sensory receptors associated with skeletal striated muscles (spindles, Golgi tendon organs), less so from joints, and is combined with cutaneous receptors signalling skin stretch and pressure.[41,43] Proprioception does not provide any particular sensations, but provides knowledge of the position and movement of our limbs and body.[41] If there is any sensation, this usually relates to a difference between what is expected and what has actually occurred.[41] In contrast to vision and vestibular sensation, loss of proprioception is instantly devastating for motor and postural control.[65] For example, in a rare case of large-fibre sensory neuropathy, the individual (I. W.) has no sensation of cutaneous light touch and no movement/position sense below the neck: without vision he has no knowledge of where his limbs and body are in space.[60] Following this loss, motor control, posture, movement and learning new control have only been possible when deliberately using direct vision of the limbs for guidance and forward planning.[65,66]

Estimation of body configuration and motion is a multimodal process integrating proprioception, vision and vestibular input.[54] The proprioceptive organs,

particularly the muscle spindles, form a 'proprioceptive chain' crossing all articulations between the eyes, feet and hands which functionally links the eye muscles to the foot and hand muscles.[43,67-69] Along the proprioceptive–kinematic chain, information accumulates from the source of sensory information to the mass segment whose location needs to be controlled. For postural control, the head and ground (or other supporting surface) source two lines of accumulating sensory information:

- Head-referenced information: Proprioception is essential for extracting body motion from visual and vestibular sensation of head movement.[54] The main mass of the body lies within or close to the trunk and the primary articulation defining trunk location from the head is the neck. Proprioception of the neck is substantial and well connected with the vestibular and visual system[68,70-73] and provides the first, most predictive estimate of body location. This estimate of body location is improved through proprioception of additional joints along the extended proprioceptive-kinematic chain.

- Ground-referenced information: Proprioception alone can extract body motion relative to the ground or other supporting surface. When supported only on the ground through the feet, the primary articulation defining body location is the ankle joints, and during free standing, ankle rotation alone provides a good estimate of centre of mass location,[7,8] which is improved through adding knowledge of articulations further along the chain from the ground reference. Consequently, proprioception of ankle rotation is highly sensitive (~0.1 degree).[56] Single joint muscles crossing the ankle such as the soleus and to a lesser extent the tibialis anterior are richly endowed with muscle spindles.[7,74,75]

To summarize, vision (with eye proprioception) and vestibular sensation give movement of the head, and movement of the body requires measurement of neck rotation. Movement of the body can be measured directly relative to the ground. For both of these proprioception is vital.

Pressure registered through the feet signals the mean location and strength of the contact support force. During free-standing postural control, accelerations are low and the ground contact force position signals the anterior–posterior and mediolateral location of the gravitational force vector and thus of the whole body centre of mass position. Thus, under normal conditions, sensation through the sole contributes to estimation of the centre of mass location relative to the foot. This estimate is important, since balance requires maintaining the centre of mass within the base of support.[76]

Proprioception provides knowledge of the kinematic chain. In unconstrained movements, proprioceptive information provides relatively accurate estimates of limb position. So-called active proprioception, in which the person moves their own limb, does not provide better estimates of limb position than passive proprioception in which the limb is moved for the participant.[77] During multijoint movement,[78] proprioceptive information is thought to be used in the translation of higher-level movement goals into joint-based motor commands[55] and also to provide local reflexive stabilization of joints.[79-81]

However, there are limits to the accuracy of proprioception, particularly for slow changes in position.[41] Muscle spindles are highly sensitive to change in muscle length and like most sensory cells tend to habituate to constant conditions that limit their capability to sense absolute values of joint angles.[41] Tendon compliance, which is high under postural conditions of low forces, and muscle slack, dependent on the previous history of contraction, both mean that muscle length and change in muscle length can be poorly related to joint angle.[6,7,41,74,82,83] Thixotropy, namely the tendency of muscle to become stiff when still,[84,85] means that joint rotation transmits less effectively into muscle length change under postural conditions, and this is compounded by the changes in muscle length caused by fluctuating muscle activity which can be an order of magnitude larger than those caused by joint rotation.[6,74] The sense of position, as identified by position-matching tasks, shows that proprioception can be substantially disturbed by the previous history of movement, contraction, muscle slack, thixotropy and exercise.[41] Proprioception becomes markedly less sensitive during co-activation across joints[41] and passive spindles are more sensitive to movements than when fusimotor neurons are contracting.[41,74,86] During voluntary muscle contraction skeletal-motor and fusimotor neurons contract together ('α-γ co-activation'). Hence these findings are at odds with the common view that proprioception is more accurate under active than passive conditions.[41] These factors, very well reviewed by Proske and Gandevia,[41] highlight three main facts: (a) proprioception provides limited absolute accuracy; (b) sense of limb position is more complex than simple measurement of joint angles through sensory organs; and (c) accuracy of proprioception is influenced by motor control (e.g. co-activation, activity). To illustrate (b), the perceptual sense of ownership (i.e. distinguishing our own body from the external world) depends primarily on proprioception, but is also highly plastic given appropriate stimuli.[41] Expectation of position through central sense of effort and prior experience are integral to the sense of position.[41] The effect of (c) is that the current postural control strategy has consequences for the quality of position sense, which thus influences motor planning, translation of higher-level movement goals into joint-based motor commands and therefore motor control. This is a feedback loop, a dynamic system, in which quality of position sense can be amplified or diminished over time.

Perception

The main point of this section is to emphasize the increasingly accepted idea that prior personal experience influences sensory analysis of sensory information.[87,88] The postural task is to control configuration appropriately with respect to perception of the environment and the current intentions of the person within that environment. Perception is not solely determined by the input from our senses but it is strongly influenced by our expectations.[29] As introduced by Kok and colleagues,[29] many perceptual illusions are explained as the result of prior knowledge of probable external sensory input influencing perceptual inference: we expect light to come from above rather than below, faces to be convex and not concave, and objects in the world to move slowly rather than fast. Illusions aside, we easily forget that our perception does not provide an absolute impression of the sensory world. We cannot tickle ourself because our prior knowledge of our action cancels the self-generated sensation of tickle.[89] If we support the dead weight of an external body part such as an arm or leg, these are surprisingly heavy, yet we do not sense our own weight which is cancelled by our prior expectation. Perhaps only when emerging from the swimming pool when our expectation has partially adapted, do we partially sense our weight. We tend to perceive difference from expectation rather than sensory information directly.[41,89]

It might be thought this Bayesian process of combining prior belief with sensory input to create a perception is confined to higher-order neural areas. However, data show that prior expectations can modify sensory representations in the early visual cortex[29] and even in the retina.[90] Prior expectations modify sensory processing at the earliest stages by affecting not only the amplitude of neural responses or their sharpness, but also by changing the contents of sensory representations.[91] In other words, prior expectations affect what is represented, rather than just how well things are represented.[29]

With respect to the control of posture, perception of the current environment concerns more than configuration alone. This element is missed in analyses that view postural control as only a low-level dedicated control of configuration isolated from wider perceptual factors. Asking people to stand 'naturally' for a photograph is an easy way to demonstrate the influence of perceptual factors on postural control. In an increasingly established paradigm,[92-96] the effect of these perceptual factors is illustrated by experiments in which the perceived risk to life is manipulated by comparing postural control at exposed height with control at ground level. At exposed height, the altered visual environment changes the visual input necessary for the control of balance: the distance to visual targets increases, decreasing visual sensitivity of postural sway with the consequence that postural sway increases.[47,52] However, at height, awareness of risk also influences visual input even to the extent that spatial dimensions perceived as dangerous are perceived to be greater than they are.[97-99] Experiment has shown that in response to postural threat, knowledge of danger rather than current visual environment was the dominant cause of cautious gait and elevated physiological arousal.[95] The disturbing control of locomotion, balance and autonomic response occurred at a level that integrates cognition and prior experience with sensory input.[95] This disturbed control results in changes of sustained postural configuration as well as higher levels of co-activation and greater restriction of movement.[94,95,100]

However, while sensory input through vision and proprioception are both modifiable by perceptual factors, the same appears not to be true for the vestibular system.[94] Galvanic vestibular stimulation of participants who were highly motivated to minimize sway because they were perturbed at height, showed little change in the initial, pure vestibular response, even though there were strong differences in the later response that integrates balance-relevant sensory feedback from all modalities. Pure vestibular sensory input and the immediate reflexive response appears to lie largely outside of cognitive and emotive control.[101] Unlike somewhat ambiguous signals from the other senses (e.g. vision, proprioception), the semicircular canals provide an unambiguous signal of head rotation.[58] It is probably important for survival that these vestibular reflexes cannot be interfered with. The reflexive vestibular-balance responses can be trusted even though fearful participants may not trust their own mechanisms.[94]

Generation of Action Possibilities

Sensory analysis provides the information needed to regulate motor output. In the context of postural control, people normally think of reflexes as being the underlying and primitive mechanism that transforms sensory input into motor output. Reflexes provide rapid, environmentally triggered responses similar in kind and easily mistaken for habitual automated habitual responses.[102] The biological process of decision making and adaptation involves generation of multiple possibilities, selection, and reinforcement of selections which are rewarded by valued outcomes. Mechanisms implementing this process of decision making extend through vertebrates,[103] invertebrates,[104] even to the level of individual cells.[105] Thus biological mechanisms of decision making are just as primitive as reflexes.[104] Neurophysiological recording shows that sensory analysis converges to the simultaneous, active representation in the frontal cortex of multiple possibilities for action.[106-108] Action possibilities include representations for movement, thought, simple or complex action, control priorities or cognitive processes

which are maintained weakly within the prefrontal and premotor cortex (Fig. 4-4).[22,35,106,107] If selected for expression, these parallel action possibilities have the possibility of being amplified by corresponding columns within the thalamus.[35]

Selection

Consistent with all vertebrates,[103,109] the human nervous system contains centralized mechanisms for switching between alternative possibilities for motor control. Anatomically and functionally, there is convergence of analysed sensorimotor input, contextual, perceptual and motivational input into and through the basal ganglia.[109] Input to the basal ganglia from all major sources, the cerebral cortex, limbic structures and the thalamus are topographically ordered.[109,110] Inputs to ventromedial sectors come from structures in which competing behavioural goals may be represented (prefrontal cortex, amygdala, hippocampus), while the connections of dorsolateral sectors are from regions that guide movements (e.g. sensory and motor cortex) (Fig. 4-4). As summarized by Redgrave,[109] basal ganglia outputs contact regions of the thalamus that project back to those regions of cortex providing original inputs. Similarly, basal ganglia outputs to the brainstem tend to target those regions that provide indirect input to the basal ganglia (Fig. 4-5). Projections from the basal ganglia output nuclei to the thalamus and brainstem are also topographically ordered. Neurons in the basal ganglia output nuclei have high tonic firing rates (40–80 Hz). This activity ensures that target regions of the thalamus and brainstem are maintained under a tight and relatively constant inhibitory control. Reduction of inhibitory output releases associated target regions in the thalamus and brainstem (e.g. superior colliculus) from normal inhibitory control.[23,35,109] Topologically, in a spiral architecture using successive connections between the

FIGURE 4-4 ■ Access of basal ganglia to motivational, cognitive and motor regions for selection and reinforcement learning. The basal ganglia are a group of interconnected subcortical nuclei that represent one of the brain's fundamental processing units. Interacting corticostriatal circuits contribute to action selection at various levels of analysis. Coloured projections reflect subsystems associated with value/motivation (red), working memory and cognitive control (green), procedural and habit learning (blue), and contextual influences of episodic memory (orange). Sub-regions within the basal ganglia (*BG*) act as gates to facilitate or suppress actions represented in frontal cortex. These include parallel circuits linking the BG with motivational, cognitive, and motor regions within the prefrontal cortex (*PFC*). Recurrent connections within the PFC support active maintenance of working memory (*WM*). Cognitive states in dorsolateral PFC (*dlPFC*) can influence action selection via projections to the circuit linking BG with the motor cortex. Dopamine (*DA*) drives incremental reinforcement learning in all BG regions, supporting adaptive behaviours as a function of experience. For colour version see Plate 2. (Reproduced from Frank.[22])

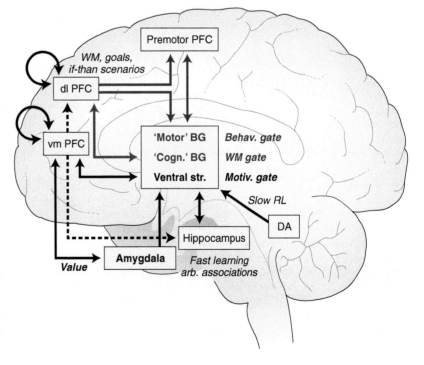

Cortical loops

Subcortical loops

FIGURE 4-5 ■ Cortical and subcortical sensorimotor loops through the basal ganglia. **(A)** For corticobasal ganglia loops the position of the thalamic relay is on the return arm of the loop. **(B)** In the case of all subcortical loops the position of the thalamic relay is on the input side of the loop. Predominantly excitatory regions and connections are shown in red while inhibitory regions and connections are blue. *Thal,* Thalamus; *SN/GP,* Substantia nigra/globus pallidus. For colour version see Plate 2. (Reproduced from Redgrave.[109])

limbic, associative and sensorimotor territories, the basal ganglia are organized to allow progressive selection of an overall goal, actions to achieve a selected goal and movements to achieve a selected action.[103,109,111]

The basal ganglia act as a system that dynamically and adaptively gates information flow in the frontal cortex, and from the frontal cortex to the motor system.[35,36,109] The basal ganglia are richly anatomically connected to the frontal cortex and the thalamocortical motor system via several distinct but partly overlapping loops.[22,35] Through hyper-direct, indirect and direct pathways, this system provides centralized mechanisms for generalized inhibition, specific inhibition and specific facilitation of action possibilities represented in the frontal cortex (Fig. 4-6).[22,35,103,112] As described by Cohen and Frank,[35] the basal ganglia system does not directly select which action to 'consider', but instead modulates the activity of already active representations in cortex. This functionality enables the cortex to weakly represent multiple potential actions in parallel; the one that first receives a 'go' signal from basal ganglia output is then provided with sufficient additional excitation to be executed. Lateral inhibition within thalamus and cortex act to suppress competing responses once the winning response has been selected by the basal ganglia circuitry.[22,35]

Mechanisms of response selection also lie within the prefrontal and premotor cortex.[113,114] While these mechanisms are the subject of much current research, a general conclusion is that together, these striatal (basal ganglia) and prefrontal systems provide both selection and reinforcement learning (i.e. progressive facilitation of those responses which achieve valued outcomes and progressive inhibition of those responses which achieve undesired outcomes).[22,35,102] While selection and reinforcement of rewarded selections is associated with the basal ganglia system, refinement and adaptation of the possibilities available for selection is associated with the cerebellum within cortico–cerebellar–cortico loops that match equivalent cortico–basal ganglia–cortico loops (Fig. 4-7).[36]

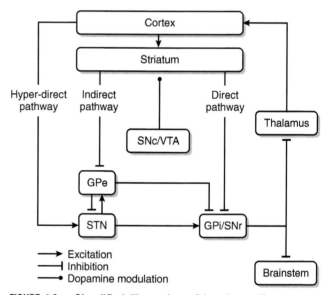

FIGURE 4-6 ■ Simplified illustration of basal ganglia anatomy based on a primate brain. The basal ganglia comprise two principal input nuclei, the striatum and the subthalamic nucleus (*STN*), and two principal output nuclei, the substantia nigra pars reticulata (*SNr*) and the internal globus pallidus (*GPi*) (primates). The external globus pallidus (*GPe*) is principally an intrinsic structure that receives most of its afferents from and provides efferent connections to other basal ganglia nuclei. Finally, dopaminergic neurones in substantia nigra (pars compacta) (*SNc*) and the adjacent ventral tegmental area (*VTA*) provide other basal ganglia nuclei, principally the striatum, with important modulatory signals.[109] The hyper-direct, direct and indirect pathways from the striatum have net effects of generalized inhibition, specific disinhibition and specific inhibition on the cortex, respectively. (Reproduced with modification from Yin and Knowlton.[102])

During learning, humans select responses flexibly depending on whether the anticipated outcome is desirable. With reinforcement of selections that are rewarded, responses can become habitual. With sufficient facilitation, corticocortical associations can become sufficiently strong to elicit automatized transcortical responses even

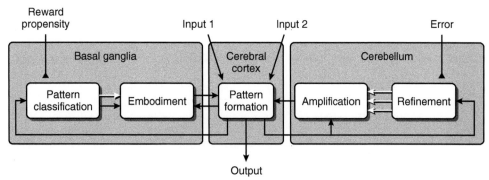

FIGURE 4-7 ■ Complementary basal ganglia and cerebellar loops for selection-reinforcement learning and optimization. An individual cortical area together with its loops through basal ganglia and cerebellum form a powerful computational structure that has been dubbed a distributed processing module (DPM).[115] DPMs communicate with each other via the cortical–cortical connections. There are on the order of a hundred DPMs in the human brain, forming a large-scale neural network. The figure shows the selection (classification) and refinement operations posited for each DPM. Net excitatory pathways are shown with closed arrows, net inhibitory pathways with open arrows and the grey diamonds signify neuromodulatory and training inputs. (Reproduced from Houk et al.[36])

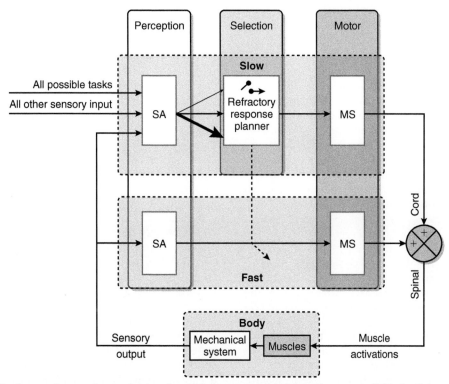

FIGURE 4-8 ■ Overall scheme of sensorimotor integration. For postural control there is an overall feedback loop relating perception, selection and motor control. Perception requires sensory analysis integrating all sensory modalities with prior experience (*SA*). Acting through central pathways such as the basal ganglia loops, selections are made. Recent evidence suggests selection converges to a serial process with a maximum rate of two to four selections per second (Refractory Response Planner).[23] The motor system (*MS*) translates selected goals, actions, movements and control priorities into coordinated motor output. Within a slow feedback loop restricted to the voluntary bandwidth of control (2 Hz) the motor system generates coordinated motor responses sequentially from each new selection. With a fast loop restricted to a higher bandwidth (>10 Hz) acting through transcortical, brain stem and spinal pathways, the motor system uses selected parameters to modulate habitual-reflexive feedback.[23,37,123]

before striatal gating signals occur, thus bypassing the basal ganglia loop (see Fig. 4-5).[22,102,116-119] Functionally, physiological reflexes, reflexes formed through operant conditioning, and habitual responses share the same characteristic of being elicited rapidly by environmental stimuli without regard to the current value of the outcome. Hence these are described collectively as habitual reflexive[22,102] and in the overall scheme of sensorimotor integration are implemented through the fast feedback loop (Fig. 4-8).

Selection represents executive function. This executive function is required for choosing postural goals, control priorities and movements required to maintain those goals.[28] The configuration to be maintained, or parameters such as peripheral feedback thresholds which determine the resulting configuration, are selected. Implicit or explicit choices are made between different control priorities. For example, does the selected control allow flexible adjustment of configuration, or does it minimize movement at the ankle, knee and hip joints?

Evidence supports a normal tendency is to allow sway within safe limits and minimize muscular effort.[9] However, normal standing conceals a large inter-individual range in leg control strategies. Commonly, leg configuration is maintained stiffly.[120] Less commonly, a bilateral, low-stiffness, energy-absorbing strategy utilizing the available degrees of freedom is shown.[120] These inter-individual differences indicate the range of possibilities available for progression with development and skill acquisition, and also for decline with age, disease, injury, and fear. Consistent with feedback around the perception–selection–motor loop (see Fig. 4-1), it is suggested that the individual coordination strategy has diagnostic and prognostic potential in relation to perceptual–posture–movement–fall interactions.[100,120]

Recent emerging evidence shows how executive function is required for ongoing adjustments in the maintenance of posture. Experimentation demonstrates substantial refractoriness up to 0.5 seconds in the implementation of postural tasks such as adjusting the position of the body and maintaining balance.[23,28,121] Refractoriness is the increased delay in selecting and forming one response before the previous selection and formation of the previous response has been completed.[23] The implication is that for postural control, sensory input converges to a sequential single channel process involving optimization, selection and temporal inhibition of alternative responses prior to motor output.[23,28] In the overall scheme of sensorimotor integration (Fig. 4-8), refractoriness (selection) occurs through the slow loop. This evidence highlights the fact that control of posture requires operation of the slow intentional feedback loop.[23]

MOTOR CONTROL

The executive selection process produces parameters which relate to the chosen tasks (e.g. standing, standing and looking, standing, looking and pointing, or standing, looking, pointing and talking). The motor system generates coordinated patterns of muscle inhibition and activation through approximately 700 distinct muscles or muscular regions acting across multiple joints.[122]

As shown in Figure 4-8, the motor system operates through fast and slow feedback loops.[22,102,119] The slow, intentional feedback loop is characterized by refractoriness.[23,28,121] To reiterate this key point, refractoriness is the increased delay in selecting and forming one response before the previous selection has been completed.[23] Refractoriness is absent from the fast, automatic feedback loop.

The Fast Loop

Much accumulated evidence summarized by Pruszynski and Scott[27] demonstrates the power and sophistication of transcortical reflexes which are a class of fast-acting responses, of latency (~60–120 ms), triggered by integrated environmental stimuli including joint rotations, visual, cutaneous and vestibular sensations. Pathways mediating these responses pass through the cortex and are influenced by many brain regions, including the cerebellum, posterior parietal cortex and frontal cortex.[27]

These responses are modulated by preceding factors, including explicit external instructions, the implicit behavioural context including the current posture and task goals, and by the external environment including the direction of the gravitational-acceleration vector and location of objects (Fig. 4-9).[27] These responses are environmentally triggered, without taking consequences into account within the feedback loop: they are reflexive in the sense of having environmental causality according to previously made choices. These responses are coherent with environmental stimuli to a frequency of 10 Hz or more.[124] The fast loop corresponds to automated, habitual and reflexive control.[22,35,102] Although functional, the fast loop alone is not adequate to reject disturbance, is highly variable and is not fully sustained.[125] Fully adequate, accurate and sustained control requires the combined operation of both fast and slow feedback loops.

The Slow Loop

The slow loop corresponds to intentional control limited to the low bandwidth of 1–2 Hz.[13,28,37,121,123,126] Within this bandwidth there is flexibility within the feedback loop to reselect the control priorities, goals, internal and external constraints at a maximum rate of two to four times per second.[15,23,28,37,121,123,127] There is recent evidence that reselection and execution of postural goals proceeds as a sequential process along a single channel of control.[28,121] The slow loop ensures that control of posture can be voluntarily reprogrammed whenever necessary. For example, when balance is challenged unexpectedly precipitating a fall, the fast system provides response within 60–120 ms, and the slow system allows intentional response within 180 ms.[23,126] When habitual control is perceived to have undesirable consequences, habitual control can be inhibited and reprogrammed.[128] It is hypothesized that this slow loop passes through the basal ganglia.[22,23,28,119] The relative contribution of the slow and fast loops is currently a matter of research and debate, though evidence is emerging that the slow loop is dominant in postural balance as well as visually guided manual control.[23,28,37,121,129] The hallmark of the slow loop is that it explains power within motor output signals coherent with unpredictable disturbances limited to below 1–2 Hz and this accounts for the majority of power in postural control.[13,23]

The motor system receives integrated sensory input from the vestibular nuclei and different sensory areas of the cerebral cortex such as the posterior parietal cortex. From the selection processes, the motor system also receives the task-related parameters which tell the motor system what kind of coordination, feedback control and muscles synergies to generate. The motor system includes more preliminary organizing function within motor parts of the basal ganglia system, the supplementary motor area, the premotor cortex and cerebellum, and influences muscle activations through the pyramidal and extrapyramidal systems.[130] The pyramidal motor system transmits directly from the motor cortex, through upper motor neurons within the corticospinal tract. Upper motor neurons terminate within the anterior horn of the spinal cord mostly on interneurons and to a lesser extent directly

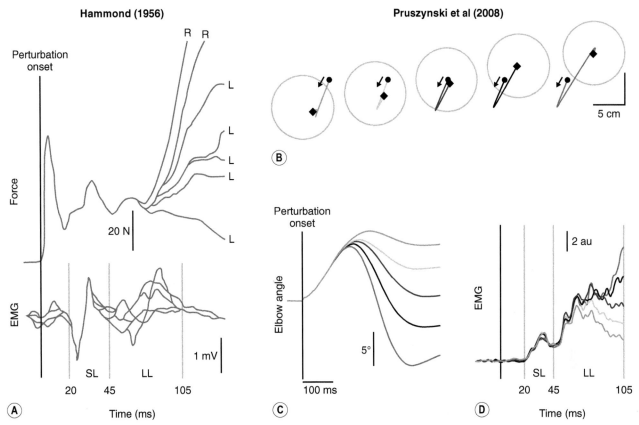

FIGURE 4-9 ■ Modulation of fast motor response by prior subject intent. (**A**) Example of how subjects can categorically modulate the long-latency (transcortical) stretch response according to verbal instruction. Subjects were verbally instructed to respond to a mechanical perturbation with one of two verbal instructions ('resist'/'let go'). The upper panel depicts force traces from individual trials aligned on perturbation onset and labelled according to the instruction. The bottom panel is the corresponding muscle activity, which shows modulation in the long-latency stretch response (*LL*) but not the short-latency (spinal) stretch response (*SL*). (**B**) Example of how subjects can continuously modulate their long-latency stretch response in accordance with spatial target position. Subjects were instructed to respond to an unpredictable mechanical perturbation by placing their hand inside one of the five presented spatial targets. Each plot represents exemplar hand kinematics as a function of target position. Subjects began each trial at the filled black circle, and the black diamond indicated final hand position. The small arrows indicate the approximate direction of motion caused by the perturbation. (**C**) Temporal kinematics for the elbow joint aligned on perturbation onset. (**D**) Pooled EMG aligned on perturbation onset and normalised to pre-perturbation muscle activity. Note that the long-latency stretch response exhibits graded modulation as a function of target position. For colour version see Plate 3. (Reproduced from Pruszynski and Scott.[27])

on lower motor neurons. Lower motor neurons directly innervate muscles as motor units. The pyramidal system is concerned specifically with discrete voluntary skilled movements, such as precise movement of the fingers and toes. The more ancient extrapyramidal motor system includes all motor tracts other than the corticospinal (pyramidal) tract, including parts of the rubrospinal, reticulospinal, vestibulospinal and tectospinal tracts. The rubrospinal tract, thought to be small in humans compared with primates, is responsible for large muscle movement as well as fine motor control, and it terminates primarily in the cervical spinal cord, suggesting that it functions in upper limb, but not in lower limb, control. The reticulospinal tract descends from the reticular formation in two tracts, medullary and pontine, to act on the motor neurons supplying the trunk and proximal limb muscles. It functions to coordinate automatic movements of locomotion and posture, facilitate and inhibit voluntary movement and influence muscle tone. The vestibulospinal tract originates in the vestibular nuclei, receives additional input from the vestibulocerebellum, and projects down to the lumbar spinal cord. It helps to

control posture by innervating extensor muscles in the legs and trunk muscles.[130]

While the motor system is complex, there is structure and organization to the generation of motor output. Firstly, while motor output is executed through multiple muscles crossing multiple joints, the motor output achieves a small number of concurrent goals: thus motor output is organized along a small number of synergistic patterns of muscle activation related to the small number of concurrent task goals.[28,131-133] There is increasing evidence that motor output is constructed from a repertoire of motor primitives which are stored in the cortex, brain stem and spinal cord for retrieval and use in the generation of movements.[19,20,108,132,134-137] Secondly, there is temporal organization to motor output. Activation of muscles proceeds sequentially from proximal reference or stabilizing segments to distal segments. This principle is observed in the so-called anticipatory postural adjustments where, for example, activation of leg and trunk muscles precedes activation of arm muscles in reaching movements.[138-140] The ground provides the reference or stabilizing segment. During reaching movements activation proceeds temporally from the trunk to the end of the arm.[141] The trunk–head axis provides the reference-stabilizing segment. During balance perturbations involving sudden translation of the floor, activation proceeds temporally from the leg to the trunk,[142] and in this case the ground provides the reference or stabilizing segment. These observations support the idea that posture is prior to movement. Posture is prior to movement both temporally and hierarchically in that control of the reference segment precedes and sets the boundary conditions for control of the end segments. Thus for control of the hands, head, vocal organs and internal respiratory muscles there is a kinematic basis to the observation[143] that control of the trunk–head axis is primary. For balance relative to the ground, there is a basis in which control of the legs is primary.

To summarize (Fig. 4-8), two levels of mechanism work together within a main perception–selection–motor feedback loop. The slow system acting through central selection and optimization pathways (e.g. basal ganglia, premotor and prefrontal cortex, cerebellum) allows online sequential planning, selection and temporal inhibition of alternative possibilities up to a maximum rate of two to four events per second. The fast system acting through transcortical, brain stem and spinal pathways allows implementation of coordinated habitual, reflexive responses to environmental stimuli with a latency as low as 50–100 ms according to preselected goals.

PRINCIPLES APPLICABLE FOR PHYSIOTHERAPEUTIC PRACTICE

Sensorimotor integration occurs at the level of the whole system. While understanding of sensorimotor integration is still evolving, we can consider principles relevant to preventing decline and improving function.

Postural control can be considered as a perception–selection–motor feedback loop (see Fig. 4-1). Perception relevant to postural control integrates prior personal experience with sensory information from the eyes, ears, proprioception and skin. Prior experience biases sensory information: thus postural control is sensitive to expectations including fears of what is required. Furthermore, postural control is likely highly facilitated, proceeding automatically from environmental stimuli without current evaluation of the consequences of the control adopted.

The selected postural control has consequences. For example, increased co-activation limits proprioceptive sensitivity.[41] Reduced quality of position sense will impair the translation of higher-level movement goals into joint-based motor commands. Increased joint stiffness limits possibilities for adjusting balance such as when required to prevent a fall.[120,144] Restriction of joint movement limits the amount, variability and asynchronicity of information gained through joint movement, and thus limits motor learning including the possibility for learning highly differentiated, skilled and economical control.[145] Unvaried, repetitive, synchronous control in which attention is paid to the task is known to cause poor even harmful adaptation within the nervous system, including reduced differentiation of sensory receptive fields and

eventually symptoms of focal dystonia.[146,147] If the biomechanical loading on bone and soft tissue are inappropriate, then wear, tear, compression, stretch, inflammation and inappropriate regeneration are likely.[148-150] These consequences are subject to feedback through the perception–selection–motor-perception feedback loop. Feedback acts to cumulatively amplify or diminish consequences (symptoms). This process can explain the evolution through time of postural problems, fear of falling and problems consequent on poor postural control. If the individual believes their *in*appropriate control is the right solution (misconception), they increase their inappropriate response to worsening symptoms: that provides destructive (mathematically positive) feedback. Thus two factors determine the progression of symptoms: (a) the concept the person has of their own control; and (b) whether that control is highly facilitated (automatic) or flexible (intentional).[128]

Within the sensorimotor loop (see Fig. 4-1), the motor and sensory processes proceed automatically. Thus there are two possibilities for re-education leading to improved function. First, individuals can be given new information. External feedback of postural and motor control can provide new input, either verbally, by educative manipulation, or using visual-audio-haptic technology.[128] Discussion and reformulation of perceptions can generate new possibilities for thought and movement. However, if postural control is so facilitated that selection proceeds automatically before striatal selection processes can intervene, then change is unlikely. Hence transfer of control from the fast to the slow loop is required to allow postural control to reformulate along more constructive lines.[143] This transfer requires training targeted at improving inhibition of highly facilitated postural control.[128] This training may be more effective if it targets areas early in the natural temporal kinematic progression of control.

To summarize, restoration of function related to sensorimotor integration requires that neurophysiological and neuromuscular mechanisms are working, and beyond that requires re-education of the central processes of perception and selection which drive postural control.

Acknowledgements

Appreciation is offered to Martin Lakie, Alison Loram and Cornelis van de Kamp for their invaluable feedback improving this chapter and additionally to Peter Gawthrop and Henrik Gollee for their collaborative contribution to the advances in understanding sensorimotor integration.

REFERENCES

1. MacConaill MA, Basmajian JV. Muscles and Movements: A Basis for Human Kinesiology. New York: Krieger; 1977. p. 400.
2. Loram ID, Maganaris CN, Lakie M. The passive, human calf muscles in relation to standing: the non-linear decrease from short range to long range stiffness. J Physiol 2007;584(Pt 2):661–75. PubMed PMID: 17823209. Pubmed Central PMCID: 2277155.
3. Kelton IW, Wright RD. The mechanism of easy standing by man. Aust J Exp Biol Med 1949;27:505. PubMed PMID: http://www.nature.com/icb/journal/v27/n5/abs/icb194949a.html.
4. Loram ID, Maganaris CN, Lakie M. The passive, human calf muscles in relation to standing: the short range stiffness lies in the

contractile component. J Physiol 2007;584(Pt 2):677–92. PubMed PMID: 17823208. Pubmed Central PMCID: 2277144.

5. Basmajian JV, De Luca C. Muscles Alive : Their Functions Revealed by Electromyography. Baltimore: Williams & Wilkins; 1985.

6. Di Giulio I, Maganaris CN, Baltzopoulos V, et al. The proprioceptive and agonist roles of gastrocnemius, soleus and tibialis anterior muscles in maintaining human upright posture. J Physiol 2009;587(Pt 10):2399–416. PubMed PMID: 19289550. Pubmed Central PMCID: 2697307.

7. Loram ID, Maganaris CN, Lakie M. Active, non-spring-like muscle movements in human postural sway: how might paradoxical changes in muscle length be produced? J Physiol 2005;564 (Pt 1):281–93. PubMed PMID: 15661825. Pubmed Central PMCID: 1456051.

8. Loram ID, Lakie M. Direct measurement of human ankle stiffness during quiet standing: the intrinsic mechanical stiffness is insufficient for stability. J Physiol 2002;545(Pt 3):1041–53. PubMed PMID: 12482906. Pubmed Central PMCID: 2290720.

9. Kiemel T, Zhang Y, Jeka JJ. Identification of neural feedback for upright stance in humans: Stabilisation rather than sway minimization. J Neurosci 2011;31(42):15144–53. PubMed PMID: 22178153.

10. Kiemel T, Elahi AJ, Jeka JJ. Identification of the plant for upright stance in humans: multiple movement patterns from a single neural strategy. J Neurophysiol 2008;100(6):3394–406. PubMed PMID: 18829854.

11. Casadio M, Morasso PG, Sanguineti V. Direct measurement of ankle stiffness during quiet standing: implications for control modelling and clinical application. Gait Posture 2005;21(4):410. PubMed PMID: 15886131.

12. Magnus R. Der Korperstellung. Berlin: Springer; 1924.

13. Peterka RJ. Sensorimotor integration in human postural control. J Neurophysiol 2002;88(3):1097. PubMed PMID: 12205132.

14. Loram ID. Mechanisms for human balancing of an inverted pendulum using the ankle strategy [PhD]. University of Birmingham; 2003.

15. Loram ID, Lakie M. Human balancing of an inverted pendulum: position control by small, ballistic-like, throw and catch movements. J Physiol 2002;540(Pt 3):1111–24. PubMed PMID: 11986396. Pubmed Central PMCID: 2290269.

16. Asai Y, Tasaka Y, Nomura K, et al. A model of postural control in quiet standing: Robust compensation of delay-induced instability using intermittent activation of feedback control. PLoS ONE 2009;4(7):PubMed PMID: 19584944.

17. Ronco E, Arsan T, Gawthrop PJ. Open-loop intermittent feedback control: Practical continuous-time GPC. IEE Pmc.-Contml Theory Appl 1999;146(5):426–34. PubMed PMID: 10.1049/ip-cta:19990504.

18. Roh J, Cheung VCK, Bizzi E. Modules in the brain stem and spinal cord underlying motor behaviors. J Neurophysiol 2011;106(3):1363–78. PubMed PMID: 21653716.

19. Flash T, Hochner B. Motor primitives in vertebrates and invertebrates. Curr Opin Neurobiol 2005;15(6):660–6. PubMed PMID: 16275056.

20. Hardwick RM, Rottschy C, Miall RC, et al. A quantitative meta-analysis and review of motor learning in the human brain. Neuroimage 2013;67:283–97. PubMed PMID: 23194819. English.

21. Bernstein NA, Latash LL, Turvey MT. On Dexterity and its Development. Mahwah: New Jersey Lawrence Erlbaum Associates; 1996. p. 3.

22. Frank MJ. Computational models of motivated action selection in corticostriatal circuits. Curr Opin Neurobiol 2011;21(3):381–6. PubMed PMID: 21498067.

23. Loram I, van de Kamp C, Lakie M, et al. Does the motor system need intermittent control?. Exerc Sport Sci Rev 2014;42:117. PubMed PMID 24819544: DOI 10.1249/JES.0000000000000018.

24. Gawthrop P, Loram I, Lakie M, et al. Intermittent control: a computational theory of human control. Biol Cybern 2011;104(1–2):31–51. PubMed PMID: 21327829. WOS:000287851400003.

25. Sherrington CS. Integrative action of the nervous system. Cambridge: Cambridge University Press; 1947.

26. Sherrington CS. Integrative action of the nervous system. London: Constable; 1906.

27. Pruszynski JA, Scott SH. Optimal feedback control and the long-latency stretch response. Exp Brain Res 2012;218(3):341–59. PubMed PMID: 22370742.

28. Van De Kamp C, Gawthrop P, Gollee H, et al. Interfacing sensory input with motor output: does the control architecture converge to a serial process along a single channel? Front Comput Neurosci 2013;7:[2013-May-9]; English.

29. Kok P, Brouwer GJ, van Gerven MAJ, et al. Prior expectations bias sensory representations in visual cortex. J Neurosci 2013; 33(41):16275–84. PubMed PMID: 24107959.

30. Berniker M, Kording K. Bayesian approaches to sensory integration for motor control. Wiley Interdisciplinary Reviews-Cognitive Science 2011;2(4):419–28. WOS:000298176400006.

31. Bays PM, Wolpert DM. Computational principles of sensorimotor control that minimise uncertainty and variability. J Physiol 2007;578(Pt 2):387–96. PubMed PMID: 17008369.

32. Butz MV, Belardinelli A, Ehrenfeld S. Modeling body state-dependent multisensory integration. Cogn Process 2012;13:S113–16. PubMed PMID: 22806661.

33. Angelaki DE, Gu Y, DeAngelis GC. Visual and vestibular cue integration for heading perception in extrastriate visual cortex. J Physiol 2011;589(4):825–33. PubMed PMID: 20679353.

34. Fetsch CR, Turner AH, DeAngelis GC, et al. Dynamic reweighting of visual and vestibular cues during self-motion perception. J Neurosci 2009;29(49):15601–12. PubMed PMID: 20007484.

35. Cohen MX, Frank MJ. Neurocomputational models of basal ganglia function in learning, memory and choice. Behav Brain Res 2009;199(1):141–56.

36. Houk JC, Bastianen C, Fansler D, et al. Action selection and refinement in subcortical loops through basal ganglia and cerebellum. Philos Trans R Soc Lond B Biol Sci 2007;362(1485):1573–83. PubMed PMID: 17428771.

37. van de Kamp C, Gawthrop PJ, Gollee H, et al. Refractoriness in sustained visuo-manual control: Is the refractory duration intrinsic or does it depend on external system properties? PLoS Comput Biol 2013;9(1):e1002843.

38. Scott SH. Optimal feedback control and the neural basis of volitional motor control. Nat Rev Neurosci 2004;5(7):532–46.

39. Kording KP, Wolpert DM. Probabilistic mechanisms in sensorimotor control. Novartis Found Symp 2006;270:191–8, discussion 198–202, 232–7. PubMed PMID: 16649715.

40. Kording KP, Wolpert DM. Bayesian integration in sensorimotor learning. Nature 2004;427(6971):244–7. PubMed PMID: 14724638.

41. Proske U, Gandevia SC. The proprioceptive senses: their roles in signalling body shape, body position and movement, and muscle force. Physiol Rev 2012;92(4):1651–97. [Epub 2012/10/18]; PubMed PMID: 23073629. eng.

42. Shadmehr R, Mussa-Ivaldi S. Biological learning and control: How the brain builds representations, predicts events, and makes decisions. Cambridge, MA, USA: MIT Press; 2012.

43. Proske U, Gandevia SC. The kinaesthetic senses. J Physiol 2009;587(17):4139–46. PubMed PMID: 19581378.

44. van der Kooij H, Jacobs R, Koopman B, et al. An adaptive model of sensory integration in a dynamic environment applied to human stance control. Biol Cybern 2001;84(2):103–15. PubMed PMID: 11205347.

45. Stein BE, Stanford TR. Multisensory integration: current issues from the perspective of the single neuron. Nat Rev Neurosci 2008;9(4):255–66. PubMed PMID: 18354398.

46. Carpenter RHS. Neurophysiology. 3rd ed. London: Hodder Arnold; 1995.

47. Paulus WM, Straube A, Brandt T. Visual stabilisation of posture – physiological stimulus characteristics and clinical aspects. Brain 1984;107(DEC):1143–63. PubMed PMID: 6509312.

48. Peterka RJ, Benolken MS. Role of somatosensory and vestibular cues in attenuating visually induced human postural sway. Exp Brain Res 1995;105(1):101–10. PubMed PMID: 7589307.

49. Paulus W, Straube A, Brandt TH. Visual postural performance after loss of somatosensory and vestibular function. J Neurol Neurosurg Psychiatry 1987;50(11):1542–5. PubMed PMID: 3501001.

50. Foster EC, Sveistrup H, Woollacott MH. Transitions in visual proprioception: A cross-sectional developmental study of the effect of visual flow on postural control. J Mot Behav 1996; 28(2):101–12. PubMed PMID: 12529212.

51. Lee D, Aronson E. Visual proprioceptive control of standing in human infants. Percept Psychophys 1974;15(3):529–32. English.

52. Paulus W, Straube A, Krafczyk S, et al. Differential-effects of retinal target displacement, changing size and changing disparity

in the control of anterior posterior and lateral body sway. Exp Brain Res 1989;78(2):243–52. PubMed PMID: 2599035.

53. Paulus WM, Straube A, Brandt T. Visual stabilisation of posture: physiological stimulus characteristics and clinical aspects. Brain 1984;107:1143. PubMed PMID: 6509312.

54. Graziano MSA. Where is my arm? The relative role of vision and proprioception in the neuronal representation of limb position. Proc Natl Acad Sci U S A 1999;96(18):10418–21. PubMed PMID: 10468623.

55. Sober SJ, Sabes PN. Multisensory integration during motor planning. J Neurosci 2003;23(18):6982–92. PubMed PMID: 12904459.

56. Fitzpatrick R, McCloskey DI. Proprioceptive, visual and vestibular thresholds for the perception of sway during standing in humans. J Physiol 1994;478(Pt 1):173. PubMed PMID: 7965833.

57. Cathers I, Day BL, Fitzpatrick RC. Otolith and canal reflexes in human standing. J Physiol 2005;563(1):229. PubMed PMID: 15618274.

58. Fitzpatrick RC, Day BL. Probing the human vestibular system with galvanic stimulation. J Appl Physiol 2004;96(6):2301. PubMed PMID: 15133017.

59. Wardman DL, Taylor JL, Fitzpatrick RC. Effects of galvanic vestibular stimulation on human posture and perception while standing. J Physiol 2003;551(3):1033. PubMed PMID: 12865505.

60. Day BL, Cole J. Vestibular-evoked postural responses in the absence of somatosensory information. Brain 2002;125:2081–8. PubMed PMID: 12183353.

61. Creath R, Kiemel T, Horak F, et al. The role of vestibular and somatosensory systems in intersegmental control of upright stance. J Vestib Res 2008;18(1):39–49. PubMed PMID: 18776597.

62. Buchanan JJ, Horak FB. Vestibular loss disrupts control of head and trunk on a sinusoidally moving platform. J Vestib Res 2001;11(6):371. PubMed PMID: 12446963.

63. Allum JH, Honegger F, Schicks H. The influence of a bilateral peripheral vestibular deficit on postural synergies. J Vestib Res 1994;4(1):49–70. PubMed PMID: MEDLINE:8186863.

64. Black FO, Wade SW, Nashner LM. What is the minimal vestibular function required for compensation? Am J Otol 1996;17(3):401. PubMed PMID: 8817017.

65. Cole J. Pride and a Daily Marathon The MIT Press. 1995.

66. Cole JD, Sedgwick EM. The perceptions of force and of movement in a man without large myelinated sensory afferents below the neck. J Physiol 1992;449:503–15. PubMed PMID: 1522522.

67. Kavounoudias A, Gilhodes JC, Roll R, et al. From balance regulation to body orientation: two goals for muscle proprioceptive information processing? Exp Brain Res 1999;124(1):80–8. PubMed PMID: 9928792.

68. Roll R, Velay JL, Roll JP. Eye and neck proprioceptive messages contribute to the spatial coding of retinal input in visually oriented activities. Exp Brain Res 1991;85(2):423–31. PubMed PMID: 1893990.

69. Karnath HO. Subjective body orientation in neglect and the interactive contribution of neck muscle proprioception and vestibular stimulation. Brain 1994;117:1001–12. PubMed PMID: 7953584.

70. Armstrong B, McNair P, Taylor D. Head and neck position sense. Sports Med 2008;38(2):101–17. [Epub 2008/01/19]; PubMed PMID: 18201114. eng.

71. Ivanenko YP, Grasso R, Lacquaniti F. Effect of gaze on postural responses to neck proprioceptive and vestibular stimulation in humans (vol 519, pg 301, 1999). J Physiol 1999;519(3):923. PubMed PMID: 10432359.

72. Taylor JL, McCloskey DI. Proprioception in the neck. Exp Brain Res 1988;70(2):351–60. [Epub 1988/01/01]; PubMed PMID: 3384037. eng.

73. Karnath HO, Sievering D, Fetter M. The interactive contribution of neck muscle proprioception and vestibular stimulation to subjective straight ahead orientation in man. Exp Brain Res 1994;101(1):140–6. PubMed PMID: 7843292.

74. Loram ID, Lakie M, Di Giulio I, et al. The consequences of short-range stiffness and fluctuating muscle activity for proprioception of postural joint rotations: the relevance to human standing. J Neurophysiol 2009;102(1):460–74. PubMed PMID: 19420127.

75. Voss H. [Tabulation of the absolute and relative muscular spindle numbers in human skeletal musculature]. Anat Anz 1971;129(5):562–72. PubMed PMID: 4260484. Tabelle der absoluten und relativen Muskelspindelzahlen der menschlichen Skelettmuskulatur.

76. Kavounoudias A, Roll R, Roll JP. Foot sole and ankle muscle inputs contribute jointly to human erect posture regulation. J Physiol 2001;532(3):869. PubMed PMID: 11313452.

77. Capaday C, Darling WG, Stanek K, et al. Pointing to oneself: active versus passive proprioception revisited and implications for internal models of motor system function. Exp Brain Res 2013;229(2):171–80. PubMed PMID: 23756602.

78. Sainburg RL, Ghilardi MF, Poizner H, et al. Control of limb dynamics in normal subjects and patients without proprioception. J Neurophysiol 1995;73(2):820–35. PubMed PMID: 7760137.

79. Riemann BL, Lephart SM. The sensorimotor system, part I: The physiologic basis of functional joint stability. J Athl Train 2002; 37(1):71–9. PubMed PMID: 16558670.

80. Mergner T. A neurological view on reactive human stance control. Ann Rev Control 2010;34(2):177–98. PubMed PMID: WOS: 000285491500001.

81. Mergner T, Maurer C, Peterka RJ. A multisensory posture control model of human upright stance. In: Prablanc C, Pelisson D, Rossetti Y, editors. Neural Control of Space Coding and Action Production. Progress in Brain Research. 1422003. 2003. p. 189–99.

82. Loram ID, Maganaris CN, Lakie M. Paradoxical muscle movement during postural control. Med Sci Sports Exerc 2009; 41(1):198–204. PubMed PMID: 19092688.

83. Loram ID, Maganaris CN, Lakie M. Paradoxical muscle movement in human standing. J Physiol 2004;556(Pt 3):683–9. PubMed PMID: 15047776. Pubmed Central PMCID: 1664994.

84. Lakie M, Walsh EG, Wright GW. Resonance at the wrist demonstrated by the use of a torque motor: an instrumental analysis of muscle tone in man. J Physiol 1984;353:265–85. PubMed PMID: 6481624.

85. Lakie M, Vernooij CA, Osborne TM, et al. The resonant component of human physiological hand tremor is altered by slow voluntary movements. J Physiol 2012;590(10):2471–83. PubMed PMID: 22431335.

86. Wise AK, Gregory JE, Proske U. The responses of muscle spindles to small, slow movements in passive muscle and during fusimotor activity. Brain Res 1999;821(1):87–94. [Epub 1999/03/05]; PubMed PMID: 10064791. English.

87. Kersten D, Mamassian P, Yuille A. Object perception as Bayesian inference. Annu Rev Psychol 2004;55:271–304. PubMed PMID: 14744217. English.

88. Helmholtz H. Handbuch der physiologischen optik. Leipzig: L. Voss; 1867.

89. Bays PM, Wolpert DM, Flanagan JR. Perception of the consequences of self-action is temporally tuned and event driven. Curr Biol 2005;15(12):1125–8. PubMed PMID: 15964278.

90. Tong F, Meng M, Blake R. Neural bases of binocular rivalry. Trends Cogn Sci 2006;10(11):502–11. PubMed PMID: 16997612.

91. Murray SO, Boyaci H, Kersten D. The representation of perceived angular size in human primary visual cortex. Nat Neurosci 2006;9(3):429–34. PubMed PMID: 16462737.

92. Adkin AL, Frank JS, Carpenter MG, et al. Fear of falling modifies anticipatory postural control. Exp Brain Res 2002;143(2):160. PubMed PMID: 11880892.

93. Carpenter MG, Frank JS, Silcher CP. Surface height effects on postural control: a hypothesis for a stiffness strategy for stance. J Vestib Res 1999;9(4):277. PubMed PMID: 10472040.

94. Osler CJ, Tersteeg MCA, Reynolds RF, et al. Postural threat differentially affects the feedforward and feedback components of the vestibular-evoked balance response. Eur J Neurosci 2013;38(8): 3239–47.

95. Tersteeg MCA, Marple-Horvat DE, Loram ID. Cautious gait in relation to knowledge and vision of height: is altered visual information the dominant influence? J Neurophysiol 2012; 107(10):2686–91. PubMed PMID: 22378173.

96. Carpenter MG, Frank JS, Silcher CP, et al. The influence of postural threat on the control of upright stance. Exp Brain Res 2001;138(2):210. PubMed PMID: 11417462.

97. Stefanucci JK, Proffitt DR. The roles of altitude and fear in the perception of height. J Exp Psychol Hum Percept Perform 2009;35(2):424–38. PubMed PMID: 19331498.

98. Clerkin EM, Cody MW, Stefanucci JK, et al. Imagery and fear influence height perception. J Anxiety Disord 2009;23(3):381–6. PubMed PMID: 19162437.

99. Stefanucci JK, Storbeck J. Don't look down: Emotional arousal elevates height perception. J Exp Psychol Gen 2009;138(1):131–45. PubMed PMID: 19203173.

100. Tersteeg M. Locomotion and stance at height [PhD]. Manchester: Manchester Metropolitan University; 2012.
101. Guerraz M, Day BL. Expectation and the vestibular control of balance. J Cognit Neurosci 2005;17(3):463–9. PubMed PMID: 15814005.
102. Yin HH, Knowlton BJ. The role of the basal ganglia in habit formation. Nat Rev Neurosci 2006;7(6):464–76.
103. Redgrave P, Prescott TJ, Gurney K. The basal ganglia: a vertebrate solution to the selection problem? Neuroscience 1999;89(4):1009–23. [Epub 1999/06/11]; PubMed PMID: 10362291. eng.
104. Brembs B. Towards a scientific concept of free will as a biological trait: spontaneous actions and decision-making in invertebrates. Proceedings of the Royal Society B: Biological Sciences 2010;[2010 December 15].
105. Balazsi G, van Oudenaarden A, Collins JJ. Cellular decision making and biological noise: from microbes to mammals. Cell 2011;144(6):910–25. [Epub 2011/03/19]; PubMed PMID: 21414483. Pubmed Central PMCID: PMC3068611, eng.
106. Cisek P, Kalaska JF. Neural correlates of reaching decisions in dorsal premotor cortex: Specification of multiple direction choices and final selection of action. Neuron 2005;45(5):801–14. PubMed PMID: 15748854.
107. Cisek P. Integrated neural processes for defining potential actions and deciding between them: A computational model. J Neurosci 2006;26(38):9761–70. PubMed PMID: 16988047.
108. Rizzolatti G, Luppino G. The cortical motor system. Neuron 2001;31(6):889–901. PubMed PMID: 11580891.
109. Redgrave P. Basal ganglia. J Scholarpedia 2007;2(6):1825.
110. Voorn P, Vanderschuren L, Groenewegen HJ, et al. Putting a spin on the dorsal-ventral divide of the striatum. Trends Neurosci 2004;27(8):468–74. PubMed PMID: 15271494.
111. Haber SN, Fudge JL, McFarland NR. Striatonigrostriatal pathways in primates form an ascending spiral from the shell to the dorsolateral striatum. J Neurosci 2000;20(6):2369–82. PubMed PMID: 10704511.
112. Mink JW. The basal ganglia: focused selection and inhibition of competing motor programs. Prog Neurobiol 1996;50(4):381–425. [Epub 1996/11/01]; PubMed PMID: 9004351. eng.
113. Jiang YH, Kanwisher N. Common neural substrates for response selection across modalities and mapping paradigms. J Cognit Neurosci 2003;15(8):1080–94. PubMed PMID: 14709228.
114. Dux PE, Ivanoff J, Asplund CL, et al. Isolation of a central bottleneck of information processing with time-resolved fMRI. Neuron 2006;52(6):1109–20. PubMed PMID: 17178412.
115. Houk J. Models of basal ganglia. Scholarpedia 2007;2(10):1633.
116. Beiser DG, Hua SE, Houk JC. Network models of the basal ganglia. Curr Opin Neurobiol 1997;7(2):185–90. PubMed PMID: 9142759.
117. Frank MJ. Dynamic Dopamine Modulation in the Basal Ganglia: A Neurocomputational Account of Cognitive Deficits in Medicated and Nonmedicated Parkinsonism. J Cognit Neurosci 2005; 17(1):51–72. [2005/01/01].
118. Frank MJ, Claus ED. Anatomy of a decision: Striato-orbitofrontal interactions in reinforcement learning, decision making, and reversal. Psychol Rev 2006;113(2):300–26. PubMed PMID: 16637763.
119. Ashby FG, Ennis JM, Spiering BJ. A neurobiological theory of automaticity in perceptual categorisation. Psychol Rev 2007; 114(3):632–56. PubMed PMID: 17638499.
120. Di Giulio I, Baltzopoulos V, Managanaris CN, et al. Human standing: does the control strategy pre-program a rigid knee? J Appl Physiol 2013;2013.
121. Van de Kamp C, Gawthrop P, Gollee H, et al., editors. Refractoriness in a whole-body human balance task. Trondheim, Norway: ISPGR; 2012.
122. Tortora, Gerard, Grabowski. Principles of Anatomy and Physiology. Harper Collins College Publishers; 1996.
123. Loram ID, Gollee H, Lakie M, et al. Human control of an inverted pendulum: Is continuous control necessary? Is intermittent control effective? Is intermittent control physiological? J Physiol 2011;589(2):307–24. PubMed PMID: 21098004.
124. Evans CM, Fellows SJ, Rack PM, et al. Response of the normal human ankle joint to imposed sinusoidal movements. J Physiol 1983;344(1):483. PubMed PMID: 6655591.
125. Marsden CD, Merton PA, Morton HB, et al. Reliability and efficacy of the long-latency stretch reflex in the human thumb. J Physiol 1981;316(JUL):47–60. PubMed PMID: 7320877.
126. Loram ID, Lakie M, Gawthrop PJ. Visual control of stable and unstable loads: what is the feedback delay and extent of linear time-invariant control? J Physiol 2009;587(Pt 6):1343–65. PubMed PMID: 19171654. Pubmed Central PMCID: 2675002.
127. Loram ID, Maganaris CN, Lakie M. Human postural sway results from frequent, ballistic bias impulses by soleus and gastrocnemius. J Physiol 2005;564(Pt 1):295–311. PubMed PMID: 15661824. Pubmed Central PMCID: 1456055.
128. Loram A. A scientific investigation into violin playing: diagnosis of musculo-kinematic coordination patterns and methodology for reducing interference with performance [MSc Dissertation]. London: UCL/MMU; 2013.
129. Loram ID, van de Kamp C, Gollee H, et al. Identification of intermittent control in man and machine. J R Soc Interface 2012;9(74):2070–84. PubMed PMID: 22491973.
130. Kandel E, Schwartz J, Jessell T. Principles of Neural Science. 4th ed. New York: McGraw-Hill; 2000.
131. Castelo Oliveira AS, Gizzi L, Kersting UG, et al. Modular organisation of balance control following perturbations during walking. J Neurophysiol 2012;108(7):1895–906. PubMed PMID: 22773783.
132. Delis I, Chiovetto E, Berret B. On the origins of modularity in motor control. J Neurosci 2010;30(22):7451–2. PubMed PMID: 20519519.
133. Latash ML. Motor synergies and the equilibrium-point hypothesis. Motor Control 2010;14(3):294–322. PubMed PMID: 20702893.
134. Hart CB, Giszter SF. A neural basis for motor primitives in the spinal cord. J Neurosci 2010;30(4):1322–36. PubMed PMID: 20107059.
135. Lockhart DB, Ting LH. Optimal sensorimotor transformations for balance. Nat Neurosci 2007;10(10):1329–36. PubMed PMID: 17873869.
136. Chvatal SA, Macpherson JM, Torres-Oviedo G, et al. Absence of postural muscle synergies for balance after spinal cord transection. J Neurophysiol 2013;110(6):1301–10. PubMed PMID: 23803327.
137. Bizzi E, Cheung VC. The neural origin of muscle synergies. Front Comput Neurosci 2013;7:[2013-April-29]; English.
138. Belen'kii VE, Gurfinkel VS. Pal'tsev EI. [Control elements of voluntary movements]. Biofizika 1967;12(1):135–41. PubMed PMID: 5623488.
139. Krishnan V, Aruin AS, Latash ML. Two stages and three components of the postural preparation to action. Exp Brain Res 2011;212(1):47–63. PubMed PMID: 21537967.
140. Ahmed AA, Wolpert DM. Transfer of dynamic learning across postures. J Neurophysiol 2009;102(5):2816–24. PubMed PMID: 19710374.
141. Vandenberghe A, Bosmans L, De Schutter J, et al. Quantifying individual muscle contribution to three-dimensional reaching tasks. Gait Posture 2012;35(4):579–84. PubMed PMID: 22410130.
142. Horak FB, Nashner LM. Central programming of postural movements – Adaptation to altered support-surface configurations. j neurophysiol 1986;55(6):1369. pubmed pmid: 3734861.
143. Door B. Towards perfect posture. London. Orion 2003;155.
144. Loram I, editor. Control Strategy in Postural-manual Interactions: is the Priority Posture or Configuration? Natal, Brazil: ISB; 2013.
145. Seidler RD. Neural correlates of motor learning, transfer of learning, and learning to learn. Exerc Sport Sci Rev 2010; 38(1):3–9. doi:10.1097/JES.0b013e3181c5cce7.
146. Blake DT, Byl NN, Cheung S, et al. Sensory representation abnormalities that parallel focal hand dystonia in a primate model. Somatosens Mot Res 2002;19(4):347–57. PubMed PMID: 12590836.
147. Byl NN, Merzenich MM, Jenkins WM. A primate genesis model of focal dystonia and repetitive strain injury: I. Learning-induced dedifferentiation of the representation of the hand in the primary somatosensory cortex in adult monkeys. Neurology 1996;47(2):508–20. [Epub 1996/08/01]; PubMed PMID: 8757029. eng.
148. Cailliet R. Cailliet R, editor. Soft Tissue Pain and Disability. 3rd ed. Philadelphia: Davis; 1996.
149. Cailliet R. Cailliet R, editor. Neck and Arm Pain. 3rd ed. Philadelphia: FA Davis Company; 1991.
150. Cailliet R. Low Back Pain Syndrome. 4th ed. Philadelphia: F.A.Davis Company; 1988. p. 34.

CHAPTER 5

MOTOR CONTROL AND MOTOR LEARNING

Natalie Mrachacz-Kersting • Peter Stubbs • Sabata Gervasio

INTRODUCTION

From the basic idea to move, to the planning and execution of movement, the nervous system must achieve the feat of activating the muscles that produce the selected movement and control these movements in an appropriate temporal and spatial manner. Temporal precision refers to the onset and offset of activity, whereas the spatial aspects relate to the resulting excursions of the bony attachments such that meaningful movements are produced, accounting for the environmental conditions, the position of the body within the environment and the cognitive and physical abilities of the individual. In doing so, the nervous system must choose between approximately 640 muscles and 360 joints and provide the appropriate combination of these to produce the desired outcome. There are often a number of ways to produce the desired outcome (degrees of freedom). For example, a soccer player may be required to pass the ball under a variety of conditions but the final goal remains the same. Specifically in the context of rehabilitation where skills such as walking need to be retrained, the question arises: What is normal? The problem of redundancy in relation to patients may be perceived as an advantage, since it allows flexibility when the degrees of freedom are reduced. However, it may also be associated with non-optimal (mal)adaptive strategies limiting the efficiency/normality of the movement.

To study motor control is to appreciate the degrees of freedom problem and the strategies the body, brain and mind employ to overcome these problems. An additional complication in the study of motor control arises from the way that any movement may be initiated or controlled once commenced. Evidence supports the notion of at least two types of control: (a) open loop or feed forward which generally implies no sensory feedback; and (b) closed loop or feedback which has sensory feedback as part of the controller system.

Open-loop control systems encompass fast, ballistic movements where no time is available to receive, extract and evaluate the sensory feedback resulting from the movement. In such a system it is assumed that sensory information is absent; however, sensory information is conveyed to higher centres in the resting state providing relevant information about the position of the joints, limbs and the individual as a whole in the environment. Without such knowledge, the nervous system would be unable to correctly select the appropriate motor programme to execute the desired movement. Furthermore, higher centres have a certain expectation of the appropriate sensory information that should be generated when a particular motor programme is executed. This is well documented by the fact that artificially induced reflexes are differently modulated within and across tasks. Closed-loop control systems are based on the assumption that sensory feedback is part of the control system. Thus, the feedback is used by the central nervous system (CNS) to continuously adjust movement parameters and ensure that the final goal is achieved. Despite these distinctions, most movement patterns are more complex than 'open' or 'closed' systems and therefore may not be solely part of an open- or closed-looped control system.

In an attempt to understand how an individual generates a movement that by nature is constrained by factors within the individual (structural or functional, e.g. body weight, shape, height, emotional and cognitive states), the environment (gravity, temperature, wind, etc.) and the task (e.g. goal of the task, implements to be manipulated, rules of the game, etc.), theories of motor control have been developed. Such theories could aid the practitioner to understand the variables that affect motor skill performance and through this provide a basis for effective development and implementation of rehabilitation strategies.

THEORIES OF MOTOR CONTROL

1. *Reflex theory*: Reflexes are generally perceived as stereotypical events where a specific stimulus leads to a specific response (i.e. when the patellar tendon is tapped by a hammer, the lower leg extends). It is now understood that reflexes are not as invariant as originally perceived, as the same sensory stimulus may produce a different behaviour depending on the context and task. Sir Charles Sherrington suggested that reflexes are the building blocks of complex behaviours. However, research on deafferented animals as well as humans has demonstrated that it is possible to control movement without sensory feedback.[1,2] This does not undermine the importance of local reflex circuits, as we know they are integrated into complex behaviour and thus form an integral part of movement control.

2. *Hierarchical theory*: Hughlings Jackson believed that higher centres within the nervous system control the lower centres and a top-down approach governs all movement. It is now generally acknowledged that although spinal reflexes are under the influence

of higher structures (e.g. modulation of reflexes during tasks), the sensory information that triggered the reflex is fed back to the higher centres that adjust their output. A multisegmental control exists where each level within the nervous system can act on the other levels.

3. *Motor programming theory*: According to Lashley a motor program is '… a generalized schemata of action which determines the sequence of specific acts'.[3] He spent his career searching for the place within the cerebral cortex where the memory trace for movement resides and, demonstrated in seminal laboratory experiments on rats, that memory (and learning) was impaired in direct proportion to the degree of cerebral cortex destroyed.[4,5] Richard Schmidt refined Lashley's initial ideas by proposing a generalized motor programme that controls classes of actions rather than individual movements. For example, if a person writes their name using the right or left hand, foot or even mouth, the generalized motor programme allows one to perform these tasks such that any person inspecting the written word would recognize the person's handwriting. The generalized motor programme represents a pattern of a movement containing fixed elements (invariant features such as relative time of phases of a movement that remain the same from trial to trial) and flexible elements (parameters that are adjusted depending on the demands of the specific situation, e.g. the speed of a movement). During learning (or relearning) of movement skills, the individual considers four pieces of information to develop a schema: (a) the initial conditions (start of the movement); (b) the response parameters (speed, size, etc.); (c) sensory consequences of the movement; and (d) the response outcome.

4. *Dynamic systems theory*: Nikolai Bernstein believed that there is not one solution for one movement problem, rather a movement pattern is produced as a function of the changing constraints placed upon it – these are the structural, environmental and task constraints mentioned previously. Constraints act as control parameters when they lead to any change in the movement. Control parameters (e.g. direction, force, speed and perceptual information) are variables that move the system (you) into a new attractor state. The acquisition of motor skills can be seen as finding the optimum values accounting for control parameters (constraints) that will meet the demand of the task for each individual. For example, following an injury to the lower leg, the patient will display a given gait pattern as a result of the constraints imposed on the system. The leg strength of the patient serves as a control parameter. As the leg of the patient becomes stronger there are changes in the walking pattern meaning that the increases in leg strength have caused a phase shift and a new gait (attractor state) self-organizes.

Currently, the opinions on which theory will prevail are divided. Some contend that aspects of the motor programme theory will be subsumed into the dynamic systems theory. However, at this point, the motor programming theory is still the predominate theory of motor control.[6,7]

In the following sections, several recent and new aspects relating to motor control and motor learning will be presented that are intended to complement the existing knowledge. Motor control and motor learning can occur at cortical, subcortical and spinal levels, and sensory information is often required for motor control and learning to occur. More specifically, three broad concepts will be examined. (a) Sensory feedback from muscle, tendon and cutaneous receptors forms an integral part of normal voluntary movement and is integrated with higher levels of control. (b) Sensory feedback as part of a reflex loop is not fixed and can be conditioned to allow improved voluntary control in both healthy and impaired populations. The necessity for higher-level input to allow these changes will be presented. (c) Sensory feedback from receptors forms an integral part, not only in the execution of already learned movements, but as a key component in the relearning and acquisition of new motor skills following a CNS insult or musculoskeletal injury.

SENSORY FEEDBACK AS AN INTEGRAL PART OF MOTOR CONTROL

It has been known for a long time that proprioceptive feedback contributes to the activation of muscles and thus the control of movement in both animals and humans. Proprioceptors encompass a group of sensory receptors, including muscle spindles, Golgi tendon organs, joint and skin receptors, that convey knowledge about the position of our limbs to the higher centres that integrate the acquired sensory information and select the correct motor programme for task execution. Thus, even though proprioceptive feedback may be too slow to adjust an ongoing fast ballistic movement, such as a tennis serve, it is a necessary part of the initial motor planning. Therefore there are elements of feedforward and feedback control required in movement control.

An example of this is when we pick up an object. In this case we are able to exert the correct force such that the object is not crushed or slips from our hands. We are able to determine the pre-controlled motor programme based on vision (for the opening of the hand to grip) and prior experience allowing us to apply an initial force (feedforward control) and then adjust this force based on the immediate characteristics of the object itself (feedback control). When subjects grip large objects, they apply more force than comparatively smaller objects of the same weight, based on previous experience. Despite this, subjects perceive the smaller object, of the same weight, as being heavier, but once the object is lifted, the grip force is modified based on the characteristics of the object itself. When an object with a rough lifting surface is lifted, it is gripped with less force than an object of the same mass but with a slippery surface. In addition, the force is modulated such that the object is gripped with a force slightly greater than the force in which the object will be dropped (see Johnsson & Westling[8] for a review). This is likely due to feedback mechanisms arising from peripheral receptors in the hand. In these examples, both feedforward and feedback control contribute to motor planning and motor control. Under normal conditions, a simple task such as picking up an object can be achieved with little thought and concentration. When there is a lack of feedback such as in patients with large fibre neuropathy, and subsequently impaired movement control, accuracy and adaptability to alterations in the environmental constraints are diminished.[9,10] However, some degree of movement persists in these patients even in the absence of visual feedback (often used as a compensatory mechanism). Rothwell et al.[10] investigated a patient with impaired sensory control, largely confined to the sensory fibres, and noted that the patient may retain the ability to produce different levels of force when asked.[10] The patient was as accurate as normal subjects when performing fast ballistic movements of the thumb, although only when he had received prior training using visual feedback. In addition, since the patient was not successful at everyday living tasks (e.g. holding objects such as pens, cups, coins, buttoning his shirt, judging weights of objects if his eyes were closed), it is questionable whether he would have been able to perform as well on such ballistic movements if the environmental constraints were altered.

SENSORY FEEDBACK DURING LOCOMOTION

During walking, sensory feedback from muscle receptors and tendon organs is required for (a) normal movement control and (b) generating appropriate reactions following an unexpected disturbance such as an obstacle or uneven ground surface. Many studies investigating sensory feedback in humans use electrical stimulation and base conclusions on motor control and motor learning on the reaction of the muscle following this. However, electrically stimulating the muscle is not representative of a true 'physiological' stimulus. Sinkjær and colleagues[11] created a specialized actuator system that mechanically stretches the ankle joint, allowing the assessment of motor control and motor learning following a 'physiological' stretch of the muscle during walking.

This actuator (Fig. 5-1)[11] was attached to the ankle joint of subjects in such a way that they could walk freely. When a sudden plantarflexion movement was applied during the stance phase of gait, thus unloading the soleus (SOL) muscle, the electromyographic (EMG) activity of the SOL was significantly reduced (Fig. 5-2B) while there was no effect on the antagonist tibialis anterior (Fig. 5.2C).[12] This was the first indication that sensory feedback arising from tendon organs or muscle afferents forms part of the normal activation of that muscle, up to 50% depending on the phase of the gait cycle. Subsequent publications from that group provided further conclusive evidence to show that force-sensitive feedback from group Ib afferents contributes to the normal locomotor muscle activity during the stance phase of walking.[13–16] This group also investigated the role of small changes in the ankle angle. Using the unique actuator system, small enhancements and reductions of the ankle joint may be imposed that are within the natural variability of the ankle angular movements from one

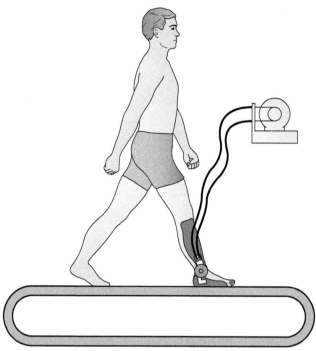

FIGURE 5-1 ■ The actuator system developed by Andersen and Sinkjær is attached to the subject via specialized casts. The subject can move his/her ankle joint freely and the actuator can be programmed to suddenly extend or flex the ankle joint at any time during the gait cycle.

step cycle to the next (Fig. 5-3A). These small adjustments do not result in a synchronized reflex response, but rather in small enhancements or reductions in the EMG signal of the SOL (Fig. 5-3B). It became evident that group Ia afferents are responsible for the increased muscle activity during slight dorsiflexion enhancements imposed such as occurs when walking up an incline,[17] whereas group II afferents are the main contributors to the decrements in activity seen during the imposed reduction movements.[18]

As we have just described how homonymous feedback contributes to the activation of the muscle itself during walking, likewise, following an unexpected disturbance, proprioceptive feedback is used to adjust the activity of the muscle(s) of the same limb,[15,19] opposite limb,[20–23] and between lower and upper limbs.[24] This mechanism allows the body to make the necessary adjustments enabling the body to remain upright (and not fall).

It is well known that afferent feedback produces interlimb reflexes that are relevant for postural stability.[25] For instance, when a unilateral rotation of the hip or knee joint is imposed during walking, bilateral responses in the leg muscles are observed. It was suggested that the purpose of these responses is to restore normal physiological movement following the perturbation.[26] Studies involving other unilateral perturbations, such as treadmill acceleration or deceleration (while one leg is on the treadmill) or peripheral nerve electrical stimulation, have reported bilateral muscle responses that are specific to the type of perturbation and dependent on when the perturbation occurs during the gait cycle.[27] Functionality is often inferred based on the observations in the EMG

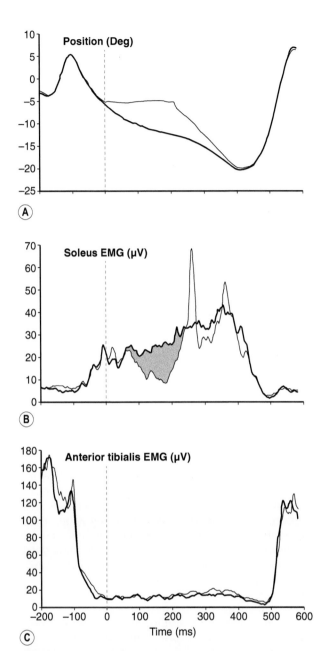

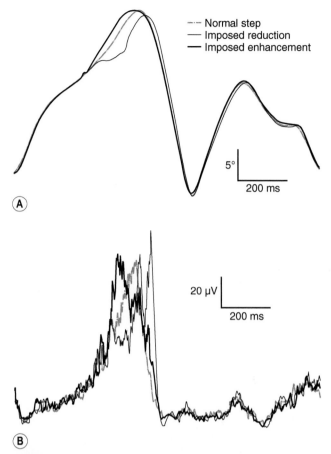

FIGURE 5-2 ■ **(A)** The position of the ankle joint under normal (thick trace) and sudden plantarflexion (thin trace) conditions during walking. The resulting electromyographic activity of the **(B)** soleus and **(C)** tibialis anterior.

FIGURE 5-3 ■ **(A)** The position of the ankle joint under normal (black trace), sudden imposed reduction (light grey trace) or enhancement (dark grey trace). **(B)** The resulting electromyographic activity of the soleus shows no reflex response but rather reduced or enhanced activity.

activity; however, the reflex action on the basis of muscle activity and actual joint function may not be correlated. To alleviate this, studies further investigate the kinematics and kinetics following joint perturbations and again infer function and dysfunction from these. However, most of these studies lack relevance to current clinical practice and are therefore inaccessible to many clinicians. Recently, we have applied a novel method to investigate changes in the centre of pressure (CoP) after evoking interlimb reflexes. These measures are frequently used in clinics to evaluate balance and postural control[28] and therefore increase relevance of this type of research to the clinician and clinical populations.

We have observed that the stimulation of the tibial nerve of one leg (at the popliteal fossa) at the end of the swing phase, elicited a facilitatory response in the contralateral gastrocnemius lateralis (Fig. 5-4A).[22] Recordings from pressure-sensitive insoles inserted into the shoe of the subject revealed that this response elicited a shift of the CoP under the contralateral foot toward the medial and anterior direction (Fig. 5.4B and C), and consequently increased the pressure at the level of the first metatarsal head. The stance phase of the stimulated leg was significantly shorter in the step following the stimulation. The crossed responses observed in the triceps surae might therefore be a method to accelerate the propulsion phase of the contralateral leg and prepare it for a faster step in the event that the stimulated leg is not able to sustain the body. This result provides direct evidence of the role of interlimb reflexes in postural control and dynamic stability.

Afferent feedback and its role within reflex pathways was for a long time considered to be non-modifiable. Thus, although afferent feedback is modulated during different tasks, it was thought that all conditions being equal, the response observed would be similar in latency and magnitude. It was through some observations on animals by Di Gorgio[29,30] that led Wolpaw and colleagues[31] to the idea that reflex pathways could be trained

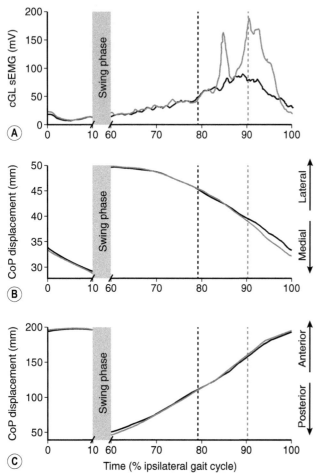

FIGURE 5-4 ■ Gastrocnemius lateralis EMG (**A**), centre of pressure (CoP) displacement under the contralateral foot in the medial–lateral (**B**) and in the anterior–posterior direction (**C**) for n = 1 subject. Grey and black traces indicate data when a stimulation occurred and the control condition (no stimulation) respectively. After the stimulation, indicated by the dashed black line, a short-latency facilitation was observed in the gastrocnemius EMG, followed by a medial anterior shift of the CoP. The onset of the shift in CoP is indicated by the dashed grey line.

and that the spinal cord, much like the brain, was capable of learning.

SENSORY FEEDBACK AS PART OF A REFLEX LOOP IS NOT STEREOTYPED

Wolpaw and colleagues (see Wolpaw[32] for a review) have demonstrated that training of a simple reflex pathway, such as the electrically evoked H-reflex, in animal preparations, can significantly alter the response to the stimulus – either increasing or decreasing the reflex depending on the protocol implemented. This is accompanied by significant alterations in function as observed in lesioned animals.[32] For example, when the H-reflex was down-conditioned, such that over time the reflex excitability was trained to decrease, the activity of the SOL during locomotion was reduced, whereas when it is up-conditioned the activity was increased.[33] In 2009, Wolpaw and colleagues applied this type of training to healthy

control subjects and patients with spinal cord injuries, and showed that in humans, as in animals, the H-reflex pathway could be altered.[34] The alterations in the H-reflex size also lead to functionally beneficial alterations in the modulation of the SOL activity during dynamic activities in both the healthy and individuals with spinal cord injuries.[34,35] This latter result is of particular importance when considering the role that reflexes have during dynamic movements (as outlined in the previous section). Here, reflexes not only contribute to the overall stiffness of a joint, but their function changes dynamically throughout activities such as walking, running and sprinting. For example, the ankle extensors are stretched under the weight of the body during the stance phase of locomotion and the stretch reflex may assist the force production during this phase. The muscles are also stretched during the early swing phase, and without suppression of this reflex, the stretch reflex could extend the ankle and may cause foot drop.[36-39] Appropriate phase-dependent modulation of spinal reflexes is thus necessary during dynamic tasks. Training these reflexes as described above, is a completely novel approach as a possible therapeutic intervention in humans, despite 30 years of successful animal studies.[32,40-43]

Recent studies have investigated whether it is possible to also condition the stretch reflex of the SOL, as shown for the human biceps brachii muscle.[44-46] This stretch reflex is more 'physiological' when compared to the electrically evoked H-reflex. In particular, this work evaluated whether the alteration in the size of the stretch reflex has functional implications for healthy subjects. The protocol of this work is depicted in Figure 5-5. Ankle dorsiflexion movements were imposed using a unique ankle perturbator while the subjects were seated (Fig. 5-6A). The activity of the SOL was quantified by the amount of EMG (bottom trace of Fig. 5-5). Generally, three bursts of activity can be visualized that are termed the short-, medium- and long-latency reflex (or M1, M2 and M3 in some studies). After six baseline sections, subjects were required to either up- or down-condition the short-latency component in the following 24 conditioning sessions (Fig. 5-6). A screen placed in front of the subject provided visual feedback (shown as bars) relating to the activity level of the SOL and the size of the SOL stretch reflex following each imposed ankle dorsiflexion stretch (Fig. 5-6B). The shaded areas in the figure represent the window in which the SOL background activity and the stretch reflex size must be maintained by the subject. During control trials, this area is set as large as possible as the subject is not training to modify the size. For a successful conditioning trial, the bar is depicted as green while unsuccessful trials result in a red bar.

Following up-conditioning, the size of the SOL stretch reflex is significantly enhanced while it is significantly decreased following down-conditioning (Fig. 5-6B). Importantly, this alteration also led to modifications in tasks unrelated to the training. For example, subjects were asked to perform drop jumps from a 30 cm height, landing on one foot and the excursion of the CoP was quantified (Fig. 5-7). Subjects trained to up-condition the SOL stretch reflex decreased their CoP excursion from touchdown for a duration of 1 minute.

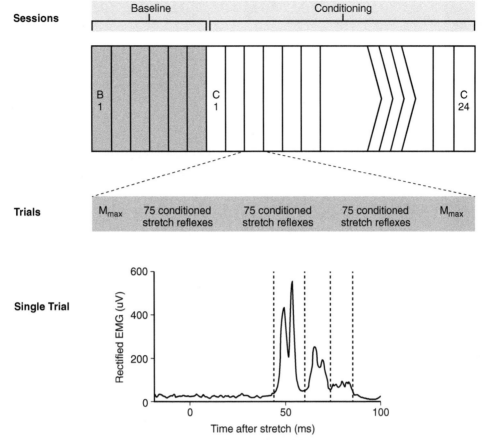

FIGURE 5-5 ■ The protocol. Subjects attend six baseline sessions during which they are exposed to 245 single trials consisting of imposed ankle dorsiflexion movements. They only receive feedback on the background level of soleus activity which they maintain at approximately 5% of the maximum activation. In the following 24 sessions, subjects are conditioned to either increase (up-condition) or decrease (down-condition) the size of the soleus stretch reflex following the imposed ankle dorsiflexions. The activity of the soleus muscle following a single imposed dorsiflexion is depicted in the lower trace. Several peaks may be seen that are separated by the vertical dashed lines. Subjects receive feedback on only the first burst.

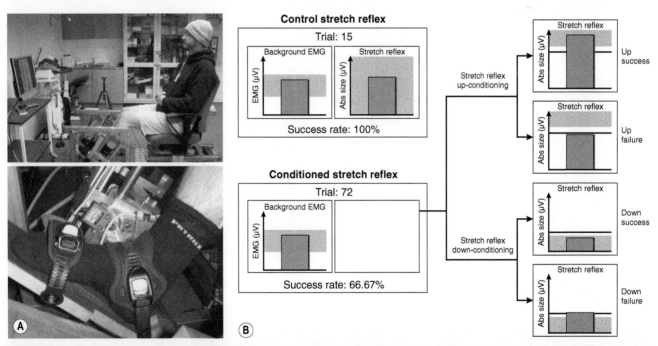

FIGURE 5-6 ■ **(A)** The unique ankle perturbator. Subjects are seated comfortably with both feet on separate foot plates. The enlarged figure on the left visualizes the foot position and fixation. A screen placed in front of the subject provides feedback to the subject relating to both the activity level of the soleus muscle as well as on the size of the soleus stretch reflex following each imposed ankle dorsiflexion. **(B)** The visual feedback on the screen is comprised of two parts, the background EMG and the stretch reflex size both shown as bars. The shaded areas represent the window in which the soleus background activity and the stretch reflex size must be maintained by the subject. During control trials, this area is set as large as possible since the subject is not training to modify the size. During up-conditioning trials, this area is above a criterion level based on the baseline sessions while for the down-conditioning trials it is below this criterion level. When the subject has a successful conditioning trial, the bar is depicted as green (light grey in the figure) while unsuccessful trials result in a red (dark grey in the figure) bar. This provides for immediate feedback to the subject for each single trial performed.

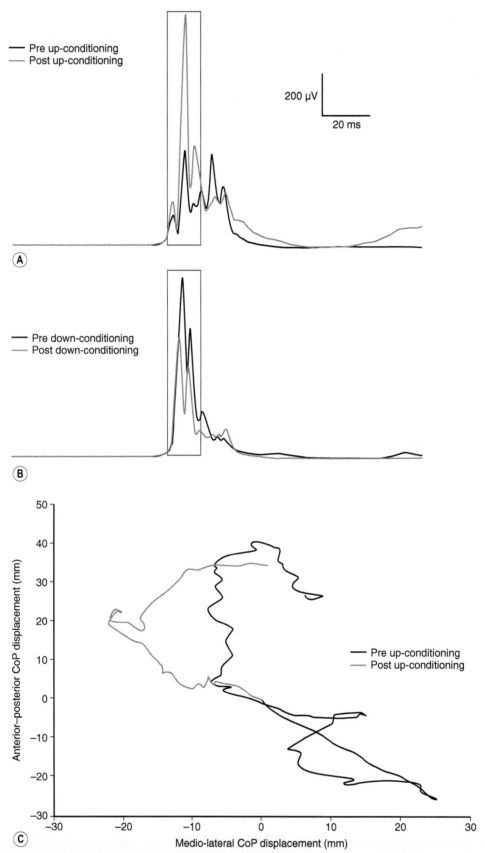

FIGURE 5-7 ■ **(A)** The soleus stretch reflex prior to (black trace) and following (grey trace) 24 sessions of up-conditioning. The grey shaded area represents the duration of the short-latency component of the soleus stretch reflex which was the target for the conditioning, **(B)** as in (A) but following 24 sessions of down-conditioning. **(C)** Excursions of the centre of pressure (CoP) during landing on one leg from a height of 50 cm. Data are the best of three trials in *n* = 1 prior to (black trace) and following (grey trace) up-conditioning.

This indicates an improved balance control. The functional benefits from conditioning the H-reflex and the stretch reflex continue to be explored. The indications are strong that this type of intervention can provide an alternative strategy for improved motor control following musculoskeletal injury. However, despite the success of conditioning reflexes in both human and animal studies, exact mechanisms causing up- and down-regulation are unknown and more research is required to investigate the underlying neural mechanisms involved.

SENSORY FEEDBACK IS A KEY COMPONENT IN MOTOR (RE)LEARNING

Chronic Pain States

The mechanisms of chronic musculoskeletal pain are not fully understood, and thus management of chronic musculoskeletal pain is often sub-optimal. One of the reasons for such a mismatch is the fact that facilitations in the CNS pain mechanisms are not accounted for. CNS structures play a key role in the development and experience of chronic pain resulting from conditions (e.g. lateral epicondylalgia).[47] Human pain models have been developed to mimic chronic pain states and we now know that significant maladaptive plasticity (i.e. negative alterations in the connections within the brain) occurs in a chronic musculoskeletal pain state. This may detrimentally alter motor control affecting the activation of the CNS.[48–50] Imaging studies[51,52] have contributed to the localization of brain areas affected by pain and those that are altered through application of treatments. However, these techniques often have a poor temporal resolution, require large and expensive equipment and confine the patient to a restricted environment such that occurrence of pain under dynamic conditions cannot be investigated. A recent review highlighted several non-pharmacological treatments designed to restore normal brain function concomitantly with a reduction of chronic pain.[53] These include repetitive transcranial magnetic stimulation, transcranial direct current stimulation and neurofeedback. The central idea behind restoring brain activity patterns is to avoid maladaptive alterations that may lead to secondary problems (i.e. altered movement patterns when performing a task that will induce pain in other areas thus adding to the problem rather than relieving it).

In order to retrain the brain and induce a relearning of the correct movement patterns (and thereby reverse maladaptive cortical reorganization), the mechanisms behind learning need to be satisfied. The current belief is that plasticity can only be induced appropriately if the relevant neural structures are activated in a correlated manner ('neurons that fire together, wire together').[54] As such, any treatment targeting the final output stage of the brain to activate the muscles that produce the movement (e.g. the motor cortex) must be designed so that the correct temporal activation is satisfied. Repetitive transcranial magnetic stimulation and transcranial direct current stimulation have a poor spatial target resolution such that many brain areas surrounding the target area are activated upon stimulation.[55] On the contrary,

neurofeedback methods allow the user to control his/her own brain activity by using immediate visual feedback on their respective brain state (by electroencephalographic [EEG] recordings). EEG activity of the user is measured continuously while he/she imagines performing a specific task (also called motor imagery) that normally leads to a painful sensation (e.g. reaching movement if the condition is lateral epicondylalgia). During motor imagery, the brain activity is shown to the user via a screen and he/she is instructed to control specific brain waves known to be altered during the experience of pain as a form of maladaptive plasticity. The correct level of brain activation is rewarded in two ways: (a) the user receives immediate positive visual feedback on their performance; and (b) pain sensation is reduced. Thus neurofeedback may reverse maladaptive plasticity as the user learns to modulate his/her brain activity.

In order to successfully use neurofeedback methods, it is imperative to understand which signals are affected during chronic musculoskeletal pain. Studies investigating EEG oscillations in central neuropathic pain[56,57] and musculoskeletal pain[58] have been restricted to resting state EEG or motor imagery. However, the effect on the EEG waves when the person is performing the task may be different. In addition, motor imagery can enhance pain and thus may not be as useful when treating patients with chronic pain resulting from musculoskeletal problems such as lateral epicondylalgia. Performing the movement may in these cases be more appropriate.

Central Nervous System Lesions

The Hebbian rule of associativity has also been applied to retrain patients following a CNS lesion. For instance, chronic stroke patients were asked to attempt a simple dorsiflexion movement of the ankle joint and the related electrical activity over the motor cortex was recorded using scalp electrodes.[59] The signal in this case is characterized by a slow negative potential (Fig. 5-7), termed movement-related cortical potential, which is generated in every movement or imagined movement, though in the latter case it is of smaller amplitude. It has been shown that when a peripheral stimulus is timed such that the afferent volley (the sensory feedback) arrives during the peak negative phase, which, represents the time of movement onset, plasticity is induced. Thus in both healthy[60,61] and chronic stroke patients,[59] the pairing of motor attempt or imagination and peripheral nerve stimulation lead to significant enhancements in the output of motor cortex to the target muscle, as assessed by changes in the amplitude of the motor evoked potential following non-invasive transcranial magnetic stimulation (TMS). In chronic stroke patients, an enhancement in dynamic task performance such as walking speed and foot tapping frequency accompanies the alterations in motor evoked potential size[59] (Fig. 5-8)

A recent study investigated if task imagination can be temporally combined with afferent information generated by a passive movement to alter M1 output.[62] Thus, in this case, both the peripheral input and the central command are generated by a physiological activation of the relevant neural structures. Subjects were asked to

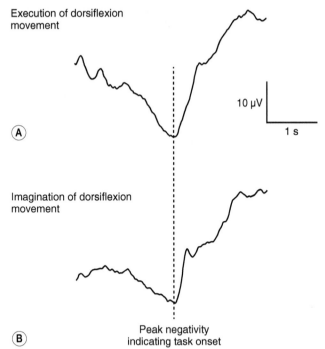

Execution of dorsiflexion movement

10 µV

1 s

(A)

Imagination of dorsiflexion movement

(B)

Peak negativity indicating task onset

FIGURE 5-8 ■ Scalp recordings over the vertex using non-invasive electrodes. The movement-related cortical potential during (**A**) execution and (**B**) imagination of a simple dorsiflexion task. The most negative peak, signals the onset of task execution (vertical dashed line). Data are the average of 50 consecutive trials in $n = 1$.

self-select when to imagine the task which was detected by a computerized algorithm. Once the algorithm detected that a movement was being imagined, it triggered a motorized orthotic device that passively moved the joint as if the movement had been executed rather than imagined. The detection accuracy of the algorithm was approximately 73%, thus not all imagined trials resulted in a subsequent movement by the orthosis; yet the motor evoked potential increased significantly following only 50 imaginations and remained enhanced 30 minutes after the cessation of the intervention. The study thus demonstrates that significant learning is possible even if the correlation between two inputs is not always given. The question arises: How many correlated repetitions are required to ensure long-term potentiation (LTP)-like changes are induced? This is not an easy question as a variety of protocols have been implemented and these lack consistency in, amongst other things, parameters such as the number of repetitions (for a review see Ziemann et al.[63]). These may be beneficial in subjects with musculoskeletal conditions that lack the strength to perform a movement properly.

Nevertheless, the most recent studies imply that afferent input in combination with central commands either elicited naturally or through artificial means, lead to motor learning. This is not to infer that techniques using either only afferent feedback (e.g. functional electrical stimulation, dual motor point stimulation) or central input (e.g. repetitive transcranial magnetic stimulation, theta burst stimulation) have no effect on plasticity. However, in the past few years, clinical trials suggest that a multimodal approach where afferent feedback is combined with modalities that have a central component and require the patient's conscious attention are more successful at inducing permanent improvements in function compared to any single method applied alone.[64–67]

CONCLUSIONS

Motor learning and control is a complex topic and many studies are being conducted to induce motor learning and improve motor control. Although previous research has investigated simple movements with non-physiological stimuli, with the advent of more sophisticated technologies for the assessment and interpretation of movement, we are now moving into the realm in which more complex movements are being altered or retrained for longer periods of time. This will therefore have implications in rehabilitation, motor learning and motor unlearning (in the case where people have adapted pathologically following an injury). Due to the number of methods used to induce motor learning and assess motor control, it is difficult to know which is best and if one should be used preferentially over another. The limits of the clinical setting, the abilities and preferences of the patient as well as the knowledge and skills of the clinician will dictate the most feasible treatment regimen. When is it best to treat the patient? What is the optimal dosage for maximal benefit? Will the effects be maintained for weeks, months or permanently following the intervention? When is the neural system most capable of recovery? What medication should be taken/avoided to assist in motor learning? A lot of these questions require long-term studies using clinical trials that are both time consuming and expensive. Further research and larger clinical trials are required to consolidate and disseminate the research that has been and continues to be conducted in this area.

REFERENCES

1. Grillner S. Locomotion in vertebrates: central mechanisms and reflex interaction. Physiol Rev 1975;55(2):247–304.
2. Pearson KG, Misiaszek JE, Hulliger M. Chemical ablation of sensory afferents in the walking system of the cat abolishes the capacity for functional recovery after peripheral nerve lesions. Exp Brain Res 2003;150(1):50–60.
3. Lashley K. The problem of serial order in behaviour. In: Jeffress LA, editor. Cerebral Mechanisms in Behaviour. New York: Wiley; 1951. p. 112–31.
4. Franz SI, Lashley KS. The retention of habits by the rat after destruction of the frontal portion of the cerebrum. Psychobiol 1917;1(1):3–18.
5. Passingham RE, Stephan KE, Kotter R. The anatomical basis of functional localisation in the cortex. Nat Rev Neurosci 2002;3(8):606–16.
6. Li KY. Examining contemporary motor control theories from the perspective of degrees of freedom. Aust Occup Ther J 2013;60(2):138–43.
7. Magill R, Anderson D. Motor Learning and Control: Concepts and Applications. 10th ed. Singapore: McGraw-Hill Education; 2011.
8. Johnsson R, Westling G. Afferent signals during manipulative tasks in humans. In: O Franzen JW, editor. Information Processing in the Somatosensory System. Macmillan Press; 1991. p. 25–48.
9. Sanes JN, Mauritz KH, Evarts EV, et al. Motor deficits in patients with large-fibre sensory neuropathy. Proc Natl Acad Sci U S A 1984;81(3):979–82.
10. Rothwell JC, Traub MM, Day BL, et al. Manual motor performance in a deafferented man. Brain 1982;105(Pt 3):515–42.

11. Andersen JB, Sinkjær T. An actuator system for investigating electrophysiological and biomechanical features around the human ankle joint during gait. IEEE Trans Rehabil Eng 1995;3(4): 299–306.

12. Sinkjær T, Andersen JB, Ladouceur M, et al. Major role for sensory feedback in soleus EMG activity in the stance phase of walking in man. J Physiol 2000;523(Pt 3):817–27.

13. Mazzaro N, Grey MJ, Sinkjær T, et al. Lack of on-going adaptations in the soleus muscle activity during walking in patients affected by large-fibre neuropathy. J Neurophysiol 2005;93(6): 3075–85.

14. Grey MJ, Nielsen JB, Mazzaro N, et al. Positive force feedback in human walking. J Physiol 2007;581(1):99–105.

15. af Klint R, Cronin NJ, Ishikawa M, et al. Afferent contribution to locomotor muscle activity during unconstrained overground human walking: an analysis of triceps surae muscle fascicles. J Neurophysiol 2010;103(3):1262–74.

16. af Klint R, Mazzaro N, Nielsen JB, et al. Load rather than length sensitive feedback contributes to soleus muscle activity during human treadmill walking. J Neurophysiol 2010;103(5):2747–56.

17. Mazzaro N, Grey MJ, Sinkjær T. Contribution of afferent feedback to the soleus muscle activity during human locomotion. J Neurophysiol 2005;93(1):167–77.

18. Mazzaro N, Grey M, do Nascimento O, et al. Afferent-mediated modulation of the soleus muscle activity during the stance phase of human walking. Exp Brain Res 2006;173(4):713–23.

19. af Klint R, Nielsen JB, Cole J, et al. Within-step modulation of leg muscle activity by afferent feedback in human walking. J Physiol 2008;586(19):4643–8.

20. Stubbs PW, Mrachacz-Kersting N. Short-latency crossed inhibitory responses in the human soleus muscle. J Neurophysiol 2009;102(6):3596–605.

21. Stubbs PW, Nielsen JF, Sinkjær T, et al. Phase modulation of the short-latency crossed spinal response in the human soleus muscle. J Neurophysiol 2011;105(2):503–11.

22. Gervasio S, Farina D, Sinkjær T, et al. Crossed reflex reversal during human locomotion. J Neurophysiol 2013;109(9):2335–44.

23. Stevenson AJ, Geertsen SS, Andersen JB, et al. Interlimb communication to the knee flexors during walking in humans. J Physiol 2013;591(Pt 19):4921–35.

24. Zehr EP, Haridas C. Modulation of cutaneous reflexes in arm muscles during walking: further evidence of similar control mechanisms for rhythmic human arm and leg movements. Exp Brain Res 2003;149(2):260–6.

25. Dietz V. Do human bipeds use quadrupedal coordination? Trends Neurosci 2002;25(9):462–7.

26. Dietz V, Colombo G, Muller R. Single joint perturbation during gait: neuronal control of movement trajectory. Exp Brain Res 2004;158(3):308–16.

27. Berger W, Dietz V, Quintern J. Corrective reactions to stumbling in man: Neuronal co-ordination of bilateral leg muscle activity during gait. J Physiol 1984;357:109–25.

28. Palmieri R, Ingersoll C, Stone M, et al. Centre-of-pressure parameters used in the assessment of postural control. J Sport Rehabil 2002;11:51–66.

29. DiGiorgio A. Azione del cervelletto-neocerebellum-sul tono posturale degli arti e localizzazioni cerebellari dell'animale rombencefalico. Arch Fisiol 1942;42:25–79.

30. DiGiorgio A. Persistenza nell'animale spinale, di asymmetrie posturali e motorie di origine cerebellare: I, II, III. Arch Fisiol 1929; 27:518–80.

31. Wolpaw JR. Activity-dependent spinal cord plasticity in health and disease. Annu Rev Neurosci 2001;24(1):807–43.

32. Wolpaw JR. Spinal cord plasticity in acquisition and maintenance of motor skills. Acta Physiol 2007;189(2):155–69.

33. Chen Y, Chen XY, Jakeman LB, et al. The interaction of a new motor skill and an old one: H-reflex conditioning and locomotion in rats. J Neurosci 2005;25(29):6898–906.

34. Thompson AK, Chen XY, Wolpaw JR. Acquisition of a simple motor skill: Task-dependent adaptation plus long-term change in the human soleus H-reflex. J Neurosci 2009;29(18):5784–92.

35. Thompson A, Abel BM, Wolpaw JR. Soleus H-reflex modulation during locomotion in people with chronic incomplete spinal cord injury. Abstract Viewer/Itinerary Planner. San Diego: Society for Neuroscience; 2010. Online.; San Diego 2010 p. Program Number 82.11.

36. Capaday C, Stein RB. Difference in the amplitude of the human soleus H reflex during walking and running. J Physiol 1987;392: 513–22.

37. Capaday C, Stein RB. Amplitude modulation of the soleus H-reflex in the human during walking and standing. J Neurosci 1986;6(5): 1308–13.

38. Schneider C, Lavoie BA, Capaday C. On the origin of the soleus H-reflex modulation pattern during human walking and its task-dependent differences. J Neurophysiol 2000;83(5):2881–90.

39. Nielsen JF, Andersen JB, Barbeau H, et al. Input-output properties of the soleus stretch reflex in spastic stroke patients and healthy subjects during walking. Neurorehabilitation 1998;10:151–66.

40. Wolpaw JR. Operant conditioning of primate spinal reflexes: the H-reflex. J Neurophysiol 1987;57(2):443–59.

41. Wolpaw JR, O'Keefe JA. Adaptive plasticity in the primate spinal stretch reflex: evidence for a two-phase process. J Neurosci 1984;4(11):2718–24.

42. Chen XY, Wolpaw JR. Operant conditioning of H-reflex in freely moving rats. J Neurophysiol 1995;73(1):411–15.

43. Wolpaw JR, Lee CL. Memory traces in primate spinal cord produced by operant conditioning of H-reflex. J Neurophysiol 1989;61(3):563–72.

44. Wolf SL, Segal RL. Conditioning of the spinal stretch reflex: implications for rehabilitation. Phys Ther 1990;70(10):652–6.

45. Segal RL, Wolf SL, Catlin PA, et al. Uncoupling of human short and long latency stretch reflex responses with operant conditioning. Restor Neurol Neurosci 2000;17(1):17–22.

46. Wolf SL, Segal RL. Reducing human biceps brachii spinal stretch reflex magnitude. J Neurophysiol 1996;75(4):1637–46.

47. Coombes BK, Bisset L, Vicenzino B. A new integrative model of lateral epicondylalgia. Br J Sports Med 2009;43(4):252–8.

48. Schabrun SM, Jones E, Kloster J, et al. Temporal association between changes in primary sensory cortex and corticomotor output during muscle pain. Neuroscience 2013;235:159–64.

49. Schabrun SM, Hodges PW. Muscle pain differentially modulates short interval intracortical inhibition and intracortical facilitation in primary motor cortex. J Pain 2012;13(2):187–94.

50. Graven-Nielsen T, Arendt-Nielsen L. Assessment of mechanisms in localised and widespread musculoskeletal pain. Nat Rev Rheumatol 2010;6(10):599–606.

51. Wiech K, Preissl H, Birbaumer N. Neuroimaging of chronic pain: phantom limb and musculoskeletal pain. Scand J Rheumatol Suppl 2000;113:13–18.

52. Wiech K, Preissl H, Birbaumer N. [Neural networks and pain processing. New insights from imaging techniques]. Anaesthesist 2001;50(1):2–12.

53. Jensen MP, Hakimian S, Sherlin LH, et al. New insights into neuromodulatory approaches for the treatment of pain. J Pain 2008; 9(3):193–9.

54. Hebb DO. The Organisation of Behaviour: A Neuropsychological Theory. Mahwah, NJ: Lawrence Erlbaum Associates Inc; 1949.

55. Lontis ER, Voigt M, Struijk JJ. Focality assessment in transcranial magnetic stimulation with double and cone coils. J Clin Neurophysiol 2006;23(5):462–71.

56. Vuckovic A, Hasan MA, Fraser M, et al. Dynamic oscillatory signatures of central neuropathic pain in spinal cord injury. J Pain 2014;15(6):645–55.

57. Michels L, Moazami-Goudarzi M, Jeanmonod D. Correlations between EEG and clinical outcome in chronic neuropathic pain: surgical effects and treatment resistance. Brain Imaging Behav 2011;5(4):329–48.

58. Chang PF, Arendt-Nielsen L, Graven-Nielsen T, et al. Psychophysical and EEG responses to repeated experimental muscle pain in humans: pain intensity encodes EEG activity. Brain Res Bull 2003;59(6):533–43.

59. Mrachacz-Kersting N, Niazi IK, Jiang N, et al. A novel brain-computer interface for chronic stroke patients. ICNR Conference, Nov 2012; Toledo, Spain, 2012.

60. Mrachacz-Kersting N, Kristensen SR, Niazi IK, et al. Precise temporal association between cortical potentials evoked by motor imagination and afference induces cortical plasticity. J Physiol 2012;590(Pt 7):1669–82.

61. Niazi IK, Mrachacz-Kersting N, Jiang N, et al. Peripheral electrical stimulation triggered by self-paced detection of motor intention enhances motor evoked potentials. IEEE Trans Neural Syst Rehabil Eng 2012;20(4):595–604.

62. Xu R, Jiang N, Mrachacz-Kersting N, et al. An EEG controlled motorised ankle-foot orthosis induces neural plasticity with minimal training. IEEE Trans Biomed Eng 2014;61(7):2092–101.

63. Ziemann U, Paulus W, Nitsche MA, et al. Consensus: Motor cortex plasticity protocols. Brain Stimulation 2008;1(3):164–82.

64. Daly JJ, Zimbelman J, Roenigk KL, et al. Recovery of coordinated gait: Randomized controlled stroke trial of functional electrical stimulation (FES) versus no FES, with weight-supported treadmill and over-ground training. Neurorehabil Neural Repair 2011; 25(7):588–96.

65. Turner DL, Murguialday AR, Birbaumer N, et al. Neurophysiology of robot-mediated training and therapy: A perspective for future use in clinical populations. Front Neurol 2013;4.

66. Hubli M, Dietz V. The physiological basis of neurorehabilitation–locomotor training after spinal cord injury. J Neuroengineering Rehabil 2013;10:5.

67. Belda-Lois JM, Mena-del HS, Bermejo-Bosch I, et al. Rehabilitation of gait after stroke: a review towards a top-down approach. J Neuroeng Rehabil 2011;8:66.

CHAPTER 6

INTERACTION BETWEEN PAIN AND SENSORIMOTOR CONTROL

Paul Hodges • Deborah Falla

INTRODUCTION

Changes in sensorimotor control are an almost obligatory feature of musculoskeletal conditions. Evidence for modification of motor and/or sensory functions has been reported for a broad array of conditions, and these changes have become common targets for rehabilitation. It has been assumed that sensorimotor changes are relevant for the development, perpetuation or recurrence of pain and/or injury. It is timely to reflect on this assumption.

Current evidence suggests that sensorimotor changes may be both a cause and a consequence of pain and/or injury, and the relevance of these changes for symptoms varies between individuals. For some it may be a major factor and the key target for treatment, whereas for others it may be an epiphenomenon (i.e. present, but without impact on the clinical condition). Although early theories proposed stereotypical changes in sensorimotor function, it is apparent that individual variation is a characteristic of most musculoskeletal conditions. This is observed in experimental conditions[1-3] and in the identification of subgroups in clinical practice.[4,5] The aim of this chapter is to present the state-of-the-art understanding of sensorimotor control and to review how and why it changes in musculoskeletal conditions. This requires consideration of an overarching theory to explain sensorimotor dysfunction to aid conceptualization of the relevance of sensorimotor control for pain and recovery.

SENSORIMOTOR DYSFUNCTION IN MUSCULOSKELETAL PAIN

Sensorimotor Control

Sensorimotor control refers to all of the sensory and motor elements that underpin an individual's potential to move in, interact with and experience the environment.[6] It includes the output that arises from any element of the nervous system that contributes to motor function, from the spinal cord to the deep brain structures (e.g. basal ganglia), brain stem, cerebellum and cortex. It includes any sensory input that contributes to interpretation of the position and movement of the body, features of the environment, and the body's interaction with the environment. It includes all of the central processing involved in interpretation of motor requirements, planning of appropriate responses and interpretation of the success of output. This interaction between input, output and processing is impacted by emotions, experiences and context, which is particularly pertinent to consider when attempts are made to understand the function of the sensorimotor system in a person experiencing pain. As a consequence of the breadth and scope of sensorimotor control it is somewhat overwhelming to consider, in a patient sitting in front of you, how and where the sensorimotor system might be modified, whether this can be changed, and where to start. A starting point is to consider the nature of the presenting sensorimotor change (e.g. poor ability to detect motion or inability to activate a muscle) and then, in combination with an understanding of optimal sensorimotor control and clinical reasoning, build a clinical hypothesis to explain the patient's presentation.

Out of the complexity of sensorimotor control arise several key issues that are particularly relevant when addressing musculoskeletal conditions (Box 6-1). A first principle is that movements generally involve components that are *task directed* and components that are *postural*, but the relative importance varies between functions.[7,8] When throwing a ball, the arm action to propel the ball requires postural control of the axioscapular region and trunk as both a stable base for the limb muscles to generate torque as well as to maintain orientation of the segments with respect to each other, and of the body with respect to gravity/environment. The division between postural and task-orientated elements of movement can be blurred;[9] in running, activity of the trunk muscles is necessary for progression through space and postural control. Pain could impact on the task-directed or postural component, or both.

A second key principle is that function requires a *balance between movement and stiffness*.[10] The relative importance placed on each varies between tasks (gait requires movement of the spine for shock absorption, load transfer and energy minimization,[11] whereas lifting 100 kg from the floor requires restriction of spine movement[12]), but all tasks require some element of each. Even maintenance of a static upright standing posture involves some movement (e.g. small movements occur in conjunction with breathing to counteract the disturbance from the mechanics of breathing when standing erect).[13,14] Pain and injury may be characterized by too much stiffness or too much movement, depending on the patient, the function or the context (e.g. whether the environment is threatening).[15]

A third principle is that the overall motor function depends on the interaction between the *passive elements, active system* and *sensor/controller*. As defined by Panjabi,[16] all are important for maintenance of control as each contributes to stiffness and guidance of movement. Modification of any element will have repercussions for sensorimotor control and the interaction between them is necessary to consider when building a clinical picture of a patient's presentation. For instance, change in passive stiffness of a joint will necessitate changes in motor control (e.g. increased ankle stiffness will require changes in coordination of the knee, hip and spine to enable gait), changes in the capacity of a muscle to generate force will require compensation elsewhere (e.g. rapid atrophy of multifidus may underlie changes in activation of other back muscles to compensate or a change in position to enable greater contribution by passive elements[1,17]), and changes in motor control strategy have repercussions for the other systems (e.g. enhanced muscle co-contraction, potentially related to fear of pain, requires compensation at other segments[18]).

A fourth principle is that motor function is inherently *variable*. There are multiple ways to achieve a goal involving different combinations of muscle activity, different coordination between body segments and multiple possible control strategies.[19,20] This redundancy (multiple ways to achieve the same outcome) has both positive and negative aspects. Variability can be helpful as variation in movement 'shares' the load around structures so that one tissue is not repeatedly loaded,[20] it enables compensation when one option is no longer available[21] and it allows trial and error, which is required for learning.[22] These processes are compromised and may underpin problems if variation is limited. If variation is excessive it can be a problem if it leads to lack of control, or if it leads to an option that achieves the task's goal but with an unnecessary cost (e.g. increased energy demand or greater tissue load[20]). Thus, both too little and too much variation may be harmful.

A fifth principle is that the *sensory system includes redundancy* (information about movement and position is available from more than one source). The nervous system relies on multiple sources of sensory information, and places 'weight' or emphasis on the most trustworthy source.[23] This provides opportunity for the nervous system to reweight to an alternative source when one is no longer available, but can also lead to problems if it relies on an inaccurate source.

The sixth and potentially most important feature of sensorimotor control is that of *individual variation*. No two individuals use their body in the same way and this variation is particularly apparent in the presence of pain and injury.[1] Although many aspects of motor function may be fundamentally similar between individuals, many are not and depend on the individual's anatomy/biomechanics (e.g. anthropometry, muscle fibres, fascial network, mass, muscle strength), the individual's experience and exposure to movements/environments, and the influence of an individual's psychosocial/cognitive features (e.g. perceived capacity of their body, motivation, experiences, beliefs about the consequence of a movement). In the presence of pain, what is 'ideal' for one person may not be so for another. Although some clustering of features may be present, and different patient subgroups or phenotypes have been identified that provide guidance for selection of treatments,[5,24] within these subgroups there is large potential for variation.[25]

Consideration of these key principles of sensorimotor control assists interpretation of the changes in motor control identified in people with pain and injury. The following section outlines the breadth of changes that have been reported and builds a conceptual model to understand and reconcile these changes.

Relationship Between Pain, Injury and Sensorimotor Dysfunction

Sensorimotor changes in the presence of pain and/or injury present across a spectrum from subtle changes in sharing of load between synergist muscles[1,3] or the distribution of activity within a muscle,[26,27] to a complete avoidance of movement or function;[28] from a subtle change in threshold to perceive a sensory input[29] to a complete reorganization of the sensory representation of the body segment[30] (Fig. 6-1). Early models predicted a systematic increase in muscle activity to protect a painful region with subsequent pain provoked by muscle ischaemia secondary to the muscle 'spasm' (vicious cycle theory[31]), or a reduced amplitude of movement or force secondary to a systematic reduction of excitability of muscles that produce a painful movement and increased excitability of the antagonist muscles (pain adaptation theory[32]). Although there are examples that support these hypotheses, these models fail to explain the diversity and complexity of individual change in sensorimotor control. New theories have been developed that consider the key principles of sensorimotor control and are inclusive of not only the individual variation in sensorimotor dysfunction in pain and injury, but also the potential role of these changes in development and/or perpetuation of pain and injury (Fig. 6-1).[15,33]

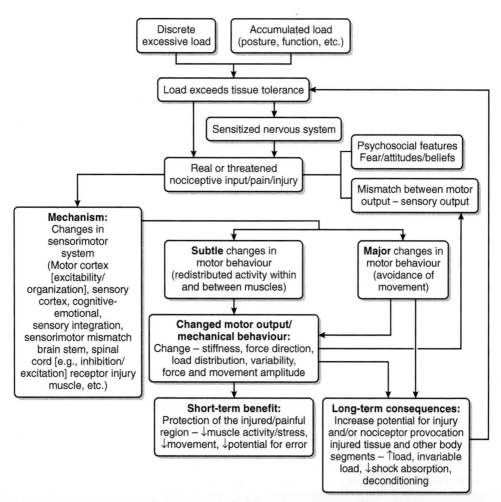

FIGURE 6-1 ■ Contemporary theory of interaction between pain, injury and motor adaptation. Changes in sensorimotor control can be a cause or outcome of injury and/or nociceptor discharge/pain. Initial tissue damage may be caused by a major loading event or repeated lower loading. Changes in sensorimotor control that range from subtle modification of movement to complete avoidance of function can be mediated by a range of mechanisms at multiple sites in the sensory and motor systems. The variable and individual specific modified sensorimotor control can have positive (often short-term outcomes aimed at immediate relief and protection) and negative outcomes (often longer-term changes) and these can underlie persistence and recurrence of pain.

Pain and/or Injury: The Cause or Consequence of Sensorimotor Dysfunction

The initial mechanisms for development of injury and/or pain are diverse and can include a single event that overloads the tissues, or an accumulation of load that exceeds the capacity of the tissues over time.[34] Whether an individual develops injury/pain from an event depends on the load, the frequency and the individual's tissue qualities (Fig. 6-1). Trauma can initiate this process when tissue tolerance is exceeded by a single high load (e.g. whiplash injury[35]) or repetitive cyclical low load (e.g. repetitive trunk flexion leads to an inflammatory response in spine ligaments[36]). Injury to the tissue has several important and diverse consequences. It may become a source of peripheral nociceptive input. Peripheral effects such as inflammation and central mechanisms may underpin sensitization of this input.[37] It may not only compromise the passive or active control of the injured region if the trauma has led to failure of ligaments or muscle injury (e.g. torn anterior cruciate ligament), but also affect sensory function if the sensory receptors or the tissue in which they are located is damaged.[38–40] It may change the control of movement either at a spinal level (e.g. reflex inhibition secondary to modified afferent input[41]) or higher centres (e.g. selection of a solution to protect the injured segment[1]).

Sensorimotor deficits could contribute to the development of injury/pain if, for example: (a) the strategy of movement/muscle activation involves components that load the tissues excessively (e.g. compromised activation of the medial vasti muscles leading to sub-optimal control of patella glide[42]); (b) the muscles are unable to meet or sustain the requirement of the task leading to sub-optimal tissue loading (e.g. lack of endurance of multifidus in rowers with back pain[43]); (c) inaccurate sensory information about the movement leading to inaccurate control (e.g. Brumagne et al.[23]); or (d) the movement involves too much (e.g. greater stride-to-stride variability, representing increased fluctuations in dynamic thoracic and pelvic oscillations in low back pain[44]) or too little variability (e.g. low variation of leg kinematics predicts injury in runners[20]). There are many other examples. A range of possible factors could lead to sub-optimal sensorimotor behaviour, which subsequently presents as a risk factor for development of injury/pain. At the trunk this could include modified demand of respiratory[45] and continence functions[46] of the trunk muscles with a subsequent effect on the quality of spine control. Other options include habitual postures or movement patterns (e.g. early lumbar rotation during hip rotation[47]), or modified function induced by the environment (e.g. repetitive use of a device[48]).

There are alternative theories regarding the relationship between sensorimotor changes and pain. For instance, several authors argue that the experience of pain may result from mismatch between the sensory input regarding a body part or a movement and the movement or position that is expected.[49] Such mismatch could arise from modification of the internal representation of the body (body schema), afferent information from the periphery,[50,51] or corrupted motor output[52] or motor organization.[53] Although the exact mechanisms are as yet unclear, it has been speculated that such mismatch may underlie neurodegenerative change and pain.[54]

It is also important to note that the original mechanism for a person to develop injury and pain in the first instance may be different from the reason that it is maintained. Although excessive load from a traumatic event or sub-optimal mechanics from less than ideal sensorimotor control may be the initial stimulus for tissue damage, nociceptive input and pain, the mechanism(s) underpinning the persistence or recurrence of pain may be very different. There will be cases where nociceptive input and load continue to be relevant, with peripheral nociceptive input continuing to drive the experience of pain.[55] Peripheral nociceptive input can maintain central sensitization.[56] In these cases continued sensorimotor dysfunction is likely to have direct relevance for recovery. The alternative is that persistence and recurrence may be mediated by psychosocial issues (e.g. catastrophization and worker support are factors in the transition to chronicity in back pain,[57] and moderate post-traumatic stress symptoms predict poor outcome following a whiplash injury[58]), central and peripheral sensitization,[37] or the development of secondary issues from sub-optimal tissue loading related to the 'new' movement pattern adopted after the initial exposure to nociceptive input/pain (e.g. development of back pain secondary to modified gait in low limb injury[59]). In these cases tissue load and nociceptive input from the initial injury may have little to do with maintenance of the pain state, and treatment is more likely to be effective if it is targeted to other issues.

Regardless of whether changes in sensorimotor control are the cause or consequence of pain, when a patient presents for management of their clinical condition this is most commonly motivated by the presence of pain and they have already entered the cycle with pain reinforcing sensorimotor dysfunction or motivating new adaptations, and sensorimotor dysfunction reinforcing sub-optimal loading on the originally injured tissues or those of other body regions as a consequence of compensatory mechanisms.

Sensorimotor Dysfunction in Pain and/or Injury Across a Spectrum from 'Subtle' to 'Major' Adaptations

Why are pain and movement linked? In the presence of acute injury and/or pain, if the nervous system concludes there is a threat to the tissues, then movement is the primary mechanism by which the nervous system can react to reduce that threat. This motor adaptation may be as simple as a flexor withdrawal reflex to move away from a noxious input,[60] or as complex as a change in movement pattern of the whole body to compensate for the reduced contribution by the painful segment (e.g. hip external rotation, decreased stance time and trunk lateral flexion to avoid loading the ankle in dorsiflexion during stance after an ankle sprain). Such changes may be relevant in the *short term* when there is potential risk to the tissue as it heals. Although early theories predicted a systematic and uniform increase or decrease in activity,[31,32] clinical observations and more recent experimental evidence point to individual variation in response from 'subtle' to 'major' adaptations (Fig. 6-1).[15]

Some individuals modify their movement in a *major* way such as the complete avoidance of a movement or function, or avoidance of participation in activity.[28] Although this change in behaviour ultimately achieves a similar goal to that achieved by the more subtle adaptations (i.e. unloading of the painful or injured tissue), the underlying mechanisms are likely to be different. There is considerable literature linking these major avoidant strategies to a range of psychosocial features such as catastrophizing and fear avoidance.[28,61]

At the other end of the spectrum are more *subtle* changes in the manner in which movement/forces are produced in the presence of pain and/or injury. Such protective adaptations can be characterized by redistribution of muscle activity to enhance stability (e.g. enhanced muscle co-contraction in back pain (Fig. 6-2),[1] neck pain[62] and knee osteoarthritis[63]), redistribution of muscle activity within and between muscles to change distribution of load on structures (Fig. 6-3)[3] or modify the direction of force (Fig. 6-3),[64] reduced variability to limit the potential for error,[48,65,66] unloading of a limb,[67] reduced force/movement amplitude,[68] increased motion at adjacent joints to compensate for reduced movement of the injured part,[17,18] redistribution of muscle activity away from a painful region,[69] failure to redistribute muscle activity when it is normally present to compensate for fatigue (Fig. 6-4),[17] and more deterministic (less random) structure of the variability in accessory (non-task-related) angular movement,[70] which indicates less random variability in the underlying muscle activation pattern (Fig. 6-5).

Redistribution of muscle activity is particularly common in musculoskeletal conditions of the spine, which is a region with many muscles available for function.[10] As a component of this redistribution of activity, there is substantial evidence for reduced activation of the deeper muscles such as transversus abdominis[52,71] and multifidus[72,73] in the lumbar region, and the deep cervical flexor and extensor muscles in the neck.[74,75] These muscles

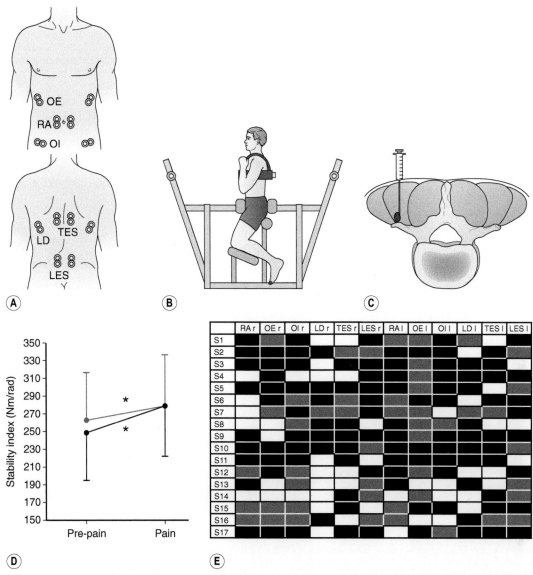

FIGURE 6-2 ■ Muscle activity is redistributed during acute pain to increase spine protection, but the pattern varies between individuals. **(A)** Recordings of electromyography (EMG) were made with 12 pairs of surface electrodes to record from superficial muscle sites. **(B)** Healthy participants moved slowly forwards and backwards in a semi-seated position. **(C)** Trials were performed before and during acute pain that was induced by injection of hypertonic saline into the longissimus muscle. **(D)** Stability of the spine (estimated using an EMG-driven mathematical model) was increased during pain. **(E)** Changes in EMG are shown individually for 12 muscles in 17 participants. Black indicates increased EMG during pain, grey indicates decreased EMG, white indicates no change. Although there was a net increase in spine stability during pain **(D)**, this was achieved by individual specific patterns of modulation of EMG activity. Each person used a different solution to protect the painful region. *l*, Left; *LD*, Latissimus dorsi; *LES*, Lumbar erector spinae; *OE*, Obliquus externus abdominis; *OI*, Obliquus internus abdominis; *r*, Right; *RA*, Rectus abdominis; *TES*, Thoracic erector spinae. (Figure redrawn from data from Hodges et al.[1])

have a unique capacity to contribute to control of intersegmental motion by virtue of their segmental attachments (enabling fine intersegmental control[76–79]) and limited torque-generating capacity (enabling control throughout range of motion without compromising dynamic function[76,80]). Reduced contribution of the deeper muscles to spine control is characterized by delayed activation;[52,73,81] reduced activation[71,74] and replacement of the usual tonic activation with phasic bursts of activity.[82] Reduced activation of deeper muscles is commonly associated with augmented activity of other muscles,[83,84] although the pattern of activation is highly variable between individuals.[1] Within this variation, there

is some evidence for a high prevalence of increased activation of the sternocleidomastoid muscle in neck pain,[85] and obliquus externus abdominis and/or long erector spinae in low back pain,[21,86,87] but this is not universal. Although a review of the back pain literature could identify no consistent patterns,[84] a recent study with experimentally induced acute low back pain showed that despite the variation in muscle activation, all but a few participants had a net increase in activity that resulted in augmented stability (estimated from an EMG-driven model) (Fig. 6-2).[1] This observation is consistent with the proposal that the nervous system adapts to acute pain with a strategy for protection and implies that some order can

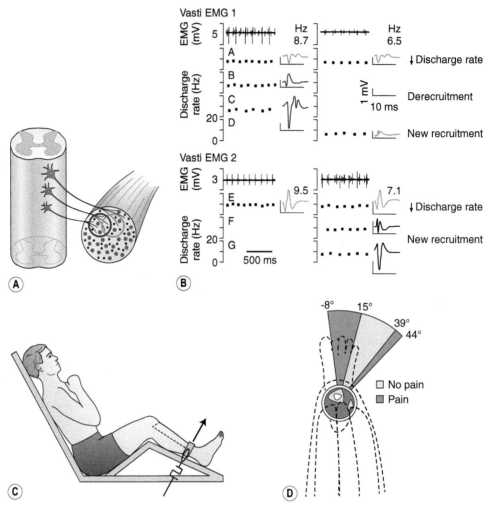

FIGURE 6-3 ■ Redistribution of muscle activity in acute pain. (**A**) During acute pain activity of motor units is redistributed within and between muscles. (**B**) Fine-wire electromyography (EMG) recordings are shown during contractions performed at identical force before (left) and during (right) pain for two recording sites in the vasti muscles. The time of discharge of individual motor units is displayed below the raw EMG recordings. The template for each unit is shown. Pain led to redistribution of activity of the motor units. Units A and E discharged at a slower rate during pain. Units B and C stopped discharging during pain and units F and G, which were not active prior to pain, began to discharge only during pain. These changes indicate that the participant maintained the force output of the muscle, by using a different population of motor units (i.e. redistribution of activity within a muscle). (**C**) Knee extension task. (**D**) The direction of force used by the participants to match the force during contractions with and without pain differed between trials. During pain, participants generated force more medially or laterally than in the pain-free trials. For colour version see Plate 4. (A, B Redrawn from data from Tucker et al.;[26] C, D redrawn from data from Tucker et al.[64])

be found amongst the variation that is characteristic of the motor adaptation present in people with spinal pain.

In other regions of the body there is substantial evidence for modified or redistributed muscle activity. There are too many examples to summarize here. Some typical examples include changes such as delayed reaction time of ankle evertor muscles in ankle sprain,[88] delayed activation of gluteus medius during stair-stepping in patellofemoral pain,[89] delayed activation of subscapularis during arm movement in shoulder pain,[90] and reduced activity of the extensor carpi radialis brevis associated with gripping in patients with lateral epicondylagia (Heales et al. 2014, unpublished data).

Each of the examples presented above is thought to change the loading on the painful tissues, although there is limited direct evidence of mechanical factors to test this hypothesis. Recent work with direct measurement of

muscle stress using ultrasound elastography techniques indicates that unloading of a painful tissue is not always achieved, and depends on the task (unloading of painful tissues is more likely in more complex tasks that involve a greater number of body segments[91]) and appears to differ between body regions.[91]

Why do different individuals adopt different strategies? The answer to this question has not been resolved, but it may relate to different functional histories, experiences with pain, or habitual postures/movement patterns. The adopted patterns of activity are likely to relate to the clinical subgroups that have been identified by several groups.[5,24] Recent work[3] shows that some people use the same muscle synergies during multijoint planar reaching tasks in non-painful and painful conditions, which is consistent with the observation that some people perform a particular task in a more stereotyped manner than

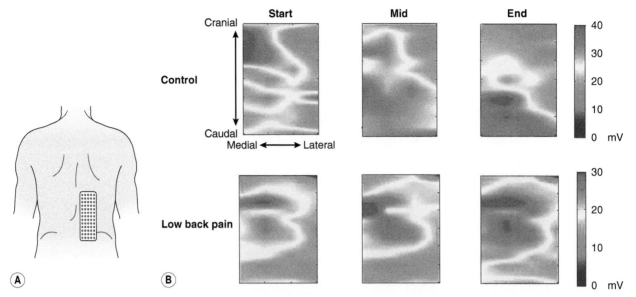

FIGURE 6-4 ■ Reduced redistribution of muscle activation in low back pain. Although healthy individuals redistribute muscle activity to maintain the motor output in the presence of fatigue, this is not observed in people with low back pain. **(A)** A 13 × 5 grid of electromyography electrodes was placed over the lumbar erector spinae in a group of healthy controls and people with chronic low back pain to assess the spatial distribution of erector spinae activity and change in the distribution during performance of a repetitive lifting task for ~200 second. **(B)** Representative topographical maps of the root mean square EMG amplitude from the right lumbar erector spinae muscle for a person with low back pain and a control. EMG maps are shown for the start, mid and end of a repetitive lifting task. Areas of blue correspond to low EMG amplitude and dark red to high EMG amplitude. Note the shift (redistribution) of activity in the caudal direction as the task progresses but for the control subject only. For colour version see Plate 5. (Reprinted with permission from Falla et al.[17])

others.[65] Those individuals with less variable motor programmes seem to be those more prone to develop pain as they overuse the same strategy rather than taking advantage of the redundancy of the motor system.

Sensorimotor Adaptations Provide a Short-Term Solution, but have Potential Long-Term Consequences

What is the outcome of the adaptation in sensorimotor control? As indicated above, adapted motor behaviour is presumed to enhance protection of the injured/painful tissue,[15] although the manner in which this is achieved differs between conditions and between individuals.[1] A major issue is that although the adaptation has potential benefits in the *short term* (either to change load and protect the injured/potentially injured tissue, or to meet the requirement of the nervous system to take action[92]) there are potential *long-term* consequences. This could arise for a number of reasons (see below, Fig. 6-6).

Sensorimotor adaptation could contribute to further tissue damage as a result of actual changes to loading of the lesioned tissues or to loading of other tissues of the same or related body parts. This could arise if the adaptation to protect the painful part leads to; increased load (e.g. increased muscle activity in people with back pain increases load on the spine during lifting,[94] and greater co-activation of the neck muscles during neck[62,95] and upper limb[96] tasks may increase compressive loading on the cervical spine) (Fig. 6-6), reduced movement for shock absorption (e.g. delayed spinal motion in back pain leads to greater perturbation from arm movement;[97]

Fig. 6-6), increased injury risk (e.g. compromised balance underpinning greater falls risk secondary to increased trunk stiffness[93]), or decreased load sharing (e.g. reduced movement variation during function in neck-shoulder pain;[48] Fig. 6-6). A recent study also demonstrated delayed activation of neck muscles in people with chronic neck pain in response to rapid, unanticipated full-body perturbations (resembling slipping or tripping), suggesting that the cervical spine may be vulnerable to further strain/injury under such conditions due to inadequate muscle support.[98]

Persistence of the motor adaptation could also underpin reduced 'confidence' regarding the injured part, thus promoting disuse or modified use of the body part. That is, the adapted motor behaviour could interact with psychosocial issues and feed into the fear-avoidance cycle.[28] For example, patients with low back pain may reduce their velocity of movement as a protective-guarding behaviour against excessive force and loading, and ensuing pain. A recent study confirmed an association between the angular velocity of trunk movement and psychological features including fear of movement, pain catastrophizing and anxiety which supports this notion.[99]

The redistribution of activity between muscles could also lead to problems if the adapted solution leads to disuse of specific muscles that provide a unique contribution to joint control. One key example is that, although enhanced activation of larger, more superficial muscles of the neck and back is common in the presence of pain and may enhance protection, these muscles generally lack segmental attachments to the spine and have a limited capacity to fine-tune control of intersegmental motion.[100]

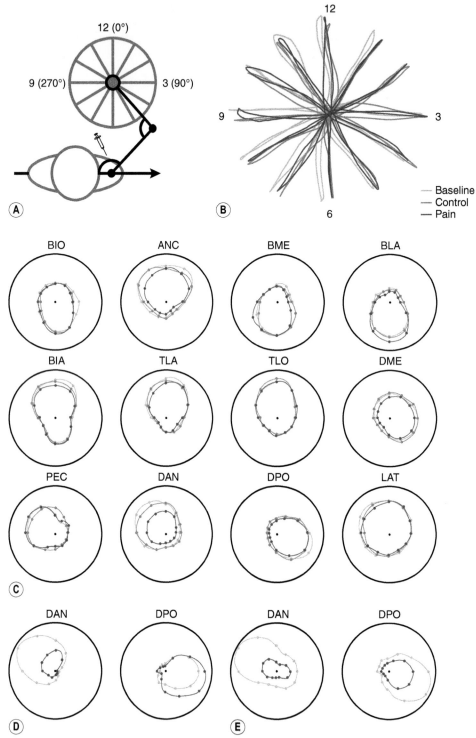

FIGURE 6-5 ■ Changes in muscle activity vary between individuals when challenged by pain, with no few consistent changes across participants. **(A)** Pain-free volunteers (*n*=8) performed multijoint reaching in the horizontal plane using a manipulandum, with the starting point at the centre of the circle. The subject had to reach the 12 targets depicted in A with each reaching movement lasting 1 second followed by a 5 second rest period at the target position before returning to the centre point over 1 second. Subjects performed the task at baseline, and following the injection of isotonic (control) and hypertonic (painful) saline. Saline was injected into the right anterior deltoid (*DAN*) muscle. **(B)** Representative example of endpoint trajectories recorded from one subject during the baseline (blue), control (magenta), and painful (red) conditions. Note that pain did not affect the kinematics of this controlled task. **(C)** Directional tuning of the EMG envelope peak value recorded from 12 muscles during the baseline (blue), the control (magenta), and pain (red) conditions. The 'shrinking' of the pain curves of the DAN muscle was due to a consistent decrease of the EMG activity of this muscle across subjects. Other muscles also change their activity, however the direction of change was different across subjects, demonstrating the variability in subject response. For example, the activity of the posterior deltoid (*DPO*), increased during pain in three subjects while it decreased in five subjects, so that on average it was unchanged. **(D)** Representative data from a single subject showing a decrease in DAN activity with a simultaneous increase in DPO activity during pain. **(E)** In contrast, representative data from another subject shows that decreased DAN activity occurred together with a decrease in DPO activity during pain. *ANC*, Anconeus; *BIA*, Brachialis; *BIO*, Brachioradialis; *BLA*, Lateral head of the biceps brachii; *BME*, Medial head of the biceps brachii; *DME*, Medial deltoid; *LAT*, Latissimus dorsi; *PEC*, Pectoralis major; *TLA*, Lateral head of the triceps brachii; *TLO*, Long head of the triceps brachii. For colour version see Plate 6. (Reprinted with permission from Muceli et al.[3])

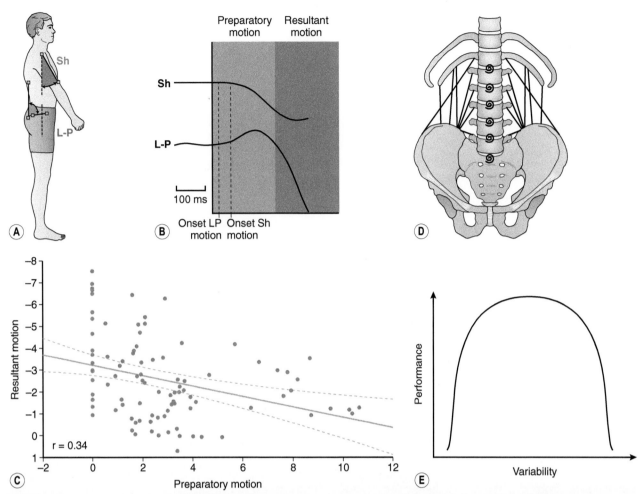

FIGURE 6-6 ■ Potential mechanisms for long-term consequences of motor adaptation with pain and injury. **(A–C)** Absence of movement to prepare the spine for the perturbation from the reactive forces induced by arm movement leads to exaggerated disturbance to the spine. **(A)** Shoulder (*Sh*) and lumbopelvic (*LP*) motion were measured with motion sensors. **(B)** Spine movement in the direction opposite to the reactive forces (preparatory motion) is initiated prior to the movement of the arm. Resultant motion is the motion resulting from the reactive moments. **(C)** Individuals with less preparatory motion are more likely to have a large resultant motion. If the adaptation with pain and injury reduces movement this would reduce the potential for motion to dampen imposed forces. **(D)** Increased co-contraction to protect the spine would have the negative consequence of increased compressive load on the spine, potentially accelerating tissue changes. **(E)** Both too little and too much variability of movement have negative consequences for the quality of performance. If variation is too low, this will compromise sharing of load between structures and compromise potential to learn and change. (A–C Redrawn from data from Mok et al.[93])

Redistribution of activity to these muscles, at the expense of the deeper muscles that provide this control could be problematic in the long term.[15] Exaggerated intersegmental motion may be linked to tissue load and pain, as evidenced by larger intersegmental translation during trunk motion in spondylolisthesis[100] and increased intersegmental rotation at the time of pain provocation in a weight-lifting effort.[12]

Why is sensorimotor adaptation maintained beyond when it is necessary? There are several possible explanations. Firstly, although nociceptive stimulation and pain is a motivator to adapt, recovery from pain might not motivate a return to the initial strategy. Secondly, it may not be possible to return to the initial sensorimotor control strategy. This could be because adaptation to body structures precludes recovery (e.g. changes in muscle capacity [muscle fibre changes in neck and back muscles,[101–103] changes in muscle fatigability[104]], or

changes in joint/muscle mobility [relative flexibility,[105] muscle length changes,[106] consolidated swelling, joint trauma, osteophytes, etc.]). Thirdly, dysfunction[23] or absence of sensory information[107] may preclude resolution of adaptation. Fourthly, in some cases it may not be possible or optimal to return to the pre-injury sensorimotor control, as a modified solution may be required to compensate for the injured tissues (e.g. modified knee muscle control following complete anterior cruciate ligament rupture[108]). Finally, lack of resolution of the adaptation may be underpinned by the more complex issues related to the physiology of persistent pain. Pain is a nonlinear system (that is, pain experienced by an individual is not linearly related to the nociceptive input from the periphery) and the experience of pain does not linearly relate to the threat to the tissues. This may be because of sensitization[37] and/or modified cognitive emotional mechanisms.[109] As a result, the adaptation to pain may be *greater* than what is required, the adaptation may persist for *longer* than is required (i.e. the time for tissue healing may have passed and the requirement for protection is no longer present) or the adaptation may be completely *inappropriate* (i.e. the nervous system may perceive the need to protect the tissues in a manner that is not relevant for the injury or in the absence of injury). In each case a different clinical strategy may be required to resolve the adaptation, and this may not be possible or desirable (if some degree of maintenance of the adaptation is required for compensation) in all individuals. The key message is that although the adaptation may be necessary in the short term, in the long term it may become part of the problem.

Mechanisms for Sensorimotor Changes in Musculoskeletal Conditions

The diverse array of sensorimotor changes in musculoskeletal conditions could be mediated by an equally diverse array of mechanisms. Potential mechanisms can be broadly defined as primarily motor or sensory, or related to the cognitive/emotional aspects of pain. The following sections outline some of the most established mechanisms.

Sensory System Mechanisms. Absent, reduced or inaccurate sensory input will compromise sensorimotor control. Any compromise to normal afferent information regarding position or movement of the body will affect the potential for accurate control.[38] Function of the sensory system can be compromised at multiple points along its path from the *receptor* to higher *supraspinal* sensory functions. The most obvious source of sensory dysfunction is direct trauma to the sensory receptors or the tissues in which they are located.[38,40] Complete or partial rupture of a ligament, intervertebral disc, or other structure not only compromises the mechanical contribution to control, but also removes or compromises afferent input.[39] Injury, inflammation and oedema may also compromise the responsiveness of receptors. In the presence of tissue damage, afferent discharge from mechanoreceptors can induce pain (e.g. muscle mechanoreceptor excitation is painful in the presence of eccentric muscle damage).[110] Plasticity in spinal cord circuits underpinning central sensitization,[37] such as the modification of function of the wide-dynamic range cells that converge input from multiple afferent sources, might also modify the utility of information provided by sensory afferents. Further, muscle spindles receive sympathetic innervation,[111] increased sympathetic drive could modulate the discharge of these receptors either through an action exerted on the receptors themselves or on their primary afferent neurons.[112]

Abnormal sensory input can affect motor function at a spinal level. Effects include modification of reflex modulation of muscle activation, such as the stretch reflex, which may be augmented by greater sensitivity of the muscle spindles in the presence of inflammatory mediators,[113] or compromised in the presence of muscle damage. Muscle activation is also modulated by afferent activity from receptors in the skin,[114] ligaments,[115] annulus

fibrosis of the intervertebral disc,[116] and tendon and this could be altered by injury and/or pain.

There is evidence of modification of the sensory integration at higher centres, which may mediate inaccurate interpretation of sensory input or reduce responsiveness to sensory information.[23] In terms of the latter, the nervous system can reduce the reliance on a particular source of sensory information (sensory reweighting). For instance, although vibration of the back muscles induces the perception of muscle stretch in pain-free individuals and leads to initiation of a postural adjustment if applied in standing, in people with back pain this is substantially reduced despite the fact that injury to all muscle spindles is unlikely.[23] There is also considerable emerging evidence for reorganization of sensory representations in the primary sensory cortex (e.g. shift of the representation of the back region in people with low back pain,[30] and smudging of cortical representations of independent fingers in focal dystonia associated with difficulty to move the fingers independently[117]), distortion of the body schema,[118] and modified cortical integration.[119]

Reduced, enhanced or distorted afferent input or inaccurate integration of sensory information will also affect the *planning* and *organization* of motor behaviours at higher centres. Inaccurate sensory input or representation of the body and/or environment has the potential to distort any process that depends on the interpretation of position or movement of the body. This could have the potential to affect planning and control of any class of motor activity including voluntary movements, postural adjustments, and motor learning processes. Although there is some evidence that acute pain interferes with motor learning,[120] if performance of the training task is controlled interference with learning is less apparent.[121] Recent evidence indicates limited interference with learning, but compromised retention of learning.[122] In persistent pain states, with accompanying distorted body schema and sensory integration, there is likely to be greater interference with learning.

In summary, many of the distorted motor behaviours identified in musculoskeletal conditions could be mediated, at least in part, by dysfunction on the sensory side of the sensorimotor equation. Although injury to the receptors may not be amenable to rehabilitation, the utilization and integration of sensory information, distortion of the body schema and compensation with alternative sources of feedback may be modifiable.

Motor System Mechanisms. Like the sensory system, sensorimotor changes can be mediated by changes at any level of the motor system from the spinal cord to the motor cortex and beyond. Most research has focused on the spinal cord and primary motor cortex as these are the most accessible to non-invasive investigation. In the spinal cord there is substantial evidence of reflex inhibition (which involves an important sensory component) following injury to joint structures such as the joint capsule and ligaments.[115] Reflex inhibition involves reduced excitation of motoneurons (primarily to extensor muscles) that is mediated by afferent input at a single level of the spinal cord.[115] There can be concomitant excitation of flexor muscle motoneuron pools.[115] The source of afferent input is unclear, but occurs in the absence of nociceptive input.[41] Reflex inhibition appears counterintuitive – it reduces the activity of the muscles that could protect the joint – but is consistently observed for limb joint lesions and can explain reduced excitability of inputs to multifidus after intervertebral disc lesion[123] and facet joint infusion.[116] Reflex inhibition may serve to reduce joint load, although this occurs in a manner that interferes with function (e.g. 'giving way' of the knee with effusion).

Although early theories of adaptation to pain predicted uniform inhibition[32] or excitation[31] of a painful muscle at a spinal or brainstem level, nociceptive afferents have both excitatory and inhibitory effects on motoneurons in animals.[124] In humans, the discharge rate of motoneurons within a single muscle can simultaneously increase and decrease leading to redistribution of activity[26] and this observation is corroborated by recent evidence of differential effects on excitability of motoneurons identified using novel experimental methods.[125]

As stated earlier, changes in the muscle, the effector organ of the motor system, are common in many musculoskeletal conditions. These changes (e.g. atrophy,[72,126] fatty infiltration,[127,128] decreased endurance,[129] changes in muscle fibre type proportion[101,103]) might be secondary to disuse as a result of general physical inactivity (e.g. avoidance of activity secondary to fear[28]), reflex inhibition,[41] or reduced (gravitational) load.[130] Recent work has highlighted alternative mechanisms such as a potential role of pro-inflammatory cytokines.[101] Tumor necrosis factor is expressed after disc lesion and plays a role in regulation of muscle fibres[131] and could explain changes in muscle fibre distribution after injury.[101]

Using transcranial magnetic stimulation, the representations of specific muscles at the motor cortex have been found to be modified in people with persistent low back (e.g. convergence of cortical representations of long and short back muscles,[132] posterolateral shift of representation of transversus abdominis;[53] Fig. 6-7) and elbow pain (loss of the multiple peaks of excitability in the cortical representation of wrist extensor muscles in lateral epicondylalgia.[133] There is some evidence that cortical changes are related to behaviour. For instance, shift of the cortical representation of transversus abdominis is correlated with delayed activation of the muscle in an arm movement task.[53] Although difficult to test or confirm, the posterolateral shift might be secondary to expansion of representation of other trunk muscles involved in a protective response. Consistent with this argument, the excitability of inputs to the more superficial oblique abdominal muscles is increased in acute pain.[134] The 'smudged' cortical representation of the extensor muscles is consistent with the loss of differential control of these muscles in back pain,[73] and could be interpreted as a strategy to simplify the protection of the back. Other studies of excitability of the corticospinal path (which is affected by excitability at the cortex and spinal cord) show increases and decreases depending on the muscle[123,135,136] and the effects at the cortex and spinal cord may be opposite.[123,135]

Considerable current work has been focused *not* on the anatomical sites of dysfunction, but the potential role of changes in motor planning. This has been inferred from motor behaviours. It has been assumed that the change in motor behaviour to one that protects the painful region, is not a simple consequence of a change in 'excitability' or 'representation', but a purposeful modification of the planning of behaviour to meet a new goal (i.e. protection).[15] The basic premise is that the central regions involved in planning and initiation of motor behaviours (premotor, frontal, somatosensory areas, limbic system) modify the coordination of muscle to achieve this new goal. Changes in activation of these areas have been reported in brain imaging studies during pain.[137] Modification of the pattern of muscle activity initiated in advance of a movement[52] is consistent with this proposal. Furthermore, when people with either neck or low back pain perform rapid arm movements, the activation of the deep muscles adopts a direction-specific response, which contrasts the response observed in healthy individuals.[52,81] This indicates the change in activation is not simply a delay that could be explained by factors such as decreased motoneuron excitability, but rather, consistent with the change in the strategy used by the central nervous system to control the spine.

Changes in movement variability also appear to reflect the objective to adapt control to protect – during pain, variability initially increases which concurs with a search for a new solution, and then decreases as a new solution is identified.[48,65] Further work is required to clarify the processes involved in the changed behaviour. If this process aims to find a new solution, it is not surprising that this could be affected by cognitive emotional aspects of pain such as catastrophization and kinesiophobia, both of which would be expected to up-regulate the adaptation to further enhance protection (see below).

In summary, motor processes are adapted at multiple levels of the nervous system and these changes could be both complementary and opposing. What is observed in a patient will be a complex interplay of these processes and there is potential for clinical interventions that target *different* components of the nervous system (e.g. techniques to change excitability at the spinal cord, or motor learning to change control at higher centres) to have relevance for recovery.

Interaction with Psychosocial Factors. Although it is well recognized that musculoskeletal conditions have biological, psychological and social elements,[138] to varying degrees, these are often considered in isolation. As stated above, there is enormous potential for interaction between psychosocial features and the biological mechanisms that underpin sensorimotor changes. From one perspective, psychosocial features may amplify the motor adaptation, which may lead to both greater muscle activity or altered movement for protection (e.g. relationship between increased erector spinae muscle activity and kinesiophobia at the end range of trunk flexion[61] and the association between reduced angular velocity of trunk movement and kinesiophobia, pain catastrophizing and

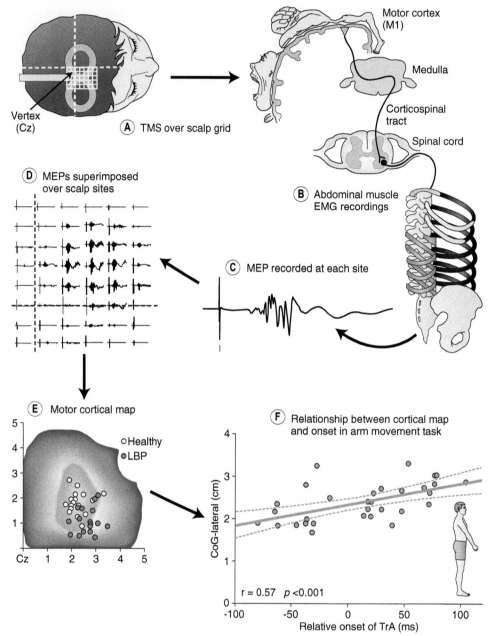

FIGURE 6-7 ■ Changes in motor cortex organization in low back pain. **(A)** Transcranial magnetic stimulation (*TMS*) was applied according to a grid over the motor cortex to stimulate the corticospinal pathway. **(B)** Electromyography was recorded from the transversus abdominis (*TrA*) muscle. **(C)** Motor evoked potentials (*MEP*) were recorded from stimuli applied at each point on the grid. **(D)** The amplitude of MEPs is larger when stimulation is applied to the cortical region with neural input to the muscle. **(E)** The gradient from low (blue) to high (light green) MEP amplitude is shown relative to the vertex (*Cz*). White/blue dots indicate the centre of the region with input to TrA in healthy participants, and the grey/orange indicates that for people with a history of LBP. The centre is positioned further posterior and lateral in the LBP group, providing evidence of reorganization of the motor cortex. **(F)** The degree of reorganization was correlated with the delay of the onset of activation of TrA EMG during an arm movement task. For colour version see Plate 7.

anxiety[99]) and more profound avoidance of activity and participation.[28] From a different perspective, cognitive emotional aspects of pain drive central sensitization, which underpins changes in excitability of sensory pathways, nociceptive and otherwise,[37] and this may modulate many of the sensory mechanisms for adapted sensorimotor control.

CONCLUSIONS

It is clear from the current state of the literature that there is diversity in the manner in which the sensorimotor system is modified in pain and this is underpinned by mechanisms that involve multiple regions of the nervous system. Although it is unquestionable that sensorimotor control is affected, the key challenge facing clinical intervention is to decide how sensorimotor changes relate to an individual patient's presentation, which aspects of sensorimotor control require management, and how this might be best achieved for the patient.

Acknowledgements

PH is supported by a Senior Principal Research Fellowship from the National Health and Medical Research Council (NHMRC) of Australia.

REFERENCES

1. Hodges PW, Coppieters MW, MacDonald D, et al. New insight into motor adaptation to pain revealed by a combination of modelling and empirical approaches. Eur J Pain 2013;17:1138–46.
2. Hodges PW, Moseley GL, Gabrielsson A, et al. Experimental muscle pain changes feedforward postural responses of the trunk muscles. Exp Brain Res 2003;151:262–71.
3. Muceli S, Falla D, Farina D. Reorganization of muscle synergies during multidirectional reaching in the horizontal plane with experimental muscle pain. J Neurophysiol 2014;111(8): 1615–30.
4. Van Dillen LR, Sahrmann SA, Norton BJ, et al. Reliability of physical examination items used for classification of patients with low back pain. Phys Ther 1998;78:979–88.
5. O'Sullivan P. Diagnosis and classification of chronic low back pain disorders: maladaptive movement and motor control impairments as underlying mechanism. Man Ther 2005;10:242–55.
6. Shumway-Cooke A, Woollacott MH. Motor Control. Baltimore: Williams and Wilkins; 1995.
7. Massion J. Postural changes accompanying voluntary movements. Normal and pathological aspects. Human Neurobiol 1984;2: 261–7.
8. Hodges PW, Richardson CA. Feedforward contraction of transversus abdominis is not influenced by the direction of arm movement. Exp Brain Res 1997;114:362–70.
9. Hodges PW, Cresswell AG, Thorstensson A. Preparatory trunk motion accompanies rapid upper limb movement. Exp Brain Res 1999;124:69–79.
10. Hodges P, Cholewicki J. Functional control of the spine. In: Vleeming A, Mooney V, Stoeckarteditors R, editors. Movement, Stability and Lumbopelvic Pain. Edinburgh: Elsevier; 2007.
11. Saunders SW, Schache A, Rath D, et al. Changes in three dimensional lumbo-pelvic kinematics and trunk muscle activity with speed and mode of locomotion. Clin Biomech 2005;20:784–93.
12. Cholewicki J, McGill SM. Mechanical stability of the *in vivo* lumbar spine: implications for injury and chronic low back pain. Clin Biomech 1996;11:1–15.
13. Gurfinkel V, Kots Y, Paltsev E, et al. The compensation of respiratory disturbances of erect posture of man as an example of the organisation of interarticular interaction. In: Gelfand I, Gurfinkel V, Formin S, et al., editors. Models of the Structural Functional Organisation of Certain Biological Systems. Cambridge, Mass: MIT Press; 1971. p. 382–95.
14. Hodges P, Gurfinkel VS, Brumagne S, et al. Coexistence of stability and mobility in postural control: evidence from postural compensation for respiration. Exp Brain Res 2002;144:293–302.
15. Hodges PW, Tucker K. Moving differently in pain: a new theory to explain the adaptation to pain. Pain 2011;152:S90–8.
16. Panjabi MM. The stabilizing system of the spine. Part I. Function, dysfunction, adaptation, and enhancement. J Spinal Disord 1992;5:383–9.
17. Falla D, Gizzi L, Tschapek M, et al. Reduced task-induced variations in the distribution of activity across back muscle regions in individuals with low back pain. Pain 2014;155(5):944–53.
18. Smith M, Coppieters MW, Hodges PW. Effect of experimentally induced low back pain on postural sway with breathing. Exp Brain Res 2005;166:109–17.
19. Bernstein N. The Co-Ordination and Regulation of Movements. Oxford: Pergamon Press; 1967.
20. Hamill J, van Emmerik RE, Heiderscheit BC, et al. A dynamical systems approach to lower extremity running injuries. Clin Biomech 1999;14:297–308.
21. Moseley GL, Hodges PW. Are the changes in postural control associated with low back pain caused by pain interference? Clin J Pain 2005;21:323–9.
22. Wu HG, Miyamoto YR, Gonzalez Castro LN, et al. Temporal structure of motor variability is dynamically regulated and predicts motor learning ability. Nature Neurosci 2014;17:312–21.
23. Brumagne S, Cordo P, Verschueren S. Proprioceptive weighting changes in persons with low back pain and elderly persons during upright standing. Neurosci Lett 2004;366:63–6.
24. Van Dillen LR, Sahrmann SA, Norton BJ, et al. Movement system impairment-based categories for low back pain: stage 1 validation. J Orthopaed Sports Phys Ther 2003;33:126–42.
25. Karayannis NV, Jull GA, Hodges PW. Physiotherapy movement based classification approaches to low back pain: comparison of subgroups through review and developer/expert survey. BMC Musculoskelet Disord 2012;13:24.
26. Tucker K, Butler J, Graven-Nielsen T, et al. Motor unit recruitment strategies are altered during deep-tissue pain. J Neurosci 2009;29:10820–6.
27. Falla D, Arendt-Nielsen L, Farina D. The pain-induced change in relative activation of upper trapezius muscle regions is independent of the site of noxious stimulation. Clin Neurophysiol 2009;120:150–7.
28. Vlaeyen JW, Linton SJ. Fear-avoidance and its consequences in chronic musculoskeletal pain: a state of the art. Pain 2000;85: 317–32.
29. Garn SN, Newton RA. Kinesthetic awareness in subjects with multiple ankle sprains. Phys Ther 1988;68:1667–71.
30. Flor H, Braun C, Elbert T, et al. Extensive reorganization of primary somatosensory cortex in chronic back pain patients. Neurosci Lett 1997;224:5–8.
31. Roland M. A critical review of the evidence for a pain-spasm-pain cycle in spinal disorders. Clin Biomech 1986;1:102–9.
32. Lund JP, Donga R, Widmer CG, et al. The pain-adaptation model: a discussion of the relationship between chronic musculoskeletal pain and motor activity. Can J Physiol Pharmacol 1991;69:683–94.
33. Murray GM, Peck CC. Orofacial pain and jaw muscle activity: a new model. J Orofac Pain 2007;21:263–78.
34. Dye SF. The knee as a biologic transmission with an envelope of function: a theory. Clin Orthopaed Rel Res 1996;10–18.
35. Ito S, Ivancic PC, Panjabi MM, et al. Soft tissue injury threshold during simulated whiplash: a biomechanical investigation. Spine 2004;29:979–87.
36. D'Ambrosia P, King K, Davidson B, et al. Pro-inflammatory cytokines expression increases following low- and high-magnitude cyclic loading of lumbar ligaments. Eur Spine J 2010;19:1330–9.
37. Woolf CJ. Central sensitization: implications for the diagnosis and treatment of pain. Pain 2011;152:S2–15.
38. Panjabi M. A hypothesis of chronic back pain: ligament subfailure injuries lead to muscle control dysfunction. Eur Spine J 2006;15:668–76.
39. Johansson H, Sjolander P, Sojka P. A sensory role for the cruciate ligaments. Clin Orthopaed Rel Res 1991;268:161–78.
40. Dolan P, Adams MA. Time-dependent mechanisms that impair muscle protection of the spine. In: Hodges PW, Cholewicki J, van Dieeneditors J, editors. Spinal Control: The Rehabilitation of Back Pain. Edinburgh: Churchill Livingstone; 2013.
41. Stokes M, Young A. The contribution of reflex inhibition to arthrogenous muscle weakness. Clin Sci 1984;67:7–14.
42. Van Tiggelen D, Cowan S, Coorevits P, et al. Delayed vastus medialis obliquus to vastus lateralis onset timing contributes to the development of patellofemoral pain in previously healthy men: a prospective study. Am J Sports Med 2009;37:1099–105.
43. Roy SH, DeLuca CJ, Snyder-Mackler L, et al. Fatigue, recovery, and low back pain in varsity rowers. Med Sci Sports Exerc 1990;22:463–9.
44. Vogt L, Pfeifer K, Portscher M, et al. Influences of nonspecific low back pain on three-dimensional lumbar spine kinematics in locomotion. Spine 2001;26:1910–19.

45. Hodges PW, Heijnen I, Gandevia SC. Reduced postural activity of the diaphragm in humans when respiratory demand is increased. J Physiol 2001;537:999–1008.

46. Smith M, Coppieters M, Hodges PW. Postural response of the pelvic floor and abdominal muscles in women with and without incontinence. Neurourol Urodyn 2007;26:377–85.

47. Scholtes SA, Gombatto SP, Van Dillen LR. Differences in lumbopelvic motion between people with and people without low back pain during two lower limb movement tests. Clin Biomech 2009;24:7–12.

48. Madeleine P, Mathiassen SE, Arendt-Nielsen L. Changes in the degree of motor variability associated with experimental and chronic neck-shoulder pain during a standardised repetitive arm movement. Exp Brain Res 2008;185:689–98.

49. McCabe CS, Haigh RC, Halligan PW, et al. Simulating sensory-motor incongruence in healthy volunteers: implications for a cortical model of pain. Rheumatol 2005;44:509–16.

50. Brumagne S, Cordo P, Lysens R, et al. The role of paraspinal muscle spindles in lumbosacral position sense in individuals with and without low back pain. Spine 2000;25:989–94.

51. Luomajoki H, Moseley GL. Tactile acuity and lumbopelvic motor control in patients with back pain and healthy controls. Br J Sports Med 2011;45:437–40.

52. Hodges PW, Richardson CA. Inefficient muscular stabilisation of the lumbar spine associated with low back pain: a motor control evaluation of transversus abdominis. Spine 1996;21:2640–50.

53. Tsao H, Galea MP, Hodges PW. Reorganization of the motor cortex is associated with postural control deficits in recurrent low back pain. Brain 2008;131:2161–71.

54. Wand BM, O'Connell NE. Chronic non-specific low back pain – sub-groups or a single mechanism? BMC Musculoskel Disord 2008;9:11.

55. Smart KM, Blake C, Staines A, et al. Mechanisms-based classifications of musculoskeletal pain: part 3 of 3: symptoms and signs of nociceptive pain in patients with low back (+/- leg) pain. Man Ther 2012;17:352–7.

56. Gracely RH, Lynch SA, Bennett GJ. Painful neuropathy: altered central processing maintained dynamically by peripheral input. Pain 1992;51:175–94.

57. Picavet HS, Vlaeyen JW, Schouten JS. Pain catastrophizing and kinesiophobia: predictors of chronic low back pain. Am J Epidemiol 2002;156:1028–34.

58. Sterling M, Jull G, Vicenzino B, et al. Physical and psychological factors predict outcome following whiplash injury. Pain 2005;114:141–8.

59. Nadler SF, Malanga GA, DePrince M, et al. The relationship between lower extremity injury, low back pain, and hip muscle strength in male and female collegiate athletes. Clin J Sport Med 2000;10:89–97.

60. Clarke RW, Harris J. The organization of motor responses to noxious stimuli. Brain Res Brain Res Rev 2004;46:163–72.

61. Watson PJ, Booker CK. Evidence for the role of psychological factors in abnormal paraspinal activity in patients with chronic low back pain. J Musculo Pain 1997;5:41–56.

62. Lindstrom R, Schomacher J, Farina D, et al. Association between neck muscle coactivation, pain, and strength in women with neck pain. Man Ther 2011;16:80–6.

63. Hubley-Kozey C, Deluzio K, Dunbar M. Muscle co-activation patterns during walking in those with severe knee osteoarthritis. Clin Biomech 2008;23:71–80.

64. Tucker KJ, Hodges PW. Changes in motor unit recruitment strategy during pain alters force direction. Eur J Pain 2010;14:932–8.

65. Moseley GL, Hodges PW. Reduced variability of postural strategy prevents normalisation of motor changes induced by back pain – a risk factor for chronic trouble? Behav Neurosci 2006;120:474–6.

66. Bergin MJ, Tucker KJ, Vicenzino B, et al. Does movement variability increase or decrease when a simple wrist task is performed during acute wrist extensor muscle pain? Eur J Appl Physiol 2014;114:385–93.

67. Hug F, Hodges PW, Salomoni SE, et al. Insight into motor adaptation to pain from between-leg compensation. Eur J Appl Physiol 2014;114(5):1057–65.

68. Svensson P, Arendt-Nielsen L, Houe L. Sensory-motor interactions of human experimental unilateral jaw muscle pain: a quantitative analysis. Pain 1995;64:241–9.

69. Madeleine P, Leclerc F, Arendt-Nielsen L, et al. Experimental muscle pain changes the spatial distribution of upper trapezius muscle activity during sustained contraction. Clin Neurophysiol 2006;117:2436–45.

70. Dideriksen JL, Gizzi L, Petzke F, et al. Deterministic accessory spinal movement in functional tasks characterizes individuals with low back pain. Clin Neurophysiol 2013;125:1663–8.

71. Ferreira P, Ferreira M, Hodges P. Changes recruitment of the abdominal muscles in people with low back pain: ultrasound measurement of muscle activity. Spine 2004;29:2560–6.

72. Hides JA, Stokes MJ, Saide M, et al. Evidence of lumbar multifidus muscle wasting ipsilateral to symptoms in patients with acute/subacute low back pain. Spine 1994;19:165–77.

73. MacDonald D, Moseley GL, Hodges PW. Why do some patients keep hurting their back? Evidence of ongoing back muscle dysfunction during remission from recurrent back pain. Pain 2009;142:183–8.

74. Falla DL, Jull GA, Hodges PW. Patients with neck pain demonstrate reduced electromyographic activity of the deep cervical flexor muscles during performance of the craniocervical flexion test. Spine 2004;29:2108–14.

75. Schomacher J, Farina D, Lindstroem R, et al. Chronic trauma-induced neck pain impairs the neural control of the deep semispinalis cervicis muscle. Clin Neurophysiol 2012;123:1403–8.

76. Hodges P, Kaigle Holm A, Holm S, et al. Intervertebral stiffness of the spine is increased by evoked contraction of transversus abdominis and the diaphragm: in vivo porcine studies. Spine 2003;28:2594–601.

77. Anderson JS, Hsu AW, Vasavada AN. Morphology, architecture, and biomechanics of human cervical multifidus. Spine 2005;30:E86–91.

78. Ward SR, Kim CW, Eng CM, et al. Architectural analysis and intraoperative measurements demonstrate the unique design of the multifidus muscle for lumbar spine stability. J Bone Joint Surg Am 2009;91:176–85.

79. Boyd-Clark LC, Briggs CA, Galea MP. Comparative histochemical composition of muscle fibres in a pre- and a postvertebral muscle of the cervical spine. J Anat 2001;199:709–16.

80. Kaigle AM, Holm SH, Hansson TH. 1997 Volvo Award winner in biomechanical studies. Kinematic behaviour of the porcine lumbar spine: a chronic lesion model. Spine 1997;22:2796–806.

81. Falla D, Jull G, Hodges PW. Feedforward activity of the cervical flexor muscles during voluntary arm movements is delayed in chronic neck pain. Exp Brain Res 2004;157:43–8.

82. Saunders S, Coppieters M, Hodges P. Reduced tonic activity of the deep trunk muscle during locomotion in people with low back pain. In: Proceedings of World Congress of Low Back and Pelvic Pain. Melbourne, Australia; 2004.

83. Ng JK, Richardson CA, Parnianpour M, et al. EMG activity of trunk muscles and torque output during isometric axial rotation exertion: a comparison between back pain patients and matched controls. J Orthop Res 2002;20:112–21.

84. van Dieen JH, Selen LP, Cholewicki J. Trunk muscle activation in low-back pain patients, an analysis of the literature. J Electromyogr Kinesiol 2003;13:333–51.

85. Jull G, Kristjansson E, Dall'Alba P. Impairment in the cervical flexors: a comparison of whiplash and insidious onset neck pain patients. Man Ther 2004;9:89–94.

86. Arendt-Nielsen L, Graven-Nielsen T, Svarrer H, et al. The influence of low back pain on muscle activity and coordination during gait: a clinical and experimental study. Pain 1996;64:231–40.

87. O'Sullivan PB, Beales DJ, Beetham JA, et al. Altered motor control strategies in subjects with sacroiliac joint pain during the active straight-leg-raise test. Spine 2002;27:E1–8.

88. Lofvenberg R, Karrholm J, Sundelin G, et al. Prolonged reaction time in patients with chronic lateral instability of the ankle. Am J Sports Med 1995;23:414–17.

89. Cowan SM, Crossley KM, Bennell KL. Altered hip and trunk muscle function in individuals with patellofemoral pain. Brit J Sports Med 2009;43:584–8.

90. Hess SA, Richardson C, Darnell R, et al. Timing of rotator cuff activation during shoulder external rotation in throwers with and without symptoms of pain. J Orthop Sports Phys Ther 2005;35:812–20.

91. Hug F, Hodges PW, Tucker KJ. Task dependency of motor adaptations to an acute noxious stimulation. J Neurophysiol 2014;111:2298–306.
92. Moseley GL. Trunk muscle control and back pain: Chicken, egg, neither or both? In: Hodges PW, Cholewicki J, van Dieeneditors J, editors. Spinal Control: The Rehabilitation of Back Pain. Edinburgh: Elsevier; 2013.
93. Mok NW, Brauer SG, Hodges PW. Failure to use movement in postural strategies leads to increased spinal displacement in low back pain. Spine 2007;32:E537–43.
94. Marras WS, Davis KG, Ferguson SA, et al. Spine loading characteristics of patients with low back pain compared with asymptomatic individuals. Spine 2001;26:2566–74.
95. Fernandez-de-las-Penas C, Falla D, Arendt-Nielsen L, et al. Cervical muscle co-activation in isometric contractions is enhanced in chronic tension-type headache patients. Cephalalgia 2008;28: 744–51.
96. Johnston V, Jull G, Darnell R, et al. Alterations in cervical muscle activity in functional and stressful tasks in female office workers with neck pain. Eur J Appl Physiol 2008;103:253–64.
97. Mok N, Brauer S, Hodges P. Changes in lumbar movement in people with low back pain are related to compromised balance. Spine 2011;36:E45–52.
98. Boudreau SA, Falla D. Chronic neck pain alters muscle activation patterns to sudden movements. Exp Brain Res 2014;232: 2011–20.
99. Vaisy M, Gizzi L, Petzke F, et al. Estimation of lumbar spine functional movement in low back pain. In: Proceedings of Schmerzkongress. 2013.
100. Crisco JJ, Panjabi MM. The intersegmental and multisegmental muscles of the lumbar spine: a biomechanical model comparing lateral stabilising potential. Spine 1991;7:793–9.
101. Hodges PW, James G, Blomster L, et al. Can pro-inflammatory cytokine gene expression explain multifidus muscle fibre changes after an intervertebral disc lesion? Spine 2014;39(13):1010–17.
102. Mannion AF. Fibre type characteristics and function of the human paraspinal muscles: normal values and changes in association with low back pain. J Electromyogr Kinesiol 1999;9:363–77.
103. Uhlig Y, Weber BR, Grob D, et al. Fibre composition and fibre transformations in neck muscles of patients with dysfunction of the cervical spine. J Orthop Res 1995;13:240–9.
104. Falla D, Jull G, Rainoldi A, et al. Neck flexor muscle fatigue is side specific in patients with unilateral neck pain. Eur J Pain 2004;8:71–7.
105. Van Dillen LR, McDonnell MK, Fleming DA, et al. Effect of knee and hip position on hip extension range of motion in individuals with and without low back pain. J Orthop Sports Phys Ther 2000;30:307–16.
106. Janda V. Muscles, central nervous motor regulation and back problems. In: Korreditor IM, editor. The Neurobiologic Mechanisms in Manipulative Therapy. New York: Plenium Press; 1978. p. 27–41.
107. Courtney C, Rine RM, Kroll P. Central somatosensory changes and altered muscle synergies in subjects with anterior cruciate ligament deficiency. Gait Posture 2005;22:69–74.
108. Bryant AL, Newton RU, Steele J. Successful feed-forward strategies following ACL injury and reconstruction. J Electromyogr Kinesiol 2009;19:988–97.
109. Moseley GL. Reconceptualising pain according to its underlying biology. Phys Ther Rev 2007;12:169–78.
110. Weerakkody NS, Whitehead NP, Canny BJ, et al. Large-fibre mechanoreceptors contribute to muscle soreness after eccentric exercise. J Pain 2001;2:209–19.
111. Barker D, Saito M. Autonomic innervation of receptors and muscle fibres in cat skeletal muscle. Proc Royal Soc Lond Series B 1981;212:317–32.
112. Passatore M, Roatta S. Influence of sympathetic nervous system on sensorimotor function: whiplash associated disorders (WAD) as a model. Eur J Appl Physiol 2006;98:423–49.
113. Pedersen J, Sjolander P, Wenngren BI, et al. Increased intramuscular concentration of bradykinin increases the static fusimotor drive to muscle spindles in neck muscles of the cat. Pain 1997;70:83–91.
114. McNulty PA, Turker KS, Macefield VG. Evidence for strong synaptic coupling between single tactile afferents and motoneurones supplying the human hand. J Physiol 1999;518:883–93.
115. Ekholm J, Eklund G, Skoglund S. On the reflex effects from the knee joint of the cat. Acta Physiol Scand 1960;50:167–74.
116. Indahl A, Kaigle AM, Reikeras O, et al. Interaction between the porcine lumbar intervertebral disc, zygapophysial joints, and paraspinal muscles. Spine 1997;22:2834–40.
117. Byl NN, Merzenich MM, Cheung S, et al. A primate model for studying focal dystonia and repetitive strain injury: effects on the primary somatosensory cortex. Phys Ther 1997;77:269–84.
118. Bray H, Moseley GL. Disrupted working body schema of the trunk in people with back pain. Br J Sports Med 2011;45: 168–73.
119. Schabrun SM, Jones E, Kloster J, et al. Temporal association between changes in primary sensory cortex and corticomotor output during muscle pain. Neurosci 2013;235:159–64.
120. Boudreau S, Romaniello A, Wang K, et al. The effects of intra-oral pain on motor cortex neuroplasticity associated with short-term novel tongue-protrusion training in humans. Pain 2007;132:169–78.
121. Ingham D, Tucker KJ, Tsao H, et al. The effect of pain on training-induced plasticity of the corticomotor system. Eur J Pain 2011;15:1028–34.
122. Bouffard J, Bouyer LJ, Roy JS, et al. Tonic pain experienced during locomotor training impairs retention despite normal performance during acquisition. J Neurosci 2014;34(28):9190–5.
123. Hodges PW, Galea MP, Holm S, et al. Corticomotor excitability of back muscles is affected by intervertebral disc lesion in pigs. Eur J Neurosci 2009;29:1490–500.
124. Kniffki KD, Schomburg ED, Steffens H. Synaptic effects from chemically activated fine muscle afferents upon alpha-motoneurones in decerebrate and spinal cats. Brain Res 1981;206: 361–70.
125. Hodges PW, Tucker K, Garland SJ, et al. Non-uniform effects of nociceptive input to motorneurons during experimental pain. In: Proceedings of International Motoneuron Meeting. Sydney, Australia; 2012.
126. Jull G, Amiri M, Bullock-Saxton J, et al. Cervical musculoskeletal impairment in frequent intermittent headache. Part 1: subjects with single headaches. Cephalalgia 2007;27:793–802.
127. Alaranta H, Tallroth K, Soukka A, et al. Fat content of lumbar extensor muscles in low back disability: a radiographic and clinical comparison. J Spinal Disord 1993;6:137–40.
128. Elliott J, Jull G, Noteboom JT, et al. Fatty infiltration in the cervical extensor muscles in persistent whiplash-associated disorders: a magnetic resonance imaging analysis. Spine 2006;31:E847–55.
129. Biering-Sørensen F. Physical measurements as risk indicators for low-back trouble over a one year period. Spine 1984;9:106–19.
130. Hides JA, Belavy DL, Stanton W, et al. Magnetic resonance imaging assessment of trunk muscles during prolonged bed rest. Spine 2007;32:1687–92.
131. Li YP, Schwartz RJ. TNF-alpha regulates early differentiation of C2C12 myoblasts in an autocrine fashion. FASEB J 2001;15: 1413–15.
132. Tsao H, Danneels LA, Hodges PW. ISSLS prize winner: smudging the motor brain in young adults with recurrent low back pain. Spine 2011;36:1721–7.
133. Schabrun SM, Hodges PW, Vicenzino B, et al. Novel adaptations in motor cortical maps: The relationship to persistent elbow pain. Med Sci Sports Exerc 2014;[Epub ahead of print].
134. Tsao H, Tucker KJ, Hodges PW. Changes in excitability of corticomotor inputs to the trunk muscles during experimentally-induced acute low back pain. Neurosci 2011;181:127–33.
135. Martin PG, Weerakkody N, Gandevia SC, et al. Group III and IV muscle afferents differentially affect the motor cortex and motoneurones in humans. J Physiol 2008;586:1277–89.
136. Le Pera D, Graven-Nielsen T, Valeriani M, et al. Inhibition of motor system excitability at cortical and spinal level by tonic muscle pain. Clin Neurophysiol 2001;112:1633–41.
137. Fomberstein K, Qadri S, Ramani R. Functional MRI and pain. Curr Opin Anaesthesiol 2013;[Epub ahead of print].
138. Waddell G. The Back Pain Revolution. Edinburgh: Churchill Livingstone; 1998.

CHAPTER 7

NEUROMUSCULAR ADAPTATIONS TO EXERCISE

Ross Pollock • Stephen Harridge

INTRODUCTION

Performing regular exercise is the single most effective method of maintaining health. It also results in a myriad of adaptations in the cardiovascular, respiratory and neuromuscular systems that can improve physical performance. The focus of this chapter is on the adaptations that occur in the neuromuscular system as a result of exercise. While it is beyond the scope of this chapter to provide a detailed description of muscle structure and function, we give a short introduction to provide context for discussions of exercise-induced adaptations.

Skeletal Muscle

Movement is ultimately facilitated by the action of our skeletal muscles which are responsible for converting the chemical energy stored in the bonds of adenosine triphosphate (ATP) into mechanical work and, like all machines, into heat. All of our muscles, depending on size, are made up of thousands and in some cases hundreds of thousands of elongated cells, known as muscle fibres which are wrapped in a connective tissue sheath (epimysium) comprising the protein collagen. Structurally, each muscle is divided into smaller units called 'fascicles', which are groups or bundles of fibres surrounded by a layer of thick connective tissue (perimysium), while each fibre is surrounded by a fine layer of connective tissue (endomysium). A single muscle fibre consists of a number of myofibrils lying in parallel with the long axis of the muscle. Each myofibril contains myofilaments consisting primarily of the contractile proteins actin and myosin. The myofibril is made up of a number of sarcomeres that lie in series and repeat along the length of the myofibril demarcated by Z-lines. Myosin and actin filaments are arranged such that the two filaments interdigitate and overlap, with muscle contracting and shortening through the interaction of myosin cross-bridges cyclically attaching, rotating and detaching from the actin filament. This process is powered by the hydrolysis of ATP as it breaks down to ADP (adenosine diphosphate), with the removal of the inorganic phosphate (P_i) bond being associated with the 'power stroke' of the cross-bridge as it rotates and acts on actin causing force generation and movement.

Neural Control of Muscle Contraction

At the level of voluntary control, the smallest functional unit that can be activated is the motor unit (MU). A MU is a single α-motoneuron and all the muscle fibres that it innervates. When a contraction is initiated in the motor cortex of the brain a depolarizing electrical current (action potential) is transmitted along the axon of the motoneuron and its branches, and at the neuromuscular junction a neurotransmitter (acetylcholine) is released resulting in the propagation of the action potential along the muscle fibre. This depolarization spreads into the muscle fibre through invaginations in the muscle membrane (T-tubules) which causes the sarcoplasmic reticulum to open ryanodine-binding channels allowing the diffusion of calcium (Ca^{2+}) into the cytoplasm. Ca^{2+} binds to troponin, a regulatory protein coupled to tropomyosin on the actin filament. The result of Ca^{2+} binding is a conformational change of the tropomyosin molecule causing binding sites on actin to be revealed, allowing cross-bridges to bind to actin and exert force. The control of voluntary force levels is determined by two basic mechanisms: (a) the recruitment/de-recruitment of motor units and (b) the rate of action potential firing by each motor unit to regulate Ca^{2+} concentration within each cell.

Muscle Function

Understanding the relationship between muscle force/power and velocity (Fig. 7-1A) helps put into context the functional adaptations that can occur as a result of exercise training. The strength of a muscle is defined as the force (or torque) generated about a joint during a maximum isometric contraction. Power is the rate at which a muscle does mechanical work and is determined by the product of the force of a contraction and velocity of shortening (concentric contraction). Any bodily action that involves movement therefore requires the generation of power, with no power being generated during an isometric contraction where no movement occurs. The maximal velocity of shortening is a point when force is zero (which does not occur in natural movements as there is always some loading on the muscle) representing the maximal rate of cross-bridge turnover. Finally, Figure 7-1A depicts the situation where a muscle is active, but rather than shortening is being forcibly lengthened (eccentric contraction). This stretching of muscle results

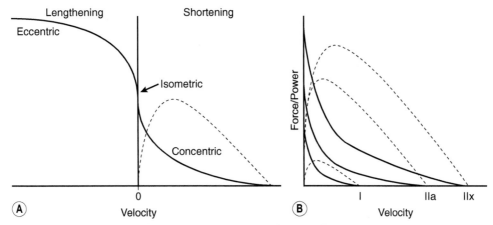

FIGURE 7-1 ■ **(A)** Schematic representation of the relationship between force (solid line)/power (dashed line) and velocity for muscle shortening (concentric), lengthening (eccentric) and static (isometric) contractions. **(B)** The force and power–velocity relationships for slow (type I) and the two types of fast (type IIa and IIx) fibres.

in the performance of negative work where it acts as a brake. Here the cross-bridges have their elastic elements stretched and the muscle is able to bear higher forces than it can during isometric or shortening contractions.

Muscle Fibre Types

Muscle fibres are not homogeneous entities and can be broadly classified into two main groups based on their contractile speed; type I (slow) or type II (fast) (Fig. 7-1B). Compared to type II fibres, type I fibres exhibit lower levels of isometric force production per unit area, demonstrate a longer time to contract and relax from a single electrical impulse (a twitch), have lower maximal speeds of shortening, but are more resistant to fatigue. This aspect is made possible by the fact that they possess more mitochondria (the organelles responsible for the generation of ATP through aerobic metabolism) and have a higher potential for aerobic metabolism. They contain the slowest cycling cross-bridges (containing myosin heavy chain isoform-I, MHC-I). Type II fibres can be further subdivided into type IIa and IIx (formally known as IIb and sometimes IId).[1] Type IIa fibres (containing MHC-IIa), have a high contractile speed and are moderately fatigue-resistant. These fibres are sometimes termed 'fast-oxidative' fibres. Type IIx fibres, the fastest to contract (contain MHC-IIa), exhibit little fatigue resistance and possess few mitochondria. These fibres have a higher potential for generating ATP through anaerobic (glycolytic) pathways. Each muscle comprises a mixture of fibre types (Fig. 7-2), but with a distribution favouring type I fibres in postural muscles such as the soleus and type II fibres dominating muscles such as the triceps brachii of the arm.[2] It is this heterogeneity in muscle composition that allows us to be able to generate explosive power when needed in some situations and yet have some resistance to fatigue in others.

Adaptation to Exercise: The Overload Principle

Improvement and adaptation to exercise rely on the overload principle. Overloading the muscular system, whether

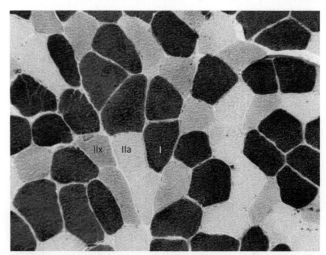

FIGURE 7-2 ■ Muscle biopsy sample taken from vastus lateralis, sectioned and processed using myosin ATPase histochemistry following preincubation at pH4.5. Type I (dark), type IIa (light). Fibres with a more intermediate stain are likely to contain MHC-IIx isoforms, either alone or more commonly co-expressing with MHC-IIA.

mechanically or metabolically, will result in specific and different adaptations that can improve performance. The magnitude of the adaptation is dependent on the type, intensity, frequency and duration of exercise. In addition to these factors there is emerging evidence that as well as an initial level of fitness, there are genetic influences which determine the body's responsiveness (responders and non-responders) to given training intervention.[3]

The mode of exercise performed is an important factor in determining the type and magnitude of adaptation. For example, if endurance training (high-repetition low-load contractions) is undertaken there will be specific changes in muscle which targets aerobic metabolism and improved fatigue resistance. By contrast, high-resistance strength training (low repetition with high-load contractions) causes muscle to adapt by increasing myofibrillar protein synthesis, such that muscle size, strength and power all may increase. Even within the context of either strength or endurance training it is important to consider the specific type of exercise being performed. The principle of specificity dictates that in regard to targeting particular adaptations 'specific exercise elicits specific adaptations creating specific training effects'.[4] For example, the most effective way to increase and improve endurance running performance is through running not cycling or swimming training, even though each mode elicits general adaptations in muscle and cardiorespiratory fitness.

While it is acknowledged that exercise represents both a continuum of types and intensities, for clarity in regard to describing the means by which adaptation occurs, we will consider two types that represent the two ends of the exercise spectrum. These are the adaptations that occur due to high-resistance strength training and those due to endurance training.

ADAPTATIONS TO HIGH-RESISTANCE STRENGTH TRAINING

Progressive resistance training refers to any type of training which, through muscular contraction, aims to increase the strength, power and size of skeletal muscle. These improvements in general rely on the overload principle in which strength is improved and muscle growth stimulated by working a muscle near to its maximal force-generating capacity. While it is not the purpose of this chapter to provide practical details of the myriad of training regimens used, a typical programme might involve lifting and lowering a weight 6–12 times (repetitions), with this being repeated 3–4 times (sets) and using loads which are equivalent to approximately 70–80% of the maximum weight that can be lifted once (1-RM). For optimal improvements in strength the intensity (how much weight is lifted) should be progressively increased over the course of the training programme so as to maintain a level of overload.

Muscle is particularly sensitive to mechanical signals with overload resulting in strength and mass gains. However, the reverse is also true with limb immobilization, bed-rest and exposure to a microgravity environment where unloading results in significant losses in muscle mass and function. The specificity of high-resistance strength training is highlighted by the fact that gains in the amount of weight that can be lifted are markedly greater than the increase in force produced during a maximum voluntary isometric contraction of the same muscle when measured in the laboratory, which in turn is greater than the gain in muscle mass.[5] At first it appears reasonable to assume that increases in the amount of weight lifted and isometric strength would be due to increases in the size (hypertrophy) of the muscle. However, it is widely acknowledged that improvements, particularly in the initial phases, are primarily due to adaptations in the central nervous system. Typical resistance training programmes last between 8–20 weeks with increases in strength occurring as early as 2 weeks, with muscle hypertrophy only becoming apparent after 6–8 weeks of training.[6] The relative time course of neural adaptations and hypertrophy to increased muscle strength is summarized in Figure 7-3.

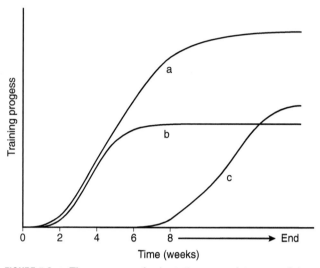

FIGURE 7-3 ■ Time course of adaptation to resistance training. a, Strength improvements; b, neural adaptations; and c, hypertrophy.

Neural Adaptations

Initial studies investigating neural adaptations to resistance training suggested that increased central drive contributed to strength gains as evidenced by increased electromyographic activity of muscles measured from surface electrodes placed over the muscle belly. Such adaptations have been confirmed in studies investigating the V-wave and H-reflex that are evoked by submaximal and supramaximal electrical stimulation of a nerve (e.g. tibial nerve exciting the soleus) giving an estimate of the excitability of the motoneuron pool and transmission efficiency of Ia afferent synapses (presynaptic inhibition). It was found that 14 weeks of resistance training increased the amplitude of the V-wave and H-reflex, indicating an enhanced neural drive in the corticospinal pathways and increased excitability of the α-motoneuron.[7] Taken together these findings indicate that there is an enhanced drive from the higher centres of the brain after resistance training, which are partly responsible for the improvements in strength observed. There may also be an increased MU synchronization (several MUs firing at similar times),[8] a decrease in the force threshold at which MUs are recruited,[9] an increase in MU firing rates[10] and a decrease in the level of co-activation of antagonist muscles[11] after training. The latter is likely to be mediated by inhibitory effects on agonist inhibitory interneurons, excitation of Golgi tendon interneurons or directly from central drive from the motor pathways.[12]

Muscular Adaptations

Although the initial gains in strength are primarily related to neural mechanisms it is well known that skeletal muscle will ultimately adapt to mechanical overload by increasing its size. As is explained below, resistance training triggers various signalling mechanisms that initiate the creation of new proteins and enlargement of muscle fibre/cell size. This is the prime, if not sole, means by which a muscle as a whole hypertrophies, with little evidence to show an increase in the number of muscle fibres (hyperplasia) occurring.[13]

When measured at the whole muscle level with high-resolution magnetic resonance imaging, increases in the anatomical cross-section area of the quadriceps average about 10% after 12–14 weeks of training.[14] In addition, changes in muscle architecture can also be observed. Ultrasound imaging has shown changes in the angle of fibre pennation, which reflects the angle at which fibres are aligned in regard to their insertion to aponeuroses. This affects force output by determining physiological cross-section area (where the cross-section area is determined perpendicular to the line of pull of muscle fibres) and by altering the line of pull of muscle fibres.

At the cellular level, hypertrophy can be seen in all fibre types, although type II fibres appear to have a greater propensity for hypertrophy than type I.[14] The patterns of activity during resistance training and preferential effect on the fast twitch fibres might suggest the possibility of a slow-to-fast transformation in fibre phenotype. However, while there is little evidence of change in relative proportions of the two fibre types, there is good evidence to show that there is in fact a decrease in the number of type IIx fibres accompanied by an increase in type IIa fibres.[15] That said, a selective hypertrophy of type II relative to type I fibres will alter the contractile protein profile of the muscle as a whole, as relatively more of the muscle would be occupied by the fast MHC-II isoforms. This is functionally important as evidence from human single-fibre studies suggests that as well as having a high speed of shortening, fast fibres are inherently stronger (greater force per unit area or 'specific force'). In other words, a given enlargement of a fast twitch fibre should have a proportionately greater effect on strength and power than the same growth of a slow twitch fibre.

Muscle Protein Synthesis

It is clear that muscle is sensitive to the loads placed on it during training. Muscle is a dynamic system with proteins being synthesized and degraded. For a muscle to grow this balance between synthesis and degradation needs to be altered by either increasing the rate at which protein is synthesized, decreasing the rate at which it is degraded or a combination of both. Using tracer techniques, where labelled amino acids (such as [1-^{13}C] leucine) are infused into volunteers and their rate of incorporation into muscle determined, it has been possible to measure objectively protein synthesis in response to exercise and feeding. Determining the rate of protein breakdown is more challenging and requires the measurement of a tracer in blood across a limb. To summarize a number of studies, the following is known about human muscle protein turnover. Muscle protein synthesis is ~0.04% per hour in the fasted state. Muscle, particularly myofibrillar, protein synthesis is stimulated by both exercise and feeding. Following resistance training muscle protein synthesis increases twofold to fivefold post exercise.[16,17] Increases in protein synthesis occur 1–2 hours post exercise; however, when in the fed state they can remain elevated for 48–72 hours.[18,19] This increase in protein synthesis post exercise is also accompanied by an

elevated protein breakdown.[18] However, in a fed state protein synthesis is greater than breakdown which, coupled with the shorter time course of protein breakdown (<24 hours),[18] results in a net gain in protein. The accumulated effect of this process over multiple exercise bouts results in a net gain in protein and therefore muscle growth.

It is apparent from the findings discussed above that adaptations to muscle are dependent on nutrient availability. By altering the availability of certain nutrients it is possible to modulate the immediate protein breakdown and synthesis response post exercise (Fig. 7-4). Resistance training and amino acid ingestion can both increase protein synthesis with an even greater effect present when both are combined.[20] The consumption of protein post exercise also promotes protein synthesis while simultaneously suppressing breakdown. The suppression of protein breakdown post exercise in the fed state is further enhanced by the associated increase in insulin levels,[21] highlighting the importance of adequate nutrition to maximize the benefits of resistance training.

What is the mechanism by which muscle protein synthesis is regulated? Muscle anabolism is regulated inside the muscle cell by the Akt/mTOR signalling pathway[22] as depicted in Figure 7.5. It is also referred to as the canonical insulin-like growth factor 1 (IGF-1) pathway, where at the top activation is triggered by the binding of IGF-1 to a receptor which activates a cascade of steps regulating the initiation, elongation and termination of proteins in the synthetic process. A detailed review of this pathway is beyond the scope of this chapter; suffice to say that IGF-1 is not actually essential for this process.[23] Indeed, activation of mTOR is initiated through the amino acid, leucine, independent of other signals, explaining how muscle protein synthesis can be increased as a result of feeding. While it is tempting to view feeding as the way to increase muscle protein synthesis without exercise, it is known that the gains are transient and that the muscle becomes resistant ('full') to further increases in muscle protein synthesis with additional feeding.[24] Interestingly, there has been a 'scaling down' in the nutritional requirements needed to initiate protein synthesis. Initially, it was observed that feeding of a mixed meal would stimulate protein synthesis. Subsequently it was suggested that ingestion of protein alone followed by just essential amino acids and finally then just the amino acid leucine would be sufficient to initiate protein synthesis. More recently, it has now been shown that one specific metabolite of leucine, β-hydroxyl-β-methylbutyrate, is sufficient to activate the anabolic pathway.[25]

Satellite Cells

The growth and repair of all skeletal muscle is inextricably linked to the action of a group of muscle stem cells known as 'satellite cells'. Muscle is a post-mitotic tissue, meaning that muscle fibres have exited the cell cycle and are no longer capable of further division. Thus, for repair they rely on their resident stem cells. These specialized cells are located in a niche between the basal lamina and the sarcolemma of a muscle fibre. When satellite cells are activated by damage and/or sufficient exercise, these cells

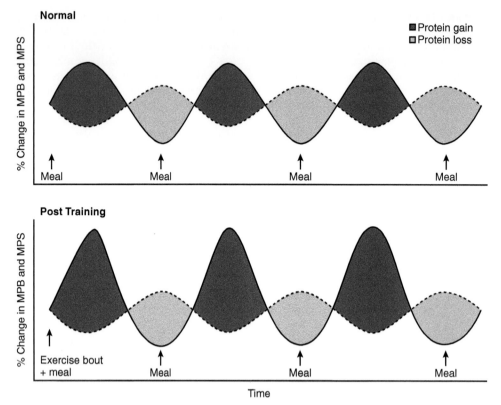

FIGURE 7-4 ■ Schematic of muscle protein synthesis (*MPS*; solid line) and muscle protein breakdown (*MPB*; dashed line) in the normal state and after performing a bout of exercise. Highlighted areas indicate either a net gain in muscle protein or net loss of muscle protein. Note the greater increase in muscle protein synthesis in the fed state post exercise.

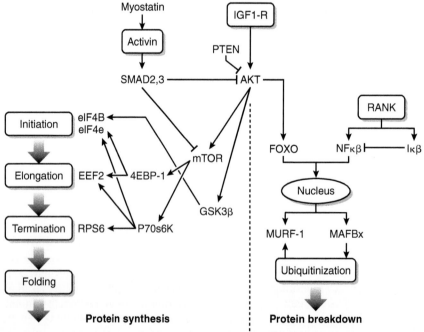

FIGURE 7-5 ■ The Akt/mTOR signalling pathway showing the intracellular regulation of muscle anabolism and catabolism.

proliferate, differentiate and fuse to an existing myofibre, forming new contractile proteins and repair damage. The effect of resistance training on satellite cells is indicated by an increase in their number within 4 days of training.[26] When resistance training is continued over a prolonged period satellite cell numbers may increase by ~30% and remain elevated even if training is stopped.[27]

In addition to acting as a means by which muscles can repair themselves following damage, another important role of satellite cells is the donation of their nuclei to act as post-mitotic nuclei in the growing muscle fibre. Muscle fibres are large cells with multiple nuclei, each of which is responsible for the maintenance of a certain volume of cytoplasm within the muscle fibre. In order for hypertrophy to occur, the myonuclear domain (the volume of cytoplasm that a nucleus can 'manage', i.e. the DNA to protein ratio) must be maintained within a certain limit.[28] In human muscle the 'ceiling' of the myonuclear domain has been estimated to be ~2000 μm^2 in cross section.[29] The theory is that if the myonuclear domain is below this value then increased rates of transcription can result in hypertrophy without the need for additional nuclei. However, as this ceiling value is approached, an increase in the number of nuclei is required.[30]

Hormonal Influences

The milieu surrounding and influencing a muscle in response to resistance training is intricate and in addition to mechanical and nutritional factors, a hormonally complex environment is created. Here we give a brief description of a few of those implicated in the hypertrophic process.

Testosterone

Testosterone is secreted from the Leydig cells of the testes in males. It is responsible for the increased muscularity seen in males at puberty and forms the basis of the anabolic steroids used by some athletes and body builders to increase muscle mass. Despite many years of hearsay about the purported effects of anabolic steroids, the first randomized controlled trial showing the efficacy of pharmacological doses of testosterone was not published until the mid-nineties.[31] Testosterone has subsequently been shown to increase muscle fibre size, satellite cell and myonuclear number in a dose-dependent manner.[32] Conversely, when testosterone production is pharmacologically blocked there is an inhibition of the acute exercise-induced increase in testosterone and an attenuation in the exercise-induced hypertrophic response.[33] Working through the androgen receptors within the cell the exact mechanisms of its action are not fully clear. The effects of testosterone may be related to its role in satellite cell entry into the cell cycle and differentiation or its influence on the IGF-1 system.[34,35]

Growth Hormone/Insulin-Like Growth Factor 1

The second hormonal system relevant to the regulation of muscle mass is the growth hormone (GH)/IGF-1 axis. GH is secreted by the anterior pituitary gland where it acts on the liver to stimulate the synthesis of IGF-1. As can be seen from the Figure 7.5 IGF-1 acts as an initiator molecule of this anabolic cascade. However, rather than circulating levels of IGF-1, it seems that IGF-1 produced locally by muscle for autocrine and paracrine actions is the most critical for muscle hypertrophy. In rodent studies, both localized infusion and genetically induced overexpression of IGF-1 result in hypertrophy.[36,37] IGF-1 is a 70-amino-acid peptide and its gene comprises five exons and two promoter regions. Alternative splicing of pre-mRNA results in the creation of E peptides (e.g. mechano growth factor, MGF) that may have different and specialized functions in muscle repair and adaptation.[38] In humans, circulating IGF-1 can be increased with administration of recombinant growth hormone (rhGH). rhGH is an effective clinical treatment for both GH-deficient adults and children, which led to its use as a potential doping agent in sport. However, laboratory trials have not shown convincing effects on muscle protein synthesis or growth over that induced by exercise training alone,[39] and the roles of both GH and IGF-1 in muscle growth in adults remain unclear.

Myostatin

A final factor to consider in this section is the growth factor, myostatin (or growth differentiation factor 8). This growth factor secreted by muscle works differently to testosterone or IGF-1, in that it acts to suppress muscle growth. It was discovered in 1997 through analysis of samples obtained from Belgium Blue cattle that demonstrated a highly hypertrophied (double-muscled) phenotype.[40] A mutation in the myostatin gene was discovered and causal effects of myostatin were shown in genetically modified mice which had the myostatin gene experimentally knocked out and were characterized by a highly hypertrophied phenotype.[41] A case report of a child exhibiting a highly hypertrophied phenotype related to a mutation in the myostatin gene[42] provided evidence in humans of its role in the regulation of muscle mass. Myostatin works as a negative regulator of muscle mass and it is thus not surprising that resistance training has been shown to result in its down-regulation[43] (i.e. the brake on growth inhibition is being taken off). Myostatin works through the Smad signalling pathway, but its interaction with the anabolic Akt/mTOR pathway can be seen in Figure 7.5.

These are only three of the factors that may influence muscle. We have described studies where muscle growth is facilitated by pharmacological administration of GH or testosterone and indeed impaired by use of a pharmacological inhibitor of testosterone, but on a final note it is worth discussing the recent study by West and co-workers.[44] Subjects undertook strength training of the elbow flexor muscles, but used prior leg exercise to instigate physiologically elevated levels of GH, IGFI and testosterone, thereby creating a physiologically induced hormonally enhanced environment. Interestingly, while these were elevated threefold to tenfold above the resting condition, the elbow flexors showed no greater increase in muscle mass or strength compared to training in the resting normal hormonal environment. This suggested that exercise-induced elevations of these hormones within the normal physiological range do not enhance muscle anabolism, adding weight to the argument that local factors regulating muscle protein synthesis are the most important in a non-pharmacological context.

ENDURANCE TRAINING

In contrast to resistance training, which is focused on increasing muscle mass strength and power, endurance training is targeted at increasing muscle fatigue resistance for exercise of longer durations. Fatigue can be defined as 'a loss in the capacity for developing force and/or velocity of a muscle, resulting from muscular activity under load and which is reversible by rest'.[45] Performance in endurance activities is reliant on the body's ability to generate ATP at a sufficient rate through aerobic respiration, a process which requires interaction of the neuromuscular, cardiovascular and respiratory systems. While adaptations in the cardiovascular system are particularly important, the focus here will be on the local adaptations that occur in skeletal muscle. Ultimately, endurance training improves the oxidative capacity and metabolic efficiency of skeletal muscle. It does this through adaptations in oxygen utilization (mitochondrial biogenesis), oxygen delivery (angiogenesis) and local substrate availability.

Mitochondrial Adaptations

In regard to oxygen utilization, mitochondria are organelles responsible for the generation of the majority of the cell's supply of ATP through aerobic respiration and thus have been termed 'the power house' of the cell. Numerous studies have shown that endurance training can increase the volume and number of mitochondria with the magnitude of these changes relating to the frequency and intensity of training.[46] The advantage of an increased number and size of mitochondria is that the proportion of pyruvate formed during glycolysis passing into the mitochondria for oxidative phosphorylation is increased with less used for the production of lactate and its by-products (e.g. H^+). Lactate accumulation in the circulation is interpreted as the point where aerobic metabolism is no longer able to supply the metabolic demands of the working muscles. After training, the blood lactate–workload relationship is shifted to the right such that the exercise intensity at which lactate begins to accumulate (the lactate threshold) is increased. In other words, the exercise intensity, which can be sustained through reliance primarily on aerobic metabolism, is higher. While it has been known for many years that these adaptations in oxygen delivery and utilization occur, the mechanisms driving these changes have not been so well understood.

Mitochondria are interesting and unique organelles in that they comprise both nuclear and mitochondrial DNA requiring complex mechanisms to construct and remodel them. One of the key regulators identified in the encoding of both nuclear and mitochondrial proteins is a transcription factor named peroxisome proliferator-activated receptor gamma co-activator 1α (PGC-1α).[47] Within 2 hours of a single bout of endurance exercise the PGC-1α gene transcription is elevated tenfold,[48] with the resulting increase in expression initiating mitochondrial biogenesis. A rapid increase in mitochondrial proteins occurs prior to increased expression of PGC-1α suggesting that activation of PGC-1α mediates the initial phase of mitochondrial biogenesis while the delayed increase in PGC-1α protein may sustain and enhance it.[49] This initial phase is likely to be mediated by the movement of PGC-1α from the cytosol into the nucleus of the cell via the activity of a number of enzymes such as AMPK, CamK and p38 MAPK which are up-regulated as a result of endurance exercise. Upon entering the nucleus PGC-1α co-activates transcription factors including nuclear respiratory factor and mitochondrial transcription factor A that regulate the expression of mitochondrial proteins resulting in mitochondrial biogenesis.[50]

Angiogenesis

In regard to oxygen delivery, it is the network of capillaries that run adjacent to muscle fibres which is responsible for allowing the diffusive exchange of gases, substrates and metabolites between the circulation and the working muscle fibres. As with the adaptations in mitochondria, it is well known that endurance exercise results in the growth of new capillaries, a process known as 'angiogenesis', with an increase of ~20% being found after as little as 8 weeks of training in both type I and II fibres.[51] A number of factors contribute to exercise-induced angiogenesis, of which the most important is the regulatory protein vascular endothelial growth factor (VEGF) which has a strong effect on endothelial cell division.[52] A single bout of endurance exercise elevates VEGF mRNA content in the working muscle,[53] while repeated bouts of exercise lead to a greater expression of VEGF protein[54] and subsequent capillary formation. Exercise-induced increases in VEGF are stimulated by a number of events which include increased shear stress as a result of increased blood flow,[55] elevated AMPK and local tissue hypoxia elevating the transcription factor HIF-1-alpha. While the total cardiac output is increased following endurance training, through a left ventricular hypertrophy-mediated increase in stroke volume, at the local tissue level increase in capillary density serves to increase the mean transit time for a given arterial blood flow, facilitating diffusion and thus oxygen delivery and CO_2 removal.

Substrate Utilization

The primary fuel sources used during submaximal exercise are carbohydrate (predominantly muscle glycogen) and fats (both local lipid deposits and circulating fatty acids). The oxidation of protein contributes minor amounts to fuel utilization and only becomes significant in times of energy crisis. One of the key adaptations to endurance training is that for a given level of submaximal exercise the contribution of fatty acid oxidation to the total energy requirement increases with a marked increase in the muscle's ability to utilize intramuscular triglycerides as the primary fuel source.[56] Training results in fibres storing both more glycogen, in the form of granules, and a greater number of intramuscular lipid droplets in contact with the mitochondria.[57] Improved fatty acid oxidation is beneficial to endurance athletes as it helps conserve or 'spare' muscle glycogen stores, which are more important during exercise of a higher intensity. Circulating blood glucose acts as another important fuel source during exercise, and is taken up into muscle through action of glucose transporter 4 with evidence that the content of this protein is increased as a result of endurance training.

Can We Switch Muscle Fibre Types?

As discussed earlier, muscle fibres can be classified on the basis of a number of different parameters (twitch time, myosin isoform composition, ATPase activity, fatigability and their metabolic properties). Usually, fibre types are discussed in relation to their ATPase activity/MHC isoform content. On this basis a number of studies have tried to establish the effect of endurance training on the relative proportions of type I and type II fibres. While it has long been recognized that high-level endurance athletes have a greater proportion of type I than type II fibres[58] than non-athletes, with the opposite being true of sprint athletes, this cross-sectional approach does not provide clear evidence that this is a result of endurance training. Indeed, it is known from studies of monozygotic and dizygotic twins that there is a large genetic component in establishing muscle phenotype.[59] It could be that people with a higher percentage of these slow twitch fibres preferentially participate in endurance activities because they are more naturally talented in this regard and find it easier. In general, it is assumed that there is little change in fibre type with endurance training although there will be a transformation from type IIx to type IIa, as indeed there is for power and strength training.[60] The evidence for a type II to type I fibre-type transformation has come from animal studies which have employed long-term chronic low-frequency electrical stimulation regimens rather than voluntary exercise.[61] However, the adaptations that result in an increased potential for increased aerobic metabolism can occur readily in all fibre types and do not require a switching of the molecular motor (i.e. the myosin cross-bridge). Thus the classification of muscle becomes more blurred following endurance training, with fibres still maintaining their given myosin isoform content, but markedly changing their metabolic properties and ability to resist fatigue.

Neural Adaptations

As with resistance training, endurance training results in adaptations to the neural system. In contrast to resistance training MU discharge rate decreases[10] while a slower rate of decline in MU conduction velocity during sustained contractions is found after endurance training.[62] In addition, endurance training has been found to increase the excitability of the H-reflex pathway[63] suggesting the recruitment threshold of the motoneuron to Ia afferent input has been lowered, while the difference in thresholds between motoneurons has decreased (i.e increased recruitment gain).[64,65] It is likely that these responses reflect adaptations that improve fatigue resistance thereby enhancing endurance performance. Indeed the specificity of adaptations to a particular activity (e.g. cycling versus running) can, in part, be explained by the different patterns of motor unit activation that are required by the same muscles undertaking different activities.

SUMMARY

Muscle is highly malleable tissue adapting to changes in both the mechanical and metabolic signals that result from exercise (Table 7-1). On the one hand resistance training induces a number of adaptations not only in skeletal muscle, but also the neural network that result in gains in strength, power and muscle size. This type of exercise results in increases in myofibrillar muscle protein synthesis and activation of the satellite cells to facilitate a hypertrophic adaptation of muscle to the loads placed upon them. In contrast, rather than increasing the strength of muscular contractions, endurance training exerts its influence by improving the aerobic capacity of muscle fibres. The main factors that allow this are the increased capillary network to facilitate local oxygen delivery and an increase in the size and number of mitochondria to facilitate oxygen utilization enabling a greater

TABLE 7-1	Summary of the Broad Changes that are Associated with the Two Extremes of Training: High Resistance Compared to Endurance Training	
	Resistance Training	Endurance Training
Functional adaptations:		
Strength and power	↑	↔
Fatigue resistance	↔	↑
Muscular adaptations:		
Muscle size	↑	↔
Fibre switching	IIx→IIa	IIx→IIa→I(?)
Muscle protein synthesis	↑ Myofibrillar fraction	↑ Mitochondrial fraction
Mitochondria volume/oxidative enzyme activity	↔	↑
Capillary network	↔/↓	↑
Neural adaptations:		
Central drive	↑	↔
MU synchronization	↑	↔
MU recruitment threshold	↓	↓
MU firing rate	↑	↓
Antagonist co-activation	↓	↔

MU, Motor unit.

ATP production through aerobic metabolism. All of these changes require a complex interaction of signalling events, our understanding of which has been aided by the rapid advances there have been in recent years in muscle molecular and cell biology.

REFERENCES

1. Schiaffino S, Reggiani C. Fibre types in mammalian skeletal muscles. Physiol Rev 2011;91:1447–531.
2. Harridge SDR, Bottinelli R, Canepari M, et al. Whole-muscle and single-fibre contractile properties and myosin heavy chain isoforms in humans. Pflugers Arch J Physiol 1996;432:913–20.
3. Bouchard C, Rankinen T. Individual differences in response to regular physical activity. Med Sci Sports Exerc 2001;33:S446–51.
4. McArdle W, Katch F, Katch V. Exercise Physiology: Energy, Nutrition, and Human Performance. 8th ed. Philidelphia: Lippincott, Williams & Wilkins; 2014.
5. Jones DA, Rutherford OM, Parker DF. Physiological changes in skeletal muscle as a result of strength training. Exp Physiol 1989; 74:233–56.
6. Sale D. Neural adaptations to resistance training. Med Sci Sports Exerc 1988;20:S135–45.
7. Aagaard P, Simonsen E, Andersen J, et al. Neural adaptation to resistance training: changes in evoked V-wave and H-reflex responses. J Appl Physiol 2002;92:2309–18.
8. Pucci AR, Griffin L, Cafarelli E. Maximal motor unit firing rates during isometric resistance training in men. Exp Physiol 2006;91: 171–8.
9. Van Cutsem M, Duchateau J, Hainaut K. Changes in single motor unit behaviour contribute to the increase in contraction speed after dynamic training in humans. J Physiol 1998;513:295–305.
10. Vila-Chã C, Falla D, Farina D. Motor unit behaviour during submaximal contractions following six weeks of either endurance or strength training. J Appl Physiol 2010;109:1455–66.
11. Häkkinen K, Alen M, Kraemer WJ, et al. Neuromuscular adaptations during concurrent strength and endurance training versus strength training. Eur J Appl Physiol Appl Physiol 2003;89: 42–52.
12. Carolan B, Cafarelli E. Adaptations in coactivation after isometric resistance training. J Appl Physiol 1992;73:911–17.
13. McCall GE, Byrnes WC, Dickinson A, et al. Muscle fibre hypertrophy, hyperplasia, and capillary density in college men after resistance training. J Appl Physiol 2004;81:2004–12.
14. Aagaard P, Andersen J, Dyhre-Poulsen P, et al. A mechanism for increased contractile strength of human pennate muscle in response to strength training: changes in muscle architecture. J Physiol 2001;534:613–23.
15. Andersen J, Aagaard P. Myosin heavy chain IIX overshoot in human skeletal muscle. Muscle Nerve 2000;23:1095–104.
16. Burd N, West DWD, Staples AW, et al. Low-load high volume resistance exercise stimulates muscle protein synthesis more than high-load low volume resistance exercise in young men. PLoS ONE 2010;5:e12033.
17. Phillips SM, Tipton KD, Ferrando AA, et al. Resistance training reduces the acute exercise-induced increase in muscle protein turnover. Am J Physiol 1999;276:E118–24.
18. Phillips SM, Tipton KD, Aarsland A, et al. Mixed muscle protein synthesis and breakdown after resistance exercise in humans. Am J Physiol 1997;273:E99–107.
19. Kumar V, Selby A, Rankin D, et al. Age-related differences in the dose-response relationship of muscle protein synthesis to resistance exercise in young and old men. J Physiol 2009;587:211–17.
20. Tipton KD, Ferrando AA, Phillips SM, et al. Postexercise net protein synthesis in human muscle from orally administered amino acids. Am J Physiol Physiol 1999;276:E628–34.
21. Hawley JA, Burke LM, Phillips SM, et al. Nutritional modulation of training-induced skeletal muscle adaptations. J Appl Physiol 2011;110:834–45.
22. Rommel C, Bodine SC, Clarke BA, et al. Mediation of IGF-1-induced skeletal myotube hypertrophy by PI(3)K/Akt/mTOR and PI(3)K/Akt/GSK3 pathways. Nat Cell Biol 2001;3:1009–13.
23. Fernández AM, Dupont J, Farrar RP, et al. Muscle-specific inactivation of the IGF-I receptor induces compensatory hyperplasia in skeletal muscle. J Clin Invest 2002;109:347–55.
24. Cuthbertson D, Smith K, Babraj J, et al. Anabolic signalling deficits underlie amino acid resistance of wasting, ageing muscle. FASEB J 2005;19:422–4.
25. Wilkinson DJ, Hossain T, Hill DS, et al. Effects of leucine and its metabolite β-hydroxy-β-methylbutyrate on human skeletal muscle protein metabolism. J Physiol 2013;591:2911–23.
26. Crameri RM, Langberg H, Magnusson P, et al. Changes in satellite cells in human skeletal muscle after a single bout of high intensity exercise. J Physiol 2004;558:333–40.
27. Kadi F, Schjerling P, Andersen LL, et al. The effects of heavy resistance training and detraining on satellite cells in human skeletal muscles. J Physiol 2004;558:1005–12.
28. Kadi F, Eriksson A, Holmner S, et al. Cellular adaptation of the trapezius muscle in strength-trained athletes. Histochem Cell Biol 1999;111:189–95.
29. Petrella JK, Kim J, Cross JM, et al. Efficacy of myonuclear addition may explain differential myofiber growth among resistance-trained young and older men and women. Am J Endocrinol Metab 2006;291:E937–46.
30. Kadi F, Charifi N, Denis C, et al. The behaviour of satellite cells in response to exercise: what have we learned from human studies? Pflugers Arch 2005;451:319–27.
31. Bhasin S, Storer TW, Berman N, et al. The effects of supraphysiologic doses of testosterone on muscle size and strength in normal men. N Engl J Med 1996;335:1–7.
32. Sinha-Hikim I, Roth SM, Lee MI, et al. Testosterone-induced muscle hypertrophy is associated with an increase in satellite cell number in healthy, young men. Am J Physiol Endocrinol Metab 2003;285:E197–205.
33. Kvorning T, Andersen M, Brixen K, et al. Suppression of endogenous testosterone production attenuates the response to strength training: a randomized, placebo-controlled, and blinded intervention study. Am J Physiol Endocrinol Metab 2006;291:1325–32.
34. Goldspink G. Loss of muscle strength during ageing studied at the gene level. Rejuvenation Res 2007;10:397–405.
35. Sinha-Hikim I, Cornford M, Gaytan H, et al. Effects of testosterone supplementation on skeletal muscle fibre hypertrophy and satellite cells in community-dwelling older men. J Clin Endocrinol Metab 2006;91:3024–33.
36. Musarò A, McCullagh K, Paul A, et al. Localized Igf-1 transgene expression sustains hypertrophy and regeneration in senescent skeletal muscle. Nat Genet 2001;27:195–200.
37. Adams G, McCue S. Localized infusion of IGF-I results in skeletal muscle hypertrophy in rats. J Appl Physiol 1998;84:1716–22.
38. Velloso CP, Harridge SDR. Insulin-like growth factor-I E peptides: implications for ageing skeletal muscle. Scand J Med Sci Sports 2010;20:20–7.
39. Yarasheski K. Growth hormone effects on metabolism, body composition, muscle mass, and strength. Exerc Sport Sci Rev 1994;22: 285–312.
40. Grobet L, Martin L, Poncelet D, et al. A deletion in the bovine myostatin gene causes the double-muscled phenotype in cattle. Nat Genet 1997;17:71–4.
41. McPherron A, Lawler A, Lee S. Regulation of skeletal muscle mass in mice by a new TGF-beta superfamily member. Nature 1997;387: 83–90.
42. Schuelke M, Wagner K, Stolz L, et al. Myostatin mutation associated with gross muscle hypertrophy in a child. N Engl J Med 2004;350:1–30.
43. Roth SM, Martel GF, Ferrell RE, et al. Myostatin gene expression is reduced in humans with heavy-resistance strength training: a brief communication. Exp Biol Med 2003;228:706–9.
44. West DWD, Burd NA, Tang JE, et al. Elevations in ostensibly anabolic hormones with resistance exercise enhance neither training-induced muscle hypertrophy nor strength of the elbow flexors. J Appl Physiol 2010;108:60–7.
45. NHLBI Workshop Summary. NHLBI Workshop summary. Respiratory muscle fatigue. Report of the Respiratory Muscle Fatigue Workshop Group. Am Rev Respir Dis 1990;142:474–80.
46. Hickson RC. Skeletal muscle cytochrome c and myoglobin, endurance, and frequency of training skeletal muscle cytochrome c and myoglobin, endurance, and frequency of training. J Appl Physiol 1981;51:746–9.
47. Lin J, Wu H, Tarr P, et al. Transcriptional co-activator PGC-1 a drives the formation of slow-twitch muscle fibres. Nature 2002;418:797–801.

48. Pilegaard H, Saltin B, Neufer PD. Exercise induces transient transcriptional activation of the PGC-1 gene in human skeletal muscle. J Physiol 2003;546:851–8.

49. Wright DC, Han D-H, Garcia-Roves PM, et al. Exercise-induced mitochondrial biogenesis begins before the increase in muscle PGC-1a expression. J Biol Chem 2007;282:194–9.

50. Holloszy JO. Regulation by exercise of skeletal muscle content of mitochondria and GLUT4. J Physiol Pharmacol 2008;59(Suppl. 7):5–18.

51. Ingjer F. Effects of endurance training on muscle fibre ATP-ase activity, capillary supply and mitochondrial content in man. J Physiol 1979;294:419–32.

52. Bloor C. Angiogenesis during exercise and training. Angiogenesis 2005;8:263–71.

53. Richardson RS, Wagner H, Mudaliar SRD, et al. Human VEGF gene expression in skeletal muscle: effect of acute normoxic and hypoxic exercise. Am J Physiol – Hear Circ Physiol 1999;277: H2247–52.

54. Gustafsson T, Knutsson A, Puntschart A, et al. Increased expression of vascular endothelial growth factor in human skeletal muscle in response to short-term one-legged exercise training. Pflugers Arch 2002;444:752–9.

55. Brown M, Hudlicka O. Modulation of physiological angiogenesis in skeletal muscle by mechanical forces: involvment of VEGF and metalloproteinases. Angiogenesis 2003;6:1–14.

56. Martin W 3rd. Effect of endurance training on fatty acid metabolism during whole body exercise. Med Sci Sport Exerc 1997; 29:635–9.

57. Tarnopolsky MA, Rennie CD, Robertshaw HA, et al. Influence of endurance exercise training and sex on intramyocellular lipid and mitochondrial ultrastructure, substrate use, and mitochondrial enzyme activity. Am J Physiol Regul Integr Comp Physiol 2007;292:R1271–8.

58. Ricoy J, Encinas A, Cabello A, et al. Histochemical study of the vastus lateralis muscle fibre types of athletes. J Physiol Biochem 1998;54:41–7.

59. Komi P, Viitasalo J, Havu M, et al. Skeletal muscle fibres and muscle enzyme activities in monozygous and dizygous twins of both sexes. Acta Physiol Scand 1977;100:385–92.

60. Andersen P, Henriksson J. Training induced changes in the subgroups of human type II skeletal muscle fibres. Acta Physiol Scand 1977;99:123–5.

61. Pette D, Vrbova G. Adaptation of mammalian skeletal muscle fibers to chronic electrical stimulation. Rev Physiol Biochem 1992; 120:115–202.

62. Vila-Chã C, Falla D, Correia MV, et al. Adjustments in motor unit properties during fatiguing contractions after training. Med Sci Sports Exerc 2012;44:616–24.

63. Vila-Chã C, Falla D, Correia MV, et al. Changes in H reflex and V wave following short-term endurance and strength training. J Appl Physiol 2012;112:54–63.

64. Kernell D, Hultborn H. Synaptic effects on recruitment gain: a mechanism of importance for the input-output relations of motoneurone pools? Brain Res 1990;507:176–9.

65. Maffiuletti N, Martin A, Babault N, et al. Electrical and mechanical H(max)-to-M(max) ratio in power- and endurance-trained athletes. J Appl Physiol 2001;90:3–9.

CHAPTER 8

The Peripheral Nervous System and its Compromise in Entrapment Neuropathies

Annina Schmid

INTRODUCTION

The nervous system is an intricate network of interconnected systems of neuronal and non-neuronal cells that relay messages between the periphery, spinal cord and brain. This chapter will focus on the peripheral nervous system (including the sensory ganglia) which contains motor, sensory and sympathetic neurons that travel in close proximity within the same nerve trunk. Peripheral neurons are the largest cells of the body, spanning up to 100 cm (e.g. motor neurons of the sciatic nerve). This extraordinary length not only permits communication between the periphery and the central nervous system, but it also means that neurons need specific anatomical and physiological properties to cater for their length. Given the extensive length of peripheral nerves and their unique anatomy and physiology, it is not surprising that nerve injuries cause symptoms and signs that are distinct from other musculoskeletal conditions. Typically, these include a mix of gain and loss of function such as motor (e.g. weakness) and sympathetic signs (e.g. impaired sweating), as well as sensory symptoms and signs such as numbness, paraesthesia, dysaesthesia, allodynia, hyperalgesia and neuropathic pain (for taxonomy see IASP[1]) in the innervation territory of the affected nerve. Nerve injuries can also lead to increased sensitivity of the nerve itself.[2] In contrast to pain of other origins, symptoms related to nerve injury are more severe and are associated with higher depression, anxiety and poorer quality of life.[3,4]

The most common condition affecting the peripheral nervous system is entrapment neuropathy. For instance, the prevalence of lumbar radiculopathy in the general population is ~2.2%,[4] whereas carpal tunnel syndrome (CTS) occurs in ~3.7% of people.[5] Systemic diseases such as obesity or diabetes can, however, elevate the lifetime risk of developing entrapment neuropathies to up to 85%.[6] Despite their high prevalence, the exact pathophysiology underlying entrapment neuropathies remains elusive,[7] but significant advances in neuroscience research have been made in the past decade. A better understanding of the pathophysiology may help to improve diagnostic reasoning and facilitate the design of more effective management options. Whereas the readers are directed to specialized texts for a comprehensive overview of the anatomy and physiology of the peripheral nervous system,[8,9] this chapter summarizes the normal anatomy and physiology of the peripheral nervous system with a focus on its compromise following entrapment neuropathies. Common clinical signs and symptoms are put in context with potential underlying mechanisms.

ANATOMY AND PHYSIOLOGY

Peripheral Neurons

The main functional component of peripheral neurons consists of the axon and dendrites as well as their cell body (e.g. in the dorsal root ganglion for sensory neurons). Another integral part of neurons is Schwann cells that can be myelinating or non-myelinating (see section on Schwann cells and myelin). Neurons can broadly be divided into three main groups based on anatomical and functional criteria (Fig. 8-1): thick myelinated fibres transmitting signals to and from muscles (e.g. Aα fibres) and conducting sensations such as touch and proprioception (Aβ fibres);[1] thinly myelinated fibres (Aδ fibres) transmitting nociceptive signals evoked by stimuli such as cold and pin prick;[2] and small-diameter unmyelinated nerve fibres (C fibres) subserving nociception evoked by heat or mechanical stimuli as well as innocuous temperature changes (e.g. warm detection) and itch.[3] As such, C fibres are not purely nociceptive. In fact, it has recently been suggested that C fibres may also mediate pleasant touch sensations elicited by brushing of the skin.[10] Furthermore, postganglionic sympathetic neurons are also small-diameter unmyelinated axons belonging to the C fibre category.

Whereas motor fibres are efferent and send signals from the central nervous system to target tissue (e.g. muscles), sensory afferent fibres convey information from the periphery to the central nervous system. The non-nociceptive sensory afferents originate from receptors in peripheral tissues (e.g. Meissner and Ruffini corpuscles, Merkel cells, muscle spindles). In contrast, the receptor organs of nociceptors are free nerve endings. These endings form an intricate network of fine axonal branches which contain an abundance of membrane proteins (ion channels) that respond to different chemical, mechanical and thermal stimuli and agents in the surrounding tissue.

Nociceptors can not only be subdivided according to their fibre diameter and myelination, but a more recent and more functional differentiation distinguishes their sensitivity to the type (modality) of stimulus (e.g.

mechanosensitive, heat sensitive or chemosensitive) and their response characteristics (e.g. low or high threshold) according to the type of ion channels present in their free nerve endings. Using this functional approach, four main groups of C-nociceptors can be distinguished (Table 8-1):[11] C-polymodal fibres (activated by mechanical, thermal and chemical stimuli;[1] C fibres that are activated by specific modalities (e.g. mechanonociceptors, heat nociceptors, etc.);[2] low-threshold C fibres which mediate pleasant touch;[3] and silent (sleeping) nociceptors.[4] The latter are not normally activated by thermal or mechanical stimuli, but become sensitized after exposure to inflammatory stimuli (for a review see Michaelis et al.[12]).

The distinct patterns of responsiveness of sensory neurons to different stimuli have led to the development of quantitative sensory testing, in which the functions of these different fibre domains are examined (see Chapter 20).[13] Clinicians are reminded that a standard bedside neurological examination (reflex, muscle and light touch testing) is limited to the function of large-diameter motor and sensory neurons, and does not provide any information on the functional or structural integrity of small myelinated or unmyelinated neurons, which represent the majority of neurons within a peripheral nerve.

Schwann Cells and Myelin

Whereas both myelinated and unmyelinated axons are associated with Schwann cells, only the Schwann cells of the myelinated fibres produce an insulating layer of lipids and proteins, the so-called myelin sheaths. In the peripheral nervous system, one Schwann cell produces the myelin sheath for only a short axon segment whereas oligodendrocytes can produce myelin sheaths for up to 30 axons in the central nervous system.[14] A thick myelinated sensory neuron of the human femoral nerve contains up to 500 Schwann cells.[14] The Schwann cells and the axons maintain close contact in regions called paranodes (Fig. 8-2), which are adjacent to the nodes of Ranvier. Nodes of Ranvier are the gaps between myelin sheaths. These are around 1 μm in length and expose the axon membranes to the extracellular space. A thick myelinated human femoral neuron contains around 300–500 nodes of Ranvier.[14] These nodes comprise a high density of voltage-gated sodium channels, whereas potassium channels are localized to the juxtaparanodes (the region adjacent to the paranodes) beneath the myelin.[16] Together with the myelin sheath (the internodes), this specific ion channel architecture allows saltatory action potential conduction in myelinated axons, which explains the higher conduction velocities of Aα and Aβ fibres (thick myelinated, ~70–120 m/s) followed by Aδ fibres (thinly myelinated, ~6–25 m/s) and C fibres (unmyelinated, ~1 m/s).[17] The distinct myelination and resulting difference in conduction velocity of the two nociceptor fibre types is suggested to account for the rapid, acute and sharp (Aδ) versus delayed, diffuse and dull pain evoked by noxious stimuli (C fibres).[18]

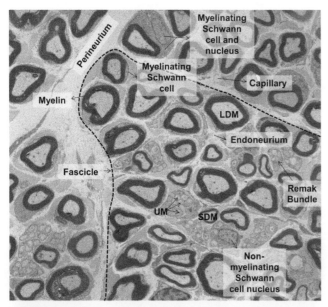

FIGURE 8-1 ■ Cross-section through a healthy peripheral nerve trunk. Electron microscope image of a normal sciatic nerve of a rat taken at 8000× magnification demonstrates the different structures present within a peripheral nerve trunk. These include the perineurium, which surrounds a fascicle, the endoneurium, large-diameter myelinated neurons (*LDM*), small-diameter myelinated neurons (*SDM*) and unmyelinated neurons (*UM*), which form Remak bundles. Several Schwann cell nuclei of both myelinating and non-myelinating Schwann cells as well as capillaries are present in this field. (Image courtesy of A/Prof Margarita Calvo, Pontificia Universidad Católica de Chile.)

TABLE 8-1	**Cutaneous Sensory Fibre Types**				
Fibre	**Myelination**	**Fibre Diameter**	**Fibre Type**	**Modality**	**%**
Aβ	Thick myelinated	Large	Slowly adapting mechanoreceptor	Touch	12
			Rapidly adapting mechanoreceptor	Touch	10
Aδ	Thinly myelinated	Smaller	Low-threshold D-hair mechanoreceptors	Touch	6
			Mechanonociceptors	Nociception	12
C	Unmyelinated	Very small	C-polymodal	Nociception	30
			C-mechanonociceptor, C-mechanoheat nociceptor; C-mechanocold nociceptor; C-heat nociceptor	Nociception	20
			C-low threshold	Pleasant touch	~5
			Silent	Nociception	~5

The table details the differentiation of cutaneous sensory nerve fibres according to their myelination properties and fibre diameters. Furthermore, the different subtypes and their sensory modalities are outlined. The percentage reflects cutaneous fibre distribution. *(Adapted from Smith and Lewin.[11])*

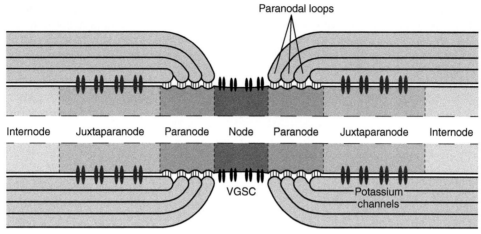

FIGURE 8-2 ■ Nodal architecture. The image depicts an axon and its myelin sheath, which have a close interaction in the paranodal region (paranodal loops). The gap between the myelin sheath is called node of Ranvier and contains an abundance of voltage-gated sodium channels (*VGSC*). In contrast, potassium channels are localized beneath the myelin sheath at the juxtaparanodes. (Figure adjusted from Poliak and Peles[15] with permission.)

Neural Connective Tissue and Its Innervation

The peripheral nervous system not only contains axons and associated Schwann cells, but also a substantial amount of connective tissue, which has an important protective function. There are three distinct connective tissue sheaths (Fig. 8-3). The endoneurium surrounds single axons and is in close contact with Schwann cells. The perineurium surrounds each nerve fascicle (bundle of axons) and consists of several layers of flat perineurial cells (epithelial-like cells) with tight junctions (see section on neural blood circulation and blood–nerve interface).[20] The perineurium has an important mechanical and physiological protective function for the nerve fascicles.[21] The epineurium is the outermost layer and surrounds all fascicles of a peripheral nerve trunk. Its thickness not only varies between individuals, but also along the nerve trunk. Generally, the epineurial tissue is thickest where a nerve passes close to a joint and thinnest in intervening regions.[22] The epineurium is loosely attached to its surrounding nerve bed but relatively fixed in regions where branches depart to innervate muscle tissue.[21] At the subarachnoidal angle of the dorsal root ganglia, the connective tissues of the peripheral nerve trunk merge with the meninges of the central nervous system. Whereas the epineurium is continuous with the dura mater, the perineurium splits to form the arachnoid layers and the root sheaths (comparable to the pia mater).[20]

Peripheral nerves also contain a small amount of adipose tissue. This is especially apparent in the sciatic nerve, whereas the nerves of the upper extremity rarely contain significant amounts of fat.[23] It has therefore been suggested that the main function of intraneural fat is protection from excessive pressure.[23]

The neural connective tissue is innervated by so-called nervi nervorum.[24] In the periphery, these run together with the nerve trunk, whereas spinal nerves, dorsal root ganglia and nerve roots are innervated by axons that project directly to the dorsal root ganglia. Some of the nervi nervorum also arise from perivascular neural plexi that surround the major blood vessels that supply the nerve trunks.[24] Nervi nervorum run longitudinally as well as spirally along the epineurium and perineurium and are also present in the endoneurium. Nervi nervorum consist of both myelinated and unmyelinated fibres and some of them end as free nerve endings,[24] which suggests a potential role as nociceptors. This proposal is further strengthened by the expression of calcitonin gene-related peptide (CGRP), peripherin or substance P in some nervi nervorum.[25,26] These neuropeptides have been implicated with nociceptors and neurogenic inflammation (see section on neurogenic inflammation).[27]

Neural Blood Circulation and Blood–Nerve Interface

Similar to other cells, neurons are highly dependent on an adequate energy supply for metabolic processes such as protein synthesis (e.g. neurotransmitters). Whereas neuron cell bodies have the greatest metabolic demand, peripheral nerve trunks also use energy for active processes including axonal transport or ion pumps to restore membrane potentials following action potential generation. In order to meet the required energy supply, the nervous system possesses an intricate blood circulation system, the vasa nervorum. The blood supply to the peripheral nervous system stems from radicular vessels that branch off blood vessels that commonly run in parallel with the major peripheral nerves (e.g. the tibial nerve together with the tibial artery and vein). The intrinsic neural blood circulation consists of longitudinally orientated epineural vessels that descend into the perineurium and ultimately pierce into the endoneurium where a dense capillary network can be found (Fig. 8-3). This network is characterized by extensive anastomoses that assure a continuous blood supply. In line with the increased metabolic demand, the capillary density and blood flow in dorsal root ganglia is greater than in peripheral nerve trunks.[28] To maintain adequate microcirculation of a nerve, a specific pressure gradient is required.[29] This gradient is characterized by the highest pressure in the arteries followed by the capillaries, the nerve fascicles, the veins and the lowest pressure in the space surrounding the nerve.[29]

In contrast to the epineurium, the endoneurial space does not contain a lymphatic system.[30] Therefore, axons, Schwann cells and other resident cells within the endoneurium are dependent on a protective interface that preserves them from potentially harmful plasma materials. This is achieved by tight junctions of the epithelium of endoneurial blood vessels and layers of perineurial cells,[20] that provide a diffusion barrier to larger molecules and restrict smaller molecules from entering the endoneurial space. As this structure not only restricts, but also regulates, the exchange of molecules between the

endoneurial space and blood vessels, it has been suggested that the term blood–nerve interface rather than blood–nerve barrier is appropriate.[20] Since the blood–nerve interface is relatively impermeable and there is a slight positive pressure in the endoneurial space, the regulated exchange of vital molecules (e.g. to maintain pH, hydrostatic pressure and ion concentrations) depends on the presence of pumps and transporters in the blood–nerve interface.[31] Another mechanism that contributes to the maintenance of the specialized microenvironment of peripheral nerves is the turnover of endoneurial fluid by a proximal to distal fluid flow whose speed is estimated to be ~3 mm per hour.[32]

In contrast to the relatively impermeable blood–nerve interface in the distal nerve trunks, the endoneurial vessels of nerve roots, dorsal root ganglia as well as

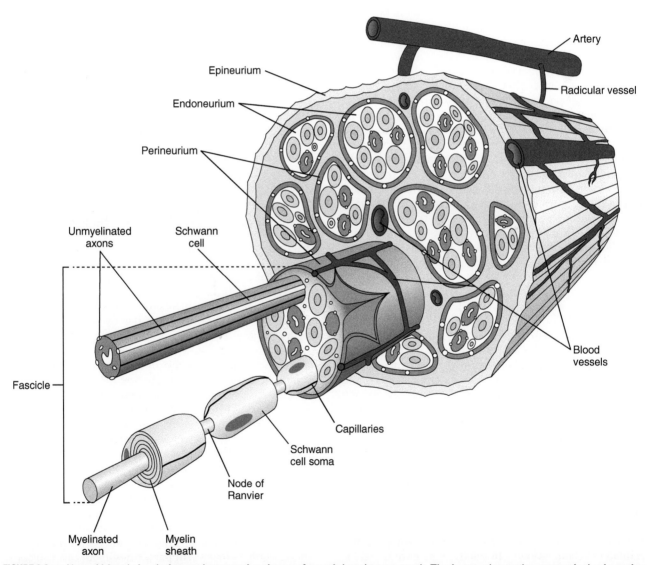

FIGURE 8-3 ■ Neural blood circulation and connective tissue of a peripheral nerve trunk. The image shows the anatomical orientation of the endoneurium which surrounds single axons and their Schwann cells, the perineurium that surrounds fascicles as well as the epineurium that surrounds all fascicles of the nerve trunk. The peripheral nerve trunk receives its blood supply from radicular vessels that branch off major extraneural arteries. The intraneural vessels form an intricate network of longitudinal epineural and perineural vessels that also pierce into the endoneurium. Note the many anastomoses that assure continuous blood supply. (Figure adjusted from[19] with permission.)

sympathetic and cranial ganglia have a fenestrated endothelium, which allows relatively free passage of molecules.[33] Furthermore, the perineurium is thinner at the subarachnoidal angle and the intercellular junctions of the nerve root sheaths are not as dense as those of the perineurium in the peripheral nerve trunk.[34] As such, these structures are not well protected from potentially harmful plasma extravasates.

Axonal Transport

In addition to the intricate blood supply, axonal transport is another system that is essential for the functioning and health of neurons. It serves the transportation of cargoes such as proteins that are produced in the neuronal cell bodies but are needed in the axons and synaptic terminals. This transport system can be divided into anterograde and retrograde transport. Anterograde transport assures the provision of structural components and new organelles such as synaptic boutons or ion channels towards the proximal and distal regions of neurons. Retrograde transport brings organelles and ligands from the synapses or peripheral nerve endings to the neuron's cell body.[21] Membranous organelles (e.g. receptors, neurotransmitters, mitochondria) are usually transported by fast axonal transport (~400 mm/day) whereas cytoskeletal proteins and peptides (e.g. CGRP) are transported by slow axonal transport (~0.2–2.5 mm/day).[35] The transport of these cargoes occurs along longitudinally orientated, hollow microtubules, which serve as rails for the transport within axons.[21] Within these microtubules, specific molecular motors (kinesin and dynein families) bind to the cargoes and transport them along the axons and dendrites.[21] These motors use energy (e.g. ATP), which makes axonal transport an active process. This is why the previously used term 'axonal flow' has been replaced with 'transport', which implies a more active process.

The Immune Cells of the Nervous System

The immune system operates to defend an organism against foreign proteins such as infectious microbes,[36] but it also plays an important role in the clearance of the body's own tissue debris. Circulating immune cells in the blood freely enter most tissues of the body. The blood–nerve interface, however, limits trafficking of immune cells into the nervous system. Nevertheless, a small number of resident immune cells can be found within the peripheral nervous system and its connective tissues. These cells include mast cells, macrophages, dendritic cells and lymphocytes, which assume a surveillance function within the peripheral nerve. The complement system, which consists of around 30 different plasma proteins, is also a major component of the immune system that once activated induces destruction of pathogens and facilitates inflammation.[37] In addition to immune cells, some cells such as Schwann cells and satellite glial cells in the dorsal root ganglia can acquire an immune modulatory function. Within the central nervous system, perivascular cells and glial cells (astrocytes and microglia) are immune-competent.

Central Nervous System

The peripheral nervous system is well connected with the central nervous system. Even though we anatomically differentiate these two systems, they form a functional entity that cannot be separated. Due to the focus of this chapter on the peripheral nervous system, readers are referred to other texts detailing the anatomy and physiology of the central nervous system.[8,9]

PATHOPHYSIOLOGY OF ENTRAPMENT NEUROPATHIES

Whereas the exact aetiology of entrapment neuropathies remains elusive and is most likely multifactorial, there is an established link with increased extraneural pressures.[38,39] These pressures may lead to ischaemia with resulting functional changes. Structural compromise of neural components may ensue in some patients. Presumably, the relative contribution of functional and structural changes to the pathophysiology of entrapment neuropathies is a matter of disease severity or progression. This part of the chapter summarizes the available evidence on the impact of entrapment neuropathies on the previously outlined anatomical and physiological aspects of the peripheral nervous system. Rather than discussing the changes triggered by acute and severe experimental nerve injuries (which may be distinct from entrapment neuropathies), focus will be placed on the growing evidence from animal models of chronic mild nerve compression and patients with entrapment neuropathies.

Entrapment Neuropathies and Ischaemia

Entrapment neuropathies are thought to lead to changes in intraneural blood flow by reversal of the pressure gradient necessary to assure adequate blood supply. Animal models demonstrate that extraneural pressures as low as 20–30 mmHg disrupt intraneural venous circulation and pressures of 40–50 mmHg suppress arteriolar and capillary blood flow.[40] In patients with entrapment neuropathies, extraneural pressure is elevated. In CTS for instance, the mean pressure in the carpal tunnel is over 30 mmHg in neutral wrist positions[38,41] and rises up to 250 mmHg in end-range wrist positions.[38,42] In patients with lumbar disc herniations, comparably high pressures of over 50 mmHg were measured around the affected nerve roots with some patients exhibiting pressures as high as 250 mmHg.[39] Such elevated pressures – especially if present for prolonged periods of time – will be sufficient to reverse the normal pressure gradient,[29] causing obstruction of venous return with subsequent intraneural circulatory slowing and oedema formation.

Transient ischaemia is a common finding in patients with entrapment neuropathies. It not only explains the classic position-dependent paraesthesia, but can also contribute to the reproduction of symptoms during provocative manoeuvres such as Phalen's or reverse Phalen's test for CTS or Spurling's test for cervical radiculopathy. The typical exacerbation of symptoms at night that resolves upon gentle movement can also be attributed to ischaemia. The physiological nocturnal decrease of blood pressure and related drop in intraneural blood flow[43] can reverse the pressure gradient, which induces ischaemia with subsequent changes in metabolic activity and ectopic firing. Venous distension itself may also contribute to the pain experience by activating venous afferents.[44]

In mild entrapment neuropathies, ischaemia may be present in the absence of structural changes. This is apparent by the immediate relief of symptoms after surgery in some patients.[45] Prolonged or repetitive compression and ischaemia can, however, initiate downstream effects including demyelination (see section entitled entrapment neuropathies cause demyelination) or a compromise of the blood–nerve interface.[46,47] This may lead to an influx of inflammatory cells (see section on the role of the immune system in entrapment neuropathies) and plasma macromolecules, which elevates the osmolality of endoneurial fluid with subsequent oedema formation. A decrease in endoneurial fluid flow due to mechanical compression and the absence of a lymphatic system may further challenge the evacuation of intraneural oedema.[48] Clinically, the presence of oedema in entrapment neuropathies is apparent by an enlargement of the compressed nerves[49,50] as well as by increases in signal intensity on specialized magnetic resonance sequences.[51–53]

If prolonged, oedema can eventually lead to intraneural and extraneural fibrotic changes affecting the connective as well as adipose tissues.[54] Neural fibrosis has been found both in radiculopathies[55] as well as entrapments of peripheral nerve trunks (e.g. cubital and carpal tunnel syndrome).[56,57] It can be speculated that extraneural fibrotic changes may underlie the impaired gliding ability of compressed nerves in relation to their surrounding tissues such as is found in patients with CTS.[58–60] However, such biomechanical changes are unlikely to be the only mechanism underlying signs of increased nerve sensitivity during neurodynamic testing (e.g. provocation of symptoms, change in symptoms by moving joints at some distance from the symptomatic area [structural differentiation], and potentially reduced range of motion). Rather, a plethora of neurophysiological changes leading to increased neural mechanosensitivity may account for positive neurodynamic tests in patients with entrapment neuropathies. Some of these neurophysiological changes are discussed below.

Entrapment Neuropathies Cause Demyelination

Focal demyelination is considered a hallmark of nerve entrapments.[54] It is thought to be responsible for the characteristic slowing of nerve conduction,[61] although ischaemia alone is also capable of inducing conduction block.[62,63] Demyelination is a typical downstream effect of prolonged ischaemia that leads to Schwann cell dysfunction,[64] but it can also be attributed to mechanical deformation[65] or a cytotoxic environment due to processes such as inflammation (see section on the role of the immune system in entrapment neuropathies). Histological data from animal models of mild nerve compression[66–68] and from patients with entrapment neuropathies[69–71] confirm focal demyelination and remyelination with intra-fascicular fibrosis and connective tissue thickening. Similar histological findings have, however, also been identified in asymptomatic individuals at common entrapment sites.[72,73] This suggests that such focal histological changes alone do not necessarily lead to symptoms.

In addition to focal demyelination, there is recent evidence that myelin changes extend beyond the lesion site. This is supported by demyelination of the tibial nerve following focal mild nerve compression of the sciatic nerve in rats[67] as well as by the presence of elongated nodes of Ranvier in skin biopsies taken over 9 cm beyond the compression site in patients with CTS (Fig. 8-4).[74] As mentioned above, nodes of Ranvier have a specific configuration of ion channels. After severe experimental nerve injury, the gene expression of electrosensitive, mechanosensitive and chemosensitive channels changes in the cell bodies of sensory neurons.[75,76] Since ion channels are more easily inserted into the membrane at demyelinated sites and the neuronal cell body, modifications of ion channel configuration are prevalent at these sites.[77–80] Changes can include both down- and up-regulation of certain channels as well as expression of novel channels. These ion channel changes have been implicated in spontaneous ectopic generation of action potentials.[81,82] Since action potentials are normally only transmitted but not initiated along the axon or their cell bodies, these sites are called abnormal impulse generating sites. There is preliminary evidence that experimental

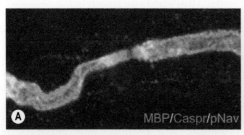
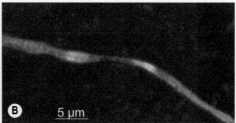

FIGURE 8-4 ■ Patients with CTS have elongated nodes of Ranvier. **(A)** Normal nodal architecture of a dermal myelinated fibre shown by a distinct band of voltage-gated sodium channels (*pNav*, blue) located in the middle of the gap between the myelin sheaths (green, myelin basic protein [*MBP*]). Paranodes are stained with contactin associated protein (*Caspr*, red). **(B)** A dermal myelinated fibre of a patient with carpal tunnel syndrome demonstrating an elongated node with an increased gap between the myelin sheaths. Voltage-gated sodium channels are dispersed within the elongated node. For colour version see Plate 8.

mild nerve compression is sufficient to induce a de novo expression of specific voltage-gated sodium channels in the injured neurons.[83] We have recently confirmed this in patients with CTS, who demonstrated changes in the localization of voltage-gated sodium channels within elongated nodes in their skin[74] (Fig. 8-4). Furthermore, threshold tracking has previously revealed sensory axon hyperexcitability in patients with CTS.[84] This is a specialized neurophysiological technique that provides information on the excitability (hyper or hypo) of axons that are presumably caused by changes in ion channels.[85] If confirmed in other studies, changes to the configuration of ion channels in entrapment neuropathies may not only underlie the ectopic activity (e.g. paraesthesia, Tinel's sign, nerve mechanosensitivity upon palpation), but may also impair normal saltatory impulse conduction, which manifests itself by the characteristic slowing or block of nerve conduction upon electrodiagnostic testing.[61,62]

Entrapment Neuropathies Affect Both Large- and Small-Diameter Nerve Fibres

It is commonly believed that entrapment neuropathies predominantly affect the large myelinated fibres (e.g. demyelination, axon damage)[54,86] and that small axons are relatively resistant to compression.[86] Indeed, numbness to light touch within the innervation territory of the affected nerve or nerve root is common and indicative of Aβ fibre dysfunction. Furthermore, motor axons can be compromised in patients with severe entrapment neuropathies as apparent by muscle atrophy (e.g. thenar atrophy in CTS) or paresis (e.g. foot drop in lumbar radiculopathy). Clinical diagnosis of suspected entrapment neuropathy therefore largely relies on large fibre tests. For instance, the guidelines on the diagnosis of CTS by the American Association of Orthopedic Surgeons mention two point discrimination, Semmes-Weinstein monofilaments, vibrometry and texture discriminations as sensory tests to diagnose CTS.[87] These tests exclusively evaluate the large myelinated fibres and no mention is made of tests evaluating small fibre function. Similarly, the guidelines for the diagnosis and treatment of cervical radiculopathy focus on tests for large fibres (e.g. reflexes, muscle strength, light touch sensation) and only mention one study where pin prick was tested.[88] Electrodiagnostic testing, which exclusively examines the function of large myelinated sensory and motor axons is also commonly used to diagnose and classify patients with entrapment neuropathies.[89] Its correlation with patients' symptoms and functional deficit is, however, often poor.[90] Furthermore, electrodiagnosis and bedside neurological examination are within normal limits in a subgroup of patients with symptoms indicative of entrapment neuropathy.[91,92] This suggests that other factors apart from large fibre (functional or structural) compromise are at play in patients with entrapment neuropathies.

In contrast to common beliefs that small fibres are relatively resistant to compression,[86] a predominant compromise of small axons with structural sparing of large axons (apart from their demyelination) was apparent in

an animal model of mild nerve compression.[67] There is a growing body of clinical evidence that small fibres are affected in patients with entrapment neuropathies. For instance, most studies using quantitative sensory testing suggest loss of function of small myelinated and unmyelinated fibres (deficit in cold and warm detection) in both lumbar and cervical radiculopathy as well as CTS.[74,92-96] Furthermore, several studies find significant alterations of sympathetic axon function in patients with CTS and radiculopathy[97-102] and laser-evoked brain potentials (mediated by Aδ and C fibres) are reduced in patients with CTS.[103]

It has been confirmed that small fibres are not only compromised in their function, but also in their structural integrity in patients with entrapment neuropathies.[74,104] This is apparent by a striking loss of epidermal nerve fibres in the skin of patients with CTS (Fig. 8-5). The density of these free nerve endings (exclusively C and Aδ fibres) can be quantified in skin biopsies using specific markers for axonal proteins (immunohistochemistry). A loss of small epidermal axons has previously been implicated with more severe neuropathic pain conditions such as diabetes mellitus[105] or HIV-associated neuropathy,[106] but the underlying mechanisms remain elusive. Potentially, ischaemia[64] or prolonged exposure to inflammation may induce changes in axonal integrity (see section on the role of the immune system in entrapment neuropathies).[107]

The impact of the identified loss of small fibres on diagnosis and management of entrapment neuropathies remains to be further explored. Interestingly though, preliminary data in patients with symptoms indicative of CTS but normal neurophysiology suggest that small axon dysfunction or loss may precede changes in electrodiagnostic testing.[74,93] These findings suggest that (early) diagnosis of entrapment neuropathies should include tests for small fibre function. Clinical small fibre tests include simple bedside neurological tests (e.g. evaluation of pin prick sensitivity, cold and warm detection) as well as more equipment-intensive examinations such as quantitative sensory testing, sympathetic reflex testing, laser or heat-evoked brain potentials or skin biopsies. Further research is required to evaluate the utility and diagnostic performance of small fibre tests in patients with entrapment neuropathies.

The Role of the Immune System in Entrapment Neuropathies

It is well established that the immune system plays a pivotal role in severe peripheral nerve injuries and neuropathic pain (for reviews see references 108–111). There is growing evidence that the immune system also contributes to signs and symptoms in entrapment neuropathies. It is well known that experimental exposure of nerve roots to nucleus pulposus material induces a local immune inflammation within nerve roots.[112,113] Similarly, experimental mild peripheral nerve compression activates immune cells locally[67,114] (Fig. 8-6A). Influx of blood-borne immune cells is facilitated by a compromise of the protective blood–nerve interface.[47] Furthermore, myelin

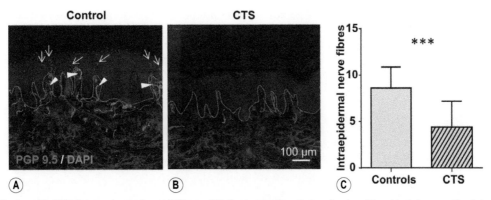

FIGURE 8-5 ■ Patients with CTS have a loss of small fibres. **(A)** Cross-section through a healthy skin taken on the lateropalmar aspect of the second digit. The dermal–epidermal junction is marked with a faint line with the epidermis located on top. Axons are stained with protein gene product 9.5 (a panaxonal marker, red) and cell nuclei are stained with DAPI (blue). There is an abundancy of nerve fibres in the subepidermal plexus as well as inside papillae (arrowheads). Many small fibres pierce the dermal–epidermal junction (arrows). **(B)** Skin of an age- and gender-matched patient with carpal tunnel syndrome (CTS) demonstrates a clear loss of intraepidermal nerve fibres and a less dense subepidermal plexus. **(C)** Graph confirms a substantial loss of intraepidermal nerve fibres (per mm epidermis) in patients with CTS ($p < 0.0001$, mean and standard deviations). For colour version see Plate 8.

and axon debris contributes to recruitment and activation of neutrophils, mast cells and phagocytic macrophages,[115] which in turn trigger a complex cascade that leads to immune cell activation (Fig. 8-7). Upon their activation, immune cells release a plethora of pro-inflammatory mediators (e.g. cytokines, prostaglandins). Immunocompetent cells such as Schwann cells also ingest myelin[115] and subsequently release pro-inflammatory and chemotactic factors that attract other immune cells.[117] Pro-inflammatory mediators lower the firing threshold of both mechanosensitive and nociceptive neurons[118–120] and can activate silent nociceptors.[12] As such, intraneural inflammation is another mechanism that can explain evoked (e.g. palpation, provocation tests such as Spurling, Phalens' or neurodynamic tests) and spontaneous pain or paraesthesia in patients with entrapment neuropathies. Together with ischaemia, it may also account for the nocturnal exacerbation of symptoms. The presence of an inflammatory component is supported by the beneficial short-term effect of anti-inflammatory medication (nonsteroidal and steroidal) in patients with radiculopathies or entrapment neuropathies of peripheral nerve trunks.[121,122]

In addition to intraneural inflammation, mild nerve compression also induces an inflammatory reaction in the connective tissue sheaths (Fig. 8-6B). If exposed to an inflammatory environment, the nervi nervorum in the connective tissue increase their mechanosensitivity.[123] It has therefore been postulated that the nervi nervorum may contribute to heightened nerve sensitivity or pain (upon palpation, provocative manoeuvres and neurodynamic tests) even if nerve conduction (electrodiagnostic tests and bedside neurological examination) is preserved.[124]

Interestingly, the activation of immune and immune-competent cells is not restricted to the lesion site, but can be found in associated dorsal root ganglia after peripheral nerve compression[67] (Fig. 8-8) or nerve root compromise.[112] Immune cell influx into the dorsal root ganglia is facilitated by the fenestrated epithelia of local blood

vessels, which limit the protective function of the blood–nerve interface at this level. Animal models of radiculopathy also demonstrate an activation of glial cells in the dorsal horn of the spinal cord,[125–127] whereas such a reaction seems to require more severe injuries to the peripheral nerve trunk.[67,128,129] Prolonged nerve root injuries or severe peripheral nerve injuries may also activate glial cells in the contralateral dorsal horn.[126,127,130] Such remote immune inflammation in areas where both injured and non-injured neurons lie in close proximity may increase the excitability of intact neurons that originate from sites distant to the actual injury. The resulting hyperexcitability of intact neurons could explain the clinically observed extradermatomal and extraterritorial pain and hyperalgesia that are commonly observed in patients with entrapment neuropathies.[131–133]

Apart from inducing neuronal hyperexcitability, pro-inflammatory cytokines and other substances associated with activated immune cells (e.g. neurotoxic oxygen radicals and proteolytic enzymes) can induce mitochondrial damage. Since mitochondria are vital energy sources for neurons and Schwann cells (e.g. for ion pumps, axonal transport, myelination), their dysfunction and the resulting energy shortage leads to demyelination and neuronal degeneration.[107,134] Whereas the effect of inflammation on small peripheral axon integrity has not specifically been examined, immune cell infiltration of the central nervous system such as in multiple sclerosis can induce axonal damage,[67] particularly of small-calibre axons.[68] Further studies are, however, needed to reveal whether inflammation is a potential explanation for small axon loss in patients with entrapment neuropathies.

Neurogenic Inflammation

In peripheral sensory neurons, action potentials normally travel towards the central nervous system (orthodromic). Upon activation and sensitization of nociceptive C fibres, however, action potentials can also travel towards the

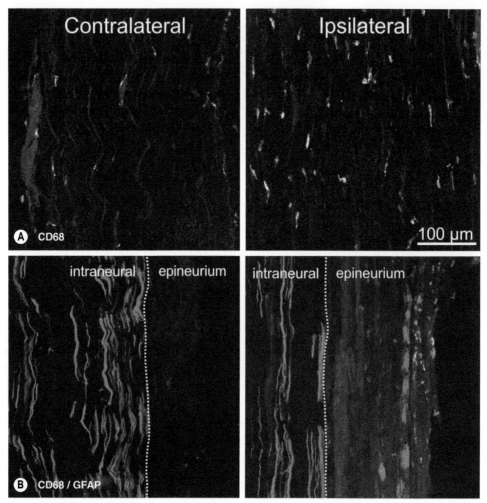

FIGURE 8-6 ■ Experimental mild nerve compression induces a local immune-inflammatory reaction intraneurally as well as in connective tissue. Longitudinal sections through non-operated (left) and mildly compressed (right) sciatic nerves of rats. **(A)** Top panel shows the presence of resident CD68+ macrophages in a non-operated nerve (left) and an intraneural activation and recruitment of macrophages beneath a mild nerve compression (right). **(B)** The activation and recruitment of CD68+ macrophages (red) within the epineurium following mild nerve compression (right) compared to a healthy nerve (left). Schwann cells are stained in green with glial fibrillary acid protein (GFAP). For colour version see Plate 9.

axon branches of the peripheral free nerve endings (antidromic). These antidromic impulses lead to the release of vasoactive and inflammatory mediators in a subgroup of small fibres (peptidergic fibres).[135] In humans, these fibres include mechano-insensitive C-nociceptors but not polymodal C fibres as is the case in animal models.[136] Human microdialysis experiments suggest that the main mediator is the potent vasodilator CGRP whereas the contribution of substance P (a vasodilator and activator of mast cells) seems minor.[137] This phenomenon is called neurogenic inflammation and if present in the skin of patients with entrapment neuropathies, it may be visible by a slight reddening, increase in temperature or trophic changes in the corresponding dermatome or peripheral nerve territory. Neurogenic inflammation may also be present in deeper tissues including the connective tissue of the nervous system, where nervi nervorum have been shown to secrete CGRP.[138] Neurogenic inflammation

within the connective tissue of the peripheral nervous system is another mechanism that may explain heightened nerve mechanosensitivity.

Experimental Mild Nerve Compression Impairs Axonal Transport

Nerve or nerve root compression can affect both the slow and fast retrograde and anterograde axonal transports as shown by radioactive labelling of the transported proteins.[139–143] In animals, pressures on nerves as low as 20 mmHg are sufficient to impair axonal transport.[141] Even though direct comparison with humans warrants caution, the extraneural pressures observed in patients with entrapment neuropathies are well above this critical experimental threshold.[38,39] In addition to mechanical factors, inflammation also impairs axonal transport.[144] Experimental blockage of axonal transport results in

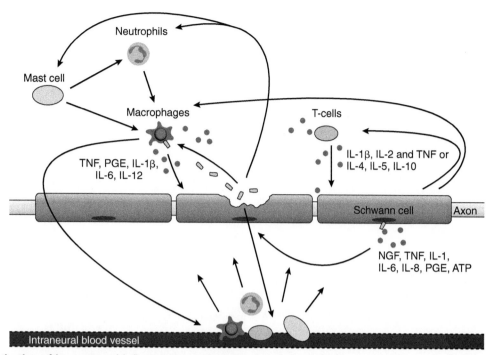

FIGURE 8-7 ■ Activation of immune and inflammatory cells at the site of a peripheral nerve injury. A peripheral nerve lesion leads to an early activation of mast cells and neutrophils, which release chemicals that activate resident macrophages. The macrophages phagocytose axonal or myelin debris and secrete pro-inflammatory substances that sensitize axons or attract other immune cells. A breakdown of the blood–nerve interface by physical damage or substances released by immune cells leads to an additional influx of blood-borne immune cells. Schwann cells also ingest myelin and subsequently release pro-inflammatory chemicals. Both Schwann cells and macrophages signal T cells, some of which will also secrete inflammatory chemicals. This complex cascade leads to a local inflammatory environment that lowers the firing threshold of axons and contributes to neuropathic pain. *ATP*, Adenosine triphosphate; *IL*, Interleukin; *NGF*, Nerve growth factor; *PGE*, Prostaglandin; *TNF-α*, Tumour necrosis factor α. (Figure adapted from Schmid et al.[116] with permission.)

increased nerve mechanosensitivity,[145] presumably by the accumulation and insertion of ion channels at the lesion site. Impaired axonal transport may thus contribute to the heightened neural mechanosensitivity in patients with entrapment neuropathies.

Axonal transport gained a lot of interest in the context of the double crush syndrome. This syndrome was first described by Upton and McComas,[146] who hypothesized that single axons having been compressed at one site become especially susceptible to damage at another site. In a recent Delphi survey, axonal transport was rated as one of the most plausible mechanisms to explain the occurrence of dual nerve disorders.[147] Impaired axonal transport may indeed contribute to the development of dual nerve disorders along the same axonal pathway (e.g. tarsal tunnel syndrome and piriformis syndrome). However, the major criticism concerns the proposition that the peripheral axons and the dorsal nerve roots have separate axonal transport systems,[148] making axonal transport unlikely to account for the most common combination of dual nerve disorders (cervical radiculopathy and CTS). Furthermore, impaired axonal transport cannot explain dual nerve disorders in two distinct peripheral nerves such as the frequently observed ulnar neuropathy in the presence of CTS.[148] Therefore, other mechanisms

in addition to impaired axonal transport have to be considered to explain the occurrence of dual nerve disorders. Readers are referred to Schmid et al (149)[149] for further reading.

Central Nervous System Changes

Since the peripheral and central nervous system form a functional entity, injuries of peripheral nerves inevitably initiate central changes, which are beyond the scope of this chapter. Central changes following severe nerve injury include, but are not limited to, immunoinflammatory reactions at the level of the spinal cord or higher pain centres,[126,127,149,150] central sensitization[151] and changes to cortical representations.[152–155] Furthermore, psychosocial factors can be associated with peripheral nerve injuries. The exact nature of central nervous system changes in patients with entrapment neuropathies remains to be explored. If present, central changes together with changes in the dorsal root ganglia may contribute to the frequently observed spread of symptoms to anatomically unrelated areas (e.g. extraterritorial paraesthesia or pain in the ulnar nerve area in CTS or non-dermatomal pain in patients with radiculopathies).[132,156]

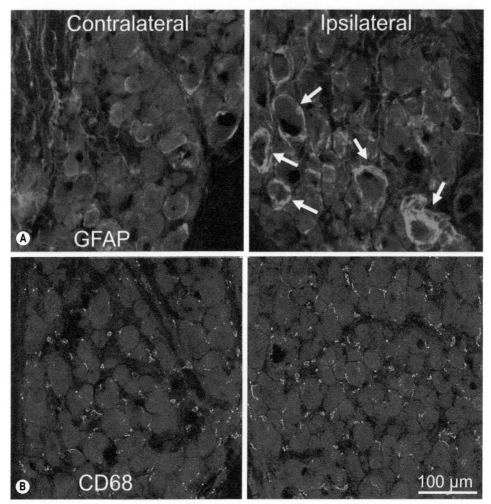

FIGURE 8-8 ■ Experimental mild nerve compression induces an immunoinflammatory reaction in dorsal root ganglia. **(A)** Satellite glia cells (glial fibrillary acid protein, GFAP) in longitudinal sections of L5 dorsal root ganglia contralateral (top left) and ipsilateral (top right) to a mild chronic compression of the sciatic nerve in rats (top right). Arrows indicate satellite glia cell proliferation as apparent by the formation of multilayer rings around sensory neuron cell bodies. **(B)** Macrophage recruitment is apparent by more abundant CD68 (macrophage) staining in a L5 dorsal root ganglion on the ipsilateral side of a mild experimental nerve compression (bottom right).

SUMMARY

This chapter summarized the anatomy and physiology of the peripheral nervous system with a focus on the evidence for its compromise following entrapment neuropathies. It should be noted that these pathophysiological mechanisms do not follow a defined time course or cascade. Rather, the above outlined mechanisms (and future research will undoubtedly unveil many more) interact in a complex manner (Fig. 8-9). In addition, some mechanisms may be absent or negligible in some patients and more prominent in others. The complex interaction and heterogeneity of the pathophysiology not only explains the diverse symptoms and signs in patients with the same diagnosis, but also why examining and treating entrapment neuropathies remains a challenge for clinicians. An enhanced knowledge of the pathophysiology may facilitate diagnostic clinical reasoning, which may improve the understanding of the mechanisms at play in individual patients. Future research will shed light on the diagnostic performance of tests to differentiate these mechanisms. In the meantime, clinicians are advised to incorporate them in their clinical reasoning framework. A better understanding of the pathophysiology is a crucial first step in our vision to provide mechanism-based interventions and to design and implement effective management strategies, which are beyond the scope of this chapter.

Acknowledgement

I would like to dedicate this chapter to Max Zusman, who continues to be a great inspiration to so many of us.

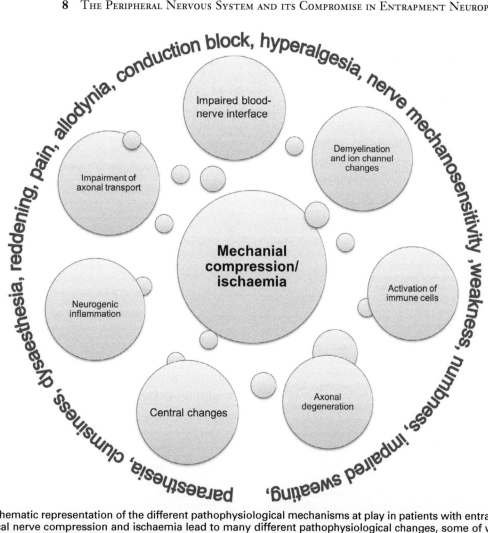

FIGURE 8-9 ■ Schematic representation of the different pathophysiological mechanisms at play in patients with entrapment neuropathies. Mechanical nerve compression and ischaemia lead to many different pathophysiological changes, some of which have been discussed in this chapter. There is a complex interaction between these mechanisms (e.g. immune cell activation may lead to axonal degeneration; impaired axonal transport may lead to ion channel changes) and future research will most certainly unveil more interactions. The presence and predominance of the various mechanisms varies however between patients. This explains the heterogeneous clinical presentation of patients, which is represented by the outer circle containing a wide variety of symptoms and signs present in patients with entrapment neuropathies.

REFERENCES

1. Merskey H, Bogduk N, editors. Part III: Pain Terms, A Current List with Definitions and Notes on Usage. Classification of Chronic Pain. 2nd ed. IASP Task Force on Taxonomy. Seattle: IASP Press; 1994. p. 209–14.
2. Hall TM, Elvey RL. Nerve trunk pain: physical diagnosis and treatment. Man Ther 1999;4(2):63–73.
3. Attal N, Lanteri-Minet M, Laurent B, et al. The specific disease burden of neuropathic pain: results of a French nationwide survey. Pain 2011;152(12):2836–43.
4. Younes M, Bejia I, Aguir Z, et al. Prevalence and risk factors of disk-related sciatica in an urban population in Tunisia. Joint Bone Spine 2006;73(5):538–42.
5. Papanicolaou GD, McCabe SJ, Firrell J. The prevalence and characteristics of nerve compression symptoms in the general population. J Hand Surg [Am] 2001;26(3):460–6.
6. Singh R, Gamble G, Cundy T. Lifetime risk of symptomatic carpal tunnel syndrome in Type 1 diabetes. Diabet Med 2005; 22(5):625–30.
7. Bland JD. Carpal tunnel syndrome. Curr Opin Neurol 2005; 18(5):581–5.
8. Kandel ER, Schwartz J, Jessell TM, et al. Principles of Neural Science. New York: McGrath-Hill; 2012.
9. Gould DJ, Fix JD. Neuroanatomy. Philadelphia, Pennsylvania: Lippincott Wiliams & Wilkins; 2013.
10. Loken LS, Wessberg J, Morrison I, et al. Coding of pleasant touch by unmyelinated afferents in humans. Nat Neurosci 2009;12(5): 547–8.
11. Smith ES, Lewin GR. Nociceptors: a phylogenetic view. J Comp Physiol A Neuroethol Sens Neural Behav Physiol 2009;195(12): 1089–106.
12. Michaelis M, Habler HJ, Jaenig W. Silent afferents: a separate class of primary afferents? Clin Exp Pharmacol Physiol 1996;23(2): 99–105.
13. Rolke R, Magerl W, Campbell KA, et al. Quantitative sensory testing: a comprehensive protocol for clinical trials. Eur J Pain 2006;10(1):77–88.
14. Zhu DQ, Zhu Y, Qiao K, et al. Proximally evoked soleus H-reflex to S1 nerve root stimulation in sensory neuronopathies (ganglion-opathies). Muscle Nerve 2013;48(5):814–16.
15. Poliak S, Peles E. The local differentiation of myelinated axons at nodes of Ranvier. Nat Rev Neurosci 2003;4(12):968–80.
16. Rasband MN, Trimmer JS. Developmental clustering of ion channels at and near the node of Ranvier. Dev Biol 2001;236(1): 5–16.
17. Julius D, Basbaum AI. Molecular mechanisms of nociception. Nature 2001;413(6852):203–10.
18. Basbaum AI, Jessell TM. Part V. Pain. In: Kandel ER, Schwartz JH, Jessell TM, editors. Principles of Neuroscience. New York: McGraw-Hill; 2000. p. 472–91.

19. Ransom R. Organization of the nervous system. In: Boron WF, Boulapaep EL, editors. A Cellular and Molecular Approach. Saunders; 2009. p. 267–88.

20. Weerasuriya A, Mizisin AP. The blood-nerve barrier: structure and functional significance. Methods Mol Biol 2011;686:149–73.

21. Sunderland S. The connective tissues of peripheral nerves. Brain 1965;88(4):841–54.

22. Sunderland S, Bradley KC. The cross-sectional area of peripheral nerve trunks devoted to nerve fibers. Brain 1949;72(3):428–49.

23. Sunderland S. The adipose tissue of peripheral nerves. Brain 1945;68:118–22.

24. Hromada J. On the nerve supply of the connective tissue of some peripheral nervous system components. Acta Anat 1963;55: 343–51.

25. Lincoln J, Milner P, Appenzeller O, et al. Innervation of normal human sural and optic nerves by noradrenaline- and peptide-containing nervi vasorum and nervorum: effect of diabetes and alcoholism. Brain Res 1993;632(1–2):48–56.

26. Bove GM, Light AR. Calcitonin gene-related peptide and peripherin immunoreactivity in nerve sheaths. Somatosens Mot Res 1995;12(1):49–57.

27. McDonald DM, Bowden JJ, Baluk P, et al. Neurogenic inflammation. A model for studying efferent actions of sensory nerves. Adv Exp Med Biol 1996;410:453–62.

28. McManis PG, Schmelzer JD, Zollman PJ, et al. Blood flow and autoregulation in somatic and autonomic ganglia. Comparison with sciatic nerve. Brain 1997;120(Pt 3):445–9.

29. Sunderland S. The nerve lesion in the carpal tunnel syndrome. J Neurol Neurosurg Psychiatry 1976;39(7):615–26.

30. Sunderland S. Nerves and Nerve Injury. Edinburgh: Churchill Livingstone; 1978.

31. Allt G, Lawrenson JG. The blood-nerve barrier: enzymes, transporters and receptors – a comparison with the blood-brain barrier. Brain Res Bull 2000;52(1):1–12.

32. Mellick R, Cavanagh JB. Longitudinal movement of radioiodinated albumin within extravascular spaces of peripheral nerves following three systems of experimental trauma. J Neurol Neurosurg Psychiatry 1967;30(5):458–63.

33. Arvidson B. A study of the perineurial diffusion barrier of a peripheral ganglion. Acta Neuropathol 1979;46(1–2):139–44.

34. McCabe JS, Low FN. The subarachnoid angle: an area of transition in peripheral nerve. Anat Rec 1969;164(1):15–33.

35. Grafstein B, Forman DS. Intracellular transport in neurons. Physiol Rev 1980;60(4):1167–283.

36. Abbas AK, Lichtman AH, Pillai S. Cellular and Molecular Immunology. 6th ed. Philadelphia: Saunders Elsevier; 2007.

37. Janeway C. Janeway's Immunobiology. In: Murphy K, Travers P, Walport M, editors. 7th ed. New York: Garland Science, Taylor & Francis Group; 2008.

38. Gelberman RH, Hergenroeder PT, Hargens AR, et al. The carpal tunnel syndrome. A study of carpal canal pressures. J Bone Joint Surg Am 1981;63(3):380–3.

39. Takahashi K, Shima I, Porter RW. Nerve root pressure in lumbar disc herniation. Spine 1999;24(19):2003–6.

40. Rydevik B, Lundborg G, Bagge U. Effects of graded compression on intraneural blood blow. An in vivo study on rabbit tibial nerve. J Hand Surg 1981;6(1):3–12.

41. Coppieters MW, Schmid AB, Kubler PA, et al. Description, reliability and validity of a novel method to measure carpal tunnel pressure in patients with carpal tunnel syndrome. Man Ther 2012;17(6):589–92.

42. Seradge H, Jia YC, Owens W. In vivo measurement of carpal tunnel pressure in the functioning hand. J Hand Surg 1995; 20(5):855–9.

43. Low PA, Tuck RR. Effects of changes of blood pressure, respiratory acidosis and hypoxia on blood flow in the sciatic nerve of the rat. J Physiol 1984;347:513–24.

44. Sumikawa K, Sakai T, Ono T. Peripheral vascular pain. Nippon Rinsho 2001;59(9):1733–7.

45. Werner RA, Andary M. Carpal tunnel syndrome: pathophysiology and clinical neurophysiology. Clin Neurophysiol 2002;113(9): 1373–81.

46. Mackinnon SE, Dellon AL, Hudson AR, et al. Chronic nerve compression – an experimental model in the rat. Ann Plast Surg 1984;13(2):112–20.

47. Yoshii Y, Nishiura Y, Terui N, et al. The effects of repetitive compression on nerve conduction and blood flow in the rabbit sciatic nerve. J Hand Surg Eur Vol 2010;35(4): 269–78.

48. Mizisin AP, Weerasuriya A. Homeostatic regulation of the endoneurial microenvironment during development, aging and in response to trauma, disease and toxic insult. Acta Neuropathol 2011;121(3):291–312.

49. Nakamichi KI, Tachibana S. Enlarged median nerve in idiopathic carpal tunnel syndrome. Muscle Nerve 2000;23(11):1713–18.

50. Yoon JS, Walker FO, Cartwright MS. Ulnar neuropathy with normal electrodiagnosis and abnormal nerve ultrasound. Arch Phys Med Rehabil 2010;91(2):318–20.

51. Cudlip SA, Howe FA, Clifton A, et al. Magnetic resonance neurography studies of the median nerve before and after carpal tunnel decompression. J Neurosurg 2002;96(6):1046–51.

52. Sirvanci M, Kara B, Duran C, et al. Value of perineural edema/inflammation detected by fat saturation sequences in lumbar magnetic resonance imaging of patients with unilateral sciatica. Acta Radiol 2009;50(2):205–11.

53. Lewis AM, Layzer R, Engstrom JW, et al. Magnetic resonance neurography in extraspinal sciatica. Arch Neurol 2006;63(10): 1469–72.

54. Mackinnon SE. Pathophysiology of nerve compression. Hand Clin 2002;18(2):231–41.

55. Ido K, Urushidani H. Fibrous adhesive entrapment of lumbosacral nerve roots as a cause of sciatica. Spinal Cord 2001;39(5):269–73.

56. Abzug JM, Jacoby SM, Osterman AL. Surgical options for recalcitrant carpal tunnel syndrome with perineural fibrosis. Hand (N Y) 2012;7(1):23–9.

57. Chhabra A, Wadhwa V, Thakkar RS, et al. Recurrent ulnar nerve entrapment at the elbow: correlation of surgical findings and 3-Tesla magnetic resonance neurography. Can J Plast Surg – J Can de Chir Plast 2013;21(3):186–9.

58. Erel E, Dilley A, Greening J, et al. Longitudinal sliding of the median nerve in patients with carpal tunnel syndrome. J Hand Surg [Br] 2003;28(5):439–43.

59. Wang Y, Filius A, Zhao C, et al. Altered median nerve deformation and transverse displacement during wrist movement in patients with carpal tunnel syndrome. Acad Radiol 2014;21(4):472–80.

60. Hough AD, Moore AP, Jones MP. Reduced longitudinal excursion of the median nerve in carpal tunnel syndrome. Arch Phys Med Rehabil 2007;88(5):569–76.

61. Mallik A, Weir AI. Nerve conduction studies: essentials and pitfalls in practice. J Neurol Neurosurg Psychiatry 2005;76(Suppl. 2):ii23–31.

62. Kiernan MC, Mogyoros I, Burke D. Conduction block in carpal tunnel syndrome. Brain 1999;122(5):933–41.

63. Cappelen-Smith C, Lin CS, Burke D. Activity-dependent hyperpolarization and impulse conduction in motor axons in patients with carpal tunnel syndrome. Brain 2003;126(4):1001–8.

64. Nukada H, Powell HC, Myers RR. Spatial distribution of nerve injury after occlusion of individual major vessels in rat sciatic nerves. J Neuropathol Exp Neurol 1993;52(5):452–9.

65. Lin MY, Frieboes LS, Forootan M, et al. Biophysical stimulation induces demyelination via an integrin-dependent mechanism. Ann Neurol 2012;72(1):112–23.

66. O'Brien JP, Mackinnon SE, MacLean AR, et al. A model of chronic nerve compression in the rat. Ann Plast Surg 1987; 19(5):430–5.

67. Schmid AB, Coppieters MW, Ruitenberg MJ, et al. Local and remote immune-mediated inflammation after mild peripheral nerve compression in rats. J Neuropathol Exp Neurol 2013; 72(7):662–80.

68. Gupta R, Rowshan K, Chao T, et al. Chronic nerve compression induces local demyelination and remyelination in a rat model of carpal tunnel syndrome. Exp Neurol 2004;187(2):500–8.

69. Foix C, Marie P. Atrophie isolée de l'éminence thénar d'origine névritique. Rôle du ligament annulaire antérieur du carpe dans la pathogénie de la lésion. Rev Neurol 1913;26:647–8.

70. Neary D. The pathology of ulnar nerve compression in men. Neuropathol Appl Neurobiol 1975;1:69–88.

71. Mackinnon SE, Dellon AL, Hudson AR, et al. Chronic human nerve compression–a histological assessment. Neuropathol Appl Neurobiol 1986;12(6):547–65.

72. Jefferson D, Eames RA. Subclinical entrapment of the lateral femoral cutaneous nerve: an autopsy study. Muscle Nerve 1979;2(2):145–54.

73. Neary D, Ochoa J, Gilliatt RW. Sub-clinical entrapment neuropathy in man. J Neurol Sci 1975;24(3):283–98.

74. Schmid AB, Bland JD, Bhat MA, et al. The relationship of nerve fibre pathology to sensory function in entrapment neuropathy. Brain 2014;137(Pt 12):3186–99.

75. Pertin M, Ji RR, Berta T, et al. Upregulation of the voltage-gated sodium channel beta2 subunit in neuropathic pain models: characterization of expression in injured and non-injured primary sensory neurons. J Neurosci 2005;25(47):10970–80.

76. Kim DS, Choi JO, Rim HD, et al. Downregulation of voltage-gated potassium channel alpha gene expression in dorsal root ganglia following chronic constriction injury of the rat sciatic nerve. Brain Res Mol Brain Res 2002;105(1-2):146–52.

77. Liu X, Zhou JL, Chung K, et al. Ion channels associated with the ectopic discharges generated after segmental spinal nerve injury in the rat. Brain Res 2001;900(1):119–27.

78. Jiang YQ, Xing GG, Wang SL, et al. Axonal accumulation of hyperpolarization-activated cyclic nucleotide-gated cation channels contributes to mechanical allodynia after peripheral nerve injury in rat. Pain 2008;137(3):495–506.

79. Drummond PD, Drummond ES, Dawson LF, et al. Upregulation of alpha1-adrenoceptors on cutaneous nerve fibres after partial sciatic nerve ligation and in complex regional pain syndrome type II. Pain 2014;155(3):606–16.

80. England JD, Gamboni F, Ferguson MA, et al. Sodium channels accumulate at the tips of injured axons. Muscle Nerve 1994;17(6): 593–8.

81. Amir R, Michaelis M, Devor M. Membrane potential oscillations in dorsal root ganglion neurons: role in normal electrogenesis and neuropathic pain. J Neurosci 1999;19(19):8589–96.

82. Chen Y, Devor M. Ectopic mechanosensitivity in injured sensory axons arises from the site of spontaneous electrogenesis. Eur J Pain 1998;2(2):165–78.

83. Frieboes LR, Palispis WA, Gupta R. Nerve compression activates selective nociceptive pathways and upregulates peripheral sodium channel expression in Schwann cells. J Orthop Res 2010; 28(6):753–61.

84. Han SE, Lin CS, Boland RA, et al. Nerve compression, membrane excitability, and symptoms of carpal tunnel syndrome. Muscle Nerve 2011;44(3):402–9.

85. Z'Graggen WJ, Bostock H. Nerve membrane excitability testing. Eur J Anaesthesiol Suppl 2008;42:68–72.

86. Dahlin LB, Shyu BC, Danielsen N, et al. Effects of nerve compression or ischaemia on conduction properties of myelinated and non-myelinated nerve fibres. An experimental study in the rabbit common peroneal nerve. Acta Physiol Scand 1989;136(1): 97–105.

87. American Academy of Orthopedic Surgeons (AAOS). Clinical Practice Guideline on the Diagnosis of Carpal Tunnel Syndrome. AAOS: Rosemont, IL. 2007.

88. Bono CM, Ghiselli G, Gilbert TJ, et al. An evidence-based clinical guideline for the diagnosis and treatment of cervical radiculopathy from degenerative disorders. Spine J 2011;11(1):64–72.

89. Werner RA. Electrodiagnostic evaluation of carpal tunnel syndrome and ulnar neuropathies. PM & R 2013;5(Suppl. 5):S14–21.

90. Longstaff L, Milner RH, O'Sullivan S, et al. Carpal tunnel syndrome: the correlation between outcome, symptoms and nerve conduction study findings. J Hand Surg [Br] 2001;26(5):475–80.

91. Koyuncuoglu HR, Kutluhan S, Yesildag A, et al. The value of ultrasonographic measurement in carpal tunnel syndrome in patients with negative electrodiagnostic tests. Eur J Radiol 2005;56(3):365–9.

92. Witt JC, Hentz JG, Stevens JC. Carpal tunnel syndrome with normal nerve conduction studies. Muscle Nerve 2004;29(4): 515–22.

93. Tamburin S, Cacciatori C, Praitano ML, et al. Median nerve small- and large-fiber damage in carpal tunnel syndrome: a quantitative sensory testing study. J Pain 2010;12(2):205–12.

94. Chien A, Eliav E, Sterling M. Whiplash (grade II) and cervical radiculopathy share a similar sensory presentation: an investigation using quantitative sensory testing. Clin J Pain 2008; 24(7):595–603.

95. Tampin B, Slater H, Hall T, et al. Quantitative sensory testing somatosensory profiles in patients with cervical radiculopathy are distinct from those in patients with nonspecific neck-arm pain. Pain 2012;153(12):2403–14.

96. Samuelsson L, Lundin A. Thermal quantitative sensory testing in lumbar disc herniation. Eur Spine J 2002;11(1):71–5.

97. Wilder-Smith EP, Fook-Chong S, Chew SE, et al. Vasomotor dysfunction in carpal tunnel syndrome. Muscle Nerve 2003; 28(5):582–6.

98. Kiylioglu N. Sympathetic skin response and axon counting in carpal tunnel syndrome. J Clin Neurophysiol 2007;24(5):424, author reply.

99. Kuwabara S, Tamura N, Yamanaka Y, et al. Sympathetic sweat responses and skin vasomotor reflexes in carpal tunnel syndrome. Clin Neurol Neurosurg 2008;110(7):691–5.

100. Kiylioglu N, Akyol A, Guney E, et al. Sympathetic skin response in idiopathic and diabetic carpal tunnel syndrome. Clin Neurol Neurosurg 2005;108(1):1–7.

101. Reddeppa S, Bulusu K, Chand PR, et al. The sympathetic skin response in carpal tunnel syndrome. Auton Neurosci 2000; 84(3):119–21.

102. Erdem Tilki H, Coskun M, Unal Akdemir N, et al. Axon count and sympathetic skin responses in lumbosacral radiculopathy. J Clin Neurol 2014;10(1):10–16.

103. Arendt-Nielsen L, Gregersen H, Toft E, et al. Involvement of thin afferents in carpal tunnel syndrome: evaluated quantitatively by argon laser stimulation. Muscle Nerve 1991;14(6): 508–14.

104. Ramieri G, Stella M, Calcagni M, et al. An immunohistochemical study on cutaneous sensory receptors after chronic median nerve compression in man. Acta Anat 1995;152(3):224–9.

105. Casanova-Molla J, Morales M, Planas-Rigol E, et al. Epidermal Langerhans cells in small fiber neuropathies. Pain 2012;153(5): 982–9.

106. Martinez V, Fletcher D, Martin F, et al. Small fibre impairment predicts neuropathic pain in Guillain-Barre syndrome. Pain 2010;151(1):53–60.

107. Bradl M, Lassmann H. Progressive multiple sclerosis. Semin Immunopathol 2009;31(4):455–65.

108. Watkins LR, Maier SF. Beyond neurons: evidence that immune and glial cells contribute to pathological pain states. Physiol Rev 2002;82(4):981–1011.

109. Wieseler-Frank J, Maier SF, Watkins LR. Immune-to-brain communication dynamically modulates pain: physiological and pathological consequences. Brain Behav Immun 2005;19(2):104–11.

110. Thacker MA, Clark AK, Marchand F, et al. Pathophysiology of peripheral neuropathic pain: immune cells and molecules. Anesth Analg 2007;105(3):838–47.

111. Moalem G, Tracey DJ. Immune and inflammatory mechanisms in neuropathic pain. Brain Res Rev 2006;51(2):240–64.

112. Otoshi K, Kikuchi S, Konno S, et al. The reactions of glial cells and endoneurial macrophages in the dorsal root ganglion and their contribution to pain-related behavior after application of nucleus pulposus onto the nerve root in rats. Spine 2010; 35(3):264–71.

113. Shamji MF, Allen KD, So S, et al. Gait abnormalities and inflammatory cytokines in an autologous nucleus pulposus model of radiculopathy. Spine 2009;34(7):648–54.

114. Gupta R, Channual JC. Spatiotemporal pattern of macrophage recruitment after chronic nerve compression injury. J Neurotrauma 2006;23(2):216–26.

115. Hirata K, Kawabuchi M. Myelin phagocytosis by macrophages and nonmacrophages during Wallerian degeneration. Microsc Res Tech 2002;57(6):541–7.

116. Schmid AB, Nee RJ, Coppieters MW. Reappraising entrapment neuropathies – mechanisms, diagnosis and management. Man Ther 2013;18(6):449–57.

117. Tofaris GK, Patterson PH, Jessen KR, et al. Denervated Schwann cells attract macrophages by secretion of leukemia inhibitory factor (LIF) and monocyte chemoattractant protein-1 in a process regulated by interleukin-6 and LIF. J Neurosci 2002;22(15): 6696–703.

118. Sorkin LS, Xiao WH, Wagner R, et al. Tumour necrosis factor-alpha induces ectopic activity in nociceptive primary afferent fibres. Neuroscience 1997;81(1):255–62.

119. Grossmann L, Gorodetskaya N, Baron R, et al. Enhancement of ectopic discharge in regenerating A- and C-fibers by inflammatory mediators. J Neurophysiol 2009;101(6):2762–74.

120. Takebayashi T, Cavanaugh JM, Cuneyt Ozaktay A, et al. Effect of nucleus pulposus on the neural activity of dorsal root ganglion. Spine 2001;26(8):940–5.

121. Marshall S, Tardif G, Ashworth N. Local corticosteroid injection for carpal tunnel syndrome. Cochrane Database Syst Rev 2007;(2):CD001554.

122. Benoist M, Boulu P, Hayem G. Epidural steroid injections in the management of low-back pain with radiculopathy: an update of their efficacy and safety. Eur Spine J 2012;21(2):204–13.

123. Bove GM, Ransil BJ, Lin HC, et al. Inflammation induces ectopic mechanical sensitivity in axons of nociceptors innervating deep tissues. J Neurophysiol 2003;90(3):1949–55.

124. Asbury AK, Fields HL. Pain due to peripheral nerve damage: an hypothesis. Neurology 1984;34(12):1587–90.

125. Takahata S, Takebayashi T, Terasima Y, et al. Activation of glial cells in the spinal cord of a model of lumbar radiculopathy. J Orthop Sci 2011;16(3):313–20.

126. Rothman SM, Nicholson KJ, Winkelstein BA. Time-dependent mechanics and measures of glial activation and behavioral sensitivity in a rodent model of radiculopathy. J Neurotrauma 2010;27(5):803–14.

127. Rothman SM, Winkelstein BA. Chemical and mechanical nerve root insults induce differential behavioral sensitivity and glial activation that are enhanced in combination. Brain Res 2007;1181:30–43.

128. Hu P, Bembrick AL, Keay KA, et al. Immune cell involvement in dorsal root ganglia and spinal cord after chronic constriction or transection of the rat sciatic nerve. Brain Behav Immun 2007;21(5):599–616.

129. Hu P, McLachlan EM. Macrophage and lymphocyte invasion of dorsal root ganglia after peripheral nerve lesions in the rat. Neuroscience 2002;112(1):23–38.

130. Koltzenburg M, Wall PD, McMahon SB. Does the right side know what the left is doing? Trends Neurosci 1999;22(3):122–7.

131. Caliandro P, La Torre G, Aprile I, et al. Distribution of paresthesias in carpal tunnel syndrome reflects the degree of nerve damage at wrist. Clin Neurophysiol 2006;117(1):228–31.

132. Murphy DR, Hurwitz EL, Gerrard JK, et al. Pain patterns and descriptions in patients with radicular pain: does the pain necessarily follow a specific dermatome? Chiropr Osteopat 2009;17:9.

133. Zanette G, Cacciatori C, Tamburin S. Central sensitization in carpal tunnel syndrome with extraterritorial spread of sensory symptoms. Pain 2010;148(2):227–36.

134. Viader A, Golden JP, Baloh RH, et al. Schwann cell mitochondrial metabolism supports long-term axonal survival and peripheral nerve function. J Neurosci 2011;31(28):10128–40.

135. Szolcsanyi J. Capsaicin-sensitive sensory nerve terminals with local and systemic efferent functions: facts and scopes of an unorthodox neuroregulatory mechanism. Prog Brain Res 1996;113:343–59.

136. Schmelz M, Michael K, Weidner C, et al. Which nerve fibers mediate the axon reflex flare in human skin? Neuroreport 2000;11(3):645–8.

137. Schmelz M, Luz O, Averbeck B, et al. Plasma extravasation and neuropeptide release in human skin as measured by intradermal microdialysis. Neurosci Lett 1997;230(2):117–20.

138. Sauer SK, Bove GM, Averbeck B, et al. Rat peripheral nerve components release calcitonin gene-related peptide and prostaglandin E2 in response to noxious stimuli: evidence that nervi nervorum are nociceptors. Neuroscience 1999;92(1):319–25.

139. Kobayashi S, Kokubo Y, Uchida K, et al. Effect of lumbar nerve root compression on primary sensory neurons and their central branches: changes in the nociceptive neuropeptides substance P and somatostatin. Spine 2005;30(3):276–82.

140. Dahlin LB, McLean WG. Effects of graded experimental compression on slow and fast axonal transport in rabbit vagus nerve. J Neurol Sci 1986;72(1):19–30.

141. Dahlin LB, Rydevik B, McLean WG, et al. Changes in fast axonal transport during experimental nerve compression at low pressures. Exp Neurol 1984;84(1):29–36.

142. Dahlin LB, Sjostrand J, McLean WG. Graded inhibition of retrograde axonal transport by compression of rabbit vagus nerve. J Neurol Sci 1986;76(2–3):221–30.

143. Ando Y. Experimental study on chronic entrapment neuropathy. Nippon Seikeigeka Gakkai Zasshi 1990;64(7):633–47.

144. Armstrong BD, Hu Z, Abad C, et al. Induction of neuropeptide gene expression and blockade of retrograde transport in facial motor neurons following local peripheral nerve inflammation in severe combined immunodeficiency and BALB/C mice. Neuroscience 2004;129(1):93–9.

145. Dilley A, Bove GM. Disruption of axoplasmic transport induces mechanical sensitivity in intact rat C-fibre nociceptor axons. J Physiol 2008;586(2):593–604.

146. Upton AR, McComas AJ. The double crush in nerve entrapment syndromes. Lancet 1973;2(7825):359–62.

147. Schmid AB, Coppieters MW. The double crush syndrome revisited – a Delphi study to reveal current expert views on mechanisms underlying dual nerve disorders. Man Ther 2011;16(6):557–62.

148. Morgan G, Wilbourn AJ. Cervical radiculopathy and coexisting distal entrapment neuropathies: double-crush syndromes? Neurology 1998;50(1):78–83.

149. Mor D, Bembrick AL, Austin PJ, et al. Evidence for cellular injury in the midbrain of rats following chronic constriction injury of the sciatic nerve. J Chem Neuroanat 2011;41(3):158–69.

150. LeBlanc BW, Zerah ML, Kadasi LM, et al. Minocycline injection in the ventral posterolateral thalamus reverses microglial reactivity and thermal hyperalgesia secondary to sciatic neuropathy. Neurosci Lett 2011;498(2):138–42.

151. Latremoliere A, Woolf CJ. Central sensitization: a generator of pain hypersensitivity by central neural plasticity. J Pain 2009;10(9):895–926.

152. Druschky K, Kaltenhauser M, Hummel C, et al. Alteration of the somatosensory cortical map in peripheral mononeuropathy due to carpal tunnel syndrome. Neuroreport 2000;11(17):3925–30.

153. Napadow V, Kettner N, Ryan A, et al. Somatosensory cortical plasticity in carpal tunnel syndrome–a cross-sectional fMRI evaluation. Neuroimage 2006;31(2):520–30.

154. Napadow V, Kettner N, Liu J, et al. Hypothalamus and amygdala response to acupuncture stimuli in carpal tunnel syndrome. Pain 2007.

155. Tecchio F, Padua L, Aprile I, et al. Carpal tunnel syndrome modifies sensory hand cortical somatotopy: a MEG study. Hum Brain Mapp 2002;17(1):28–36.

156. Nora DB, Becker J, Ehlers JA, et al. Clinical features of 1039 patients with neurophysiological diagnosis of carpal tunnel syndrome. Clin Neurol Neurosurg 2004;107(1):64–9.

FUNCTIONAL ANATOMY

CHAPTER 9.1 ■ THE CERVICAL SPINE

Gail Forrester-Gale • Ioannis Paneris

INTRODUCTION

The following chapter aims to review and highlight the key anatomical and biomechanical features of the craniocervical region that are relevant to and support clinical practice.

The occiput, atlas, axis and surrounding soft tissues are collectively referred to as the craniocervical region. It is a unique spinal region that exhibits highly specialized anatomy and considerable mobility in comparison to other spinal regions. Of particular note are the atypical, modified vertebrae (the atlas and axis), the absence of intervertebral discs, the presence of an odontoid peg and the configuration of double convex joints bilaterally at the C1–C2 articulation.[1]

The atlas (C1) and axis (C2) together with the occiput form a unique triad of articulations referred to as the occipito–atlantoaxial (O-AA) complex. This complex is responsible for approximately one-third or 20° of the total cervical sagittal plane movements of flexion and extension.[2–8] In vivo movement analysis studies report that 4–7° of flexion and 17–21° of extension occur across this complex with the majority of this movement occurring specifically at the atlanto-occipital joint (C0-C1).[4–8] The atlanto-occipital joint (A-O joint) configuration is specifically designed to facilitate upper cervical flexion and extension (retraction and protraction). The lack of intervertebral disc along with the congruous joint surfaces, which are long and thin and orientated in a posterior–anterior direction, facilitate the nodding movement of the head on neck.[2,5,8]

Clinically, in situations where craniocervical spine (CCS) pain is associated with movements of upper cervical flexion and extension, the A-O joint should be a primary consideration in terms of assessment and treatment.

Axial rotation is the largest range of motion available across the O-AA complex.[1] Studies consistently show that the atlanto-axial joint (A-A joint; Fig. 9-1) provides 60% of the total cervical rotation, which amounts to approximately 38–56° to each side.[1,5,9–11] This is unsurprising,

as anatomically the A-A joint is specifically designed for rotation. It has a central pivot joint between the odontoid peg and the osseoligamentous ring formed by the transverse ligament and anterior arch of the atlas, double convex joints bilaterally and it lacks an intervertebral disc.[1,12,13] In addition to its large range of rotation, in vivo studies on asymptomatic subjects have shown that the A-A joint plays a key role in the initiation of cervical rotation.[9,14] Cervical rotation has been shown to start at the C1–C2 level and to continue sequentially down the cervical spine with each joint moving only once the preceding joint has completed its range of movement.[1,14]

CRANIOCERVICAL-COUPLED MOVEMENTS AND CLINICAL IMPLICATIONS

Alongside movement analysis studies exploring the range and direction of CCS mobility, there is a growing body of evidence from in vivo three-dimensional computed tomography (3D CT) scan studies demonstrating the coupling of movements occurring in the CCS.[15–19] A recent study by Salem et al. carried out on 20

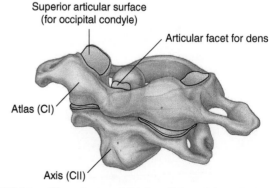

FIGURE 9-1 ■ The atlanto-axial joint. (Adapted from Drake et al. Grey's Anatomy for Students. Edinburgh: Churchill Livingstone; 2005.)

Superior articular surface (for occipital condyle)

Articular facet for dens

Atlas (CI)

Axis (CII)

asymptomatic participants used up-to-date imaging techniques (3D CT kinematic analysis) to explore the coupled motion patterns of the CCS in maximal axial rotation.[1] This study found that rotation in the CCS was consistently coupled with contralateral lateral flexion, which is in contrast to the ipsilateral coupling pattern found in the sub-axial cervical spine.[20]

SYNOVIAL FOLDS IN THE CRANIOCERVICAL SPINE

The synovial folds of the CCS are formed by wedge-shaped folds of synovial membrane.[21-24] They have an abundant vascular network and are innervated.[21,25] The composition of the synovial folds varies across the craniocervical region possibly due to the different amounts of mechanical stress they are subjected to at each level. The synovial folds found at the A-O joint do not project between the joint surfaces and are therefore unlikely to be exposed to mechanical stresses. They are composed of adipose-type synovial membrane. The synovial folds of the A-A articulation, however, project as far as 5 mm between the articular surfaces and will therefore be exposed to mechanical stresses. They are formed of a stronger more fibrous type of synovial membrane.[21,24,25]

The synovial folds have been suggested to perform various functions in the CCS. They have been described as 'passive space fillers' serving to fill non-congruent areas of the joint and thus enhance joint congruity and stability. They may also help to protect or lubricate the articular surfaces and assist in weight bearing or shock absorption.[21] Additionally, the CCS synovial folds may have a proprioceptive role providing mechanosensory information important for sensorimotor control in the upper cervical spine.[25]

THE ANATOMY OF CRANIOCERVICAL STABILITY AND CLINICAL IMPLICATIONS

CCS stability is provided through a combination of mechanical restraint from the ligamentous system and sensorimotor control from the neuromuscular system.[26-33]

Ligamentous System

The chief mechanical restraints of the craniocervical region are generally recognized as the transverse and alar ligaments with other ligaments such as the tectorial membrane, capsular ligaments, ligamentum flavum, A-A ligaments, ligamentum nuchea, posterior atlanto-occipital membranes and atlanto-axial membranes acting as secondary stabilizers (Fig. 9-2).[15,17,34-36]

Clinical Anatomy and Biomechanics of the Alar Ligaments

There is consensus in the literature that the alar ligaments provide the main passive restraints to contralateral axial rotation and lateral flexion across the O-AA complex.[16,17,37,38] They are strong, collagenous cords approximately 1 cm in length, which run from the posterolateral aspect of the odontoid peg to the medial surface of the occipital condyles.[15] Due to their posterior attachment on the odontoid peg, they are wound around the process during contralateral axial rotation and become maximally tightened at 90° cervical rotation. Further stretch can be added to these ligaments with the addition of upper cervical flexion.[16,17,34]

Clinical Anatomy and Biomechanics of the Transverse Ligament and Relevance to Clinical Testing

Magnetic resonance imaging (MRI) studies on healthy participants have confirmed findings from cadaveric studies that the transverse ligament is a broad collagenous band, approximately 2.5 mm thick, which extends across the atlantal ring directly behind the odontoid peg and attaches to the medial aspect of each lateral mass of the atlas.[16,31] It acts like a sling and serves to hold the odontoid peg against the anterior arch of the atlas. In this way it restricts forward translation of the atlas in relation to the axis particularly during movements of cervical flexion.[35,39]

Clinical Anatomy and Biomechanics of the Tectorial Membrane and Relevance to Clinical Testing

Combined findings from in vitro cadaveric studies and in vivo MRI scan studies concur that the tectorial membrane is a broad fibroelastic band, approximately 5–7.5 cm in length, 1.5–3 cm in width and 1–1.5 mm thick.[37,40] Recent anatomical and radiological studies have confirmed that it originates on the posterior surface of the C2 body and runs vertically upwards, as a specialized cranial continuation of the posterior longitudinal ligament, attaching to the basilar grove of the occipital bone.[35,37] It is adherent to the anterio superior dura mater that may be of clinical relevance in patients with whiplash-associated disorder (WAD) or other disorders presenting with head, neck or facial pain and altered response to neurodynamic testing such as passive neck flexion.[36,40-42] The tectorial membrane becomes taught at 15° of craniocervical flexion; however, anatomical studies suggest that its primary role is not to limit craniocervical flexion but to prevent posterior migration of the odontoid peg into the cervical spinal canal.[37,40] Due to its high elastin content it is thought that the membrane acts as a hammock, stretching and tightening over the odontoid peg in craniocervical flexion thus assisting the transverse ligament in preventing a posterior movement of the odontoid peg into the spinal canal and preventing impingement of the peg onto the spinal cord.[36,40]

Craniocervical Muscles and Their Clinical Significance

The key muscles acting directly on the CCS are the suboccipital muscle (SOM) group posteriorly and the craniocervical flexor (CCF) muscle group anteriorly.

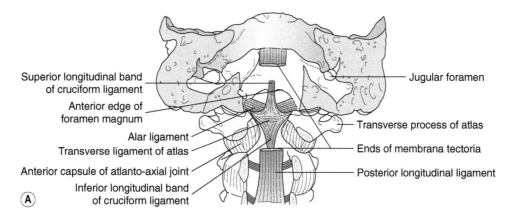

Superior longitudinal band of cruciform ligament
Anterior edge of foramen magnum
Alar ligament
Transverse ligament of atlas
Anterior capsule of atlanto-axial joint
Inferior longitudinal band of cruciform ligament
Jugular foramen
Transverse process of atlas
Ends of membrana tectoria
Posterior longitudinal ligament

(A)

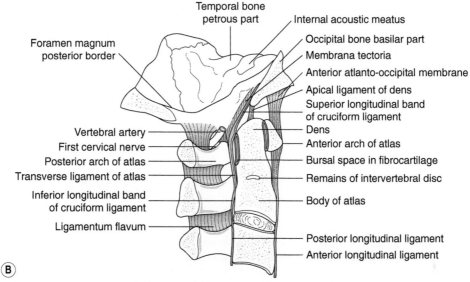

Temporal bone petrous part
Internal acoustic meatus
Foramen magnum posterior border
Occipital bone basilar part
Membrana tectoria
Anterior atlanto-occipital membrane
Apical ligament of dens
Superior longitudinal band of cruciform ligament
Vertebral artery
First cervical nerve
Posterior arch of atlas
Transverse ligament of atlas
Inferior longitudinal band of cruciform ligament
Ligamentum flavum
Dens
Anterior arch of atlas
Bursal space in fibrocartilage
Remains of intervertebral disc
Body of atlas
Posterior longitudinal ligament
Anterior longitudinal ligament

(B)

FIGURE 9-2 ■ The craniocervical ligamentous system.

Both groups are composed of short, deep segmental muscles that largely function to provide segmental control and support to the craniocervical joints.[18,43–46] Both muscle groups have been shown to contain a high density of muscle receptors, particularly muscle spindles, with the largest concentration of muscle spindles being found in the SOM.[18,19,46–48] This would suggest that both these muscle groups are likely to act primarily as sensory receptors monitoring and controlling the position, direction, amplitude and velocity of craniocervical joint movement and therefore have an important role in the maintenance of dynamic stability in the CCS. In addition, afferent information from the SOM and CCF muscle spindles is integrated with information from the vestibular and visual apparatus via the vestibular nuclei and is thus involved in various postural reflexes in the control of balance.[49–51]

The CCF muscle group include longus capitis (LCap), rectus capitis anterior (RCA), rectus capitus lateralis (RCL) and longus colli (Fig. 9-3). The first three muscles all have an attachment in the CCS. LCap arises from the transverse processes of the third to sixth cervical vertebrae and ascends to insert onto the inferior surface of the occiput. It is narrow subaxially but broad and thick in the CCS.[3,13,44]

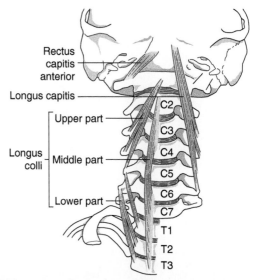

Rectus capitis anterior
Longus capitis
Upper part
Longus colli
Middle part
Lower part
C2
C3
C4
C5
C6
C7
T1
T2
T3

FIGURE 9-3 ■ The craniocervical flexor muscle group. (Adapted from Palastanga et al. Anatomy and Human Movement. Edinburgh: Churchill Livingstone; 2006.)

The RCA muscle is a short, flat muscle, situated immediately behind the upper part of the LCap. It arises from the anterior surface of the lateral mass of the atlas, and passes obliquely upward and medially to insert on the inferior surface of the occiput in front of the foramen magnum. The RCL is another short, flat muscle, which arises from the upper surface of the transverse process of the atlas, and is inserted onto the undersurface of the jugular process of the occiput.[3,13,51-53]

Acting as a group, the CCF muscle group provides support to the cervical lordosis and segmental stability to the cervical spine as a whole. RCA and LCap in particular provide stability to the upper cervical motion segments.[54] In addition to their proprioceptive role, they serve to produce flexion of the upper cervical spine or a nodding movement of the head on the neck.[55]

The SOM group includes rectus capitis posterior major (RCPmajor), rectus capitis posterior minor (RCPminor), obliqus capitis superior (OCS) and obliqus capitis inferior (OCI) (Fig. 9-4).[13,52,53]

RCPminor is stated to be the only muscle with a direct attachment to the atlas (C1). It is documented to arise from the posterior arch of the atlas (C1) and to insert onto the occipital bone below the inferior nuchal line lateral to the midline and medial to RCPmajor.[20]

The RCPmajor muscle is commonly cited to arise from the spinous process of the axis (C2) and to ascend to its insertion on the lateral part of the inferior nuchal line of the occiput.[13] However, Scali et al. carried out an anatomical and histological study on 11 cadavers primarily to explore the atlanto-axial interspace.[56] They found in all 11 cadavers examined that the RCPmajor muscle was firmly attached to the spinous process of the atlas (C1). It would therefore appear that both RCPmajor and RCPminor have an attachment onto the atlas (C1).

The main actions of RCPmajor and RCPminor are extension, side flexion and rotation of the O-AA joint complex. However, studies have shown that both muscles, in particular the RCPminor, have a high density of muscle spindles suggesting that they have a more important role in CCS proprioception than in movement and may help to stabilize the atlas in relation to the occiput.[18,19,47] This has been supported by a recent electromyographic study on RCPminor muscles that demonstrated activity in the muscle with the head in a neutral position but significantly increased activity with the head in a retracted position.[46]

Anatomical connections between the anterior surfaces of RCPmajor and RCPminor muscles and the posterior cervical spinal dura mater through fibrous connective tissue or myodural bridges have been consistently reported.[56-58] These connections may provide a form of anchorage for the dura mater but more importantly, due to findings of proprioceptive fibres throughout the myodural connections, are believed to be involved in the monitoring and controlling of dural tension during flexion and extension movements of the head and neck.[46,56] Additionally, the fibrous bridge may provide proprioceptive information regarding the position of the AO and AA joints to help prevent infolding of the pain-sensitive dura mater during head and neck movements.[46,56] Clinically, the myodural bridges between the SOM and the cervical spinal dura may be of relevance in relation to cervicogenic headache.[46,56,59-61]

The OCS is a small muscle arising from the lateral mass of the atlas (C1) ascending to attach onto the lateral half of the inferior nuchal line on the occiput. It acts at the A-O joint to extend and side flex the head. The OCI muscle is the larger of the two oblique craniocervical muscles. It lies deep to semispinalis capitus, arising from the apex of the spinous process of the axis (C2) and passing laterally and upwards to insert on the posterior aspect of the transverse process of the atlas (C1). It is responsible for rotation of the A-A joint.[13] Similarly to RCPmajor and RCPminor, both OCS and OCI have a high density of Golgi tendon organs and muscle spindles indicating that proprioception is likely to be the primary role of these and indeed all the SOM allowing for accurate positioning of the head on the neck.

MID TO LOW CERVICAL SPINE

Although the first, second and seventh vertebrae have special features, the rest of the vertebrae of the cervical spine are almost identical with the sixth having only minor distinguishing features.[62]

The Vertebral Body

The typical vertebra consists of two parts: the vertebral body and the vertebral arch. The body of the typical vertebra is a relatively small and broad mass of trabecular, spongy bone covered by a layer of cortical bone.[63] The shape of the cervical vertebral body is oval with the transverse diameter being greater than the anteroposterior diameter and height.[63] The cervical intervertebral joints are saddle-shaped and they consist of two concavities facing each other at 90°.[64] The opposing surfaces of the

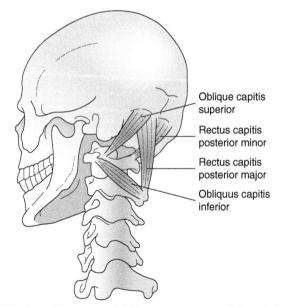

Oblique capitis superior

Rectus capitis posterior minor

Rectus capitis posterior major

Obliquus capitis inferior

FIGURE 9-4 ■ The suboccipital muscle group. (Adapted from Middleditch & Oliver. Functional Anatomy of the Spine. Edinburgh: Butterworth Heinnemann; 2005.)

vertebral bodies are gently curved in the sagittal plane with the anterior part of the vertebra sloping downwards partially overlapping the anterior surface of the intervertebral disc. The superior surface of the vertebral body is also curved on the coronal plane forming a concavity of which its sides are the uncinate processes.[62]

The uncinate processes are projections that arise from most of the circumference of the upper margin of the vertebral body of C3 to C7. Although the uncinate processes are present in utero, they start to enlarge gradually between the ages of 9 to 14 years reaching their maximum height.[63,65] In mature spines the uncinate processes articulate with the superior vertebra at its incisures forming the uncovertebral joints or joints of Luschka. The size of the uncinate processes varies slightly from level to level. Their average height ranges from 3–6.1 mm and the anteroposterior length from 5–8.3 mm,[66] and they are significantly higher at C4 to C6 compares to C3 and C7 levels.[67]

The uncinate processes and the uncovertebral joints limit side flexion of the cervical spine and stabilize the intervertebral disc in the coronal plane during axial rotation.[5] The uncovertebral joints play a stabilizing role primarily in extension and side flexion followed by torsion.[68] The uncinate processes, by forming the saddle shape of the superior surface of the vertebra, working together with the zygapophyseal joints dictate the coupling movement of side flexion and ipsilateral rotation of the vertebrae of the low cervical spine on an the axis perpendicular to the plane of the facet joints.[64,69]

The Vertebral Arch

The vertebral arch consists of the pedicles and the laminae. The pedicles are short, projecting posterolaterally and arising midway between the discal surfaces of the vertebral bodies making the superior and inferior vertebral notches of similar depth. The laminae are longer and thinner and project posteromedially. They have a thinner superior border compared to the inferior and they are slightly curved. The junction of the laminar forms the spinous process which is short and bifid and the two tubercles being often of unequal size.

The junction of the pedicle with the ipsilateral lamina bulges laterally forming the superior and inferior articular processes. The articulations between the superior and inferior processes (facet or zygapophyseal joints) form the articular pillar (lateral mass) on each side. The superior articular processes are flat, oval-shaped and face superoposteriorly. Small morphological differences exist for the superior articular processes of the C3 which, in addition to facing superiorly and posteriorly, also face medially to about 40°. Also, the superior articular facets of C3 lie slightly inferiorly in relation to their vertebral body compared to the rest of the typical cervical levels.[64] This morphological specificity of the superior processes of the C3 lead to alteration of the biomechanical behaviour at the C2–C3 level. Indeed, the expected coupling of ipsilateral rotation and side flexion does not seem to exist at this level. The medial orientation on the facets at this level serves to minimize rotation, thus stabilizing the C2 during rotational movements of the neck.[14] On average

a contralateral rotation and side flexion pattern seem to take place on C2.[64] The orientation of the superior facets in relation to the transverse plane seems to change gradually from posteromedially at C3 to posterolaterally at C7 to T1. However this change could be either gradual or sudden and the level of change of the orientation was not constant, occurring at any level of the lower cervical spine with the most common being the level of C5–C6.[70] The shape of the superior articular facets gradually changes from almost circular at the level of C3, to oval with an elongated transverse diameter at C7.[70]

The cervical zygapophyseal joints were found to be the most common source of pain after whiplash injury.[71] This could be due to the mechanical compressional and shear forces applied to the dorsal part of the joints during this form of impact.[72-74] Further, the absence of articular cartilage, especially at the dorsal part of the joint, could lead to impingement and bone to bone contact and trauma.[75] The facet joint capsule consists of bundles of dense, regularly arranged, collagen fibres, containing elongated nuclei of fibroblasts and loose connective tissue with areas of adipose-like tissue.[76,77] Fibroblasts with ovoid and round nuclei are found within the loose connective tissue.[76] The capsule of the lower cervical spine is also covered by an average of 22.4% by muscle fibres, possibly by the semispinalis and multifidi, suggesting a potential path for loading of the facet capsule.[78] A number of animal and human cadaveric studies have verified the presence of mechanoreceptors and nociceptors in the capsules of the cervical facet joints.[76,77,79-81] The dorsal part of the cervical facet joint is innervated by the dorsal ramus via its middle branch.[41]

Intra-articular inclusions, or synovial folds, are present in the majority of the zygapophyseal joints. Because of the location, to the ventral and dorsal parts of the joints, it has been hypothesized that they act as space fillers protecting the parts of the cartilage that become exposed during translatory movements by maintaining a film of synovial fluid between themselves and the cartilage. In addition, and due to their fibrous consistency, it has also been hypothesized that meniscoids could play a role in mechanical stress distribution.[82] Although, an earlier study has indicated that intra-articular meniscoids are features of cervical spine in the first two decades of life,[83] more recent cadaveric studies have confirmed their presence in the majority of facet joints of cervical spines of advanced age.[82,84]

Ligaments

The main ligaments that are associated with the intervertebral and zygapophyseal joints are the anterior longitudinal ligament, the posterior longitudinal ligament and the ligamentum flavum.

The anterior longitudinal ligament (ALL) is attached to the anterior surfaces of the vertebral bodies and discs.[62] The ALL is comprised of four layers with distinguishable patterns of attachment.[85] The fibres of the superficial layer of the ALL run longitudinally crossing several segments and they are attached to the central areas of the anterior surfaces of the vertebral bodies. They cover roughly the middle two-quarters of the anterior vertebral bodies and, in contrast to the upper cervical levels, at the lower cervical segments the fibres of the ALL are less densely packed and the ligament expands laterally. The fibres of the second layer also run longitudinally. At this layer the fibres cover one intervertebral disc and attach to the anterior surfaces of the inferior and superior vertebrae but never further than half way up or down that surface. The fibres of the third layer are similar to the ones of the second one in orientation, but these fibres are shorter, covering one intervertebral disc and attaching just cranial of caudal to the margins of the adjacent vertebrae. The fibres of the fourth layer are of more alar disposition. They arise from the anterior surface of the vertebra above, close to its inferior margin, and passing inferiorly and laterally insert to the vertebra below just inferiorly to its superior margin. The most lateral of these fibres reach the summit of the uncinate processes.[85]

The posterior longitudinal ligament (PLL) covers the entire posterior surface of the vertebral bodies in the vertebral canal, attaching to the central posterior surfaces of the vertebral bodies and has three distinct layers.[85] The superficial layer contains longitudinal fibres that bridge three to four vertebrae and lateral extensions that extend inferolaterally from the central band to cross an intervertebral disc and attach to the base of the pedicle one or two levels below.[85] The fibres of the intermediate layer are longitudinal, span only one intervertebral disc and occupy a narrow area close to the midline of the posterior surface of the vertebral body. The deep layer consists of fibres that cover one intervertebral disc and arise from the inferior margin of the cephalad vertebra and extend inferiorly and laterally to the superior margin of the caudal vertebrae. The most lateral fibres extend in an alar fashion to the posterior end of the base of the uncinate process.[85] In the cervical spine the ALL and the deep layer of the PPL are continuous, surrounding the entire vertebral body while the superficial layer of the PPL surrounds the dura matter, nerve root and the vertebral artery suggesting a dual role for this structure: as a conventional ligament; and as a protective membrane for the soft tissues inside the vertebral canal.[86]

The ligamentum flavum (LF) connects the laminae of the adjacent vertebra and extends from the facet joint capsules to the point where the laminae fuse to form the spines.[62] In the low cervical spine the majority of ligamenta flava do not fuse at the midline,[87] leaving gaps that admit veins connecting the internal and posterior external venous plexuses.[62] The LF consists of yellow elastic and collagen fibres that are longitudinal in orientation connecting the anterior surface and lower margin of the lamina above to the posterior surface and upper margin of the lamina below. At the cervical spine the LF is thin, broad and long and it limits separation of the laminae in flexion and assists restoration of the neutral posture after flexion.[62] The LF becomes thinner in cervical flexion and thicker and shortened in extension protruding in the spinal canal to an average of 3.25 mm approximately.[88] At the levels of C6–C7 and C7–T1 the LF is uniquely thick in extension, which may predispose to cord compression.

From the rest of the ligaments of the cervical spine, the ligamentum nuchae (LN) commands the most attention, especially in the mid and low cervical segments. Despite the fact that in most anatomical texts the LN is described as a ligament homologous to the supraspinous and interspinous ligaments, the LN is not a ligament but a structure that consists of a dorsal nuchal raphe and a midline fascial septum.[89] The dorsal raphe and the ventral fascial portions of the LN are a single entity and consist of muscular aponeurotic fibres and in the mid-cervical spine; they are derived from the trapezius and splenius capitis. The aponeurotic fibres decussate at the midline, forming a triangular body representing the dorsal raphe which becomes progressively larger caudally with a progressive increase in aponeurotic fibres. The decussate fibres then project ventrally to attach to the spinous processes of the C2 to C5 vertebrae forming the ventral portion of the LN. At the C6, C7 levels the two portions of the LN are not distinguishable and the LN is formed by horizontal aponeurotic fibres of the trapezius, rhomboideus minor, serratus posterior minor and splenius capitis.[90]

The Intervertebral Disc

The intervertebral disc of the cervical spine shows distinct morphological and histological differences to the rest of the discs of the spinal column. The intervertebral disc consists of the nucleus pulposus and the annulus fibrosus as in the rest of the sections of the spine. However, the nucleus pulposus at birth constitutes no more than 25% of the entire disc and quickly changes from gelatinous to fibrocartilagenous in consistency by the middle of the second decade of life.[65]

The annulus fibrosus has a crescentic form anteriorly with a thick anterior part in the sagittal plane, which becomes progressively thinner when traced to the uncinate processes. The posterior part consists only of a thin layer of collagen fibres. The anterior part of the annulus is covered by a thin layer of collagen fibres. This is a transitional layer between the deepest layers of the anterior longitudinal ligament and the annulus. The fibres of the transitional layer pass inferiorly and diverge laterally, whereas more laterally they pass inferiorly and laterally in a more alar disposition attaching to the edges of the vertebral bodies. The fibres of the annulus fibrosus proper arise laterally from the apex and anterior surface of the uncinate process and the superior part of the inferior disc and run medially to insert on the inferior surface of the vertebrae above. Towards the midline the fibres interweave with the fibres coming from the opposite side. Deeper layers of the annulus progressively originate closer to the midline maintaining the interweaving pattern. At its deepest (2–3 mm), the fibres of the annulus are embedded with proteoglycans to form a fibrocartilagenous mass increasingly becoming less laminated, forming the nucleus of the disc.[85] The posterior part of the annulus is about 1 mm thin and covers a small posteromedial section. Its fibres run vertically between the facing surfaces of the adjacent vertebral bodies. The rest of the posterior fibrocartilagenous core to the uncus either side is covered by periosteofascial tissue.[65,85]

The Intervertebral Foramina and Spinal Nerves

The cervical spinal nerves exit the spinal cord in an oblique orientation towards their respective neural foramen.[91] The intervertebral foramen is shaped as a funnel with its narrowest part medially and its borders are comprised by the pedicles of the superior and inferior vertebrae, the facet joint posteriorly and the disc and uncovertebral joint anteriorly.[91,92] The foramina are also larger in the upper cervical spine becoming gradually narrower at lower levels with the narrowest at the C7–T1 level.[91] The anatomical cadaveric study of Tanaka et al.[92] provided significant findings regarding the anatomy of the cervical nerve roots that have clinical implications. The spinal nerve is comprised of the ventral and dorsal nerve roots. The ventral nerve root lies caudal to the dorsal root and courses along the caudal border of the dorsal nerve root in the intervertebral foramen. The ventral root is approximately two-thirds the size of the dorsal root.

Further, at the level of C4-C5 intervertebral foramen the majority of the C5 nerve roots are situated caudal or just anterior to the intervertebral disc. The majority of the C6 and C7 nerve roots lie cephalad to the intervertebral disc while the vast majority of the C8 nerve roots have no contact with the disc. Furthermore, below the level of C5 the nerve rootlets, which comprise the ventral and dorsal nerve roots, pass downwards with increased obliquity reaching their corresponding intervertebral foramina, with the dorsal rootlets of C5, C6 and C7 forming a number of intra-dural connections. The consequence is that whichever nerve root is going to be compressed, the dorsal, the ventral or perhaps both, depends upon the compressing structure (disc, superior facet joint or ligamentum flavum) and its anatomical relationship to the nerve root. In addition, the course of the rootlets and the interconnections between the dorsal rootlets can explain the spread of clinical signs and symptoms in more than one nerve root from disc herniations, as well as the variation and overlapping sensory symptoms cause by nerve root compression.[92]

The spinal nerves at the lower cervical spine have significant connective tissue attachments posteriorly to the medial end of the intervertebral foramina, the capsules of the zygapophyseal joints, the periosteum of the inferior pedicles and anteriorly to the vertebral bodies, the intervertebral discs and the posterior longitudinal ligament.[93] All the above structures are innervated by the sinuvertebral nerve (intervertebral discs, posterior longitudinal ligament and ventrolateral spinal canal periosteum) and by the cervical dorsal ramus (zygapophyseal joints). The potential of those structures to evoke pain could render the findings of the neural tension tests more difficult to interpret.[93]

REFERENCES

1. Salem W, Lenders C, Mathieu J, et al. In vivo three-dimensional kinematics of the cervical spine during maximal axial rotation. Man Ther 2013;18:339–44.
2. Chancey V, Ottaviano D, Myers B, et al. A kinematic and anthropometric study of the upper cervical spine and the occipital condyles. J Biomech 2007;40:1953–9.
3. Jull G, Sterling M, Falla D, et al. Whiplash, Headache and Neck Pain. Research-Based Direction for Physical Therapists. Edinburgh: Churchill Livingstone; 2008.
4. Amiri M, Jull G, Bullock-Saxton J. Measurement of upper cervical flexion and extension with the 3-space fastrak measurement system: a repeatability study. J Man Manip Ther 2003;11(4):198–203.
5. Panjabi M, Crisco J, Vasavada A, et al. Mechanical properties of the human cervical spine as shown by three-dimensional load displacement curves. Spine 2001;26(24):2692–700.
6. Ordway N, Seymour R, Donelson R, et al. Cervical flexion, extension, protrusion and retraction: a radiographic segmental analysis. Spine 1999;24(3):240–7.
7. Panjabi M, Dvorak J, Duranceau J, et al. Three-dimensional movements of the upper cervical spine. Spine 1988;13(7):726–30.
8. Bogduk N, Mercer S. Biomechanics of the cervical spine. I: normal kinematics. Clin Biomech 2000;15:633–48.
9. Ishii T, Mukai Y, Hosono N, et al. Kinematics of the cervical spine in rotation in vivo three-dimensional analysis. Spine 2004;29(7):139–44.
10. Iai H, Moriya H, Goto S, et al. Three-dimensional motion analysis of the upper cervical spine during axial rotation. Spine 1993;18(16):2388–92.
11. Mimura M, Moriya H, Watanabe T, et al. Three dimensional motion analysis of the cervical spine with special reference to axial rotation. Spine 1989;14(11):1135–9.
12. Palastanga N, Field D, Soames R. Anatomy and Human Movement. Structure and Function. 5th ed. Butterworth Heinnemann, Elsevier; 2006.
13. Standring S. Gray's Anatomy. 40th ed. Churchill Livingstone; 2008.
14. Hino H, Abumi K, Kanayama M, et al. Dynamic motion analysis of normal and unstable cervical spines using cineradiography. An in vivo study. Spine 1999;24(2):163–8.
15. Crisco J, Panjabi M, Dvorak J. A model of the alar ligaments of the upper cervical spine in axial rotation. J Biomech 1991;24(7):607–14.
16. Dvorak J, Schneider E, Saldinger P, et al. Biomechanics of the craniocervical region; the alar and transverse ligaments. J Orthop Res 1988;6:452–61.
17. Dvorak J, Panajabi M. Functional anatomy of the alar ligaments. Spine 1987;12(2):183–9.
18. McPartland J, Brodeur R. Rectus capitus posterior minor: a small but important suboccipital muscle. J Bodyw Mov Ther 1999;3(1):30–5.
19. Boyd Clark L, Briggs C, Galea M. Comparative histochemical composition of muscle fibres in a pre and post-vertebral muscle of the cervical spine. J Anat 2001;199:709–16.
20. Cook C, Hegedus E, Showalter C, et al. Coupling behaviour of the cervical spine: a systematic review of the literature. J Manipulative Physiol Ther 2006;29(7):570–5.
21. Mercer S, Bogduk N. Intra-articular inclusions of the cervical synovial joints. Br J Rheumatol 1993;32(8):705–10.
22. Friedrich K, Reiter G, Pretterklieber M, et al. Reference data for in vivo MRI properties of meniscoids in the cervical zygapophyseal joints. Spine 2008;33(21):E778–83.
23. Webb A, Darekar A, Sampson M, et al. Synoival folds of the lateral atlanto-axial joints: in vivo quantitative assessment using MRI in healthy volunteers. Spine 2009;34(19):E697–702.
24. Tang X, Liu L, Yang H, et al. Anatomic study of the synovial folds of the O-AA joints. Clin Anat 2007;20(4):376–81.
25. Inami S, Shiga T, Tsujino A, et al. Immunohistochemical demonstration of nerve fibres in the synovial folds of the human cervical facet joint. J Orthop Res 2001;19:593–6.
26. Goel V, Winterbottom J, Schulte K, et al. Ligamentous laxity across C0-C1-C2 complex. Axial torque-rotation characteristics until failure. Spine 1990;15(10):990–6.
27. Panjabi M, Dvorak J, Duranceau J, et al. Three-dimensional movements of the upper cervical spine. Spine 1988;13(7):726–30.
28. Panjabi M. The stabilising system of the spine. Part I. Function, dysfunction, adaptation and enhancement. J Spinal Disord 1992a;5(4):383–9.
29. Panjabi M. The stabilising system of the spine. Part II. Neutral zone and instability hypothesis. J Spinal Disord 1992b;5(4):390–7.

30. Panjabi M, Abumi K, Duranceau J, et al. Spinal stability and inter-segmental muscle forces: a biomechanical model. Spine 1989;14:194–200.
31. Panjabi M, Lydon C, Vasavada A, et al. On the understanding of clinical instability. Spine 1994;19(23):2642–50.
32. Panjabi M, Cholewicki J, Nibu K, et al. Critical load of the human cervical spine: an in vitro experimental study. Clin Biomech 1998;13:11–17.
33. Brolin K, Halldin P. Development of a finite model of the upper cervical spine in a parameter study of ligament characteristics. Spine 2004;29(4):376–85.
34. Goel V, Winterbottom J, Schulte K, et al. Ligamentous laxity across C0-C1-C2 complex. Axial torque-rotation characteristics until failure. Spine 1990;15(10):990–6.
35. Krakenes J, Kaale B, Nordli H, et al. MR analysis of the transverse ligament in the late stage of whiplash injury. Acta Radiol 2003; 44:637–44.
36. Krakenes J, Kaale B, Moen G, et al. MR analysis of the tectorial and posterior antlanto-occipital membranes in the late stage of whiplash injury. Neuroradiology 2003;45:585–91.
37. Krakenes J, Kaale B. Magnetic resonance imaging assessment of craniovertebral ligaments and membranes after whiplash trauma. Spine 2006;31(24):2820–6.
38. Dvorak J, Hayek J, Zehnder R. CT-functional diagnostics of the rotatory instability of the upper cervical spine: 2. An evaluation on healthy adults and patients with suspected instability. Spine 1987;12:726–31.
39. Dickman C, Mamourian A, Sonntag V, et al. Magnetic resonance imaging of the transverse atlantal ligament for the evaluation of atlantoaxial instability. J Neurosurg 1991;75:221–7.
40. Tubbs S, Kelly D, Humphrey R, et al. The tectorial membrane: anatomical, biomechanical and histological analysis. Clin Anat 2007;20:382–6.
41. Krakenes J, Kaale B, Rorvik J, et al. MRI assessment of normal ligamentous structures in the craniovertebral junction. Neuroradiology 2001;43:1089–97.
42. Kaale B, Krakenes J, Albreksten G, et al. Whiplash associated disorders impairment rating: neck disability index score according to severity of MR-findings of ligaments and membranes in the upper cervical spine. J Neurotrauma 2005;22(4):466–75.
43. Schomacher J, Falla D. Function and structure of the deep cervical extensor muscles in patients with neck pain. Man Ther 2013;18: 360–6.
44. Falla D. Unravelling the complexity of muscle impairment in chronic neck pain. Man Ther 2004;9(3):125–33.
45. Jull G, Falla D, Treleaven J, et al. A therapeutic exercise approach for cervical disorders. In: Boyling J, Palastanga N, editors. Grieves' Modern Manual Therapy. 3rd ed. Edinburgh: Churchill Livingstone; 2004.
46. Hallgren R, Pierce S, Prokop L, et al. EMG activity of rectus capitus posterior minor muscles associated with voluntary head retraction. Spine 2014;14:104–12.
47. Boyd Clark L, Briggs C, Galea M. Muscle spindle distribution, morphology and density in longus colli and multifidus muscles of the cervical spine. Spine 2002;27(7):694–701.
48. Kettler A, Hartwig E, Schultheib L, et al. Mechanically stimulated muscle forces strongly stabilise intact and injured upper cervical spine specimens. J Biomech 2002;35:339–46.
49. Armstrong B, McNair P, Taylor D. Head and neck position sense. Sports Med 2008;38(2):101–17.
50. Treleaven J. Sensorimotor disturbances in neck disorders affecting postural stability, head and eye movement control. Man Ther 2008;13(1):2–11.
51. Kristjansson, E. The Cervical spine and proprioception. In: Boyling J, Jull G, editors. Grieve's Modern Manual Therapy. 3rd ed. Churchill Livingstone; 2004.
52. Middleditch A, Oliver J. Functional Anatomy of the Spine. 2nd ed. Edinburgh: Elsevier Butterworth Heinnemann; 2005.
53. Taylor J, Twomey L. Functional and applied anatomy of the cervical. In: Spine IN, Grant R, editors. Physical Therapy of the Cervical and Thoracic Spine. 3rd ed. New York: Churchill Livingstone; 2002.
54. O'Leary S, Falla D, Jull G. The relationship between superficial muscle activity during the craniocervical flexion test and clinical features in patients with chronic neck pain. Man Ther 2011; 16:452–5.
55. Kelly M, Cardy N, Melvin E, et al. The craniocervical flexion test: an investigation of performance in young asymptomatic subjects. Man Ther 2013;18:83–6.
56. Scali F, Pontell M, Enix D, et al. Histological analysis of the rectus capitus posterior major's myodural bridge. Spine J 2013;13: 558–63.
57. Hack G, Koritzer R, Walker L. Anatomic relation between the rectus capitus posterior minor muscle and the dura mater. Spine 1995;20:2484–6.
58. Scali F, Marsili E, Pontell M. Anatomical connection between the rectus capitis posterior major and the dura mater. Spine 2011; 36:E1612–14.
59. Alix M, Bates D. A proposed etiology of cervicogenic headache: the neurophysiological basis and anatomic relationship between the dura mater and rectus capitis minor muscle. J Manipulative Physiol Ther 1999;22:534–9.
60. Hack G, Hallgren R. Chronic headache relief after section of sub-occipital muscle dural connections: a case report. Headache 2004;44:84–9.
61. Haldeman S, Dagenais S. Cervicogenic headaches: a critical review. Spine J 2001;1(1):31–46.
62. Standring S. Standring S, editor. Gray's Anatomy. The Anatomical Basis of Clinical Practice. 39th ed. Oxford: Elsevier, Churchill Livingstone; 2005.
63. Levangie PK, Norkin CC. Joint Structure and Function. A Comprehensive Analysis. 3ed ed. Philadelphia: F. A. Davis Company; 2001.
64. Bogduk N, Mercer S. Biomechanics of the cervical spine. I: normal kinematics. Clin Biomech (Bristol, Avon) 2000;15(9):633–48. [Epub 2000/08/18].
65. Mercer SR, Jull GA. Morphology of the cervical intervertebral disc: implications for McKenzie's model of the disc derangement syndrome. Man Ther 1996;1(2):76–81.
66. Tubbs RS, Rompala OJ, Verma K, et al. Analysis of the uncinate processes of the cervical spine: an anatomical study. J Neurosurg Spine 2012;16(4):402–7. [Epub 2012/01/24].
67. Ebraheim NA, Lu J, Biyani A, et al. Anatomic considerations for uncovertebral involvement in cervical spondylosis. Clin Orthop Relat Res 1997;334:200–6. [Epub 1997/01/01].
68. Kotani Y, McNulty PS, Abumi K, et al. The role of anteromedial foraminotomy and the uncovertebral joints in the stability of the cervical spine. A biomechanical study. Spine (Phila Pa 1976) 1998;23(14):1559–65. [Epub 1998/07/31].
69. Penning L. Differences in anatomy, motion, development and aging of the upper and lower cervical disk segments. Clin Biomech 1988;3(1):37–47.
70. Pal GP, Routal RV, Saggu SK. The orientation of the articular facets of the zygapophyseal joints at the cervical and upper thoracic region. J Anat 2001;198(Pt 4):431–41. [Epub 2001/05/01].
71. Barnsley L, Lord SM, Wallis BJ, et al. The prevalence of chronic cervical zygapophysial joint pain after whiplash. Spine (Phila Pa 1976) 1995;20(1):20–5, discussion 6. [Epub 1995/01/01].
72. Bogduk N, Yoganandan N. Biomechanics of the cervical spine Part 3: minor injuries. Clin Biomech (Bristol, Avon) 2001;16(4):267–75. [Epub 2001/05/19].
73. Stemper BD, Yoganandan N, Pintar FA. Gender dependent cervical spine segmental kinematics during whiplash. J Biomech 2003; 36(9):1281–9. [Epub 2003/08/02].
74. Stemper BD, Yoganandan N, Pintar FA. Gender- and region-dependent local facet joint kinematics in rear impact: implications in whiplash injury. Spine (Phila Pa 1976) 2004;29(16):1764–71. [Epub 2004/08/11].
75. Yoganandan N, Knowles SA, Maiman DJ, et al. Anatomic study of the morphology of human cervical facet joint. Spine (Phila Pa 1976) 2003;28(20):2317–23. [Epub 2003/10/16].
76. Kallakuri S, Singh A, Chen C, et al. Demonstration of substance P, calcitonin gene-related peptide, and protein gene product 9.5 containing nerve fibers in human cervical facet joint capsules. Spine (Phila Pa 1976) 2004;29(11):1182–6. [Epub 2004/05/29].
77. Kallakuri S, Li Y, Chen C, et al. Innervation of cervical ventral facet joint capsule: histological evidence. World J Orthop 2012;3(2):10–14. [Epub 2012/04/04].
78. Winkelstein BA, McLendon RE, Barbir A, et al. An anatomical investigation of the human cervical facet capsule, quantifying

muscle insertion area. J Anat 2001;198(Pt 4):455–61. [Epub 2001/05/01].

79. Chen C, Lu Y, Kallakuri S, et al. Distribution of A-delta and C-fiber receptors in the cervical facet joint capsule and their response to stretch. J Bone Joint Surg 2006;88(8):1807–16. [Epub 2006/08/03].

80. Fukui S, Ohseto K, Shiotani M, et al. Referred pain distribution of the cervical zygapophyseal joints and cervical dorsal rami. Pain 1996;68(1):79–83. [Epub 1996/11/01].

81. McLain RF. Mechanoreceptor endings in human cervical facet joints. Spine 1994;19(5):495–501. [Epub 1994/03/01].

82. Mercer S, Bogduk N. Intra-articular inclusions of the cervical synovial joints. Br J Rheumatol 1993;32(8):705–10.

83. Fletcher G, Haughton VM, Ho KC, et al. Age-related changes in the cervical facet joints: studies with cryomicrotomy, MR, and CT. Am J Roentgenol 1990;154(4):817–20. [Epub 1990/04/01].

84. Inami S, Kaneoka K, Hayashi K, et al. Types of synovial fold in the cervical facet joint. J Orthop Sci 2000;5(5):475–80. [Epub 2001/02/17].

85. Mercer S, Bogduk N. The ligaments and annulus fibrosus of human adult cervical intervertebral discs. Spine 1999;24(7):619–26, discussion 27–8.

86. Hayashi K, Yabuki T, Kurokawa T, et al. The anterior and the posterior longitudinal ligaments of the lower cervical spine. J Anat 1977;124(Pt 3):633–6. [Epub 1977/12/01].

87. Lirk P, Kolbitsch C, Putz G, et al. Cervical and high thoracic ligamentum flavum frequently fails to fuse in the midline. Anesthesiology 2003;99(6):1387–90. [Epub 2003/11/26].

88. Jia LS, Shen QA, Chen DY, et al. Dynamic changes of the cervical ligamental flavum in hyperextension – hyperflexion movement and their measurements. Chin Med J 1990;103(1):66–70. [Epub 1990/01/01].

89. Mercer SR, Bogduk N. Clinical anatomy of ligamentum nuchae. Clin Anat 2003;16(6):484–93. [Epub 2003/10/21].

90. Johnson GM, Zhang M, Jones DG. The fine connective tissue architecture of the human ligamentum nuchae. Spine 2000;25(1): 5–9. [Epub 2000/01/27].

91. Caridi JM, Pumberger M, Hughes AP. Cervical radiculopathy: a review. HSS J 2011;7(3):265–72. [Epub 2012/10/02].

92. Tanaka N, Fujimoto Y, An HS, et al. The anatomic relation among the nerve roots, intervertebral foramina, and intervertebral discs of the cervical spine. Spine 2000;25(3):286–91. [Epub 2000/03/07].

93. Moses A, Carman J. Anatomy of the cervical spine: implications for the upper limb tension test. Aust J Physiother 1996;42(1):31–5. [Epub 1996/01/01].

CHAPTER 9.2 ■ LUMBAR SPINE

Michael Adams • Patricia Dolan

THE VERTEBRAL COLUMN

The lumbar vertebral column provides a semi-rigid axis for the body, one that enables upright stance and which provides attachment points for muscles to move the limbs. It also protects the spinal cord within the bony vertebral foramina. This segmented column can bend and twist because its rigid vertebrae are separated by deformable intervertebral discs (Fig. 9-5). However, only small movements are permitted between individual vertebrae: typically 13° of combined flexion and extension, 4° of lateral bending to each side, and 1–2° of axial rotation (Fig. 9-6). Movements are greater in the cervical spine, and less in the thoracic spine, largely because of differing proportions in the heights of discs and vertebral bodies. Vertebral bodies grow in height faster than intervertebral discs, causing spinal mobility to decrease during the growth period. Further decreases in spinal mobility after skeletal maturity are largely attributable to biochemical changes in collagen which stiffen spinal tissues.

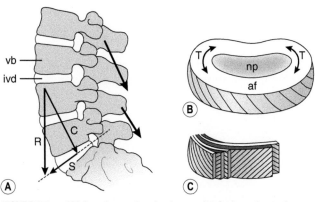

FIGURE 9-5 ■ **(A)** Lumbar spine in the sagittal plane (anterior on left) showing intervertebral discs (*ivd*) between the vertebral bodies (*vb*). Bold arrows indicate muscle forces on the spine, which can be summed to a resultant force (*R*) with compressive (*C*) and shear (*S*) components. **(B)** Intervertebral discs have a soft nucleus pulposus (*np*) surrounded by a fibrous annulus fibrosus (*af*). Spinal compression increases the fluid pressure in the nucleus, and generates tension (*T*) in the annulus. **(C)** Exploded view of annulus, showing its lamellar structure, with alternating orientation of collagen fibres.

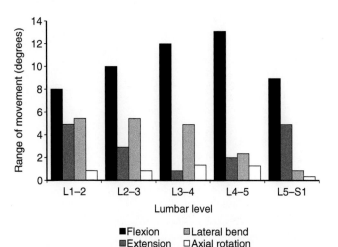

FIGURE 9-6 ■ Ranges of normal movement at each lumbar level. Note that the combined range of flexion and extension is approximately constant at different lumbar levels. Values for lateral bending and axial rotation are averaged for movements to the left and right. Data from bilateral radiographs of healthy young men standing upright. (Adapted from: The Biomechanics of Back Pain, published by Churchill Livingstone.[1])

Postnatal development of a thoracic kyphosis, and a cervical and lumbar lordosis, leads to the familiar S-shape of the adult spine. These sagittal plane curves play a role in shock absorption and energy conservation during locomotion, because they increase when the body sinks down in mid-stride, and decrease when the body rises at toe-off. Spinal ligaments, discs and (especially) tendons of the trunk muscles all resist changes in spinal curvature, storing energy as they are deformed, and releasing it later in the gait cycle.[1] The effect is similar to the action of flexing the knees when landing from a jump: stretched muscles and tendons oppose rapid knee flexion and soften the landing.

LUMBAR VERTEBRAE

The Vertebral Body

This short cylindrical bone lies between adjacent intervertebral discs, and primarily resists compressive forces acting down the long axis of the spine (Fig. 9-5). It is mostly trabecular bone, with a thin shell of cortical bone that is perforated on the superior and inferior surfaces ('endplates') in order to facilitate nutrient transport into the discs.[2] Vertebral body trabeculae are predominantly parallel, or at right angles, to the spine's long axis (Fig. 9-7), but parasagittal sections show that trabeculae also arch in from the pedicles to provide additional support for the endplates. These curved trabeculae appear to reinforce the inferior endplate more than the superior, because the superior endplate is more easily injured.[3] The vertebral body has a rich blood supply, and nerves have been identified within it, including close to the endplates.[4]

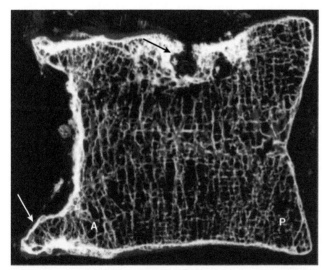

FIGURE 9-7 ■ Radiograph of a mid-sagittal plane slice of a human lumbar vertebral body. In the mid-sagittal plane, trabeculae are mostly orientated vertically or horizontally, and the anterior cortex (on the left) is thicker than the posterior. Note two common features of elderly vertebrae: a large Schmorl's node adjacent to the upper endplate (black arrow), and large outgrowths ('osteophytes') around the superior and inferior margins of the anterior cortex (white arrow). (Adapted from: The Biomechanics of Back Pain, published by Churchill Livingstone.[1])

Neural Arch

The neural arch, which is mostly cortical bone, contains more than 50% of the mineral content of a typical vertebra. It protects the spinal cord in a ring of bone, while its processes act as attachment points for muscles and ligaments to effect and limit spinal movements, respectively. The ends of the spinous and transverse processes are cartilaginous during childhood, contributing to enhanced spinal mobility. Conversely they can be sites of bony hypertrophy in old age, when they contribute to reduced mobility and to kyphosis.

Apophyseal Joints

Two plane synovial joints regulate movement between adjacent vertebrae and help to stabilize the spine. The cartilage-covered articular surfaces are oblique in both the sagittal and transverse planes, and this obliquity varies with spinal level (Fig. 9-8). Apophyseal ('facet') joints primarily resist forward shear and axial rotation between vertebrae, but under certain circumstances (see below) they resist compression also.

INTERVERTEBRAL DISCS

These pads of fibrocartilage allow small intervertebral movements, and serve to distribute compressive loading evenly on to the vertebral bodies, even when the spine is flexed or extended.

Nucleus Pulposus

The central amorphous nucleus pulposus (Fig. 9-9A) comprises a soft gel of water-binding proteoglycan molecules which is so soft and deformable that it behaves mechanically like a pressurized fluid (Fig. 9-9B). A loose network of very fine collagen type II fibrils binds the nucleus together, and anchors it to adjacent annulus and endplates.[5]

Annulus Fibrosus

The nucleus is surrounded by concentric lamellae (layers) of the annulus fibrosus, which are mostly composed of

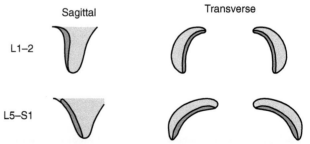

FIGURE 9-8 ■ Orientation of the articular surfaces (shaded) of lumbar apophyseal joints varies gradually with spinal level, from L1–L2 to L5–S1, both in the sagittal plane and in the transverse (horizontal) plane. (Adapted from: The Biomechanics of Back Pain, published by Churchill Livingstone.[1])

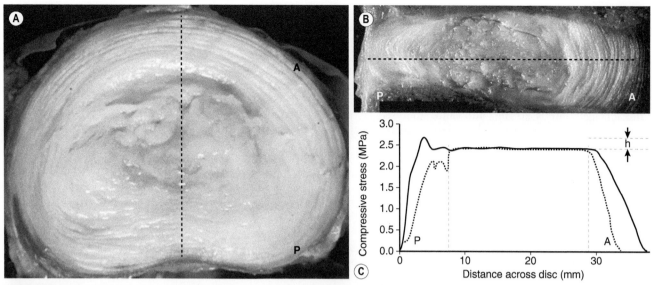

FIGURE 9-9 ■ **(A)** Photograph of a typical middle-aged intervertebral disc sectioned in the transverse plane (*A*, anterior; *P*, posterior). The dashed line indicates the mid-sagittal diameter. **(B)** A similar disc sectioned in the mid-sagittal plane. **(C)** Distribution of compressive stress measured across the mid-sagittal diameter of a similar disc. Note that in the central region of the disc, bounded by the vertical dashed lines, horizontal and vertical stresses (shown by broken and solid graphs respectively) are very similar. Small stress concentrations (*h*) are common in the posterior annulus. (Adapted from: The Biomechanics of Back Pain, published by Churchill Livingstone.[1])

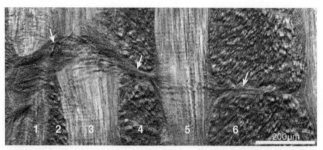

FIGURE 9-10 ■ In the annulus fibrosus of intervertebral discs, several adjacent lamellae (numbered) are bound together in the radial direction by 'translamellar bridges' (arrows) which are probably made of collagen. Photograph of a sheep disc sectioned in a para-sagittal plane. (Reproduced with permission from Schollum et al.[6])

coarse fibres of collagen type I, embedded in a hydrated proteoglycan matrix. Collagen fibres within each lamella run obliquely from bone to bone, with the fibre orientation alternating in successive lamellae (Fig. 9-5C). This arrangement, together with radially directed 'translamellar bridges' (Fig. 9-10), which bind adjacent lamellae together, ensures that any cracks developing in the annulus do not easily spread in a radial direction, so that the tissue is extremely tough.[7] Spinal compression creates a high fluid pressure in the disc nucleus, which is resisted by a tensile 'hoop' stress in the annulus lamellae (Fig. 9-5B). In addition, the annulus is stiff enough to resist compression in its own right. Collagen fibres in the outer lamellae are strongly anchored to the adjacent vertebrae, but in the inner annulus they merely envelop the nucleus. During flexion movements, the posterior annulus can be stretched vertically by more than 50%,[8] but discs are effectively protected from excessive bending, twisting

and shearing movements by intervertebral ligaments and by the neural arch.[1]

Vertebral Endplates

Central regions of the perforated cortical bone endplate of the vertebral body are weakly bonded to a thin layer of hyaline cartilage on the disc side. This cartilage, which resembles articular cartilage, is more rigid than annulus and does not normally swell. It serves as a biological filter which restricts movements of large molecules into the disc, and also the expulsion of water from the disc nucleus when it is compressed.[2]

Internal Mechanical Function of Intervertebral Discs

Internal disc function has been investigated by pulling a miniature pressure transducer along the mid-sagittal diameter of loaded cadaveric discs.[9] These measurements confirm that the nucleus *and* inner annulus do indeed behave like a fluid (Fig. 9-9B). However, with advancing age, the fluid-like region shrinks, and localized concentrations of compressive stress develop in the annulus.

Blood and Nerve Supply

Intervertebral discs are the largest avascular structures in the human body, and consequent nutrient transport problems limit cell density to very low levels, particularly in the adult nucleus.[10] Nerves are found within the discs of infants, but they retreat in early childhood, and in the adult do not normally penetrate more than 1–3 mm into the peripheral annulus.

INTERVERTEBRAL LIGAMENTS

Longitudinal Ligaments

The anterior and posterior longitudinal ligaments bind together adjacent vertebrae, covering the anterior and posterior surfaces of the disc and vertebral bodies. The anterior ligament is strong, and helps to resist spinal extension, but the posterior ligament is mechanically weak and probably functions mainly as a 'nerve net' to sense changes (such as bulging) in the underlying disc.

Ligamentum Flavum

The ligamentum flavum, which joins the laminae of adjacent neural arches, is comprised mainly of elastin, which allows it to be stretched by up to 80% before failure. This ligament is pre-stressed in all postures except hyperextension, and habitual tension within the ligament acts in conjunction with pre-stress in the annulus fibrosus to provide intrinsic spinal stability in bending.

Supraspinous and Interspinous Ligaments

These ligaments join adjacent spinous processes, and are mechanically coupled to each other. They provide minimal resistance to small flexion movements, but in full flexion they become taut and are the first structures to be damaged in hyperflexion.[11]

Iliolumbar Ligaments

By joining the transverse processes of lower lumbar vertebrae to the ilia, these ligaments help to stabilize L5 (especially) within the pelvis.

MUSCLES OF THE LUMBAR SPINE

Anterolateral Muscles

Psoas major originates from the anterolateral surfaces of the lumbar vertebral bodies and passes over the rim of the pelvis to the lesser trochanter. As well as flexing the hip, it compresses and stabilizes the upright lumbar spine.

Quadratus lumborum arises from the anterior aspect of the transverse processes and twelfth rib to insert on to the ilium. It is essentially a muscle of respiration, but can also move the lumbar spine into lateral bending.

Back Muscles

True 'back muscles' are innervated by the posterior rami of the spinal nerves, and lie posterior to the transverse processes. They can be classified into three groups: intersegmental, short polysegmental and long polysegmental.

Intersegmental Back Muscles

Several small and deep back muscles join adjacent vertebrae, including the interspinales between the spinous processes, and intertransversarii between the transverse processes. They are weak but contain a particularly high density of muscle spindles, which probably enables them to play a major role in proprioception and the subtle control of movements and postures.

Short Polysegmental Back Muscles

These are exemplified by multifidus, a deep medial muscle which extends from the lumbar spinous process at each level to insert onto the mammillary processes of lower vertebrae and on to the sacrum and ilium. Because it has a long lever arm posterior to the centre of rotation in the intervertebral discs,[12] multifidus is a powerful extensor of the lumbar spine, and largely determines lumbar lordosis.

Long Polysegmental Back Muscles

These are typified by the three large back muscles which comprise the 'erector spinae' group: iliocostalis lies most lateral and superficial, longissimus is more medial, and spinalis is most medial and deep (although diminished in the lumbar spine). They arise from the laminae, transverse processes and ribs at several spinal levels, and insert on to other spinal levels, and to the pelvis. The erector spinae are powerful extensors of the whole spine and play a major role in the lifting of heavy weights. All of these strong back muscles have a high proportion of large type I ('endurance') fibres, which enable the muscles to maintain spinal posture for long periods of time.

Other Muscles Relevant to the Lumbar Spine

Four layers of abdominal muscles (transversus abdominis, rectus abdominis, internal obliques and external obliques) move and stabilize the trunk. More distant muscles such as latissimus dorsi and the gluteals also affect the lumbar spine because they attach to the lumbodorsal fascia, a strong collagenous sheet which lies superficial to the back muscles and which can be employed to help extend the spine from a flexed position.[13]

REFERENCES

1. Adams M, Bogduk N, Burton K, et al. The Biomechanics of Back Pain. 3rd ed. Edinburgh: Churchill Livingstone; 2013.
2. Rodriguez AG, Slichter CK, Acosta FL, et al. Human disc nucleus properties and vertebral endplate permeability. Spine (Phila Pa 1976) 2011;36(7):512–20. [Epub 2011/01/18]; PubMed PMID: 21240044. Pubmed Central PMCID: 3062730.
3. Zhao FD, Pollintine P, Hole BD, et al. Vertebral fractures usually affect the cranial endplate because it is thinner and supported by less-dense trabecular bone. Bone 2009;44(2):372–9. PubMed PMID: 19049912. eng.
4. Fields AJ, Liebenberg EC, Lotz JC. Innervation of pathologies in the lumbar vertebral end plate and intervertebral disc. Spine J 2013;PubMed PMID: 24139753.
5. Wade KR, Robertson PA, Broom ND. On how nucleus-endplate integration is achieved at the fibrillar level in the ovine lumbar disc. J Anat 2012;221(1):39–46. [Epub 2012/04/27. eng]; PubMed PMID: 22533741.

6. Schollum ML, Robertson PA, Broom ND. A microstructural investigation of intervertebral disc lamellar connectivity: detailed analysis of the translamellar bridges. J Anat 2009;214(6):805–16. [Epub 2009/06/23. eng]; PubMed PMID: 19538627.

7. Green TP, Adams MA, Dolan P. Tensile properties of the annulus fibrosus II. Ultimate tensile strength and fatigue life. Eur Spine J 1993;2(4):209–14. PubMed PMID: 20058407.

8. Adams MA, Hutton WC. Prolapsed intervertebral disc. A hyperflexion injury 1981 Volvo Award in Basic Science. Spine 1982;7(3):184–91. PubMed PMID: 0007112236.

9. Adams MA, McNally DS, Dolan P. 'Stress' distributions inside intervertebral discs. The effects of age and degeneration. J Bone Joint Surg Br 1996;78(6):965–72. PubMed PMID: 0008951017.

10. Hastreiter D, Ozuna RM, Spector M. Regional variations in certain cellular characteristics in human lumbar intervertebral discs, including the presence of alpha-smooth muscle actin. J Orthop Res 2001;19(4):597–604. PubMed PMID: 11518268.

11. Adams MA, Hutton WC, Stott JR. The resistance to flexion of the lumbar intervertebral joint. Spine 1980;5(3):245–53. PubMed PMID: 0007394664.

12. Pearcy MJ, Bogduk N. Instantaneous axes of rotation of the lumbar intervertebral joints. Spine 1988;13(9):1033–41. PubMed PMID: 0003206297.

13. Dolan P, Mannion AF, Adams MA. Passive tissues help the back muscles to generate extensor moments during lifting. J Biomech 1994;27(8):1077–85. PubMed PMID: 0008089162.

TENDON AND TENDINOPATHY

CHAPTER **10.1** ■ TENDON AND TENDON PATHOLOGY
Hazel Screen

INTRODUCTION AND TENDON FUNCTION

Tendons perform the primary role of connecting muscle to bone to facilitate motion. At first glance, these passive, collagen-rich tissues appear to be very simple rope-like structures. However, as we delve further into their mechanobiology, we discover that this view is far too simplistic. Structure and material properties are not universal across tendons, but are optimized to enable different types of tendons to effectively perform their varied functional roles within the musculoskeletal system.[1] As a clinician, it may therefore not be appropriate to treat all tendons in the same manner, and knowledge of how tendon structure and function are optimized becomes critical to understanding and treating injuries and diseases effectively. As our understanding of the differences between tendons evolves, we can begin looking for opportunities to target treatment modalities towards specific types of tendon or even types of injury, based on an understanding of the basic science of these conditions.

In connecting muscle and bone, tendons provide a passive linkage to ensure that active muscle contraction results in joint movement. Including a tendon in the muscle-to-bone connection is vital for a number of reasons. Firstly, muscle is compliant whereas bone is very stiff. Tendon provides a graduated change in material characteristics between these extremes, minimizing the development of areas of stress concentration where failure is likely to occur.[2] Secondly, to provide active contraction, muscles are often quite bulky, particularly when they must generate significant power. The role of the tendon in this instance is to move the muscle belly away from its point of action.[3] This creates space, but also allows the tendon to work like a lever arm, moving the point of action away from the centre of rotation, thereby reducing the forces required for movement, much like a spanner when manipulating a nut.

Beyond these universal functions, specific tendons, aided by their individual material properties, assist movement in different ways. Tendons such as the flexor and extensor tendons in our hands are subjected to low stresses and strains, but must modulate muscle contraction with extreme precision to allow us to perform intricate activities such as writing. They must be reasonably inextensible, so muscle contraction is transferred fully and precisely to the fingers, yet must provide a degree of damping in the system so our movements are not jerky but finely controlled.[4] This functional role contrasts heavily with that of a tendon such as the Achilles. The Achilles must withstand multiples of body weight when we walk or run, and act as part of the locomotory system to help propel us forward. It must act like a spring, stretching when it is loaded before recoiling to return energy to the system as we push off, thereby improving locomotory efficiency.[5] While tendons, such as the Achilles, must be sufficiently stiff to enable efficient force transfer to the skeleton, they must also incorporate a degree of elasticity to enable them to stretch and store energy.[6,7]

Tendons such as the Achilles and patellar are termed energy-storing tendons, whereas those in the hand are referred to as positional tendons. While the hand tendons and Achilles provide examples of extreme functional requirements, many tendons require a combination of these properties, and must find an appropriate balance between elasticity for energy storage and stiffness for efficient force transfer. Creating these opposing functional requirements necessitates subtle structural and compositional differences between tendons to provide appropriate mechanical behaviour;[8] such differences may also result in differences in the mechanisms of damage or injury between these tendons.

COMPOSITION AND STRUCTURE

It is staggering to appreciate that the tendon extracellular matrix, as in all biological materials, is made entirely from the tissue's resident cells. The cellular component only constitutes approximately 10% of the dry weight in mature tendon, with the predominant cell type termed the tenocyte.[9] While tenocyte phenotype remains poorly understood, it is known that tenocytes are sensitive to the mechanical loading environment they perceive during tendon use, and control tendon structure, composition and health at least partly in response to these stimuli.[10] Understanding the important chemical and mechanical stimuli that govern tenocyte metabolism, and harnessing these to promote healthy matrix production or repair, is subsequently a key area of interest in tendon basic science research.

The general structure of tendon extracellular matrix (ECM) was first described in the late 1970s in the seminal work of Kastelic and co-workers.[11] Tendon ECM is typically 60–90% type I collagen, arranged in a series of hierarchical levels. The smallest structural unit is the nanoscale individual collagen molecule and these cross-link together to build collagen fibrils, in the order of 50–500 nm diameter. Collagen fibrils aggregate into fibres, then fascicles, and finally the whole tendon, with the collagen at each of these hierarchical levels interspersed with a proteoglycan-rich matrix (Fig. 10-1A). The highly aligned, hierarchical organization of collagen is responsible for the exceptional tensile strength of tendon. Tendon also contains approximately 0.5–3%

elastin, 2–5% proteoglycans and small amounts of a range of other types of collagens[12,13] (Fig. 10-1B). While these proteins are far less abundant than collagen type I, they may still play important roles, with elastin known to provide high elasticity and proteoglycans responsible for imbibing water and resisting compressive strains or providing lubrication. A range of other glycoproteins have been reported in different tendons in varying amounts, but no clear structural roles have been identified for most of these additional proteins to date.

From a materials science perspective, the tendon ECM may be described as a fibre-composite material. Fibre composites are made by combining two distinct materials together, where each material is known as a phase; the fibre material makes the 'fibre' phase, and the secondary material surrounding them makes another phase known as the 'matrix' phase. The 'fibres' of a fibre composite are strong under tension and reinforce the material, whereas the surrounding 'matrix' is usually more ductile, holding the 'fibres' together and helping them to share or distribute the applied loads.[14] Fibre-composite materials are in common use, examples include steel-reinforced concrete and carbon fibre. They provide a number of advantages over single-phase

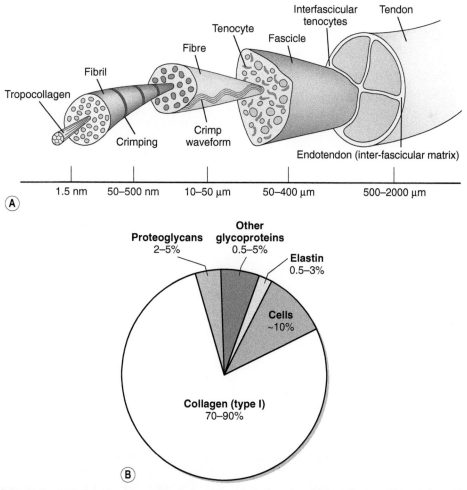

FIGURE 10-1 ■ **(A)** Schematic depicting the hierarchical structure of tendon, in which collagen units are bound together by either crosslinks or non-collagenous matrix at multiple hierarchical levels, to make a fibre-composite material with outstanding tensile strength. **(B)** Tendon composition varies according to the functional role of the tendon, but the composition of the majority of tendons is within the ranges outlined in the pie chart.

materials, as they combine the properties of both constituent parts, allowing material to both be light weight and strong. They also have good fatigue resistance, as damage in one area cannot easily propagate through the whole material because the 'fibres' of the composite are all separate entities.

When considering tendon from a materials science perspective as a fibre composite, the aligned collagen units constitute the 'fibres' and the surrounding proteoglycan-rich phase the 'matrix'. As such, tendon is effectively a multilevel fibre-composite material, as there is a fibre-composite arrangement (collagen units surrounded by matrix) at every level of its hierarchical structure. It is easy to get confused with the terminology as, from a biological perspective, the term fibre is also used to describe a single level of the tendon hierarchy. Indeed, to add to the confusion, different terms are also regularly used by different research groups to describe each level of the tendon collagen hierarchy, so care must be taken when reviewing the literature to be clear to what the text is referring. In this text, quotation marks around the word fibre denote the more generic materials science use of the word.

MECHANICAL BEHAVIOUR

There have been numerous investigations into the mechanical properties of tendons. Typically a tendon is pulled to failure, recording how much force is required to stretch the tissue, and how much it stretches before it breaks. This is shown graphically in a force-extension curve (Fig. 10-2A), and the stiffness can be found from the slope of the curve, where a steeper curve denotes a stiffer tendon. While these data are useful, they are not only dependent on the properties of the tendon, but also the size of the piece of tendon tested (intuitively, it takes more force to break a thicker sample, simply because it is thicker), so data are usually normalized and presented as a stress–strain curve, which specifically describes the properties of the tissue itself (Fig. 10-2B). The term modulus is then used for the gradient of the curve, so modulus is simply a normalized stiffness measure, taking into account dimensions of the test sample.

The three-stage shape to the tendon stress–strain curve is typical of the mechanical behaviour of many of our soft tissues, although compared to other tissues such

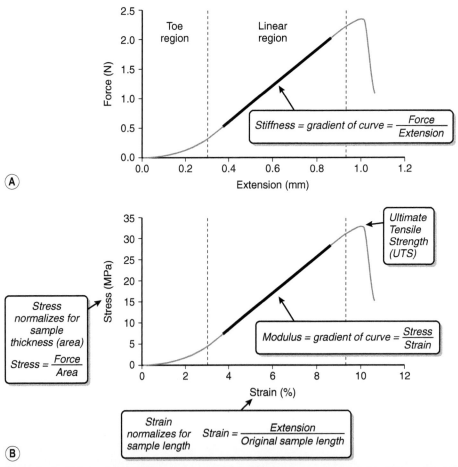

FIGURE 10-2 ■ **(A)** Schematic depicting a typical force–extension curve for a tendon pulled apart to failure. The data show how much force is required to stretch the tendon until it breaks. The gradient of the force–extension curves denotes the stiffness of the sample. A steeper gradient would denote a stiffer sample, where more force was required to extend the sample. **(B)** The force–extension data can be normalized for sample dimensions and shown as a stress–strain curve. The stress–strain characteristics of a material are thus independent of the test sample size, so the stress–strain curve describes the generic material behaviour. The gradient of the stress–strain curve is referred to as the modulus.

TABLE 10-1 **The mechanical properties of a range of different tendons**

Tendon Type	Modulus (MPa)	Ultimate Tensile Strength (MPa)	Authors	Ref
Ovine plantaris tendon (energy storing)	1650 ± 290	90 ± 12	Bennett et al. (1986)	17
Wallaby tail tendon (positional)	1662 ± 105	107 ± 19	Bennett et al. (1986)	17
Equine superficial digital flexor tendon (energy storing)	614 ± 115	115 ± 24	Thorpe et al. (2011)	18
Equine common digital extensor tendon (positional)	1012 ± 154	157 ± 34	Thorpe et al. (2011)	18
Rat tail tendon (positional)	663 ± 167	47 ± 8.4	Screen et al. (2004)	15
Rat Achilles tendon (energy storing)	400 ± 50	40 ± 6	Netti et al. (1996)	19
Human Achilles tendon (energy storing)	816 ± 218	71 ± 17	Wren et al. (2001)	20
Human hamstring tendon (energy storing)	362 ± 21	87 ± 13	Butler et al. (1984), Schechtman et al. (2000)	21,22

The modulus and ultimate tensile strength are reported in MPa (as described in Fig. 10-2).

as skin, tendon has a high failure stress and modulus (Table 10-1). The low stiffness behaviour we can see within the toe region results from the alignment and organization of collagen in the loading direction, in addition to straightening of the collagen fibres, which display a periodic crimp pattern in the unstressed state.[15,16] With further applied strain, the stiffness of the tendon increases rapidly, in what is commonly referred to as the linear region. With all the collagen straightened and aligned in the loading direction, the large increase in stiffness in this region reflects the direct loading of the tendon structure. The stress–strain behaviour of the tendon is then reasonably linear until close to failure, at which point material microrupture leads to a steady drop in stiffness, as the fibres pull apart and the sample fails.[2]

Modulus or stiffness values for tendon are generally reported from the linear region, and most tendons probably operate within this region during physiological loading. Positional tendons, which experience very small loads in use, are stiffer (high moduli), but probably only just encounter sufficient load to operate in the linear region, whereas energy-storing tendons are more extensible and are often loaded to values close to the absolute failure stress of the tissue, explaining their significantly high risk of injury[23,24] (Fig. 10-3). In order to facilitate these different load requirements and mechanical characteristics, the mechanisms by which positional and energy-storing tendons extend through the linear region also differ. Tendons with a more positional function appear to stretch predominantly through sliding between collagen fibrils and fibres.[25] This sliding is governed by the proteoglycan-rich matrix between these collagen units, which creates the more viscoelastic and damped behaviour required in positional tendons such as the digital extensor and flexor tendons of the hand, and possibly the rotator cuff. By contrast, recent data indicate that there is very little viscous sliding behaviour between fibres and fibrils in energy-storing tendons such as the Achilles and patella. Instead, the fascicles are helically

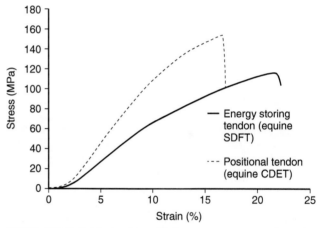

FIGURE 10-3 ■ Typical stress–strain curves, contrasting the mechanical behaviour of the energy-storing equine superior digital extensor tendon (SDFT) and the positional equine common digital extensor tendon (CDET). The high failure strain and reduced stiffness of the energy-storing tendon is important to facilitate its energy-storing role.

arranged like individual springs, and when the tendon is stretched, the springs can stretch to store energy and recoil very effectively.[26] In energy-storing tendons, sliding occurs predominantly between fascicles and is more elastic in nature, with recent data indicating that fascicle sliding may be critical for energy-storing function[18] (Fig. 10-4). While these data are very recent, and further work is necessary to fully understand the important structural differences between tendon types, they do highlight the importance of taking a tendon-specific, or at least tendon-function-specific, approach to considering an injury. Some data suggest that the specific high-strain mechanisms in energy-storing tendons (both fascicle sliding and helical arrangement) reduce in efficacy as tendon ages, coinciding with an increased injury risk.[27,28] If factors such as reduced fascicle sliding are implicated in increased tendon injury risk, it may be

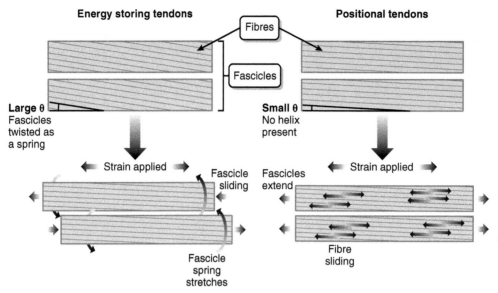

FIGURE 10-4 ■ Energy-storing and positional tendons meet their different mechanical requirements though differences in their structure and how it responds to applied strain. Energy-storing tendons extend through stretching or unwinding of the helical organization in their fascicles, so the fascicles act like springs (see the large θ, denoting a larger twist to the resting fibre arrangement). The fascicles also slide past one another to enable the high strains seen in these tendons. By contrast, positional tendons have little twist in the resting configuration (small θ) and instead extend through sliding between adjacent collagen fibres within fascicles.

possible to develop more targeted treatments to directly treat these mechanical and structural changes.

TENDON INJURIES AND REPAIR

Despite our increased understanding of normal tendon structure and function, there remains a surprising dearth of knowledge concerning tendon pathophysiology. This lack of knowledge reflects not just the complexities associated with tendon diseases, but also the difficulties in exploring these during the early stages of disease development. We do not know if the pain signals alerting a patient to tendon damage are delayed relative to injury onset, and it is rare to perform any immediate invasive protocol to assess injury post diagnosis.

There is a suggestion that the processes leading to sudden tendon rupture are different to those involved in the development of tendinopathic conditions,[29] but it is also quite possible that the development of tendinopathy differs between tendon types. Sudden tendon ruptures tend to occur in people who have been largely pain-free in the lead up to injury, whereas tendinopathic patients present with significant, often debilitating pain, but the condition rarely progresses to rupture.[30] Understanding of pain mechanisms is currently very limited and it is uncertain if the different presentation of these conditions indicates different underlying pathophysiologies, or if the pain associated with tendinopathy simply prevents additional overuse and damage accumulation in this condition. For a tendon to rupture it must already be structurally compromised; however, these injuries have only ever been viewed post rupture, so the nature of early tendon deterioration and structural compromise remains unknown. In tendinopathic tendon, classic reports of the condition describe a highly disordered tendon matrix

containing increased levels of collagen type III, proteoglycans and water, with increased vasculature but no signs of inflammation[29,31,32] (Fig. 10-5 compares healthy and tendinopathic tendon sections). However, while these findings have led to a strong leaning towards diagnoses of tendinosis, this perspective has been derived from the analysis of tendons months after the initiation of the disease, and provides little insight into the early development of the condition.

It seems highly likely that tendon pathogenesis will involve an interplay between localized overuse matrix damage, and a cell-mediated response to the loading conditions. Various animal models have been adopted to investigate the interplay of these factors in early tendinopathy.[34] These generally report that cyclic overuse of tendon results in disruption of the tendon matrix, and an increase in cell number and a rounding of the cells, alongside an up-regulation of various catabolic proteinases.[35-38] However, the order in which these processes are initiated and how they progress to the aetiology reported in long-term degenerate tendinopathy remains unknown, and significantly more work is necessary if the aetiology of tendinopathy is to be established. Current theories suggest that the up-regulation of various matrix proteases in early tendinopathy may be accompanied by an inflammatory response, a cellular attempt to turnover and repair the tendon.[39-42] The increase in cell number is additionally thought to occur as a result of infiltration of inflammatory cells to the injured site.[41] Such a repair response fits with the concept that tendon pathology is a continuum in which early-stage reactive tendinopathy may correlate with minimal local damage that can be effectively repaired by the cells, whereas excess overload can imbalance any repair attempts and lead to an inappropriate cell metabolic response and more significant matrix breakdown.[43]

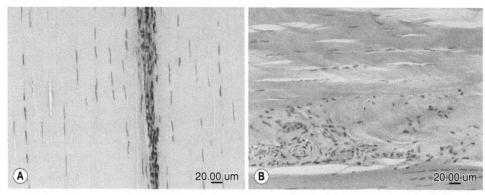

FIGURE 10-5 ■ Histological sections, viewed with a Nikon Eclipse 80i, from the energy-storing equine superior digital extensor tendon. Images compare (**A**) a healthy tendon and (**B**) a tendinopathic tendon. Note the aligned and ordered matrix in the healthy tendon, and clearly differentiated interfascicular matrix. By contrast, the tendinopathic sample shows the disordered matrix, rounded cells and increased cellularity. For colour version see Plate 10. (Photographs taken in Professor Peter Clegg's laboratory, University of Liverpool.[33])

Fibre-composite theory indicates that tendon damage will initiate in the non-collagenous matrix components,[44] hence the fraying of collagen seen in late-stage chronic tendinopathy is likely a later phenomenon, quite possibly cell-mediated in nature. Indeed, the turnover of non-collagenous matrix is substantially faster than that of collagenous matrix in tendon,[45] with some studies indicating that the half-life of tendon collagen is hundreds of years, so is barely altered in normal healthy mature tendon.[46] Furthermore, the turnover of non-collagenous matrix is faster in more highly loaded energy-storing tendons, suggesting it may provide an important mechanism by which tendons can manage and repair injuries before they propagate.[45] With fascicle sliding currently proposed as a key mechanism facilitating tendon extension in energy-storing tendons, the non-collagenous matrix between fascicles is an interesting target for further study.

With such limited understanding of the initiation and development of tendinopathic conditions, it is perhaps unsurprising that so many treatment options for tendon conditions have been proposed. However, as we begin to identify the structural and functional differences between tendons in health, it becomes less surprising that a one-size-fits-all approach is ineffective in treating tendinopathies.[47] All of the intrinsic and extrinsic factors which may lead to tendinopathy must be considered, with epigenetics and ageing also currently of prominent interest in establishing disease risk.[47] Studies are now focusing on tendon overload or fatigue damage development in different types of tendon, and how ageing alters matrix structure and increases injury risk. Hopefully new opportunities for targeting treatments will soon be forthcoming.

REFERENCES

1. Ker RF. Mechanics of tendon, from an engineering perspective. Int J Fatigue 2007;29(6):1001–9.
2. Woo SL. Mechanical properties of tendons and ligaments. I. Quasi-static and nonlinear viscoelastic properties. Biorheology 1982;19(3):385–96.
3. Zajac FE. Muscle and tendon – properties, models, scaling, and application to biomechanics and motor control. Crit Rev Biomed Eng 1989;17(4):359–411.
4. Lin TW, Cardenas L, Soslowsky LJ. Biomechanics of tendon injury and repair. J Biomech 2004;37(6):865–77.
5. Wilson AM, McGuigan MP, Su A, et al. Horses damp the spring in their step. Nature 2001;414(6866):895–9.
6. Alexander RM. Energy-saving mechanisms in walking and running. J Exp Biol 1991;160:55–69.
7. Alexander RM. Tendon elasticity and muscle function. Comp Biochem Physiol A Mol Integr Physiol 2002;133(4):1001–11.
8. Batson EL, Paramour RJ, Smith TJ, et al. Are the material properties and matrix composition of equine flexor and extensor tendons determined by their functions? Equine Vet J 2003;35(3):314–18.
9. Elliott DH. Structure and function of mammalian tendon. Biol Rev Camb Philos Soc 1965;40:392–421.
10. Banes AJ, Horesovsky G, Larson C, et al. Mechanical load stimulates expression of novel genes in vivo and in vitro in avian flexor tendon cells. Osteoarthritis Cartilage 1999;7(1):141–53.
11. Kastelic J, Galeski A, Baer E. The multicomposite structure of tendon. Connect Tissue Res 1978;6(1):11–23.
12. Kannus P. Structure of the tendon connective tissue. Scand J Med Sci Sports 2000;10(6):312–20.
13. Woo SL, Debski RE, Zeminski J, et al. Injury and repair of ligaments and tendons. Annu Rev Biomed Eng 2000;2:83–118.
14. Martin JW. Composite materials. In: Martin JW, editor. Materials for Engineering. ed 3. Woodhead Publishing Ltd; 2006.
15. Screen HRC, Lee DA, Bader DL, et al. An investigation into the effects of the hierarchical structure of tendon fascicles on micromechanical properties. J Eng Med 2004;218(2):109–19.
16. Atkinson TS, Ewers BJ, Haut RC. The tensile and stress relaxation responses of human patellar tendon varies with specimen cross-sectional area. J Biomech 1999;32(9):907–14.
17. Bennett MB, Ker RF, Dimery NJ, et al. Mechanical-properties of various mammalian tendons. J Zool 1986;209:537–48.
18. Thorpe CT, Udeze CP, Birch HL, et al. Specialization of tendon mechanical properties results from interfascicular differences. J R Soc Interface 2012;9(76):3108–17.
19. Netti P, DAmore A, Ronca D, et al. Structure-mechanical properties relationship of natural tendons and ligaments. J Mater Sci-Mater M 1996;7(9):525–30.
20. Wren TA, Yerby SA, Beaupre GS, et al. Mechanical properties of the human achilles tendon. Clin Biomech (Bristol, Avon) 2001;16(3):245–51.
21. Butler DL, Grood ES, Noyes FR, et al. Effects of structure and strain measurement technique on the material properties of young human tendons and fascia. J Biomech 1984;17(8):579–96.
22. Schechtman H, Bader DL. Fatigue damage of human tendons. J Biomech 2002;35(3):347–53.
23. Biewener AA. Muscle-tendon stresses and elastic energy storage during locomotion in the horse. Comp Biochem Physiol B Biochem Mol Biol 1998;120(1):73–87.
24. Birch HL, Thorpe CT, Rumian AP. Specialisation of extracellular matrix for function in tendons and ligaments. Muscles Ligaments Tendons J 2013;3(1):12–22.
25. Cheng VWT, Screen HRC. The micro-structural strain response of tendon. J Mater Sci 2007;42(21):8957–65.
26. Thorpe CT, Klemt C, Riley GP, et al. Helical sub-structures in energy-storing tendons provide a possible mechanism for efficient energy storage and return. Acta Biomater 2013;9(8):7948–56.

27. Thorpe CT, Riley G, Birch HL, et al. Fascicles from energy-storing tendons show an age-specific response to cyclic fatigue loading. J R Soc Interface 2014;11(92):20131058.

28. Thorpe CT, Udeze CP, Birch HL, et al. Capacity for sliding between tendon fascicles decreases with ageing in injury prone equine tendons: a possible mechanism for age-related tendinopathy? Eur Cell Mater 2013;25:48–60.

29. Riley G. Tendinopathy–from basic science to treatment. Nat Clin Pract Rheumatol 2008;4(2):82–9.

30. Sharma P, Maffulli N. Tendon injury and tendinopathy: healing and repair. J Bone Joint Surg Am 2005;87(1):187–202.

31. Jones GC, Corps AN, Pennington CJ, et al. Expression profiling of metalloproteinases and tissue inhibitors of metalloproteinases in normal and degenerate human achilles tendon. Arthritis Rheum 2006;54(3):832–42.

32. Khan KM, Cook JL, Kannus P, et al. Time to abandon the 'tendinitis' myth. BMJ 2002;324(7338):626–7.

33. Clegg PD, Strassburg S, Smith RK. Cell phenotypic variation in normal and damaged tendon. Int J Exp Pathol 2007;88(4):227–35.

34. Lake SP, Ansorge HL, Soslowsky LJ. Animal models of tendinopathy. Disabil Rehabil 2008;30(20–22):1530–41.

35. Fung DT, Wang VM, Andarawis-Puri N, et al. Early response to tendon fatigue damage accumulation in a novel in vivo model. J Biomech 2010;43(2):274–9.

36. Sun HB, Andarawis-Puri N, Li Y, et al. Cycle-dependent matrix remodeling gene expression response in fatigue-loaded rat patellar tendons. J Orthop Res 2010;28(10):1380–6.

37. Shepherd JH, Screen HR. Fatigue loading of tendon. Int J Exp Pathol 2013;94(4):260–70.

38. Sereysky JB, Andarawis-Puri N, Jepsen KJ, et al. Structural and mechanical effects of in vivo fatigue damage induction on murine tendon. J Orthop Res 2012;30(6):965–72.

39. Legerlotz K, Jones ER, Screen HR, et al. Increased expression of IL-6 family members in tendon pathology. Rheumatology 2012;51(7):1161–5.

40. Legerlotz K, Jones GC, Screen HR, et al. Cyclic loading of tendon fascicles using a novel fatigue loading system increases interleukin-6 expression by tenocytes. Scand J Med Sci Sports 2013;23(1):31–7.

41. Dakin SG, Dudhia J, Smith RK. Science in brief: resolving tendon inflammation. A new perspective. Equine Vet J Jul 2013;45(4):398–400.

42. Scott A. The fundamental role of inflammation in tendon injury. Curr Med Res Opin 2013;29(Suppl. 2):3–6.

43. Cook JL, Purdam CR. Is tendon pathology a continuum? A pathology model to explain the clinical presentation of load-induced tendinopathy. Br J Sports Med 2009;43(6):409–16.

44. Shepherd JH, Legerlotz K, Demirci T, et al. Functionally distinct tendon fascicles exhibit different creep and stress relaxation behaviour. J Eng Med 2013;e-pub ahead of print.

45. Thorpe CT, Streeter I, Pinchbeck GL, et al. Aspartic acid racemization and collagen degradation markers reveal an accumulation of damage in tendon collagen that is enhanced with aging. J Biol Chem 2010;285(21):15674–81.

46. Heinemeier KM, Schjerling P, Heinemeier J, et al. Lack of tissue renewal in human adult Achilles tendon is revealed by nuclear bomb (14)C. FASEB J 2013;27(5):2074–9.

47. Cook J. Tendinopathy: no longer a 'one size fits all' diagnosis. Br J Sports Med 2011;45(5):385.

CHAPTER 10.2   ◼   MANAGING TENDINOPATHIES

Jill Cook • Ebonie Rio • Jeremy Lewis

INTRODUCTION

Tendinopathy is the term given to the combination of pain and loss of function originating from tendon. It is a common clinical presentation and occurs in upper and lower limb tendons. Tendinopathy is typically associated with changes in tendon structure, but not all changes result in symptoms and a loss of function. This is confusing for patients and clinicians, and as such, clinical examination currently remains the cornerstone of assessment. Changes in tendon-loading behaviour typically precede the onset of symptomatic tendinopathy and load management currently underpins the treatment for tendinopathies.

Prevalence of tendinopathy generally increases with age; ageing tissue and cumulative load increase susceptibility.[1] Lateral epicondylopathy has a reported prevalence of 1.3% in the general population,[2] but may be as high as 40% in tennis players,[3] and it is most common in the fourth and fifth decades.[2,4] An episode of lateral epicondylopathy may be prolonged and associated with episodes of recurrence.[2] Patellar tendinopathy is common in sports that involve jumping (energy storage and release) and quick changes in direction, such as occur in basketball. It is more common in younger populations, with prevalence rates reported as high as 40% in jumping athletes.[5,6]

Tendinopathy can be persistent and recalcitrant to treatment and symptoms may continue for more than 15 years.[7] Although ongoing research has resulted in a better understanding of tendinopathy management, substantial deficits in the knowledge required to treat this common musculoskeletal problem exist and managing tendinopathies remains a challenge. Chapter 10.1 highlighted differences in tendons and their function and it is clear that clinically a 'one-size-fits-all' approach is not appropriate and treatment must be individualized. A holistic approach that appreciates the individual's aspirations, and a consideration of other relevant factors such as; age, previous injuries, co-morbidities, hormonal status and lifestyle factors (e.g. smoking) need to be factored in to treatment planning.[8]

TENDON PATHOLOGY

Tendon structure is complex and the process that leads to tendon pathology is controversial. Chapter 10.1 has comprehensively covered normal tendon and tendon pathology; however, additional clinical and imaging factors need to be considered. Firstly, as described in Chapter 10.1, tendon pathology may not be uniform and there may be discrete regions of pathology within a tendon that are surrounded by normal tendon. Secondly, there are pathological variations between different tendons, for example, patellar tendinopathy tends to develop well-defined areas of pathology, whereas the Achilles may demonstrate quite diffuse pathology. Thirdly, and as mentioned, pathological changes observed within tendons do not always correlate with symptoms.

Pure tendinopathy (within the body of the tendon) occurs most commonly in the mid-Achilles tendon region. Tensile overload is the key driver of tendon pathology, and energy storage (rapid tendon lengthening) and release loads are particularly stressful for tendon.[9] The use of a tendon like a spring (stretch and release) occurs in many vocational and athletic activities to reduce the metabolic demand of high-speed movement. This is exemplified in the Achilles during activities involving sprinting and jumping. Normally, tendon structure can sustain these loads, and Chapter 10.1 describes the sliding between helically arranged fascicles during energy storage.

Most other tendons develop pathology at the complex bone–tendon junction, excess tensile, compressive or shear loads (and combinations) can induce pathology. The bone–tendon junction is designed to transition mechanical load between the more flexible tendon and stiffer bone. This complex structure is called the enthesis organ[10] where compression of the tendon against the bone proximal to the insertion protects the insertion and improves the mechanical advantage of the tendon.[11] The compression is ameliorated by fibrocartilage within the tendon and on the bone, and bursae are typically present between the tendon and bone.[12]

Excessive compressive load at the insertion causes change within the enthesis organ, increasing pathology in the tendon and possible inflammation in the bursa. It is a clinical homily that symptomatic bursitis is part of compressive insertional tendinopathy and should be managed as a tendinopathy and not as an isolated bursitis. For example, trochanteric and subacromial bursal injections should not be seen as a standalone treatment but should be considered as part of the staged management of gluteal and rotator cuff tendinopathy.[13,14]

Tendons where compressive loads have a role in tendinopathy include the Achilles insertion, hamstring origin, gluteal medius and minimus, tibialis posterior, peroneals and adductor tendons. In the upper limb the rotator cuff tendons are susceptible to compressive tendinopathy. It is important to note that the site of compression can be immediately before the insertion or quite distant from it, as is the case with the peroneal tendon and tibialis posterior. During extremes of shoulder movement, compression may occur within the structurally independent parallel fascicles of the rotator cuff tendons.[15] The compression proximal to the tendon insertion is not true of all tendons; patellar and elbow tendinopathy do not have an obvious compressive site. The tip of the patella[16] and the fat pad[17] have been proposed as potential compressive structures in the patellar tendon, but their involvement is not confirmed.

Pathoaetiology

The transition from structurally normal tendon to structurally degenerative tendon is well described in animal models, with a cell-initiated process that affects the ECM.[18] Uncertainty exists if this process is identical in humans and remains the subject of ongoing debate due in part to the differences between small animal and human tendons. Small animals have different anatomical architecture, different metabolic rates and different capacity to repair tendon. There is also the challenge of translating knowledge from large quadrapedal animal models such as equine tendon to bipedal humans.

There are several hypothetical models to describe the transition from normal tendon to pathology. The models can be divided into: (a) the cell models, where the cell is the first response to overload; and (b) collagen-tearing models, where the initial injury occurs in the ECM. The cell model was first proposed by Leadbetter[19] and developed further in the continuum model.[20] The continuum model proposes that the cells detect overload and respond by increased proteoglycan production that progressively separates and then disrupts the collagen matrix, leaving potential for vessel ingrowth. Tendon pain has not been fully integrated into this pathology model but is likely to occur in the early reactive phase or in a reactive on degenerative presentation where the remaining normal part of the tendon that is loadbearing is overloaded as the area of the pathology fails to absorb and transfer load.

Conversely, the collagen-tearing models propose a variable response after collagen tearing, including inflammation,[21] pain, failed healing[22] and degeneration. Pain is integrated into these models, however the link to common clinical presentation is not always obvious, and the cause of pain in tendons throughout the various stages of pathology has not yet been identified.

Definitive evidence of an inflammatory process, in the traditional sense, is lacking at any stage of tendon pathology. There has been recent interest in inflammation having a role in tendon pathology[23] and the literature and evidence in this complicated area remains uncertain and incomplete. One area of confusion is semantics, particularly the definition of inflammation, and the presence of what substances, cells or processes indicate inflammation. It is important to note that tendon pain is not consistent with a triphasic inflammatory process, so clinicians should consider avoiding therapies such as absolute rest, ice and anti-inflammatory medications as definitive treatments for tendinopathy.

It is important to emphasize that current understanding of the structural, cellular and chemical changes that occur in pain-free and painful tendons is poor. Most importantly, how pathology and pain are linked is not clear.

Source of Tendon Pain

Pain is the primary reason people with tendinopathy present to clinicians. This is true for the young athlete experiencing tendinopathy for the first time or for someone with a long history of tendon symptoms. Both seek resolution of pain but we currently know little about the origin of the pain, and if it differs in these clinical examples and in different tendons.

Pain is an output from the central nervous system (CNS), which may or may not be associated with a physiological nociceptive input caused by tissue disruption. Persistent symptoms often indicate that there are changes within the CNS which are contributing to a chronic pain state. The clinical features of tendinopathy include tenderness to palpation (primary hyperalgesia), well-localized pain, impaired function but no spreading of pain (secondary hyperalgesia) regardless of the length of time of symptoms and variable evidence of local and more distant sensory change. This indicates that physiological (tissue protecting) and pathophysiological (functional changes within the nervous system) pain are present in tendinopathy.

The evidence for local nociceptive input is strong as tendon pain typically has a transient on/off nature closely linked with loading. It appears that tendon pain serves to protect the injured tendon. However, many features of tendon pain, such as its tendency for chronicity and the fact that pain during rehabilitation is sometimes encouraged[24] and may not be deleterious,[25] demonstrate that it is more complex than local tissue damage. To add to this complexity, there may be differences in upper and lower limb tendons, as well as between energy storage and positional tendons.

Furthermore, the source of pain in tendons cannot currently be seen on tendon imaging, as there is an inconsistent relationship between pain and pathological changes identified on imaging. Tendons demonstrating little tissue disruption on imaging may still be associated with pain.[26] Neither ECM change[27] nor neovascularization[28,29] has been consistently linked to pain. Similarly, severe pathology that progresses to tendon rupture may never have caused symptoms.[30] Lastly recovery, defined by improvement in the experience of pain and return to activity, also correlates poorly with imaging.[31]

The source of local nociception may include changes in tendon biochemistry, the tendon cell or nerve. Early-stage tendinopathy may have profound biochemical and cell changes but little neural ingrowth; conversely, degenerative tendons may have areas of acellularity and less biochemical involvement but an increase in the nerve supply.[32] Furthermore, the nerve supply is not uniform throughout tendon, and in fact there appear to be few neural structures within tendon even when it is pathological.[33] Most of the nerve supply appears to be peritendinous so it is possible that pathology may occur within the tendon, without the CNS receiving any nociceptive input, potentially explaining asymptomatic tendinopathy.

There is some evidence for CNS modulation in tendinopathy; multiple studies have demonstrated alterations in sensory response, both at the site of tendon pain and at other body sites.[34,35] Changes to brain and spinal cord excitability and cortical reorganization may occur with tendon pain.[36] This may explain the poor correlation between local tendon imaging changes and symptoms.[37] Modulation of neural activity may occur at the spinal cord and cortical levels; input (nociception) may be either up-regulated or down-regulated to produce variable outputs (motor/muscle activation and pain). Ongoing research into the contribution from, and the changes to, the CNS in tendon pain are required.

What Causes Tendon to Become Painful?

Unusual or unaccustomed load on tendon is associated with onset of pain, but why change in load results in pain or where the pain is coming from remains unknown. However, many people place high loads on tendons and never experience symptoms, even in the presence of tendon pathology. This reinforces the fact that tendon injury and tendon pain are a result of a complex interaction of intrinsic and extrinsic factors, as well as biopsychosocial factors. The experience of pain is unique for each individual and is based around the context of the experience, alterations to sensory integration and motor changes.[38]

ASSESSMENT

A thorough history is mandatory when assessing someone with tendinopathy. The priority is to identify recent tendon overload and current aggravating activities. Changes in loading may be very subtle, especially in athletes where a simple change in running shoe may bring on Achilles tendon symptoms. Similarly, a change in working height, speed of activity, weight or resistance of equipment may provoke rotator cuff and lateral elbow tendinopathy. It is important to identify previous episodes of tendon pain, their cause, what treatments were received and the response to treatment.

Assessment should enquire about pain and pain behaviour. Tendon pain commonly is reported as being maximal 24 hours after the aggravating activity. However, each tendon has its own classic pain behaviour, for example Achilles tendinopathy will be associated with morning stiffness and pain, patellar and hamstring tendinopathy with pain on sitting. In the upper limb, pain associated with lateral epicondylopathy commonly increases with wrist extension and the rotator cuff (especially the supraspinatus and infraspinatus) is typically painful in shoulder external rotation (often with shoulder elevation). Due to difficulties in achieving a definitive diagnosis, other causes of pain in these regions need to be considered.

Questioning is required pertaining to risk factors that may heighten the tendon's response to load, or contribute to a low baseline capacity of the tendon, making it more vulnerable to loading. Factors such as gender, age, obesity and systemic conditions (such as diabetes and menopause) may also influence the response to treatment. These conditions may sometimes be undiagnosed and in many cases require referral for investigation. Lifestyle factors such as smoking behaviour need to be identified.

The level of the clinical examination will be determined by the responses gained in the interview, as the history will indicate tendon irritability and capacity. Someone who is older and generally inactive presenting with substantial pain when the tendon is first loaded, will not be examined to the same level or in the same way as a younger athlete with mild pain, experienced after extreme activity. Clinical reasoning skills will determine the appropriate level of examination for the individual patient.

Key features of physical examination include determining the area of pain. Typically, tendon pain should be localized and require no more than two fingers to demonstrate the area. Bursal involvement in some tendinopathies, such as in rotator cuff and gluteus medius tendinopathies, may have a more extensive pain distribution. However, extensive pain distribution that does not change with increasing load should trigger suspicion for an alternative or coexisting condition.

Examination may reveal muscle wasting in the affected muscle–tendon unit and this may extend to regions above and below the affected tendon. In the lower limb, it is necessary to assess how the person absorbs and transfers load in both single leg and bilateral activities. In the upper limb it is important to determine how load is transferred from the lower limb to the upper limb, especially in explosive activities such as pitching in baseball and serving in tennis. Local tendon assessment involves graded loading of the involved tendon and examination is complete when sufficient information about tendon pain and capacity has been obtained. Although commonly used clinically, tendon palpation may not be informative[39] and more research is needed.

Imaging is frequently used as a diagnostic tool in tendinopathy, and will demonstrate the extent of the pathology and determine if there are any associated structural abnormalities such as peritendinopathy or bursal thickening. Its application in clinical reasoning currently remains limited due to the poor relationship between structural pathology and pain. Recent advances in ultrasound imaging such as ultrasound tissue characterization that can produce relative quantities of four echotypes that have been correlated with tendon pathology may improve the utility of imaging in clinical diagnosis.[40] Ruling the tendon in or out as the source of symptoms should still be primarily based on the patient's history and clinical examination.

MANAGEMENT OF TENDINOPATHY

The management of tendinopathy is primarily determined by the clinical presentation, the risk factor profile of the individual and an appreciation of, but limited reliance on, any imaging findings. Tendon rehabilitation should always be specific to the person and their functional level.

Patient education and appropriate loading strategies are essential in successful management. Patient education should include explanation that while excessive load is the likely initiating factor it is also load that will reduce pain and improve function. Therapeutic load must be administered carefully and in a graduated and controlled fashion. Education must reinforce that treating a tendinopathy demands the same respect as fracture healing. No-one would consider serving in tennis with a broken humerus, or running on a fractured tibia. Equally, tendon rehabilitation must be given time and be carefully planned.

The key to rehabilitation is a graduated exercise-loading programme. Initially consider isometric contractions as this type of muscle contraction may reduce tendon pain. This may be followed by muscle strengthening involving heavy slow-resistance training (considering all relevant muscles within the kinetic chain).[41] The next stage involves increasing load on the tendon by incrementally introducing speed and finally energy storage loads. When designing a rehabilitation programme, time

between exercise sessions should be considered, and the 24-hour pain response following loading will guide progression. Three to four days between sessions may initially be important when introducing increases in speed, especially in substantially deconditioned tendon.

Endurance and compression loads should be included as tolerated but usually not in the initial stages of management as they can be provocative. Eccentric loading is inherent in all these stages, but the authors do not use it as an isolated treatment.

Lifestyle management is a critical component of tendon rehabilitation, as many people with tendon pain are unable to exercise effectively. Excess weight, insulin resistance or diabetes, high cholesterol, poor diet and smoking can all affect the recovery of a tendon and treatment should include discussion and education of these important issues.

Treatments such as massage of the muscle, electrotherapy and taping or bracing may be considered as adjuncts to a load-based rehabilitation, but they should not be the main focus of management. Frictions over the tendon, heavy stretching and excessive loading will all be detrimental to a tendon, especially in the early stages of rehabilitation.

There is no quick-fix solution and adequate time and care must be given to restore the tendon to the optimal level.

CONCLUSION

Tendinopathy is a common yet complex musculoskeletal problem. Assessment requires a thorough history to ascertain the loading and individual factors that contributed to symptoms and a detailed physical evaluation to guide load-based rehabilitation. Patient education is an essential component of tendon rehabilitation.

The presence of tendon pain 24 hours after loading should guide rehabilitation as opposed to pain on palpation or pain during exercise. The role of the CNS in the modulation of tendon pain is gaining increasing interest and assessment of the contribution of the CNS may be an important consideration.

Rehabilitation must be graded, commencing with isometric loads to reduce tendon pain, followed by progression through strength, power and sports- and activity-specific function. However, the progression needs to be adjusted to reflect the goals of the specific individual and the capacity of the tendon.

REFERENCES

1. Kujala UM, Sarna S, Kaprio J. Cumulative incidence of achilles tendon rupture and tendinopathy in male former elite athletes. Clin J Sport Med 2005;15(3):133–5.
2. Hamilton PG. The prevalence of humeral epicondylitis: a survey in general practice. J R Coll Gen Pract 1986;36(291):464–5.
3. Gruchow HW, Pelletier D. An epidemiologic study of tennis elbow. Incidence, recurrence, and effectiveness of prevention strategies. Am J Sports Med 1979;7(4):234–8. [Epub 1979/07/01].
4. Shiri R, Viikari-Juntura E, Varonen H, et al. Prevalence and determinants of lateral and medial epicondylitis: a population study. Am J Epidemiol 2006;164(11):1065–74.
5. Ferretti A. Epidemiology of jumper's knee. Sports Med 1986;3(4):289–95.

6. Lian O, Engebretsen L, Bahr R. Prevalence of jumper's knee among elite athletes from different sports: a cross-sectional study. Am J Sports Med 2005;33(4):561–7.

7. Kettunen J, Kvist M, Alanen E, et al. Long-term prognosis for jumper's knee in male athletes. Am J Sports Med 2002;30(5):689–92.

8. Holmes GB, Lin J. Etiologic factors associated with symptomatic achilles tendinopathy. Foot Ankle Int 2006;27(11):952–9. [Epub 2006/12/06].

9. Soslowsky LJ, Thomopoulos S, Esmail A, et al. Rotator cuff tendinosis in an animal model: role of extrinsic and overuse factors. Ann Biomed Eng 2002;30(8):1057–63.

10. Benjamin M, Moriggl B, Brenner E, et al. The 'enthesis organ' Concept. Why enthesopathies may not present as focal insertional disorders. Arthritis Rheum 2004;50(10):3306–13.

11. Cook J, Purdam C. Is compressive load a factor in the development of tendinopathy? Br J Sports Med 2012;46(3):163–8.

12. Rufai A, Ralphs J, Benjamin M. Structure and histopathology of the insertional region of the human Achilles tendon. J Orthop Res 1995;13(4):585–93.

13. Lewis JS. Subacromial impingement syndrome: a musculoskeletal condition or a clinical illusion? Phys Ther Rev 2011;16(5):388–98.

14. Fearon AM, Scarvell JM, Neeman T, et al. Greater trochanteric pain syndrome: defining the clinical syndrome. Br J Sports Med 2013;47(10):649–53. [Epub 2012/09/18].

15. Lewis JS. Rotator cuff tendinopathy. Br J Sports Med 2009;43(4):236–41. [Epub 2008/09/20].

16. Johnson DP. Arthroscopic surgery for patellar tendinitis: a new technique. Arthroscopy 1998;14(Suppl. 1):S44.

17. Culvenor A, Cook JL, Warden SJ, et al. Infrapatellar fat pad size, but not patellar alignment, is associated with patellar tendinopathy. Scand J Med Sci Sports 2011;21(6):e405–11.

18. Scott A, Cook JL, Hart DA, et al. Tenocyte responses to mechanical loading in vivo: a role for local insulin-like growth factor 1 signaling in early tendinosis in rats. Arthritis Rheum 2007;56(3):871–81.

19. Leadbetter WB. Cell-matrix response in tendon injury. Clin Sports Med 1992;11(3):533–78.

20. Cook J, Purdam C. Is tendon pathology a continuum? Br J Sports Med 2009;43(6):409–16.

21. Abate M, Silbernagel KG, Siljeholm C, et al. Pathogenesis of tendinopathies: inflammation or degeneration? Arthritis Res Ther 2009;11(3):235.

22. Fu S, Rolf C, Cheuk Y, et al. Deciphering the pathogenesis of tendinopathy: a three-stage process. Sports Med Arthrosc Rehabil Ther 2010;2(1):30.

23. Rees JD, Stride M, Scott A. Tendons – time to revisit inflammation. Br J Sports Med 2014;48(21):1553–7.

24. Alfredson H, Pietila T, Jonsson P, et al. Heavy-load eccentric calf muscle training for the treatment of chronic Achilles tendinosis. Am J Sports Med 1998;26(3):360–6.

25. Silbernagel KG, Thomee R, Eriksson BI, et al. Continued sports activity, using a pain-monitoring model, during rehabilitation in patients with Achilles tendinopathy: a randomized controlled study. Am J Sports Med 2007;35(6):897–906.

26. Malliaras P, Cook J. Patellar tendons with normal imaging and pain: change in imaging and pain status over a volleyball season. Clin J Sport Med 2006;16(5):388–91.

27. Cook JL, Khan KM, Harcourt PR, et al. Patellar tendon ultrasonography in asymptomatic active athletes reveals hypoechoic regions: a study of 320 tendons. Victorian Institute of Sport Tendon Study Group. Clin J Sport Med 1998;8(2):73–7.

28. Lewis JS, Raza SA, Pilcher J, et al. The prevalence of neovascularity in patients clinically diagnosed with rotator cuff tendinopathy. BMC Musculoskelet Disord 2009;10(1):163.

29. Wilde B, Havill A, Priestley L, et al. The efficacy of sclerosing injections in the treatment of painful tendinopathy. Phys Ther Rev 2011;16(4):244–60.

30. Kannus P, Jozsa L. Histopathological changes preceding spontaneous rupture of a tendon. A controlled study of 891 patients. J Bone Joint Surg Am 1991;73(10):1507–25.

31. de Vos RJ, Weir A, Tol JL, et al. No effects of PRP on ultrasonographic tendon structure and neovascularisation in chronic midportion Achilles tendinopathy. Br J Sports Med 2011;387–92.

32. Rio E, Moseley L, Purdam C, et al. The pain of tendinopathy: physiological or pathophysiological? Sports Med 2013;1–15.

33. Bjur D, Alfredson HK, Forsgren S. The innervation pattern of the human Achilles tendon: studies of the normal and tendinosis tendon with markers for general and sensory innervation. Cell Tissue Res 2005;320(1):201–6.

34. Slater H, Gibson W, Graven-Nielsen T. Sensory responses to mechanically and chemically induced tendon pain in healthy subjects. Eur J Pain 2011;15(2):146–52.

35. van Wilgen CP, Konopka KH, Keizer D, et al. Do patients with chronic patellar tendinopathy have an altered somatosensory profile? – A Quantitative Sensory Testing (QST) study. Scand J Med Sci Sports 2013;23(2):149–55.

36. Ngomo S, Mercier C, Roy J-S. Cortical mapping of the infraspinatus muscle in healthy individuals. BMC Neurosci 2013;14(1):52.

37. Lewis JS. Rotator cuff tendinopathy/subacromial impingement syndrome: is it time for a new method of assessment? Br J Sports Med 2009;43(4):259–64. [Epub 2008/10/08].

38. Coombes BK, Bisset L, Vicenzino B. A new integrative model of lateral epicondylalgia. Br J Sports Med 2009;43(4):252–8.

39. Cook J, Khan K, Kiss S, et al. Reproducibility and clinical utility of tendon palpation to detect patellar tendinopathy in young basketball players. Br J Sports Med 2001;35:65–9.

40. van Schie H, de Vos R, de Jonge S, et al. Ultrasonographic tissue characterisation of human Achilles tendons: quantification of tendon structure through a novel non-invasive approach. Br J Sports Med 2010;44(16):1153–9.

41. Kongsgaard M, Kovanen V, Aagaard P, et al. Corticosteroid injections, eccentric decline squat training and heavy slow resistance training in patellar tendinopathy. Scand J Med Sci Sports 2009;19(6):790–802.

CHAPTER 11

LIFESTYLE AND MUSCULOSKELETAL HEALTH

Elizabeth Dean • Anne Söderlund

INTRODUCTION

Musculoskeletal conditions are non-communicable disorders (NCDs) that are the most common conditions treated by physiotherapists.[1] They also remain the most common causes of physical disability and pain globally.[2,3] Health-related quality of life associated with musculoskeletal conditions including back pain has been reported to be comparable to that in individuals with chronic conditions such as complicated diabetes and terminal cancer.[4] This chapter synthesizes the evidence supporting the associations between patients' lifestyle practices such as smoking, diet and exercise that underlie modifiable NCDs. It describes how these practices affect musculoskeletal health with special attention to back pain. Lastly, this chapter addresses how musculoskeletal disability may impact lifestyle-related health behaviours such as; smoking, nutrition, activity, sleep quality, and anxiety and stress, further compromising back pain.

Health-based physiotherapy practice refers to maximizing a person's overall health through healthy living to help address the presenting complaint as well as maximize long-term health and well-being.[1] By so doing, the physiotherapist may reduce the patient's risk factors for lifestyle-related conditions and their severity.[5]

To assess the status of health-based practice within the profession and develop a global strategic plan, two physiotherapy summits on global health have been convened. The goal of the first summit in 2007 was to examine the findings of global health surveillance initiatives and synthesize the findings with respect to implications for contemporary physiotherapy practice.[1] The second summit in 2011 developed a global action plan for integrating health promotion as a clinical competency into entry-level physiotherapy education, research and practice.[5]

The evidence supporting these initiatives and also underpinning this chapter includes:

1. Physiotherapists have adopted the International Classification of Functioning, Disability and Health (ICF) globally,[6] which is holistic and person-centred, and predicated on the World Health Organization's global definition of health[7] (Fig. 11-1 and Box 11-1).
2. Physiotherapists espouse best, evidence-based practice.
3. Healthy living (e.g. not smoking, healthy diet, healthy weight, minimal periods of prolonged sitting, regular physical activity, optimal sleep and manageable stress) is the best evidence-based means of maximizing health and preventing, reversing as well as managing chronic lifestyle-related conditions.
4. Lifestyle behaviour change, a non-pharmacologic intervention, is the basis for promoting patients' overall health as well as maximizing conventional physiotherapy outcomes.
5. Physiotherapists are the leading established health professionals who primarily exploit non-pharmacologic interventions.

Based on these lines of support, physiotherapists have a professional responsibility to implement health-based physiotherapy consistent with the established definition of health promotion (Box 11-2), and serve as a resource and model for other health professionals. Given the escalating epidemic of NCDs worldwide[8–10] in conjunction with that of disability from musculoskeletal conditions, the majority of patients seen by physiotherapists likely have one or more risk factors for lifestyle-related conditions.

Extending the content of this chapter, Chapter 37 describes the clinical implications of lifestyle behaviours on musculoskeletal health. It describes basic assessment and outcome evaluation tools, and evidence-based strategies and interventions that may be integrated into physiotherapy practice, with a view to minimizing the patient's musculoskeletal complaints and maximizing health overall.

NON-COMMUNICABLE DISEASES AND EVIDENCE-INFORMED ORTHOPAEDIC PHYSIOTHERAPY

The findings of a United Nations high-level meeting on NCDs were reported recently in a special issue of The Lancet.[12–14] This publication re-iterated multiple World Health Reports concerning the urgency around preventing and, in some cases, reversing ischaemic heart disease, smoking-related conditions, hypertension, stroke, type 2 diabetes mellitus and cancer. The report concluded that there needs to be a concerted effort on the part of health professionals to address these largely preventable conditions clinically, as well as those involved in health services delivery and health policy. These initiatives are consistent with long-standing recommendations from the World Health Organization.[12] To do its part in addressing NCDs, the World Confederation for Physical Therapy has published several position statements related to health promotion, particularly physical activity.

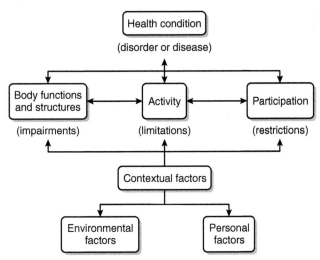

FIGURE 11-1 ■ The International Classification of Functioning, Disability and Health. (World Health Organization, 2001).[6]

BOX 11-1   Definition of Health

World Health Organization Definition of Health (1948)

'Health is a state of complete physical, mental and social wellbeing and not merely the absence of disease or infirmity'

SOURCE: *World Health Organization. Definition of health. Available at: www.who.int/about/definition/en/print.html. Accessed 1/20/2014.*[7]

BOX 11-2   Definition of Health Promotion

Health as Conceptualized in The Ottawa Charter for Health Promotion (1986)

Health is 'a resource for everyday life, not the objective of living; it is a positive concept emphasising social and physical resources as well as physical and mental capacity'.

'Health promotion is the process of enabling people to increase control over, and to improve, their health.'

SOURCE: *The Ottawa Charter for Health Promotion. First International Conference on Health Promotion, Ottawa, 21 November 1986. Available at: http://www.who.int/healthpromotion/conferences/previous/ottawa/en/. Accessed 1/14/2014.*[11]

The relationship between lifestyle behaviours and NCDs is unequivocal. Table 11-1 summarizes the evidence linking lifestyle practices with six leading NCDs. Although ischaemic heart disease can manifest as or contribute to back pain, several risk factors for back pain are those for heart disease (e.g. smoking, obesity, sedentary lifestyle and stress) as well as other lifestyle-related conditions.[15,16] Physiotherapists should play a major role in health education (i.e. smoking cessation; healthy nutrition; weight control; increasing physical activity; improving sleep hygiene; and reduction of anxiety, depression and stress).

Musculoskeletal health and back pain, its resolution and likelihood of recurrence, may be improved with lifestyle-related health changes.[17,18] People with chronic conditions including chronic back pain have a greater prevalence of smoking, weight gain, inactivity, and depressive symptoms and stress, compared with people without such conditions.[19] Lifestyle-related health practices (beyond ergonomic practices) can impact musculoskeletal health status, specifically, positive health practices may prevent back pain; and unhealthy practices may contribute to back pain, worsen it or impair treatment response. Experiencing chronic back pain may have variable effects in patients. Patients who smoke may smoke more, patients may eat un-nutritious foods for comfort, and they may sit longer and be less physically active in general, have poorer sleep, and experience more anxiety and stress. On the other hand, back pain may be an incentive for the patient to improve one or more adverse lifestyle-related health behaviours under the guidance of the physiotherapist, with the added benefit of improving health overall. Various factors contribute to back pain, thus the physiotherapist through systematic assessment can examine the degree to which lifestyle-related health practices impact a patient's back pain and how these may need to be addressed with or without conventional physiotherapy interventions.

Evidence supporting such relationships with respect to shoulder conditions may have implications for spinal conditions. Associations have been reported, for example, between smoking, body mass and type 2 diabetes mellitus and shoulder pain.[20,21] Further, lifestyle-related co-morbidity negatively impacts pre-operative pain and general health status reported by patients with rotator cuff tears.[22] Research is needed to elucidate these associations in relation to medical and surgical management of orthopaedic conditions such as back pain.

Finally, sex differences have been reported with respect to the presentation of low back pain and its management.[23] Women are particularly affected by low back pain and have a worse prognosis than men. Although women have been reported to adhere to healthy living practices more than men, they may benefit from greater attention to lifestyle practices to help mitigate their signs and symptoms. Men appear to be more active than women, yet men's health disadvantage is related to smoking and being overweight.[24] Given the relationship between back pain and impaired bone health, the role of lifestyle and its impact on bone health in both women and men warrants greater attention.[25]

SMOKING AND MUSCULOSKELETAL HEALTH

Deleterious Effects of Smoking

Smoking is deleterious to the musculoskeletal system.[26–28] Best documented are the effects of long-term smoking on bone thinning and fracture. The underlying mechanism has been related to altered bone metabolism and reduced blood flow given nicotine is a powerful vasoconstrictor. Further, bone loss can be accelerated in people who have been exposed chronically to second-hand smoke during their growing years. The onset of menopause is accelerated in female smokers, and in turn, increased age-related bone loss. Risk of fracture increases the longer a person smokes and smoking delays healing

TABLE 11-1 **Lifestyle-Related Conditions and Their Modifiable Risk Factors**

Risk Factor	Cardiovascular (Ischaemic Heart Disease and Hypertension) and Peripheral Vascular Disease	Chronic Obstructive Lung Disease	Stroke	Type 2 Diabetes Mellitus	Cancer	Osteoporosis
Smoking	X	X	X	X	X*	X
Physical inactivity	X		X	X	X	X
Obesity	X	X	X	X	X	
Nutrition	X	X	X	X	X	X
High blood pressure	X		X	X		
Dietary fat†/blood lipids	X		X	X	X	
Elevated glucose levels	X		X	X	X	
Alcohol‡	X		?	X	X	X

*An increased risk of all-cause cancer. Smoking is not only related to cancer of the nose, mouth, airways, and lungs; smoking increases the risk of all-cause cancer.
†Partially saturated, saturated, and trans fats are the most injurious to health.
‡Alcohol can be protective in moderate quantities, red wine in particular.
Sources:
Goldstein LB, Bushnell CD, Adams RJ, et al. Guidelines for the primary prevention of stroke: a guideline for healthcare professionals from the American Heart Association/American Stroke Association. Stroke 2011;42(2):517–84. doi: 10.1161/STR.0b013e3181fcb238. Epub 2010 Dec 2.
Canadian Heart and Stroke Foundation. Available from: http://www.heartandstroke.com/site/c.iklQLcMWJtE/b.2796497/k.BF8B/Home.htm. Accessed 1/14/2014.
Harvard School of Public Health. Your Disease Risk Initiative. Available from: http://www.yourdiseaserisk.wustl.edu/YDRDefault.aspx ?ScreenControl=YDRGeneral&ScreenName=YDRAbout. Accessed 1/14/2014.

and increases complications both of fractures and trauma related to a back condition. Smoking is often associated with drinking coffee and alcohol. Both long-term high caffeine and alcohol consumption have been implicated in bone density loss.

Smoking contributes to the onset of or aggravates the progression of back pain and arthritis.[26] Smokers have been reported to have a lower pain threshold (women's lower than men's) and experience more intense pain (dose dependent) in relation to musculoskeletal conditions as well as other conditions, than former smokers and non-smokers.[29,30] Both smoking early in life and over many years increase the probability of experiencing frequent pain over one's life.

The extent to which exercise as well as smoking cessation can restore bone density and overall bone health in smokers remains unknown. Compelling findings from animal studies suggest that prolonged exercise may offset the damaging effects of smoking on lung function and this effect may be mediated through exercise-induced anti-oxidant production.[31] It appears that the oxidant-induced injury associated with smoking may have a reversible component. Research is warranted to establish whether such an effect can be observed in other organ systems.

Beneficial Effects of Quitting Smoking

Individuals who have never smoked are likely to experience less back pain over the course of their lives.[26] The multisystem benefits of quitting smoking are substantial and these benefits can be powerful incentives for people to quit smoking when they are ready to do so.

Smoking cessation improves musculoskeletal health primarily by maintaining bone density and maximizing vascular perfusion of tissue for its nutrition, healing and repair, and augmenting systemic and local immune and anti-inflammatory responses.[32] Quitting smoking can lower the rate of bone loss and fractures, but may take several years to be reduced to the rate of non-smokers.[33] The benefits of smoking cessation on bone health have been documented with respect to improved outcomes after orthopaedic surgery including faster wound healing, reduced complications and reduced hospital stay.[34]

NUTRITION AND MUSCULOSKELETAL HEALTH

The relationship between musculoskeletal health and nutrition has been best documented in relation to malnutrition in children, athletic performance and in relation to age-related musculoskeletal changes, particularly those related to hormonal changes in the life cycles of women (menstruation, pregnancy and menopause).[35]

Commensurate with globalization, the consequences of the Western diet are now being realized with the prevalence of NCDs in high-income countries, and increasingly in middle- and low-income countries.[8] Criticism has been lodged against the promoters of established food pyramids given their apparent role in contributing to the prevalence of NCDs. The role of lobby groups in the development of nutritional guidelines has been a matter of contention in the United States.[36] Plant-based nutritional regimens including the Mediterranean diet have the highest level of evidence supporting their health-protective anti-inflammatory benefits[37,38] and health outcomes overall.

In contemporary society, people may eat for comfort and emotional support rather than biological needs.[39] Typically, comfort foods tend to be high in fat, sugar and salt, and lack nutrition. Living with a chronic condition may contribute to such eating patterns and may negatively impact recovery from injury or illness.

Bone Mineralization

Bone health begins in childhood and depends on balanced nutrition, regular physical activity throughout life and not smoking. In Western countries lifestyle practices including smoking, poor nutritional choices and inactivity are common, and contribute to reduced bone density and mass, and osteoporosis. Low bone mineral density is not only a red flag for osteoporosis, but a risk factor for cardiovascular disease which has implications for the prescription of exercise for back problems and monitoring during prescribed therapeutic exercise.[40]

A key index of bone health with respect to mass and density is calcium balance.[41] Western lifestyle practices contribute to calcium negative balance. Interestingly, guidelines for maintaining calcium balance, most frequently focus on calcium loading, e.g. supplementation, rather than striving for optimal calcium balance by reducing calcium loss. Although a requisite amount of calcium is required for healthy physiological function, the depletion of calcium through sedentary living, caffeine and alcohol consumption, smoking and possibly animal protein consumption has been well documented.[42,43]

Body Composition

Body composition and mass impact bone musculoskeletal health directly and indirectly. High body mass impairs the constituents of bone that are most important for bone strength and fracture protection.[44] Although counterintuitive, bone loading due to excess body mass is not necessarily protective against fractures. With respect to an indirect effect on musculoskeletal health, increased mass limits a person's capacity to be active (biomechanically and energetically). Inactivity can be further compounded by obesity-related conditions such as ischaemic heart disease, hypertension and type 2 diabetes mellitus. Chronic pain and obesity have been associated. Lifestyle behaviour change is recommended as a primary intervention to lose weight, thereby improving a patient's function and quality of life.[45] If surgery is indicated, people who are obese have increased likelihood of poor post-operative outcomes compared with people of healthy weight.[46]

Chronic Systemic Low-Grade Inflammation

Comparable to other chronic lifestyle-related conditions, obesity is associated with chronic systemic low-grade inflammation (CSLGI).[47–49] CSLGI is a physiological stress reaction to pathological insults often associated with chronic lifestyle-related conditions.[50] The CSLGI that is associated with obesity may be mitigated with physical activity.[51] Whether such low-grade inflammation predisposes people who are obese to pain and disability warrants elucidation.

Pain Threshold

The relationship between obesity and pain threshold is an area of both clinical and research interest. A recent study of over 2000 Chinese men reported that pressure pain threshold was reduced in those individuals with greater abdominal girths and who were less active than those with healthy girths.[52] Guneli and colleagues[53] observed that lean people are less susceptible, and obese people are more susceptible, to pain based on the activation of circulating ghrelin. They hypothesized that ghrelin, a hormone directly related to body mass index and obesity, is involved in the obesity–pain relationship.

Immunity and Immune Response

Musculoskeletal complaints are hallmarked by soft tissue trauma and local inflammation which trigger an anti-inflammatory response. The quality of this response largely depends on a person's health status, in particular nutritional status. Biomarkers for CSLGI can be elevated in people with localized inflammation.[54] Conversely, the role of CSLGI in local inflammation and pain in response to tissue injury is less clear.

Obesity

The causes of and contributors to the obesity epidemic are multifactorial. Food choices that are calorie dense versus nutrient dense are principal contributors. Typical Western diets remain high in animal protein, refined grains, sugar, fat and salt content, and low in terms of servings of vegetables, fruit and whole grains. The combination of low activity and the Western diet is a deadly one contributing to the current lifestyle-related conditions including overweight/obesity.[55,56] Overweight/obesity impacts every organ system, directly or indirectly.[57] With respect to the musculoskeletal system, obesity increases the risk of hyperuricemia and gout,[58] osteoarthritis of the hips and knees[59] and back pain.[60,61] In addition, obesity is related to immobility[62] which further contributes to musculoskeletal disability and delayed therapeutic response and recovery.

Weight loss has been proposed as a means of offsetting back pain in people who are obese.[63] Further studies are needed to elucidate the relationship between body mass and spine health. Although the association of body mass and the need for total joint replacement has been argued to be related to inactivity associated with pain limitations from degenerative processes of joints, this supposition does not appear to be supported. Body weight appears to increase after total joint replacement surgery from pre-operative levels or remain unchanged.[64]

Finally, being overweight or obese is more likely to be associated with one or more lifestyle-related risk factors, for one or more lifestyle-related conditions.[65] Managing the physiotherapy musculoskeletal needs of patients who are obese requires detailed multisystem and behavioural assessment and monitoring and targeted treatment prescription. Management needs to be informed by the multisystem assessment findings as well as the assessment of the patient's musculoskeletal complaint. It is possible that addressing the lifestyle-related risk factors could yield the best long-term physiotherapy musculoskeletal outcome and minimize recurrence of the presenting complaint.

INACTIVITY/ACTIVITY AND MUSCULOSKELETAL HEALTH

The relationship between activity and musculoskeletal health can be viewed in two ways. Firstly, a sedentary lifestyle is deleterious to musculoskeletal health,[66] in addition to being an independent risk factor for NCDs[60] including cardiometabolic syndrome.[67-69] Joint surfaces may degenerate due to reduced synovial fluid production that protects joint surfaces.[70] Secondly, this risk factor persists even in individuals who are exercising routinely based on recommended guidelines but have patterns of prolonged periods of inactivity during the day.

Deleterious Effects of Inactivity

The Western lifestyle tends to be sedentary, i.e. characterized by prolonged periods of inactivity, even in those individuals who participate in structured exercise regularly (participate in moderately intense physical activity three to five times a week, for 20 to 40 minutes). Prolonged periods of inactivity are an independent risk factor for cardiometabolic disease[71,72] and back problems.[73] Inactivity has been associated with the prevalence of back complaints, with many of the risk factors of back pain being those of cardiovascular disease.[74] This association has important implications for the management of back pain in terms of prescribing healthy living practices to minimize back complaints and their recurrence, as well as maximizing the outcomes of traditional physiotherapy for back complaints. In addition, people with cardiovascular risk or manifestations of the signs and symptoms of cardiovascular disease warrant related assessment and monitoring during exercise.

A sedentary lifestyle along with smoking and unhealthy weight contributes to premature ageing. The mechanism has been associated with shortening of telomere length.[75] Telomere length is further compromised with oxidative stress and inflammation associated with unhealthy lifestyles leading to NCDs.[50,75]

Because of the hazards of sedentary living, researchers have focused not only on volume of physical activity, but also have been interested in quantifying sedentary activity. Tudor-Locke and colleagues recently quantified daily inactivity based on a step-defined sedentary lifestyle index: <5000 steps/day.[76] The use of such a marker could be useful in the musculoskeletal assessment of people with disabilities such as back pain, and as an outcome evaluation tool.

Beneficial Effects of Regular Physical Activity

Regular physical activity is unequivocally associated with positive health status and outcomes of multisystem function including musculoskeletal health.[77] That regular physical activity throughout the day is protective of musculoskeletal health is well established and is highly recommended for protection against bone impairment secondary to chronic conditions and potentially medications to manage them (e.g. corticosteroids). In response

to this evidence, standing offices and treadmill workstations are being promoted to break-up periods of prolonged sitting during the work day.[78]

Current guidelines for physical activity are 150 minutes of moderately intense activity per week.[79] The effect size of this relatively low level of exercise is substantial. Such levels of activity are consistent with positive health, reduced morbidity and improved response to health care management, particularly as people age.[4,80] Not only is 'tolerable' activity now recommended in standards of practice for even acute back pain,[81] but it may also reduce pain-related anxiety and depression particularly if the pain becomes chronic.[82]

Like those with other chronic conditions, people with chronic back pain walk less and are generally less physically active than people without such conditions. McDonough and co-workers recently reported that people with low back pain can increase their walking daily over 8 weeks, in a pedometer-driven walking programme.[83] The programme was reported to be safe, able to reduce disability and pain, and increase function.

SLEEP AND MUSCULOSKELETAL HEALTH

Regular sleep is biologically necessary for physiological restoration. Most adults require an average of 8 to 10 hours of sleep a night for optimal health and well-being with periods of intermittent rapid eye movement (REM), yet they report often falling short of this.[84] Young people tend to report having substantially fewer hours of sleep compared with older people who are more likely to complain of poor-quality sleep (unable to fall asleep, or unable to fall back to sleep if awakened during the night).[85] The impact of sleep deprivation on health is substantial, affecting a person physically, psychologically and cognitively. For children, poor sleep impacts physical and social development. Inadequate or disturbed and irregular sleep such as in shift workers is associated with illness and injury.[86]

Deleterious Effects of Sleep Deprivation

Insomnia and sleep deprivation are common in Western society.[87] Sleep deprivation can exist independently of the complaint the patient presents to the physiotherapist, or can be a consequence of that complaint. Recent studies have reported that at least 50% of patients with low back pain report symptoms of insomnia.[88,89] Insomnia is associated with fatigue, cognitive impairment, mood disturbance, anxiety and depression[90] leading to functional impairments and accidents.[87]

People with pain have been reported to sleep less well, and when they sleep better, they report less pain.[86] Insomnia can adversely affect an individual's experience of pain through decreasing pain threshold and tolerance.[91,92] Hyperalgesia associated with sleep deprivation[93] has been reported in people in the absence of a health condition. Affective pain ratings and health anxiety have been reported to be the best predictors of insomnia severity, amounting to 30% of the total variance, even when pain intensity is controlled.[94]

Tissue injury related to the stress of sleep deprivation has been proposed to be mediated by impaired immune response and potentially free radical production.[95] REM sleep deprivation, specifically, has been associated with an increase in free radical induced damage in blood shown by increased plasma malondialdehyde levels. Animal studies have shown an increase in plasma malondialdehyde level as the duration of sleep deprivation increased.[96] Increased malondialdehyde can be attributed to an increase in free radical formation and damage, as the duration of REM sleep deprivation increases. Regular REM sleep therefore is essential to minimize free radical formation and consequent tissue irritation.

Finally, people who are chronically sleep deprived have poorer immunity than those who are rested,[95] thus they tend to have higher infection rates. Healing may be impaired due to CSLGI, an index of an impaired immune response which is independently associated with poor sleep, a risk factor for heart disease and stroke.[97]

Beneficial Effects of Optimal Sleep

When a person has optimal sleep, both cognitive and physical function are improved, and overall constitutionality is stronger. Importantly, the person is restored physically so has the capacity to physically exert him- or herself. He or she has a greater capacity for healing and repair, and greater resistance to infection due to stronger immunity. When pathological factors are ruled out, optimal sleep is best achieved through regular sleep hygiene habits and regularity of sleep, place and conditions.[84,98]

Sleep alone may improve physical and functional performance. A striking example is that of figure skater, Sarah Hughes. Following a long plateau of unchanged performance, Sarah increased her sleep by two hours a night based on the work of Maas,[99,100] whereupon she achieved Olympic gold in 2002. This observation has implications for physiotherapists whose priority is also maximal functional capacity in their patients.

MENTAL HEALTH AND MUSCULOSKELETAL HEALTH

The relationship between musculoskeletal health and mental health is bidirectional. People with mental health challenges may be more susceptible to physical health issues including musculoskeletal problems,[101] and people with musculoskeletal problems often experience anxiety and depression,[102] which can reduce pain threshold, further increasing disability.[103]

Deleterious Effects of Mental III Health

The literature related to the relationship between musculoskeletal health and mental health largely focuses on the adverse health and lifestyles of people with mental health challenges, which may secondarily affect the musculoskeletal system, e.g. smoking, inactivity and poor nutritional options and choices, and inactivity. People

with such challenges include those who are anxious or exhibit depressive symptoms as well as those with pathological conditions such as clinical depression, schizophrenia and psychosis. These individuals tend to smoke more, eat less well, are less active, and may consume more alcohol and use recreational drugs more than those without mental health conditions.[104,105]

Chronic health issues such as chronic pain are well known to affect mental health, i.e. they can contribute to anxiety, depression and stress.[106] Depression influences the course of low back pain.[107] Six weeks after shoulder pain onset, for example, assessment of concurrent depressive symptoms has been advised, in order for these to be identified and addressed, thereby potentially augmenting therapeutic outcome and recovery.

Beneficial Effects of Mental Hygiene

Mental hygiene refers to the promotion and preservation of mental health. Mental hygiene may not necessarily prevent musculoskeletal problems, but good mental health may improve a person's self-efficacy, resilience and resources to manage their problems and associated musculoskeletal disability. Of particular relevance to the physiotherapist is the role of physical exercise in preserving and improving depressive symptoms. People who are inactive report poorer emotional and mental health compared with active people, thus inactivity can compound the mental health consequences of chronic conditions such as back pain. Structured exercise on the other hand can improve emotional and mental health, thereby offsetting impaired mental health associated with chronic conditions.[108] Strategies such as cognitive behaviour therapy may have a role in the management of such disability, and can be adapted to the physiotherapy context.

CONCLUSION

Patients with musculoskeletal conditions including back pain typically complain of discomfort/pain, loss of functional capacity, and reduced capacity to perform daily activities, all of which can interfere with their health-related quality of life. This chapter describes how lifestyle-related health behaviours (beyond ergonomic and biomechanical corrections) may cause or contribute to these complaints, their severity and frequency. This chapter introduced physiotherapists to the evidence supporting that musculoskeletal health is influenced by lifestyle factors including smoking; nutrition; overweight and obesity; inactivity; sleep deprivation; and anxiety, depression and stress. It also describes how musculoskeletal ill health, in turn, can increase negative health behaviours such as smoking, sub-optimal nutrition, obesity, inactivity, poor sleep, and anxiety, depression and stress.

Beyond the scope of this chapter are important issues such as alcohol and drug abuse. Given their detriment to health and interference with a patient's capacity to follow treatment recommendations, these behaviours warrant being assessed and followed, even when these are being managed primarily by other health professionals.

REFERENCES

1. Dean E, Al-Obaidi S, De Andrade AD, et al. The first physical therapy summit on global health: implications and recommendations for the 21st century. Physiother Theory Pract 2011;27(8): 531–47.
2. Mody GM, Brooks PM. Improving musculoskeletal health: global issues. Best Pract Res Clin Rheumatol 2012;26(2): 237–49.
3. Vos T, Flaxman AD, Naghavi M, et al. Years lived with disability (YLDs) for 1160 sequelae of 289 diseases and injuries 1990–2010: a systematic analysis for the Global Burden of Disease Study 2010. Lancet 2012;380(9859):2163–96.
4. Taylor W. Musculoskeletal pain in the adult New Zealand population: prevalence and impact. N Z Med J 2005;118(1221): U1629.
5. Dean E, Dornelas de Andrade A, O'Donoghue G, et al. The second physical therapy summit on global health: developing an action plan to promote health in daily practice and reduce the burden of non-communicable diseases. Physiother Theory Pract 2013;Ahead of print. Available from: <http://www.unboundmedicine.com/medline/citation/24252072/The _Second_Physical_Therapy_Summit_on_Global_Health:_devel oping_an_action_plan_to_promote_health_in_daily_practice_ and_reduce_the_burden_of_non_communicable_diseases>.
6. International Classification of Functioning, Disability and Health 2001 [Internet]. Geneva, Switzerland: World Health Organization; 2001 Available from: <http://rehabmalaysia.org/ wp-content/uploads/2011/12/4-International-Classification-of-Functioning-Disability-and-Health.pdf>; [cited 2014 Jan 20.].
7. WHO. Definition of Health 1948 [Internet]. Geneva, Switzerland: World Health Organization; 2003 Available from: <http:// www.who.int/about/definition/en/print.html>; [cited 2014 Jan 20.].
8. WHO. Priority noncommunicable diseases and conditions [Internet]. Geneva, Switzerland: World Health Organization; Available from: <http://www.wpro.who.int/health_research/docu ments/dhs_hr_health_in_asia_and_the_pacific_13_chapter _8_priority_noncommunicable_diseases_and_disorders.pdf>; [cited 2014 Jan 20].
9. Bloom DE, Cafiero ET, Jané-Llopis E, et al. The Global Economic Burden of Noncommunicable Diseases [Internet]. Geneva, Switzerland: World Economic Forum; 2011 Sept Available from: <http://www3.weforum.org/docs/WEF_Harvard_HE_ GlobalEconomicBurdenNonCommunicableDiseases_2011.pdf>; [cited 2014 Jan 20.].
10. Final draft of the global NCD action plan 2013–2020 [Internet]. Geneva, Switzerland: World Health Organization; 2013 Available from: <http://ncdalliance.org/sites/default/files/rfiles/WHO%20 Global%20NCD%20Action%20Plan%202013-2020.pdf>; [cited 2014 Jan 20.].
11. The Ottawa Charter for Health Promotion. First International Conference on Health Promotion, Ottawa, 21 November 1986 [Internet]. World Health Organization; 2014 Available from: <http://www.who.int/healthpromotion/conferences/previous/ ottawa/en/>; [cited 2014 Feb 22].
12. Beaglehole R, Yach D. Globalisation and the prevention and control of non-communicable disease: the neglected chronic diseases of adults. Lancet 2003;362(9387):903–8.
13. Beaglehole R, Bonita R, Alleyne G, et al. UN high-level meeting on non-communicable diseases: addressing four questions. Lancet 2011;378(9789):449–55.
14. Research: UN summit on non-communicable diseases [Internet]. GHD-NET Available from: <http://www.ghd-net.org/negoti ations/un-summit-non-communicable-diseases/research>; [cited 2014 Jan 20.].
15. Kauppila LI. Atherosclerosis and disc degeneration/low-back pain: a systematic review. Eur J Vasc Endovasc Surg 2009;37(6): 661–70.
16. Zhu K, Devine A, Dick IM, et al. Association of back pain frequency with mortality, coronary heart events, mobility, and quality of life in elderly women. Spine 2007;32(18):2012–18.
17. Yildirim Y, Gunay S, Karadibak D. Identifying factors associated with low back pain among employees working at a package producing industry. J Back Musculoskelet Rehabil 2014;27(1): 25–32.
18. Notarnicola A, Fischetti F, Maccagnano G, et al. Daily pilates exercise or inactivity for patients with low back pain: a clinical prospective observational study. Eur J Phys Rehabil Med 2014;28(6):372–9.
19. Huan HC, Chang HJ, Lin KC, et al. A closer examination of the interaction among risk factors for low back pain. Am J Health Promot 2013;Forthcoming.
20. Rechardt M, Shiri R, Karppinen J, et al. Lifestyle and metabolic factors in relation to shoulder pain and rotator cuff tendinitis: a population-based study. BMC Musculoskelet Disord 2010;11(1): 165.
21. Viikari-Juntura E, Shiri R, Solovieva S, et al. Risk factors of atherosclerosis and shoulder pain – is there an association? A systematic review. Eur J Pain 2008;12(4):412–26.
22. Tashjian RZ, Henn RF, Kang L, et al. The effect of comorbidity on self-assessed function in patients with a chronic rotator cuff tear. J Bone Joint Surg Am 2004;86-A(2):355–62.
23. Chenot J, Becker A, Leonhardt C, et al. Sex differences in presentation, course, and management of low back pain in primary care. Clin J Pain 2008;24(7):578–84.
24. Ross CE, Bird CE. Sex stratification and health lifestyle: consequences for men's and women's perceived health. J Health Soc Behav 1994;35(2):161–78.
25. Briggs AM, Straker LM, Wark JD. Bone health and back pain: what do we know and where should we go? Osteoporosis Int 2009;20(2):209–19.
26. Abate M, Vanni D, Pantalone A, et al. Cigarette smoking and musculoskeletal disorders. Muscles Ligaments Tendons J 2013; 3(2):63–9.
27. A clinical practice guideline for treating tobacco use and dependence: 2008 Update. A US public health service report. Am J Prev Med 2008;35(2):158–76.
28. Ending the tobacco epidemic | HHS.gov [Internet]. Washington, D.C.: US Department of Health and Human Services Available from: <http://www.hhs.gov/ash/initiatives/tobacco/>; [cited 2014 Jan 20.].
29. Pisinger C, Aadahl M, Toft U, et al. The association between active and passive smoking and frequent pain in a general population. Eur J Pain 2011;15(1):77–83.
30. Pulvers K, Hood A, Limas EF, et al. Female smokers show lower pain tolerance in a physical distress task. Addict Behav 2012; 37(10):1167–70.
31. Al-Obaidi S, Mathew TC, Dean E. Exercise may offset nicotine-induced injury in lung tissue: a preliminary histological study based on a rat model. Exp Lung Res 2012;38(4):211–21.
32. CDC – fact sheet – health effects of cigarette smoking – smoking & tobacco use [Internet]. Atlanta, GA: Centers for Disease Control and Prevention; 2013 Available from: <http:// www.cdc.gov/tobacco/data_statistics/fact_sheets/health_effects/ effects_cig_smoking/>; [updated 2013 Dec 17; cited 2014 Jan 20.].
33. Smoking and bone health [Internet]. Bethesda, MD: NIH Osteoporosis and Related Bone Diseases National Resource Center; 2012 Available from: <http://www.niams.nih.gov/Health_Info/ Bone/Osteoporosis/Conditions_Behaviors/bone_smoking.asp>; [cited 2014 Jan 20.].
34. Lindström D, Azodi OS, Wladis A, et al. Effects of a perioperative smoking cessation intervention on postoperative complications. Ann Surg 2008;248(5):739–45.
35. Morgan SL. Nutrition and bone: it is more than calcium and vitamin D. Womens Health 2009;5(6):727–37.
36. Nestle M. Food lobbies, the food pyramid, and U.S. nutrition policy. Int J Health Serv 1993;23(3):483–96.
37. Pitsavos C, Panagiotakos DB, Chrysohoou C, et al. The effect of the combination of Mediterranean diet and leisure time physical activity on the risk of developing acute coronary syndromes, in hypertensive subjects. J Hum Hypertens 2002;16(7):517–24.
38. Polidori MC. Antioxidant micronutrients in the prevention of age-related diseases. J Postgrad Med 2003;49(3):229–35.
39. Cleobury L, Tapper K. Reasons for eating 'unhealthy' snacks in overweight and obese males and females. J Hum Nutr Diet 2013;doi:10.1111/jhn.12169.
40. Broussard DL, Magnus JH. Coronary heart disease risk and bone mineral density among U.S. women and men. J Womens Health 2008;17(3):479–90.
41. Peacock M. Calcium metabolism in health and disease. Clin J Am Soc Nephrol 2010;5(Suppl. 1):S23–30.

42. Calvez J, Poupin N, Chesneau C, et al. Protein intake, calcium balance and health consequences. Eur J Clin Nutr 2012;66(3): 281–95.
43. Ward EM. Osteoporosis diet dangers: foods to avoid [Internet]. Web MD; 2008 Available from: <http://www.webmd.com/osteoporosis/living-with-osteoporosis-7/diet-dangers>; [cited 2014 Jan 20.].
44. Madeira E, Mafort TT, Madeira M, et al. Lean mass as a predictor of bone density and microarchitecture in adult obese individuals with metabolic syndrome. Bone 2014;59:89–92.
45. Arranz L, Rafecas M, Alegre C. Effects of obesity on function and quality of life in chronic pain conditions. Curr Rheumatol Rep 2014;16(1):390.
46. Liljensoe A, Lauersen JO, Soballe K, et al. Overweight preoperatively impairs clinical outcome after knee arthroplasty: a cohort study of 197 patients 3–5 years after surgery. Acta Orthop 2013; 84(4):392–7.
47. Hulsmans M, Geeraert B, De Keyzer D, et al. Interleukin-1 receptor-associated kinase-3 is a key inhibitor of inflammation in obesity and metabolic syndrome. PLoS ONE 2012;7(1): e30414.
48. Issa RI, Griffin TM. Pathobiology of obesity and osteoarthritis: integrating biomechanics and inflammation. Pathobiol Aging Age Relat Dis 2012;2(2012):17470.
49. Stienstra R, Duval C, Muller M, et al. PPARs, obesity, and inflammation. PPAR Res 2007;95974.
50. Dean E, Gormsen Hansen R. Prescribing optimal nutrition and physical activity as 'first-line' interventions for best practice management of chronic low-grade inflammation associated with osteoarthritis: evidence synthesis. Arthritis 2012;560634.
51. Wärnberg J, Cunningham K, Romeo J, et al. Physical activity, exercise and low-grade systemic inflammation. Proc Nutr Soc 2010;69(03):400–6.
52. Zhang Y, Zhang S, Gao Y, et al. Factors associated with the pressure pain threshold in healthy Chinese men. Pain Med 2013;14(9):1291–300.
53. Guneli E, Gumustekin M, Ates M. Possible involvement of ghrelin on pain threshold in obesity. Med Hypotheses 2010;74(3): 452–4.
54. Shiri R, Viikari-Juntura E, Varonen H, et al. Prevalence and determinants of lateral and medial epicondylitis: a population study. Am J Epidemiol 2006;164(11):1065–74.
55. WHO. Physical inactivity a leading cause of disease and disability, warns WHO [Internet]. World Health Organization; 2002 Available from: <http://www.who.int/mediacentre/news/releases/release23/en/index.html>; [updated 2014; cited 2014 Jan 20.].
56. Obesity: preventing and managing the global epidemic. Report of a WHO consultation. World Health Organ Tech Rep Ser 2000; 894:i-xii, 1–253.
57. Kushner RF. Road Maps for Clinical Practice: Case Studies in Disease Prevention and Health Promotion-Assessment and Management of Adult Obesity: A Primer for Physicians [Internet]. Atlanta, GA: American Medical Association; 2003 Available from: <www.yaleruddcenter.org/resources/upload/docs/what/bias/AMAprimerforobesitycommunication.pdf>; [cited 2014 Jan 20.].
58. DeMarco MA, Maynard JW, Huizinga MM, et al. Obesity and younger age at gout onset in a community-based cohort. Arthritis Care Res (Hoboken) 2011;63(8):1108–14.
59. Mezhov V, Ciccutini FM, Hanna FS, et al. Does obesity affect knee cartilage? A systematic review of magnetic resonance imaging data. Obes Rev 2014;15(2):143–57.
60. Paulis WD, Silva S, Koes BW, et al. Overweight and obesity are associated with musculoskeletal complaints as early as childhood: a systematic review. Obes Rev 2014;15(1):52–67.
61. Seaman DR. Body mass index and musculoskeletal pain: is there a connection? Chiropr Man Therap 2013;21(1):15.
62. Bierma-Zeinstra SM, Koes BW. Risk factors and prognostic factors of hip and knee osteoarthritis. Nat Clin Pract Rheumatol 2007;3(2):78–85.
63. Woolner J, Dean E. Status of weight reduction as an intervention in physical therapy management of low back pain: systematic review and implications. Eur J Physiother 2013;15(2): 46–55.
64. Kandil A, Novicoff W, Browne J. Obesity and total joint arthroplasty: do patients lose weight following surgery? Phys Sportsmed 2013;41(2):34–7.
65. Schuit AJ, van Loon AJ, Tijhuis M, et al. Clustering of lifestyle risk factors in a general adult population. Prev Med 2002;35(3): 219–24.
66. Whedon GD. Disuse osteoporosis: physiological aspects. Calcif Tissue Int 1984;36(Suppl. 1).S146–50.
67. Henson J, Yates T, Biddle SJ, et al. Associations of objectively measured sedentary behaviour and physical activity with markers of cardiometabolic health. Diabetologia 2013;56(5):1012–20.
68. Stamatakis E, Hamer M, Mishra GD. Early adulthood television viewing and cardiometabolic risk profiles in early middle age: results from a population, prospective cohort study. Diabetologia 2012;55(2):311–20.
69. Thorp AA, Healy GN, Owen N, et al. Deleterious associations of sitting time and television viewing time with cardiometabolic risk biomarkers: Australian Diabetes, Obesity and Lifestyle (AusDiab) study 2004–2005. Diabetes Care 2010;33(2):327–34.
70. Hootman JM, Macera CA, Ham SA, et al. Physical activity levels among the general US adult population and in adults with and without arthritis. Arthritis Rheum 2003;49(1):129–35.
71. Celis-Morales CA, Perez-Bravo F, Ibanez L, et al. Objective vs. self-reported physical activity and sedentary time: effects of measurement method on relationships with risk biomarkers. PLoS ONE 2012;7(5):e36345.
72. Gennuso KP, Gangnon RE, Matthews CE, et al. Sedentary behavior, physical activity, and markers of health in older adults. Med Sci Sports Exerc 2013;45(8):1493–500.
73. Socio-demographic and lifestyle correlates of obesity: technical report on the secondary analyses using the 2000–2001 Canadian Community Health Survey. Canadian Population Health Initiative [Internet]. Ottawa, ON: Canadian Institute for Health Information; 2005 Available from: <https://secure.cihi.ca/estore/productFamily.htm?pf=PFC538&lang=en&media=0>; [cited 2014 Jan 20.].
74. Smuck M, Kao M, Brar N, et al. Does physical activity influence the relationship between low back pain and obesity? Spine J 2014;14(2):209–16.
75. Cherkas LF, Hunkin JL, Kato BS, et al. The association between physical activity in leisure time and leukocyte telomere length. Arch Intern Med 2008;168(2):154–8.
76. Tudor-Locke C, Craig CL, Thyfault JP, et al. A step-defined sedentary lifestyle index. Appl Physiol Nutr Metab 2013;38(2): 100–14.
77. Vuori I. Exercise and physical health: musculoskeletal health and functional capabilities. Res Q Exerc Sport 1995;66(4):276–85.
78. Tudor-Locke C, Schuna JM, Frensham LJ, et al. Changing the way we work: elevating energy expenditure with workstation alternatives. Int J Obes 2014;38(6):755–65.
79. 2008 physical activity guidelines for Americans [Internet]. Washington, D.C.: US Department of Health and Human Services; 2013 Available from: <http://www.health.gov/paguidelines/guidelines/default.aspx#toc>; [updated 2013 Nov 3; cited 2014 Jan 20.].
80. Warburton DE, Nicol CW, Bredin SS. Prescribing exercise as preventive therapy. CMAJ 2006;174(7):961–74.
81. Delitto A, George SZ, Van Dillen LR, et al. Low back pain: clinical practice guidelines linked to the International Classification of Functioning. J Orthop Sports Phys Ther 2012;42(4):A1–57.
82. Coombes JS, Law J, Lancashire B, et al. 'Exercise is medicine': curbing the burden of chronic disease and physical inactivity. Asia Pac J Public Health 2013;Forthcoming.
83. McDonough SM, Tully MA, Boyd A, et al. Pedometer-driven walking for chronic low back pain: a feasibility randomized controlled trial. Clin J Pain 2013;29(11):972–81.
84. Coren S. Sleep health and its assessment and management in physical therapy practice: the evidence. Physiother Theory Pract 2009;25(5–6):442–52.
85. Ohayon MM, Carskadon MA, Guilleminault C, et al. Meta-analysis of quantitative sleep parameters from childhood to old age in healthy individuals: developing normative sleep values across the human lifespan. Sleep 2004;27(7):1255–73.
86. Shift work & sleep [Internet]. Arlington, VA: National Sleep Foundation; 2013 Available from: <http://www.sleepfoundation.org/article/sleep-topics/shift-work-and-sleep>; [cited 2014 Feb 12.].
87. Morin CM, Benca R. Chronic insomnia. Lancet 2012;379(9821): 1129–41.

88. van de Water AT, Eadie J, Hurley DA. Investigation of sleep disturbance in chronic low back pain: an age- and gender-matched case-control study over a 7-night period. Man Ther 2011;16(6): 550–6.

89. O'Donoghue GM, Fox N, Heneghan C, et al. Objective and subjective assessment of sleep in chronic low back pain patients compared with healthy age and gender matched controls: a pilot study. BMC Musculoskelet Disord 2009;10:122.

90. Neckelmann D, Mykletun A, Dahl AA. Chronic insomnia as a risk factor for developing anxiety and depression. Sleep 2007;30(7): 873–80.

91. Haack M, Scott-Sutherland J, Santangelo G, et al. Pain sensitivity and modulation in primary insomnia. Eur J Pain 2012;16(4): 522–33.

92. Kundermann B, Krieg JC, Schreiber W, et al. The effect of sleep deprivation on pain. Pain Res Manag 2004;9(1):25–32.

93. Schuh-Hofer S, Wodarski R, Pfau DB, et al. One night of total sleep deprivation promotes a state of generalized hyperalgesia: a surrogate pain model to study the relationship of insomnia and pain. Pain 2013;154(9):1613–21.

94. Tang NK, Wright KJ, Salkovskis PM. Prevalence and correlates of clinical insomnia co-occurring with chronic back pain. J Sleep Res 2007;16(1):85–95.

95. Ackermann K, Revell VL, Lao O, et al. Diurnal rhythms in blood cell populations and the effect of acute sleep deprivation in healthy young men. Sleep 2012;35(7):933–40.

96. Thamaraiselvi K, Mathangi DC, Subhashini AS. Effect of increase in duration of REM sleep deprivation on lipid peroxidation. Int J Biol Med Res 2012;3(2):1754–9.

97. Simpson N, Dinges DF. Sleep and inflammation. Nutr Rev 2007;65(12 Pt 2):S244–52.

98. Coren S. Sleep Thieves. New York, NY: Free Press; 1996.

99. Maas JB. Power Sleep. New York, NY: Harper Collins Publishers Inc.; 1999.

100. Maas JB, FeldmanHall O, Boyles K. Power sleep and peak performance [Internet]. Health and Fitness; March 2003 Available from: <http://www.usfsa.org/Content/parentsarticles/Health%20Fitness_March03.pdf>; [cited 2014 Feb 12.].

101. Interventions to improve cardiovascular risk factors in people with serious mental illness – executive summary | AHRQ Effective Health Care Program [Internet]. Rockville, MD: Agency for Healthcare Research and Quality; 2013 Apr 22 Available from: <http://effectivehealthcare.ahrq.gov/index.cfm/search-for-guides-reviews-and-reports/?productid=1464&pageaction=displayproduct>; [cited 2014 Feb 12.].

102. Lloyd C, Waghorn G, McHugh C. Musculoskeletal disorders and comorbid depression: implications for practice. Aust Occup Ther J 2008;55(1):23–9.

103. Marazziti D, Castrogiovanni P, Rossi A, et al. Pain threshold is reduced in depression. Int J Neuropsychopharmacol 1998;1(1): 45–8.

104. Centers for Disease Control and Prevention. Prevalence of disabilities and associated health conditions among adults – United States, 1999. JAMA 2001;285(12):1571–2.

105. Galletly CA, Foley DL, Waterreus A, et al. Cardiometabolic risk factors in people with psychotic disorders: the second Australian national survey of psychosis. Aust N Z J Psychiatry 2012;46(8): 753–61.

106. Krishnan KRR, France RD, Pelton S, et al. Chronic pain and depression. II: symptoms of anxiety in chronic low back pain patients and their relationship to subtypes of depression. Pain 1985;22(3):289–94.

107. Melloh M, Elfering A, Käser A, et al. Depression impacts the course of recovery in patients with acute low-back pain. Behav Med 2013;39(3):80–9.

108. Eriksson S, Gard G. Physical exercise and depression. Phys Ther Rev 2011;16(4):261–8.

CHAPTER 12

AGEING AND THE MUSCULOSKELETAL SYSTEM

Christopher McCarthy • Aubrey Monie • Kevin Singer

This chapter is divided into two sections. Section one describes some of the physiological mechanisms of ageing, to introduce the reader to the changes we face when dealing with the ageing musculoskeletal system. The second section details the more specific changes ageing brings to the axial spine.

AGEING OF THE MUSCULOSKELETAL SYSTEM

Ageing is the declining ability to respond to stress and by virtue of the increasing homoeostatic imbalance and incidence of pathology, death remains the ultimate consequence of ageing.[1] There are a number of theories regarding ageing, with a quick reference list displayed in Table 12-1. For a more detailed overview of this area please consider the excellent review by Weinert and Timiras published in 2003.[2]

Numerous hypotheses regarding the diminishing function of cells with time exist. Mechanisms that have been proposed to be life- and/or function-limiting for cells include cumulative oxidative damage to proteins, accumulation of mutations and genomic instability, glycation of proteins and telomere (the protective region of the chromosome) dysfunction.[1] Ageing of tissues is accompanied by increases in genome rearrangements and mutations, which may cause cell senescence and/or apoptosis (programmed cell death). Cell senescence refers to the temporal decrements in the ability of cells to replicate, repair and maintain tissue, and is induced by both cell-intrinsic and cell-extrinsic mechanisms.[1]

The cellular senescence theory of ageing (1965) describes a process where there is a limit to the number of cell divisions normal human cells can undergo in culture. This 'limit in replicative capacity' occurs after a characteristic number of cell divisions and results in terminally arrested cells with altered physiology.[2] Classical descriptions of cell senescence most often refer to the loss of the ability of mitotic cells to further divide in culture after a period of 30–40 population doublings. However, cell senescence appears to be much more complex than simple cell-cycle arrest occurring after a finite number of cell divisions. More recently, attention has been drawn to other forms of cell senescence sometimes referred to as 'extrinsic' or 'stress-induced' senescence as opposed to the intrinsic senescence resulting from replication.[3,4] Stress-induced senescence can occur from diverse stimuli including oxidative damage, activated oncogenes and chronic inflammation.[4] Stress-induced senescence due to oxidative stress fits well with one of the long-standing theories of ageing that suggests that free radicals could be mediators of ageing.[5]

Ageing Joints

Oxidative damage from the chronic production of endogenous reactive oxygen species and free radicals has been associated with ageing in various human tissues and has long been thought to play a central role in the ageing process.[5] Increased production of reactive oxygen species leads to oxidative stress, a condition within cells where the amount of reactive oxygen species exceeds the antioxidant capacity of the cell. Human articular chondrocytes can actively produce reactive oxygen species and have been found to increase directly with age.[5,6]

Some of the changes observed in ageing joints and their contribution to the development of osteoarthritis are detailed in Table 12-2.

Ageing Muscles

In both young and aged skeletal muscle, it has been shown that oxidative stress increases in response to unloading (lack of activity/immobilization) and may have an important role in mediating muscle atrophy.[8] Decline of muscle mass is primarily due to type II fibre atrophy and loss of muscle fibre numbers. Increased variability in fibre size, accumulation of scattered and angulated fibres and expansion of extracellular matrix are characteristic to muscle atrophy.[8,9] The rate of muscle loss has been estimated to range from 1–2% per year past the age of 50, 25% in persons under the age of 70 and 40% of those older than 80 years are sarcopenic.[10] Significant loss of myofibrils results in an increased negative nitrogen balance which exacerbates reductions in strength and endurance.[11]

With advancing age, muscles display 'hybrid' muscle fibre characteristics. Ageing muscle demonstrates selective loss of fast motoneurons, leading to 'orphan' fast twitch muscle fibres that are adopted by the relatively more abundant slow motor units. These fibres partially convert to slow twitch fibres, ending with a hybrid phenotype showing the characteristics of both fast and slow fibres.[11] When, fast type II muscle fibres are incorporated into slow motor units (and eventually turned into a hybrid fibre), there are irregularities in the size distribution of motor units. This, in turn, affects motor accuracy, especially with low force movements, as the recruitment order does not adjust well to the previously small motor

TABLE 12-1   Theories of Ageing

Biological Level/Theory	Description
Evolutionary	
Mutation accumulation	Mutations that affect health at older ages are not selected against
Disposable soma	Somatic cells are maintained only to ensure continued reproductive success; after reproduction, soma becomes disposable
Antagonistic pleiotropy	Genes beneficial at younger age become deleterious at older ages
Molecular	
Gene regulation	Ageing is caused by changes in the expression of genes regulating both development and ageing
Codon restriction	Fidelity/accuracy of mRNA translation is impaired due to inability to decode codons in mRNA
Error catastrophe	Decline in fidelity of gene expression with ageing results in increased fraction of abnormal proteins
Somatic mutation	Molecular damage accumulates, primarily to DNA/genetic material
Dysdifferentiation	Gradual accumulation of random molecular damage impairs regulation of gene expression
Cellular	
Cellular senescence-Telomere theory	Phenotypes of ageing are caused by an increase in frequency of senescent cells. Senescence may result from telomere loss (replicative senescence) or cell stress (cellular senescence)
Free radical	Oxidative metabolism produces highly reactive free radicals that subsequently damage lipids, protein and DNA
Wear-and-tear	Accumulation of normal injury
Apoptosis	Programmed cell death from genetic events or genome crisis
System	
Neuroendocrine	Alterations in neuroendocrine control of homoeostasis results in ageing-related physiological changes
Immunologic	Decline of immune function with ageing results in decreased incidence of infectious diseases but increased incidence of autoimmunity
Rate-of-living	Assumes a fixed amount of metabolic potential for every living organism (live fast, die young)

From the review by Weinert and Timiras 2003.[2]

TABLE 12-2   Ageing and Its Contribution to Osteoarthritis

Ageing Change	Contribution to Osteoarthritis
Accumulation of cells exhibiting the senescent secretory phenotype	Increased cytokine and MMP production stimulates matrix degradation
Oxidative stress/damage	Increased susceptibility to cell death and reduced matrix synthesis
Decreased levels of growth factors and decreased growth factor responsiveness	Reduced matrix synthesis and repair
Increased AGE formation	Brittle tissue with increased fatigue failure
Reduced aggrecan size and cartilage hydration and increased collagen cleavage	Reduced resiliency and tensile strength
Increased matrix calcification	Altered mechanical properties and potential activation of inflammatory signalling

MMP, Matrix metalloproteinases; AGE, Advanced glycation end-products.
From Shane and Loeser (2010).[7]

units having grown bigger and stronger, and is one of the main reasons that motor and locomotor skills deteriorate with age.[12]

Ageing Nervous System

In the central nervous system there are age-related reductions in the total number of brain cells and fibres and the organization of fibres within the brain's white matter in addition to the reduction to the large diameter (A-beta proprioceptive) fibres in peripheral nerves.[11] In addition to reductions in the number of fast myelinated fibres, within the nerve the speed of signal conduction within the axon also reduces with age.[13] Neuromuscular junctions have been shown to demonstrate age-related reductions in size and speed of conduction, thereby reducing the efficiency of efferent transmission to the muscles.[10] These widespread physiological changes have been shown to result in poorer performance on cognitive and motor tests.[14,15]

Ageing, Falling and Pain

Rates of falls among community-living, generally healthy elderly people (age ≥65) are of the order of (0.3–1.6 per person annually), with about 5% of these resulting in a fracture or hospitalization. Fall rates rise steadily with age and are about doubled for persons aged >75 years. Persons living in long-term care institutions have much higher fall rates (0.6–3.6 annually). Falls among those in institutions also tend to result in more serious complications; with 10–25% of such falls resulting in fracture or laceration. It is often reported that older adults experience greater prevalence of pain, greater pain intensity and pain at more sites than younger adults.[15,16]

It has long been thought that the increase in the prevalence of pain among older adults is partly due to the progressive musculoskeletal degeneration that accompanies ageing. Another explanation for increased pain in older populations has been that ageing is associated with greater sensitivity to painful stimuli that results from changes in the structure and function of the nociceptive system.[17]

Ageing and the Beneficial Effects of Movement

It is thought that mechanical forces are important regulators of several biological functions, with mechanical signals having been shown to mediate the development of a variety of tissues (e.g. skeletal muscle, bone, cartilage).[18,19] Mechanical signals can affect diverse cellular processes including cell growth, differentiation, cellular migration, gene expression, protein synthesis and apoptosis.[18,19] Given the potential importance that mechanical signalling functions have in maintaining cellular homoeostasis, it is likely that changes in mechanotransduction may also play a role in the pathophysiology of disease.[19] Recent data strongly support this, as it is recognized that many aspects of sarcopenia may be related to alteration in cellular mechanotransduction.[19] The ability of cells involved in the musculoskeletal system to sense, process and respond to mechanical stimuli deteriorates with age and that these changes may be involved in the aetiology of ageing-associated disease.[20] Encouragingly, movement quantity, quality, locality and intensity are relatively modifiable influences and are certainly influences within the scope of the manual therapists. The influence of mechanotransduction on tissue health and the symptoms of ageing are exciting areas for future research, particularly for those of us involved in the provision and prescription of therapeutic movement.

THE AGEING SPINE

Most individuals achieve old age with some evidence of degenerative or pathological changes in spinal joints, which reflect the interactions between: genetics, occupation, lifestyle, nutrition, trauma and destiny. Most published reviews on the health of the spine are seen through the prism of clinical perspectives, with an absence of large-scale, long time-lapse epidemiological surveys to discern patterns and to test predictions. Post-mortem surveys and large radiological population-based studies[21,22,23] agree that spinal degenerative and age changes have an extremely high prevalence in adult populations. Of late, subtle differences in disc degeneration patterns are being realized as genomic sequencing emerges as an investigatory tool.[24] In the current era of Western society, osteoporosis is acutely studied given the cost and morbidity associated with the declining bone mineral health of the axial skeleton and its attendant fracture risk. This trend is not surprising, as over the last 100 years developed societies have evolved from physically demanding occupations to becoming increasingly urbanized and inactive. The call to add physical activity to counter the epidemic of poor lifestyle choices (i.e. inactivity, smoking, poor nutrition) has become urgent given the projected cost and negative health outcomes for society.[25]

Our biology uses both ageing and degeneration strategies to constrain the musculoskeletal system against further injury or damage. In the case of the spine, which serves the principal objectives of mobility, stability and protection of neural elements, overload or dynamic loading strains can induce a spectrum of either local or regional trauma and degenerative changes. Consequently, this chapter draws upon literature that represents both age-related and degeneration models, and their outcomes for the axial skeleton.

Normal physiological strains are well accommodated by each functional mobile segment, which comprises an intervertebral disc (IVD) with an anulus fibrosus and nucleus pulposus, and the vertebral end-plates (VEP). Paired synovial zygapophysial joints link both vertebrae posteriorly and articulate closely to regulate both load and movement of the segment. Applied moments from muscle actions and axial compressive loads may be coupled with shear, bending (rotations) and torsion about the long axis of the spine, which are in turn moderated by the unique geometry of the segment's zygapophysial and ligamentous anatomy (Fig. 12-1). Inertial strains from dynamic loading, even several times body weight, may also be tolerated by the spine given its unique capacity to attenuate energy.[26] The regional response to loading is reflected in different patterns of injury or degeneration.

Vertebral bone adapts to loading by the cyclic remodelling which is optimal by the third decade of life and declines variously thereafter.[27] Loss of trabecular connectivity, endocortical bone trabeculation and intracortical porosity are the late stages of remodelling. VEP collapse occurs due to trabecular bone fragility, with vertebral body fracture the clinical end-point in some cases. IVD degeneration is considered a normal process of ageing, but may be precipitated by multiple factors including genetic, anatomical, mechanical (occupational, overload, torsion, vibration), cell-mediated molecular cascades, trauma, infection and toxins as major influences to disc health[28-30] (Fig. 12-2).

Osteoarthritis of the spine develops as a consequence of the natural ageing process coupled with attrition, and is associated with a degenerative cascade that may involve

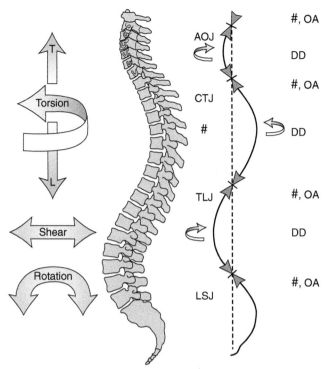

FIGURE 12-1 ■ The regional patterns of injury and degeneration in the spine. *AOJ*, Atlanto-occipital joint; *CTJ*, Cervicothoracic joint; *DD*, Disc degeneration/Disc disease?; *L*, Lumbar; *LSJ*, Lumbosacral joint; *OA*, Osteoarthritis; *T*, Thoracic; *TLJ*, Thoraco-lumbar joint;. #, these sites along the column are disposed to trauma and fracture.

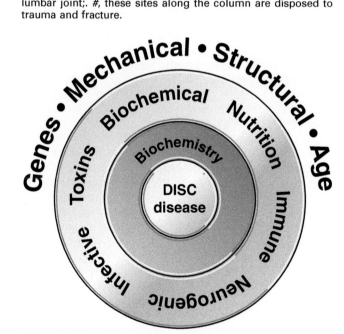

FIGURE 12-2 ■ The influences on the intervertebral disc associated with ageing.

the discrete elements or an entire functional mobile segment, individually or regionally.[31,32]

The IVD is essentially aneural apart from the peripheral superficial outer third, although with injury to the disc, vascular ingrowth associated with repair may contribute vasomotor nerves.[33] The disc is also avascular, apart from the peripheral annulus, with a reliance upon nutritional substances transported via diffusion across the

VEPs[34] or through vessels that communicate directly with the outer annular layers. Consequently, disruption to either system occurring through normal ageing, surgical intervention, spinal deformity or trauma can disrupt and lengthen the pathways of nutritional support to the disc and is presumed to contribute to subsequent disc degeneration. The consequence of either ageing or injury to the functional mobile segment may be degeneration of its elements with initial progressive increase in strain tolerance beyond the normal, which may progress to increased segmental mobility. One mechanical response to such changes, particularly affecting the stability and function of the IVD, is spondylosis, initiated through osteogenic stimulation in the junctional region between the VEP periphery and the annulus, resulting in the early formation of osteophytes.[35] Experimentally induced osteoarthrosis of the paired zygapophysial joints has been associated with anular rim lesions of the IVD.[36] The posterior paired costotransverse and costovertebral zygapophysial joints are true synovial joints invested with hyaline articular cartilage, a capsule and synovium. These joints contribute stability of the respective segment(s) and facilitate respiratory excursions of the thorax and regional mobility within the vertebral column, respectively. Each may respond to overload with degenerative patterns of synovial joints characterized by mechanical changes of the articular cartilage. Subchondral bone sclerosis, fissuring and detachment of the cartilage, and marginal joint osteophytosis may follow changes in the IVD, particularly a loss of vertical height which in turn alters the mechanical alignment of the respective superior and inferior articular processes of the posterior joints. Bumper fibrocartilage formations at the joint margin are associated with evidence of articular cartilage degeneration and fissuring, ossification of the ligamentum flavum, and reactive hyperplasia at the posterior joint margins. A further consequence of degenerative changes leading to altered morphology of the IVD and vertebral bodies is the response by the spinal ligaments. With progressive deformation of the segment, ligaments may demonstrate buckling and, in response to exaggerated segmental motion strains, subsequent hypertrophic changes may contribute to stenotic change within the vertebral and intervertebral canals.[37] Ossification within the ligamentum flavum may occur as a consequence of degeneration of the articular triad, although this tends to predominate in the region of the lower thoracic and upper lumbar segments.[38]

Patterns of spinal degeneration and age changes become evident when merged onto a common model of the axial skeleton; the mobile cervical and lumbar segments, and their respective stiffer transitional junctions display different trends. The general pattern is for spinal motion to decline in all directions with age, and this feature is illustrated with the combined movement examination assessment for the lumbar spine (Fig. 12-3). Where segmental mobility is greatest degeneration of the disc and facet joints dominate. In the case of the bony thorax, focal changes are seen at the respective costovertebral joint articulations of the first and last ribs, a consequence of transferring large torques from the musculature of the neck and trunk, respectively. When one

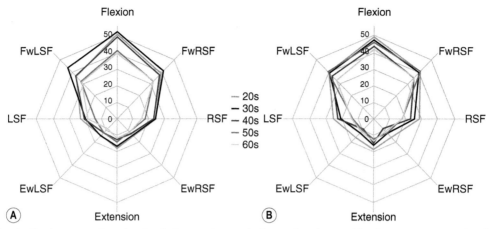

FIGURE 12-3 ■ The decline in range of motion in all planes, observed when using the combined movement examination of the lumbar spine. F, flexion; FwRSF, flexion with right side flexion; RSF, right side flexion; EwRSF, extension with right side flexion; E, extension; EwLSF, extension with left side flexion; LSF, left side flexion; FwLSF, flexion with left side flexion; For colour version see Plate 11.

considers the complete vertebral column as a multisegmented curved rod, with physiological inflexions that cross the neutral axis line, the literature presents evidence of different responses to stress accumulations at points of both maximum and minimum change in curve. The segments adjacent to the transitional junctions, having less relative motion, are designed more for stability and represent locations where axial compressive load is greater, the change in spinal curvature is least and where arthrosis of these synovial joints is found. In contrast, where the curvature away from the neutral axis line is maximum, as in the middle region of the lordosis and kyphosis, respectively, and where bending, torsion and shear stresses are relatively higher, the trend is for greater disc degeneration (see Fig. 12-1).

The major degenerative conditions reviewed in this chapter include osteoporosis and anomalies of spinal curvature, and changes that arise secondary to trauma. Inflammatory disease of the spine is excluded from this discussion; the interested reader is directed to the compilation by Klippel and Dieppe[39] for a comprehensive review. Degenerative conditions that principally have a spinal manifestation may involve all elements of the functional mobile segment, either singularly as in the case of early IVD degeneration, or across the joint complex, exemplified by late zygapophysial joint arthrosis coincident with IVD degeneration.[40,41]

Disc Degeneration

Literature describing the incidence of disc degeneration throughout the vertebral column concentrates predominantly on the lumbar and cervical regions of the spine.[42] From post-mortem studies, discs with altered vascularity during the second decade of life show precursor changes to early degeneration.[43] The pathway of age-related degeneration change has been described as compromised nutrition, loss of viable cells, cell senescence, post-translational modification of matrix proteins, accumulation of degraded matrix molecules, a reduction in pH levels that may impede cell function and ultimately induce cell death, and finally fatigue failure of the matrix.[44] The

highest prevalence of disc degeneration is in the mid-cervical, mid-thoracic and mid-lumbar discs as these regions show a marked degree of reactive changes of the vertebral bodies with marginal osteophyte formation (Fig. 12-4). Early post-mortem studies by von Lushka[45] demonstrated a large proportion of cervical discs with fissures and clefts. This was considered to be a normal characteristic of the region, with complete transverse clefts extending across and into the region of the uncovertebral joints found in the middle of healthy cervical discs on coronal section.[46] From similar post-mortem reviews of the thoracic spine, the most severely affected discs are located predominantly within the middle segments, peaking between T6–T7, with a greater incidence in males.[47] Given the tendency to axial plane segmental motion in the mid-thoracic spine, reported in the classic paper by Gregersen and Lucas,[48] such degenerative changes may relate to the large rotation strains imposed upon these segments. Investigations by Farfan et al.[49] into the effects of torsion on lumbar IVDs concluded that relatively small rotation strains >2° per segment induced potential injury in the anulus fibrosus. The pattern of age-related decline in anterior disc height in men typifies the disc ageing process associated with senile kyphosis whereby the cumulative effects of axial loading and torsional stresses result in degeneration of the anterior anulus and osteophytosis.[21] In females, however, loading through the anterior aspect of the kyphotic curve is more likely to produce progressive change of the vertebral bodies, causing the wedge deformity commonly associated with spinal osteoporosis.[50] Mechanically, the middle vertebral segments are predisposed to greater axial compressive and bending moments, due to their position within the apex of the thoracic kyphosis.[51]

Osteophytosis

Osteophyte formation and its associated IVD degeneration has been recognized as an attempt to distribute force more uniformly across the VEPs to achieve stress reduction on the segment.[52] Where thoracolumbar disc degeneration is present, marginal osteophyte formation of the

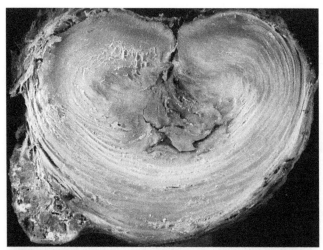
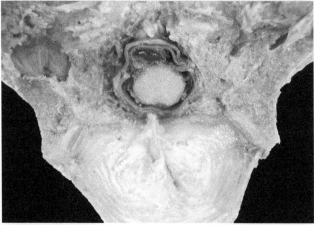

FIGURE 12-4 ■ Macroscopic view of the L2–L3 (top) and T10–T11 (bottom) discs sectioned in the horizontal plane of two elderly cases to highlight disc herniation and advanced degeneration. The T10–T11 section depicts a central disc prolapse deforming the anterior dural sac. At L2–L3, age-related changes are demonstrated in the form of the large right-sided anterolateral osteophyte and advanced disintegration of the nucleus. A central fissure is evident through the posterior anulus.

vertebral body is frequently seen.[22,35] This pattern of excess bone formation, commonly referred to as spondylosis deformans, is seen in approximately 60% of women and 80% of men.[21] The degree of intervertebral space narrowing and subsequent tilting of the vertebral bodies, resulting from disc degeneration, often determines the extent and the type of marginal osteophytes.[53] In summary, the segments that appear susceptible to osteophytes are often the most mobile regions with the higher levels of disc degeneration, or where local stress may be accumulated.

Vertebral End-Plate Lesions and Schmorl's Nodes

The vertebral end-plate is a membrane of tissue comprising hyaline cartilage and a 0.5-mm-thin trabecular layer at the discovertebral junction.[54] Its role is to mediate axial compressive load applied to the IVD and permit transfer of this energy within the subchondral and cancellous bone of the vertebral body. Physiological axial loading, as

occurs with gait, acts as a 'pump' to assist diffusion of nutrients within the vascular vertebral body across the VEP and into/away from the disc. Abrupt or fatigue axial loading of the spine may cause localized failure of the VEP resulting in either a frank sharply demarcated vertebral intra-osseous prolapse, often termed a Schmorl's node, or marked irregularity of the end-plate. The repair process for both lesions often results in bony sclerosis which can significantly impair the normal nutrient exchange to the IVD by reducing the effectiveness of this diffusion pathway. Schmorl's nodes have been reported to occur during the late teens,[55] with lesions as frequent in the young as in the older individual.[21] Cadaveric studies of lumbar spines have indicated that Schmorl's nodes develop at an early age and can exhibit advanced degenerative changes.[35] Schmorl's nodes are found most commonly in males and are considered to be related to a genetic disposition, strenuous occupations[21] or sports involving dynamic and violent axial loading as might occur with a heavy landing in flexion.[55] Most authors agree that the inferior end-plate is more susceptible to infraction[53,56] which implies that the VEP fails under compression (Fig. 12-5).

Zygapophysial and Costovertebral Joint Degeneration

There appear to be specific sites within the spine where preferential degeneration of the synovial joints occur. The upper and lower segments of the thoracic region show a tendency for zygapophysial and costovertebral joint degeneration.[57,58,59] Similar trends for osteophytic remodelling of the zygapophysial joints of the lumbosacral junction have been reported.[60,61] This may be due to the design of these elements that provide stability and protection in contrast to the adjacent mobile segments which show a correspondingly higher frequency of disc disease[62] (see Fig. 12-1). The development of osteophytes and eventual bony fusion of costovertebral and costo-transverse joints in aged vertebral columns was also noted by Schmorl and Junghans[21] in their extensive survey of spinal pathology. The cervicothoracic junction and thoracolumbar junction represent transitional areas between mobile and relatively immobile regions of the spine. At the cervicothoracic junction, Boyle et al.[63,64] found evident IVD and VEP changes, along with osteophytic formation that were more pronounced in the mobile segments immediately above the transition. The upper thoracic region and thoracic cage acted to impede intersegmental motion and thus safeguard these levels from marked degeneration.[64] At the thoracolumbar junction, Malmivaara et al.[53] demonstrated that particular pathologies tended to be concentrated at each segment. The T10–T11 segment was characterized by disc degeneration, vertebral body osteophytosis and Schmorl's nodes; the T11–T12 segment tended to show both anterior and posterior degeneration, involving zygapophysial and costovertebral joints, while the T12–L1 joint was characterized primarily by posterior joint degeneration. A comparison of zygapophysial joint orientation with degenerative findings suggested that the posterior elements play a significant role in resisting torsional loads.

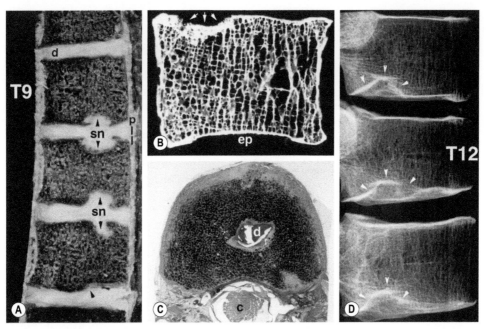

FIGURE 12-5 ■ **(A)** Intravertebral protrusions, or Schmorl's nodes, are depicted from several views to highlight their location and extent. They may project cranially and/or caudally through the vertebral end-plate (arrows). End-plate irregularities are typically in the lower thoracic spine, as represented by the inferior end-plate of T11 (arrow). **(B)** A depression on the superior end-plate of a 2-mm-thick bone section from T11 with slight sclerosing of the end-plate compared with the regular thin inferior end-plate. **(C)** A central Schmorl's node at T12 in a 100-mm-thick horizontal histological section shows disc material surrounded by sclerotic bony margins. **(D)** Multiple Schmorl's nodes are shown at the thoracolumbar junction, all approximately in the same location and affecting the inferior vertebral end-plate, a characteristic of Scheuermann's disease. *c,* Spinal cord; *d,* Disc; *ep,* End-plate; *pll,* Posterior longitudinal ligament; *sn,* Schmorl's nodes. (Adapted from Singer 2000.[47])

Asymmetry in the zygapophysial joint orientation tended to result in degenerative changes occurring mostly on the sagittal facing facet,[53] an observation originally made by Farfan et al.[49] at the lumbosacral junction.

Degenerative Spinal Curvature Anomalies

Idiopathic scoliosis involves a lateral curvature of the spine that is introduced through a disturbance in the longitudinal growth of the spine. It may occur early in the growth of the child and particularly during the early adolescent years.[65] Four main curve patterns have been identified: thoracic, lumbar, thoracolumbar and double major curves. Each of these curvature patterns has its own characteristics and predictable end-point.[65] It is well accepted that the severity of the scoliosis can continue to progress through the life span.[66,67] Disc degeneration is known to develop due to the often extreme compression and ipsilateral tension strains experienced within wedged scoliotic IVDs. A cascade of degenerative changes occur in advanced scoliosis due to the attempt to stabilize against the increasingly asymmetric mechanical loads induced by this deformity (Fig. 12-6).

Osteoporosis and Osteoporotic Fracture

Osteoporosis is an endocrine disease characterized by decreased bone mass and micro-architectural deterioration of bone, which may lead to bone fragility and subsequently to an increased rate of fracture. Although resorption of bone follows the normal process of ageing,

it may be induced through disordered metabolism and is accelerated following menopause in women.[68] A gender difference in bone fragility emerges due to the dynamic change in relationship between the mechanics of load transfer and the margins of safety. Males accumulate more periosteal bone than females, with a corresponding increase in vertebral cross-sectional area which confers a relatively higher load-bearing capability such that reductions in bone strength are less dramatic than seen in women. During ageing, this ratio is disturbed and fracture risk increases as the stress on bone begins to approximate its strength. Twenty per cent of postmenopausal women have a stress-to-strength ratio imbalance, whereas only 2–3% of men are at risk of fracture due to the greater preservation of bone strength.[69] The epidemiology of osteoporosis is well known whereby the risk factors of age, gender and racial contributors to bone loss and corresponding fracture risk increase exponentially with age. For the thoracic spine, one in four women over the age of 60 years will show at least one vertebral body fracture on radiographic examination, while the incidence increases to 100% in women over 80 years of age;[70] for men, there is a decade offset before osteopenia and osteoporosis develops.[71] The mid-thoracic segments are the most vulnerable to osteoporotic collapse or progressive wedge deformity due to the mechanical disadvantage of these segments situated within the apex of the thoracic kyphosis.[47] The second peak for thoracic osteoporotic fracture is at the thoracolumbar junction where more rapid loading of the thoracic spine can induce a hinging of the stiffened thorax on the upper lumbar spine. These

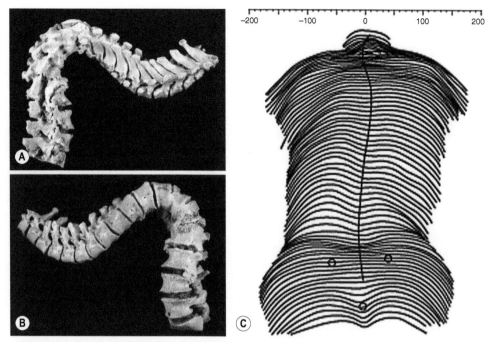

FIGURE 12-6 ■ An elderly macerated spinal column depicting severe kyphoscoliosis and marked osteophytic fusion across several segments within the region of the thoracolumbar transition, depicted from the **(A)** posterior and **(B)** anterior aspect. Note the remarkable osseous degeneration and remodelling. **(C)** A surface contour image of a marked scoliosis in an elderly woman, showing the typical rib hump appearance and asymmetry of the thoracic cage.

more dynamic loads may be sufficient to cause marked wedge compression fractures. Degenerative change to the IVD is not common in osteoporosis, suggesting a sparing of the IVD despite the vertebral body deformation.

Intervertebral Disc Prolapse

Clinically, the regions susceptible to prolapse of the intervertebral disc and the resulting disc degeneration typically are those with higher levels of mobility within the mid to lower cervical region and lower lumbar segments.[42] What is not often appreciated is the high frequency of macroscopic discal prolapse within the thoracic region[47] (see Fig. 12-4) with the T11–T12 level most commonly involved. This trend may be due to the relatively greater disc height and volume at this region, coupled with localization of torsional forces that can occur immediately above the level of thoracolumbar junction transition. Markolf[72] proposed that the eleventh and twelfth thoracic vertebrae represented a site of structural weakness for stresses in the vertebral column, due to the reduced constraint of the ribcage and the change in zygapophysial joint morphology that facilitated rotation above the transitional levels and impeded it below. The implication of disc prolapse is mechanical decompression of the nucleus, fissuring of the annulus and the cascade of changes that follow this injury.[44]

Summary

The human spine contributes a large proportion of the musculoskeletal presentations seen in manual therapy practice. This chapter has reviewed the effect of age on the human spine, including those degenerative processes that are secondary to metabolic disease, spinal deformity or trauma. Ageing of the spine is not merely a chronological process, as remodelling and repair follow such insults as trauma, disease, deformity or surgery and reflects a biological strategy to stabilize against further segment damage from imposed loads.[73] While ageing is an unavoidable certainty, skeletal loading remains a critical requirement for optimal function. Loading the musculoskeletal system throughout its dynamic range, over the lifespan, is crucial for sustaining not just musculoskeletal health but health in general.

REFERENCES

1. Carrington JL. Ageing bone and cartilage: cross-cutting issues. Biochem Biophys Res Commun 2005;328(3):700–8.
2. Weinert BT, Timiras PS. Invited review: theories of ageing. J Appl Physiol (1985) 2003;95(4):1706–16.
3. DelCarlo M, Loeser RF. Chondrocyte cell death mediated by reactive oxygen species-dependent activation of PKC-betaI. Am J Physiol Cell Physiol 2006;290(3):C802–11.
4. Loeser RF. Ageing and osteoarthritis: the role of chondrocyte senescence and ageing changes in the cartilage matrix. Osteoarthritis Cartilage 2009;17(8):971–9.
5. Loeser RF. The effects of ageing on the development of osteoarthritis. HSS J 2012;8(1):18–19.
6. Loeser RF. Age-related changes in the musculoskeletal system and the development of osteoarthritis. Clin Geriatr Med 2010;26(3):371–86.
7. Shane AA, Loeser RF. Why is osteoarthritis an age-related disease? Best Pract Res Clin Rheumatol 2010;24(1):15–26.
8. Seene T, Kaasik P, Riso EM. Review on ageing, unloading and reloading: changes in skeletal muscle quantity and quality. Arch Gerontol Geriatr 2012;54(2):374–80.
9. Seene T, Kaasik P. Role of exercise therapy in prevention of decline in ageing muscle function: glucocorticoid myopathy and unloading. J Ageing Res 2012;2012:172492.

10. Kaya RD, Nakazawa M, Hoffman RL, et al. Interrelationship between muscle strength, motor units, and ageing. Exp Gerontol 2013;48(9):920–5.

11. Jokl P. The biology of ageing muscle: quantitative versus qualitative findings of performance capacity and age. In: Nelson C, Dwyer AP, editors. The Ageing Musculoskeletal System. Toronto: The Collamore Press; 1984. p. 49–58.

12. Hausdorff JM, Levy BR, Wei JY. The power of ageism on physical function of older persons: reversibility of age-related gait changes. J Am Geriatr Soc 1999;47(11):1346–9.

13. Mittal KR, Logmani FH. Age-related reduction in 8th cervical ventral nerve root myelinated fiber diameters and numbers in man. J Gerontol 1987;42(1):8–10.

14. Hausdorff JM, Edelberg HK, Cudkowicz ME, et al. The relationship between gait changes and falls. J Am Geriatr Soc 1997;45(11):1406.

15. Rubenstein LZ. Falls in older people: epidemiology, risk factors and strategies for prevention. Age Ageing 2006;35(Suppl. 2):ii37–41.

16. Rubenstein LZ, Josephson KR. The epidemiology of falls and syncope. Clin Geriatr Med 2002;18(2):141–58.

17. Cruz-Almeida Y, Black ML, Christou EA, et al. Site-specific differences in the association between plantar tactile perception and mobility function in older adults. Front Ageing Neurosci 2014;6:68.

18. Duncan RL, Turner CH. Mechanotransduction and the functional response of bone to mechanical strain. Calcif Tissue Int 1995;57(5):344–58.

19. Shwartz Y, Blitz E, Zelzer E. One load to rule them all: mechanical control of the musculoskeletal system in development and ageing. Differentiation 2013;86(3):104–11.

20. Isermann P, Lammerding J. Nuclear mechanics and mechanotransduction in health and disease. Curr Biol 2013;23(24):R1113–21.

21. Schmorl G, Junghanns H. The Human Spine in Health and Disease. New York Grune and Stratton; 1971.

22. Lawrence JS. Rheumatism in Populations. London: William Heinemann Medical Books; 1977.

23. Prescher A. Anatomy and pathology of the ageing spine. Eur J Radiol 1998;27(3):181–95.

24. Colombier P, Clouet J, Hamel O, et al. The lumbar intervertebral disc: from embryonic development to degeneration. Joint Bone Spine 2014;81(2):125–9. [Epub 2013/08/13].

25. Trost SG, Blair SN, Khan KM. Physical inactivity remains the greatest public health problem of the 21st century: evidence, improved methods and solutions using the '7 investments that work' as a framework. Br J Sports Med 2014;48(3):169–70.

26. Adams MA, Bogduk N, Burton K, et al. The Biomechanics of Back Pain. Edinburgh: Churchill Livingstone; 2013.

27. Tobias JH, Gould V, Brunton L, et al. Physical activity and bone: may the force be with you. Front Endocrinol 2014;5:20. [Epub 2014/03/14].

28. Battie MC, Videman T, Kaprio J, et al. The twin spine study: contributions to a changing view of disc degeneration. Spine J 2009;9(1):47–59. [Epub 2008/12/30].

29. Gopal D, Ho AL, Shah A, et al. Molecular basis of intervertebral disc degeneration. Adv Exp Med Biol 2012;760:114–33. [Epub 2013/01/03].

30. Neidlinger-Wilke C, Galbusera F, Pratsinis H, et al. Mechanical loading of the intervertebral disc: from the macroscopic to the cellular level. Eur Spine J 2014;23(Suppl. 3):S333–43.

31. Laplante BL, DePalma MJ. Spine osteoarthritis. PM & R 2012;4(Suppl. 5):S28–36. [Epub 2012/06/01].

32. Vo N, Niedernhofer LJ, Nasto LA, et al. An overview of underlying causes and animal models for the study of age-related degenerative disorders of the spine and synovial joints. J Orthop Res 2013;31(6):831–7.

33. Palmgren T, Gronblad M, Virri J, et al. An immunohistochemical study of nerve structures in the anulus fibrosus of human normal lumbar intervertebral discs. Spine 1999;24(20):2075–9.

34. Dolan P, Luo J, Pollintine P, et al. Intervertebral disc decompression following endplate damage implications for disc degeneration depend on spinal level and age. Spine 2013;38(17):1473–81.

35. Vernon-Roberts B, Pirie CJ. Degenerative changes in intervertebral disks of lumbar spine and their sequelae. Rheumatol Rehabil 1977;16(1):13–21.

36. Osti OL, Vernonroberts B, Moore R, et al. Annular tears and disk degeneration in the lumbar spine – a postmortem study of 135 disks. J Bone Joint Surg Br 1992;74(5):678–82.

37. Weinstein P, Ehni G, Wilson C. Clinical features of lumbar spondylosis and stenosis. In: Weinstein PREG, Wilson CB, editors. Lumbar Spondylosis, Diagnosis, Management and Surgical Treatment. Chicago: Year Book; 1977.

38. Maigne JY, Ayral X, Guerin-Surville H. Frequency and size of ossifications in the caudal attachments of the ligamentum flavum of the thoracic spine. Role of rotatory strains in their development. An anatomic study of 121 spines. Surg Radiol Anat: SRA 1992;14(2):119–24. [Epub 1992/01/01].

39. Klippel JH, Dieppe PA. Rheumatology. London: Mosby; 2008.

40. Oegema TR Jr, Bradford DS. The inter-relationship of facet joint osteoarthritis and degenerative disc disease. Br J Rheumatol 1991;30(Suppl. 1):16–20.

41. Fujiwara A, Lim TH, An HS, et al. The effect of disc degeneration and facet joint osteoarthritis on the segmental flexibility of the lumbar spine. Spine 2000;25(23):3036–44. [Epub 2001/01/06].

42. Kramer J. Intervertebral disk diseases. Causes, Diagnosis, Treatment and Prophylaxis. Stuttgart: Georg Thieme Verlag; 1990.

43. Boos N, Weissbach S, Rohrbach H, et al. Classification of age-related changes in lumbar intervertebral discs: 2002 Volvo Award in Basic Science. Spine 2002;27(23):2631–44. [Epub 2002/12/04].

44. Buckwalter JA. Ageing and degeneration of the human intervertebral disc. Spine 1995;20(11):1307–14. [Epub 1995/06/01].

45. von Luschka H. Die Halbbgelenke des Menschlichen Körpers. Berlin: Druck und Verlag von Georg Reimer; 1858.

46. Tenhave H, Eulderink F. Degenerative changes in the cervical-spine and their relationship to its mobility. J Pathol 1980;132(2):133–59.

47. Singer KP. Pathology of the thoracic spine. In: Giles LGF, Singer KP, editors. Clinical Anatomy and Management of Thoracic Spine Pain. Oxford: Butterworth Heinemann; 2000. p. 63–82.

48. Gregersen GG, Lucas DB. An in vivo study of the axial rotation of the human thoracolumbar spine. J Bone Joint Surg Am 1967;49(2):247–62. [Epub 1967/03/01].

49. Farfan HF, Cossette JW, Robertson GH, et al. The effects of torsion on the lumbar intervertebral joints: the role of torsion in the production of disc degeneration. J Bone Joint Surg 1970;52(3):468–97. [Epub 1970/04/01].

50. Goh S, Price RI, Leedman PJ, et al. The relative influence of vertebral body and intervertebral disc shape on thoracic kyphosis. Clin Biomech 1999;14(7):439–48. [Epub 1999/10/16].

51. Singer K, Edmondston S, Day R, et al. Prediction of thoracic and lumbar vertebral body compressive strength – correlations with bone-mineral density and vertebral region. Bone 1995;17(2):167–74.

52. Nathan H. Osteophytes of the vertebral column – An anatomical study of their development according to age, race, and sex with considerations as to their etiology and significance. J Bone Joint Surg 1962;44(2):243–68.

53. Malmivaara A, Videman T, Kuosma E, et al. Facet joint orientation, facet and costovertebral joint osteoarthrosis, disc degeneration, vertebral body osteophytosis, and Schmorl's nodes in the thoracolumbar junctional region of cadaveric spines. Spine 1987;12(5):458–63. [Epub 1987/06/01].

54. Grignon B, Grignon Y, Mainard D, et al. The structure of the cartilaginous end-plates in elder people. Surg Radiol Anat 2000;22(1):13–19. [Epub 2000/06/23].

55. Fisk JW, Baigent ML, Hill PD. Scheuermann's disease. Clinical and radiological survey of 17 and 18 year olds. Am J Phys Med 1984;63(1):18–30. [Epub 1984/02/01].

56. Yasuma T, Saito S, Kihara K. Schmorls nodes – correlation of X-ray and histological-findings in postmortem specimens. Acta Pathol Jpn 1988;38(6):723–33.

57. Shore LR. On osteo-arthritis in the dorsal intervertebral joints – A study in morbid anatomy. Br J Surg 1935;22(88):833–49.

58. Shore LR. Some examples of disease of the vertebral column found in skeletons of ancient Egypt – A contribution to palaeopathology. Br J Surg 1935;22(94):256–62.

59. Nathan H, Robin GC, Weinberg H, et al. Costovertebral joints anatomical-clinical observations in arthritis. Arthritis Rheum 1964;7(3):228–40.

60. Cihak R. Variations of lumbosacral joints and their morphogenesis. Acta Univ Carol [Med] (Praha) 1970;16(1):145–65.

61. Resnick D. Degenerative diseases of the vertebral column. Radiology 1985;156(1):3–14.

62. Resnick D, Niwayama G. Diffuse idiopathic skeletal hyperostosis (DISH): ankylosing hyperostosis of Forestier and Rotes-Querol. In: Resnick D, editor. Diagnosis of Bone and Joint Disorders. Philadelphia: Saunders; 1995. p. 1463–508.

63. Boyle JJW, Singer KP, Milne N. Pathoanatomy of the intervertebral discs at the cervicothoracic junction. Man Ther 1998;3:72–7.

64. Boyle JWW, Milne N, Singer KP. Clinical anatomy of the cervicothoracic junction. In: Singer LGK, editor. Clinical Anatomy and Management of Cervical Spine Pain. Oxford: Butterworth Heinemann; 1998. p. 40–52.

65. Weinstein SL. Adolescent idiopathic scoliosis: prevalence and natural history. In: Weinstein S, editor. The Pediatric Spine. New York: Raven; 1994. p. 463–78.

66. Ascani E, Bartolozzi P, Logroscino CA, et al. Natural history of untreated idiopathic scoliosis after skeletal maturity. Spine 1986;11(8):784–9. [Epub 1986/10/01].

67. Gillespy T 3rd, Gillespy T Jr, Revak CS. Progressive senile scoliosis: seven cases of increasing spinal curves in elderly patients. Skeletal Radiol 1985;13(4):280–6. [Epub 1985/01/01].

68. Kanis JA. Textbook of Osteoporosis. Oxford: Blackwell Science; 1996.

69. Seeman E. During ageing, men lose less bone than women because they gain more periosteal bone, not because they resorb less endosteal bone. Calcif Tissue Int 2001;69(4):205–8.

70. Melton JL. Epidemiology of fractures. In: Melton LRJ, editor. Osteoporosis: Etiology, Diagnosis, and Management. Philadelphia: Lippincott-Raven; 1995. p. 225–47.

71. Seeman E. The dilemma of osteoporosis in men. Am J Med 1995;98:S76–88.

72. Markolf KL. Deformation of the thoracolumbar intervertebral joints in response to external loads: a biomechanical study using autopsy material. J Bone Joint Surg Am 1972;54(3):511–33. [Epub 1972/04/01].

73. Kirkaldy-Willis WH, Farfan HF. Instability of the lumbar spine. Clin Orthop Relat Res 1982;165:110–23. [Epub 1982/05/01].

SECTION 2.2

ADVANCES IN MEASUREMENT METHODS

Physiotherapists have always been diligent in their attempts to quantify methods of assessment, measurement and patient outcomes in the area of musculoskeletal pain, both in the clinical environment as well as in research. In recent times, significant technological advances have been made in many areas, including those that measure central nervous system functioning, imaging of various musculoskeletal structures, quantifying movement and muscle function, as well as being able to effectively measure the effects of physiotherapy treatment and patient outcomes. This section will bring together new developments in these areas and their implications for musculoskeletal physiotherapy practice and future research.

The state of the art in the measurement of the mechanics of human movement is presented with a focus on data provided by optoelectronic stereophotogrammetric systems, magnetic and inertial measurement units, and force platforms. Imaging techniques are then explored. New developments in ultrasound imaging are outlined including both real-time ultrasound imaging as a safe and relatively inexpensive means of examining various structures including muscle, nerves and tendons, as well as rehabilitative ultrasound imaging used by physiotherapists for assessment and biofeedback purposes. New research findings of changes in musculoskeletal tissues that both conventional and more advanced MRI imaging provide are then discussed. Here technology is progressing at a rapid pace and providing information about tissue morphology that has not been possible previously. The use of fMRI to gain an increased

understanding of the representation of pain in the brain is discussed and interactions between musculoskeletal therapies and central pain processing are considered. This technology has advanced the knowledge of central nociceptive processes but its use comes with some caveats that will be discussed. Also discussed is investigation of the brain's functioning and interconnections using the technology of transcranial magnetic stimulation (TMS).

Electromyography (EMG) has been used for a long time in physiotherapy research, but significant advances in the use, acquisition, analysis and interpretation of EMG data have been made and these, along with their clinical implications, are presented in this section. However, EMG cannot provide information about the load on various structures during movement and the use of computational modelling, the only viable possibility for estimating the forces inside the human body is therefore also presented. The section then moves to the evaluation of the sensory and nociceptive systems using quantitative sensory testing. Although physiotherapists have used sensory tests in simple forms for many years, the now greater understanding of nociceptive processing and neuropathic pain demands more rigorous assessment techniques like detailed quantitative sensory testing.

The final chapter in this section, but by far not the least important, will discuss the current state of play regarding patient-centred outcome measures and their importance in being able to determine change in a patient's health status. This forms the basis for important evaluation of physiotherapy interventions.

CHAPTER 13

MOVEMENT ANALYSIS

Aurelio Cappozzo • Andrea Cereatti • Valentina Camomilla •
Claudia Mazzà • Giuseppe Vannozzi

INTRODUCTION

Quantitative movement analysis, through measurement (see also Chapters 15 and 17) and computational modelling (see Chapter 19), provides information on functions of the locomotor sub-systems and on the overall strategy of motor activity. These outcomes contribute to the understanding of the key factors that affect internal loading and thus injury, tissue degeneration or regeneration, as well as motor control and its adaptation, energy consumption and fatigue. Quantitative subject-specific analysis can be effectively used in prevention, early diagnosis (e.g. monitoring of functional status in the elderly, specific workers or athletes), intervention (e.g. prognosis, therapeutic programming, workplace optimization, physical training) and for quantifying outcomes. Advanced movement analysis technology may be used for the implementation of real-time biofeedback (virtual reality) both in rehabilitation and training (institutionalized or not).

In this chapter, which aims to provide the reader with a picture of the state of the art in the measurement of the mechanics of human movement, the attention will be focused on data provided by optoelectronic stereophotogrammetric systems, magnetic and inertial measurement units and force platforms.

A MECHANICAL MODEL OF THE MUSCULOSKELETAL SYSTEM

A thorough understanding of the way in which an individual moves is typically obtained through a mechanical model of the portion of the musculoskeletal system (MSS) under analysis, which would represent a trade-off between tractability and accuracy of the end results (Fig. 13-1). Normally, this model is made of links, which represent the bony segments, connected through spherical hinges (three degrees of freedom) located in points approximating the joint centres of rotation. An anatomical set of axes (anatomical frame) is associated to each link (Fig. 13-1A). For each joint, out of the six axes associated with the two bones involved, three axes are chosen as joint axes. Normally these axes, which are not necessarily orthogonal, are the mediolateral axis of the proximal bone and the anteroposterior and longitudinal axes of the distal bone (Fig. 13-1B). The rotation angles about these axes are used to describe joint kinematics. Each of these rotations is assumed to be controlled by a muscle-equivalent rotational motor acting about the corresponding joint axis. Consequently, muscle activity about a joint is described through the couple (Fig. 13-1B) and power supplied by each of those motors.

In summary, the mechanics of a joint during movement is described using the time histories of three angles, three couples and three powers. If, at a given joint, one rotation angle prevails the other two to the extent that these are either irrelevant to the analysis or their estimate is unreliable, then that joint may be represented with a cylindrical (one degree of freedom) hinge (Fig. 13-1A).

The above-illustrated model neglects the linear displacements that occur between adjacent bones in some joints. This is acceptable on the grounds that the amplitude of these displacements is too small to be accurately estimated with the experimental methodologies dealt with herein and illustrated below. This limitation may be overcome using three-dimensional videofluoroscopy or dynamic magnetic resonance imaging that are cumbersome techniques and grant relatively small measurement volumes, allowing the analysis of one joint at a time, normally during movements on the spot.[1,2]

While analysing a motor task, relevant events are detected and their time of occurrence marked (event markers) on the time axis of the graphs reporting the time history of the mechanical variables of interest. This is done, for instance, to identify cycles or phases within the observed task that help data interpretability and comparison. Typical examples are events such as initial contact (or heel strike) and final contact (or toe-off) of each foot during walking, which define the gait cycle and the stance, swing and double-support phases. These events are detected either using ad hoc sensors (mostly on–off pressure sensors or accelerometers mounted under and on the foot, respectively), or they are extracted from the time histories of estimated mechanical variables.

MOTION CAPTURE

The basic information for the analysis of human movement, in terms of joint mechanics, dwells in the data that allow for the reconstruction in-silico (through computer processing) of each bone of interest. These data include bone morphology and position and orientation relative to a laboratory-embedded Cartesian set of axes (global frame), in each sampled instant of time during the execution of the analysed motor act. The combination of position and orientation of a set of axes is referred to as pose.

After having associated a bone-embedded frame to each bone (Fig. 13-2A), the reconstruction is achieved in the six phases depicted in Fig. 13-2B–G.[3]

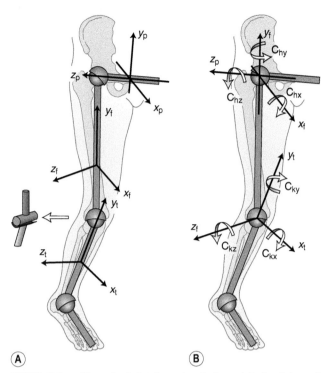

(A)   (B)

FIGURE 13-1 ■ Musculoskeletal mechanical model of pelvis and lower limb. **(A)** Anatomical frames of femur and tibia. **(B)** Hip joint axes made of the mediolateral axis of the pelvis (z_p), anteroposterior axis of the femur (x_f), and longitudinal axis of the femur (y_f); knee joint axes made of the mediolateral axis of the femur (z_t), anteroposterior axis of the tibia (x_t), and longitudinal axis of the tibia (y_t); the couples of the three muscle-equivalent motors acting at the hip and at the knee (C_{hx}, C_{hy}, C_{hz} and C_{kx}, C_{ky}, C_{kz}, respectively).

The kinematic quantities required to drive the MSS model described above are normally recorded either using optoelectronic stereophotogrammetry (video systems) or magnetic and inertial measurement units.

Stereophotogrammetry

Optoelectronic stereophotogrammetry is, to date, the most widely used and accurate solution for measuring skeletal kinematics. It is made of a number of video cameras, connected to a computer, the fields of view of which intersect defining the measurement volume. This system provides the position (Cartesian coordinates) of markers, either emitting or retro-reflecting light, relative to a global frame. This is done through mathematical operators that receive the two-dimensional coordinates of the marker images, measured on the image plane of at least two cameras at any given instant of time, and parameters that describe the location in space and optical features of the cameras. These parameters are obtained through the calibration of the stereophotogrammetric system.

Three or more non-aligned physical markers (marker cluster) are attached to the skin above the bone of interest, either directly or through a plaque or a wand,[4] complying with the technical requirements illustrated in Figure 13-3. In the intent to minimize the number of physical markers to be tracked, some of them may be

substituted with virtual markers. A virtual marker corresponds to a point assumed to be in common between two adjacent bones (Fig. 13-3B,C): if the pose of one bony segment is successfully reconstructed, the position time history of the virtual marker, which belongs to this segment, can be obtained and used to reconstruct the pose of the second body segment as if it were a physical marker.[5] The reconstructed positions in the global frame of the markers and a mathematical estimator are used to construct a local set of axes (or technical frame) and determine its pose relative to the global frame. The technical frame is not rigidly associated with the bone because reconstructed marker positions are affected by inaccuracies due to experimental errors[6] and because the markers move with respect to the underlying bone, due to soft tissue deformation and sliding (soft tissue artefact[7,8]). After the data are processed so as to minimize the propagation of the above errors, the technical frame is taken as an estimate of the bone-embedded frame (Fig. 13-3).

Having carried out the above-illustrated procedures, the pose of the estimated bone-embedded frame, relative to the global frame, of each bone of interest in each sampled instant of time is available (Fig. 13-2E).

Markers may be located on a body segment without any reference to the anatomy, thus, normally, their local position is not repeatable, both intra- and inter-subjects. As a consequence, the obtained bone-embedded frame might result in an equally not repeatable relationship with the morphology of the bone. This repeatability issue calls for the execution of another procedure referred to as anatomical calibration (Fig. 13-2B–D).[3,9] The digital model of the bone of interest may be defined at different levels of resolution, which depend on the number of points used to describe the bone external surface. The minimum number of these points is three, as imposed by the possibility of constructing the anatomical frame of the bone involved, which is essential for proceeding in the analysis. A larger number of points may allow a more realistic rendering of the bone in-silico representation. The bone digital model is hence constructed with reference to a morphology frame that depends on the methodology used. Consequently, the pose of that frame in the bone-embedded frame must also be acquired to allow further registration between the two frames (Fig. 13-2B–D). This is done by recording the position of selected points (either anatomical landmarks or markers) both in the morphology frame and in the bone-embedded frame.

A high-resolution digital model of the bone may be acquired using medical imaging (e.g. magnetic resonance), but this is rarely possible. An alternative approach is the estimate of the model using subject-specific partial information and population statistical information. Subject-specific information may be as minimal as the position of palpable anatomical landmarks (e.g. with reference to the femur: greater trochanter, medial and lateral epicondyles) determined using stereophotogrammetry. To these points, internal anatomical landmarks may be added when non-invasively identifiable. A typical example in this respect is the centre of the femoral head that can be assumed to coincide with the centre of rotation of the femur relative to the pelvic bone. As such,

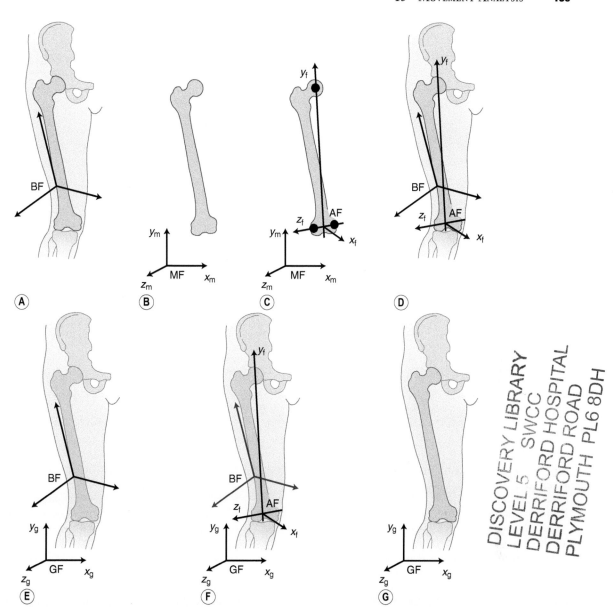

FIGURE 13-2 ■ In-silico reconstruction of a bone during movement. **(A)** An arbitrary bone-embedded frame (BF) is defined. Time invariant parameters are determined during an anatomical calibration procedure. **(B)** A digital model of the bone is acquired in a morphology frame (MF). **(C)** Morphological features and/or anatomical landmarks of the bone are identified and an anatomical frame of the bone (AF) is constructed using them. **(D)** A mathematical operator that would allow the placement of the AF relative to the BF (registration operator) is determined. In each sampled instant of time during movement the following motion capture procedures are carried out: **(E)** the pose of the BF in the global frame (GF) is reconstructed during movement using a motion capture technology; **(F)** given the pose of the BF, the pose of the AF is determined using the registration operator and then the latter frame is associated to the MSS mechanical model depicted in Figure 13-1; **(G)** the bone digital model given in the AF can eventually be represented in-silico as observed from the GF using a chosen rendering approach.

this point is identifiable through an ad hoc experiment during which a hip circumduction is reconstructed using stereophotogrammetry.[10] Although with a lower accuracy, the position of this anatomical landmark in the pelvic anatomical frame can also be determined using predictive equations.[9] Another and more sophisticated way of gathering partial bone morphological information is through two planar X-rays of the bone. This method is made applicable by X-ray imaging technology performed at a low dose and with an expanded dynamic range that allows for whole-body scanning.[11]

Whatever the method used to measure the morphology, the position of an adequate number of anatomical landmarks must be made available to allow the construction of a bone anatomical frame (Fig. 13-2C). This must be achievable with the maximum possible repeatability, because the value of the variables used to describe joint mechanics strongly depends on position and orientation of the set of axes used.[9] For the same reason relevant, standardized, definitions must be adopted.

One of the axes of an anatomical frame is sometimes determined using a functional approach,[12] similar to the

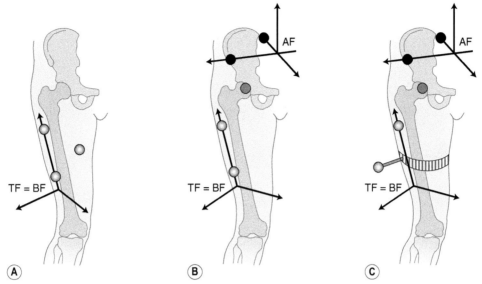

FIGURE 13-3 ■ Marker set-up. **(A)** A minimum of three markers is attached to the segment skin in positions where the soft tissue artefact is minimal, in order that each marker is visible to at least two cameras in any given instant of time, and so as to maximize the relative distance between markers. A number of markers greater than three may be beneficial to the reduction of experimental error propagation to the end results. **(B)** Some time virtual markers are used:[4,5,9] the illustrated example refers to the hip joint centre of rotation determined in the pelvic anatomical frame (AF), using either a functional approach or a prediction model, and associated to the femur. **(C)** With reference to upper and lower limbs, due to their morphology, markers are at a short distance from the body segment longitudinal axis; this means that internal–external rotations of the segment cause small linear displacements of the marker and, because of this, are prone to large relative errors, which propagate to the orientation about that axis. In the attempt to minimize this effect, markers are sometime mounted on wands as shown in this figure. BF, Bone-embedded frame; MF, Morphology frame.

one previously described and used for the determination of the hip joint centre of rotation. This may be done when the bone ends with a joint that has a dominant rotational degree of freedom for which a mean axis of rotation may be defined with sufficient accuracy using stereophotogrammetry (normally the flexion–extension axis). Other examples are the elbow, the knee and the ankle. Given this axis, at least an additional anatomical landmark is required to construct the anatomical frame.

In order to construct the MSS model, the centres of the relevant joints must be identified. Normally, the location of these points is determined using their geometrical relationship with respect to the available anatomical landmarks (e.g. for the knee, the mid-point between the lateral and medial femoral epicondyles; for the ankle, the mid-point between the lateral and medial malleoli), or using a functional approach as with the hip joint.

Magnetic and Inertial Measurement Units

Miniature magnetic and inertial measurement units (MIMU), embedding a microprocessor and often endowed with wireless communication technology, are an increasingly popular alternative to stereophotogrammetry for three-dimensional human movement analysis.[13,14] A MIMU comprises a three-axes linear accelerometer and angular rate sensors, and a three-axes magnetometer. The physical quantities provided by each sensor are measured with respect to the axis of a unit-embedded technical frame generally aligned with the edges of the unit case. Through algorithms able to fuse the redundant information available and compensate for sensor noise and drift,

the three-dimensional orientation of the technical frame relative to a global frame is provided. Although, as with the skin markers, the MIMU is subject to soft tissue artefacts, the technical frame is usually assumed to coincide with a bone-embedded frame (Fig. 13-2E). No literature is as yet available dealing with the compensation of this artefact while using MIMUs.

As opposed to stereophotogrammetry, MIMUs do not supply reliable positional information. Thus, the MSS model is driven only by the orientation of the body segments and is unable to displace in space. This means that this motion capture technology is effectively applicable only for joint kinematics (that is, for relative rotational motion) and not for joint kinetics studies. In fact, normally the inertial forces due to linear accelerations, necessary for the estimate of kinetic quantities, cannot be determined. However, this is made possible when the instantaneous position of at least one point of the MSS model is known. This is the case, for instance, when that point is stationary, as when the base of support is fixed.

Regarding the anatomical calibration, a straightforward (but rarely sufficiently accurate) solution is to manually align the MIMU case, with observationally detected anatomical planes and axes of the underlying bony segment, thus aligning technical and anatomical frames. An alternative solution for anatomical frame identification is based on a functional approach.[15–17] A subject is asked to perform a joint movement about an anatomical axis. The orientation of this axis coincides with the direction of the mean angular velocity vector measured by the MIMU attached to the body segment of interest. A second axis of the anatomical frame can be defined using the acceleration vector measured by the MIMU during a known resting posture (the gravitational acceleration), in which the MIMU acts as an inclinometer. The anatomical frame of the body segment under analysis can also be identified using a specifically designed calibration device consisting of a rod carrying two mobile pointers perpendicular to it.[18] The rod carries a MIMU that provides the orientation relative to the technical frame of the line joining the tips of the pointers. Using this device the orientation of lines passing through palpable anatomical landmarks and, therefore, an anatomical frame can be determined (Fig. 13-2D). If a digital model of the bone involved in the analysis is available, then this may be reconstructed in-silico following the same procedure described for stereophotogrammetry (Fig. 13-2G).

An important limitation of MIMUs is that, for a reliable use of the magnetic sensor outputs, the Earth's magnetic field must be uniform. This occurs rarely due to the common presence of ferromagnetic materials in, or in the vicinity of, the measurement volume. Thus, under average indoor conditions, when the measurement volume exceeds a cubic metre, great care must be taken not to put at risk the reliability of the results. Better results can be expected when the measurements are performed outdoors.

MEASURE OF EXTERNAL FORCES

External forces represent the interaction of the human body, or portion of it, with the planet Earth and, through contact, with other bodies. These are the gravitational forces and the reaction forces, respectively. The former forces may be represented by a resultant force vector (weight), acting downward along the gravity line and applied to the centre of gravity, which for all practical purposes coincides with the centre of mass, of the body segment or ensemble of body segments under analysis. The reaction forces act through a surface of contact and are distributed over it. Their resultant may be represented using a force vector passing through an arbitrarily chosen point and a couple vector (resultant load).

The subject-specific mass and position of the centre of mass of a single body segment (that, together with the mass moments of inertia, are referred to as the segment's inertial parameters) may be estimated using either data provided by medical imaging technologies,[19] with the obvious utilizability limits, or through predictive mathematical[20] or geometrical models[21] that use easy to make anthropometric measurements.

The reaction resultant load is measured using dynamometers. These provide six signals: three force and three couple components relative to a technical frame embedded in the dynamometer. A typical example of dynamometer used in human movement analysis is the so-named force-plate, used to measure the resultant reaction load exchanged between feet and floor (Fig. 13-4A). When analysing locomotor acts or stationary postures, the trajectory of the centre of pressure, defined in Figure 13-4B, is also used in a stand-alone fashion for motor function assessment.

JOINT MECHANICS

Joint Kinematics

After the pose of the anatomical frames of two adjacent bones has been estimated, in a given instant of time during movement, the three angles that describe their relative orientation can be determined. These angles measure the three rotations that the distal anatomical frame must undergo to move from an orientation aligned with that of the proximal anatomical frame to its current orientation. By convention,[22] these rotations are assumed to occur sequentially, first around the mediolateral axis of the proximal bone, then about the anteroposterior and finally about the longitudinal axis of the distal bone (Fig. 13-1B). Given this definition, for most joints, the resulting angles may be termed flexion–extension, abduction–adduction and internal–external rotation, respectively (Fig. 13-5A). Given their definition, these angles strongly depend on the orientation of the axes used. In particular, it is important to be aware of the fact that, when one angle prevails in amplitude, even a slight misorientation of the axes involved causes large relative errors on the smaller angles (this effect is named

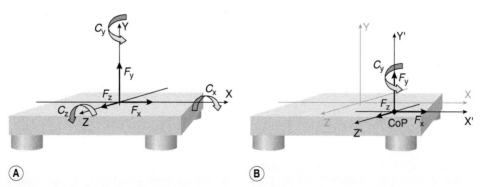

(A) **(B)**

FIGURE 13-4 ■ Force-plate. **(A)** The force-plate embedded system of axes (technical frame, TF: X, Y, Z), the three scalar components of the reaction resultant force, and the three scalar components of the reaction resultant couple relative to the force-plate TF (i.e. output of the measuring instrument) are represented. **(B)** The resultant reaction force and couple components are represented relative to a force-plate TF (X', Y', Z') the origin of which is located in the centre of pressure (CoP). This is the pierce point on the force-plate surface of the resultant of the distributed reaction force component orthogonal to the surface. When using this representation of the reaction resultant load, only the component of the couple along the vertical axis is different from zero.

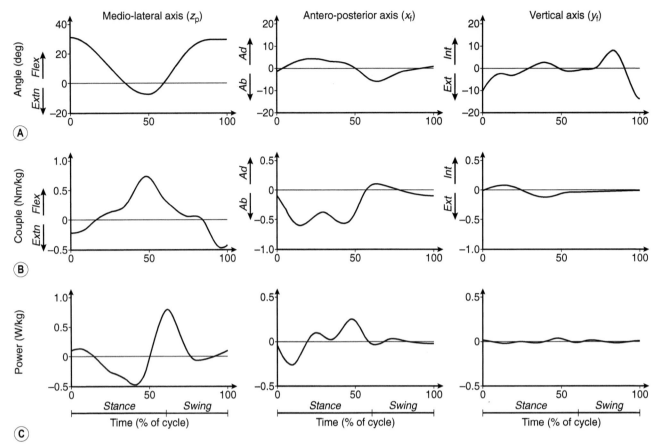

FIGURE 13-5 ■ Example of joint mechanics quantitative description. The hip mechanics during level walking of a male adult able-bodied volunteer is taken as a paradigmatic case: **(A)** kinematics; **(B)** muscle-equivalent couples (normalized with respect to body mass); and **(C)** muscle-equivalent powers (normalized with respect to body mass). Stance and swing phases are indicated. z_p: mediolateral axis of the pelvis; x_f and y_f: anteroposterior axis and longitudinal axes of the femur, respectively (see Fig. 13-1B). *Ab*, Abduction; *Ad*, Adduction; *Extn*, Extension; *Flex*, Flexion; *Ext*, External; *Int*, Internal.

cross-talk). As a consequence, results, for instance, relative to abduction–adduction and internal–external rotation of the knee during walking or running must be taken with great caution. When these circumstances occur, it may be advisable to modify the MSS model and substitute the spherical hinge involved with a cylindrical hinge that accounts only for the largest rotation (Fig. 13-1A).

Joint Kinetics

If, in a given instant of time during movement, the pose of the anatomical frame in the global frame of the underlying bone and the inertial parameters are known for each body segment involved in the analysis, and the resultant reaction loads have been obtained, then the couples and related powers of the muscle-equivalent motors embedded in the MSS model can be estimated.[23] The relevant mathematical procedure is based on Newton's equations of motion applied to the locomotor system MSS model (solution of the inverse dynamics problem) and entails the estimate of linear and angular velocities and accelerations. Of course, all vector quantities must be represented in the same global frame. This, for instance, means that the relative pose of the technical frame of a dynamometer, such as a force-plate, and the global frame used when

acquiring kinematic data through stereophotogrammetry or MIMUs, must be determined and measured forces and couples represented in the latter frame (Fig. 13-5B,C).

The most critical stages of the above-mentioned estimation procedure are, depending on the experimental data source, the single or double differentiation or integration of noisy data and, of course, the discrepancy of the MSS model of the locomotor system from reality. In the latter respect, the accuracy with which the joint centres are located in the relevant anatomical frames and the assumption that they will not move with respect to them have the greatest impact on the end results.[24]

FUTURE DEVELOPMENTS

The potential of quantitative movement analysis in professional decision-making and intervention practice, as illustrated in the Introduction to this chapter, is fully recognized. Nevertheless, several issues currently limit its full application. Firstly, the experimental and analytical protocols used in most movement analysis laboratories were introduced some 30 years ago and do not exploit the full potential of current technologies. They provide results with precision and accuracy that are insufficient to answer many of the questions posed by scientists and professionals. Nevertheless, these remain virtually the only protocols implemented in marketed software packages. Secondly, presently available computational models of the neuromusculoskeletal system encounter difficulties in incorporating the characteristics of a specific subject. Finally, as mentioned in the previous sections, the metrics to be used when assessing motor function calls for refinement.

Overcoming the above-mentioned limitations requires the creation of new techniques and knowledge through the fusion of contributions from past and ongoing research, development programmes, as well as fostering novel conceptual approaches.

REFERENCES

1. Borotikara BS, Sipprell WH III, Wiblea EE, et al. A methodology to accurately quantify patellofemoral cartilage contact kinematics by combining 3D image shape registration and cine-PC MRI velocity data. J Biomech 2007;45(6):1117–22.
2. Zhu Z, Li G. An automatic 2D-3D image matching method for reproducing spatial knee joint positions using single or dual fluoroscopic images. Comput Method Biomec 2012;15(11):1245–56.
3. Cappozzo A, Della Croce U, Leardini A, et al. Human movement analysis using stereophotogrammetry. Part 1: theoretical background. Gait Posture 2005;21(2):186–96.
4. Davis RB, Ounpuu S, Tyburski D, et al. A gait analysis data collection and reduction technique. Human Mov Sci 1991; 10(5):575–87.
5. Kadaba MP, Ramakrishnan HK, Wootten ME. Measurement of lower extremity kinematics during level walking. J Orthop Res 1990;8(3):383–92.
6. Chiari L, Della Croce U, Leardini A, et al. Human movement analysis using stereophotogrammetry. Part 2: instrumental errors. Gait Posture 2005;21(2):197–211.
7. Leardini A, Chiari L, Della Croce U, et al. Human movement analysis using stereophotogrammetry. Part 3. Soft tissue artifact assessment and compensation. Gait Posture 2005;21(2):212–25.
8. Peters A, Galna B, Sangeux M, et al. Quantification of soft tissue artifact in lower limb human motion analysis: a systematic review. Gait Posture 2010;31(1):1–8.
9. Della Croce U, Leardini A, Chiari L, et al. Human movement analysis using stereophotogrammetry. Part 4: assessment of anatomical landmark misplacement and its effects on joint kinematics. Gait Posture 2005;21(2):226–37.
10. Camomilla V, Cereatti A, Vannozzi G, et al. An optimized protocol for hip joint centre determination using the functional method. J Biomech 2006;39(6):1096–106.
11. McKenna C, Wade R, Faria R, et al. EOS 2D/3D X-ray imaging system: a systematic review and economic evaluation. Health Technol Asses 2012;16(14):1–188.
12. Ehrig RM, Taylor WR, Duda GN, et al. A survey of formal methods for determining functional joint axes. J Biomech 2007; 40(10):2150–7.
13. Aminian K. Monitoring human movement with body-fixed sensors and its clinical application. In: Begg R, Palaniswami M, editors. Computational Intelligence for Movement Sciences. Hershey, PA: Idea Group Pub; 2006. p. 101–38.
14. Luinge HJ, Veltink PH. Measuring orientation of human body segments using miniature gyroscopes and accelerometers. Med Biol Eng Comput 2005;43(2):273–82.
15. Cutti AG, Ferrari A, Garofalo P, et al. 'Outwalk': a protocol for clinical gait analysis based on inertial and magnetic sensors. Med Biol Eng Comput 2010;48(1):17–25.
16. O'Donovan KJ, Kamnik R, O'Keeffe DT, et al. An inertial and magnetic sensor based technique for joint angle measurement. J Biomech 2007;40(12):2604–11.
17. Luinge HJ, Veltink PH, Baten CTM. Ambulatory measurement of arm orientation. J Biomech 2007;40(1):78–85.
18. Picerno P, Cereatti A, Cappozzo A. Joint kinematics estimate using wearable inertial and magnetic sensing modules. Gait Posture 2008;28(4):588–95.
19. Mungiole M, Martin PE. Estimating segment inertial properties: comparison of magnetic resonance imaging with existing methods. J Biomech 1990;23(10):1039–46.
20. de Leva P. Adjustments to Zatsiorsky-Seluyanov's segment inertia parameters. J Biomech 1996;29(9):1223–30.
21. Yeadon MR. The simulation of aerial movement – ii. a mathematical inertia model of the human body. J Biomech 1990;23(1): 67–74.
22. Grood ES, Suntay WJ. A joint coordinate system for the clinical description of three-dimensional motions: application to the knee. J Biomech Eng-T ASME 1983;105(2):136–44.
23. Zatsiorsky VM. Kinetics of Human Motion. Champaign, IL: Human Kinetics; 2002.
24. Riemer R, Hsiao-Wecksler ET, Zhang X. Uncertainties in inverse dynamics solutions: a comprehensive analysis and an application to gait. Gait Posture 2008;27(4):578–88.

CHAPTER 14

New Developments in Ultrasound Imaging in Physiotherapy Practice and Research

Alan Hough • Maria Stokes

INTRODUCTION

Real-time ultrasound imaging (USI) is a safe, portable, objective and relatively inexpensive means of examining muscle, nerves, tendons and structures (e.g. the bladder) in research and clinical settings. The term rehabilitative ultrasound imaging (RUSI) was introduced in 2006 to define use by physiotherapists for assessment and bio-feedback purposes.[1] Other uses of USI in physiotherapy, such as tissue motion techniques and imaging nerves, fit logically with and extend the boundaries of RUSI, but they are also used by physiologists and sports scientists so it would not be appropriate to restrict such uses to the term RUSI.

Physiotherapists also use diagnostic USI of musculoskeletal injuries but this requires different skills and training.[2] This chapter focuses on non-diagnostic USI and the reader is directed to other sources for diagnostic USI.[3–5] Distinction between the two USI applications is important, as there are implications for practice, including observing professional boundaries.[6] Training pathways and guidelines for musculoskeletal diagnostic imaging are well established[7] and are open to physiotherapists (http://www.bmus.org), whereas training for RUSI is in its infancy. This chapter gives a brief overview of existing uses of RUSI and emerging applications.

TYPES OF ULTRASOUND IMAGING AND TECHNICAL CONSIDERATIONS

There are several modes of ultrasound imaging used in health care (not all available on each machine), as outlined in Table 14-1.

When imaging muscle, depending on its depth, frequencies of between 5.0 and 7.5 MHz are often used.[6] For peripheral nerves, linear transducers with frequencies between 7.5 and 15 MHz or higher are preferable.[8] Resolution is lost with lower frequencies. As a general guide:
- The *deeper* the structure, the *lower* the *frequency*.
- The more *superficial* the structure the *higher* the *frequency*.

For details on technical aspects, see Kremkau.[5]

An extended field of view for imaging large muscles or length of fibres/tissues can be achieved in various ways. A wide transducer (large footprint) can be used but these are not available for all types of scanner. A stand-off pad of gel can be placed between the skin and transducer to increase the field of view. A recent advance in technology is panoramic ultrasound, which extends the view by building up a composite scan as the operator moves the transducer over the area of interest.[9] This is similar to the way compound scanners (now obsolete) are used to enable a cross-sectional area view of large muscles to be measured (e.g. quadriceps);[10] panoramic scanning is now achieved using much more compact equipment.

ASSESSMENT OF MUSCLE MORPHOMETRY AND MORPHOLOGY (ARCHITECTURE)

Morphology is the evaluation of muscle structure (architecture) and morphometry is the measurement of morphological features, such as muscle thickness (depth), cross-sectional area, volume and fibre length and pennation angles. More dynamic imaging involves assessing changes in these features during contraction and the impact on associated structures (e.g. the bladder), and tissue movement and deformation (using high-frame rate USI and elastography).

The most common measure of muscle size is its thickness, as it can be made more rapidly and reliably measured than cross-sectional area. The relatively small size of transducers means that whole-muscle cross-section can only be imaged in very few muscles (e.g. multifidus).[6]

Much of the RUSI literature has focused on lumbar multifidus[11] and the anterolateral abdominal muscles (transversus abdominis [TrA], external and internal oblique)[12] due to their role in stabilizing the lumbar spine.[13] Other muscles include: facial, cervical (semispinalis capitis, deep posterior group), trapezius, rectus abdominis and inter-recti distance, hip flexors (psoas) and abductor (gluteus medius and minimus) muscles, pelvic floor muscles, quadriceps, posterior and anterior tibial

TABLE 14-1 **Types of Ultrasound Imaging**

Mode	Description and Application
A-Mode (amplitude mode)	Shows amplitude of ultrasound echoes over time. Available on specialized systems used in ophthalmology
B-Mode (brightness mode)	A plane is scanned through the body and presented as a two-dimensional anatomical greyscale image. Most common mode utilized in rehabilitative and musculoskeletal ultrasound (Fig. 14-1A; see also Figs 14-2 to 14-4)
M-Mode (motion Mode)	Displays depth displacement of tissue (vertical axis) over time (horizontal axis). Typically used to show motion of cardiac structures, but has been used to indicate abdominal muscle activity (see Fig. 14-1B)
Colour Doppler	Colour-coded velocity information superimposed on a B-mode image. Typically used to visualize blood velocity and flow characteristics (see Fig. 14-1C)
Pulsed-wave (PW) Doppler	Doppler information sampled from a small selected region (sample volume) and displayed usually as velocity (vertical axis) over time (horizontal axis). Used to quantify blood velocity and flow characteristics (see Fig. 14-1D)
Tissue Doppler	Basic colour or PW Doppler modes with parameters adjusted to measure tissue velocity, displacement and strain. Typically used in cardiac muscle applications
Power Doppler	Colour-coded blood flow intensity information superimposed on a B-mode image. Greater sensitivity to slow flow that can provide an index of relative tissue perfusion and neovascularity. Potential applications in rheumatology and tendinopathies
3D and 4D modes	Multiple B-mode images can be captured and reconstructed to produce 3D volume images. Advanced 3D transducers provide a rapid electronic sweep of the ultrasound beam over the region of interest that allows 3D reconstruction and display in real-time, where it is known as 4D ultrasound. Most extensive applications to date have been in obstetrics, but has wide potential application

3D, Three-dimensional; *4D*, Four-dimensional.

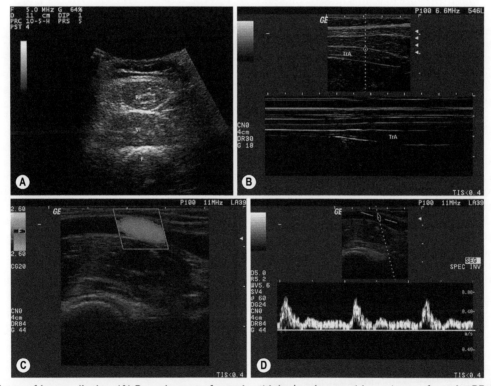

FIGURE 14-1 ■ Types of image display. (**A**) B-mode scan of anterior thigh showing quadriceps (rectus femoris, *RF* and vastus intermedius, *VI*) above the femur (*F*). (**B**) B-/M-mode scan of lateral abdominal muscles during a contraction, showing thickening of transversus abdominis (TrA). The upper image is B-mode, whereas the lower timeline trace is M-mode. (**C**) Colour Doppler and (**D**) pulsed-wave (spectral) Doppler of the brachial artery. For colour version see Plate 12.

muscles.[6] The effects of ageing[10] and exercise programmes[14] on muscle size can be assessed with USI.

Contracted Muscles

Measurement of contracting muscle may be more sensitive for discriminating between health and pathology than resting muscle.[15,16] The TrA can be tested during voluntary activity (e.g. abdominal drawing in manoeuvre) or automatic activity (e.g. active straight leg raise) test.[13,14,17] When TrA contracts and shortens the anterior abdominal fascia slides/glides in a lateral direction and this movement is reduced in patients with low back pain.[14]

Relationship Between Muscle Size and Strength

The size of resting muscle is of potential value for predicting force-generating capacity when strength measurements are either not possible or appropriate due to pain or instability of structures. However, the relationship between size and strength varies between muscles and cannot be assumed to show high correlation.[10,18]

Perimuscular Connective Tissue Thickness

A study by Whittaker et al.[19] has highlighted the importance of measuring connective tissue as well as muscle thickness. They found that greater thickness of muscle boundaries of the anterolateral abdominal muscles, as well as the inter-recti distance, in patients with lumbopelvic pain compared with healthy controls. These findings may reflect altered loading due to wasting of the rectus abdominis (RA) muscle.

Validity of USI Against Other Imaging Techniques and Electromyography

The validity of USI for measuring muscle size has been tested in various muscles against magnetic resonance imaging, which is considered the gold standard. There is general agreement that USI provides accurate measurements under static conditions at rest[20] and also during contraction.[21] However, most studies have been restricted to small groups of young, healthy participants and studies are needed in older healthy groups and patient populations to confirm validity.

The correlation between changes in muscle thickness during contraction has been studied using force and electromyography. Increases in muscle thickness during contraction are not proportional to changes in force above about 30% of maximal force, as demonstrated by a curvilinear relationship for TrA[22] and lumbar multifidus[23] Conversely, McMeeken et al.[24] found a linear relationship for TrA, but there were methodological differences between studies.

Reliability

Any assessment tool must be robust enough to produce similar results on different occasions, so that any changes observed are not due to measurement error. Different types of reliability examined for USI include intra-rater reliability/repeatability within the same images, on different images taken within the same session and images taken on different days. The latter is the most clinically relevant scenario, as the complete scanning procedure as well as scan interpretation and measurement technique are being tested. Inter-rater reliability has also been examined between two or more investigators and between experienced and novice investigators. The wealth of literature cannot be covered here, but it indicates that USI is reliable for measuring various muscles. Most studies are on the abdominal and lumbar multifidus muscles (see systematic reviews by Hebert et al.[25] and Costa et al.[26]) and studies have begun to include patient groups (e.g. Koppenhaver et al.[27]). Reliability of measuring muscle fascicle length and pennation angle,[28] as well as measuring nerves has been demonstrated in several studies.[29–32]

Despite the lower reliability of thickness change with contraction than resting thickness, the former is a better indicator of dysfunction (e.g. in back pain[33]). Lateral glide may also be a better indicator of muscle dysfunction than resting thickness.[14,33]

The remainder of the chapter is dedicated to dynamic USI, specifically biofeedback that is used clinically, and measurement of motion, currently used primarily in research but with clinical potential.

BIOFEEDBACK OF MUSCLE FUNCTION

According to a recent survey, 81% of physiotherapists using USI use it as a biofeedback tool to aid rehabilitation.[34] Studies have shown benefit from using USI for biofeedback, for example the ability to contract multifidus in healthy participants[35] improved, learning to contract the pelvic floor muscles was achieved within five minutes of training,[36] and USI reduced the number of trials needed to perform the abdominal hollowing exercise in people with[37] and without[38] low back pain. However, Teyhen et al.[39] did not find the same effect of RUSI to enhance the ability of their group of patients with low back pain to perform the same exercise. Given the increasing recognition of the importance of motor relearning, randomized controlled trials are needed to determine the role of RUSI as a biofeedback tool in rehabilitation. The split-screen facility on a scanner can be useful for comparing the change in muscle thickness from rest to contraction, as illustrated for multifidus and the lateral abdominals in Figure 14-2.

MEASURING TISSUE MOTION AND MECHANICAL PROPERTIES OF MUSCLE–TENDON UNIT

A great strength of USI is that it provides a non-invasive means for quantifying tissue motion in vivo.[5,40] This has led to its use in rehabilitation research as a tool to estimate the motion of muscles, tendons and nerves associated with active and passive movements. By measuring tissue displacement and strain it is possible to gain

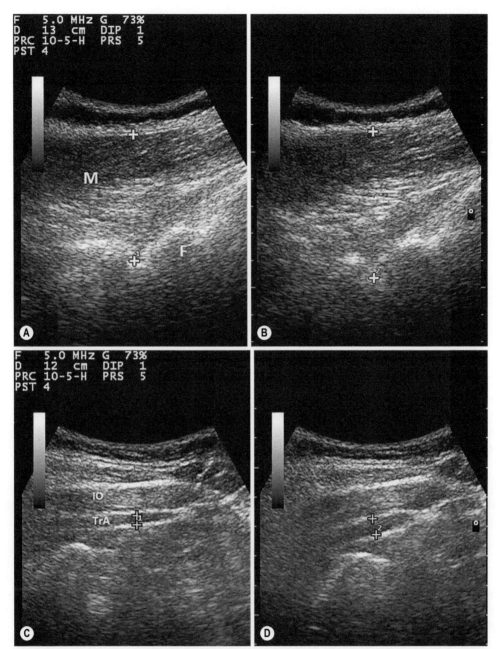

FIGURE 14-2 ■ Split-screen facility used for biofeedback. Sagittal view of lumbar multifidus (*M*) above the facet (*F*) joints (**A**) at rest and (**B**) during contraction; note the increase in thickness measured by on-screen cursors (46.6 mm to 54 mm). Transverse view of the lateral abdominal muscles (**C**) at rest and (**D**) during contraction; note the thickening of transversus abdominis (*TrA*) and internal oblique (*IO*) muscles.

insights into the mechanical properties of the tissues in response to loading in both health and disease.

Movement of structures can be estimated using B-mode (brightness mode) images taken before and after an active or passive movement. Measurements can be made using electronic callipers on the ultrasound system or in image measurement software on exported images or cine clips. This basic B-mode image analysis approach has proved useful in several research areas, for example measurement of transverse plane motion and deformation of the median nerve in studies exploring aetiological factors in carpal tunnel syndrome[41,42] and dynamic changes in acromio–humeral distance under varying conditions.[43,44]

Valid and reliable measurement of muscle architectural features such as fascicle length and pennation angles using B-mode ultrasound (Fig. 14-3[28]) has enabled identification of changes in these features under varying loading conditions and comparison between population groups.[45–48] Furthermore, by tracking displacement of myofascial anatomical landmarks in combination with force measurements, it is possible to estimate mechanical properties of the muscle–tendon unit.[49,50]

The literature using USI to measure muscle architectural features and mechanical properties is extensive and detailed discussion is beyond the scope of this chapter. The interested reader is directed to Magnusson et al.[51] for an excellent discussion of the strengths and

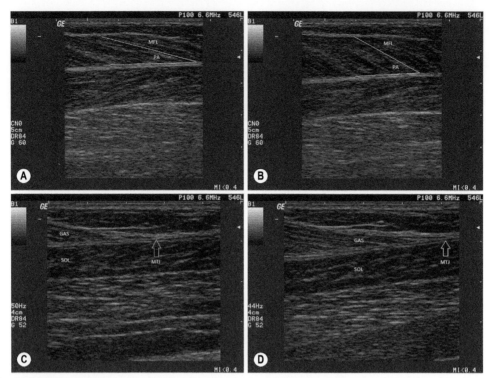

FIGURE 14-3 ■ Sagittal view of triceps surae, illustrating muscle fascicle length (*MFL*) and pennation angle (*PA*) (**A**) at rest and (**B**) during isometric contraction. Distal displacement of the musculotendinous junction (*MTJ*) of gastrocnemius (**C**) and (**D**) during ankle dorsiflexion indicates lengthening of the muscle. *GAS*, Gastrocnemius muscle; *SOL*, Soleus muscle.

limitations of the general approach, and to Cronin et al.[52] for a review of USI measures of muscle–tendon complex during walking. In addition, Magnusson et al.[53] provides a thorough overview of how USI and other approaches have enhanced our understanding of in vivo tendon function.

M-MODE

M-mode (motion mode) ultrasound provides an alternative to B-mode for tracking tissue motion.[5] In M-mode, a single selected scan line is used to display depth changes of tissue over time. A potential benefit of M-mode is that several seconds of motion data can be displayed and measured from a single image, and for this reason it has been suggested as an alternative to B-mode for measuring abdominal wall muscle activity.[54] High-frame rate M-mode could also provide a non-invasive alternative to needle electromyography for detecting the onset of deep muscle activity.[55] A major limitation of this mode is that it displays one-dimensional movement only (away or towards the ultrasound beam).

MOTION TRACKING USING TISSUE DOPPLER AND B-MODE SPECKLE TRACKING

When tracking tissue motion in the absence of distinct anatomical landmarks, for example when trying to measure longitudinal motion of peripheral nerves or free tendon, relying on visual tracking of movement is challenging (Fig. 14-4). Several approaches have been developed to assist in such circumstances, including those based on tissue Doppler principles and B-mode speckle tracking; as explained below.

Tissue Doppler Imaging (TDI)

While Doppler ultrasound modes are primarily used in the measurement of blood flow characteristics,[5] it is possible to modify the technique to detect tissue motion.[56] Studies using TDI-based approaches have been used to measure longitudinal motion of tendons and nerves[57,58] and for detection of onset of muscle activity.[55,59] TDI-based approaches are well suited to tracking fast tissue motion, and good reliability and validity have been reported for some applications.[59–62] There are potential limitations for detecting slow tissue movement[63] and measures may be open to substantial error, in particular due to the angle dependence of this approach.[57] A major limitation to the basic TDI approach is that it assumes movement in one dimension only. Specialized 'vector Doppler' systems have been developed that can resolve two-dimensional movement of muscles and tendons[64] but this option is not typically available on ultrasound systems.

B-Mode Speckle Tracking

B-mode speckle tracking techniques overcome the one-dimensional and angle dependence limitations of TDI-based approaches.[65] The basic principles of this approach involve the capture of a B-mode image sequence of the tissue movement of interest. The image sequence is then analysed using tracking software that typically requires

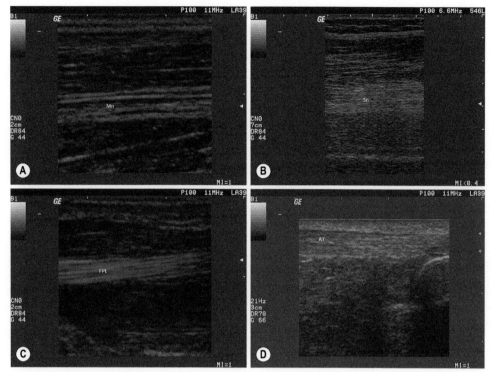

FIGURE 14-4 ■ Typical appearance of peripheral nerves and free tendons in longitudinal section: **(A)** median nerve; **(B)** sciatic nerve; **(C)** flexor pollicis longus tendon; and **(D)** Achilles tendon. Note the apparent lack of clear anatomical landmarks that could be visually tracked during longitudinal movement. Also note the reduced ultrasound resolution of the more deeply placed sciatic nerve compared to the more superficial median nerve.

the operator to select points or regions of interest within the first frame of the image sequence. The grey-scale ('speckle') patterns within the selected regions are then tracked from frame to frame using a mathematical matching algorithm that finds the best match in subsequent frames and enables estimation of the displacement of the tissue in two dimensions.[40]

The technique has been developed to allow concurrent measurement of both longitudinal and superficial/deep movement of nerves and tendons.[66,67] An extensive series of studies using this approach on upper and lower limb peripheral nerves have substantially enhanced our knowledge and understanding of in vivo nerve dynamics in healthy and patient populations.[68–71] The approach has also been applied to continuously track muscle fascicle movement as a non-invasive method for monitoring neuromotor activity in posture and locomotion,[72] and to facilitate studies exploring mechanical properties and behaviour of muscle.[73]

Relative motion between adjacent structures can also be measured (e.g. between the median nerve, flexor tendons and/or subsynovial connective tissue at the carpal tunnel). Identification of relative movement ratios with the consequent potential for shear force development may be relevant in the aetiology of entrapment syndromes[74] and tendinopathy.[75] Differential strain within layers of the same tendon under loading has also been identified using speckle tracking.[76]

The validity of B-mode speckle tracking for measuring displacement under well-controlled laboratory conditions is typically reported as high.[66,67,72] The primary threat to validity in vivo is when the tissue of interest

moves out of the ultrasound beam plane,[72] although three-dimensional tracking techniques could address this problem.[77] The success of the technique is also dependent on the quality of the image sequence captured, which may be influenced by several factors, including depth of the structure imaged (see Figs 14-4A and 14-4B). For more detailed discussion of technical aspects of B-mode speckle tracking and related approaches for measuring displacement, the interested reader is directed to the papers by Korstanje et al.,[67] Loram et al.[72] and Revell et al.[78]

Developing a valid B-mode speckle tracking system for measuring local strain is more challenging.[79] While there is evidence supporting the validity of this approach in tendons,[80] caution is required due to some inherent limitations.[81] Refinements to the standard B-mode approach have been recommended to better capture local strain.[79] However, there are a range of existing techniques known as 'elastography' that should be well suited to the measurement of local strain and mechanical properties in neuromusculoskeletal tissues.

ELASTOGRAPHY

The basic principle common to all ultrasound-based elastography approaches is that ultrasound is used to detect the tissue response to perturbation that is either generated externally (e.g. by manual compression) or internally (e.g. by muscle contraction). Primarily developed for use in cardiac and tumour detection applications, musculoskeletal elastography applications are emerging.[82,83]

Perhaps the most familiar elastography approach uses manual compression of the tissues (via the transducer) as the perturbing source. The deformation of the compressed tissues is captured by the ultrasound and is displayed as a colour-coded map of relative tissue stiffness, where localized areas of greater stiffness (e.g. tumours) can be identified. The estimation of deformation is based on correlation techniques similar to B-mode speckle tracking but the raw ultrasound data are used, which provides higher spatial and temporal resolution. Several studies have explored the potential of this approach in the assessment of tendon health, where identification of regions of relatively reduced stiffness may be indicative of tendinopathy.[84] Variations on the basic technique include using a controlled longitudinal stretching to provide a more functional loading source for tendon applications,[85] and controlled electrical stimulation of muscle to standardize force applications.[86]

An early form of elastography used tissue Doppler to detect the response to low-frequency vibration ('sono-elasticity imaging'[87]). An example of this approach is the 'Doppler imaging of vibrations' developed to provide a measure of sacroiliac joint laxity.[88,89] Vibration is applied to the ilium anteriorly, and the resultant relative movement of the ilium and sacrum posteriorly at the sacroiliac joint is captured by tissue Doppler and used to provide an index of sacroiliac joint laxity. Studies using Doppler imaging of vibrations have informed assessment and management of pregnancy-related pelvic girdle pain,[90] and the approach has potential in other musculoskeletal applications, for example in the assessment of myofascial trigger points.[91]

More recently a range of 'dynamic' elastography techniques using a single ultrasound transducer without the need for an external vibration source or manual compression force have been developed.[82] These techniques, which include supersonic shear wave imaging, are still considered to be at an evaluative stage[83] but they have the potential to provide a more repeatable and quantifiable measure of tissue mechanical properties.[82,83]

FUTURE DIRECTIONS

The USI applications most readily available for routine clinical use and research are visual biofeedback and static measurements of tissue characteristics from B-mode images. These areas were included in the original definition of RUSI in 2006. More recent uses of tissue motion techniques require more sophisticated equipment and software, and are less well developed than the earlier RUSI techniques. The extended field of view provided by panoramic ultrasound is a major advance for enabling the size of large muscles to be viewed and measured, as well as length of tendons and nerves. As use of this specific facility becomes more widespread, it will greatly enhance research into the clinical utility of ultrasound. Similarly, three-dimensional ultrasound provides more accurate and realistic assessments, particularly during motion of tissues, as out-of-plane activity is not captured by two-dimensional imaging. The use of power Doppler ultrasound (see Table 14-1) to detect changes in tissue vascularity is another developing area with research and clinical potential, for example in the assessment of tendinopathies.[92]

The predominant use of USI in physiotherapy has been for musculoskeletal conditions, but since changes in the musculoskeletal system can occur in other conditions (e.g. respiratory and neurological disorders) USI is potentially useful. For example, USI of the diaphragm may provide a complimentary technique for assessing respiratory function,[93] the gastrocnemius muscle after stroke[94] and wrist extensors in tetraplegic patients.[95] Mechanical properties using USI motion tracking techniques have been studied in patients with stroke,[96] cerebral palsy[97] and multiple sclerosis.[98] The response of muscles to exercise programmes in patients with neurological conditions could be monitored using USI.

All uses of USI in physiotherapy need standardized imaging protocols, with evidence of validity and reliability, as well as normal reference values for comparison with clinical cohorts. The tissue motion techniques, in particular, require further development to make them more accessible, affordable and user friendly. Randomized controlled trials are needed to provide evidence of the clinical and cost effectiveness of using USI to enhance clinical practice, both for aiding assessment and rehabilitation through biofeedback. Uses in research to investigate mechanisms of dysfunction and recovery also warrant further exploration.

The ultimate goal is for USI to become a routine tool in physiotherapy. For this aim to be achieved, formal training programmes are needed that are recognized by therapists' national professional bodies and medical disciplines. Eventually, basic USI training would become part of the undergraduate curriculum, both as a teaching tool to aid teaching structural and functional anatomy and as a clinical tool for assessment and biofeedback. Postgraduate training for specific clinical applications and research would be needed. Education programmes will remain a challenge until uptake of USI becomes more widespread, to provide the infrastructure to support practical training.

REFERENCES

1. Teyhen DS. Rehabilitative Ultrasound Imaging Symposium, May 8–10, 2006, San Antonio, Texas. J Orthop Sports Phys Ther 2006;36:A-1–17.
2. Chhem RK, Kaplan PA, Dussault RG. Ultrasonography of the musculoskeletal system. Radiol Clin North Am 1994;32:275–89.
3. WHO. Training in diagnostic ultrasound: essentials, principles and standards. Report of a WHO Study Group. World Health Organ Tech Rep Ser 1998;875:i–46, back cover.
4. Van Holsbeeck M, Introcaso JH. Musculoskeletal Ultrasound, 2nd edn. St Louis, MO, USA: Mosby; 2001. p. 648.
5. Kremkau FW. Diagnostic Ultrasound, Principles and Instruments, 7th edn. London: Saunders; 2005. p. 126, 142, 159.
6. Whittaker JL, Teyhen DS, Elliott JM, et al. Rehabilitative ultrasound imaging: understanding the technology and its applications. J Orthop Sports Phys Ther 2007;37:434–49.
7. Boyce S, Murray A, Jeffrey M. A review of musculoskeletal ultrasound training guidelines and recommendations for sport and exercise medicine physicians. Ultrasound 2013;21:155–8.
8. Thain LMF, Downey DB. Sonography of peripheral nerves: technique, anatomy, and pathology. Ultrasound Q 2002;18:225–45.
9. Ryan ED, Rosenberg JG, Scharville MJ, et al. Test-retest reliability and the minimal detectable change for Achilles tendon length: a

panoramic ultrasound assessment. Ultrasound Med Biol 2013; 39(12):2488–91.

10. Young A, Stokes M, Crowe M. The size and strength of the quadriceps muscles of old and young men. Clin Physiol 1985;5: 145–54.

11. Stokes M, Hides J, Elliott J, et al. Rehabilitative ultrasound imaging of the posterior paraspinal muscles. J Orthop Sports Phys Ther 2007;37(10):581–95.

12. Teyhen DS, Gill NW, Whittaker JL, et al. Rehabilitative ultrasound imaging of the abdominal muscles. J Orthop Sports Phys Ther 2007;37(8):450–66.

13. Hodges PW, Moseley GL. Pain and motor control of the lumbopelvic region: effect and possible mechanisms. J Electromyogr Kinesiol 2003;13:361–70.

14. Hides JA, Stanton WR, Wilson SJ, et al. Retraining motor control of abdominal muscles among elite cricketers with low back pain. Scand J Med Sci Sports 2010;20:834–42.

15. Teyhen DS, Bluemle LN, Dolbeer JA, et al. Changes in lateral abdominal muscle thickness during the abdominal drawing-in maneuver in those with lumbopelvic pain. J Orthop Sports Phys Ther 2009;39(11):791–8.

16. Teyhen DS, Williamson JN, Carlson NH, et al. Ultrasound characteristics of the deep abdominal muscles during the active straight leg raise test. Arch Phys Med Rehabil 2009;90:761–7.

17. Whittaker JL, Thompson JA, Teyhen DS, et al. Rehabilitative ultrasound imaging of pelvic floor muscle function. J Orthop Sports Phys Ther 2007;37:487–98.

18. Kanehisa H, Ikegawa S, Fukunaga T. Comparison of muscle cross-sectional area and strength between untrained women and men. Eur J Appl Physiol Occup Physiol 1994;68:148–54.

19. Whittaker JL, Warner MB, Stokes M. Comparison of the sonographic features of the abdominal wall muscles and connective tissues in individuals with and without lumbopelvic pain. J Orthop Sports Phys Ther 2013;43:11–19.

20. Hides JA, Richardson CA, Jull GA. Magnetic resonance imaging and ultrasonography of the lumbar multifidus muscle. Comparison of two different modalities. Spine 1995;20:54–8.

21. Hides J, Wilson S, Stanton W, et al. An MRI investigation into the function of the transversus abdominis muscle during 'drawing-in' of the abdominal wall. Spine 2006;31:E175–8.

22. Hodges PW, Pengel LHM, Herbert RD, et al. Measurement of muscle contraction with ultrasound imaging. Muscle Nerve 2003; 27(6):682–92.

23. Kiesel KB, Uhl TL, Underwood FB, et al. Measurement of lumbar multifidus muscle contraction with rehabilitative ultrasound imaging. Man Ther 2007;12:161–6.

24. McMeeken JM, Beith ID, Newham DJ, et al. The relationship between EMG and change in thickness of transversus abdominis. Clin Biomech 2004;19(4):337–42.

25. Hebert JJ, Koppenhaver SL, Parent EC, et al. A systematic review of the reliability of rehabilitative ultrasound imaging for the quantitative assessment of the abdominal and lumbar trunk muscles. Spine 2009;34:E848–56.

26. Costa LOP, Maher CG, Latimer J, et al. Reproducibility of rehabilitative ultrasound imaging for the measurement of abdominal muscle activity: a systematic review. Phys Ther 2009;89: 756–69.

27. Koppenhaver SL, Hebert JJ, Parent EC, et al. Rehabilitative ultrasound imaging is a valid measure of trunk muscle size and activation during most isometric sub-maximal contractions: a systematic review. Aus J Physiotherapy 2009;55:153–69.

28. Kwah LK, Pinto RZ, Diong J, et al. Reliability and validity of ultrasound measurements of muscle fascicle length and pennation in humans: a systematic review. J App Physiol 2013;114:761–9.

29. Cartwright MS, Demar S, Griffin LP, et al. Validity and reliability of nerve and muscle ultrasound. Muscle Nerve 2013;47: 515–21.

30. Impink BG, Gagnon D, Collinger JL, et al. Repeatability of ultrasonographic median nerve measures. Muscle Nerve 2010;41: 767–73.

31. Tagliafico A, Cadoni A, Fisci E, et al. Reliability of side-to-side ultrasound cross-sectional area measurements of lower extremity nerves in healthy subjects. Muscle Nerve 2012;46:717–22.

32. Tagliafico A, Martinoli C. Reliability of side-to-side sonographic cross-sectional area measurements of upper extremity nerves in healthy volunteers. J Ultrasound Med 2013;32:457–62.

33. Wong AYL, Parent EC, Funabashi M, et al. Do various baseline characteristics of transversus abdominis and lumbar multifidus predict clinical outcomes in nonspecific low back pain? A systematic review. Pain 2013;154:2589–602.

34. Potter CL, Cairns MC, Stokes MJ. Use of ultrasound imaging by physiotherapists: a pilot study to survey use, skills and training. Man Ther 2012;17:39–46.

35. Van K, Hides JA, Richardson CA. The use of real-time ultrasound imaging for biofeedback of lumbar multifidus muscle contraction in healthy subjects. J Orthop Sports Phys Ther 2006;36:920–5.

36. Dietz HP, Wilson PD, Clarke B. The use of perineal ultrasound to quantify levator activity and teach pelvic floor muscle exercises. Int Urogynecol J Pelvic Floor Dysfunct 2001;12:166–8, discussion 168–9.

37. Worth S, Henry S, Bunn J. Real-time ultrasound feedback and abdominal hollowing exercises for people with low back pain. NZ J Physiother 2007;35:4–11.

38. Henry SM, Westervelt KC. The use of real-time ultrasound feedback in teaching abdominal hollowing exercises to healthy subjects. J Orthop Sports Phys Ther 2005;35:338–45.

39. Teyhen DS, Miltenberger CE, Deiters HM, et al. The use of ultrasound imaging of the abdominal drawing-in maneuver in subjects with low back pain. J Orthop Sports Phys Ther 2005;35: 346–55.

40. Anderson T, McDicken WN. Measurement of tissue motion. Proc Inst Mech Eng [H] 1999;213:181–91.

41. Yoshii Y, Ishii T, Tung W-L, et al. Median nerve deformation and displacement in the carpal tunnel during finger motion. J Orthop Res 2013;31:1876–80.

42. van Doesburg MHM, Henderson J, Yoshii Y, et al. Median nerve deformation in differential finger motions: ultrasonographic comparison of carpal tunnel syndrome patients and healthy controls. J Orthop Res 2012;30:643–8.

43. Seitz AL, McClure PW, Lynch SS, et al. Effects of scapular dyskinesis and scapular assistance test on subacromial space during static arm elevation. J Shoulder Elbow Surg 2012;21:631–40.

44. Luque-Suarez A, Navarro-Ledesma S, Petocz P, et al. Short term effects of kinesiotaping on acromiohumeral distance in asymptomatic subjects: a randomised controlled trial. Man Ther 2013;18: 573–7.

45. Kubo K, Kanehisa H, Fukunaga T. Gender differences in the viscoelastic properties of tendon structures. Eur J Appl Physiol 2003;88:520–6.

46. Narici MV, Binzoni T, Hiltbrand E, et al. In vivo human gastrocnemius architecture with changing joint angle at rest and during graded isometric contraction. J Physiol 1996;496:287–97.

47. Narici MV, Maganaris CN, Reeves ND, et al. Effect of aging on human muscle architecture. J App Physiol 2003;95:2229–34.

48. Burgess KE, Graham-Smith P, Pearson SJ. Effect of acute tensile loading on gender-specific tendon structural and mechanical properties. J Orthop Res 2009;27:510–16.

49. Fukashiro S, Itoh M, Ichinose Y, et al. Ultrasonography gives directly but noninvasively elastic characteristic of human tendon in vivo. Eur J Appl Physiol Occup Physiol 1995;71:555–7.

50. Maganaris CN, Paul JP. In vivo human tendon mechanical properties. J Physiol 1999;521:307–13.

51. Magnusson SP, Aagaard P, Dyhre-Poulsen P, et al. Load-displacement properties of the human triceps surae aponeurosis in vivo. J Physiol 2001;531:277–88.

52. Cronin NJ, af Klint R, Grey MJ, et al. Ultrasonography as a tool to study afferent feedback from the muscle-tendon complex during human walking. J Electromyogr Kinesiol 2011;21:197–207.

53. Magnusson SP, Narici MV, Maganaris CN, et al. Human tendon behaviour and adaptation, in vivo. J Physiol 2008;586:71–81.

54. Bunce SM, Hough AD, Moore AP. Measurement of abdominal muscle thickness using M-mode ultrasound imaging during functional activities. Man Ther 2004;9:41–4.

55. Vasseljen O, Fladmark AM, Westad C, et al. Onset in abdominal muscles recorded simultaneously by ultrasound imaging and intramuscular electromyography. J Electromyogr Kinesiol 2009;19: e23–31.

56. Heimdal A. Technical principles of tissue velocity and strain imaging methods. In: Marwick TH, Yu C-M, Sun JP, editors. Myocardial Imaging: Tissue Doppler and Speckle Tracking. Oxford, UK: Blackwell Scientific Publications: Oxford; 2007. p. 3–16.

57. Hough AD, Moore AP, Jones MP. Reduced longitudinal excursion of the median nerve in carpal tunnel syndrome. Arch Phys Med Rehabil 2007;88:569–76.

58. Soeters JNM, Roebroeck ME, Holland WP, et al. Reliability of tendon excursion measurements in patients using a color Doppler imaging system. J Hand Surg [Am] 2004;29:581–6.

59. Pulkovski N, Schenk P, Maffiuletti NA, et al. Tissue Doppler imaging for detecting onset of muscle activity. Muscle Nerve 2008;37:638–49.

60. Holland WP, Buyruk HM, Hoorn E, et al. Tendon displacement assessment by pulsed Doppler tissue imaging: validation with a reciprocating string test target. Ultrasound Med Biol 1999;25:1229–39.

61. Hough AD, Moore AP, Jones MP. Peripheral nerve motion measurement with spectral Doppler sonography: a reliability study. J Hand Surg [Br] 2000;25:585–9.

62. Mannion AF, Pulkovski N, Schenk P, et al. A new method for the noninvasive determination of abdominal muscle feedforward activity based on tissue velocity information from tissue Doppler imaging. J Appl Physiol 2008;104:1192–201.

63. Oh S, Belohlavek M, Zhao C. Detection of differential gliding characteristics of the flexor digitorum superficialis tendon and subsynovial connective tissue using color Doppler sonographic imaging. J Ultrasound Med 2007;26:149–55.

64. Eranki A, Bellini L, Prosser L, et al., editors. Measurement of tendon velocities using vector tissue Doppler imaging: a feasibility study. Buenos Aires, Argentina: Annual International Conference of the IEEE Engineering in Medicine and Biology Society; 2010, 31st August-4th September.

65. Bohs LN, Trahey GE. A novel method for angle independent ultrasonic imaging. IEEE Trans Biomed Eng 1991;38:280–6.

66. Dilley A, Greening J, Lynn B, et al. The use of cross-correlation analysis between high-frequency ultrasound images to measure longitudinal median nerve movement. Ultrasound Med Biol 2001;27:1211–18.

67. Korstanje J-WH, Selles RW, Stam HJ, et al. Development and validation of ultrasound speckle tracking to quantify tendon displacement. J Biomech 2010;43:1373–9.

68. Boyd BS, Gray AT, Dilley A, et al. The pattern of tibial nerve excursion with active ankle dorsiflexion is different in older people with diabetes mellitus. Clin Biomech 2012;27:967–71.

69. Dilley A, Lynn B, Greening J, et al. Quantitative in vivo studies of median nerve sliding in response to wrist, elbow, shoulder and neck movements. Clin Biomech 2003;18:899–907.

70. Ellis RF, Hing WA, McNair PJ. Comparison of different neural mobilization exercises upon longitudinal sciatic nerve movement: an in-vivo study utilizing ultrasound imaging. J Orthop Sports Phys Ther 2012;42:667–75.

71. Ridehalgh C, Moore A, Hough AD. Normative sciatic nerve excursion during a modified straight leg raise test. Man Ther 2013;19:59–64.

72. Loram ID, Maganaris CN, Lakie M. Use of ultrasound to make noninvasive in vivo measurement of continuous changes in human muscle contractile length. J Appl Physiol 2006;100:1311–23.

73. Herbert RD, Clarke J, Kwah LK, et al. In vivo passive mechanical behaviour of muscle fascicles and tendons in human gastrocnemius muscle-tendon units. J Physiol 2011;589:5257–67.

74. Korstanje J-WH, Scheltens-De Boer M, Blok JH, et al. Ultrasonographic assessment of longitudinal median nerve and hand flexor tendon dynamics in carpal tunnel syndrome. Muscle Nerve 2012;45:721–9.

75. Tian M, Herbert RD, Hoang PD, et al. Myofascial force transmission between the human soleus and gastrocnemius muscles during passive knee motion. J Appl Physiol 2012;113:517.

76. Arndt A, Bengtsson A-S, Peolsson M, et al. Non-uniform displacement within the Achilles tendon during passive ankle joint motion. Knee Surg Sports Traumatol Arthrosc 2011;20:1868–74.

77. Harris EJ, Miller NR, Bamber JC, et al. Speckle tracking in a phantom and feature-based tracking in liver in the presence of respiratory motion using 4D ultrasound. Phys Med Biol 2010;55:3363–80.

78. Revell JD, Mirmehdi M, McNally DS. Musculoskeletal motion flow fields using hierarchical variable-sized block matching in ultrasonographic video sequences. J Biomech 2004;37:511–22.

79. Revell JD, Mirmehdi M, McNally D. Computer vision elastography: speckle adaptive motion estimation for elastography using ultrasound sequences. IEEE Trans Med Imaging 2005;24:755–66.

80. Brown PG, Alsousou J, Thompson M, et al. Ultrasound strain imaging measurement in Achilles tendons as a measure of healing from rupture with controlled ankle motion. J Biomech 2012;45:S402.

81. Slagmolen P, Scheys L, D'Hooge J, et al. Letter: In regard to: 'In vivo strain analysis of the intact supraspinatus tendon by ultrasound speckles tracking imaging' (J Orthop Res 2011;29:1931–7). J Orthop Res 2012;29:1–3.

82. Gennisson J-L, Deffieux T, Fink M, et al. Ultrasound elastography: principles and techniques. Diagn Interv Imag 2013;94:487–95.

83. Wu C-H, Chen W-S, Park G-Y, et al. Musculoskeletal sonoelastography: a focused review of its diagnostic applications for evaluating tendons and fascia. J Med Ultrasound 2012;20:79–86.

84. De Zordo T, Fink C, Feuchtner GM, et al. Real-time sonoelastography findings in healthy Achilles tendons. AJR Am J Roentgenol 2009;193:W134–8.

85. Brown PG, Alsousou J, Cooper A, et al. The AutoQual ultrasound elastography method for quantitative assessment of lateral strain in post-rupture Achilles tendons. J Biomech 2013;46:2695–700.

86. Lopata RGP, van Dijk JP, Pillen S, et al. Dynamic imaging of skeletal muscle contraction in three orthogonal directions. J Appl Physiol 2010;109:906–14.

87. Parker KJ, Doyley MM, Rubens DJ. Imaging the elastic properties of tissue: the 20 year perspective. Phys Med Biol 2011;56:R1–29.

88. Buyruk HM, Stam HJ, Snijders CJ, et al. Measurement of sacroiliac joint stiffness in peripartum pelvic pain patients with Doppler imaging of vibrations (DIV). Eur J Obstet Gynecol Reprod Biol 1999;83:159–63.

89. de Groot M, Spoor CW, Snijders CJ. Critical notes on the technique of Doppler imaging of vibrations (DIV). Ultrasound Med Biol 2004;30:363–7.

90. Mens JMA, Damen L, Snijders CJ, et al. The mechanical effect of a pelvic belt in patients with pregnancy-related pelvic pain. Clin Biomech 2006;21:122–7.

91. Ballyns JJ, Turo D, Otto P, et al. Office-based elastographic technique for quantifying mechanical properties of skeletal muscle. J Ultrasound Med 2012;31:1209–19.

92. McCreesh KM, Riley SJ, Crotty JM. Neovascularity in patellar tendinopathy and the response to eccentric training: a case report using power Doppler ultrasound. Man Ther 2013;18:602–5.

93. Harper CJ, Shahgholi L, Cieslak K, et al. Variability in diaphragm motion during normal breathing, assessed with B-mode ultrasound. J Orthop Sports Phys Ther 2013;43:927–31.

94. Cho KH, Lee HJ, Lee WH. Reliability of rehabilitative ultrasound imaging for the medial gastrocnemius muscle in poststroke patients. Clin Physiol Funct Imaging 2014;34:26–31.

95. Gorgey AS, Timmons MK, Michener LA, et al. Intra-rater reliability of ultrasound imaging of wrist extensor muscles in patients with tetraplegia. PM R 2014;6:127–33.

96. Zhao H, Ren Y, Wu Y-N, et al. Ultrasonic evaluations of Achilles tendon mechanical properties poststroke. J Appl Physiol 2009;106:843–9.

97. Zhao H, Wu Y-N, Hwang M, et al. Changes of calf muscle-tendon biomechanical properties induced by passive-stretching and active-movement training in children with cerebral palsy. J Appl Physiol 2011;111:435–42.

98. Hoang P, Saboisky JP, Gandevia SC, et al. Passive mechanical properties of gastrocnemius in people with multiple sclerosis. Clin Biomech 2009;24:291.

CHAPTER 15

ADVANCES IN MAGNETIC RESONANCE IMAGING (MRI) MEASURES

James Elliott • Graham Galloway • Barbara Cagnie • Katie McMahon

INTRODUCTION

Magnetic resonance imaging (MRI) provides a map of the distribution of hydrogen atoms, principally in water and fat molecules, through the use of radiofrequency pulses and static and changing magnetic fields to produce anatomical images of the body. Different tissue types and pathologies have their own signature.[1] MRI does not use ionizing radiation, making it particularly useful in monitoring longitudinal management of injury and disease. MRI provides excellent soft tissue definition with a range of contrasts that allow for a non-invasive visualization of tissues and abnormalities in multiple planes. Although still evolving and more expensive compared to other imaging modalities (e.g. computed tomography, radiography and ultrasound), MRI is being used increasingly to identify tissue changes at the microscopic, metabolic and macroscopic levels to determine any of the following: (a) the severity and extent of injury or a disease process; (b) progress and response to treatments; (c) a specific underlying pathological cause and location; or (d) when specific tissues are affected.[2]

MRI has long been an important tool for evaluating the musculoskeletal system.[2] There are many examples where MRI is used in the diagnosis of relevant musculoskeletal disease/injury,[3–8] thus helping to direct appropriate treatment. There are not always consistent findings of patho-anatomical lesions that are related to the clinical symptoms. However, advancing MRI technologies are providing mechanistic, diagnostic and possibly therapeutic-based information.[9–25] These advancing technologies are providing a glimpse into the physiological, cognitive and affective processes[26] that may be associated with poor functional recovery and chronic pain-related disability in high-risk patients. The following chapter will explore how MRI is being used (and may be used) in neuromusculoskeletal research, what is being measured with various applications, and its uses and limitations.

MRI CONTRASTS

It is first necessary to understand the fundamental area of MRI contrasts. There are a range of MRI contrasts, which highlight different processes. Contrast between different tissues in MRI is dependent on a combination of the concentration of the protons and their molecular environment. The greatest influences on contrast weighting[1] are the relaxation properties, which are largely dependent on molecular motion and also by the technologist selecting and setting the different sequence applications. However, the presence of relaxation agents also has an influence and these agents may be either endogenous (e.g. iron) or exogenous (e.g. gadolinium). Each family of sequences has different applications and disadvantages in musculoskeletal imaging. A brief guide to some of the terms is provided in Table 15-1. For more information, the interested reader is encouraged to refer to McMahon et al.[1] A user-friendly pocket guide to MRI acronyms across manufacturers is also available from Hitachi at http://www.hitachimed.com/idc/groups/hitachimedical/documents/supportingdocumentpdf/poc_001960.pdf.

Changing the parameters (e.g. timing) of any of the families of sequences will lead to a different contrast in target tissues (Table 15-1). When investigating vascular tissues or muscle haemorrhaging, a gradient echo sequence is preferred. However, gradient echo sequences are very sensitive to tissue interfaces, of which there are many in all joints, as well as metallic implants such as pins or screws. Their presence results in signal loss and geometric distortions in the surrounding areas. A spin echo sequence is less sensitive to disturbances in the magnetic field and is a good option for visualizing meniscal tears. There are steady-state or hybrid sequences, which offer superior muscle/blood contrast and can allow real-time imaging of joint motion.

Trabecular bone and bone marrow are brighter in proton density weighting than tendons and cortical bone. General anatomical imaging can be performed with T_1 weighting (where fat is bright and water is dark). However, if pathologies such as inflammation or fluid accumulation are suspected, T_2 weighting will most clearly reveal the extent of the effusions (Fig. 15-1). Often the fat signal is suppressed to aid in the visualization of pathological processes in a T_2-weighted image. A fat-suppressed acquisition using a short-tau inversion recovery sequence, which nulls the signal from fat, has predictive capacity to identify denervated muscles in the periphery (Fig. 15-2).[2,7]

TABLE 15-1	A Brief Guide to Different Sequences and Contrast Weightings of Clinical MRI Applications Commonly Used in Musculoskeletal Imaging	
Sequence family	Gradient echo	Sensitivity to iron-rich compounds and vascularity, but has artefacts around metal implants like pins or screws
	Spin echo	Less sensitivity to metal implants, usually slower to acquire
	Hybrid sequences (e.g. true-FISP or steady-state sequences)	Can be rapid sequences, offer great tissue/blood contrast and allow real-time imaging
Contrast weighting	T_1	Fat and meniscal tears will appear bright; fluids, muscles and tendons are grey, air and cortical bone are black
	T_2	Fluids like water and cerebrospinal fluid, as well as fat appear bright; muscle and tendons are grey, air and cortical bone are black
	T_2^*	An additional relaxation to T_2, caused by local field changes. This is very sensitive to blood oxygen level changes and vascularity
	Proton density	The more protons the tissue contains, the brighter it is
	Diffusion	Creates a sensitivity to motion within the tissue voxels, allowing the investigation of tissue microstructure

FAT/WATER SEPARATION: MACROSCOPIC STRUCTURE OF MUSCLE

Clinical observations of altered muscle structure and function on conventional MRI have been reported in patients with neuromusculoskeletal complaints, such as low back pain,[27–31] neck, head and shoulder girdle disorders,[15,17,18,20–22,32–35] radiculopathy[2,7] and peripheral neuropathies,[36] rotator cuff pathology[37] and chronic fibromyalgia.[25] Recent conventional and advanced MRI evidence from our research in Brisbane, Australia[20] and Chicago, USA (in preparation) has identified the unique early expression of neck muscle degeneration (fatty infiltrates) in patients following whiplash injury from a motor vehicle collision (MVC) who go on to develop chronic pain-related disability.[20] Such muscle changes are not present in patients with lower levels of initial pain or in patients with chronic non-traumatic neck pain,[21] suggesting traumatic factors play a role in altering the make-up and structure of the neck muscles. Furthermore, the presence of a post-traumatic stress response mediated the relationship between initial pain levels and the development of neck muscle fat.[20] While preliminary, these findings demonstrate a relationship between symptoms of post-traumatic stress disorder (a psychological disorder) and objective longitudinal MRI data for muscle degeneration (a physical pathology), suggesting multiple neuropsychobiological factors influence recovery rates following an MVC. Questions regarding more informed interventions for retarding (if not preventing) muscular degeneration remain. However, the prospect is that advanced, and currently available, MRI measures can provide spatio-temporal information on disease stage and progression. Ultimately, emerging MRI applications could be used to explore and inform interventions aimed at influencing functional recovery.

There are several MRI applications to measure the macroscopic and microscopic expression of the fat and water composition of a muscle in neuromuscular disorders.[38,39] A dual acquisition method may be used, where

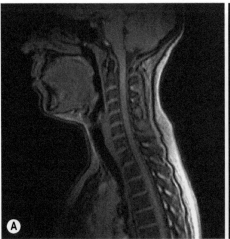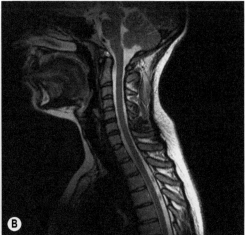

FIGURE 15-1 ■ Sagittal **(A)** T_1-weighted and **(B)** T_2-weighted magnetic resonance images of the cervical spine.

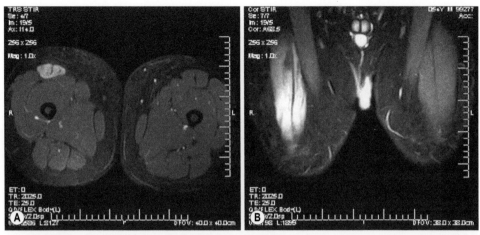

FIGURE 15-2 ■ **(A)** Axial and **(B)** coronal short-tau inversion recovery images detailing increased signal intensity suggesting denervation of the right rectus femoris muscle in a patient with lumbar spine radiculopathy due to a herniated disc at L3/4.

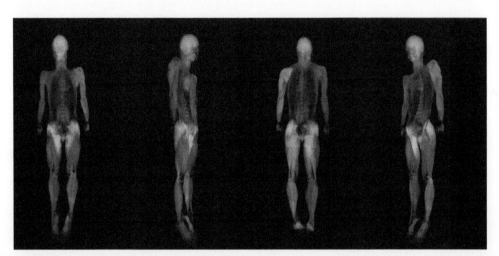

FIGURE 15-3 ■ An example of whole body magnetic resonance imaging using a three-dimensional semi-automated segmentation algorithm where the quantification of specific muscle volume and fat infiltration can be realized. For colour version see Plate 13. (Images are courtesy of Dr Olof Dahlqvist-Leinhard, Linköping University, Sweden; Advanced MR Analytics http://amraab.se/).

a fat-suppressed image (water only) and a standard image (fat and water) are collected. Subtracting the first from the second yields a fat image. This type of acquisition does suffer from its reliance on the uniform frequency of fat across the whole volume of excitation, which is often difficult to obtain especially at higher magnetic fields (3 Tesla and above). An alternative is the Dixon method,[40] where data are collected at two echo times; one when water and fat are in-phase and one when water and fat are out of phase. The data can be combined in such a way that they generate separate fat and water images. This method is susceptible to short T_2^*, which is often the case in musculoskeletal imaging. More sophisticated methods collect data from more than two echoes to improve the estimation of the fat and water images. These methods have been applied successfully in the liver and musculoskeletal application using an iterative least squares solution called IDEAL.[41] Such methodology provides foundation for rapid data acquisition of whole-body imaging[42] which has implications for studying and quantifying muscle degeneration in systemic[38,43] and other neuromusculoskeletal disorders (e.g. fibromyalgia,[25]

chronic whiplash and incomplete spinal cord injury [Elliott, manuscript in preparation]). Figure 15-3 details a semi-automated segmentation algorithm that can be used to calculate specific or whole-body muscle volume and fat infiltration in rapid fashion. Figure 15-4 demonstrates an axial fat/water separation (fat only) image of the ankle plantar and dorsiflexors in one subject with incomplete spinal cord injury and one with chronic (3 years duration) whiplash-related disability. Furthermore, recent investigation has validated such methodologies against the gold-standard biopsy with histological confirmation.[39]

MUSCLE FUNCTIONAL MRI: MICROSCOPIC ACTIVATION AND FUNCTION OF MUSCLE

Muscle functional MRI (mfMRI) offers a non-invasive method to quantify changes in muscle

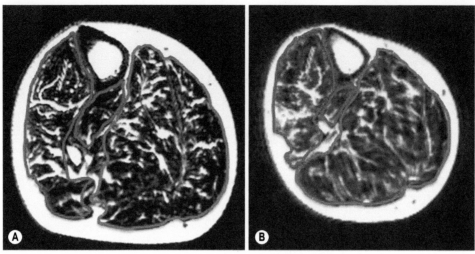

FIGURE 15-4 ▧ Magnetic resonance (fat only) image of the right plantar (*red*) and dorsiflexors (*blue*) in (**A**) subject with incomplete spinal cord injury and (**B**) subject with chronic whiplash-associated disorder. Note the increased signal throughout the plantar/ dorsiflexors in both subjects, suggestive of fatty infiltrates. Note: The posterior tibialis is highlighted in green. For colour version see Plate 13.

physiology following the performance of exercise. The mfMRI technique is based on signal intensity changes due to increases in the relaxation time (T_2) of tissue water following exercise. Specifically, exercise results in a slower decay of the muscle water transverse magnetization, which causes an enhancement in signal intensity of the activated muscles. As a consequence, activated muscles look brighter on T_2-weighted images when compared to muscles imaged in a resting state.[44] The proposed underlying physiological mechanism of this shift in T_2 relaxation time is that the influx of fluid during activity is accompanied by an accumulation of osmolites (phosphate, lactate, sodium) in the cytoplasm and their presence prolongs the relaxation time of soft-aqueous skeletal muscle.[44]

In contemporary research, mfMRI is an emerging tool for assessing the extent of muscle activation (and possibly function) following the performance of a task and for the evaluation of neuromuscular adaptations as a result of therapeutic interventions.[13,32] Some studies utilizing mfMRI have investigated muscle activity patterns during commonly prescribed clinically based exercises.[32,45–47] Other studies have evaluated muscle activity during exercise of the lower (knee extension, ankle extension and flexion, running and cycling)[48–50] and upper extremities as well as the spine.[32,46,51–53] It has been demonstrated that T_2 shifts may be useful for non-invasive inferences regarding moderate levels of muscle activity, but less valid for the lower and higher levels of activity.

There are many clinical and preliminary experimental investigations to highlight changes in muscle activation pattern as a result of pain.[14,29,32,54–57] mfMRI has also been used to non-invasively evaluate neuromuscular adaptations as a result of resistance training. However, there is a paucity of information in the literature to definitively ascribe and generalize its use to clinical assessment.[52,58]

ADVANCED TECHNIQUES: MICROSCOPIC EVALUATION OF THE MUSCLE AND NERVOUS SYSTEMS

Magnetization Transfer Ratios

Magnetization transfer ratios (MTRs) are an indirect measure of tissue stability, relying on the exchange of magnetically saturated hydrogen nuclei (protons) between solid tissue structures and free water.[59,60] MTRs have been widely studied as semi-quantitative metrics for mild and traumatic brain injury,[61,62] and peripheral neuropathy,[36] and are used clinically in diagnostic studies of neuronal degeneration in multiple sclerosis,[63] Alzheimer's disease[64–67] and Parkinson's disease.[68,69] Furthermore, MTR can be used to characterize the demyelination/ degeneration of ascending and descending spinal pathways in patients with spinal cord injury to assess prognosis.[70]

Preliminary evidence (Elliott, manuscript in preparation) suggests that the expression of muscle fatty infiltrates in the plantar and dorsiflexors (Fig. 15-4) in a small sample of patients with chronic whiplash could result from mild damage to descending white matter pathways of the cervical spinal cord as detected from the MTR data. Such data provide a foundation for further prospective investigations to quantify temporal losses in neural substrates within specific descending and ascending spinal cord pathways following traumatic spinal injuries. Figure 15-5 details magnetization transfer contrast and use of MTR in the spinal cord.

Diffusion Weighted Imaging

The microstructure of tissue can be assessed with an advanced technique known as diffusion weighted imaging (DWI). The sequences used in DWI are sensitive to the motion of intracellular and extracellular water

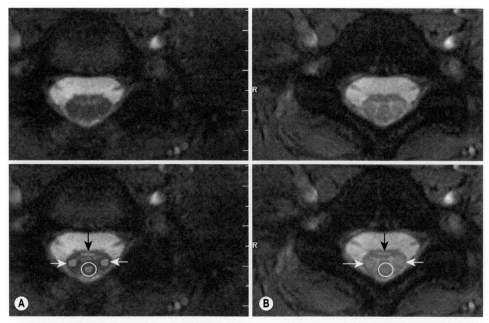

FIGURE 15-5 ■ Anatomically defined regions of interest (ROIs) on the (**A**) magnetization transfer (MT) and (**B**) non-MT-weighted image over the ventromedial and dorsolateral (green in colour plate, arrows in this figure) primarily descending motor pathways and the dorsal column (red in colour plate, circled in this figure) ascending sensory pathways of the cervical spinal cord. The non-magnetization transfer (non-MT) scan (**B**) is identical except that the MT saturation pulse is turned off and run as a separate co-registered acquisition. The MTR is calculated on a voxel-by-voxel basis using the formula of: MTR = 100*(non-MT − MT)/non-MT. For colour version see Plate 14.

molecules and provide information on changes to the boundaries within the tissue. An increase in diffusion is indicative of an increase in fluid or breakdown in cellularity (e.g. cysts or necrosis), whereas a decrease in diffusion indicates a loss of permeability in the microstructure (e.g. ischaemia and cell swelling). It is commonly used to investigate neuromusculoskeletal tumours as it allows determination of the extent of necrosis. DWI can also be used to monitor treatment progression and to estimate prognosis.[71] Emerging applications use diffusion to gauge musculature changes and therapeutic response.[19,72] For example, diffusion values can be used to investigate the loss of vertebral disc integrity in compression fractures.[72] Increased muscle diffusion values may precede electrophysiological and histological evidence of denervation.[2,73]

Functional Magnetic Resonance Imaging: Functional and Structural

Functional magnetic resonance imaging (fMRI) is the process of observing signal changes due to blood oxygenation level differences (BOLD).[74] Neuronal activity is highly correlated to blood oxygenation changes, and fMRI allows the localization of these changes, although it suffers low temporal resolution. There is a signal increase in a BOLD-sensitive sequence approximately 4.5 seconds after a cognitive challenge, in response to the haemodynamic fluctuations of active tissue. Although predominantly a neuroimaging technique for the brain, applications of fMRI to study the spinal cord are emerging. These applications sometimes use BOLD, but also use a signal enhancement by extravascular water protons,[75]

which utilizes T_2 rather than T_2^* relaxation, giving it an advantage in complex structures such as the brain and spine. Neuronal activity in the spinal cord has been mapped in response to normal processing of stimuli such as thermal changes and motor tasks, as well as the effect of trauma and disease processes.[76]

From a clinical perspective, spinal cord fMRI data may be used in clinical trials to provide information on the site of action, efficacy and mechanisms of treatments, and may prove valuable in the diagnosis of diseases afflicting the peripheral and central nervous systems.[77] Such knowledge will greatly expand our understanding of the peripheral and central nervous system and the pathophysiological mechanisms underlying many of the common, yet enigmatic, disorders frequently assessed and managed by physiotherapists, worldwide.

As an example, thrust manipulation applied to the axial and appendicular skeleton has long been shown to improve the active range of motion, reduce self-reported pain and improve function in groups of patients with mechanical spinal and shoulder pain.[78–80] While biomechanical models have yet to explain the mechanisms by which manipulation works,[81] preliminary fMRI evidence from a thoracic spine manipulation model[82] and animal models of mobilization[83] suggests that supraspinal mechanisms may explain the attendant, albeit immediate, hypoalgesic effect. Future work, with larger datasets and different patient populations, should shed light on neurophysiological mechanisms of manipulative procedures.

Caution

fMRI is a potentially powerful method for evaluating regional brain and spinal cord activation. It can also be used to determine the connectivity or interactions between regions, either when a subject is performing an explicit task, or at rest. Numerous techniques have been proposed to acquire and analyse fMRI data with the primary aim to find an optimal combination of methods to plot activated (or deactivated) brain regions (functional) and understand relationships between them (structural). This requires the optimization of many aspects of (a) data acquisition (e.g. duration of scan, spatial resolution, spatial smoothing during pre-processing) and (b) data analysis, such as seed-based and independent component analyses. Accordingly, the reader is encouraged to be a cautious and informed consumer of the literature in regard to findings from fMRI studies and to understand the complexities of such methodologies before definitively interpreting any/all available literature. This is a call to 'talk across fences' in order to establish interdisciplinary relationships whereby challenging clinical questions can be interpreted, rigorously (and accurately) tested and translated.

MRI IN MUSCULOSKELETAL CLINICAL PRACTICE

When used appropriately, MRI studies can be a crucial component for managing a patient with a neuromusculoskeletal complaint. MRI provides objective measures of the damage to the neuromusculoskeletal system, making it an excellent tool for accurate diagnosis, improved understanding of the pathophysiology of disease and evaluating the efficacy of treatment regimens, which otherwise are often based on the patients' self-reporting of pain. MRI does not use radiation and so is non-invasive. Accordingly, it is the technique of choice for research and for longitudinal clinical studies. It is necessary to note that a subset of patients will be incompatible for MRI, as there are a number of contraindications. Depending upon the area to be imaged, these include, but are not limited to, certain pacemakers, aneurysm clips, metallic foreign bodies and claustrophobia. A full list of magnetic resonance conditional and incompatible devices can be found at www.mrisafety.com[84] and interested readers are encouraged to refer to Durbridge.[85]

Ongoing research is further defining the role of MRI in evaluating disorders of the musculoskeletal system. Nevertheless, there are some negative aspects of MRI from a clinical perspective. For example, early MRI referrals of patients with acute low back pain on the basis of self-reported pain and without any other indication generally provide little benefit and contribute to poor outcomes and often to a strong iatrogenic effect.[86-88] A patient's knowledge (or interpretation) of imaging abnormalities (e.g. a 'bulging disc') can actually decrease self-perception of health and may lead to fear avoidance and catastrophizing behaviours that may predispose people to chronicity.[89,90] Accordingly, clinicians should understand and refer to the available guidelines on appropriate use of and judicious referral for imaging.[91, 92]

Furthermore, the use of clinical pathways[93] that reduce the referral for inappropriate imaging studies, reduce costs of healthcare delivery and ultimately improve patient-centred outcomes, are all important components of patient management. In short, healthcare practitioners worldwide can play a primary-care role through participation in pathways that are based on diagnostic and patient management algorithms.[94-97] The judicious adherence to such algorithms can reduce practice variation,[96] and ensure that our patients understand both the necessity for appropriate imaging studies and the negative influence of unnecessary imaging.[98,99]

REFERENCES

1. McMahon KL, Cowin G, Galloway G. Magnetic resonance imaging: the underlying principles. J Orthop Sports Phys Ther 2011;41:806–19.
2. Fritz RC, Domroese ME, Carter GT. Physiological and anatomical basis of muscle magnetic resonance imaging. Phys Med Rehabil Clin N Am 2005;16:1033–51.
3. Bendszus M, Koltzenburg M, Wessig C, et al. Sequential MR imaging of denervated muscle: experimental study. AJNR Am J Neuroradiol 2002;23:1427–31.
4. Bendszus M, Wessig C, Reiners K, et al. MR imaging in the differential diagnosis of neurogenic foot drop. AJNR Am J Neuroradiol 2003;24:1283–9.
5. Bendszus M, Wessig C, Solymosi L, et al. MRI of peripheral nerve degeneration and regeneration: correlation with electrophysiology and histology. Exp Neurol 2004;188:171–7.
6. Bredella MA, Tirman P, Fritz RC, et al. Denervation syndromes of the shoulder girdle: MR imaging with electrophysiologic. Skeletal Radiol 1999;28:567–72.
7. Carter GT, Fritz R. Electromyographic and lower extremity short time to inversion recovery magnetic resonance imaging findings in lumbar radiculopathy. Muscle Nerve 1997;20:1191–3.
8. Wessig C, Koltzenburg M, Reiners K, et al. Muscle magnetic resonance imaging of denervation and reinnervation: correlation with electrophysiology and histology. Exp Neurol 2004;185:254–61.
9. Apkarian AV. Functional magnetic resonance imaging of pain consciousness: cortical networks of pain critically depend on what is implied by 'pain'. Curr Rev Pain 1999;3:308–15.
10. Apkarian AV, Hashmi JA, Baliki MN. Pain and the brain: specificity and plasticity of the brain in clinical chronic pain. Pain 2011;152 (Suppl. 3):S49–64.
11. Baliki MN, Geha PY, Apkarian AV. Parsing pain perception between nociceptive representation and magnitude estimation. J Neurophysiol 2009;101:875–87.
12. Baliki MN, Geha PY, Fields HL, et al. Predicting value of pain and analgesia: nucleus accumbens response to noxious stimuli changes in the presence of chronic pain. Neuron 2010;66:149–60.
13. Cagnie B, Elliott J, O'Leary S, et al. Muscle functional MRI as an imaging tool to evaluate muscle activity. J Orthop Sports Phys Ther 2011;41:896–903.
14. Cagnie B, Elliott J, O'Leary S, et al. Pain-induced changes in the activity of the cervical extensor muscles evaluated by muscle functional magnetic resonance imaging. Clin J Pain 2011;27:392–7.
15. Elliott J. Are there implications for morphological changes in neck muscles after whiplash injury? Spine 2011;36(Suppl. 25):S205–10. Review.
16. Elliott J, Cannata E, Christensen E, et al. MRI analysis of the size and shape of the oropharynx in chronic whiplash. Otolaryngol Head Neck Surg 2008;138:747–51.
17. Elliott J, Jull G, Noteboom JT, et al. Fatty infiltration in the cervical extensor muscles in persistent whiplash-associated disorders: a magnetic resonance imaging analysis. Spine 2006;31:E847–55.
18. Elliott J, Jull G, Noteboom JT, et al. MRI study of the cross-sectional area for the cervical extensor musculature in patients with persistent whiplash associated disorders (WAD). Man Ther 2008;13:258–65.
19. Elliott J, Pedler A, Beattie P, et al. Diffusion-weighted magnetic resonance imaging for the healthy cervical multifidus: a potential method for studying neck muscle physiology following spinal trauma. J Orthop Sports Phys Ther 2010;40:722–8.
20. Elliott J, Pedler A, Kenardy J, et al. The temporal development of fatty infiltrates in the neck muscles following whiplash injury: an

association with pain and posttraumatic stress. PLoS ONE 2011;6(6):e21194.

21. Elliott J, Sterling M, Noteboom JT, et al. Fatty infiltrate in the cervical extensor muscles is not a feature of chronic, insidious-onset neck pain. Clin Radiol 2008;63:681–7.

22. Elliott JM, O'Leary S, Sterling M, et al. Magnetic resonance imaging findings of fatty infiltrate in the cervical flexors in chronic whiplash. Spine 2010;35:948–54.

23. Elliott JM, Pedler AR, Cowin G, et al. Spinal cord metabolism and muscle water diffusion in whiplash. Spinal Cord 2011;50:474–6.

24. Elliott JM, Walton DM, Rademaker A, et al. Quantification of cervical spine muscle fat: a comparison between T1-weighted and multi-echo gradient echo imaging using a variable projection algorithm (VARPRO). BMC Med Imaging 2013;13:30.

25. Gerdle B, Forsgren MF, Bengtsson A, et al. Decreased muscle concentrations of ATP and PCR in the quadriceps muscle of fibromyalgia patients – A (31) P-MRS study. Eur J Pain 2013; 17:1205–15.

26. Wager TD, Atlas LY, Lindquist MA, et al. An fMRI-based neurologic signature of physical pain. N Engl J Med 2013;368: 1388–97.

27. Campbell WW, Vasconcelos O, Laine FJ. Focal atrophy of the multifidus muscle in lumbosacral radiculopathy. Muscle Nerve 1998;21:1350–1353F.

28. Danneels LA, Vanderstraeten GG, Cambier DC, et al. CT imaging of trunk muscles in chronic low back pain patients and healthy control subjects. Eur Spine J 2000;9:266–72.

29. Dickx N, Cagnie B, Achten E, et al. Changes in lumbar muscle activity because of induced muscle pain evaluated by muscle functional magnetic resonance imaging. Spine 2008;33:E983–9.

30. Kader DF, Wardlaw D, Smith FW. Correlation between the MRI changes in the lumbar multifidus muscles and leg pain. Clin Radiol 2000;55:145–9.

31. Paalanne N, Niinimäki J, Karppinen J, et al. Assessment of association between low back pain and paraspinal muscle atrophy using opposed phase magnetic resonance imaging a population-based study among young adults. Spine 2011;36:1961–8.

32. Cagnie B, Dickx N, Peeters I, et al. The use of functional MRI to evaluate cervical flexor activity during different cervical flexion exercises. J Appl Physiol 2008;104:230–5.

33. Elliott JM, Pedler AR, Jull GA, et al. Differential changes in muscle composition exist in traumatic and non-traumatic neck pain. Spine 2014;39:39–47.

34. Fernandez-de-Las-Penas C, Bueno A, Ferrando J, et al. Magnetic resonance imaging study of the morphometry of cervical extensor muscles in chronic tension-type headache. Cephalalgia 2007;27: 355–62.

35. Sheard B, Elliott J, Cagnie B, et al. Evaluating serratus anterior muscle function in neck pain using muscle functional magnetic resonance imaging. J Manipulative Physiol Ther 2012;35:629–35.

36. Sinclair CD, Morrow JM, Miranda MA, et al. Skeletal muscle MRI magnetisation transfer ratio reflects clinical severity in peripheral neuropathies. J Neurol Neurosurg Psychiatry 2012;83: 29–32.

37. Gladstone JN, Bishop JY, Lo IK, et al. Fatty infiltration and atrophy of the rotator cuff do not improve after rotator cuff repair and correlate with poor functional outcome. Am J Sports Med 2007;35:719–28.

38. Bley TA, Wieben O, Francois CJ, et al. Fat and water magnetic resonance imaging. J Magn Reson Imaging 2010;31:4–18.

39. Gaeta M, Scribano E, Mileto A, et al. Muscle fat fraction in neuromuscular disorders: dual-echo dual-flip-angle spoiled gradient-recalled MR imaging technique for quantification a feasibility study. Radiology 2011;259:487–94.

40. Dixon W. Simple proton spectroscopic imaging. Radiology 1984; 153:189–94.

41. Costa DN, Pedrosa I, McKenzie C, et al. Body MRI using IDEAL. Am J Roentgenol 2008;190:1076–84.

42. Schmidt GP, Reiser MF, Baur-Melnyk A. Whole-body imaging of the musculoskeletal system: the value of MR imaging. Skeletal Radiol 2007;36:1109–19.

43. Rönn M, Lind PM, Karlsson H, et al. Quantification of total and visceral adipose tissue in fructose-fed rats using water-fat separated single echo MRI. Obesity (Silver Spring) 2013;21:E388–95.

44. Meyer RA, Prior BM. Functional magnetic resonance imaging of muscle. Exerc Sport Sci Rev 2000;28:89–92.

45. Cagnie B, D'Hooge R, Achten E, et al. A magnetic resonance imaging investigation into the function of the deep cervical flexors during the performance of craniocervical flexion. J Manipulative Physiol Ther 2010;33:266–91.

46. Elliott JM, O'Leary SP, Cagnie B, et al. Craniocervical orientation affects muscle activation when exercising the cervical extensors in healthy subjects. Arch Phys Med Rehabil 2010;91:1418–22.

47. O'Leary S, Cagnie B, Reeve A, et al. Is there altered activity of the extensor muscles in chronic mechanical neck pain? A functional magnetic resonance imaging study. Arch Phys Med Rehabil 2011;92:929–34.

48. Jenner G, Foley JM, Cooper TG, et al. Changes in magnetic resonance images of muscle depend on exercise intensity, duration, not work. J Appl Physiol 1994;76:2119–24.

49. Kinugasa R, Akima H. Neuromuscular activation of triceps surae using muscle functional MRI and EMG. Med Sci Sports Exerc 2005;37:593–8.

50. Ono T, Higashihara A, Fukubayashi T. Hamstring functions during hip-extension exercise assessed with electromyography and magnetic resonance imaging. Res Sports Med 2011;19:42–52.

51. Conley MS, Meyer RA, Bloomberg JJ, et al. Noninvasive analysis of human neck muscle function. Spine 1995;20:2505–12.

52. Conley MS, Stone MH, Nimmons M, et al. Resistance training and human cervical muscle recruitment plasticity. J Appl Physiol 1997;83:2105–11.

53. Mayer JM, Graves JE, Clark BC, et al. The use of magnetic resonance imaging to evaluate lumbar muscle activity during trunk extension exercise at varying intensities. Spine 2005;30:2556–63.

54. Falla D, Jull G, Hodges P. Neck pain patients demonstrate reduced EMG activity of the deep cervical flexors during performance of the craniocervical flexion test. Spine 2004;29:2108–14.

55. Falla D, Bilenkij G, Jull G. Patients with chronic neck pain demonstrate altered patterns of muscle activation during performance of a functional upper limb task. Spine 2004;29:1436–40.

56. Falla D, Dall'Alba P, Rainoldi A, et al. Repeatability of surface EMG variables in the sternocleidomastoid and anterior scalene muscles. Eur J Appl Physiol 2002;87:542–9.

57. Schomacher J, Farina D, Lindstroem R, et al. Chronic trauma-induced neck pain impairs the neural control of the deep semispinalis cervicis muscle. Clin Neurophysiol 2012;123:1403–8.

58. Akima H, Ushiyama J, Kubo J, et al. Resistance training during unweighting maintains muscle size and function in human calf. Med Sci Sports Exerc 2003;35:655–62.

59. Wolff SD, Balaban RS. Magnetisation transfer contrast (MTC) and tissue water proton relaxation in vivo. Magn Reson Med 1989;10:135–44.

60. Wolff SD, Eng J, Balaban RS. Magnetisation transfer contrast: method for improving contrast in gradient-recalled-echo images. Radiology 1991;179:133–7.

61. Bagley LJ, McGowan JC, Grossman RI, et al. Magnetisation transfer imaging of traumatic brain injury. J Magn Reson Imaging 2000;11:1–8.

62. Sinson G, Bagley LJ, Cecil KM, et al. Magnetisation transfer imaging and proton MR spectroscopy in the evaluation of axonal injury: correlation with clinical outcome after traumatic brain injury. AJNR Am J Neuroradiol 2001;22:143–51.

63. Dehmeshki J, Chard DT, Leary SM, et al. The normal appearing grey matter in primary progressive multiple sclerosis: a magnetisation transfer imaging study. J Neurol 2003;250:67–74.

64. Hanyu H, Asano T, Iwamoto T, et al. Magnetisation transfer measurements of the hippocampus in patients with Alzheimer's disease, vascular dementia, and other types of dementia. AJNR Am J Neuroradiol 2000;21:1235–42.

65. Hanyu H, Asano T, Sakurai H, et al. Magnetisation transfer measurements of the hippocampus in the early diagnosis of Alzheimer's disease. J Neurol Sci 2001;188:79–84.

66. Hanyu H, Shimizu S, Tanaka Y, et al. Differences in magnetisation transfer ratios of the hippocampus between dementia with Lewy bodies and Alzheimer's disease. Neurosci Lett 2005;380:166–9.

67. Kabani NJ, Sled JG, Chertkow H. Magnetisation transfer ratio in mild cognitive impairment and dementia of Alzheimer's type. Neuroimage 2002;15:604–10.

68. Eckert T, Sailer M, Kaufmann J, et al. Differentiation of idiopathic Parkinson's disease, multiple system atrophy, progressive supranuclear palsy, and healthy controls using magnetisation transfer imaging. Neuroimage 2004;21:229–35.

69. Tambasco N, Pelliccioli GP, Chiarini P, et al. Magnetisation transfer changes of grey and white matter in Parkinson's disease. Neuroradiol 2003;45:224–30.

70. Cohen-Adad J, El Mendili MM, et al. Demyelination and degeneration in the injured human spinal cord detected with diffusion and magnetisation transfer MRI. Neuroimage 2011;55:1024–33.

71. Khoo MM, Tyler PA, Saifuddin A, et al. Diffusion-weighted imaging (DWI) in musculoskeletal MRI: a critical review. Skeletal Radiol 2011;40:665–81.

72. Beattie P. Diffusion-weighted magnetic resonance imaging of the musculoskeletal system: an emerging technology with potential to impact clinical decision making. J Orthop Sports Phys Ther 2011;41:887–95.

73. Holl N, Echaniz-Laguna A, Bierry G, et al. Diffusion-weighted MRI of denervated muscle: a clinical and experimental study. Skeletal Radiol 2008;37:1111–17.

74. Ogawa S. Finding the BOLD effect in brain images. Neuroimage 2012;62:608–9.

75. Stroman PW. Magnetic resonance imaging of neuronal function in the spinal cord: spinal fMRI. Clin Med Res 2005;3:146–56.

76. Agosta F, Valsasina P, Caputo D, et al. Tactile-associated recruitment of the cervical cord is altered in patients with multiple sclerosis. Neuroimage 2008;39:1542–8.

77. Kornelsen J, Mackey S. Potential clinical applications for spinal functional MRI. Curr Pain Headache Rep 2007;11:165–70.

78. Childs JD, Fritz JM, Flynn TW, et al. A clinical prediction rule to identify patients with low back pain most likely to benefit from spinal manipulation: a validation study. Ann Int Med 2004;141:920–8.

79. Cleland JA, Childs JD, Fritz JM, et al. Development of a clinical prediction rule for guiding treatment of a subgroup of patients with neck pain: use of thoracic spine manipulation, exercise, and patient education. Phys Ther 2007;87:9–23.

80. Mintken PE, Cleland JA, Carpenter KJ, et al. Some factors predict successful short-term outcomes in individuals with shoulder pain receiving cervicothoracic manipulation: a single-arm trial. Phys Ther 2010;90:26–42.

81. Ross JK, Bereznick DE, McGill SM. Determining cavitation location during lumbar and thoracic spinal manipulation – Is spinal manipulation accurate and specific? Spine 2004;29:1452–7.

82. Sparks C, Cleland JA, Elliott JM, et al. Using functional magnetic resonance imaging to determine if cerebral hemodynamic responses to pain change following thoracic spine thrust manipulation in healthy individuals. J Orthop Sports Phys Ther 2013;43:340–8.

83. Malisza KL, Gregorash L, Turner A, et al. Functional MRI involving painful stimulation of the ankle and the effect of physiotherapy joint mobilisation. Magn Reson Imaging 2003;21:489–96.

84. Shellock FG. Reference Manual for Magnetic Resonance Safety, Implants, and Devices. 2013 edition.

85. Durbridge G. Magnetic resonance imaging: fundamental safety issues. J Orthop Sports Phys Ther 2011;41:820–8.

86. Chou R, Fu R, Carrino JA, et al. Imaging strategies for low-back pain: systematic review and metaanalysis. Lancet 2009;373:463–72.

87. Chou R, Qaseem A, Owens DK, et al. Diagnostic imaging for low back pain: advice for high-value health care from the American College of Physicians. Ann Intern Med 2011;154:181–9.

88. Webster BS, Bauer AZ, Choi Y, et al. Iatrogenic consequences of early magnetic resonance imaging in acute, work-related, disabling low back pain. Spine 2013;38:1939–46.

89. Ash LM, Modic MT, Obuchowski NA, et al. Effects of diagnostic information, per se, on patient outcomes in acute radiculopathy and low back pain. AJNR 2008;29:1098–103.

90. Fisher ES, Welch HG. Avoiding the unintended consequences of growth in medical care: how might more be worse? JAMA 1999;281:446–53.

91. American College of Radiology Appropriateness Critera®. <http://www.acr.org/Quality-Safety/Appropriateness-Criteria>.

92. Davis PC, Wippold FJ 2nd, Brunberg JA, et al. ACR appropriateness criteria on low back pain. J Am Coll Radiol 2009;6:401–7.

93. Furhmans V. A novel plan helps hospital wean itself off pricey tests. Wall St J 2007.

94. Boissonnault WG, Goodman C. Physical therapists as diagnosticians: drawing the line on diagnosing pathology. J Orthop Sports Phys Ther 2006;36:351–3.

95. Boissonnault WG, Badke MB, Powers JM. Pursuit and implementation of hospital-based outpatient direct access to physical therapy services: an administrative case report. Phys Ther 2010;90:100–9.

96. Fritz J, Flynn TW. Autonomy in physical therapy: less is more. J Orthop Sports Phys Ther 2005;35:696–8.

97. Ross MD, Boissonnault WG. Red flags: to screen or not to screen? J Orthop Sports Phys Ther 2010;40:682–4.

98. Flynn TW, Smith B, Chou R. Appropriate use of diagnostic imaging in low back pain – a reminder that unnecessary imaging may do as much harm as good. J Orthop Sports Phys Ther 2011;41:838–46.

99. Jarvik JG, Hollingworth W, Martin B, et al. Rapid magnetic resonance imaging vs radiographs for patients with low back pain: a randomized controlled trial. JAMA 2003;289:2810–18.

CHAPTER 16

MUSCULOSKELETAL PAIN IN THE HUMAN BRAIN:

INSIGHTS FROM FUNCTIONAL BRAIN IMAGING TECHNIQUES

Michael Farrell

INTRODUCTION

Pain commonly occurs in association with musculoskeletal disorders, and can be the most important problem from the patient's perspective. The ideal way to address musculoskeletal pain is to resolve the underlying disorder, although this is not feasible in all cases and in some circumstances pain persists despite the resolution of musculoskeletal dysfunction. Musculoskeletal therapists are well placed to make a substantial contribution to the management of pain in those patients who are troubled by their symptoms in both the short and longer term. Management strategies should be grounded in an understanding of the underlying problem, and the treatment of persistent pain is no exception. Neural processes subsequent to noxious stimulation of somatic structures occur in peripheral, spinal and supraspinal components of the nervous system, but ultimately pain is a function of the brain. The objective of this chapter is to discuss the representation of pain in the brain and to consider interactions between musculoskeletal therapies and central pain processing.

THE BRAIN NETWORK FOR PAIN

Pain in humans is represented in a widely distributed brain network that reflects the multidimensional nature of the sensation.[1] Evidence from studies involving patients with brain lesions and functional brain imaging studies of healthy people and clinical groups point to a high level of integration among brain regions implicated in pain processing.[2,3] A single, critical pain region in the brain does not exist,[4] which means that lesions or antagonism of components of the pain network can change the expression of the sensation but are unlikely to eradicate pain altogether. One way to understand distributed pain processing is to ascribe functional attributes to regions incorporated in the network. In order to appreciate the neural integration requisite for pain it is first necessary to consider the functional components of the sensation.

Components of Pain Experience

The fully integrated experience of pain includes discriminative, affective and cognitive components.[5] Pain discrimination incorporates localization, intensity coding and the representation of qualitative attributes (e.g. sharp, dull, aching, etc.).[6] The affective component of pain can be a primary or secondary attribute.[7] Unpleasantness is a defining element of pain,[8] and this intrinsic component is primary to the felt state.[9,10] Autonomic responses such as changes of heart rate, blood pressure and cutaneous vasoconstriction may contribute a somatic expression to the primary unpleasantness of pain.[11] More elaborate, secondary emotional responses, such as fear or altered mood states, including anxiety and depression, are not essential for the experience of pain per se, but are common co-morbidities of persistent pain.[12] The experience of pain also involves cognitive processes including appraisal of the meaning of the sensation, which may involve memory of past experiences, and can influence behavioural and emotional responses.[13,14]

Functional Components of the Pain Network

Nociceptive inputs to the brain project from the dorsal horn via the contralateral anterolateral portion of the white matter of the spinal cord, and also arise from homologous nuclei in the brainstem receiving primary afferents from the head and face. Ascending nociceptive inputs from the spinal cord project to two principal sites in the brain: the brainstem via spinobulbar pathways and the thalamus via the spinothalamic tract.

Spinobulbar Pathways

Nociceptive inputs from the spinal cord project to nuclei in the brainstem including the periaqueductal grey (PAG) and parabrachial region. Relays from these nuclei ascend to subcortical regions, but also project to other regions in the brainstem. The two principal functions of spinobulbar pathways relevant to pain experience are descending modulation of nociceptive processing in the spinal cord and the control of autonomic responses.

The PAG is a midbrain region that has been implicated in descending modulation of dorsal horn responses to nociceptive inputs from the periphery (Fig. 16-1C). Very early electrophysiological studies and neurosurgical interventions showed that stimulation of the PAG was associated with analgesia in animals and humans.[15-17] Further animal studies established that the influence of the PAG on spinal processing was mediated via relay through the rostral ventral medulla[18] (Fig. 16-1E), and recent functional brain imaging studies have provided evidence to support a similar role for this region in humans.[19] However, descending modulation of the dorsal horn is not confined to inhibition. Stimulation of the rostral ventral medulla can lead to facilitation of nociceptive processing in the spinal cord,[20] and the rostral ventral medulla has been implicated in the development of hyperalgesia subsequent to tissue injury and inflammation.[21] Importantly, the PAG is subject to control by higher brain centres, including the prefrontal cortex.[22,23] Collectively, spinobulbospinal pathways and higher-order brain inputs to these pathways constitute a network with significant implications for the experience of pain. Contributions of this modulating network to spinal cord processing can dampen or exacerbate pain depending on a wide range of contingencies, and could provide partial explanation for the plasticity of pain reports encountered in clinical practice.

Nociceptive inputs to the parabrachial nuclei[24,25] (Fig. 16-1D) are relayed in turn to the hypothalamus and amygdala,[26-28] although these structures may also receive direct spinal nociceptive inputs. This spinoparabrachial pathway contributes to autonomic responses accompanying pain and may influence the expression of affective components of the experience.[29] The hypothalamus is a key brain region for the control of autonomic and neuroendocrine functions contributing to homoeostasis, and this region is likely to mediate pain-related responses via pathways to the PAG.[30] In addition to a role in analgesia, the PAG has been implicated in emotion-related behaviours such as flight and freezing, and is also involved in the sympatho-excitation and inhibition that can accompany these behavioural states.[31] Parabrachial inputs to the amygdala are mainly to the central part of the structure.[32] The amygdala plays a role in pain-related emotional responses, such as anxiety, and is also involved in the conditioned fear that can be enlisted by painful stimulation.[33-35] Emotional responses associated with activation in the amygdala are likely to be contingent on projections to other cortical brain regions. It is salient to note when considering musculoskeletal pain that parabrachial pathways may be especially important for the relay of nociceptive information from bone.[36]

Spinothalamic Pathways and Other Hemispheric Regions

Projections originating from the dorsal horn terminate in two main regions of the thalamus: the ventroposterior lateral nucleus and the medially located intralaminar and medial dorsal nuclei.[37] The ventroposterior lateral nucleus relays nociceptive input to the primary and secondary somatosensory cortex. Projections from the medial thalamus terminate in the cingulate cortex, insula and prefrontal cortex. A third region in the posterior part of the ventromedial thalamus may receive input from the spinothalamic tract and project to the posterior part of the insula,[38] although the role of this pathway in nociception is disputed.[39] Human functional brain imaging studies show pain activation throughout the projection sites of the ventroposterior lateral nucleus and medial thalamus, although the consistencies of these activations vary regionally. The insula and cingulate cortex are most reliably activated in association with pain, whereas activation in the primary somatosensory cortex is inconsistent[2,40] (see Fig. 16-2). Additionally, brain regions not in receipt of direct input from nociceptive thalamic nuclei also activate during the experience of pain. Pain activations in regions such as the amygdala are a consequence of bulbar inputs, whereas activations in other regions such as the basal ganglia and association cortices are dependent on corticocortical and cortico-thalamo-cortical connections or direct spinal inputs.[41,42]

Investigations in humans have provided insights into the hemispheric brain regions implicated in functional

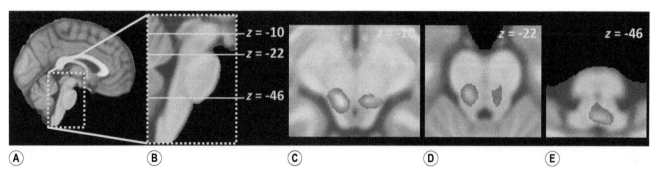

FIGURE 16-1 ■ **(A)** A midline sagittal view of the brain is provided to show the location of the brainstem, which is enclosed within the dashed box. **(B)** The brainstem outlined in panel A is enlarged and transverse lines indicate the axial level of images displayed in the remaining panels. The z-value refers to the distance in mm inferior to the anterior commissure. **(C)** An axial slice through the midbrain shows pain activations encompassing the ventrolateral regions of the periaqueductal grey. The aqueduct is visible on the image as a dark oval region at the midline between the symmetrical activations. **(D)** The parabrachial regions are incorporated within the pain activations on this axial slice at the upper level of the pons. **(E)** An axial slice through the upper (rostral) part of the medulla also cuts through the lowest portion of the pons (grey tissue highest in the panel). The pain activation overlays the midline nucleus raphe magnus, which is the human homologue of the rostroventral medulla in animals. For colour version see Plate 15.

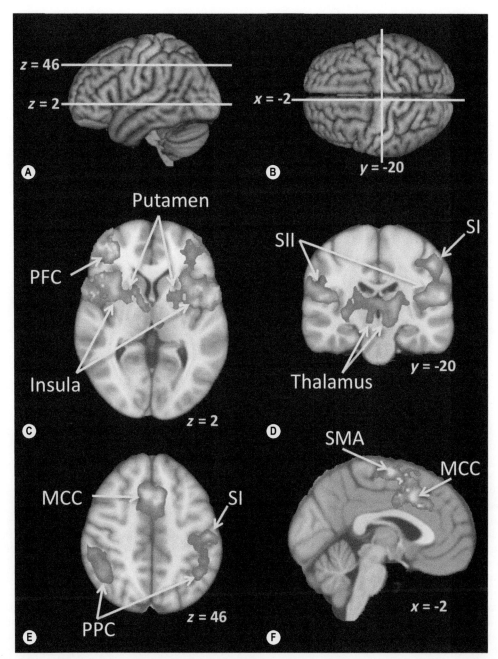

FIGURE 16-2 ■ **(A)** A three-dimensional rendering of the left hemisphere of human brain is traversed by two yellow lines that indicate the positions of axial slices shown in panels C and E. The z-values are the distances in mm of the lines above the anterior commissure. **(B)** The hemispheres are viewed from above to show the position of a sagittal slice 2 mm into the left hemisphere (x = –2) and a coronal slice 20 mm posterior to the anterior commissure (y = –20). The slices appear in panels D and F. **(C)** Pain activation commonly occurs in the insula and prefrontal cortex (*PFC*). Regions within the basal ganglia, such as the putamen can also show pain activation. **(D)** The thalamus is the projection site of inputs from the spinothalamic tract. The ventroposterior lateral nuclei of the thalamus project to the primary (*SI*) and secondary (*SII*) somatosensory cortices. **(E)** The midcingulate cortex (*MCC*) almost invariably activates in association with pain. The primary somatosensory cortex (*SI*) is less consistently activated during noxious stimulation. Pain activation in the posterior parietal cortex (*PPC*) predominates in the right hemisphere for stimuli on either side of the body, although the left PPC can also activate during pain. **(F)** The midcingulate cortex (*MCC*) is a midline structure that is proximal to, and has connections with, the supplementary motor area (*SMA*). For colour version see Plate 16.

components of the pain experience. Generally, distributed regions represent individual dimensions of the pain experience, and regions within these networks are frequently implicated in more than one functional process. Schemas have been developed to encapsulate structure/function relationships, of which a model of medial and lateral pain pathways has been most frequently espoused.[43]

This model proposes a lateral pathway incorporating the ventroposterior lateral and its projection sites in the primary and secondary somatosensory cortices that is involved in discriminative pain processes, and a medial pathway including the medial thalamus, cingulate cortex, insula and prefrontal cortex that has been ascribed with a role in the affective/motivational aspect of pain. The general tenets of medial and lateral pain pathways are sound from a neuroanatomical perspective, but the empirical data from functional brain imaging studies would suggest a high level of integration between the constituent brain regions that is not consistent with a dichotomous division of functional processes.[44] Outcomes from lesion studies and direct brain stimulation also support the proposition that the neural substrates of pain functions are best conceptualized as distributed, dynamic, interdependent activations.[3,45]

Intensity coding is a feature of almost all brain regions implicated in pain processing. For instance, studies comparing responses to varied stimulus intensities show graduated responses in thalamus, insula, and the cingulate, somatosensory and prefrontal cortices.[46,47] These outcomes are compatible with the behavioural observation that most features of pain are closely related to intensity. As pain becomes more intense it also becomes more unpleasant, more salient, more threatening and more likely to arouse anxiety, etc. However, functional brain imaging studies that manipulate stimuli in the context of matching tasks have identified a more circumscribed network involved in judgements of pain intensity. This network includes insula and prefrontal regions that are distinct from posterior parietal cortex and dorsolateral prefrontal cortex that activate in association with pain localization.[48,49] Judgements of both intensity and localization of pain are associated with activation in the cingulate cortex. Collectively, these findings resonate with findings from other sensory modalities whereby ventrally directed processes code the 'what' and a dorsal stream processes the 'where' of afferent inputs.[50]

The representation of pain unpleasantness is of considerable interest, given that this intrinsic attribute distinguishes pain from other, exteroceptive sensations like vision and hearing that do not incorporate an affective component. It is likely that processes in the brainstem, hypothalamus and amygdala contribute to the unpleasantness of pain, although it is debatable whether activation in these regions would equate with conscious experience.[7] Implicating other brain regions in the conscious experience of pain unpleasantness is difficult to do because pain unpleasantness and intensity are very closely related. There are circumstances such as the repeated application of noxious heat and hypnotic suggestion where pain intensity and unpleasantness vary independently, and in these cases the mid cingulate cortex shows activation levels that most accurately reflect variance in pain unpleasantness.[11,51] A number of other unpleasant interoceptive sensations also show this pattern of activation in the mid cingulate cortex.[52-55] Like other interoceptive sensations, the affective dimension of pain is a key attribute of the experience that increases the likelihood of adaptive behaviours compatible with tissue integrity. Consequently, it is notable that the mid cingulate cortex has established connections to motor and premotor cortices, and this circuitry may be involved in the motivation of actions that are compatible with pain avoidance or relief.[56,57]

The interaction between cognition and pain processing has received sustained attention among researchers who argue convincingly that this interplay is likely to have important implications for understanding the vagaries of clinical presentations.[4] The general approach of these studies is to manipulate participants' beliefs or expectations about the meaning or nature of pain and to identify activation in brain regions that accompany decreases or increases in pain engendered by the experimental paradigm. These studies usually find two types of response patterns. Firstly, the distributed pain network shows levels of activation that correspond with participants' reports, in that a reduction or exacerbation of pain will be associated with decreased or increased levels of activation in pain regions, which suggests that a neurobiological process is operating, as distinct from a psychologically mediated relabelling phenomenon.[58] Secondly, studies involving cognitive manipulation also show regions where activation patterns are related to modulation. Typically, these patterns are not aligned with cognitive processing, nor with pain processing, but do show an interaction between cognition and pain.[59] In other words, these activation patterns implicate regions as active contributors to the modification of pain. The network of regions implicated in pain modulation is the same for paradigms that make pain more or less intense, and incorporates the dorsolateral and ventromedial prefrontal cortices, the pregenual cingulate cortex, thalamus, PAG and rostral ventral medulla.[60] Given the established role of the PAG and the rostral ventral medulla in descending modulation of spinal processing, it would appear that thoughts about pain fundamentally change the level of nociceptive input to the brain.

THE PAIN NETWORK IN MUSCULOSKELETAL DISORDERS

The preceding discussion provided a broad outline of pain regions and functions based on studies involving experimental pain. In many respects, the processing of pain under experimental conditions is likely to recruit similar mechanisms to those that operate under clinical conditions. However, there are attributes of clinical pain that distinguish the experience from experimental pain paradigms and could potentially involve distinct neural representations. Broadly speaking, commonalities and differences between experimental and clinical pain can be considered in the contexts of evoked and spontaneous pain.

Evoked Pain in Musculoskeletal Disease

The modus operandi of many pain-processing experiments is to compare and contrast regional signals measured from the brain during the application of a noxious extrinsic stimulus versus a no-stimulus or innocuous-stimulus control.[1] Regions showing significantly increased levels of signal change during noxious stimulation compared to control stimuli are ascribed with a role in pain processing. Contrasts compatible with functional brain imaging can be applied in the context of musculoskeletal pain with varying degrees of ecological validity.

Pain responses to the same stimulus modality at a site unrelated to clinical pain can be compared between healthy people and patients with a musculoskeletal condition to assess the effects of ongoing pain on central processing of a novel stimulus. Generally, studies of this type are notably for comparable or slightly reduced pain activation in patients compared to healthy groups,[2] and this outcome may not be unexpected given that the relationship between the stimulus and the clinical condition is tenuous at best. Nevertheless, studies of this type can provide insights into other aspects of the pain experience when the experimental paradigm incorporates additional components such as manipulation of cognition or associations with mood state.

Measures of central pain processing associated with stimulation of clinically relevant sites have shown differences between patients with some clinical conditions and controls that point to plasticity of responses. The most readily apparent example of altered pain processing in a musculoskeletal condition is the impact of fibromyalgia on responses to noxious pressure. Patients with fibromyalgia show greatly enhanced activation throughout the pain network compared to healthy controls stimulated with similar levels of pressure.[61] This outcome corroborates the heightened sensitivity to pressure that is a hallmark of the disease,[62] but does not necessarily implicate central processing as a causal mechanism because an increase in central responses would also be expected if peripheral inputs were up-regulated. However, there is evidence that fibromyalgia patients show decreased pain activation in a key modulation region, the pregenual cingulate cortex, when compared to controls, suggesting an impairment of endogenous analgesia in the clinical group.[63] Similar studies involving pressure applied to the knee in people with osteoarthritis and healthy controls have not shown differences of hemispheric activation between groups.[64–66] This absence of effect is unexpected given that hyperalgesia under experimental conditions and in neuropathic pain states is associated with changes in pain processing that point to fundamental differences in the processing of pain from sensitized tissues,[67] possibly reflecting the unique implications of these inputs for physiological integrity.[68] However, studies of pain from clinically relevant sites in musculoskeletal conditions are scarce and consequently conclusions about the representation of hyperalgesia in osteoarthritis and similar conditions should await further studies.

Central Processing of Spontaneous Pain

Ongoing, spontaneous pain is the most common complaint of people with musculoskeletal conditions. Indeed, pain at rest or in association with movement among people with musculoskeletal disorders is probably the most prevalent of any type of pain in the community at large.[69] Consequently, it is not difficult to motivate studies of central processing of spontaneous musculoskeletal pain, yet experiments of this type are rarely reported. The paucity of literature relates to the mismatch between the techniques of functional brain imaging and the behaviour of spontaneous pain. As mentioned in the previous section, functional brain imaging is dependent on contrasts between different states. Spontaneous pain may not conveniently turn on and off nor vary in predictable ways

that permit meaningful tests of signal changes measured with functional brain imaging techniques. Despite these difficulties there have been a handful of studies of spontaneous musculoskeletal pain and the outcomes point to important distinctions in the representation of ongoing symptoms. Analyses based on spontaneous fluctuations of intensity in chronic back and osteoarthritis pain have identified activations in regions including the ventromedial prefrontal cortex, amygdala, nucleus accumbens and orbitofrontal cortex.[64,66,70,71] A parsimonious explanation for this medial prefrontal–limbic network activation is that the principal components of ongoing musculoskeletal pain are cognitive and emotional. The relative absence of regional activity elsewhere in the brain that typically accompanies brief experimental pain stimuli, and is likely involved in sensory discrimination, would suggest that discriminative components have less functional relevance as pain persists. The outcomes of studies of spontaneous pain await replication and expansion before definitive conclusions can be reached, but results to date would suggest that caution should be exercised when making inferences about clinical pain processing on the basis of experimental pain paradigms involving brief extrinsic stimulation.

MUSCULOSKELETAL PHYSIOTHERAPY AND PAIN PROCESSING

Commentaries advocating research into the interaction of musculoskeletal physiotherapy and central pain processing in musculoskeletal disorders regularly appear in the literature,[72–74] but unfortunately very few empirical studies have been published. Indeed, despite reasoned arguments that manual therapy is likely to recruit endogenous inhibitory circuits,[75] there have been no reports in support of this contention using imaging techniques that provide functional neuroanatomical information. The limited information regarding pain processing and musculoskeletal physiotherapy that has been published relates to behaviour-related changes and the application of transcutaneous electrical nerve stimulation (TENS).[76,77]

In addition to widespread pain and tenderness, people with fibromyalgia also demonstrate low levels of activity compared to their healthy counterparts.[78] The degree of activity impairment in fibromyalgia bears a relationship to pain sensitivity, in that the least active patients show the greatest levels of sensitivity to noxious thermal stimuli.[77] The relationship between activity and pain sensitivity extends to regional brain responses in fibromyalgia. Brain regions implicated in modulation, such as the dorsolateral prefrontal cortex, show increasing levels of activation in association with increased activity, whereas the converse relationship is evident for activation in the somatosensory cortex, possibly reflecting diminished discriminative processing in the more active patients.[77] These outcomes point to interesting interactions between motor programming and pain processing, and chapters elsewhere in this book discuss these issues in detail. Nevertheless, the association between activity and pain-related regional brain responses in people with fibromyalgia, supported by findings in other settings,[79] provides considerable impetus to explore similar processes in musculoskeletal conditions more generally.

TENS is occasionally used by musculoskeletal therapists to relieve pain, and a recent meta-analysis lends support to the device as a management strategy in musculoskeletal disorders.[80] Measurement of laser-evoked potentials in healthy people has shown that TENS is associated with an attenuation of key pain-related peaks in the electroencephalogram,[81] which supports the conclusion that the treatment can decrease levels of activation in the pain network. A similar effect of TENS has also been demonstrated using fMRI in patients with a musculoskeletal condition.[76] Additionally, the fMRI study showed increased pain-related activation in the prefrontal and posterior parietal cortices that correlated with TENS-related levels of pain relief, suggesting that the device had recruited pain modulation circuits in the patients with subacromial impingement syndrome.

CONCLUSIONS

Pain is represented in the brain by a dynamic network that subserves multiple functions requisite for integrated sensory experience. The pain network is notable for its plasticity, which is aided by caudally orientated circuits that extend beyond the brain to exert influence on the lowest levels of central nociceptive processing in the spinal cord. Musculoskeletal pain that persists may have a unique representation in the human brain that emphasizes the emotional and cognitive dimensions of pain experience. Therapists have recognized that strategies directed at pain processing have great potential in the management of musculoskeletal disorders given the demonstrable capacity of the network for endogenous modulation. Clinicians and researchers involved in musculoskeletal physiotherapy have a clear rationale to develop and test new methods that target pain processing.

REFERENCES

1. Peyron R, Laurent B, Garcia-Larrea L. Functional imaging of brain responses to pain. A review and meta-analysis (2000). Clin Neurophysiol 2000;30(5):263–88.
2. Apkarian AV, Bushnell MC, Treede RD, et al. Human brain mechanisms of pain perception and regulation in health and disease. Eur J Pain 2005;9(4):463–84.
3. Garcia-Larrea L. Insights gained into pain processing from patients with focal brain lesions. Neurosci Lett 2012;520(2):188–91.
4. Tracey I, Mantyh PW. The cerebral signature for pain perception and its modulation. Neuron 2007;55(3):377–91.
5. Melzack R, Wall PD. Pain mechanisms: a new theory. Science 1965;150(3699):971–9.
6. Melzack R, Casey KL. Sensory, motivational and central control determinants of chronic pain: A new conceptual model. In: Kenshalo DR, editor. The Skin Senses. Springfield, IL: Chas C. Thomas; 1968. p. 423–39.
7. Price DD. Psychological and neural mechanisms of the affective dimension of pain. Science 2000;288(5472):1769–72.
8. Merskey H, Bogduk N. Classification of Chronic Pain, IASP Task Force on Taxonomy. Seattle. USA: IASP Press; 1994.
9. Gracely RH, McGrath P, Dubner R. Validity and sensitivity of ratio scales of sensory and affective verbal pain descriptors: manipulation of affect by diazepam. Pain 1978;5(1):19–29.
10. Price DD, Harkins SW, Baker C. Sensory-affective relationships among different types of clinical and experimental pain. Pain 1987;28(3):297–307.
11. Rainville P, Bao QV, Chretien P. Pain-related emotions modulate experimental pain perception and autonomic responses. Pain 2005;118(3):306–18.
12. Magni G, Marchetti M, Moreschi C, et al. Chronic musculoskeletal pain and depressive symptoms in the National Health and Nutrition Examination. I. Epidemiologic follow-up study. Pain 1993; 53(2):163–8.
13. Apkarian AV, Baliki MN, Geha PY. Towards a theory of chronic pain. Prog Neurobiol 2009;87(2):81–97.
14. Turner JA, Dworkin SF, Mancl L, et al. The roles of beliefs, catastrophizing, and coping in the functioning of patients with temporomandibular disorders. Pain 2001;92(1–2):41–51.
15. Hosobuchi Y, Adams JE, Linchitz R. Pain relief by electrical stimulation of the central gray matter in humans and its reversal by naloxone. Science 1977;197(4299):183–6.
16. Mayer DJ, Wolfle TL, Akil H, et al. Analgesia from electrical stimulation in the brainstem of the rat. Science 1971;174(4016): 1351–4.
17. Reynolds DV. Surgery in the rat during electrical analgesia induced by focal brain stimulation. Science 1969;164(3878):444–5.
18. Gebhart GF. Descending modulation of pain. Neurosci Biobehav Rev 2004;27(8):729–37.
19. Eippert F, Bingel U, Schoell ED, et al. Activation of the opioidergic descending pain control system underlies placebo analgesia. Neuron 2009;63(4):533–43.
20. Zhuo M, Gebhart GF. Characterization of descending inhibition and facilitation from the nuclei reticularis gigantocellularis and gigantocellularis pars alpha in the rat. Pain 1990;42(3):337–50.
21. Urban MO, Gebhart GF. Supraspinal contributions to hyperalgesia. Proc Natl Acad Sci U S A 1999;96(14):7687–92.
22. Duncan NW, Wiebking C, Tiret B, et al. Glutamate concentration in the medial prefrontal cortex predicts resting-state cortical-subcortical functional connectivity in humans. PLoS ONE 2013; 8(4):e60312.
23. Keay KA, Bandler R. Parallel circuits mediating distinct emotional coping reactions to different types of stress. Neurosci Biobehav Rev 2001;25(7–8):669–78.
24. Bester H, Chapman V, Besson JM, et al. Physiological properties of the lamina I spinoparabrachial neurons in the rat. J Neurophysiol 2000;83(4):2239–59.
25. Bester H, Matsumoto N, Besson JM, et al. Further evidence for the involvement of the spinoparabrachial pathway in nociceptive processes: a c-Fos study in the rat. J Comp Neurol 1997;383(4): 439–58.
26. Bernard JF, Peschanski M, Besson JM. A possible spino (trigemino)-ponto-amygdaloid pathway for pain. Neurosci Lett 1989;100(1–3): 83–8.
27. Jasmin L, Burkey AR, Card JP, et al. Transneuronal labeling of a nociceptive pathway, the spino-(trigemino-)parabrachio-amygdaloid, in the rat. J Neurosci 1997;17(10):3751–65.
28. Pan B, Castro-Lopes JM, Coimbra A. Central afferent pathways conveying nociceptive input to the hypothalamic paraventricular nucleus as revealed by a combination of retrograde labeling and c-fos activation. J Comp Neurol 1999;413(1):129–45.
29. Benarroch EE. Pain-autonomic interactions: a selective review. Clin Auton Res 2001;11(6):343–9.
30. Lumb BM. Hypothalamic and midbrain circuitry that distinguishes between escapable and inescapable pain. News Physiol Sci 2004;19:22–6.
31. Bandler R, Keay KA, Floyd N, et al. Central circuits mediating patterned autonomic activity during active vs. passive emotional coping. Brain Res Bull 2000;53(1):95–104.
32. Gauriau C, Bernard JF. Pain pathways and parabrachial circuits in the rat. Exp Physiol 2002;87(2):251–8.
33. Ji G, Fu Y, Ruppert KA, et al. Pain-related anxiety-like behavior requires CRF1 receptors in the amygdala. Mol Pain 2007;3:13.
34. Neugebauer V, Li W, Bird GC, et al. The amygdala and persistent pain. Neuroscientist 2004;10(3):221–34.
35. Gao YJ, Ren WH, Zhang YQ, et al. Contributions of the anterior cingulate cortex and amygdala to pain- and fear-conditioned place avoidance in rats. Pain 2004;110(1–2):343–53.
36. Williams MC, Ivanusic JJ. Evidence for the involvement of the spinoparabrachial pathway, but not the spinothalamic tract or post-synaptic dorsal column, in acute bone nociception. Neurosci Lett 2008;443(3):246–50.

37. Hodge CJ Jr, Apkarian AV. The spinothalamic tract. Crit Rev Neurobiol 1990;5(4):363–97.

38. Craig AD, Zhang ET. Retrograde analyses of spinothalamic projections in the macaque monkey: input to posterolateral thalamus. J Comp Neurol 2006;499(6):953–64.

39. Graziano A, Jones EG. Widespread thalamic terminations of fibers arising in the superficial medullary dorsal horn of monkeys and their relation to calbindin immunoreactivity. J Neurosci 2004; 24(1):248–56.

40. Farrell MJ, Laird AR, Egan GF. Brain activity associated with painfully hot stimuli applied to the upper limb: a meta-analysis. Hum Brain Mapp 2005;25(1):129–39.

41. Cavada C, Goldman-Rakic PS. Posterior parietal cortex in rhesus monkey: I. Parcellation of areas based on distinctive limbic and sensory corticocortical connections. J Comp Neurol 1989; 287(4):393–421.

42. Chudler EH, Dong WK. The role of the basal ganglia in nociception and pain. Pain 1995;60(1):3–38.

43. Treede RD, Kenshalo DR, Gracely RH, et al. The cortical representation of pain. Pain 1999;79(2–3):105–11.

44. Brooks J, Tracey I. From nociception to pain perception: imaging the spinal and supraspinal pathways. J Anat 2005;207(1):19–33.

45. Mazzola L, Isnard J, Peyron R, et al. Stimulation of the human cortex and the experience of pain: Wilder Penfield's observations revisited. Brain 2012;135(Pt 2):631–40.

46. Coghill RC, Sang CN, Maisog JM, et al. Pain intensity processing within the human brain: a bilateral, distributed mechanism. J Neurophysiol 1999;82(4):1934–43.

47. Derbyshire SW, Jones AK, Gyulai F, et al. Pain processing during three levels of noxious stimulation produces differential patterns of central activity. Pain 1997;73(3):431–45.

48. Oshiro Y, Quevedo AS, McHaffie JG, et al. Brain mechanisms supporting discrimination of sensory features of pain: a new model. J Neurosci 2009;29(47):14924–31.

49. Lobanov OV, Quevedo AS, Hadsel MS, et al. Frontoparietal mechanisms supporting attention to location and intensity of painful stimuli. Pain 2013;154(9):1758–68.

50. Reed CL, Klatzky RL, Halgren E. What vs. where in touch: an fMRI study. Neuroimage 2005;25(3):718–26.

51. Tolle TR, Kaufmann T, Siessmeier T, et al. Region-specific encoding of sensory and affective components of pain in the human brain: a positron emission tomography correlation analysis. Ann Neurol 1999;45(1):40–7.

52. Farrell MJ, Cole LJ, Chiapoco D, et al. Neural correlates coding stimulus level and perception of capsaicin-evoked urge-to-cough in humans. Neuroimage 2012;61(4):1324–35.

53. Farrell MJ, Egan GF, Zamarripa F, et al. Unique, common, and interacting cortical correlates of thirst and pain. Proc Natl Acad Sci U S A 2006;103(7):2416–21.

54. Farrell MJ, Johnson J, McAllen R, et al. Brain activation associated with ratings of the hedonic component of thermal sensation during whole-body warming and cooling. J Therm Biol 2011;36:57–63.

55. von Leupoldt A, Sommer T, Kegat S, et al. Dyspnea and pain share emotion-related brain network. Neuroimage 2009;48(1):200–6.

56. Dum RP, Levinthal DJ, Strick PL. The spinothalamic system targets motor and sensory areas in the cerebral cortex of monkeys. J Neurosci 2009;29(45):14223–35.

57. Perini I, Bergstrand S, Morrison I. Where pain meets action in the human brain. J Neurosci 2013;33(40):15930–9.

58. Benedetti F, Mayberg HS, Wager TD, et al. Neurobiological mechanisms of the placebo effect. J Neurosci 2005;25(45): 10390–402.

59. Bantick SJ, Wise RG, Ploghaus A, et al. Imaging how attention modulates pain in humans using functional MRI. Brain 2002;125(Pt 2):310–19.

60. Tracey I. Getting the pain you expect: mechanisms of placebo, nocebo and reappraisal effects in humans. Nat Med 2010;16(11): 1277–83.

61. Gracely RH, Petzke F, Wolf JM, et al. Functional magnetic resonance imaging evidence of augmented pain processing in fibromyalgia. Arthritis Rheum 2002;46(5):1333–43.

62. Wolfe F, Clauw DJ, Fitzcharles MA, et al. The American College of Rheumatology preliminary diagnostic criteria for fibromyalgia and measurement of symptom severity. Arthritis Care Res 2010;62(5):600–10.

63. Jensen KB, Kosek E, Petzke F, et al. Evidence of dysfunctional pain inhibition in fibromyalgia reflected in rACC during provoked pain. Pain 2009;144(1–2):95–100.

64. Baliki MN, Geha PY, Jabakhanji R, et al. A preliminary fMRI study of analgesic treatment in chronic back pain and knee osteoarthritis. Mol Pain 2008;4:47.

65. Gwilym SE, Keltner JR, Warnaby CE, et al. Psychophysical and functional imaging evidence supporting the presence of central sensitization in a cohort of osteoarthritis patients. Arthritis Rheum 2009;61(9):1226–34.

66. Parks EL, Geha PY, Baliki MN, et al. Brain activity for chronic knee osteoarthritis: dissociating evoked pain from spontaneous pain. Eur J Pain 2011;15(8):843, e1–14.

67. Lanz S, Seifert F, Maihofner C. Brain activity associated with pain, hyperalgesia and allodynia: an ALE meta-analysis. J Neural Transm 2011;118(8):1139–54.

68. Lorenz J, Minoshima S, Casey KL. Keeping pain out of mind: the role of the dorsolateral prefrontal cortex in pain modulation. Brain 2003;126(Pt 5):1079–91.

69. Magni G, Caldieron C, Rigatti-Luchini S, et al. Chronic musculoskeletal pain and depressive symptoms in the general population. An analysis of the 1st National Health and Nutrition Examination Survey data. Pain 1990;43(3):299–307.

70. Howard MA, Sanders D, Krause K, et al. Alterations in resting-state regional cerebral blood flow demonstrate ongoing pain in osteoarthritis: an arterial spin-labeled magnetic resonance imaging study. Arthritis Rheum 2012;64(12):3936–46.

71. Kulkarni B, Bentley DE, Elliott R, et al. Arthritic pain is processed in brain areas concerned with emotions and fear. Arthritis Rheum 2007;56(4):1345–54.

72. Moseley GL. Pain, brain imaging and physiotherapy–opportunity is knocking. Man Ther 2008;13(6):475–7.

73. Shacklock MO. Central pain mechanisms: A new horizon in manual therapy. Aust J Physiother 1999;45(2):83–92.

74. Zusman M. Forebrain-mediated sensitization of central pain pathways: 'non-specific' pain and a new image for MT. Man Ther 2002;7(2):80–8.

75. Vicenzino B, Wright A. Managing pain: physical treatments. In: Strong J, Unruh AM, Wright A, et al., editors. Pain: a Textbook for Therapists. Edinburgh: Churchill Livingston; 2002. p. 187–206.

76. Kocyigit F, Akalin E, Gezer NS, et al. Functional magnetic resonance imaging of the effects of low-frequency transcutaneous electrical nerve stimulation on central pain modulation: a double-blind, placebo-controlled trial. Clin J Pain 2012;28(7):581–8.

77. McLoughlin MJ, Stegner AJ, Cook DB. The relationship between physical activity and brain responses to pain in fibromyalgia. J Pain 2011;12(6):640–51.

78. McLoughlin MJ, Colbert LH, Stegner AJ, et al. Are women with fibromyalgia less physically active than healthy women? Med Sci Sports Exerc 2011;43(5):905–12.

79. Villamar MF, Wivatvongvana P, Patumanond J, et al. Focal modulation of the primary motor cortex in fibromyalgia using 4×1-ring high-definition transcranial direct current stimulation (HD-tDCS): immediate and delayed analgesic effects of cathodal and anodal stimulation. J Pain 2013;14(4):371–83.

80. Johnson M, Martinson M. Efficacy of electrical nerve stimulation for chronic musculoskeletal pain: a meta-analysis of randomized controlled trials. Pain 2007;130(1–2):157–65.

81. Vassal F, Creac'h C, Convers P, et al. Modulation of laser-evoked potentials and pain perception by transcutaneous electrical nerve stimulation (TENS): a placebo-controlled study in healthy volunteers. Clin Neurophysiol 2013;124(9):1861–7.

CHAPTER 17

ADVANCES IN ELECTROMYOGRAPHY

Deborah Falla • Dario Farina

INTRODUCTION

Electromyography (EMG), a technique for the acquisition and analysis of myoelectric signals, has contributed significantly to the understanding of function and dysfunction of the neuromuscular system and has become an essential tool in modern musculoskeletal physiotherapy. The detection, recording and analysis of myoelectric signals provide a reproducible means of determining disturbances in muscle activation in patients with musculoskeletal disorders. EMG is typically applied in musculoskeletal physiotherapy for the assessment of disturbed muscle function and for monitoring changes with rehabilitation. The EMG signal provides information at several levels, such as the onset or offset of muscle activity, the progress of muscle fatigue, the intensity of muscle activation, the directional specificity of muscle activation, the spatial distribution of muscle activity and the behaviour of individual motor units. This chapter will present an overview of contemporary electrode detection systems, review fundamental methods of EMG assessment as a means of evaluating neuromuscular impairment in patients with musculoskeletal disorders, and will discuss the limitations of EMG evaluation.

ELECTRODE SYSTEMS

The electrical activity associated with the contraction of muscle fibres in motor units can be recorded using either intramuscular or non-invasive (surface) detection systems. Intramuscular EMG signals are detected with needles or wires inserted into muscles. With respect to non-invasive techniques, intramuscular EMG has greater selectivity. Depending on the type of intramuscular electrode used and its location, the recorded action potentials can be the result of the activity of a small (1–3), moderate (15–20) or large (more than 20) number of muscle fibres.[1] In neurophysiological investigations, intramuscular recordings are often used to identify the discharge times of individual motor units.[2] In this application, the shape of the action potentials is used to identify the occurrences of the discharges of the active motor units. Although surface EMG signals can also be decomposed into individual motor unit activities,[3,4] the analysis of motor unit behaviour is usually more accurate using intramuscular systems because of the high degree of selectivity. Moreover, by contrast with surface

techniques, intramuscular electromyography allows the activity of deep muscles to be recorded.

In 1929, Adrian and Bronk[2] proposed the first electrode for intramuscular EMG, the concentric needle. This needle electrode detects signals between the tip of a wire insulated in the cannula and the cannula. Other needle electrodes have since been proposed, such as a modified version of the concentric needle that comprised 12 insulated wires (array) in a slot in the cannula.[5] With this system it was possible to estimate the size of the territory of individual motor units. Contrary to needles, wire electrodes are flexible and therefore can be used with minimal discomfort for the subject. Modern types of wire electrode technology include multiple-site detection systems on flexible substrates,[6] for a well-defined and reproducible spatial arrangement of the detection points.

Classic electrodes for surface EMG detection are made of solid silver or gold, sintered silver and silver chloride, carbon, sponge saturated with electrolyte gel or conductive hydrogel. In clinical applications, gelled electrodes are preferred over dry electrodes since the presence of gel reduces the influence of movement artefacts on the signal quality. The classic recording modality for surface EMG is the bipolar derivation, in which the recorded signal is the difference between two electrodes placed on the muscle at a distance, which is typically 10–20 mm. In addition to the bipolar derivation, surface EMG can be acquired by monopolar systems or as the linear combination of the electrical activity detected by more than two electrodes. For example, the double differential system consists of three electrodes whose signals are summed with weights −1, 2 and −1 to increase the selectivity with respect to the bipolar system.

Modern electrode technology for surface EMG consists of multi-channel systems with tens to hundreds of electrodes arranged in linear arrays or bi-dimensional grids (for a recent review see Farina et al.[7]). Among the multi-channel surface EMG systems, the so-called high-density EMG is characterized by a large number of electrodes (usually in the order of hundreds), closely spaced between each other (common separation of 2.5–10 mm) (Fig. 17-1). These recordings provide a two-dimensional sampling of the electric potential distribution over a large surface area during muscle contraction.[8,9] Unlike classic bipolar EMG applications, this method provides a topographical representation of EMG amplitude, and can identify relative adaptations in the intensity of activity within regions of the muscle.[9]

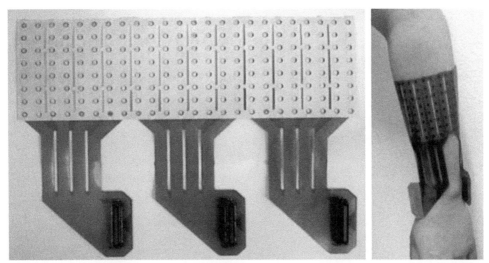

FIGURE 17-1 ■ Advances in electrode systems. Multi-channel surface EMG electrode grid containing 192 electrodes. The electrode grid provides two-dimensional sampling of the electric potential distribution over a large surface area (e.g. around the forearm) during muscle contraction.

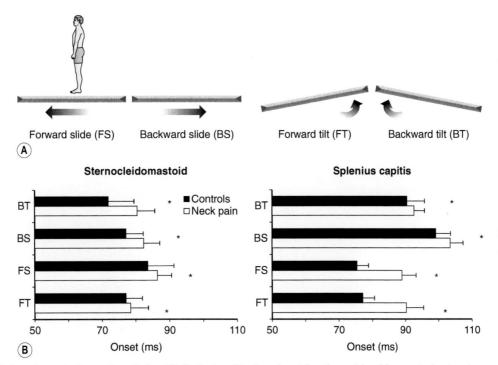

FIGURE 17-2 ■ Delayed onset of muscle activity. **(A)** Patients with chronic neck pain and healthy controls stood on a moveable platform and were exposed to randomized full body postural perturbations (8 cm forward slides, 8 cm backward slides, 10° forward tilts and 10° backward tilts). **(B)** Mean and SD of the onset of the sternocleidomastoid and splenius capitis muscles in response to the perturbations. Note the significantly (* = $P < 0.05$) delayed onset time of the neck muscles for the patients with neck pain regardless of the perturbation direction. (Reprinted with permission from Boudreau and Falla.[23])

APPLICATIONS

Timing of Muscle Activity

Detection of the onset and termination of muscle activity during tasks such as postural perturbations can be used to enhance our understanding of neuromuscular control and the impact of musculoskeletal disorders. Various methods can be employed to assess the onset and offset of EMG bursts, ranging from visual determination[10,11] to computer-based algorithms.[12,13] Studies evaluating the EMG responses of spinal muscles to postural perturbations have revealed delayed trunk muscle responses in back[14–21] and neck pain[22,23] (Fig. 17-2). Alterations in the timing of muscle activity have been identified in other musculoskeletal pain conditions such as long-standing groin pain[24] and knee pain.[25] EMG has also been applied in clinical trials to confirm that the onset of muscle activation can be enhanced via training in patients with various musculoskeletal disorders including low back pain,[26] neck pain[27] and patellofemoral pain syndrome.[28]

Myoelectric Manifestations of Fatigue

The characteristics of the surface EMG signal vary during sustained muscle contractions and these modifications are usually termed as myoelectric manifestations of muscle fatigue.[29-31] The application of EMG to monitor fatigue is common due to the immediate changes that occur in the EMG signal from the onset of the contraction which allows fatigue to be assessed during short-duration contractions.[31-33]

For the assessment of myoelectric manifestations of fatigue, linear arrays of at least four electrodes are typically applied. The most frequently monitored surface EMG variables are the mean or median power spectral frequencies, the signal amplitude estimates such as the average rectified value or root mean square, and muscle fibre conduction velocity (CV). The typical pattern observed during sustained, relatively high force contractions is a decrease in both the CV and spectral variables over time,[29,33-35] and an initial increase followed by a decrease in signal amplitude (although amplitude trends are not as consistent as the spectral and CV trends).[33,36,37]

The decrement of CV over time during sustained isometric contractions[33,38] is due to alterations of sarcolemma excitability.[39] The generation of action potentials induces cellular K^+ efflux and Na^+ and Cl^- influx, causing perturbations in the intracellular and extracellular K^+ and Na^+ gradient concentrations.[40] These alterations depolarize the sarcolemma and t-tubular membranes that reduce membrane excitability.[39] The changes in CV determine changes in the power spectral variables since CV scales the EMG power spectrum towards lower frequencies.[29,34,38,41,42] However, other factors, in addition to CV, also influence spectral variables, such as the shape of the intracellular action potential, motor unit synchronization[43-45] and progressive motor unit recruitment.[46] Despite the large number of influencing factors, the high correlation usually observed between relative changes in CV and spectral variables in isometric conditions[47-50] indicates that CV has a strong influence on spectral variables.

To analyse myoelectric manifestations of muscle fatigue in isometric conditions and allow comparison between different variables, different muscles and different subjects, a fatigue plot is usually produced.[51] The fatigue plot reports each surface EMG variable over time (duration of contraction) after normalization relative to a reference value (typically the initial value) (Fig. 17-3). As demonstrated elsewhere,[29] the fatigue plot highlights differences in myoelectric manifestations of fatigue, which might be related to different pools of activated motor units and muscle fibres.

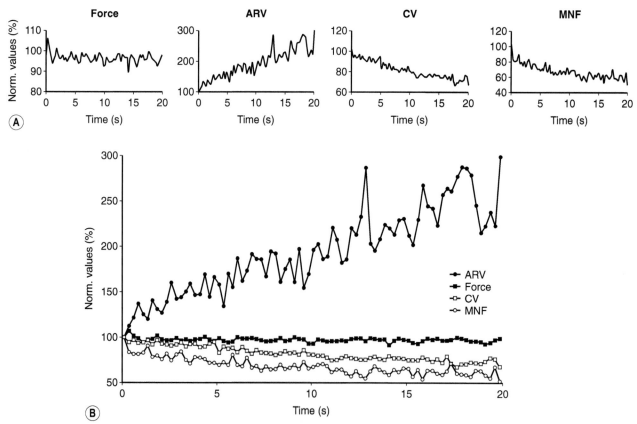

FIGURE 17-3 ■ Fatigue plot. **(A)** Individual plots of the surface EMG variables average rectified value (*ARV*), conduction velocity (*CV*), mean frequency (*MNF*) and force recorded from the anterior scalene muscle of a healthy control contracting at 25% of their maximum voluntary neck flexion force. Plots are obtained by normalizing each variable with respect to the initial value of its own regression line. **(B)** The time course of MNF, ARV, CV and force are combined to produce a 'fatigue plot'. Note that although the force is maintained constant, the signal characteristics are modified from the onset of the contraction. Myoelectric manifestations of fatigue are identified by an increase in ARV values with time and decrease in MNF and CV values.

Greater myoelectric manifestations of fatigue have been identified in a number of musculoskeletal disorders, including chronic low back and neck pain.[52–58] Moreover, it has been shown that fatigue-related EMG variables may have a diagnostic value.[59] For example, the classification of individuals with low back pain with respect to controls reached approximately 90% accuracy when the force values obtained from a maximum voluntary contraction were associated with the EMG spectral variables as features for the classification.[60]

In more recent times, the estimation of CV and alterations with fatigue have been monitored during fast dynamic contractions, in addition to isometric tasks.[61,62] Instantaneous mean power spectral frequency of the EMG signal can also be estimated with time-frequency tools[63] and used for muscle characterization in dynamic tasks.[64] However, despite the strong association between CV and spectral variables in isometric, constant force contractions, these variables are poorly related during fast dynamic tasks when the number of active motor units fluctuates over time.[65] This has been observed in several experimental conditions (e.g. in high-load dynamic contractions),[66–69] which indicates that a direct estimation of CV is necessary to monitor fatigue during dynamic activities.

EMG Amplitude

The amplitude of the surface EMG is frequently used as a measure of the intensity of muscle activity and has often been used as an indicator of muscle force. Since the surface EMG is a random signal, its amplitude cannot be estimated as the peak value but rather needs statistical estimators.[70] Among the estimators of EMG amplitude, the average rectified value and root mean square are those most often used. They correspond to the best (i.e. with minimal variability) estimators when the signal has a Gaussian (root mean square) or Laplacian (average rectified value) distribution of amplitude values. In practice, they are equivalent and often used interchangeably in applications.[70]

Although the amplitude of the surface EMG is related to the number of motor unit action potentials discharged (i.e. to the number of active units and their discharge rates), other factors influence its measure. Among these, EMG amplitude is strongly influenced by the thickness of the subcutaneous tissue, the length of the muscle fibres and their orientation with respect to the electrodes.[70] Moreover, amplitude values cannot be compared when different electrode systems or distances between electrodes are used. For these reasons, normalization of the EMG amplitude estimation is necessary for comparing data across subjects or different muscles. Normalization of the EMG amplitude is typically performed by expressing the value obtained during a sub-maximal task as a percent relative to the amplitude measured during a maximum voluntary contraction or a reference voluntary contraction. When patient populations are investigated, often a reference voluntary contraction is selected since a discrepancy in strength likely exists between patients and controls.

Numerous studies have evaluated changes in the amplitude of muscle activation in various musculoskeletal disorders. As an example, EMG studies have revealed augmented superficial neck muscle activity during isometric contractions[71–74] and functional upper limb activities[75–77] in people with neck pain. Furthermore, increased co-contraction of trunk flexor and extensor muscles has been reported when a load is released unexpectedly from the trunk[17] or during unexpected, multidirectional translation perturbations[78,79] in low back pain. In addition, increased erector spinae activity has been observed during the stride[80–82] and swing[83,84] phase of gait and bracing of the abdominal muscles is increased during an active straight leg raise.[85] On the contrary, the activity of the deep cervical flexors (longus colli, longus capitis)[71] and deep extensors (semispinalis cervicis and multifidus)[86,87] has commonly been found to be reduced in the presence of neck pain. Likewise with low back pain, the tonic activity of the deep transversus abdominis may be reduced during walking[88] and during repetitive arm movements[89] and the activity of the lumbar multifidus is decreased during trunk loading.[90]

EMG Tuning Curves

EMG tuning curves represent the intensity of muscle activity (amplitude) as a function of force direction and have been used to study activation strategies of arm and neck muscles.[91–96] When tuning curves are consistent among subjects, analysing the orientation and focus (mean direction and spread of EMG activity, respectively; defined below) of EMG tuning curves in relation to musculoskeletal mechanics has provided insight into central nervous system (CNS) control.[95]

EMG tuning curves of neck muscles have been recorded by asking subjects to perform contractions at a predefined force (e.g. 15 N of force) with continuous change in force direction in the range 0–360° in the horizontal plane[96] (Fig. 17-4A). During these circular contractions, the amplitude of the surface EMG is estimated and represented as a function of the angle of force direction. The directional activation curves represent the modulation in intensity of muscle activity with the direction of force exertion and represent a closed area when expressed in polar coordinates. The line connecting the origin with the central point (barycentre) of this area defines a directional vector, whose length is expressed as a percent of the mean average rectified value during the entire task. This normalized vector length represents the specificity of muscle activation with direction: it is equal to zero if the muscle is active in the same way in all directions and, conversely, it corresponds to 100% if the muscle is active in exclusively one direction (Fig. 17-4B).

In healthy subjects, neck muscles show well-defined preferred directions of activation that are in accordance with their anatomical position relative to the spine.[95–97] These observations suggest that the CNS copes with the anatomical complexity and redundancy of the neck muscles by developing consistent muscle synergies to generate multidirectional patterns of force.[95–97] However, recent studies have shown that patients with either whiplash-induced neck pain or idiopathic neck pain have reduced specificity of neck muscle activity with respect to asymptomatic individuals[87,96,98] (Fig. 17-4C).

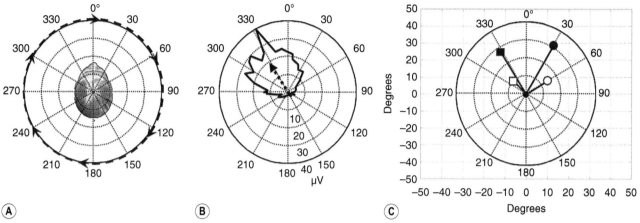

FIGURE 17-4 ■ EMG tuning curves. **(A)** The subject performs a circular contraction in the horizontal plane at a defined force with change in force direction in the range 0–360°. **(B)** During this task, the amplitude of the surface EMG is recorded and EMG tuning curves are generated. The EMG tuning curve represents the modulation in intensity of muscle activity with the direction of force exertion. The central point of the tuning curve defines a directional vector (dashed arrow), whose length is expressed as a percent of the mean EMG amplitude during the entire task. This provides an objective measure of the *directional specificity* of muscle activity. **(C)** Data for the directional vector describing the specificity of sternocleidomastoid activity during the circular contraction performed at 15 N of force. People with chronic neck pain displayed reduced values of directional specificity in the surface EMG of the sternocleidomastoid muscle bilaterally ($P < 0.05$). Control data are presented in black and patient data in white. Squares represent the left sternocleidomastoid and circles, the right sternocleidomastoid. (Reprinted with permission from Falla et al.[96])

Polar plots or EMG tuning curves are also useful to display and compare the EMG amplitude of a muscle in response to multidirectional perturbations. For example, Figure 17-5 displays polar plots of the normalized EMG amplitude of the left internal oblique, left erector spinae, tibialis anterior and gastrocnemius muscles in response to unexpected balance perturbations performed in 12 directions in a group of individuals with and without low back pain.[79] Note the increased activity in the gastrocnemius during backward perturbations (i.e. when acting as a prime mover) in the control group and increased tibialis anterior activation following perturbation directions in which the muscle would also act as a prime mover, namely perturbation directions with a forward component. In addition, the individuals with low back pain showed reduced activation of the left internal oblique in directions with either a leftward or leftward/backward component and increased left internal oblique activity during perturbations in which the left internal oblique could contribute to a hip/trunk strategy.

Distribution of Muscle Activity

Spatial heterogeneity in muscle activity has been observed from multi-channel surface EMG recordings during sustained constant-force contractions,[8,99] contractions of increasing load,[99] and during dynamic contractions,[100] which suggests a non-uniform distribution of motor units or spatial dependency in the control of motor units.[101,102]

To characterize the spatial distribution of muscle activity, two coordinates of the centroid (centre of activity) of the root mean square map (x- and y-axes coordinates for the medial–lateral and cranial–caudal direction, respectively) are typically calculated.[8] Studies in asymptomatic individuals show a change in the distribution of activity over the lumbar erector spinae muscle during a fatiguing sustained lumbar flexion contraction[103] or during repetitive lifting[104] as reflected by a shift of the centroid towards the caudal region of the lumbar spine.

Furthermore, a shift of activity towards the cranial region of the upper trapezius muscle is observed in healthy individuals during sustained shoulder abduction[8,105,106] as reflected by the change in the y-axis coordinate of the root mean square map. This response reflects a greater progressive recruitment of motor units within the cranial region of the upper trapezius muscle.[105]

Redistribution of activity within the same muscle has been shown to be functionally important to maintain motor output in the presence of altered afferent feedback (e.g. pain or fatigue).[8] This variation in activation within regions of the same muscle is potentially relevant to avoid overload of the same muscle fibres during prolonged activation and is of particular relevance for muscles commonly exposed to repetitive or sustained activation, such as the upper trapezius muscle[107] and the lumbar erector spinae.[108]

On the contrary, in the presence of either experimentally induced muscle pain[106,109,110] or clinical pain (e.g. fibromyalgia, low back pain),[104,111] the redistribution of activity to different regions of the muscle during sustained contractions is reduced (Fig. 17-6). These findings suggest that muscle pain prevents the adaptation of muscle activity during sustained or repetitive contractions as observed in non-painful conditions, which may induce overuse of similar muscle regions with fatigue.

Muscle Synergies

A long-lasting hypothesis in motor control is that the CNS adopts strategies that simplify the control of complex tasks by combining few motor modules.[112] Unit burst generators,[113] spinal force fields[114] and muscle synergies[115] have been proposed as modular elements. This hypothesis has been indirectly verified by factorization of multi-channel EMG signals (i.e. by analysing the dimensionality of EMG signals). During complex motor tasks, it can be shown that the number of non-redundant signals necessary to explain the tasks is less than the number of

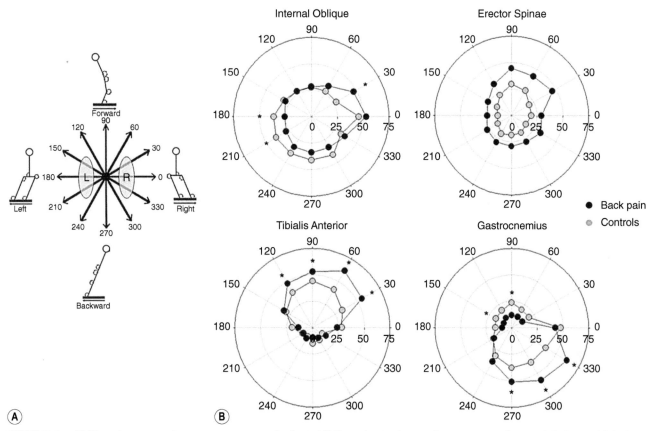

FIGURE 17-5 ■ EMG tuning curves in response to perturbations. (**A**) Experimental setup for support surface translations which shows the directions of platform perturbations with the induced body sway resulting from perturbations in the cardinal directions (i.e. left, forward, right and backward perturbations). Schematic stick figures are depicted with the subject facing to the right for the sagittal plane views and are viewed from the back for the frontal plane views. (**B**) Polar plots of the normalized EMG amplitude of the left internal oblique muscles, left erector spinae, tibialis anterior and gastrocnemius muscles in response to unexpected balance perturbations performed in 12 directions translations in a group of individuals with and without low back pain. (Reprinted with permission from Jones et al.[79])

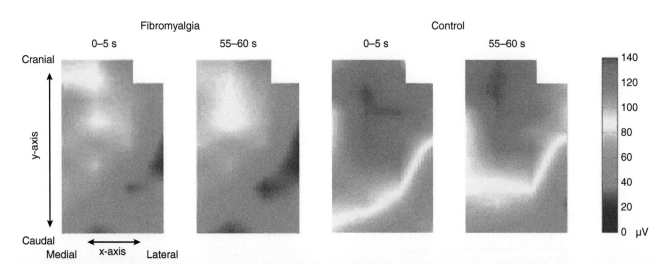

FIGURE 17-6 ■ Topographical mapping of muscle activity. Representative topographical maps (interpolation by a factor 8) of the EMG root mean square value from the right upper trapezius muscle for a person with fibromyalgia and a control subject. Maps are shown for the first and last 5 seconds of a 60-degree sustained shoulder abduction contraction. Areas of blue correspond to low EMG amplitude and dark red to high EMG amplitude. Note the shift of activity in the cranial direction as the task progresses but for the control subject only. For colour version see Plate 17. (Reprinted with permission from Falla et al.[111])

active muscles. This is due to the redundancy of the neuromuscular system.

Factorization methods, such as non-negative matrix factorization,[115] have been applied to extract the dimensionality from multi-channel EMG recordings, which are divided into so-called activation signals (in a lower dimension) and muscle synergies. The original EMG recording over multiple muscles is explained by the weighted sum (by the synergy coefficients) of the activation signals. Using this factorization analysis, it has been demonstrated, for example, that experimental muscle pain disrupts the normal synergistic muscle activation in a subject-specific way.[116]

Single Motor Unit Behaviour

The most detailed analysis of the neural control of movement from EMG signals is at the level of individual motor units. As indicated, this analysis has been possible with intramuscular EMG recording systems for more than 80

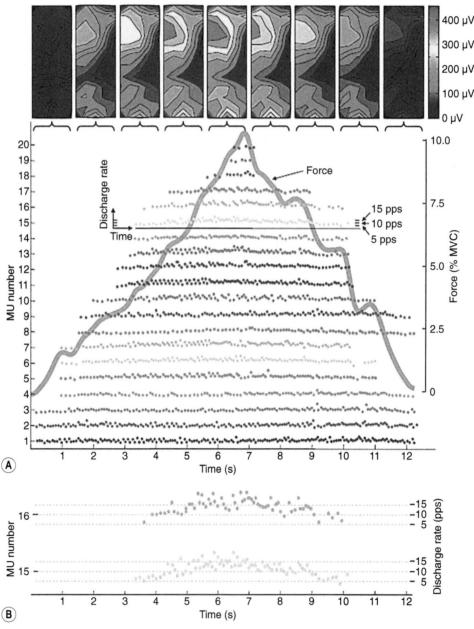

FIGURE 17-7 ■ Extraction of single motor unit discharge patterns from high-density surface EMG. **(A)** Motor unit discharge patterns during an increasing (6 seconds) and decreasing (6 seconds) force isometric contraction (to 10% of the maximum) of the abductor pollicis brevis muscle, as estimated from surface EMG recordings obtained with a 13 × 5 electrode grid. Each dot indicates a motor unit discharge at a time instant. The grey thick line represents the exerted muscle force. The upper panel depicts the root mean square EMG map under the electrode grid during the same muscle contraction. RMS values were calculated from signal epochs of 1-s duration. **(B)** The discharge times of two motor units from **(A)** are shown on a larger vertical scale to illustrate the discharge rate modulation during the contraction. MU: motor unit. For colour version see Plate 18. (Reprinted with permission from Merletti et al.[119])

years.[2] More recently, however, it has been demonstrated that the same information can be obtained from non-invasive muscle recordings, using high-density surface EMG signals (Fig. 17-7). In a series of studies, this direct approach of investigating the neural determinants of movement has been shown to be feasible and accurate.[7,117,118] These new possibilities for the extraction of information from the surface EMG have opened a new line of research in which the alterations of single motor unit behaviour can be analysed in clinical conditions and used to monitor the effects of therapies.

MONITORING CHANGE WITH REHABILITATION

EMG is frequently used as a tool to document change in neuromuscular function with rehabilitation. High levels of repeatability of normalized EMG estimates have been shown for both the neck and back muscles,[120,121] confirming the suitability of using EMG between sessions to monitor changes. EMG has been used to monitor the physiological efficacy of multiple physical therapy interventions, including exercise,[122] mobilization/manipulation[123,124] and taping.[125,126] In relation to exercise, EMG has been used to determine the most appropriate exercise to prescribe to patients,[127–130] to monitor improvement in muscle activation post-intervention[26,27,131,132] and as a tool for biofeedback with training.[133,134]

LIMITATIONS

Intramuscular EMG has the important limitation of being an invasive procedure which often precludes its use as a monitoring tool that would require multiple insertions. Moreover, it is very selective and therefore may not well represent the activity of the muscle. On the other hand, surface EMG suffers from opposite limitations due to the lack of selectivity. For example, crosstalk is an open problem in surface EMG recordings. The most appropriate method has to be chosen for each specific investigation and its limitations taken into account when interpreting the results.

CONCLUSION

EMG is a fundamental tool in musculoskeletal physiotherapy and has been successfully used for the assessment of disturbed motor control and to monitor the physiological efficacy of multiple physical therapy interventions. A number of analyses of the EMG signal can be performed to gain insight into the peripheral status of the muscle and the strategies used by the CNS to control movement and posture. This chapter has reviewed some of the most frequently applied analyses in musculoskeletal physical therapy research, including both classic methods for information extraction and more recent developments.

REFERENCES

1. Merletti R, Farina D. Analysis of intramuscular electromyogram signals. Philos Trans A Math Phys Eng Sci 2009;367:357–68.
2. Adrian ED, Bronk DW. The discharge of impulses in motor nerve fibres: Part II. The frequency of discharge in reflex and voluntary contractions. J Physiol 1929;67:i3–151.
3. Gazzoni M, Farina D, Merletti R. A new method for the extraction and classification of single motor unit action potentials from surface EMG signals. J Neurosci Methods 2004;136:165–77.
4. Holobar A, Zazula D. Correlation-based decomposition of surface electromyograms at low contraction forces. Med Biol Eng Comput 2004;42:487–95.
5. Buchthal F, Guld C, Rosenfalck P. Multielectrode study of the territory of a motor unit. Acta Physiol Scand 1957;39:83–104.
6. Farina D, Yoshida K, Stieglitz T, et al. Multi-channel thin-film electrode for intramuscular electromyographic recordings. J Appl Physiol 2008;104:821–7.
7. Farina D, Holobar A, Merletti R, et al. Decoding the neural drive to muscles from the surface electromyogram. Clin Neurophysiol 2010;121:1616–23.
8. Farina D, Leclerc F, Arendt-Nielsen L, et al. The change in spatial distribution of upper trapezius muscle activity is correlated to contraction duration. J Electromyogr Kinesiol 2008;18:16–25.
9. Zwarts MJ, Stegeman DF. Multichannel surface EMG: basic aspects and clinical utility. Muscle Nerve 2003;28:1–17.
10. Latash ML, Aruin AS, Neyman I, et al. Anticipatory postural adjustments during self inflicted and predictable perturbations in Parkinson's disease. J Neurol Neurosurg Psychiatry 1995;58:326–34.
11. Woollacott MH, von Hosten C, Rosblad B. Relation between muscle response onset and body segmental movements during postural perturbations in humans. Exp Brain Res 1988;72:593–604.
12. Karst GM, Willet GM. Onset timing of electromyographic activity in the vastus medialis oblique and vastus lateralis muscles in subjects with and without patellofemoral pain syndrome. Phys Ther 1995;75:813–23.
13. Merlo A, Farina D, Merletti R. A fast and reliable technique for muscle activity detection from surface EMG signals. IEEE Trans Biomed Eng 2003;50:316–23.
14. Hodges PW, Richardson CA. Inefficient muscular stabilization of the lumbar spine associated with low back pain. A motor control evaluation of transversus abdominis. Spine 1996;21:2640–50.
15. Hodges PW, Richardson CA. Feedforward contraction of transversus abdominis is not influenced by the direction of arm movement. Exp Brain Res 1997;114:362–70.
16. Cholewicki J, Silfies SP, Shah RA, et al. Delayed trunk muscle reflex responses increase the risk of low back injuries. Spine 2005;30:2614–20.
17. Radebold A, Cholewicki J, Panjabi MM, et al. Muscle response pattern to sudden trunk loading in healthy individuals and in patients with chronic low back pain. Spine 2000;25:947–54.
18. Reeves N, Cholewicki J, Milner T. Muscle reflex classification of low-back pain. J Electromyogr Kinesiol 2005;15:53–60.
19. Jacobs J, Henry S, Jones S, et al. A history of low back pain associated with altered electromyographic activation patterns in response to perturbations of standing balance. J Neurophysiol 2011;106:2506–14.
20. Boudreau S, Farina D, Kongstad L, et al. The relative timing of trunk muscle activation is retained in response to unanticipated postural-perturbations during acute low back pain. Exp Brain Res 2011;210:259–67.
21. MacDonald D, Moseley GL, Hodges PW. Why do some patients keep hurting their back? Evidence of ongoing back muscle dysfunction during remission from recurrent back pain. Pain 2009;142:183–8.
22. Falla D, Jull G, Hodges PW. Feedforward activity of the cervical flexor muscles during voluntary arm movements is delayed in chronic neck pain. Exp Brain Res 2004;157:43–8.
23. Boudreau S, Falla D. Chronic neck pain alters muscle activation patterns to sudden movements. Exp Brain Res 2014;232(6):2011–20.

24. Cowan SM, Schache AG, Brukner P, et al. Delayed onset of transversus abdominus in long-standing groin pain. Med Sci Sports Exerc 2004;36:2040–5.

25. Boling MC, Bolgla LA, Mattacola CG, et al. Outcomes of a weight-bearing rehabilitation program for patients diagnosed with patellofemoral pain syndrome. Arch Phys Med Rehabil 2006; 87:1428–35.

26. Tsao H, Hodges PW. Persistence of improvements in postural strategies following motor control training in people with recurrent low back pain. J Electromyogr Kinesiol 2008;18:559–67.

27. Jull G, Falla D, Vicenzino B, et al. The effect of therapeutic exercise on activation of the deep cervical flexor muscles in people with chronic neck pain. Man Ther 2009;14:696–701.

28. Cowan SM, Bennell KL, Hodges PW, et al. Simultaneous feedforward recruitment of the vasti in untrained postural tasks can be restored by physical therapy. J Orthop Res 2003;21:553–8.

29. Merletti R, Knaflitz M, De Luca CJ. Myoelectric manifestations of fatigue in voluntary and electrically elicited contractions. J Appl Physiol 1990;69:1810–20.

30. Merletti R, Rainoldi A, Farina D. Surface electromyography for noninvasive characterization of muscle. Exerc Sport Sci Rev 2001;29:20–5.

31. Merletti R, Roy S. Myoelectric and mechanical manifestations of muscle fatigue in voluntary contractions. J Orthop Sports Phys Ther 1996;24:342–53.

32. De Luca CJ. The use of the surface EMG signal for performance evaluation of back muscles. Muscle Nerve 1993;16:210–16.

33. Basmajian JV, DeLuca CJ. Muscles Alive: Their Functions Revealed by Electromyography. USA: Williams and Wilkins; 1985.

34. De Luca CJ. Myoelectrical manifestations of localized muscular fatigue in humans. Crit Rev Biomed Eng 1984;11:251–79.

35. Kramer CG, Hagg G, Kemp B. Real time measurement of muscle fatigue related changes in surface EMG. Med Biol Eng Comput 1987;25:627–30.

36. Bigland-Ritchie B, Cafarelli F, Vollestad N. Fatigue of submaximal static contractions. Acta Physiol Scand 1986;128(Suppl. 556): 137–48.

37. Moritani T, Muro M, Nagata A. Intramuscular and surface electromyogram changes during muscle fatigue. J Appl Physiol 1986;60:1179–85.

38. Brody LR, Pollock MT, Roy SH, et al. pH-induced effects on median frequency and conduction velocity of the myoelectric signal. J Appl Physiol 1991;71:1878–85.

39. Kossler F, Lange F, Caffier G, et al. External potassium and action potential propagation in rat fast and slow twitch muscles. Gen Physiol Biophys 1991;10:485–98.

40. McKenna MJ, Bangsbo J, Renaud JM. Muscle K+, Na+, and Cl disturbances and Na+-K+ pump inactivation: implications for fatigue. J Appl Physiol 2008;104:288–95.

41. Stulen FB, DeLuca CJ. Frequency parameters of the myoelectric signal as a measure of muscle conduction velocity. IEEE Trans Biomed Eng 1981;28:515–23.

42. Lindstrom L, Magnusson R, Petersen R. Muscle fatigue and action potential conduction velocity changes studied with frequency analysis of EMG signals. Electromyogr Clin Neurophysiol 1970;10:341–56.

43. Bigland-Ritchie B, Donovan EF, Roussos CS. Conduction velocity and EMG power spectrum changes in fatigue of sustained maximal efforts. J Appl Physiol 1981;51:1300–5.

44. Kleine BU, Stegeman D, Mund D, et al. Influence of motorneuron firing synchronisation on SEMG characteristics in dependence of electrode position. J Appl Physiol 2001;91:1588–99.

45. Stegeman D, Blok J, Hermens H, et al. Surface EMG models: properties and applications. J Electromyogr Kinesiol 2000;10: 313–26.

46. Gazzoni M, Farina D, Merletti R. Motor unit recruitment during constant low force and long duration muscle contractions investigated by surface electromyography. Acta Physiol Pharmacol Bulg 2001;26:67–71.

47. Milner-Brown HS, Stein RB, Yemm R. Changes in firing rate of human motor units during linearly changing voluntary contractions. J Physiol 1973;230:371–90.

48. Lindstrom L, Magnusson R. Interpretation of myoelectric power spectra: a model and its applications. Proc IEEE 1977;65: 653–62.

49. Arendt-Nielsen L, Mills KR. The relationship between mean power frequency of the EMG spectrum and muscle fibre conduction velocity. Electroencephalogr Clin Neurophysiol 1985;60: 130–4.

50. Lowery MM, Vaughan CL, Nolan PJ, et al. Spectral compression of the electromyographic signal due to decreasing muscle fiber conduction velocity. IEEE Trans Rehabil Eng 2000;8: 353–61.

51. Merletti R, Lo Conte LR. Advances in processing of surface myoelectric signals: Part 1. Med Biol Eng Comput 1995;33:362–72.

52. Falla D, Rainoldi A, Merletti R, et al. Myoelectric manifestations of sternocleidomastoid and anterior scalene muscle fatigue in chronic neck pain patients. Clin Neurophysiol 2003;114:488–95.

53. Gogia PP, Sabbahi MA. Electromyographic analysis of neck muscle fatigue in patients with osteoarthritis of the cervical spine. Spine 1994;19:502–6.

54. Roy SH, De Luca CJ, Casavant DA. Lumbar muscle fatigue and chronic lower back pain. Spine 1989;14:992–1001.

55. Kankaanpaa M, Taimelas S, Laaksonen D, et al. Back and hip extensor fatigability in chronic low back pain patients and controls. Arch Phys Med Rehabil 1998;79:412–17.

56. Elfving B, Dedering A, Nemeth G. Lumbar muscle fatigue and recovery in patients with long-term low-back trouble: electromyography and health-related factors. Clin Biomech (Bristol, Avon) 2003;18:619–30.

57. Dehner C, Schmelz A, Völker H, et al. Intramuscular pressure, tissue oxygenation, and muscle fatigue of the multifidus during isometric extension in elite rowers with low back pain. J Sport Rehabil 2009;18:572–81.

58. Sung P, Lammers A, Danial P. Different parts of erector spinae muscle fatigability in subjects with and without low back pain. Spine J 2009;9:115–20.

59. Roy SH, De Luca CJ, Emley M, et al. Classification of back muscle impairment based on the surface electromyographic signal. J Rehabil Res Dev 1997;34:405–14.

60. Candotti C, Loss J, Pressi A, et al. Electromyography for assessment of pain in low back muscles. Phys Ther 2008;88:1061–7.

61. Farina D, Pozzo M, Merlo E, et al. Assessment of average muscle fiber conduction velocity from surface EMG signals during fatiguing dynamic contractions. IEEE Trans Biomed Eng 2004; 51:1383–93.

62. Falla D, Farina D. Muscle fiber conduction velocity of the upper trapezius muscle during dynamic contraction of the upper limb in patients with chronic neck pain. Pain 2005;116:138–45.

63. Choi HI, Williams WJ. Improved time-frequency representation of multicomponent signals using exponential kernels. IEEE Trans Acoust Speech Sig Proc 1989;37:862–71.

64. Bonato P, Gagliati G, Knaflitz M. Analysis of surface myoelectric signals recorded during dynamic contractions. IEEE Eng Med Biol Mag 1996;15:102–11.

65. Farina D, Fosci M, Merletti R. Motor unit recruitment strategies investigated by surface EMG variables. J Appl Physiol 2002;92: 235–47.

66. Masuda K, Masuda T, Sadoyama T, et al. Changes in surface EMG parameters during static and dynamic fatiguing contractions. J Electromyogr Kinesiol 1999;9:39–46.

67. Merlo E, Pozzo M, Antonutto G, et al. Time-frequency analysis and estimation of muscle fiber conduction velocity from surface EMG signals during explosive dynamic contractions. J Neurosci Methods 2005;142:267–74.

68. Pozzo M, Alkner B, Norrbrand L, et al. Muscle fiber conduction velocity during concentric and eccentric actions on a flywheel exercise device. Muscle Nerve 2006;34(2):169–77.

69. Falla D, Graven-Nielsen T, Farina D. Spatial and temporal changes of upper trapezius muscle fiber conduction velocity are not predicted by surface EMG spectral analysis during a dynamic upper limb task. J Neurosci Methods 2006;156:236–41.

70. Farina D, Merletti R, Enoka RM. The extraction of neural strategies from the surface EMG. J Appl Physiol 2004;96:1486–95.

71. Falla D, Jull G, Hodges PW. Patients with neck pain demonstrate reduced electromyographic activity of the deep cervical flexor muscles during performance of the craniocervical flexion test. Spine 2004;29:2108–14.

72. Jull G, Kristjansson E, Dall'Alba P. Impairment in the cervical flexors: a comparison of whiplash and insidious onset neck pain patients. Man Ther 2004;9:89–94.

73. Chiu TT, Law E, Chiu TH. Performance of the craniocervical flexion test in subjects with and without chronic neck pain. J Orthop Sports Phys Ther 2005;35:567–71.

74. Descarreaux M, Mayrand N, Raymond J. Neuromuscular control of the head in an isometric force reproduction task: comparison of whiplash subjects and health controls. Spine J 2007;7: 647–53.

75. Szeto GP, Straker LM, O'Sullivan PB. A comparison of symptomatic and asymptomatic office workers performing monotonous keyboard work 1: neck and shoulder muscle recruitment patterns. Man Ther 2005;10:270–80.

76. Nederhand MJ, Ijzerman MJ, Hermens HJ, et al. Cervical muscle dysfunction in the chronic whiplash associated disorder grade II (WAD-II). Spine 2000;25:1938–43.

77. Falla D, Bilenkij G, Jull G. Patients with chronic neck pain demonstrate altered patterns of muscle activation during performance of a functional upper limb task. Spine 2004;29:1436–40.

78. Henry S, Hitt J, Jones S, et al. Decreased limits of stability in response to postural perturbations in subjects with low back pain. Clin Biomech (Bristol, Avon) 2006;21:881–92.

79. Jones S, Hitt J, DeSarno M, et al. Individuals with non-specific low back pain in an active episode demonstrate temporally altered torque responses and direction-specific enhanced muscle activity following unexpected balance perturbations. Exp Brain Res 2012;221:413–26.

80. van der Hulst M, Vollenbroek-Hutten M, Rietman J, et al. Back muscle activation patterns in chronic low back pain during walking: a "guarding" hypothesis. Clin J Pain 2010;26:30–7.

81. Ahern D, Follick M, Council J, et al. Reliability of lumbar paravertebral EMG assessment in chronic low back pain. Arch Phys Med Rehabil 1986;67:762–5.

82. Vogt L, Pfeifer K, Banzer W. Neuromuscular control of walking with chronic low-back pain. Man Ther 2003;8:21–8.

83. Arendt-Nielsen L, Graven-Nielsen T, Svarrer H, et al. The influence of low back pain on muscle activity and coordination during gait: a clinical and experimental study. Pain 1996;64:231–40.

84. Lamoth C, Meijer O, Daffertshofer A, et al. Effects of chronic low back pain on trunk coordination and back muscle activity during walking: changes in motor control. Eur Spine J 2006;15: 23–40.

85. O'Sullivan PB, Beales DJ, Beetham JA, et al. Altered motor control strategies in subjects with sacroiliac joint pain during the active straight-leg-raise test. Spine 2002;27:E1–8.

86. Schomacher J, Boudreau S, Petzke F, et al. Localized pressure pain sensitivity is associated with lower activation of the semispinalis cervicis muscle in patients with chronic neck pain. Clin J Pain 2013;29(10):898–906.

87. Schomacher J, Farina D, Lindstroem R, et al. Chronic traumainduced neck pain impairs the neural control of the deep semispinalis cervicis muscle. Clin Neurophysiol 2012;123:1403–8.

88. Saunders S, Rath D, Hodges P. Postural and respiratory activation of the trunk muscles changes with mode and speed of locomotion. Gait Posture 2004;20:280–90.

89. Hodges PW, Moseley GL, Gabrielsson A, et al. Experimental muscle pain changes feedforward postural responses of the trunk muscles. Exp Brain Res 2003;151:262–71.

90. MacDonald D, Moseley G, Hodges P. People with recurrent low back pain respond differently to trunk loading despite remission from symptoms. Spine (Phila Pa 1976) 2010;35:818–24.

91. Buchanan T, Rovai G, Rymer W. Strategies for muscle activation during isometric torque generation at the human elbow. J Neurophysiol 1989;62:1201–12.

92. Keshner EA, Campbell D, Katz RT, et al. Neck muscle activation patterns in humans during isometric head stabilization. Exp Brain Res 1989;75:335–44.

93. Flanders M, Soechting J. Arm muscle activation for static forces in three-dimensional space. J Neurophysiol 1990;64:1818–37.

94. van Bolhuis B, Gielen C. The relative activation of elbow-flexor muscles in isometric flexion and in flexion/extension movements. J Biomech 1997;30:803–11.

95. Vasavada AN, Peterson BW, Delp SL. Three-dimensional spatial tuning of neck muscle activation in humans. Exp Brain Res 2002;147:437–48.

96. Falla D, Lindstrom R, Rechter L, et al. Effect of pain on the modulation in discharge rate of sternocleidomastoid motor units with force direction. Clin Neurophysiol 2010;121:744–53.

97. Blouin JS, Siegmund GP, Carpenter MG, et al. Neural control of superficial and deep neck muscles in humans. J Neurophysiol 2007;98:920–8.

98. Lindstrom R, Schomacher J, Farina D, et al. Association between neck muscle co-activation, pain, and strength in women with neck pain. Man Ther 2011;16:80–6.

99. Holtermann A, Roeleveld K. EMG amplitude distribution changes over the upper trapezius muscle are similar in sustained and ramp contractions. Acta Physiol (Oxf) 2006;186:159–68.

100. Falla D, Farina D, Graven Nielsen T. Spatial dependency of trapezius muscle activity during repetitive shoulder flexion. J Electromyogr Kinesiol 2007;17:299–306.

101. Holtermann A, Roeleveld K, Karlsson JS. Inhomogeneities in muscle activation reveal motor unit recruitment. J Electromyogr Kinesiol 2005;15:131–7.

102. Falla D, Farina D. Periodic increases in force during sustained contraction reduce fatigue and facilitate spatial redistribution of trapezius muscle activity. Exp Brain Res 2007;182:99–107.

103. Tucker K, Falla D, Graven-Nielsen T, et al. Electromyographic mapping of the erector spinae muscle with varying load and during sustained contraction. J Electromyogr Kinesiol 2009;19:373–9.

104. Falla D, Gizzi L, Tschapek M, et al. Reduced task-induced variations in the distribution of activity across back muscle regions in individuals with low back pain. Pain 2014;155(5):944–53.

105. Falla D, Farina D. Non-uniform adaptation of motor unit discharge rates during sustained static contraction of the upper trapezius muscle. Exp Brain Res 2008;191:363–70.

106. Falla D, Arendt-Nielsen L, Farina D. Gender-specific adaptations of upper trapezius muscle activity to acute nociceptive stimulation. Pain 2008;138:217–25.

107. Westgaard RH. Muscle activity as a releasing factor for pain in the shoulder and neck. Cephalalgia 1999;19:251–8.

108. Andersson G, Ortengren R. Assessment of back load in assembly line work using electromyography. Ergonomics 1984;27: 1157–68.

109. Madeleine P, Leclerc F, Arendt-Nielsen L, et al. Experimental muscle pain changes the spatial distribution of upper trapezius muscle activity during sustained contraction. Clin Neurophysiol 2006;117:2436–45.

110. Falla D, Arendt-Nielsen L, Farina D. The pain-induced change in relative activation of upper trapezius muscle regions is independent of the site of noxious stimulation. Clin Neurophysiol 2009;120:150–7.

111. Falla D, Andersen H, Danneskiold-Samsøe B, et al. Adaptations of upper trapezius muscle activity during sustained contractions in women with fibromyalgia. J Electromyogr Kinesiol 2010; 20:457–64.

112. Bernstein N. The Co-ordination and Regulation of Movements. Oxford: Pergamon; 1967.

113. Grillner S. Control of locomotion in bipeds, tetrapods, and fish. In: Brooks V, editor. Handbook of Physiology. Bethesda, MD, USA: Am Physiol Soc; 1981. p. 1179–236.

114. Giszter SF, Hart CB, Silfies SP. Spinal cord modularity: evolution, development, and optimization and the possible relevance to low back pain in man. Exp Brain Res 2010;200:283–306.

115. Tresch MC, Saltiel P, Bizzi E. The construction of movement by the spinal cord. Nat Neurosci 1999;2:162–7.

116. Muceli S, Falla D, Farina D. Reorganization of muscle synergies during multidirectional reaching in the horizontal plane with experimental muscle pain. J Neurophysiol 2014;111(8):1615–30.

117. Holobar A, Minetto MA, Botter A, et al. Experimental analysis of accuracy in the identification of motor unit spike trains from high-density surface EMG. IEEE Trans Neural Syst Rehabil Eng 2010;18:221–9.

118. Holobar A, Minetto MA, Farina D. Accurate identification of motor unit discharge patterns from high-density surface EMG and validation with a novel signal-based performance metric. J Neural Eng 2014;11(1):016008.

119. Merletti R, Holobar A, Farina D. Analysis of motor units with high-density surface electromyography. J Electromyogr Kinesiol 2008;18:879–90.

120. Falla D, Dall'Alba P, Rainoldi A, et al. Repeatability of surface EMG variables in the sternocleidomastoid and anterior scalene muscles. Eur J Appl Physiol 2002;87:542–9.

121. Dankaerts W, O'Sullivan P, Burnett A, et al. Reliability of EMG measurements for trunk muscles during maximal and sub-maximal

voluntary isometric contractions in healthy controls and CLBP patients. J Electromyogr Kinesiol 2004;14:333–42.

122. Jørgensen M, Andersen L, Kirk N, et al. Muscle activity during functional coordination training: implications for strength gain and rehabilitation. J Strength Cond Res 2010;24:1732–9.

123. Ferreira M, Ferreira PH, Hodges PW. Changes in postural activity of the trunk muscles following spinal manipulative therapy. Man Ther 2007;12:240–8.

124. Krekoukias G, Petty N, Cheek L. Comparison of surface electromyographic activity of erector spinae before and after the application of central posteroanterior mobilisation on the lumbar spine. J Electromyogr Kinesiol 2009;19:39–45.

125. Greig A, Bennell K, Briggs A, et al. Postural taping decreases thoracic kyphosis but does not influence trunk muscle electromyographic activity or balance in women with osteoporosis. Man Ther 2008;13:249–57.

126. Ng G, Wong P. Patellar taping affects vastus medialis obliquus activation in subjects with patellofemoral pain before and after quadriceps muscle fatigue. Clin Rehabil 2009;23:705–13.

127. Bressel E, Dolny D, Gibbons M. Trunk muscle activity during exercises performed on land and in water. Med Sci Sports Exerc 2011;43:1927–32.

128. Okubo Y, Kaneoka K, Imai A, et al. Electromyographic analysis of transversus abdominis and lumbar multifidus using wire electrodes during lumbar stabilization exercises. J Orthop Sports Phys Ther 2010;40:743–50.

129. Schomacher J, Petzke F, Falla D. Localised resistance selectively activates the semispinalis cervicis muscle in patients with neck pain. Man Ther 2012;17:544–8.

130. Andersen L, Andersen C, Mortensen O, et al. Muscle activation and perceived loading during rehabilitation exercises: comparison of dumbbells and elastic resistance. Phys Ther 2010;90:538–49.

131. Søgaard K, Blangsted A, Nielsen P, et al. Changed activation, oxygenation, and pain response of chronically painful muscles to repetitive work after training interventions: a randomized controlled trial. Eur J Appl Physiol 2012;112:173–81.

132. Falla D, Jull G, Hodges P, et al. An endurance-strength training regime is effective in reducing myoelectric manifestations of cervical flexor muscle fatigue in females with chronic neck pain. Clin Neurophysiol 2006;117:828–37.

133. Ma C, Szeto G, Yan T, et al. Comparing biofeedback with active exercise and passive treatment for the management of work-related neck and shoulder pain: a randomized controlled trial. Arch Phys Med Rehabil 2011;92:849–58.

134. Dellve L, Ahlstrom L, Jonsson A, et al. Myofeedback training and intensive muscular strength training to decrease pain and improve work ability among female workers on long-term sick leave with neck pain: a randomized controlled trial. Int Arch Occup Environ Health 2011;84:335–46.

CHAPTER 18

Non-invasive Brain Stimulation in the Measurement and Treatment of Musculoskeletal Disorders

Siobhan Schabrun • Caroline Alexander

People have been investigating cortical connections to muscles since the 1800s by electrically stimulating the brain and watching the muscle contract. Electrical stimulation to the motor cortex is still used today. It can be applied directly to the cortex to evaluate corticospinal output during surgery or indirectly to the skull to stimulate the cortex below. However, the stimulus intensity required to overcome the resistance of the skull is high, and this is painful. This limitation was overcome and the field of brain stimulation was revolutionized when, in 1985, Barker and colleagues used a magnetic stimulator (transcranial magnetic stimulation; TMS) to induce an electrical charge in the cortex.[1] Here, a short-lasting electrical current is discharged through a wire coil inducing a magnetic field, which in turn produces a short-lasting electrical charge in underlying brain tissue (Fig. 18-1). If the coil is centred over the motor cortex, axons that synapse with corticospinal pathways are stimulated and, if the stimulus intensity is high enough to evoke an action potential, the relevant muscle will contract. This muscle twitch is called a motor evoked potential (MEP; Fig. 18-2) and can be recorded using electromyography.

TMS can be used to deliver single pulses at low frequency (approximately one every 5–6 seconds). When used in this manner, TMS is a measurement tool that can provide information about corticomotor control of movement.

SINGLE-PULSE TRANSCRANIAL MAGNETIC STIMULATION

A number of physiological measures can be made using single-pulse TMS. These include corticomotor control of a particular muscle, excitability of the corticospinal pathway, investigation of intra- and inter-cortical neural networks and the effect of pathology or treatment on corticospinal control. These investigations require knowledge of the optimal anatomical site for stimulation. In the motor cortex this site is found by locating either the 'hotspot' or the centre of gravity.[2-6] The site most easily found is the hotspot, which is defined as the scalp site that evokes an MEP of greatest amplitude in the target muscle at the lowest stimulator intensity.[7] The hotspot can be located more accurately by linking the position of the magnetic stimulator coil to an individual's brain scan;[8,9] however, this is costly and not used universally.

Cortical Representation Mapping

The hotspot is not the only site that will evoke an MEP in the target muscle. Stimulating the area around this site will also evoke the MEP. As the coil is positioned further away from the hotspot, the amplitude of the MEP will reduce until it disappears. This surface topography of the corticomotor projection to a particular muscle can be systematically mapped by moving the coil around a grid placed over the scalp[10] (Fig. 18-3). The averaged amplitude of the MEPs evoked at each scalp site creates a map of the cortical representation for a target muscle. These maps provide information on the area, excitability (volume) and amplitude-weighted centre (centre of gravity) of the corticomotor representation. The size and location of these maps have been used to explore the

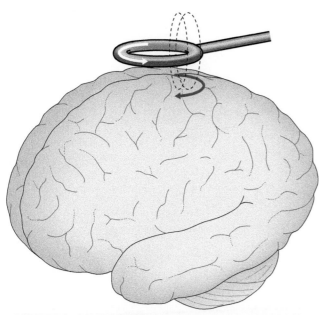

FIGURE 18-1 ■ A short-lasting electrical current (anticlockwise arrow) is discharged through a wire housed in a coil that can be of varying shapes and sizes. This induces a magnetic field (dashed lines), which in turn produces a short-lasting electrical charge in underlying brain tissue (clockwise arrow).

impact of a painful stimulus or disorders such as focal hand dystonia, lateral epicondylalgia and low back pain on brain architecture.[11-14] Of interest, early evidence suggests that non-invasive brain stimulation,[15] peripheral electrical stimulation[16] and motor retraining[17] strategies may be effective in normalizing aberrant cortical organization and improving symptoms in some clinical disorders.

Resting and Active Motor Threshold

The motor (or MEP) threshold is the lowest stimulus intensity that elicits an MEP at rest (resting motor threshold) or during muscle activation (active motor threshold). Threshold can be measured using a number of different strategies,[18-20] but resting motor threshold is most commonly defined as the stimulus intensity required to elicit an MEP at rest of approximately 100 μV in at least five of ten consecutive trials.[19] Threshold is thought to reflect neuronal membrane excitability and consequently is increased by drugs that block sodium channels.[21] Threshold is also influenced by the degree and depth of a muscle's cortical representation.[7] For instance, lower limb, paraspinal and pelvic muscles have higher motor thresholds than hand muscles. Motor thresholds also differ in some clinical disorders.[14,20,22-28] For example, resting motor threshold is increased for erector spinae in individuals with chronic low back pain,[24] for lower trapezius in non-traumatic shoulder instability[29] and following immobilization of hand muscles in healthy individuals.[28] These changes suggest a reduction in cortical excitability in these muscles in these conditions.

Motor Evoked Potential Latency

The latency of an MEP is the time between TMS pulse delivery and the onset of the evoked response in the target muscle (see Fig. 18-2). The latency is dependent on a number of factors, including the central and peripheral pathway distance, whether MEPs are recorded at rest or during contraction and the number of synapses in the pathway. Consequently, a monosynaptic pathway to a trunk muscle will have a shorter latency than a multisynaptic pathway to a lower limb muscle. MEP latency is measured at a consistent stimulus intensity (usually 1.2 or 1.5 times threshold) and the response to multiple stimuli are averaged. MEP latency has been reported as an outcome measure in healthy people and in people with musculoskeletal problems.[24,27,30,31] For example, the MEP latency of the lower trapezius is longer in individuals with non-traumatic shoulder instability than for healthy individuals,[29] suggesting a shift towards the use of alternate, more complex corticospinal pathways. Conversely, MEP latency has been reported as unchanged in individuals with chronic low back pain[24] and chronic fatigue syndrome.[30]

Motor Evoked Potential Amplitude

MEP amplitude provides a measure of the excitability of the corticomotor pathway to a target muscle, which is inclusive of both upper and lower motoneuron excitability. When used in conjunction with measures of peripheral (e.g. M-wave) and spinal (e.g. F-wave or H-reflex) excitability it can also be used to estimate

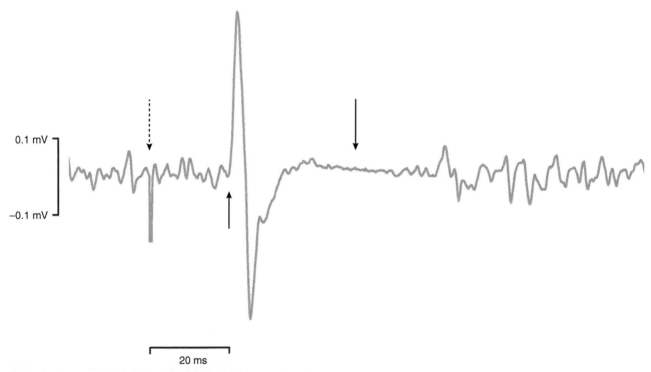

FIGURE 18-2 ■ Averaged electromyographic activity of the quadriceps muscle, which is contracting at 10% of maximum voluntary contraction. This is the result of ten stimuli over the hotspot for quadriceps, stimulating the contralateral motor cortex. The downward dashed arrow points to the stimulus artefact. The upward arrow points to the onset of the motor evoked potential (MEP). The time between the stimulus artefact and the onset of the MEP is the MEP latency. The downward arrow points to the mid part of the silent period.

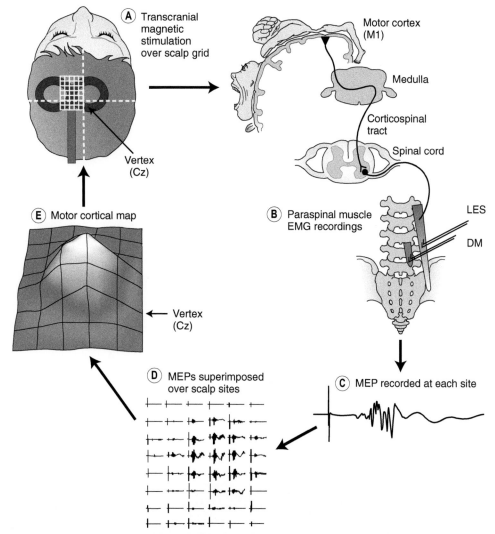

FIGURE 18-3 ▦ Mapping of the motor cortex using transcranial magnetic stimulation (TMS). **(A)** Stimuli over the motor cortex using a figure-of-eight coil excite intracortical neurons that provide synaptic input to corticospinal cells. **(B)** In this example the area of the motor cortex corresponding to the paraspinal muscles is excited and electromyographic recordings are made from short/deep fascicles of multifidius (DM) and longissimus erector spinae (LES) at the L4 spinal level. **(C)** The descending volley from the TMS pulse excites spinal motoneurons and results in a motor evoked potential (MEP), mainly in contralateral muscles. **(D)** MEPs are recorded in both muscles from TMS stimuli applied at each point on a grid placed over the scalp and aligned to the vertex (Cz). **(E)** A three-dimensional map of MEP amplitude can then be created for a muscle. (Reproduced with permission from Tsao et al 2011; Spine 2011: 36(21): 1721–7.)

changes in cortical excitability.[32] As a result, MEP amplitude is frequently used as a marker of neuroplasticity, where increased MEP amplitude is thought to reflect long-term potentiation of synaptic efficacy, and decreased MEP amplitude, long-term depression of synaptic efficacy. This measure is particularly useful for evaluating the corticomotor effects of an intervention. For instance, MEP amplitudes are reduced in healthy individuals following transcutaneous electrical nerve stimulation, suggesting a reduction in cortical excitability, and an increase in response to neuromuscular electrical stimulation, indicating that cortical excitability is enhanced.[33–35] Such findings have relevance for the use of these therapeutic techniques in clinical populations; however, the variability of MEP amplitude can be high and may require studies with large sample sizes to establish differences.

Recruitment Curves

Recruitment curves are constructed by gradually increasing or decreasing the stimulus intensity while the target muscle is maintained at rest or at a constant level of contraction. The MEP amplitude is then plotted as a function of the stimulus intensity. Figure 18-4 illustrates a typical recruitment curve that fits a sigmoid shape. In this example, the stimulus intensity is increased incrementally by 5% of the output of the magnetic stimulator and the MEP rises until full recruitment of muscle fibre is achieved. The curve plateaus once full recruitment has occurred. A number of outcome measures can be calculated from the recruitment curve.

- The peak slope of the fitted recruitment curve ($[1/b]a/4$), where a is the amplitude of the MEP at the slope's maximum and b is the slope parameter.

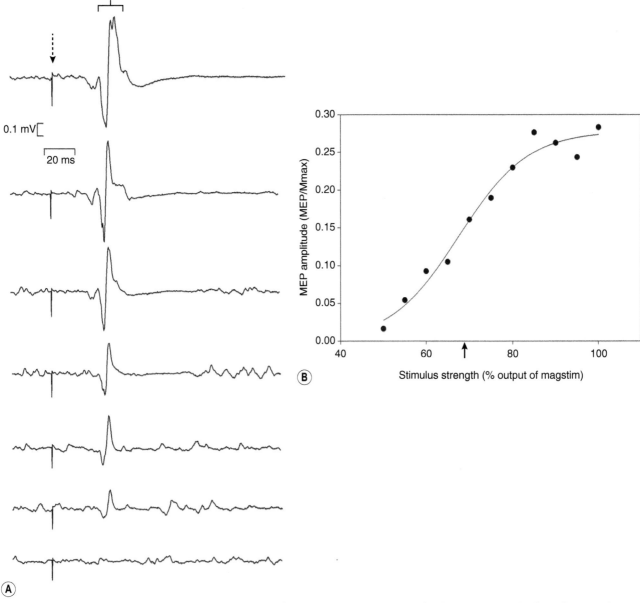

FIGURE 18-4 ■ **(A)** Averaged electromyographic activity of the quadriceps muscle, which is active at 10% of maximum voluntary contraction. Each trace is the result of three stimuli over the hotspot for quadriceps, stimulating the contralateral motor cortex at increasing stimulus intensities. The downward arrow points to the stimulus artefact. The normalized amplitude of the averaged MEPs can be plotted against stimulus intensity. **(B)** A curve can then be fitted to these points; here a sigmoid curve is fitted from which outcomes such as the stimulus intensity that evokes a response equivalent to 50% of the maximum amplitude (upward arrow), the peak slope of the curve and the peak amplitude of the curve can be calculated.

- The stimulus intensity that evokes a response equivalent to 50% of the maximum amplitude of the fitted curve (often termed x_{50}).
- The slope of the rising phase of the recruitment curve.
- The maximum MEP amplitude at the plateau (which can be normalized to the M_{max}).

These outcome measures reflect different features of the strength of corticospinal projection.[36] For example, if MEPs of equal amplitude are comparable across two groups then one interpretation is that there is no difference in excitability between groups. However, if one group exhibits a steep slope in the recruitment curve,

this implies that the maximum amplitude of the MEP can be achieved with minimum increase in stimulus intensity – a measure of recruitment gain. Conversely, if the slope is shallow it suggests that greater stimulus intensity is required to evoke a response of equal amplitude. Recruitment curves were used by Nicotra and colleagues to examine the impact of surgery on corticospinal excitability in patients with cervical myelopathy.[37] This pilot study demonstrated that the recruitment curve differed between controls and patients revealing reduced corticospinal excitability in the patient group. Many of the parameters explored had not improved three months after surgery.

Cortical Silent Period

TMS given during a voluntary muscle contraction evokes a period of electromyographic silence, termed the cortical silent period (CSP), which can be evoked at a lower threshold than the MEP and can be seen immediately after the MEP (see Fig. 18-2). Reduced electromyographic (EMG) activity is influenced in the early stage (up to 60 ms) by spinal mechanisms such as Renshaw inhibition, while the later stage is thought to be due to cortical inhibitory interneurons activated by TMS.[38-40] The duration, amplitude, gain and stimulus intensity needed to evoke the CSP are typically recorded.[41] Measures of the CSP have been found to correlate with some musculoskeletal pathologies. For example, the stimulus intensity required to evoke a CSP in erector spinae is higher in people with low back pain compared to healthy individuals and increased stimulus intensity is correlated with level of disability (Oswestry Disability Index).[24] In contrast, the CSP is reduced in the facial muscles of individuals with migraine, suggesting a possible dysfunction of cortical inhibitory interneurons in this condition.[42]

Fatigue

Motor fatigue arises from both peripheral and central sources, which can in part be explored using TMS. Here an individual is asked to maintain a brief but maximum static contraction while TMS is delivered at an intensity to achieve a maximum amplitude MEP. Any additional force evoked by the TMS over the force of the voluntary contraction is indicative of a loss of voluntary drive to the muscle (termed central fatigue). If the muscle is then worked to fatigue, any change in voluntary drive can be plotted over time.[43] These methods have been used to investigate the contribution of central mechanisms to fatigue in a range of different muscles[44-46] in response to substances such as caffeine and to a variety of pathologies.[47]

PAIRED-PULSE TRANSCRANIAL MAGNETIC STIMULATION

Paired-pulse TMS can be used to explore intracortical, intrahemispheric and interhemispheric neural networks.[48] These protocols involve a conditioning stimulus given to a relevant brain region prior to a test stimulus given to the motor cortex. Depending on the site of stimulation and interstimulus interval, a range of inhibitory and facilitatory cortical circuits can be investigated. These methods can provide information on how particular neural networks may be altered in conditions such as acute pain,[49] fibromyalgia,[23] chronic regional pain syndrome,[50] chronic low back pain[51] and fatigue,[52-54] as well as following therapeutic or training interventions.[55-57]

REPETITIVE TRANSCRANIAL MAGNETIC STIMULATION

TMS can also be used to deliver repetitive pulses at high frequencies (5–20 stimuli every seconds); in this form it is known as repetitive TMS (rTMS). A rapidly changing magnetic field induces electrical currents in underlying neurons that are capable of inducing neuroplastic effects that outlast the period of stimulation. rTMS at high frequencies (5–20 Hz) can facilitate,[58,59] and at low frequencies (0.2–1 Hz) suppress,[60] neural activity and cortical excitability. Although few studies have investigated how long these effects persist, the duration appears dependent on the length and number of rTMS trains.[61] rTMS can also be delivered in patterned trains. For example, three short, high-frequency trains of rTMS in theta-frequency (theta-burst stimulation) facilitate cortical excitability at intermittent intervals, and suppress cortical excitability when delivered continuously.[62] Thus rTMS is predominantly an intervention used to induce long-term potentiation or long-term depression-like effects in the cortex. This property of rTMS has been exploited as a treatment in psychiatric, neurological and musculoskeletal disorders (see Neuromodulation: A New Treatment Strategy in Physiotherapy section).

rTMS effects on cortical excitability can also be used to produce transient disruption of neural activity in local and remote brain regions, creating a 'virtual lesion'. This approach is widely used to study structure–function relationships in the human brain. For example, rTMS has been used to examine the relationship between cortical regions such as the primary motor cortex,[63,64] primary sensory cortex[65] or premotor areas[66,67] with function during object manipulation. Here, rTMS is applied to the relevant cortical region before or during a task. The effect of disruption to a particular cortical area on task performance is then evaluated, providing insight into the cortical control of a specific function. This information can be used to guide and inform rehabilitation.

NEUROMODULATION: A NEW TREATMENT STRATEGY IN PHYSIOTHERAPY

Electrical and magnetic stimulation techniques, such as those described above, can be used not only to measure human neural function but may also induce and enhance neuroplasticity for therapy. When used to modulate neural activity, non-invasive brain stimulation may promote adaptive, and suppress maladaptive, neural modifications ('plasticity') and may have the potential to expedite and enhance recovery. Neuromodulatory interventions can be applied in two ways: (a) as stand-alone treatments that change the resting state of the cortex or (b) as priming protocols that modulate cortical excitability in an attempt to increase the brain's receptiveness to subsequent treatments (for a review see Schabrun et al.[68]). Priming the cortex is of particular interest to physiotherapists where clinical outcomes might be enhanced by combining neuromodulation with traditional therapies such as motor retraining, peripheral electrical stimulation (e.g. transcutaneous electrical nerve stimulation, functional electrical stimulation) or pharmacological treatments. An overview of two common neuromodulatory interventions, rTMS and transcranial direct current stimulation (tDCS) is provided below.

Repetitive Transcranial Magnetic Stimulation

rTMS has been used to varying effect in the treatment of chronic pain conditions such as neuropathic pain,[69] complex regional pain syndrome,[70] fibromyalgia,[71-74] pelvic and perineal pain[75] and phantom limb pain.[76,77] The mechanisms that underpin any analgesic effect of rTMS are not yet fully understood. However, it is hypothesized that rTMS may act on intracortical networks to restore defective inhibitory mechanisms[78] and may influence endogenous opioid systems.[79] The duration of effect appears to be dependent on the frequency of rTMS application, the protocol used and the clinical condition treated. For instance, ten daily sessions of 10 Hz rTMS to the motor cortex is reported to improve pain and quality of life for up to two weeks in individuals with fibromyalgia.[73] Indeed, a recent systematic review in fibromyalgia reported a significant and lasting impact on pain reduction beyond the period of stimulation using high-frequency rTMS protocols.[80] However, evidence for the effectiveness of rTMS in other pain conditions is limited by a small number of heterogeneous studies, small effect sizes and variable findings.[81] Further work is needed to determine the clinical efficacy of this technique in chronic pain.[82]

Transcranial Direct Current Stimulation

Direct current is the uninterrupted flow of electric charge in a single direction. Also known as constant current or galvanism, the application of direct current to the human body as a therapeutic tool is not new. Physiotherapists have utilized direct current since the early 1900s for iontophoresis and wound healing.[83,84] tDCS is a contemporary direct current application that involves a weak direct current (less than 2 mA) delivered to the scalp via two surface sponge electrodes (20–35 cm^2). The current penetrates the cranium and modulates the resting membrane potential of underlying neurons. The resting membrane potential of neurons under the anode is increased, whereas the resting membrane potential of neurons under the cathode is reduced. This leads to increased or decreased neuronal firing rates[85,86] and a subsequent increase or decrease in the excitability of brain circuits. Altered cortical excitability with tDCS is thought to reflect neuroplastic processes akin to long-term potentiation and long-term depression of synaptic efficacy.[87] These effects can be observed in the brain region under the electrodes and in distant neuronal circuits.[78]

tDCS has been investigated in a variety of chronic pain conditions including low back pain,[88] pelvic pain,[89] fibromyalgia,[90,91] multiple sclerosis[92] and spinal cord injury.[93] Analgesia is thought to be produced by direct cortical effects on thalamic nuclei as well as downstream effects on the anterior cingulate cortex and upper brainstem.[94,95] Stimulation parameters have comprised an intensity of 1–2 mA, a duration of 20–30 minutes, and single through to multiple, consecutive daily treatments. The most common application is anodal tDCS to the primary motor cortex (M1). In chronic pain conditions (spinal cord injury, fibromyalgia, multiple sclerosis) pain has been reduced by 58–63% following 5 days of anodal tDCS to M1.[81] A greater number of consecutive sessions (ten as opposed to five daily sessions) produces longer-lasting effects, with pain relief lasting up to 60 days following treatment.[91] However, these findings need to be considered carefully, as a recent systematic review concluded there was still insufficient evidence from which to conclude the effectiveness of tDCS for chronic pain, and responses to tDCS are known to be highly variable between individuals.[82] Further high-quality studies are required.

SAFETY CONSIDERATIONS

Brain stimulation techniques used to measure or induce neural modifications are considered safe and painless when current safety guidelines are followed. The only absolute contraindication to TMS and rTMS is the presence of metallic hardware in close proximity to the stimulating coil.[9,19] rTMS carries a small risk of seizure induction particularly in those using pro-epileptogenic medication, are epileptic, have had brain injury or when rTMS protocols outside current safety guidelines are implemented.[9,19] The use of tDCS in healthy subjects and across a range of pathological conditions has not resulted in any significant adverse effects to date.[96] However, it must be noted that while single and multi-day applications of tDCS and rTMS appear safe, there have been few studies of prolonged periods of stimulation or investigation of long-term effects in humans.

REFERENCES

1. Barker AT, Jalinous R, Freeston IL. Non-invasive magnetic stimulation of human motor cortex. Lancet 1985;1:1106–7.
2. Borghetti D, Sartucci F, Petacchi E, et al. Transcranial magnetic stimulation mapping: a model based on spline interpolation. Brain Res Bull 2008;77:143–8.
3. MacKinnon CD, Quartarone A, Rothwell JC. Inter-hemispheric asymmetry of ipsilateral corticofugal projections to proximal muscles in humans. Exp Brain Res 2004;157:225–33.
4. Miranda PC, de Carvalho M, Conceicao I, et al. A new method for reproducible coil positioning in transcranial magnetic stimulation mapping. Electroencephalogr Clin Neurophysiol 1997;105:116–23.
5. Ridding MC, Brouwer B, Miles TS, et al. Changes in muscle responses to stimulation of the motor cortex induced by peripheral nerve stimulation in human subjects. Exp Brain Res 2000;131:135–43.
6. Uy J, Ridding MC, Miles TS. Stability of maps of human motor cortex made with transcranial magnetic stimulation. Brain Topogr 2002;14:293–7.
7. Rossini PM, Barker AT, Berardelli A, et al. Non-invasive electrical and magnetic stimulation of the brain, spinal cord and roots: basic principles and procedures for routine clinical application. Report of an IFCN committee. Electroencephalogr Clin Neurophysiol 1994;91:79–92.
8. Boroojerdi B, Foltys H, Krings T, et al. Localization of the motor hand area using transcranial magnetic stimulation and functional magnetic resonance imaging. Clin Neurophysiol 1999;110:699–704.
9. Rossi S, Hallett M, Rossini PM, et al. Safety, ethical considerations, and application guidelines for the use of transcranial magnetic stimulation in clinical practice and research. Clin Neurophysiol 2009;120:2008–39.
10. Byrnes ML, Thickbroom GW, Wilson SA, et al. The corticomotor representation of upper limb muscles in writer's cramp and changes following botulinum toxin injection. Brain 1998;121(Pt 5):977–88.

11. Krause P, Forderreuther S, Straube A. TMS motor cortical brain mapping in patients with complex regional pain syndrome type I. Clin Neurophysiol 2006;117:169–76.

12. Tsao H, Danneels L, Hodges PW. Individual fascicles of the paraspinal muscles are activated by discrete cortical networks in humans. Clin Neurophysiol 2011.

13. Tsao H, Danneels LA, Hodges PW. ISSLS prize winner: smudging the motor brain in young adults with recurrent low back pain. Spine (Phila Pa 1976) 2011;36:1721–7.

14. Tsao H, Galea MP, Hodges PW. Reorganization of the motor cortex is associated with postural control deficits in recurrent low back pain. Brain 2008;131:2161–71.

15. Schabrun SM, Jones E, Elgueta-Cancino E, et al. Targeting chronic recurrent low back pain from the top-down and the bottom-up: a combined transcranial direct current stimulation and peripheral electrical stimulation intervention. Brain Stimul 2014;7:451–9.

16. Schabrun SM, Stinear CM, Byblow WD, et al. Normalizing motor cortex representations in focal hand dystonia. Cereb Cortex 2009;19:1968–77.

17. Tsao H, Galea MP, Hodges PW. Driving plasticity in the motor cortex in recurrent low back pain. Eur J Pain 2010;14:832–9.

18. Awiszus F. On relative frequency estimation of transcranial magnetic stimulation motor threshold. Clin Neurophysiol 2012;123:2319–20.

19. Groppa S, Oliviero A, Eisen A, et al. A practical guide to diagnostic transcranial magnetic stimulation: report of an IFCN committee. Clin Neurophysiol 2012;123:858–82.

20. Qi F, Wu AD, Schweighofer N. Fast estimation of transcranial magnetic stimulation motor threshold. Brain Stimul 2011;4:50–7.

21. Ziemann U, Lonnecker S, Steinhoff BJ, et al. Effects of antiepileptic drugs on motor cortex excitability in humans: a transcranial magnetic stimulation study. Ann Neurol 1996;40:367–78.

22. Davey NJ, Puri BK, Catley M, et al. Deficit in motor performance correlates with changed corticospinal excitability in patients with chronic fatigue syndrome. Int J Clin Pract 2003;57:262–4.

23. Mhalla A, de A, Baudic S, et al. Alteration of cortical excitability in patients with fibromyalgia. Pain 2010;149:495–500.

24. Strutton PH, Theodorou S, Catley M, et al. Corticospinal excitability in patients with chronic low back pain. J Spinal Disord Tech 2005;18:420–4.

25. Strutton PH, Catley M, McGregor AH, et al. Corticospinal excitability in patients with unilateral sciatica. Neurosci Lett 2003;353:33–6.

26. Svensson P, Romaniello A, Wang K, et al. One hour of tongue-task training is associated with plasticity in corticomotor control of the human tongue musculature. Exp Brain Res 2006;173:165–73.

27. Alexander CM. Altered control of the trapezius muscle in subjects with non-traumatic shoulder instability. Clin Neurophysiol 2007;118:2664–71.

28. Facchini S, Romani M, Tinazzi M, et al. Time-related changes of excitability of the human motor system contingent upon immobilisation of the ring and little fingers. Clin Neurophysiol 2002;113:367–75.

29. Alexander CM. Altered control of the trapezius muscle in subjects with non-traumatic shoulder instability. Clin Neurophysiol 2007;118:2664–71.

30. Davey NJ, Puri BK, Nowicky AV, et al. Voluntary motor function in patients with chronic fatigue syndrome. J Psychosom Res 2001;50:17–20.

31. Romaniello A, Cruccu G, McMillan AS, et al. Effect of experimental pain from trigeminal muscle and skin on motor cortex excitability in humans. Brain Res 2000;882:120–7.

32. Davey NJ, Smith HC, Savic G, et al. Comparison of input-output patterns in the corticospinal system of normal subjects and incomplete spinal cord injured patients. Exp Brain Res 1999;127:382–90.

33. Andrews RK, Schabrun SM, Ridding MC, et al. The effect of electrical stimulation on corticospinal excitability is dependent on application duration: a same subject pre-post test design. J Neuroeng Rehabil 2013;10:51.

34. Chipchase LS, Schabrun SM, Hodges PW. Corticospinal excitability is dependent on the parameters of peripheral electric stimulation: a preliminary study. Arch Phys Med Rehabil 2011;92:1423–30.

35. Chipchase LS, Schabrun SM, Hodges PW. Peripheral electrical stimulation to induce cortical plasticity: a systematic review of stimulus parameters. Clin Neurophysiol 2011;122:456–63.

36. Boroojerdi B, Battaglia F, Muellbacher W, et al. Mechanisms influencing stimulus-response properties of the human corticospinal system. Clin Neurophysiol 2001;112:931–7.

37. Nicotra A, King NK, Catley M, et al. Evaluation of corticospinal excitability in cervical myelopathy, before and after surgery, with transcranial magnetic stimulation: a pilot study. Eur Spine J 2013;22:189–96.

38. Fecteau S, Lassonde M, Theoret H. Intrahemispheric dysfunction in primary motor cortex without corpus callosum: a transcranial magnetic stimulation study. BMC Neurol 2006;6:21.

39. Werhahn KJ, Behrang-Nia M, Bott MC, et al. Does the recruitment of excitation and inhibition in the motor cortex differ? J Clin Neurophysiol 2007;24:419–23.

40. Ziemann U, Netz J, Szelenyi A, et al. Spinal and supraspinal mechanisms contribute to the silent period in the contracting soleus muscle after transcranial magnetic stimulation of human motor cortex. Neurosci Lett 1993;156:167–71.

41. King NK, Kuppuswamy A, Strutton PH, et al. Estimation of cortical silent period following transcranial magnetic stimulation using a computerised cumulative sum method. J Neurosci Methods 2006;150:96–104.

42. Curra A, Pierelli F, Coppola G, et al. Shortened cortical silent period in facial muscles of patients with migraine. Pain 2007;132:124–31.

43. Todd G, Taylor JL, Gandevia SC. Measurement of voluntary activation of fresh and fatigued human muscles using transcranial magnetic stimulation. J Physiol 2003;551:661–71.

44. McKenzie DK, Bigland-Ritchie B, Gorman RB, et al. Central and peripheral fatigue of human diaphragm and limb muscles assessed by twitch interpolation. J Physiol 1992;454:643–56.

45. Schabrun SM, Stafford RE, Hodges PW. Anal sphincter fatigue: is the mechanism peripheral or central? Neurourol Urodyn 2011;30:1550–6.

46. Todd G, Petersen NT, Taylor JL, et al. The effect of a contralateral contraction on maximal voluntary activation and central fatigue in elbow flexor muscles. Exp Brain Res 2003;150:308–13.

47. Gruet M, Temesi J, Rupp T, et al. Stimulation of the motor cortex and corticospinal tract to assess human muscle fatigue. Neuroscience 2013;231:384–99.

48. Chen R. Interactions between inhibitory and excitatory circuits in the human motor cortex. Exp Brain Res 2004;154:1–10.

49. Schabrun SM, Hodges PW. Muscle pain differentially modulates short interval intracortical inhibition and intracortical facilitation in primary motor cortex. J Pain 2012;13:187–94.

50. Eisenberg E, Chistyakov AV, Yudashkin M, et al. Evidence for cortical hyperexcitability of the affected limb representation area in CRPS: a psychophysical and transcranial magnetic stimulation study. Pain 2005;113:99–105.

51. Masse-Alarie H, Flamand VH, Moffet H, et al. Corticomotor control of deep abdominal muscles in chronic low back pain and anticipatory postural adjustments. Exp Brain Res 2012;218:99–109.

52. Takahashi K, Maruyama A, Maeda M, et al. Unilateral grip fatigue reduces short interval intracortical inhibition in ipsilateral primary motor cortex. Clin Neurophysiol 2009;120:198–203.

53. Takahashi K, Maruyama A, Hirakoba K, et al. Fatiguing intermittent lower limb exercise influences corticospinal and corticocortical excitability in the nonexercised upper limb. Brain Stimul 2011;4:90–6.

54. Baumer T, Munchau A, Weiller C, et al. Fatigue suppresses ipsilateral intracortical facilitation. Exp Brain Res 2002;146:467–73.

55. Clark BC, Taylor JL, Hoffman RL, et al. Cast immobilization increases long-interval intracortical inhibition. Muscle Nerve 2010;42:363–72.

56. Nordstrom MA, Butler SL. Reduced intracortical inhibition and facilitation of corticospinal neurons in musicians. Exp Brain Res 2002;144:336–42.

57. Rosenkranz K, Williamon A, Rothwell JC. Motorcortical excitability and synaptic plasticity is enhanced in professional musicians. J Neurosci 2007;27:5200–6.

58. Berardelli A, Inghilleri M, Rothwell JC, et al. Facilitation of muscle evoked responses after repetitive cortical stimulation in man. Exp Brain Res 1998;122:79–84.

59. Pascual-Leone A, Valls-Sole J, Wassermann EM, et al. Responses to rapid-rate transcranial magnetic stimulation of the human motor cortex. Brain 1994;117(Pt 4):847–58.

60. Muellbacher W, Ziemann U, Boroojerdi B, et al. Effects of low-frequency transcranial magnetic stimulation on motor excitability and basic motor behavior. Clin Neurophysiol 2000;111:1002–7.

61. Fitzgerald PB, Fountain S, Daskalakis ZJ. A comprehensive review of the effects of rTMS on motor cortical excitability and inhibition. Clin Neurophysiol 2006;117:2584–96.

62. Huang YZ, Edwards MJ, Rounis E, et al. Theta burst stimulation of the human motor cortex. Neuron 2005;45:201–6.

63. Berner J, Schonfeldt-Lecuona C, Nowak DA. Sensorimotor memory for fingertip forces during object lifting: the role of the primary motor cortex. Neuropsychologia 2007;45:1931–8.

64. Nowak DA, Voss M, Huang YZ, et al. High-frequency repetitive transcranial magnetic stimulation over the hand area of the primary motor cortex disturbs predictive grip force scaling. Eur J Neurosci 2005;22:2392–6.

65. Schabrun SM, Ridding MC, Miles TS. Role of the primary motor and sensory cortex in precision grasping: a transcranial magnetic stimulation study. Eur J Neurosci 2008;27:750–6.

66. Davare M, Andres M, Cosnard G, et al. Dissociating the role of ventral and dorsal premotor cortex in precision grasping. J Neurosci 2006;26:2260–8.

67. Davare M, Andres M, Clerget E, et al. Temporal dissociation between hand shaping and grip force scaling in the anterior intra-parietal area. J Neurosci 2007;27:3974–80.

68. Schabrun SM, Chipchase LS. Priming the brain to learn: the future of therapy? Man Ther 2012;17:184–6.

69. Hosomi K, Shimokawa T, Ikoma K, et al. Daily repetitive transcra-nial magnetic stimulation of primary motor cortex for neuropathic pain: a randomized, multicenter, double-blind, crossover, sham-controlled trial. Pain 2013;154:1065–72.

70. Pleger B, Janssen F, Schwenkreis P, et al. Repetitive transcranial magnetic stimulation of the motor cortex attenuates pain percep-tion in complex regional pain syndrome type I. Neurosci Lett 2004;356:87–90.

71. Lee SJ, Kim DY, Chun MH, et al. The effect of repetitive trans-cranial magnetic stimulation on fibromyalgia: a randomized sham-controlled trial with 1-mo follow-up. Am J Phys Med Rehabil 2012;91:1077–85.

72. Mhalla A, Baudic S, Ciampi de AD, et al. Long-term maintenance of the analgesic effects of transcranial magnetic stimulation in fibromyalgia. Pain 2011;152:1478–85.

73. Passard A, Attal N, Benadhira R, et al. Effects of unilateral repeti-tive transcranial magnetic stimulation of the motor cortex on chronic widespread pain in fibromyalgia. Brain 2007;130:2661–70.

74. Sampson SM, Rome JD, Rummans TA. Slow-frequency rTMS reduces fibromyalgia pain. Pain Med 2006;7:115–18.

75. Louppe JM, Nguyen JP, Robert R, et al. Motor cortex stimulation in refractory pelvic and perineal pain: report of two successful cases. Neurourol Urodyn 2013;32:53–7.

76. Pallanti S, Di RA, Antonini S, et al. Low-frequency rTMS over right dorsolateral prefrontal cortex in the treatment of resistant depression: cognitive improvement is independent from clinical response, resting motor threshold is related to clinical response. Neuropsychobiology 2012;65:227–35.

77. Topper R, Foltys H, Meister IG, et al. Repetitive transcranial mag-netic stimulation of the parietal cortex transiently ameliorates phantom limb pain-like syndrome. Clin Neurophysiol 2003;114:1521–30.

78. Lefaucheur JP, Antal A, Ahdab R, et al. The use of repetitive trans-cranial magnetic stimulation (rTMS) and transcranial direct current stimulation (tDCS) to relieve pain. Brain Stimul 2008;1:337–44.

79. de Andrade DC, Mhalla A, Adam F, et al. Neuropharmacological basis of rTMS-induced analgesia: the role of endogenous opioids. Pain 2011;152:320–6.

80. Marlow NM, Bonilha HS, Short EB. Efficacy of transcranial direct current stimulation and repetitive transcranial magnetic stimulation for treating fibromyalgia syndrome: a systematic review. Pain Pract 2013;13:131–45.

81. Plow EB, Pascual-Leone A, Machado A. Brain stimulation in the treatment of chronic neuropathic and non-cancerous pain. J Pain 2012;13:411–24.

82. O'Connell NE, Wand BM, Marston L, et al. Non-invasive brain stimulation techniques for chronic pain. A report of a Cochrane systematic review and meta-analysis. Eur J Phys Rehabil Med 2011;47:309–26.

83. Chipchase LS, Williams MT, Robertson VJ. Factors affecting cur-riculum content and the integration of evidence-based practice in entry-level physiotherapy programs. J Allied Health 2007;36:17–23.

84. Robertson V, Ward A, Low J, et al. Electrotherapy explained. 4th ed. 2006.

85. Miranda PC, Lomarev M, Hallett M. Modeling the current distri-bution during transcranial direct current stimulation. Clin Neuro-physiol 2006;117:1623–9.

86. Wagner T, Valero-Cabre A, Pascual-Leone A. Noninvasive human brain stimulation. Annu Rev Biomed Eng 2007;9:527–65.

87. Nitsche MA, Seeber A, Frommann K, et al. Modulating parameters of excitability during and after transcranial direct current stimula-tion of the human motor cortex. J Physiol 2005;568:291–303.

88. O'Connell NE, Cossar J, Marston L, et al. Transcranial direct current stimulation of the motor cortex in the treatment of chronic nonspecific low back pain: a randomized, double-blind exploratory study. Clin J Pain 2013;29:26–34.

89. Fenton BW, Palmieri PA, Boggio P, et al. A preliminary study of transcranial direct current stimulation for the treatment of refrac-tory chronic pelvic pain. Brain Stimul 2009;2:103–7.

90. Fregni F, Gimenes R, Valle AC, et al. A randomized, sham-controlled, proof of principle study of transcranial direct current stimulation for the treatment of pain in fibromyalgia. Arthritis Rheum 2006;54:3988–98.

91. Valle A, Roizenblatt S, Botte S, et al. Efficacy of anodal transcranial direct current stimulation (tDCS) for the treatment of fibromyal-gia: results of a randomized, sham-controlled longitudinal clinical trial. J Pain Manag 2009;2:353–61.

92. Mori F, Codeca C, Kusayanagi H, et al. Effects of anodal transcra-nial direct current stimulation on chronic neuropathic pain in patients with multiple sclerosis. J Pain 2010;11:436–42.

93. Fregni F, Boggio PS, Lima MC, et al. A sham-controlled, phase II trial of transcranial direct current stimulation for the treatment of central pain in traumatic spinal cord injury. Pain 2006;122:197–209.

94. Garcia-Larrea L, Peyron R, Mertens P, et al. Electrical stimulation of motor cortex for pain control: a combined PET-scan and elec-trophysiological study. Pain 1999;83:259–73.

95. Strafella AP, Vanderwerf Y, Sadikot AF. Transcranial magnetic stimulation of the human motor cortex influences the neuronal activity of subthalamic nucleus. Eur J Neurosci 2004;20:2245–9.

96. Poreisz C, Boros K, Antal A, et al. Safety aspects of transcranial direct current stimulation concerning healthy subjects and patients. Brain Res Bull 2007;72:208–14.

CHAPTER 19

MUSCULOSKELETAL MODELLING

Mark de Zee • John Rasmussen

INTRODUCTION

Consideration of the load on the musculoskeletal system is relevant in physiotherapy for both diagnosis and treatment of musculoskeletal conditions. The first consideration is the cause of an injury that could be due to overloading of the musculoskeletal system in sports or in occupational circumstances. The next step is to modify the system via an intervention. This could be an exercise intervention which aims to change the loading of the musculoskeletal system. However, the therapist cannot quantify the load on different structures of the musculoskeletal system and will not know how or in what way an intervention changes the load. Surface electromyography (EMG) may provide an indication about the change in muscle coordination,[1] but this technique does not provide an indication about the load on different structures. Knowledge of the muscle, ligament and joint reaction forces inside the human body may help to improve clinical decision making or improve the understanding of a specific treatment. However, single muscle forces, ligament forces and joint reaction forces are extremely difficult and in many cases impossible to measure in vivo. The only viable possibility for estimating the forces inside the human body is to make use of computational modelling of the musculoskeletal system based on the laws of physics.

There are many examples in the literature where the technology of musculoskeletal modelling has been applied within areas related to physiotherapy. For example, Pontonnier et al.[2] demonstrated the use of musculoskeletal modelling in occupational health by predicting the optimal bench height for meat cutting tasks. Alkjær et al.[3] investigated the function of the cruciate ligaments during a forward lunge exercise using a musculoskeletal model. Their study indicated that the posterior cruciate ligament had an important stabilizing role in the forward lunge movement, while the anterior cruciate ligament did not have any significant mechanical function during this task. Furthermore, they showed that the gluteus maximus muscle may play a role as a knee stabilizer in addition to the hamstring muscles. Rasmussen et al.[4] demonstrated the use of musculoskeletal modelling to provide insight in to the complex relationship of chair design and seat posture on muscle activity and spinal joint forces. As a last example, Dubowsky et al.[5] estimated the shoulder joint forces during wheelchair propulsion using a musculoskeletal model of the upper limb and this model could be used to identify the optimal axle placement in order to lower the forces on the shoulder joint.

Erdemir et al.[6] wrote an extensive review describing different methods to estimate muscle forces using musculoskeletal modelling. In this chapter the focus will be on musculoskeletal modelling based on inverse dynamics and optimization. The theory behind this methodology will be explained and two examples will be given of how musculoskeletal modelling can be applied and what information can be gained from these models.

BASICS OF MUSCULOSKELETAL MODELLING BASED ON INVERSE DYNAMICS

Biomechanics, as all mechanics, is essentially based on the laws of Newton. Newton's second law states:

$$F = ma \qquad [1]$$

where F is the sum of forces acting on a body, m is the mass of the body and a is its acceleration. In spatial coordinates, F and a are three-dimensional. As with any equation, we can determine one property if the other properties are known. Let us presume that m is known. This leaves us with the following two options:

1. If we know the sum of forces, F, then we can determine the acceleration and thereby the motion.
2. If we know the motion and thereby the acceleration a, then we can determine the sum of forces that must have affected the body in order to generate the motion.

Newton's second law applies to particles and can be extended to rigid bodies and even to mechanisms (i.e. several rigid bodies connected by joints) if m is interpreted as mass moment of inertia and mass, F as moments and forces and a as angular and linear accelerations. These equations are called the Newton–Euler equations and they are much more complicated than Newton's second law, but they are essentially structured the same way and describe the same relationships between masses, forces and motions. So even for very complex mechanisms, such as the human body with its hundreds of bones, we can determine the motion if we know the forces and vice versa.

If we know the forces, we can define the motions, and if we know the motions, we can determine the forces. There is more than an academic difference to the two approaches. It is very complicated experimentally to determine all the forces acting on the human body, since many of these come from muscles that are voluntarily or involuntarily activated by the central nervous system. However, several methods are available to capture motions of living organisms, for instance by photogrammetry, so motions can be found experimentally and can be used to compute forces, whereas the opposite is complicated. In many ergonomically relevant cases, the body can be presumed to be static or analysed in certain key frames and, in this case, the kinematics of the problem is even simpler. The process of finding forces from motions is called *inverse dynamics*.

A Simple Example

Let us consider the simplified example of a lifting task as shown in Figure 19-1 and the associated free body diagram in Figure 19-2.

Despite the anatomical reality we shall consider the spinal joint as a perfect two-dimensional hinge in which two reaction force components, R_x and R_y, are working. We disregard the self-weight of the body segments and consider the system loaded only by the gravity force of the lifted load, F_g. We consider initially only the muscle force, F_m, from a branch of the erector spinae muscle.

We start by the moment equilibrium about the spinal joint:

$$F_g s_1 - F_m s_2 = 0$$
$$\Downarrow$$
$$F_m = \frac{F_g s_1}{s_2}$$

Horizontal equilibrium yields:

$$R_x - F_{mx} = 0$$
$$\Downarrow$$
$$R_x = F_{mx} = F_m \cos(\theta)$$

All that remains now is to determine R_y from vertical equilibrium:

$$R_y - F_{my} - F_g = 0$$
$$\Downarrow$$
$$R_y = F_{my} + F_g = F_m \sin(\theta) + F_g$$

Let us insert some plausible numbers:

$$\theta = 30°, s_1 = 0.5 \text{ m}, s_2 = 0.04 \text{ m}, F_g = 200 \text{ N}$$

This leads to the following forces in the system:

$$F_m = 2500 \text{ N}$$
$$R_x = 2169 \text{ N}$$
$$R_y = 1450 \text{ N}$$

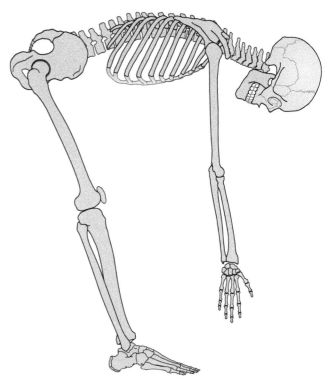

FIGURE 19-1 ■ Illustration of a lifting situation.

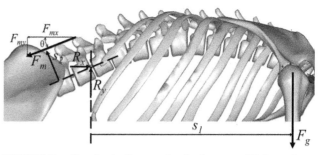

FIGURE 19-2 ■ Free body diagram for the force equilibrium about a spinal joint.

The external force of just 200 N leads to internal forces that are an order of magnitude larger, and this is typical for the human body; our internal forces are larger than most people imagine. The mechanical explanation is that the moment arms of the external forces are typically larger than the moment arms of the muscles or, in physiological terms, the moment arms of muscles correspond to the thickness of limbs while the external forces' moment arms correspond to the length of limbs. Although the strength of our tissues is substantial, injuries can occur when, for instance, we lift a heavy load.

Despite this example being static, it is in reality *inverse dynamics* in its simplest form: We know the posture and the velocity (in this case the velocity is zero) of the elements in the system, and we also know the external forces acting on the system. With this input we can compute the internal forces (i.e. the muscle force and the joint reaction force). However, we can only do this by hand if the situation is very simple. Muscle systems tend to be complicated and the spine is a good example: it is three-dimensional, it contains many degrees-of-freedom, it is actuated by many muscles, actually hundreds if we consider all the different muscle fascicles and real-life loading situations are rarely static.

Coping with such complexities requires more computational power and software systems particularly developed for the purpose. The development of physiologically realistic models for use in such systems is also a complex task. Figure 19-3 shows an example.

EXAMPLE 1: SIMULATED CHANGES IN LUMBAR MUSCLE ACTIVATION FROM A PELVIC TILT

Back pain is a complex and generally poorly understood problem, and back pain may even be associated with other types of musculoskeletal pain.[7] Numerous clinical[8–10] and experimental studies[11] have confirmed alterations in back muscle activation as a result of back pain. However, the changes of muscle activity in response to postural change are complex and for unilateral pain they are not confined to the ipsilateral side and they do not correlate with the level of pain. It is possible that pain evolves beyond the original injury through the process illustrated in Figure 19-4.

To investigate the potential for improved understanding of back pain development through musculoskeletal simulation, pelvis lateral tilt typical of one-sided back pain was imposed in small steps on an otherwise symmetrical computational model[12] of a standing individual, and the reconfiguration of muscle loads was reviewed. The pelvic tilt was accompanied by a compensatory lateral flexion of the lumbar spine in such a way that static balance of the model was maintained.

A graph of the activation development of the hundreds of spinal muscles in the model for increasing pelvis tilt is depicted in Figure 19-5.

The model shows a complex increase of muscle activation levels for the model as a result of the postural change (Fig. 19-6). The primarily affected muscle groups are branches of psoas major, quadratus lumborum and obliquus internus, where the increase of activity level is significant from 0 to more than 5%. The increase of muscle activation concerns both sides of the body.

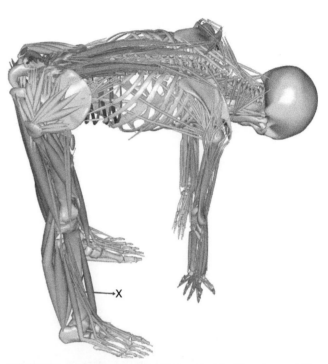

FIGURE 19-3 ■ Model of human lifting a load with spine and hip flexion. The model is developed in the AnyBody Modelling System™ and comprises more than 1000 individually activated muscles. The colour shading of the muscles indicates the level of activity. X indicates the x-direction of the global coordinate system. For colour version see Plate 19.

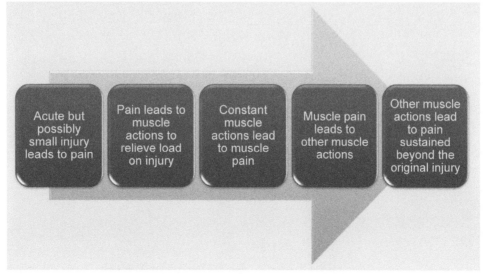

FIGURE 19-4 ■ Possible development of acute back pain.

This model shows that a relatively small asymmetrical postural change as seen in Figure 19-5 requires a complex reorganization of the muscle activation pattern. If the duration of the pain requires maintenance of the asymmetrical posture constantly, the constant loading of these muscles may lead to muscle soreness, injury and evolving pain.

EXAMPLE 2: UNDERSTANDING THE RECRUITMENT OF THE SEMISPINALIS CERVICIS MUSCLE USING MUSCULOSKELETAL MODELLING

The cervical spine is a complex structure with many degrees of freedom and complicated kinematics.[13] In

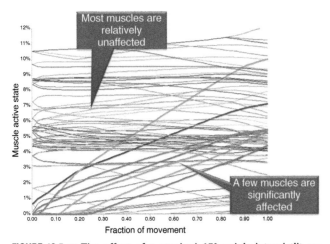

FIGURE 19-5 ■ The effect of a gradual 15° pelvic lateral tilt on muscle activation in the lumbar spine. For colour version see Plate 19.

order to be able to control the head in three-dimensional space the cervical spine has multiple muscles. Many of those muscles span several joints, which makes it very difficult to judge or predict a muscle action without performing a full multi-body analysis based on the equations of motion. Recently, Schomacher et al.[14] investigated the recruitment of semispinalis cervicis muscle at the levels of the second (C2) and fifth (C5) cervical vertebrae using intramuscular EMG during isometric neck extensions. They found significantly greater EMG amplitude at C5 than at C2. This was explained by the fact that the external moment around C5–C6 is larger than the external moment around C2–C3. One has to realize that the semispinalis cervicis is a complex muscle, with multiple fascicles that originate from the transverse processes of the upper five or six vertebrae and insert on the cervical spinous processes, with each fascicle spanning four to six segments. This makes it indeed difficult to explain precisely the mechanical action without taking the full three-dimensional multi-body analysis into account. The goal of this example is to show that the recruitment of the semispinalis cervicis can be predicted using a musculoskeletal model of the cervical spine purely based on the equations of motion and optimization principles. Moreover, it will be demonstrated that the analysis will give additional information about the loading of the cervical spine.

Description of the Cervical Spine Model and Simulation

The three-dimensional musculoskeletal model of the cervical spine was built using the AnyBody Modelling System (AnyBody Technology A/S, Aalborg, Denmark). The model consists of nine rigid segments: skull, seven cervical vertebrae and the thoracic region. The joints between the vertebrae from T1 to C2 are modelled as

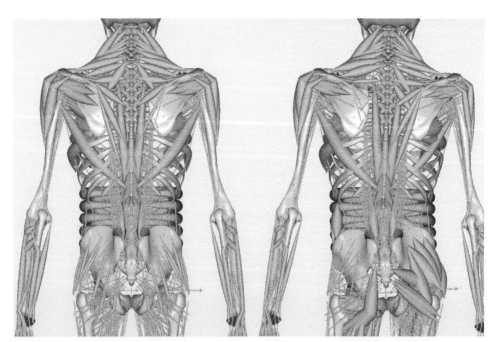

FIGURE 19-6 ■ Alteration of muscle forces (illustrated by the thickness of each fascicle) from symmetrical standing (left) to 10° pelvic lateral tilt (right). For colour version see Plate 19.

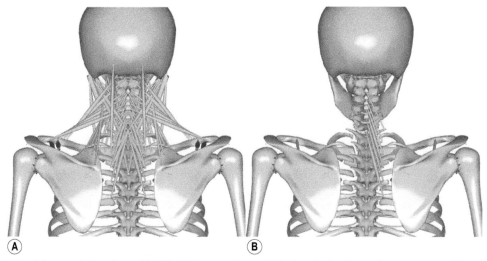

FIGURE 19-7 ■ Model of the cervical spine with (**A**) all the muscle and (**B**) the six fascicles of the semispinalis cervicis on the right side. For colour version see Plate 20.

three degrees-of-freedom spherical joints, while the joints between C2 and the skull are modelled as one degree-of-freedom revolute joints. The locations of the centres of rotations are based on the work of Amevo et al.[15] The model is equipped with 136 muscle actuators and the muscle parameters are based on the work by Van der Horst.[16] Figure 19-7A illustrates the cervical spine model and Figure 19-7B provides an illustration of how the semispinalis cervicis was implemented in the model. The semispinalis cervicis is modelled as six independent fascicles. The most cranial fascicle spans from T1 to C2, while the most caudal fascicle spans from T6 to C7. The maximal force these fascicles can produce in the model is based on their physiological cross-sectional areas and these values were based on the work by Van der Horst.[16] The physiological cross-sectional area of the semispinalis cervicis is increasing from the cranial to caudal direction starting with 0.13 cm² for the most cranial fascicle to 1.1 cm² for the most caudal fascicle.

In the simulation, the model was forced to create a ramped extension moment in 5 seconds from 0 to around 50% of the model's maximum capacity in extension. This was to mimic the ramped extension contractions in the experiments reported by Schomacher et al.[14] The activities of the different fascicles of the semispinalis cervicis were now predicted for the generation of these ramped extension moments plus the reaction forces between the vertebrae were determined. For these calculations the polynomial muscle recruitment was used with the power of three. It is assumed that all fascicles of all muscles work independently from each other.

Results

Figure 19-8 shows the predicted activity for the six fascicles of the semispinalis cervicis during the ramped extension task. It can be seen that the three caudal fascicles T6C7, T5C6 and T4C5 show much higher activity than the three cranial fascicles. The prediction also showed that the timing between the fascicles is different.

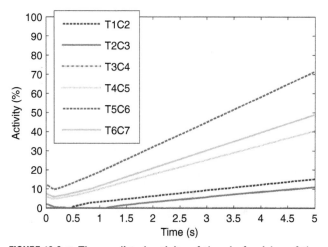

FIGURE 19-8 ■ The predicted activity of the six fascicles of the semispinalis cervicis during ramped extension. For colour version see Plate 20.

For example the fascicle T1C2 starts its activation after about 0.5 seconds while the T5C6 is active from the start.

Figure 19-9 shows the predicted absolute force levels in the fascicles of the semispinalis cervicis during the ramped extension. The difference between the caudal and cranial fascicles is now even more pronounced than when only considering the predicted activity. The cranial fascicles have small force levels below 2 N, while the highest caudal fascicle reaches 25 N.

Figure 19-10 shows the predicted reaction forces between the vertebrae. One should be aware that these forces are the products of all muscle forces around the cervical spine, and not only the semispinalis cervicis. It can be seen that the predicted forces increase from the cranial to the caudal direction with the highest force of around 700 N occurring between T1 and C7. This is a high force for a submaximal isometric neck extension contraction.

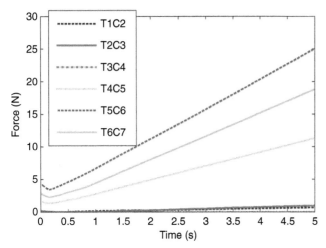

FIGURE 19-9 ■ The predicted force in the six fascicles of the semispinalis cervicis during ramped extension. For colour version see Plate 20.

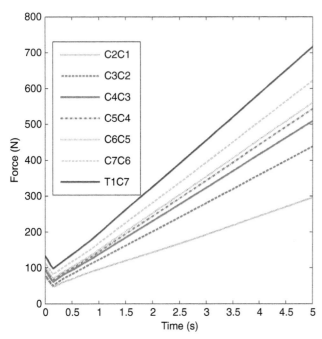

FIGURE 19-10 ■ The predicted reaction forces between the vertebrae in the cervical spine during ramped extension. For colour version see Plate 21.

The goal of this example was to demonstrate that it is possible to obtain detailed information from a relatively simple analysis, namely a ramped extension moment in 5 seconds from 0 to around 50% of the model's capacity. The model predicts varying levels of activity in the different fascicles of the semispinalis cervicis depending on the location of the fascicle. The complex experiment performed by Schomacher et al.[14] also showed that individual fascicles of the semispinalis cervicis muscle are activated partly independently. However, due to the invasive nature of this experiment (fine-wire EMG), recordings of the activity of the semispinalis cervicis were limited to two levels, the C2 and C5 levels. In contrast, the model gives information on all fascicles of the

semispinalis cervicis in addition to the many other muscles of the cervical region. It is also interesting to note that Schomacher et al.[14] observed an earlier recruitment of the caudal fascicles in comparison with the cranial fascicles during the extension contraction. The model predicted the same, but this prediction was purely based on the equilibrium equations and optimization as explained in the paragraph about the basics of musculoskeletal modelling.

The biggest advantage of a musculoskeletal model is that the output contains information which would not be possible to measure in an experimental setup. The results depicted in Figures 19-9 and 19-10 are an example of this. The absolute forces in the fascicles of the semispinalis cervicis show a clear distinction between the caudal and cranial regions. The combination of higher predicted activations and a larger cross-sectional area in the caudal region results in higher absolute forces in these fascicles. The combination of all muscle forces around the cervical spine leads to reaction forces between the cervical vertebrae. Those reaction forces are also impossible to measure in an experimental setup. The result that the highest reaction forces are between the caudal vertebrae is not surprising, since the external extension moment, which has to be balanced, increases linearly with the distance from the force vector on the skull. The model also gives an estimate of the quantity of each reaction force and shows high forces between the caudal vertebrae. This may partially explain why most disc herniations are observed in the caudal region of the cervical spine.[17]

CONCLUSION AND PERSPECTIVES

Musculoskeletal modelling is generally used for two purposes. The first purpose is to increase our understanding of the loads working in the musculoskeletal system under different circumstances, including in patients. The second purpose is the use of musculoskeletal modelling in clinical applications. As Erdemir et al.[6] already indicated, the use of musculoskeletal modelling in the clinic is still limited, but promising developments are now taking place.

One of the key requirements for using musculoskeletal modelling in the clinic is that the model resembles a certain patient. So there is a need for patient-specific modelling. Pellikaan et al.[18] showed that with a combination of imaging technology and morphing algorithms they were able to estimate subject-specific muscle attachment sites in the lower extremity in a fast and automated manner.

The second requirement for using musculoskeletal models in the clinic is the need for validation. When a model would be used for critical decisions in a treatment of a patient, the consequences of erroneous models can be very serious. Recently, Lund et al.[19] published a review about validation methods of musculoskeletal models and provided a number of recommendations. One of the recommendations is a stronger focus on trend validation. One of the promising uses of a musculoskeletal model in the clinic would be the investigation of so-called 'what if' scenarios. For example, what would happen with the reaction force in the knee if we could strengthen the vastus medialis? To answer these questions the model parameters have to interact with each other in the correct way, and this can be tested using trend validation. An example of a trend validation was the work of Pontonnier et al.[2] where they changed the bench height during simulated meat cutting tasks in a systematic way and the same was done in the model. The EMG outputs of certain shoulder muscles were then compared with the model outputs as a function of bench height.

In conclusion, musculoskeletal modelling provides a multitude of quantitative information of the loading of the musculoskeletal system; information which would otherwise be very difficult or impossible to measure in vivo. Musculoskeletal models have therefore been used extensively in research. For widespread clinical use of musculoskeletal models, further work is necessary, progress is being made both with respect to imaging technology to build patient-specific models and validation.

REFERENCES

1. Hug F. Can muscle coordination be precisely studied by surface electromyography? J Electromyogr Kinesiol 2011 2;21(1):1–12.
2. Pontonnier C, de Zee M, Samani A, et al. Strengths and limitations of a musculoskeletal model for an analysis of simulated meat cutting tasks. Appl Ergon 2014;45(3):592–600.
3. Alkjær T, Wieland MR, Andersen MS, et al. Computational modeling of a forward lunge: towards a better understanding of the function of the cruciate ligaments. J Anat 2012;221(6):590–7.
4. Rasmussen J, Tørholm S, de Zee M. Computational analysis of the influence of seat pan inclination and friction on muscle activity and spinal joint forces. Int J Ind Ergon 2009 1;39(1):52–7.
5. Dubowsky SR, Rasmussen J, Sisto SA, et al. Validation of a musculoskeletal model of wheelchair propulsion and its application to minimizing shoulder joint forces. J Biomech 2008;41(14):2981–8.
6. Erdemir A, McLean S, Herzog W, et al. Model-based estimation of muscle forces exerted during movements. Clin Biomech 2007;22(2):131–54.
7. Hartvigsen J, Natvig B, Ferreira M. Is it all about a pain in the back? Best Pract Res Clin Rheumatol 2013;10;27(5):613–23.
8. Ferreira PH, Ferreira ML, Hodges PW. Changes in recruitment of the abdominal muscles in people with low back pain. Spine 2004;29(22):2560–6.
9. Lamoth CJC, Meijer OG, Daffertshofer A, et al. Effects of chronic low back pain on trunk coordination and back muscle activity during walking: changes in motor control. Eur Spine J 2006;15(1): 23–40.
10. Lamoth C, Meijer O, Wuisman P, et al. Pelvis-thorax coordination in the transverse plane during walking in persons with nonspecific low back pain. Spine 2002;27(4):E92–9.
11. Dickx N, Cagnie B, Achten E, et al. Changes in lumbar muscle activity because of induced muscle pain evaluated by muscle functional magnetic resonance imaging. Spine 2008;33(26):E983–9.
12. de Zee M, Hansen L, Wong C, et al. A generic detailed rigid-body lumbar spine model. J Biomech 2007;40(6):1219–27.
13. Bogduk N, Mercer S. Biomechanics of the cervical spine. I: Normal kinematics. Clin Biomech 2000;15(9):633–48.
14. Schomacher J, Dideriksen JL, Farina D, et al. Recruitment of motor units in two fascicles of the semispinalis cervicis muscle. J Neurophysiol 2012;107(11):3078–85.
15. Amevo B, Worth D, Bogduk N. Instantaneous axes of rotation of the typical cervical motion segments: a study in normal volunteers. Clin Biomech 1991;6(2):111–17.
16. van der Horst MJ. Human Head Neck Response in Frontal, Lateral and Rear End Impact Loading: Modelling and Validation. Eindhoven: Technische Universiteit Eindhoven; 2002.
17. Mann E, Peterson CK, Hodler J. Degenerative marrow (modic) changes on cervical spine magnetic resonance imaging scans. Spine 2011;36(14):1081–5.
18. Pellikaan P, van der Krogt MM, Carbone V, et al. Evaluation of a morphing based method to estimate muscle attachment sites of the lower extremity. J Biomech 2014;47(5):1144–50.
19. Lund ME, de Zee M, Andersen MS, et al. On validation of multibody musculoskeletal models. Proc Inst Mech Eng [H] 2012;226(2): 82–94.

CHAPTER 20

QUANTITATIVE SENSORY TESTING: IMPLICATIONS FOR CLINICAL PRACTICE

Toby Hall • Kathy Briffa • Axel Schäfer • Brigitte Tampin • Niamh Moloney

Sensory examination is a critical component of the assessment of a wide range of clinical conditions, including musculoskeletal and neuropathic disorders. Bedside examination of the somatosensory system includes the assessment of touch/vibration/proprioception (large myelinated Aβ fibres) pinprick/blunt pressure sensitivity (small thinly myelinated Aδ and small unmyelinated C fibres), cold (Aδ fibres) and heat (C fibres) sensitivity utilizing simple equipment such as cotton wool, tuning fork, tooth pick, digital pressure, and cold and warm stimuli such as test tubes or coins (Table 20-1). Sensory loss (loss of function) and/or gain of function (hypersensitivity) would be documented; the borders of changes established and findings compared with the contralateral side if symptoms are unilateral. The bedside assessment may reveal a sensory deficit or evoke pain that can then be interpreted in the context of its location and distribution. Limitations of the bedside examination are that stimulus intensities are generally not calibrated and testing procedures are not standardized.[1]

Quantitative sensory testing (QST) is a complimentary approach that utilizes some more sophisticated equipment and standardized testing protocols to allow quantification of the stimuli applied during testing. Consequently, QST delivers more precise outcomes. It is important to recognize, however, that QST is not an objective assessment of pain or sensation, nor is it specifically diagnostic.[3] Rather, QST is a psychophysical method of assessment in which objective stimuli are applied and subjects' responses are quantified and recorded. Hence, cognitive factors may influence a patient's responses.[4] QST can also be influenced by environmental factors such as ambient temperature and noise, and methodological factors such as test protocol, instructions and application of the test.[5,6] QST can be used in research and clinical contexts.

Despite strong research interest, incorporation of QST procedures into clinical practice has been slow. This may be due to poor knowledge regarding standards for application, lack of information about its clinical utility,[1] and time-consuming procedures and costly equipment. The purpose of this chapter is to describe QST and its use in research, as well as its potential role in clinical practice.

QUANTITATIVE SENSORY TESTING

A variety of sensory stimuli can be used for QST (Table 20-1). With appropriate choice of stimuli and testing protocols QST can be used to evaluate the integrity of the entire sensory system, including thinly myelinated Aδ fibres, unmyelinated C fibres and large-diameter Aβ fibres as well as the dorsal column and spinothalamic tract,[3,7] assessing sensory pathways from the peripheral receptor to the central cortex.[2] It is unique in that it can be used to measure the function of all sensory nerve fibres as well as the peripheral and central processing of sensation.[8] It has the ability to quantify both loss and gain of sensory function, detecting even subtle changes in nociceptive pathways missed by conventional nerve conduction tests, which can only assess loss of function in large Aβ fibres.[9] As a consequence, a number of aspects of sensory function can be evaluated including the primary afferents that mediate innocuous and painful sensation, central processes that further alter the character and sensitivity of the primary afferents[10] and the clinical manifestations of peripheral and central sensitization.[4,11]

IMPORTANCE OF STANDARDIZING PROTOCOLS

A number of different QST protocols have been developed. Typically they include various mechanical and thermal stimuli testing detection and pain thresholds.[2,9,12]

In order to generate reliable QST results it is critical that the test stimulus and examination procedure are standardized and protocols strictly adhered to. Variations in technical equipment used to generate stimuli and associated factors such as the size of the stimulated area and rate of change of stimulus can influence the results and have implications for comparing data between patients and between different research groups. For these reasons normative data must be protocol-specific. Moreover, values vary according to the body site being measured and, for some parameters, there are age- and gender-related differences. It is imperative therefore that reference data used for the interpretation of test results have been collected using the *same* protocols and *well-matched* healthy controls. In many cases this means that the test laboratory must collect their own normative reference data.

The reliability of QST has been demonstrated in multiple studies.[13–18] However, it has to be acknowledged that all reliability data are protocol- and population-specific and statistical analyses vary between reliability studies, hence reliability coefficients are not necessarily comparable between studies. As with reference data, in view of

TABLE 20-1 Modalities, Receptors and Testing Methods[2]

QST Parameter	Laboratory Test	Clinical Test	Principal Receptors and Axon Type	Postulated Mechanism of Hyperalgesia/ Allodynia	Clinical Relevance
Mechanical					
Vibration threshold	Graded tuning fork or vibrometer	Tuning fork	Pacinian, Aβ	Unknown	Lemniscal
Mechanical detection thresholds	Calibrated von Frey filaments	Cotton wool	Aβ		Lemniscal
Punctate pain thresholds	Pin or calibrated sharp metal pin pricks	Toothpick	Unencapsulated, Aδ and C		Spinothalamic
Pressure pain threshold	Algometer	Analogue Algometer, thumb	Intramuscular afferents, iii and iv Aδ and C	Unknown	Spinothalamic
Dynamic mechanical	Brush, cotton wool, Q-tip	Brush, cotton wool, Q-tip	Meissner's Pacinian, hair follicle Aβ and C	Central sensitization	Lemniscal
Wind-up	Pin prick	Toothpick	Aδ	Central sensitization, reduced inhibition	Spinothalamic
Thermal					
Cold detection threshold	Computer-controlled thermotester	Thermoroller, test tubes, coins	Unencapsulated, Aδ		Spinothalamic
Warm detection threshold		Thermoroller, test tubes, coins	Unencapsulated, C		Spinothalamic
Cold pain threshold		Thermoroller, test tubes, ice cube, cold pressor test	Unencapsulated Aδ and C	Central and peripheral sensitization, reduced inhibition	Spinothalamic
Heat pain threshold		Thermoroller, test tubes	Unencapsulated Aδ and C	peripheral sensitization	Spinothalamic

QST, Quantitative sensory testing.

the specificity of QST results to testing protocols, unless published QST protocols are being adhered to strictly, it would be prudent for most groups to undertake their own well-designed reliability studies rather than assuming reliability in their hands will be comparable to published values.

In view of the specificity of results to testing parameters, the German Research Network on Neuropathic Pain (DFNS) has developed a comprehensive battery of quantitative sensory tests that combined, provide a complete somatosensory profile[17,19,20] for which there are validation and normative data accumulating in the literature.[21-23] It is comprised of seven tests that are used to measure 13 parameters. These tests are described in detail in the literature[19] and will not be reproduced in detail here; however, methods documented in this chapter are part of the DFNS protocol. The DFNS also have processes and procedures in place to train clinicians and researchers in QST in order to guarantee standardized QST between users. This could be advantageous for clinics and research facilities wishing to incorporate QST into their assessment and data collection regimens, as it would validate their use of DFNS reference data.[22] Another advantage of these protocols is that published reliability data are available for comparison.[17] Although the standardized DFNS protocol has many advantages, it must be recognized that QST is a broader concept than just one protocol and there are many valid and reliable

testing stimuli and protocols that are not part of the DFNS protocol.

TEST PARAMETERS

Mechanical Quantitative Sensory Testing

Vibration Thresholds

Vibration thresholds are typically measured by a vibrometer or Rydel-Seiffer graded tuning fork[19] (Fig. 20-1) placed against a bony point where it is left until the vibration can no longer be felt. Reduced vibration sense has been identified as an indicator for the presence of peripheral nerve damage in diabetic neuropathy,[24,25] in peripheral nerve injuries,[26,27] cervical and lumbar radiculopathies[28-32] and in patient groups with neuropathic pain.[33] Reduced vibration sense in people with non-specific neck–arm pain[34-39] was proposed to reflect the presence of a minor neuropathy.[34,35] However, the finding of widespread vibration threshold alterations in this patient population[40] suggests that altered central processing,[39] possibly secondary to pain,[41] may be an important underlying mechanism explaining this finding. Furthermore, reduced vibration sense has been documented in other musculoskeletal, non-neuropathic pain conditions such as knee and hip osteoarthritis,[42,43] temporomandibular joint disorders[44]

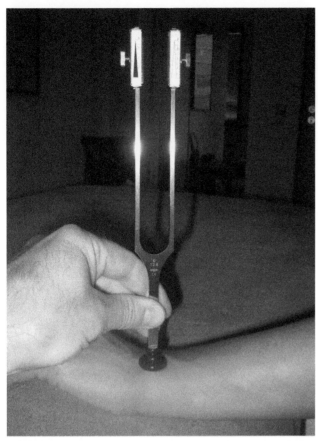

FIGURE 20-1 ■ Vibration threshold evaluation using a graded tuning fork.

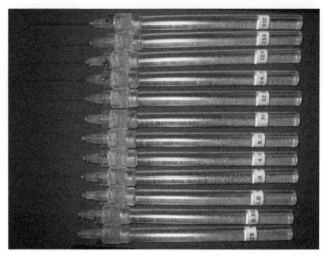

FIGURE 20-2 ■ Mechanical detection threshold evaluation using a calibrated filament.

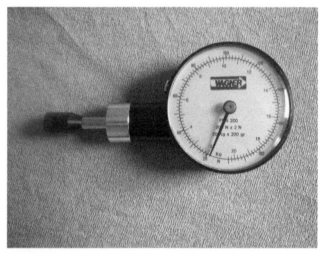

FIGURE 20-3 ■ Pressure pain threshold evaluation using a pressure algometer.

and fibromyalgia.[32,45] Therefore, any evidence of altered vibration thresholds must be interpreted within the context of the overall clinical presentation, rather than as a stand-alone method of assessment. Increased vibration sensitivity (vibration allodynia) has been reported as an indicator of altered central processing.[46]

Light Touch

Mechanical detection thresholds are measured using calibrated von Frey hairs that exert specific forces upon bending that vary according to the stiffness of the hair used (Fig. 20-2). Reduced mechanical detection can be indicative of a peripheral nerve lesion if the topographic area follows a plausible neuroanatomical distribution.[27,30–32,45,47] Elevated mechanical detection thresholds have also been found in people suffering from musculoskeletal pain disorders,[48] joint arthropathies[49] and fibromyalgia.[21,32] In this regard, tactile hypoaesthesia does not specifically indicate structural nerve fibre damage and may relate to central nervous system plasticity.[33] Careful mapping of the distribution of sensory changes may enable identification of the location of nerve injury: peripheral nerve, plexus, or nerve root.

Heightened sensitivity to light touch is referred to as mechanical allodynia that can be classified into static and dynamic mechanical allodynia, depending on which stimulus is used. Dynamic mechanical allodynia can be assessed using different degrees of soft contact force on the skin, gently brushing/stroking the skin with a cotton wisp (3 mN), a cotton wool tip (100 mN) or a brush (200–400 mN). Light touch allodynia in an area of secondary hyperalgesia is mediated by large myelinated Aβ fibres[50] and results from sensitization of nociceptive neurons in the dorsal horn due to C fibre discharge.[51–54] Dynamic mechanical allodynia is considered the hallmark sign of central sensitization.[55]

Pressure Pain Thresholds

Pressure pain thresholds are measured using a pressure algometer (Fig. 20-3). A flat probe is applied to the skin, pressure is gradually increased and the subject is asked to indicate the onset of pain. Loss of function (hypoaesthesia) as well as a gain of function (hyperalgesia) can be established. Pressure pain thresholds have been investigated in a diverse range of disorders, including non-specific neck–arm pain, cervical radiculopathy, neck pain, whiplash-associated disorder, knee osteoarthritis, patellofemoral pain, low back pain and low-back-related leg pain.[2,3,7–9,19,33,56] Increased pressure sensitivity has been found within anatomically local and distal sites in people with whiplash-associated disorders, non-specific arm pain and cervical radiculopathy when compared with asymptomatic groups.[28] Increased pressure sensitivity at a distal point may suggest widespread sensitization, while local changes alone may indicate peripheral nerve dysfunction. Interestingly, in people undergoing total knee replacement, pre-operative increased pressure pain sensitivity at a remote site (forearm), but not at the knee, showed a weak ($r = 0.37$) but significant correlation with worse pain scores using the WOMAC at 1-year follow-up.[49] Similar associations between QST measures and recovery were found across a range of different surgeries including thoracic surgery,[57] subacromial decompression[58] and herniotomy.[59]

Mechanical Pain Thresholds

Mechanical pain thresholds can be measured using calibrated weighted pinprick stimulators[19] (Fig. 20-4). The tip of the stimulator is gently placed on the skin and maintained for a duration of 2 seconds and subjects are asked to indicate if the stimulus feels sharp or blunt and/or if the stimulus is painful. Hyperalgesia to pinprick is induced by C fibre discharges and mediated by Aδ fibres (heterosynaptic facilitation),[60] leading to central sensitization to the input of A fibre nociceptors.[53] Loss of function may be indicative of neuropathy, while a gain of function may be indicative of peripheral and central sensitization.[53]

Temporal Summation of Pain (Wind-Up Ratio)

Wind-up is defined as the summation of repeated C fibre input to produce an augmented response.[61,62] Although not fully understood, it is thought that the mechanism of wind-up relates to the depolarization of neurons and the activation of the N-methyl-D-aspartate receptor.[62] This process results in the progressive increase in the action potential discharge elicited by each C fibre stimulus, such that relatively brief input can produce rapid and long-lasting changes in excitability. Wind-up can be assessed with thermal or punctate stimuli.

An example for the latter is the wind-up protocol of the DFNS. The perceived magnitude of a single pinprick stimulus is compared with that of a series of ten pinprick stimuli of the same force repeated at a rate of one per second given within the same location.[19] A pain rating is given for the first stimulus and for the series of ten pinpricks using a 0–100 scale. The pain rating of repeated pinprick stimuli is divided by the pain rating of the single stimulus to provide the wind-up ratio.

Thermal Quantitative Sensory Testing

Thermal detection and pain thresholds (cold and heat) are measured using a thermal sensory testing device (Fig. 20-5). A thermode is placed on the skin, the temperature of which can be altered ramping up and down in precise increments, typically in 1°C per second. For the measurement of detection thresholds the subject is asked to indicate when they feel a change in temperature, for pain thresholds the subject is asked to indicate as soon as the stimulus becomes painful.

Thermal QST has been investigated in many common musculoskeletal pain disorders including non-specific neck–arm pain, cervical radiculopathy, neck pain, whiplash-associated disorder, knee osteoarthritis, patellofemoral pain, low-back-related leg pain among others,[1,6–9,19,33,56] with some variation in findings.

Reduced thermal detection, indicated when the subject takes longer to feel the change of temperature, can be indicative of a loss of small nerve fibre function. Reduced thermal detection was evident on the symptomatic side in patients with cervical and lumbar radiculopathy,[29–31,63] findings suggestive of nerve root damage. However, some studies demonstrated a bilateral loss of function in patients with unilateral nerve injury.[29–31,63–65] It is hypothesized that bilateral hypoaesthesia may be mediated by peripheral nerve damage-induced central plasticity.[66] Widespread hypoaesthesia was also present in whiplash patients, suggestive of disordered central pain processing.[67]

Increased heat sensitivity implicates mechanisms of peripheral sensitization and has been demonstrated in various musculoskeletal disorders.[50,68] Cold sensitivity measured in the patient's main pain area is a common sequel of peripheral nerve injury;[27,69] however, it is not necessarily associated with the presence of pain or nerve damage, as evidenced in patients with painless nerve injuries,[69] in patients with fibromyalgia[70–72] and in patients with depression without pain.[71] Mechanisms underlying cold-evoked pain are still not fully understood and likely

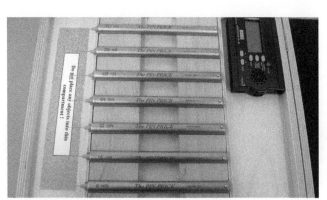

FIGURE 20-4 ■ Mechanical pain threshold evaluation.

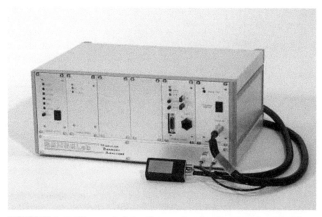

FIGURE 20-5 ■ Thermal detection and pain threshold evaluation.

include both peripheral and central nervous system mechanisms.[73–75]

TEST SITE AND INTERPRETATION OF QUANTITATIVE SENSORY TESTING DATA

QST data are usually collected in the area of maximal sensory disturbance, often the area of maximal pain, and a control area. The choice of test sites depends on the clinical question to be answered. For example, testing sensory function at the primary area of pain provides information about primary afferent function and peripheral sensitivity as well as central sensitization, whereas testing in anatomically remote areas can provide information about central sensitization and central processing.

For the assessment of neuropathic pain, sensation testing should be performed in the area of maximal pain. Dermatomal sensory loss in patients with cervical/lumbar radiculopathy is indicative of nerve root damage,[29–31] whereby sensory loss in the main pain area supports the presence of neuropathic pain.[31,33,76]

An important consideration for the interpretation of QST data and comparison of QST data between studies is the variation in both normative and patient data due to heterogeneity of participants (including age and gender) and methodological differences between studies such as the body region assessed and the specific QST protocols used.[7,19,31,32,77] The DFNS has published reference data for their protocols for the cheek, dorsum of the hand, dorsum of the foot and trunk for male and female adults in age decades from 20 to 70 years[22] and there are some reference data for children and juveniles.[23]

Furthermore, there is a lack of consensus as to what cut-off values are meaningful for the interpretation of QST data, for example what constitutes a clinically important side-to-side difference for thermal detection thresholds.[19,65] A cut-off of 15°C has been defined as cold hyperalgesia;[78] however, this score may fall within the 95% confidence interval of normative data.[22] The DFNS proposes the use of z-scores to analyse an individual's data and ascertain the presence of sensory gain or sensory loss.[7,19,31,32,77] Using this system, two standard deviations above/below the mean of reference data is considered indicative of a pathological value.

Profiling patients using QST involves analysing multiple parameters of sensory testing to evaluate the function of sensory receptors, nerve fibres and their respective pathways to determine whether patients demonstrate dominant features of loss or gain of function.[19,33] An example is shown in Figure 20-6. Subgroups of patients

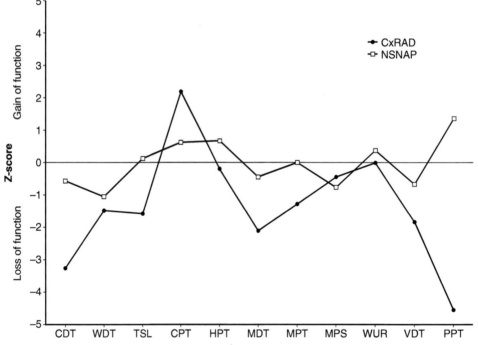

FIGURE 20-6 ■ Sensory profiling. The z-score quantitative sensory testing sensory profiles are shown for the maximal pain area in two patients presenting with neck–arm pain in the C7 dermatomal distribution. Healthy control subjects are represented by a z-score of 'zero'. The patient with cervical radiculopathy (*CxRAD*, filled circle) was characterized by sensory alterations in the maximal pain area (reduced thermal, mechanical and vibration detection and reduced pressure pain sensitivity), indicating a loss of small and large sensory nerve fibre function, suggestive of nerve root damage and the presence of neuropathic pain. The thermal, mechanical detection and pressure pain thresholds were two standard deviations below the mean of reference data. The patient also demonstrated cold hypersensitivity compared to the reference data. The QST profile of the patient with non-specific neck–arm pain (*NSNAP*, open square) did not demonstrate any loss of function, but demonstrated heightened pressure sensitivity compared to reference data. However the value was not above 2 standard deviations from the mean of reference data. *CDT,* Cold detection threshold; *CPT,* Cold pain threshold; *HPT,* Heat pain threshold; *MDT,* Mechanical detection threshold; *MPS,* Mechanical pain sensitivity; *MPT,* Mechanical pain threshold; *PPT,* Pressure pain threshold; *TSL,* Thermal sensory limen; *VDT,* Vibration detection threshold; *WDT,* Warm detection threshold; *WUR,* Wind-up ratio.

with distinct somatosensory profiles have been identified within one aetiology, illustrating the heterogeneity of pain disorders.[7,19,31,32,77] Moreover, patients with similar somatosensory profiles can be present across aetiologically different groups.[33,79] It has been proposed that these trans-aetiological profiles reflect underlying pain mechanisms and that sensory profiling may have a role in matching patients to the most appropriate interventions.[19,79]

QST is generally not recommended as a stand-alone method of assessment;[2] however, it often adds value to comprehensive assessment or as a component of a diagnostic profile. For example, quantitative thermal threshold testing combined with skin biopsy has been recommended for the assessment of small-fibre involvement in diabetic neuropathy.[2]

CLINICAL UTILITY OF QUANTITATIVE SENSORY TESTING IN PHYSIOTHERAPY

Persistent musculoskeletal pain disorders can be challenging to manage by traditional methods of physiotherapy. Systematic reviews reveal evidence of poor efficacy for physical treatments when given to patients with complex pain conditions such as whiplash-associated disorder[4] or chronic non-specific low back pain.[80] It has been suggested that this might be because of the 'washout effect'[81,82] whereby only a small subgroup of people with a specific feature-set respond to this form of intervention. This may be due to the fact that such persistent conditions comprise a constellation of different underlying mechanisms despite presenting with similar symptoms. Such symptoms may be explained by the complex interaction of a number of factors in any single pain presentation including ongoing tissue damage, psychosocial co-morbidities, peripheral and central nerve injury, and altered central processing of sensory stimuli.[83] Identifying these factors may lead to enhanced, individualized patient-focused care.[84] An example of this can be seen in a mechanism-based classification system designed to assist in the manual therapy management of low-back-related leg pain.[84] The validity of this classification system has been established through the use of QST to establish subgroups suitable for physical intervention.[85,86] Additional benefits of the use of mechanism-based classification include improved patient satisfaction through better diagnostic labelling, a clearer understanding of prognosis, and the potential for mechanism-based therapeutic interventions that would specifically target the underlying pathophysiology.[1,47–49,61] QST can assist in the interpretation of pain mechanisms underlying a patient's clinical presentation and its application should be considered in physiotherapy assessment and management of acute as well as persistent musculoskeletal pain disorders.

REFERENCES

1. Backonja MM, Attal N, Baron R, et al. Value of quantitative sensory testing in neurological and pain disorders: NeuPSIG consensus. Pain 2013;154(9):1807–19.
2. Krumova EK, Geber C, Westermann A, et al. Neuropathic pain: is quantitative sensory testing helpful? Curr Diab Rep 2012;12(4):393–402.
3. Hansson P, Backonja M, Bouhassira D. Usefulness and limitations of quantitative sensory testing: clinical and research application in neuropathic pain states. Pain 2007;129(3):256–9.
4. Wilder-Smith OH, Tassonyi E, Crul BJ, et al. Quantitative sensory testing and human surgery: effects of analgesic management on postoperative neuroplasticity. Anesthesiology 2003;98(5):1214–22.
5. Verhagen AP, Scholten-Peeters GG, van Wijngaarden S, et al. Conservative treatments for whiplash. Cochrane Database Syst Rev 2007;(2):CD003338.
6. Backonja MM, Walk D, Edwards RR, et al. Quantitative sensory testing in measurement of neuropathic pain phenomena and other sensory abnormalities. Clin J Pain 2009;25(7):641–7.
7. Meier PM, Berde CB, DiCanzio J, et al. Quantitative assessment of cutaneous thermal and vibration sensation and thermal pain detection thresholds in healthy children and adolescents. Muscle Nerve 2001;24(10):1339–45.
8. Yarnitsky D, Granot M. Chapter 27 Quantitative sensory testing. Handb Clin Neurol 2006;81:397–409.
9. Arendt-Nielsen L, Yarnitsky D. Experimental and clinical applications of quantitative sensory testing applied to skin, muscles and viscera. J Pain 2009;10(6):556–72.
10. Sang CN, Max MB, Gracely RH. Stability and reliability of detection thresholds for human A-beta and A-delta sensory afferents determined by cutaneous electrical stimulation. J Pain Symptom Manage 2003;25(1):64–73.
11. Cruccu G, Anand P, Attal N, et al. EFNS guidelines on neuropathic pain assessment. Eur J Neurol 2004;11(3):153–62.
12. Walk D, Sehgal N, Moeller-Bertram T, et al. Quantitative sensory testing and mapping: a review of nonautomated quantitative methods for examination of the patient with neuropathic pain. Clin J Pain 2009;25(7):632–40.
13. Wylde V, Palmer S, Learmonth ID, et al. Test-retest reliability of quantitative sensory testing in knee osteoarthritis and healthy participants. Osteoarthritis Cartilage 2011;19(6):655–8.
14. Wang R, Cui L, Zhou W, et al. Reliability study of thermal quantitative sensory testing in healthy Chinese. Somatosens Mot Res 2014;31(4):198–203.
15. Moloney NA, Hall TM, O'Sullivan TC, et al. Reliability of thermal quantitative sensory testing of the hand in a cohort of young, healthy adults. Muscle Nerve 2011;44(4):547–52.
16. Moloney NA, Hall TM, Doody CM. Reliability of thermal quantitative sensory testing: a systematic review. J Rehabil Res Dev 2012;49(2):191–207.
17. Geber C, Klein T, Azad S, et al. Test-retest and interobserver reliability of quantitative sensory testing according to the protocol of the German Research Network on Neuropathic Pain (DFNS): a multi-centre study. Pain 2011;152(3):548–56.
18. Felix ER, Widerstrom-Noga EG. Reliability and validity of quantitative sensory testing in persons with spinal cord injury and neuropathic pain. J Rehabil Res Dev 2009;46(1):69–83.
19. Rolke R, Baron R, Maier C, et al. Quantitative sensory testing in the German Research Network on Neuropathic Pain (DFNS): standardized protocol and reference values. Pain 2006;123(3):231–43.
20. Rolke R, Baron R, Maier C, et al. Quantitative sensory testing: a comprehensive protocol for clinical trials. Eur J Pain 2006;10(1):77–88.
21. Pfau DB, Krumova EK, Treede RD, et al. Quantitative sensory testing in the German Research Network on Neuropathic Pain (DFNS): reference data for the trunk and application in patients with chronic postherpetic neuralgia. Pain 2014;155(5):1002–15.
22. Magerl W, Krumova EK, Baron R, et al. Reference data for quantitative sensory testing (QST): refined stratification for age and a novel method for statistical comparison of group data. Pain 2010;151(3):598–605.
23. Blankenburg M, Boekens H, Hechler T, et al. Reference values for quantitative sensory testing in children and adolescents: developmental and gender differences of somatosensory perception. Pain 2010;149(1):76–88.
24. Gelber DA, Pfeifer MA, Broadstone VL, et al. Components of variance for vibratory and thermal threshold testing in normal and diabetic subjects. J Diabetes Complications 1995;9(3):170–6.
25. Martin CL, Waberski BH, Pop-Busui R, et al. Vibration perception threshold as a measure of distal symmetrical peripheral neuropathy in type 1 diabetes: results from the DCCT/EDIC study. Diabetes Care 2010;33(12):2635–41.

26. Schmid AB, Soon BT, Wasner G, et al. Can widespread hypersensitivity in carpal tunnel syndrome be substantiated if neck and arm pain are absent? Eur J Pain 2012;16(2):217–28.

27. Taylor KS, Anastakis DJ, Davis KD. Chronic pain and sensorimotor deficits following peripheral nerve injury. Pain 2010;151(3):582–91.

28. Chien A, Eliav E, Sterling M. Whiplash (grade II) and cervical radiculopathy share a similar sensory presentation: an investigation using quantitative sensory testing. Clin J Pain 2008;24(7):595–603.

29. Freynhagen R, Rolke R, Baron R, et al. Pseudoradicular and radicular low-back pain – a disease continuum rather than different entities? Answers from quantitative sensory testing. Pain 2008;135(1–2):65–74.

30. Nygaard OP, Mellgren SI. The function of sensory nerve fibers in lumbar radiculopathy. Use of quantitative sensory testing in the exploration of different populations of nerve fibers and dermatomes. Spine (Phila Pa 1976) 1998;23(3):348–52, discussion 353.

31. Tampin B, Slater H, Hall T, et al. Quantitative sensory testing somatosensory profiles in patients with cervical radiculopathy are distinct from those in patients with nonspecific neck-arm pain. Pain 2012;153(12):2403–14.

32. Tampin B, Briffa NK, Slater H. Self-reported sensory descriptors are associated with quantitative sensory testing parameters in patients with cervical radiculopathy, but not in patients with fibromyalgia. Eur J Pain 2013;17(4):621–33.

33. Maier C, Baron R, Tölle TR, et al. Quantitative sensory testing in the German Research Network on Neuropathic Pain (DFNS): somatosensory abnormalities in 1236 patients with different neuropathic pain syndromes. Pain 2010;150(3):439–50.

34. Greening J, Lynn B. Vibration sense in the upper limb in patients with repetitive strain injury and a group of at-risk office workers. Int Arch Occup Environ Health 1998;71(1):29–34.

35. Greening J, Lynn B, Leary R. Sensory and autonomic function in the hands of patients with non-specific arm pain (NSAP) and asymptomatic office workers. Pain 2003;104(1–2):275–81.

36. Jensen BR, Pilegaard M, Momsen A. Vibrotactile sense and mechanical functional state of the arm and hand among computer users compared with a control group. Int Arch Occup Environ Health 2002;75(5):332–40.

37. Laursen LH, Jepsen JR, Sjogaard G. Vibrotactile sense in patients with different upper limb disorders compared with a control group. Int Arch Occup Environ Health 2006;79(7):593–601.

38. Pilegaard M, Jensen BR. An 18-month follow-up study on vibrotactile sense, muscle strength and symptoms in computer users with and without symptoms. Int Arch Occup Environ Health 2005;78(6):486–92.

39. Tucker AT, White PD, Kosek E, et al. Comparison of vibration perception thresholds in individuals with diffuse upper limb pain and carpal tunnel syndrome. Pain 2007;127(3):263–9.

40. Moloney NA, Hall T, Doody CM. Pathophysiology in nonspecific arm pain. Physical Therapy Reviews 2011;16:321–5.

41. Apkarian AV, Stea RA, Bolanowski SJ. Heat-induced pain diminishes vibrotactile perception: a touch gate. Somatosens Mot Res 1994;11(3):259–67.

42. Shakoor N, Agrawal A, Block JA. Reduced lower extremity vibratory perception in osteoarthritis of the knee. Arthritis Rheum 2008;59(1):117–20.

43. Shakoor N, Lee KJ, Fogg LF, et al. Generalized vibratory deficits in osteoarthritis of the hip. Arthritis Rheum 2008;59(9):1237–40.

44. Hollins M, Sigurdsson A, Fillingim L, et al. Vibrotactile threshold is elevated in temporomandibular disorders. Pain 1996;67(1):89–96.

45. Koroschetz J, Rehm SE, Pontus H, et al. Quantitative sensory testing in patients suffering from fibromyalgia. Eur J Pain 2010;4(Suppl.):66.

46. Courtney CA, Kavchak AE, Lowry CD, et al. Interpreting joint pain: quantitative sensory testing in musculoskeletal management. J Orthop Sports Phys Ther 2010;40(12):818–25.

47. George SZ, Bishop MD, Bialosky JE, et al. Immediate effects of spinal manipulation on thermal pain sensitivity: an experimental study. BMC Musculoskelet Disord 2006;7:68.

48. Lewis C, Souvlis T, Sterling M. Sensory characteristics of tender points in the lower back. Man Ther 2010;15(5):451–6.

49. Wylde V, Palmer S, Learmonth ID, et al. The association between pre-operative pain sensitisation and chronic pain after knee replacement: an exploratory study. Osteoarthritis Cartilage 2013;21(9):1253–6.

50. Kilo S, Schmelz M, Koltzenburg M, et al. Different patterns of hyperalgesia induced by experimental inflammation in human skin. Brain 1994;117(Pt 2):385–96.

51. Simone DA, Sorkin LS, Oh U, et al. Neurogenic hyperalgesia: central neural correlates in responses of spinothalamic tract neurons. J Neurophysiol 1991;66(1):228–46.

52. Torebjork HE, Lundberg LE, LaMotte RH. Central changes in processing of mechanoreceptive input in capsaicin-induced secondary hyperalgesia in humans. J Physiol 1992;448:765–80.

53. Magerl W, Fuchs PN, Meyer RA, et al. Roles of capsaicin-insensitive nociceptors in cutaneous pain and secondary hyperalgesia. Brain 2001;124(Pt 9):1754–64.

54. Woolf CJ, Max MB. Mechanism-based pain diagnosis: issues for analgesic drug development. Anesthesiology 2001;95(1):241–9.

55. Woolf CJ, Mannion RJ. Neuropathic pain: aetiology, symptoms, mechanisms, and management. Lancet 1999;353(9168):1959–64.

56. Moloney N, Hall T, Doody C. Sensory hyperalgesia is characteristic of nonspecific arm pain: a comparison with cervical radiculopathy and pain-free controls. Clin J Pain 2013;29(11):948–56.

57. Yarnitsky D, Crispel Y, Eisenberg E, et al. Prediction of chronic post-operative pain: pre-operative DNIC testing identifies patients at risk. Pain 2008;138(1):22–8.

58. Gwilym SE, Oag HC, Tracey I, et al. Evidence that central sensitisation is present in patients with shoulder impingement syndrome and influences the outcome after surgery. J Bone Joint Surg Br 2011;93(4):498–502.

59. Aasvang EK, Gmaehle E, Hansen JB, et al. Predictive risk factors for persistent postherniotomy pain. Anesthesiology 2010;112(4):957–69.

60. Ziegler EA, Magerl W, Meyer RA, et al. Secondary hyperalgesia to punctate mechanical stimuli. Central sensitization to A-fibre nociceptor input. Brain 1999;122(Pt 12):2245–57.

61. Woolf CJ. Central sensitization: implications for the diagnosis and treatment of pain. Pain 2011;152(3 Suppl.):S2–15.

62. Yaksh TL, Malmber AB, editors. Central Pharmacology of Nociceptive Transmission. 3rd ed. London: Churchill Livingstone; 1994.

63. Tampin B, Slater H, Briffa NK. Neuropathic pain components are common in patients with painful cervical radiculopathy, but not in patients with nonspecific neck-arm pain. Clin J Pain 2013;29(10):846–56.

64. Jaaskelainen SK, Teerijoki-Oksa T, Forssell H. Neurophysiologic and quantitative sensory testing in the diagnosis of trigeminal neuropathy and neuropathic pain. Pain 2005;117(3):349–57.

65. Leffler AS, Hansson P, Kosek E. Somatosensory perception in patients suffering from long-term trapezius myalgia at the site overlying the most painful part of the muscle and in an area of pain referral. Eur J Pain 2003;7(3):267–76.

66. Davis KD, Taylor KS, Anastakis DJ. Nerve injury triggers changes in the brain. Neuroscientist 2011;17(4):407–22.

67. Chien A, Eliav E, Sterling M. Hypoaesthesia occurs with sensory hypersensitivity in chronic whiplash – further evidence of a neuropathic condition. Man Ther 2009;14(2):138–46.

68. Staud R, Weyl EE, Price DD, et al. Mechanical and heat hyperalgesia highly predict clinical pain intensity in patients with chronic musculoskeletal pain syndromes. J Pain 2012;13(8):725–35.

69. Kleggetveit IP, Jorum E. Large and small fiber dysfunction in peripheral nerve injuries with or without spontaneous pain. J Pain 2010;11(12):1305–10.

70. Blumenstiel K, Gerhardt A, Rolke R, et al. Quantitative sensory testing profiles in chronic back pain are distinct from those in fibromyalgia. Clin J Pain 2011;27(8):682–90.

71. Klauenberg S, Maier C, Assion HJ, et al. Depression and changed pain perception: hints for a central disinhibition mechanism. Pain 2008;140(2):332–43.

72. Pfau DB, Rolke R, Nickel R, et al. Somatosensory profiles in subgroups of patients with myogenic temporomandibular disorders and fibromyalgia syndrome. Pain 2009;147(1–3):72–83.

73. Berglund B, Harju EL, Kosek E, et al. Quantitative and qualitative perceptual analysis of cold dysesthesia and hyperalgesia in fibromyalgia. Pain 2002;96(1–2):177–87.

74. de Medinaceli L, Hurpeau J, Merle M, et al. Cold and post-traumatic pain: modeling of the peripheral nerve message. Biosystems 1997;43(3):145–67.

75. Treede RD, Meyer RA, Raja SN, et al. Peripheral and central mechanisms of cutaneous hyperalgesia. Prog Neurobiol 1992; 38(4):397–420.

76. Cruccu G, Sommer C, Anand P, et al. EFNS guidelines on neuropathic pain assessment: revised 2009. Eur J Neurol 2010; 17(8):1010–18.

77. Westermann A, Krumova EK, Pennekamp W, et al. Different underlying pain mechanisms despite identical pain characteristics: a case report of a patient with spinal cord injury. Pain 2012; 153(7):1537–40.

78. Bennett GJ. Can we distinguish between inflammatory and neuropathic pain. Pain Res Manage 2006;11(Suppl. A):11A–15A.

79. Freeman R, Baron R, Bouhassira D, et al. Sensory profiles of patients with neuropathic pain based on the neuropathic pain symptoms and signs. Pain 2014;155(2):367–76.

80. Rubinstein SM, van Middelkoop M, Assendelft WJ, et al. Spinal manipulative therapy for chronic low-back pain: an update of a Cochrane review. Spine (Phila Pa 1976) 2011;36(13):E825–46.

81. Wand BM, O'Connell NE. Chronic non-specific low back pain – sub-groups or a single mechanism? BMC Musculoskelet Disord 2008;9:11.

82. Rose S. Physical therapy diagnosis: role and function. Phys Ther 1989;69(7):535–7.

83. Curatolo M. Diagnosis of altered central pain processing. Spine (Phila Pa 1976) 2011;36(25 Suppl.):S200–4.

84. Schäfer A, Hall T, Briffa K. Classification of low back-related leg pain – a proposed patho-mechanism-based approach. Man Ther 2009;14(2):222–30.

85. Schäfer A, Hall T, Müller G, et al. Outcomes differ between subgroups of patients with low back and leg pain following neural manual therapy: a prospective cohort study. Eur Spine J 2011; 20(3):482–90.

86. Schäfer AG, Hall TM, Rolke R, et al. Low back related leg pain: An investigation of construct validity of a new classification system. J Back Musculoskelet Rehabil 2014;27(4):409–18.

CHAPTER 21

OUTCOME MEASURES IN MUSCULOSKELETAL PRACTICE

Jonathan Hill

INTRODUCTION

Outcome measures (OMs) are integral to improving quality of treatment for patients with musculoskeletal disorders (Box 21-1). Originally emerging from scientific research as robust instruments designed to objectively evaluate treatment, OMs are now rapidly gaining a pivotal position at the heart of services as part of the wider agenda to put patient needs, interests and feedback at the centre of care.[1] It is increasingly acknowledged that 'we can only be sure to improve what we can actually measure',[2] and as a consequence urgent efforts are being made to make what is important measurable and not simply what is measurable important. Patients' views about their health and quality of care are increasingly valued[1] as part of the wider re-orientation away from acute and episodic care, towards prevention, self-care, and better coordinated care.[3] The 'appropriateness' of patient-reported outcomes and their place within quality improvement initiatives has gained ascendency as the importance of the patient voice has increased. Propelled by these political changes in health care combined with the impact of the IT revolution, seismic shifts are occurring in the way OMs in musculoskeletal practice are used. OMs are more than just tools with which treatment is evaluated and the quality of care is monitored. They are now equally involved in guiding clinicians whether or not to refer someone for treatment or to enable patients to self-track their own health online. Commissioners of musculoskeletal services are insisting that outcomes are collected in order to benchmark performance, and in some sectors performance-related pay is on the horizon. For clinicians treating patients with musculoskeletal disorders, the importance of understanding OMs has therefore never been so critical.

This chapter aims to inform the reader about the complex world of OMs to ensure they are equipped to deal with this new context in which outcomes are embedded into every-day clinical practice (see Table 21-1).

TYPES OF OUTCOME MEASURES

A health outcome measure is an instrument that enables an observer to objectively evaluate an intended goal (typically an improvement in health status) from a health-care activity (treatment). Outcomes exist for a wide range of purposes and it is therefore essential to choose an instrument that has the appropriate properties for its intended use. The most commonly used outcomes in musculoskeletal practice are patient-reported outcome (PRO) measures, although some anthropometric instruments (e.g. grip strength) and examiner-completed observation lists (e.g. Berg Balance Scale) are still used. PROs are a series of questions asked of the patient in order to gauge their views of their own health status. As a consequence PROs are not entirely 'objective', but in musculoskeletal health PROs are particularly valued as personal perceptions of clinical status are considered to be at least as valid as indirect laboratory and radiographic data.[1] PROs are typically administered before and after treatment, increasingly by electronic means, and are usually distinguished from patient-reported experience measures (e.g. patient satisfaction) and measures of patient safety (e.g. accident/near-miss reporting) that are measured at a single time point. It is important to note that quality of care can be evaluated using various domains including measures of patient safety, experiences, clinical indicators as well as OMs.

When OM data from large numbers of patients are collected at two fixed time points, the mean difference between the two scores can be used to evaluate the improvements in health care achieved. In this way PROs can act as a catalyst for organizational change to raise standards. In the UK, this has already been evidenced through a National Programme of PRO reporting (http://www.ic.nhs.uk/proms) with performance reports available online.[4] These reports identify the best and worst health-care providers for four elective secondary care surgery procedures, while in The Netherlands there is for the first time an

---

BOX 21-1   Case Example

Consider Mrs Jones with a 2-year history of osteoarthritic pain in her shoulders and left knee, who is now presenting to health care with a new episode of low back pain.

- What musculoskeletal health domains should be systematically measured?
- Is the impact severe enough for her to require a course of treatment?
- Could outcome measures improve the transition of care between practitioners?
- Is it possible that she could track her own health progress over time?
- How should her outcomes be presented, who should see them and should her progress be comparable to others in a similar position?

TABLE 21-1 COSMIN Definitions of Domains, Measurement Properties and Aspects of Measurement Properties

Domain	Measurement Property	Aspect of A Measurement Property	Definition
Reliability			The degree to which the measurement is free from measurement error
Reliability (extended definition)			The extent to which scores for patients who have not changed are the same for repeated measurement under several conditions: e.g. using different sets of items from the same health-related patient-reported outcomes (HR-PRO) (internal consistency); over time (test-retest); by different persons on the same occasion (inter-rater); or by the same persons (i.e. raters or responders) on different occasions (intra-rater)
	Internal consistency		The degree of the interrelatedness among the items
	Reliability		The proportion of the total variance in the measurements which is due to 'true'[†] differences between patients
	Measurement error		The systematic and random error of a patient's score that is not attributed to true changes in the construct to be measured
Validity			The degree to which an HR-PRO instrument measures the construct(s) it purports to measure
	Content validity		The degree to which the content of an HR-PRO instrument is an adequate reflection of the construct to be measured
		Face validity	The degree to which (the items of) an HR-PRO instrument indeed looks as though it is an adequate reflection of the construct to be measured
	Construct validity		The degree to which the scores of an HR-PRO instrument are consistent with hypotheses *(for instance with regard to internal relationships, relationships to scores of other instruments, or differences between relevant groups)* based on the assumption that the HR-PRO instrument validly measures the construct to be measured
		Structural validity	The degree to which the scores of an HR-PRO instrument are an adequate reflection of the dimensionality of the construct to be measured
		Hypotheses testing	Idem Construct validity
		Cross-cultural validity	The degree to which the performance of the items on a translated or culturally adapted HR-PRO instrument are an adequate reflection of the performance of the items of the original version of the HR-PRO instrument
	Criterion validity		The degree to which the scores of an HR-PRO instrument are an adequate reflection of a 'gold standard'
Responsiveness			The ability of an HR-PRO instrument to detect change over time in the construct to be measured
	Responsiveness		Idem Responsiveness
Interpretability			Interpretability is the degree to which one can assign qualitative meaning – that is, clinical or commonly understood connotations – to an instrument's quantitative scores or change in scores

initiative being organized by the Dutch Physiotherapy Association to collect PROs for a national survey of musculoskeletal services.

Some PROs are designed as generic instruments for all health conditions such as the EuroQol[5] and SF-36[6] that measure overall health-related quality of life. There is also a plethora of instruments specific to a particular set of conditions or part of the body, for example the Oxford Knees Score.[7] The advantage of specific instruments is that they are generally more sensitive to change than generic measures, making them better able to discriminate treatment effectiveness when comparing services (benchmarking) or treatments (clinical trials). However, the advantage of generic measures is that they can be used to compare changes in health across different patient and population groups. A common current

By placing a tick in one box in each group below, please indicate which statements best describe your own health state today.

Mobility

I have no problems in walking about   ☐
I have some problems in walking about   ☐
I am confined to bed   ☐

Self-Care

I have no problems with self-care   ☐
I have some problems washing or dressing myself   ☐
I am unable to wash or dress myself   ☐

Usual Activities *(e.g., work, study, housework, family or leisure activities)*

I have no problems with performing my usual activities   ☐
I have some problems with performing my usual activities   ☐
I am unable to perform my usual activities   ☐

Pain/Discomfort

I have no pain or discomfort   ☐
I have moderate pain or discomfort   ☐
I have extreme pain or discomfort   ☐

Anxiety/Depression

I am not anxious or depressed   ☐
I am moderately anxious or depressed   ☐
I am extremely anxious or depressed   ☐

To help people say how good or bad a health state is, we have drawn a scale (rather like a thermometer) on which the best state you can imagine is marked 100 and the worst state you can imagine is marked 0.

We would like you to indicate on this scale how good or bad your own health is today, in your opinion. Please do this by drawing a line from the box below to whichever point on the scale indicates how good or bad your health state is today.

Your own
health state
today

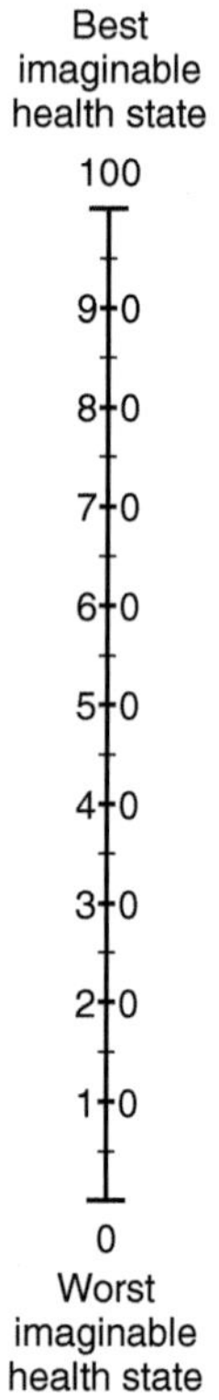

Best
imaginable
health state

100
9 0
8 0
7 0
6 0
5 0
4 0
3 0
2 0
1 0
0

Worst
imaginable
health state

FIGURE 21-1 ■ The EQ-5D. (UK (English) © 1990 EuroQol Group EQ-5D™ is a trade mark of the EuroQol Group.)

recommendation is therefore that generic and specific instruments are used in combination.[1]

The EQ-5D is one of the most commonly used generic instruments and captures quality of life from five health domains: mobility, self-care, usual activities, pain/discomfort and anxiety/depression (Fig. 21-1). The EQ-5D is known to lack responsiveness to change in musculoskeletal conditions and has therefore been superseded by the EQ-5D-5L, which offers five rather than three levels within each domain making it more sensitive to changes in health.[1]

There are literally thousands of condition-specific OMs available. One unresolved dilemma is how 'condition-specific' is specific enough, and can a broad musculoskeletal tool be used instead of something which is patho-anatomically specific? There is an obvious trade-off between clinical practicality and accuracy and often clinicians will choose more generic tools, while researchers will still want to use condition-specific measures. One recently developed and validated brief multidimensional instrument designed specifically for clinicians is the Keele Musculoskeletal Patient Reported Outcome Measure (MSK-PROM).[8] (Fig. 21-2). The MSK-PROM enables clinicians to quickly evaluate and monitor musculoskeletal health status using single questions for each health domain. The tool was developed using musculoskeletal patients and experts together to prioritize the most important health domains regarding independence from others, physical function, pain intensity, work interference, limitations in activities and roles that matter, quality of life, understanding about how to deal with the condition, anxiety/depression, overall impact and a patient-generated item about the severity of their worst symptom. To avoid duplication the MSK-PROM is designed to complement the widely used EQ-5D-5L with six additional items that considerably increase the responsiveness of the EQ-5D-5L items when used alone.[8] This brief tool is freely available for clinicians to use and ensures that health domains which matter to patients are systematically monitored.

Another key source of evidence for clinicians about which health domains should be measured in musculoskeletal practice is the International Classification of Functioning, Disability and Health (ICF: http://www.icf-research-branch.org/icf-core-sets-projects-sp-16410 24398/musculoskeletal-conditions). The ICF provides a standard classification framework based on the biopsychosocial model introduced by Engel[9] and suggests the following categories: body functions and structures, activity and participation restriction, environmental factors and personal factors. The most important health domains for a number of musculoskeletal conditions have been identified by the ICF for low back pain, chronic widespread pain, ankylosing spondylitis, osteoporosis, osteoarthritis and rheumatoid arthritis. Common domains across conditions include symptom severity (pain intensity), function (physical function, social function, work function), general well-being/quality of life, global improvement, emotional functioning, participation restriction and environmental factors such as levels of support needed, independence, relationships with family/others and patient satisfaction.

Another type of outcome is provided by patient-generated measures, such as the patient-specific function scale[10] or the MYMOP.[11] Their particular value is for goal setting and monitoring progress at a completely individual level, which tends to make them more sensitive to change than conventional measures. However, policy makers tend not to favour these types of OMs as they are less useful for group-level comparisons. It is therefore recommended that clinicians use a patient-generated measure alongside conventional OMs to get the advantages of both.[12]

There are considerable clinical benefits of using PROMs data to provide feedback at an individual level to patients and clinicians during treatment to help monitor progress. For example, in mental health services positive results have been shown from systems that use real-time outcome data to identify failing patients with rapid intervention to avoid poor response.[13] It has also been shown that using individual-level feedback to both the patient and clinician improves attendance rates and cost-effectiveness, without the need for additional clinical training or negative impact on the therapeutic process.[14] There is some evidence that formal patient monitoring tools prevent clinicians from arbitrarily modifying treatment plans without sufficient cause.[13] It seems that clinicians are sometimes tempted to modify treatment because they predict treatment failure based primarily on their perception of the therapeutic relationship rather than on actual progress.[14] It has also been reported that greater benefits are seen when progress feedback is given to clinicians and patients because this can prompt discussion that helps to empower patients about their treatment options, resulting in greater shared care planning.[15]

There are some OMs that have been specifically designed to facilitate clinical decision making such as the Orebro Musculoskeletal Pain Screening Tool.[16] This has established cut-off thresholds for provision of cognitive behavioural approaches alongside manual therapy to prevent work absence. High-quality clinical trial evidence is also available for the use of a brief questionnaire as part of a stratified care approach for low back pain that is designed to match patient profiles to treatment subgroups.[17]

Applications are increasingly being developed to facilitate easy implementation of PROs in practice. For example the Care Response System (www.care-response.com) enables clinicians and patients to collectively monitor progress and simultaneously provide aggregated service-level outcomes. A further relatively recent innovation in the use of PROs has been the development of OMs that are specifically designed to enable patients to track their own health status over time, such as 'Hows your health BC?' (http://www.howsyourhealthbc.ca/). The purposes for using OMs are therefore rapidly expanding and clinicians need to make themselves aware of such developments. However, it should be noted that research publications using these online technologies are lacking and evidence is urgently required to establish which outcomes should be monitored in musculoskeletal practice (see Box 21-2).

The Keele MSK-PROM for Monitoring Musculoskeletal Health

This questionnaire is about the health problem for which you are seeking treatment from this service. Place a **tick** in **one** box for each question below to indicate which statement best describes <u>**your view today**</u> (from 'never' to 'all the time'). Each **column** records a different treatment visit.

Q1. Needing help		Visit 1	Visit 2	Visit 3	Visit 4	Visit 5	Visit 6
How often do you need help from others because of your symptoms?							
Never	1						
Rarely	2						
Sometimes	3						
Frequently	4						
All the time	5						

Q2. Work/daily routine		Visit 1	Visit 2	Visit 3	Visit 4	Visit 5	Visit 6
How often have your symptoms interfered with your normal work/daily routine (including jobs around the house)?							
Never	1						
Rarely	2						
Sometimes	3						
Frequently	4						
All the time	5						

Q3. Activities and roles		Visit 1	Visit 2	Visit 3	Visit 4	Visit 5	Visit 6
How often are you prevented from doing activities and roles that matter to you?							
Never	1						
Rarely	2						
Sometimes	3						
Frequently	4						
All the time	5						

Q4. Severity of worst problem (e.g., sleep, fatigue, driving)		Visit 1	Visit 2	Visit 3	Visit 4	Visit 5	Visit 6
Think about the one thing you have the most difficulty with. How often are you finding this difficult?							
Never	1						
Rarely	2						
Sometimes	3						
Frequently	4						
All the time	5						

Q5. Understanding how to deal with symptoms		Visit 1	Visit 2	Visit 3	Visit 4	Visit 5	Visit 6
How often do you feel unsure about how to deal with your symptoms?							
Never	1						
Rarely	2						
Sometimes	3						
Frequently	4						
All the time	5						

Q6. Overall impact		Visit 1	Visit 2	Visit 3	Visit 4	Visit 5	Visit 6
Overall, how often do your symptoms bother you?							
Never	1						
Rarely	2						
Sometimes	3						
Frequently	4						
All the time	5						

Any and all copyrights © in Questions 1–6, their order and layout vest in Keele University (May 2013).
The tool is scored by summing all 6 items together.

FIGURE 21-2 ■ The Keele Musculoskeletal Patient Reported Outcome Measure (MSK-PROM) for monitoring musculoskeletal health.

BOX 21-2   **Useful Resources**

For more information, the following websites provide a handy source of free information, including references to key publications reporting on outcome measures.

- ProQolid (www.proqolid.org/) is a French database of instruments that is publicly accessible, with payment options for additional access
- ICF provides a standard classification framework for relevant health domains: http://www.icf-research-branch.org/icf-core-sets-projects-sp-1641024398/musculoskeletal-conditions
- The Omeract organization provides excellent advice on outcomes for use in rheumatology. http://www.omeract.org/
- Oxford University has a searchable database of relevant outcome measures: http://phi.uhce.ox.ac.uk/
- The EuroQol Group website (www.euroqol.org) provides information on the EQ-5D instruments, and a searchable references list. Users of the EQ-5D must register their studies with the EuroQol Group and respect the copyright on the instrument. However, the EQ-5D is generally free-of-charge for academic research use, and NHS users can now also use the EQ-5D under an arrangement with the Department of Health
- The International Society for Pharmacoeconomics and Outcomes Research provides useful material on patient-reported outcome methods, concepts and studies on its website: www.ispor.org/
- The UK Department of Health's PROMs webpages are located at: http://www.hscic.gov.uk/proms
- EU Musc net (http://www.eumusc.net/) provides an online facility to collect and collate information on the impact of musculoskeletal conditions across the EU Member States
- The Musculoskeletal Elf provides digested research reviews including some about outcome measures: http://www.themusculoskeletalelf.net
- The Assessment in Ankylosing Spondylitis (ASAS) group (www.asas-group.org)
- The group for research and assessment of psoriasis and psoriatic arthritis (GRAPPA) (www.grappanetwork.org)
- The OMERACT/OARSI initiative for osteoarthritis (www.oarsi.org/) and the fibromyalgia
- MAPI Research Institute (http://mapigroup.com/)
- The International Society for Quality of Life Research (http://www.isoqol.org/).

THE DEVELOPMENT AND VALIDATION OF OUTCOME MEASURES

One challenge for clinicians in choosing musculoskeletal OMs is that the methodological quality of different instruments varies considerably. The COSMIN guidelines (http://www.cosmin.nl) are an internationally agreed source of the appropriate methods required for outcome measure development and validation. They suggest that the quality of a health-related PRO can be assessed by testing an instrument's reliability, validity, responsiveness and interpretability. As mentioned in the introduction, the perceived relevance and acceptability to patients (face validity) is increasingly important in the choice of outcomes used in practice. Another key area for clinicians is the interpretability of the instrument, which is the degree

to which a tool has a qualitative meaning for clinical practice including how easy it is to score. The definitions and measurement properties of the main instrument quality domains are provided in Table 21-1 directly using the COSMIN agreed definitions.

PRACTICAL ISSUES IN COLLECTING OUTCOME MEASURES

The following practical issues are useful to agree before starting to collect OMs:

1. Set a clear purpose for gathering data, and determine the inclusion/exclusion criteria, who has an interest in the information and who is affected by your plans.
2. Decide on the timing of your measures.
3. Include some baseline case-mix adjustment factors.
4. Decide where and how the data will be collected.

Set a Clear Purpose

At the outset it is essential to decide on the purpose of collecting the outcome measure. Why do you want the information, who is needed to help, who do you want it for and which patient population is included/excluded? Gathering OMs from patients can be a little more complex than it may initially appear. To ensure reliable, rigorous evidence is obtained the process must be systematic. Patients and clinicians prefer to complete outcomes where there is a direct relevance between the measurement and clinical decision making. It is also important to consider whether the collection of OMs is constrained by a national policy, or by the service commissioner/funders. The more integrated the data collection process to routine care the better and clearly the patient population must be carefully specified.

Decide on the Timing

An important practical issue when collecting OMs is deciding when to evaluate change and the correct timing of measures. Evidence suggests that on average the natural course of common musculoskeletal conditions means patient symptom severity is at its worst at the point of initial consultation to health care.[18] This has implications for outcome measurement, as it is therefore best to obtain the initial baseline measurement as near to the first contact consultation as possible. This fact means that two equally effective musculoskeletal services measuring improvements at first appointment and at 3-month follow-up are still likely to see differences in their pooled outcome improvements if they assess patients with slightly different episode durations. For example, this might occur if one service permitted direct treatment access and the other only accepted referred patients (e.g. by their general practitioner). This is because the average episode duration (and pain severity) of patients at initial assessment in each service may systematically differ, giving the service obtaining the earliest baseline measure an advantage in achieving greater outcome improvements. There are also likely to be systematic differences if the follow-up time point is not the same with greater improvements seen with a longer gap between measured time points (until around 6 months follow-up depending on the condition). The timing of follow-up measures should therefore be considered and where possible standardized, according to the natural course of the condition and the conceptual framework for the mechanism of treatment in question.

Case-Mix Adjustment

Another important practical issue is collecting the right case-mix adjusters that enable patient outcomes to be compared between services by statistically correcting for differences in population demographics and severity. Using risk adjustment enables 'raw' PRO change scores to better reflect the outcomes achieved had the provider treated a national average case-mix of patients. This case-mix or risk adjustment ensures that comparisons between services can be made on a like-for-like basis, controlling for differences in local patient population characteristics such as age, social deprivation and co-morbidities. Methods to case-mix adjust PROs data have been published,[19] but the methodology for case-mix adjustment in musculoskeletal practice is still in its relative infancy.[20] To guide clinicians a number of commonly used case-mix adjustment factors for collection alongside baseline OMs are presented in Figure 21-3.

Musculoskeletal Case-mix Adjustment

1. How old are you (years)? ☐ 2. Gender: M ☐ F ☐ 3. Postcode ☐

4. What is your current **work** situation?

- I am **retired** ☐
- I am **not in** paid work, because of my health ☐
- I am **not in** paid work, but **not** because of my health (e.g. student) ☐
- I am **in work** and have **not** had time off work because of my health ☐
- I am **in work** having had time off in the last 3 months ☐ → ☐
- I am in work but am currently **on sick leave** because of my health ☐ → ☐

How many days off, in the last 3 months?

5. Have you come for treatment from: Your GP or nurse ☐ A&E (casualty) ☐ Other ☐ Self-referral ☐ NHS Consultant ☐

6. Which **PART of your BODY** is the **main** problem for which you are seeking treatment? (tick 1)

Shoulder	☐	Head	☐	Hip	☐
Elbow	☐	Neck	☐	Knee	☐
Wrist	☐	Back	☐	Ankle/foot	☐
Hand	☐	Multi-site pain	☐	Other	☐

7. In the last 3 months, how many times have you consulted healthcare for this problem? ☐

8. For **how long** have you had your **current** episode of this main problem?

Number of Weeks ☐ Months ☐ Years ☐

9. How much do you expect your condition will **respond** to treatment in this service?

It will get worse — It will stay the same — It will be cured

0 ☐ 1 ☐ 2 ☐ 3 ☐ 4 ☐ 5 ☐ 6 ☐ 7 ☐ 8 ☐ 9 ☐ 10 ☐

10. Do you feel that your **problem is terrible** and that **it is never going to get any better?**

Completely disagree — Completely agree

0 ☐ 1 ☐ 2 ☐ 3 ☐ 4 ☐ 5 ☐ 6 ☐ 7 ☐ 8 ☐ 9 ☐ 10 ☐

11. How would you rate your **general health** and well-being for your age?

Please do this by giving a number from 0 to 100 (where 0 = poor health, and 100 = perfect health). ☐

FIGURE 21-3 ■ Musculoskeletal case-mix adjustment.

Data Collection Method

Another practical issue is where and how to collect OMs. Due to the self-selection involved in patients' ongoing treatment attendance, less selection bias is present when data are collected outside of the clinic setting. Evidence is growing for the use of text messaging to collect clinical OMs[21] due to its strengths as increasing numbers carry their phone with them at all times, providing high response rates and data collected from the patient's natural environment. The limitations however, are that this technology is less familiar to elderly patients and that the questions have to be short with a limited number of characters. Perhaps the greatest innovation for modern data collection is with online facilities, with patients able to choose how they are contacted (e.g. by text, email or post) and its ability to present progress in real time. Such systems also empower patients to be the owners of their own data and to decide with whom they share the information. Case-mix adjustment questions are typically included and a range of reporting methods is available according to the needs of the person accessing the data. Further research is needed to identify the optimal methods to present data and to facilitate the clinical consultation using such information. Leadership from professional organizations is also required to prevent hundreds of different and incompatible systems being introduced.

ACTING ON INFORMATION

A key consideration is how you will act on the information received and how you will evaluate the impact of any changes made. The health-care context within which the information was collected (such as the type of access) and the population surveyed should be clearly defined. It is useful to examine changes in performance when surveys are repeated, for example at the same time each year. This also helps to measure the impact of any new initiatives that have been introduced. Findings can also be compared with results from others that are similar in size, type, or location to identify where strengths and weaknesses exist. Linking with other work brings many benefits and will help you to interpret your data in the light of the findings of others. A workshop with patient involvement is a good way to explore the issues and priorities in order to deliver a future quality improvement action plan (see Box 21-3).

SUMMARY

This chapter has highlighted the benefits from OMs for evaluating treatment and monitoring the quality of care for clinicians working with patients with musculoskeletal disorders. The need for outcomes that have robust measurement properties including reliability, validity and clinical 'appropriateness' using the patient's perspective has been noted. The chapter has also outlined advantages of using electronic online data collection alongside timely feedback of patient scores to improve patient care and experience. Other considerations discussed included benefits from working collectively with other organizations rather than in isolation to ensure standardization for benchmarking, particularly in respect to the OMs used, their timing and the case-mix adjusters captured. Clinicians who treat musculoskeletal disorders need to embrace this new world where OMs are embedded into routine practice to assist clinical decision making and systematically monitor treatment in order to deliver the best care possible to their patients.

BOX 21-3 **Recommendations for Choosing an Outcome Measure**

- Use patients to help chose appropriate outcome domains
- Consider whether the PROM is for primarily for research or clinical practice
- Consider at least one patient-generated item – as they are most sensitive to change
- Use a generic measure and condition-specific measure in combination
- Multidimensional measures are more feasible than unidimensional outcomes
- Measure at baseline with follow-up timed for conceptual framework of treatment
- Discuss outcomes and monitor progress with patients as a powerful treatment tool
- Aim for consistency across services to help assist benchmarking
- Collect key demographic characteristics to enable case-mix adjustment
- Try to collect some of your data from outside the clinic setting (preferably online)
- Do not forget permission is needed to use some outcome measures

REFERENCES

1. Devlin N, Appleby J. Getting the Most Out of PROMs: Putting Health Outcomes at the Heart of NHS Decision Making. London: King's Fund and Office of Health Economics; 2010. <http://www.kingsfund.org.uk/sites/files/kf/Getting-the-most-out-of-PROMs-Nancy-Devlin-John-Appleby-Kings-Fund-March-2010.pdf>.
2. Darzi A. High Quality Care For All: NHS Next Stage Review Final Report. Cm 7432. London: The Stationery Office; 2008. Available at: <www.dh.gov.uk/dr_consum_dh/groups/dh_digitalassets/@dh/@en/documents/digitalasset/dh_085828.pdf>; [accessed on 30th Dec 2011.].
3. Candace I, Chris N, Nick G, et al. Transforming our health care system: Ten priorities for commissioners. The Kings Fund. 12th May 2011. Available at: <http://www.kingsfund.org.uk/publications/articles/transforming-our-health-care-system-ten-priorities-commissioners>.
4. Health & Social Care Information Centre. Hospital Episode Statistics. <http://www.hesonline.nhs.uk/Ease/ContentServer?siteID=1937&categoryID=1295>.
5. Brooks R. EuroQol: the current state of play. Health Policy (New York) 1996;37:53–72.
6. Ware JE Jr. SF-36 Health Survey Update. Spine 2000;25:3130–9.
7. Dawson J, Fitzpatrick R, Murray D, et al. Questionnaire on the perceptions of patients about total knee replacement. J Bone Joint Surg Br 1998;80(1):63–9.
8. Hill JC, Thomas E, Hill S, et al. Development and validation of the Keele Musculoskeletal Patient Reported Outcome Measure (MSK-PROM). Abstract for The British Pain Society 2014. 2014.
9. Engel GL. The need of a new medical model: a challenge for biomedicine. Science 1977;196:129–36.

10. Stratford P, Gill C, Westaway M, et al. Assessing disability and change on individual patients: a report of a patient specific measure. Physiother Can 1995;47:258–63.

11. Paterson C. Measuring outcome in primary care: a patient-generated measure, MYMOP, compared to the SF-36 health survey. Br Med J 1996;312:1016–20.

12. McDowell I, Newell C. Measuring Health: A Guide to Rating Scales and Questionnaires. 2nd ed. New York: Oxford University Press; 1996.

13. Newnham EA, Page AC. Bridging the gap between best evidence and best practice in mental health. Clin Psychol Rev 2009;10:1016.

14. Miller SD, Duncan BL, Sorrell R, et al. The Partners for Change outcome management system. J Clin Psychol 2005;61:199–208.

15. Harmon C, Lambert MJ, Smart DW, et al. Enhancing outcome for potential treatment failures: therapist/client feedback and clinical support tools. Psychother Res 2007;17(4):379–92.

16. Linton SJ, Hallden K. Can we screen for problematic back pain? A screening questionnaire for predicting outcome in acute and subacute back pain. Clin J Pain 1998;14:209–15.

17. Hill JC, Dunn KM, Lewis M, et al. A primary care back pain screening tool: identifying patient subgroups for initial treatment. Arthritis Rheum 2008;59(5):632–41.

18. Mallen CD, Thomas E, Belcher J, et al. Point-of-care prognosis for common musculoskeletal pain in older adults. JAMA Intern Med 2013;173(12):1119–25.

19. Austin PC. An introduction to propensity score methods for reducing the effects of confounding in observational studies. Multivariate Behav Res 2011;46(3):399–424.

20. Resnik L, Liu D, Hart DL, et al. Benchmarking physical therapy clinic performance: statistical methods to enhance internal validity when using observational data. Phys Ther 2008;88:1078–87.

21. Lemeunier N, Kongsted A, Axén I. Prevalence of pain-free weeks in chiropractic subjects with low back pain – a longitudinal study using data gathered with text messages. Chiropr Man Therap 2011;19:28. doi:10.1186/2045-709X-19-28.

RESEARCH APPROACHES FOR MUSCULOSKELETAL PHYSIOTHERAPY

Research forms the basis and framework for evidence based physiotherapy practice. In order to be effective evidence based clinicians, it is important to have a broad understanding of various research approaches. The astute clinician can then critically evaluate the results of research studies and effectively integrate them into their practice as indicated. Researchers also benefit from an understanding of various research approaches; especially those not familiar to them where different approaches can often shed new light on problematic research questions.

This section will outline several research methods commonly used in studies that are relevant to musculoskeletal physiotherapy practice. First, clinical research methods to test treatment effects are presented. The randomized controlled trial is the most common design to test the effect of treatment but other less familiar designs are also discussed including cross-over, diamond and factorial designs as well as randomized withdrawal and expertise-based designs. Finally N-of-1 designs are outlined together with situations where this study approach is particularly indicated. Second, other research methods are discussed including quantitative methods which physiotherapist may be most familiar with in addition to qualitative and mixed-method designs which are becoming more common-place in musculoskeletal physiotherapy research. A key element of most research approaches is the inclusion of robust data which underpins a study's findings and this is vital regardless of the type of study being undertaken. As such, the third chapter will explore the concept of standardized data collection and the mechanisms for developing standardized data collection tools.

Finally, research is of little use if it is not effectively translated into clinical practice as well as to policy stakeholders and consumers with musculoskeletal pain. Successful translation of research is difficult and complex. The final chapter of this section will focus on relevant research methods exploring the process of improving the implementation of research findings into physiotherapy practice.

CHAPTER 22

CLINICAL RESEARCH TO TEST TREATMENT EFFECTS

Anita Gross • Charlie Goldsmith • David Walton • Joy MacDermid

INTRODUCTION

Clinical trial designs are powerful tools for ascertaining benefits, harms and patient recruitment for intervention. Numerous treatment approaches have been pronounced as having great effects only to be shown to be useless or even harmful when subject to rigorous independent empirical evaluation.[1] We will explore trial design options that optimize various objectives.

CLASSIC MULTIPLE GROUP PARALLEL DESIGN RANDOMIZED CONTROLLED TRIAL

The establishment of randomized controlled trials (RCTs) dates back to the 18th century but became a core element of health research with the advent of evidence-based medicine (practice) and is labelled one of the top ten medical advancements.[2,3] The classic format is a two-group parallel RCT (see Fig. 22-1). The Cervical Overview Group's experience[4-6] in systematically reviewing RCTs on manual therapies and exercise for neck pain confirms that challenges exist in the design and conduct of RCTs (see Table 22-1). These challenges point to the need for greater understanding of designs on the classic RCT as well as to consider both alternative RCT designs and the role for concurrent observational data collection. Figure 22-2 shows the emerging biases inherent in the manual therapy and exercise trial designs. A key source of bias that needs to be considered in trial design and interpretation is performance bias (blinding of participants and personnel); it is often impossible to blind the clinician providing hands-on manual therapy or the exercise interventions to the treatment assignment. This can be even more problematic if the treating clinician is involved in assessment of the outcomes. Hence, in such situations blinded evaluators play a critical role in reducing bias. Patient-reported outcome measures (PRO) are not directly influenced by the assessor and measures like the Numeric Rating Scale and Neck Disability Index[7] are commonly used as primary outcomes in clinical research and practice.[8] Yet self-report scales are still considered to be soft outcomes, and can be influenced by patient recall and the patient's desire to please their treating practitioner. Triangulating different categories of outcome measures as the primary outcome may help to reduce detection bias. For example, integrating soft outcomes like self-report scales with hard outcomes measure such as (a) performance-based outcomes (i.e. Fit-HaNSA,[9] Neck Walk Index[10]) where an external independent evaluator assesses the outcome; and (b) a biological measure (i.e. serum marker tests[11]) in the primary measure grouping could help manage detection bias. When using multiple outcome measures, interpretation must consider both the potential for bias and differential effects either across different types of outcomes or overtime. Reporting bias impacts the size of the effect measure most. In the manual therapy systematic reviews (Fig. 22-2, Table 22-2), 68% (mobilization[12]/77% (manipulation[12])/94% (massage[13]) of trials report on either immediate post or short-term outcomes; these are generally depicting a positive effect. There is better reporting of intermediate or long-term follow-up in exercise[4] (48%) or manual therapy/exercise[5] (42%) systematic reviews when contrasted against reviews addressing solely manual therapies (6%) (see Table 22-2), thus giving a better estimate of the effect. Finally, since many RCTs in orthopaedics have small sample sizes, the potential for imprecise estimation and flawed treatment recommendations is a primary concern. The literature also reveals a lack of utilization of designs that might be more appropriate for multimodal interventions commonly used in conservative management. Thus larger and multicentre trials with designs discussed in the next sections are needed.

THE CROSS-OVER DESIGN, DIAMOND DESIGN, FACTORIAL DESIGN AND FRACTIONAL FACTORIAL DESIGN

A *cross-over design* (Fig. 22-3) is particularly helpful when one wants to compare two active therapies and there is no response carry over between periods. The comparison between the two therapies has to overcome within-patient variation, which makes the design more precise than a two-group comparison in a single period. The model fitted to these data also assumes that there is no interaction between time or period and the therapies. In addition, the disease process should be capable of returning to baseline between the two periods, not

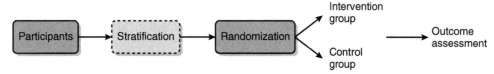

FIGURE 22-1 ■ A parallel two-group comparison randomized controlled trial design. An explanatory design aims to show that a treatment works using a placebo comparison thus testing efficacy while a pragmatic design aims to allow clinicians to make a decision by comparing the new active treatment relative to a standard treatment thus testing effectiveness. Stratification to balance key modulating factors is commonly used prior to randomization. Both primary and secondary outcomes (response variables) are measures based on identified primary and secondary trial objectives.

TABLE 22-1	Randomized Controlled Trial Design Strengths, Challenges and Opportunities for Redesign Considerations	
Strengths	**Challenges**	**Opportunities**
Appropriately designed and conducted RCT allow one to determine that a treatment causes a specific outcome Concealment of allocation and randomization results in a fair comparison by distributing potential covariates equally across comparison groups	Trials can be very expensive; there are many regulatory issues affecting trials; regulatory and ethics issues vary across countries and pose challenges for the conduct of large international randomized trials: the burden of recruitment and data collection can be difficult to integrate in clinical practice; often require dedicated research personnel that are not routinely available In trials using conservative management approaches such as manual therapy, the trials are not seeded in clearly understood 'biology'; there are difficulties with classifying spinal pain (many frameworks exist, e.g. biopsychosocial)	There are alternative research designs that can mitigate challenges by reducing sample size requirements or improving validity Research priorities need to be set to focus trials on priority questions CONSORT statement can guide trial design, CONSORT criteria are improving the reporting of trials Trial registry and Protocol publication prior to start of trial will limit reporting bias Sound 'biological' framework is needed to classify and characterize 'the disorder' being randomized and the nature and impacts of the complex interventions being tested
Analysis can be easy in simple RCT design; statistical analysis software has become more user-friendly	The definition of optimal outcome is difficult; different outcomes may be more important at different time points The definition of adverse events is difficult to adjudicate	Emerging work on defining adverse events in manual therapy may provide a frameworks[6]
Need large number of patients to minimize random errors; we need large trials of 1000 to 2000 observations or unbiased meta-analysis of moderate to large trials which collectively includes a few thousand observations	Challenges in multicentre trials contribute to a single site small trials that can fail to detect differences, produce unstable results contributing to inconsistent conclusions across trials; single sites may have unique samples that are not easily generalizable	Small trials may be needed for rare diseases If we do small trials we need better small trials: protocols avoid reporting bias; blending outcomes to reduce detection bias To perform large trials in manual therapy we need international collaboration on trials; international multicentre trials Linking into large existing databanks will reduce costs Unit of randomization is the site Web-based data collection enhances the ability to collaborate across sites
	Patients are resistant to some of the key elements of clinical research design: including that their treatment is determined by chance, the burden of follow-up, and the potential for not receiving timely treatment if they are in control group	
Balance can be achieved in prognostic factors if the trial is large enough; confounders are managed through stratification, the randomization process and design (subgroup analysis) thus patients with a better prognosis are not preferably treated	Sceptical if this balance can actually be achieved if trials are small It can be important to know which patients are most likely to benefit from certain treatments, so unless collection of data on potential effect modifiers is preplanned the study may not identify those most likely to benefit	Stratified block design can improve and mitigates confounders in design. Statistical analyses can control for effect modifiers, if measured The development of treatment based clinical prediction rules can increase the accuracy of treatment based prognosis
Compliant patients may have better prognosis, regardless of treatment; use ITT analysis; keep track of everyone, low loss to follow-up rate	Standardized measurement of treatment fidelity, co-intervention and compliance to care in rehab trials is usually inadequate In long trials for chronic disease, it is difficult to adhere to the therapy and is often polluted by co-intervention	

Continued on following page

TABLE 22-1	Randomized Controlled Trial Design Strengths, Challenges and Opportunities for Redesign Considerations (Continued)		
Strengths	**Challenges**	**Opportunities**
The use of appropriate mock procedures, hard outcome and blind adjudication of outcomes in RCTs help protect against patients who like their treatment and may report spuriously better outcomes unrelated to the mechanism of action	Trial can be done poorly: The trial is busted if it uses surrogate outcomes, soft outcomes and if end points are measured solely in the immediate post-treatment period or at short follow-up	Outcomes selection needs triangulation using self-report scale strategies; observer/performance-based outcomes with blind adjudication of outcomes; biologically based outcomes with blind adjudication of outcomes
Blinding of the practitioner (treater) and hard outcomes (morbidity, i.e. performance based) or blended evaluation of outcomes usually helps to protects against performance bias. For example, unblinded practitioners who like a treatment or are experts in a treatment might report spuriously better outcomes unrelated to the mechanism of action	Pressure to produce appealing results is especially strong in experts who prefer one approach	Expertise-based design helps balance differential treatment bias by only having experts in intervention A and experts in intervention B perform the treatments
Dosage of the intervention can easily be determined in large trials	Difficult to determine dosage since cells of care are very small	Factorial design
Benefits vs harm trade-offs can be determined. Can determine adverse event rate	Difficult to pick up adverse effects if they are rare or occur late or if the investigator does not look hard enough (or even look) for adverse outcome	
	Adverse events law suites; pay out of compensation for any adverse event not only severe adverse event; even those in control or what is part of usual clinical course require compensation for adverse events	

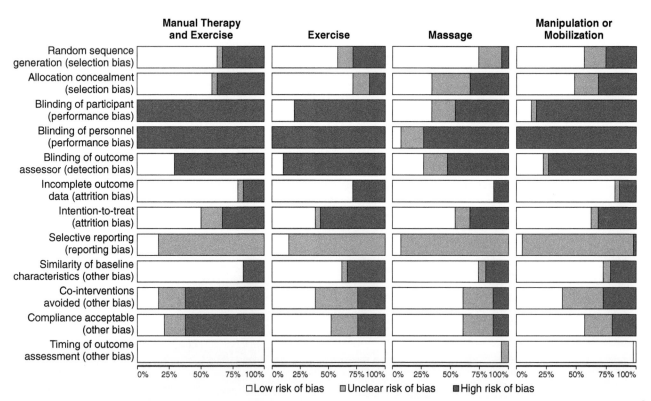

FIGURE 22-2 ■ Risk of bias from four Cochrane systematic reviews of clinical trials for neck pain on manual therapy and exercise,[5] exercise,[4] massage[13] and mobilization or manipulation.[12]

TABLE 22-2   **Reporting Bias Impacts the Size of the Effect Measure Most in the Manual Therapy Systematic Reviews**

Follow-up period	Manual therapy and exercise (*n* = 26)		Exercise (*n* = 21)		Massage (*n* = 16)		Manipulation (*n* = 39)		Mobilization (*n* = 16)	
LT	6/26	38%	6/21	29%	1/16	6%	4/39	10%	1/16	6%
IT	1/26	4%	4/21	19%	0/16	0%	5/39	13%	4/16	25%
IP or ST	15/26	58%	11/21	52%	15/16	94%	30/39	77%	11/16	68%

Positive effects are reported more often at immediate post treatment or in the short term such as 68% (mobilization[12])/77% (manipulation[12])/94% (massage[13]). There is better reporting of intermediate or long-term follow-up in exercise[4] (48%) or manual therapy plus exercise[5]>(42%) systematic reviews when contrasted against reviews addressing solely manual therapies[12] (6%), thus, giving a 'better' estimate of the true treatment effect.
IP, Immediate post treatment follow-up; *ST*, short-term follow-up; *IT*, Intermediate-term follow-up; *LT*, Long-term follow-up; *n*, number of randomized controlled trials.

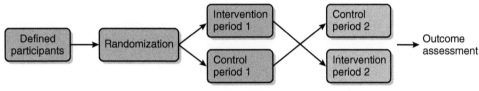
FIGURE 22-3 ■ Cross-over design.

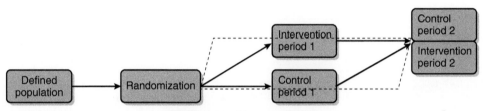
FIGURE 22-4 ■ Diamond design.

something that patients or clinicians would like to see in a chronic disease. If these assumptions cannot be reasonably assumed with the therapies and the condition being studied, this design should be avoided. If there is an interaction between time and the therapies, then the statistical literature suggests that using the first period data alone should be used for statistical inference. This means that the second period data are wasted and patients may be put at extra risk with little extra benefit.

The so-called *diamond design* (Fig. 22-4) describes the shape of the response versus time plot when the therapy being evaluated is of patient benefit in both periods; the control group has little benefit in the first period, but hopefully similar benefit during the second period as the intervention group did during the first period. If the intervention group does not receive any additional therapy during the second period, then the magnitude of the benefit lasting for the second period can be estimated. The design allows for the magnitudes of the intervention benefit in the first period to be compared to the control benefit during the second period; something not available for the single-period two-group design shown in Figure 22-1. While the diamond design takes twice as long to

conduct, it means that all patients get exposed to the new therapy being tested, an advantage over the Figure 22-1 design, as this should minimize dropouts that expect to get the new therapy. Figure 22-4 shows a plot of the response versus time type of graph for the diamond design. An example of the diamond design, however, without the plot, is shown using occupational therapy in patients with rheumatoid arthritis.[14]

The *factorial design* (Table 22-3) is a design that is useful if the therapy has many separate components. If the therapy has at least two components with at least two levels then a factorial design has groups created by multiplying the number of levels in each factor together to create the experimental groups such as shown in Table 22-3 with 4 duration levels and 3 frequency levels to create 12 experimental groups. Randomization here is to the 12 different groups. The main effects of each factor as well as all interactions are estimable from the complete factorial design with multiple replicates. Factorial designs using factors with at least three levels can also be modelled using response surface methods that allow the analyst to determine the optimal experimental conditions amongst the combination of factor levels. An example of a 2 × 2 factorial design is shown comparing a sleeping neck pillow and isometric neck exercises in patients with chronic neck pain.[15]

The *special fractional factorial design* (Table 22-4) is used when the combinations of the multiple therapies that are suggested in a factorial design may not be feasible clinically. For example, if a patient is referred to you for care, you may be uncomfortable putting patients into trial groups where the patients may not get a therapy that is proven to be efficacious. For example in a factorial design there is usually a group that gets no therapy. Suppose we have three therapies at two levels each, one of which (A) is a therapy of unknown efficacy and the other two (B, C) are therapies that many clinicians use alone or in combination. A full factorial design would have $2^3 = 8$ groups as outlined in Table 22-4.

Groups 1 and 2 contain no therapy that is proven and so many clinicians would be reluctant to put patients into these groups. On the other hand groups 3 to 8 get either therapy B or C or both. If we ran the design as a ¾

fraction of the complete factorial design as long as the proper model for the data had no interaction between therapy A and either B or C, then the main effect of factor A is still estimable, albeit with less efficiency than in the complete factorial design. Indeed the estimates would be of similar magnitude to the estimate provided by the one period – two-group design in factor A alone, yet, the patients would NOT be denied effective therapies. Hopefully, this design will minimize dropouts since all patients receive therapy of known benefit.

RANDOMIZED WITHDRAWAL AND EXPERTISE-BASED DESIGNS

The objective of the *randomized withdrawal design* (Fig. 22-5) is to assess the response to either reducing the dosage of a treatment or discontinuing it. This design is an option when either: (a) there is a chronic disease where participants have taken part in an effective therapy for a prolonged period; the goal is to determine if life-long therapy is necessary (i.e. withdrawal of maintenance chiropractic care); or (b) the efficacy of a treatment has not

---

TABLE 22-3 Factorial Design

	Number of Treatment Doses		
	Frequency (per week)		
Duration (weeks)	1	2	3
0	0	0	0
3	3	6	9
6	6	12	18
12	12	24	36

For a manual therapy (MT) dosage trial compared to standard care (i.e. exercise), if one factor has three levels (frequency per week) and the other four levels (duration of treatment in weeks), the factorial design is the product of the number of levels of the factors in the design, i.e. 3 × 4 = 12, where the 12 groups receive: (cell 1) neither of the two dosage factors = 0 times per week for 0 weeks, i.e. no MT just standard care; (cell 2) the first of the two dosage factors but not the second = standard treatment two times per week, (cell 4) the second of the two dosage factors and not the first (1 time per week for 3 weeks = 3 sessions of MT), (cell 12) both of the dosage factors (3 times a week for 12 weeks = 36 sessions of MT).

TABLE 22-4 Special Fractional Factorial Design

Group	*A*	*B*	*C*
1	No	No	No
2	Yes	No	No
3	No	Yes	No
4	Yes	Yes	No
5	No	No	Yes
6	Yes	No	Yes
7	No	Yes	Yes
8	Yes	Yes	Yes

Groups 1 and 2 contain no therapy that is proven. On the other hand groups 3 to 8 get either therapy B or C or both. If the design is run as a ¾ fraction of the complete factorial design then the main effect of factor A is still estimable, albeit with less efficiency than in the complete factorial design.

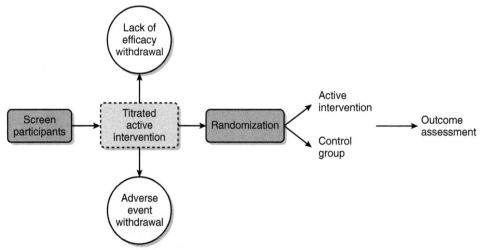

FIGURE 22-5 ■ Randomized withdrawal design.

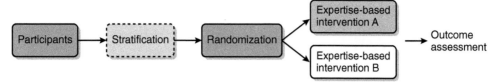

FIGURE 22-6 ■ Expertise-based design.

been conclusively shown to be beneficial (i.e. withdrawal of manual therapy from the proven combined manual therapy/exercise treatment approach; is this combination of care needed longer than in a short initial course of care?). Limitations of such designs are that a highly selected sample is assessed often having had an intervention for years while those with adverse effects will have had their therapy discontinued. The effect size in such designs is overestimated and the adverse effect underestimated.

In *expertise-based designs* (Fig. 22-6), randomization of participants to experts in intervention 'A' or experts in intervention 'B', ensures therapists perform only the procedure where they are expert. Differential expertise bias can occur in a conventional RCT when there is a disproportionate number of cases being performed by the expert in intervention 'A' compared with the expert in intervention 'B' and will bias results favouring intervention 'A'. Additionally, the unblinded clinician performing intervention 'A', an intervention that they favour, may be more meticulous in applying the procedure or subconsciously prescribe effective co-interventions. This trial design is more feasible for therapists with expertise are more willing to participate and perform only the techniques/interventions in which they are expert. Competence needs to be ensured in such trial designs. A clinician will also have ethical concerns enrolling patients into trials where they perform a technique in which they feel inexperienced (i.e. manipulation + exercise versus mobilization + exercise).

One of the challenges that occur within trials with non-pharmacologic interventions is that the skill and experience of the treatment provider is integral to the outcomes obtained. In the classic RCTs, treatment providers provide both treatments including one where they have a more experience, a preference and greater experience and the comparator which in some cases they only perform within the trial. This can contaminate the assessment of treatment efficacy. A potential solution is the expertise-based design where the patient consents to be randomized to treatment and as a result be treated by an expert clinician who can provide the treatment assigned.[16]

This has potential to provide a 'fair' comparison of the two treatment options but also has challenges in execution. The participant must consent to having their clinician determined by a random process which can be challenging if they prefer a specific person, and a pre-screening strategy is needed to consent and allocate patients. Further each site must have clinicians with experience in both treatment options. However, the benefits can include enhanced participation of clinicians and more valid comparisons. The definition of treating clinicians

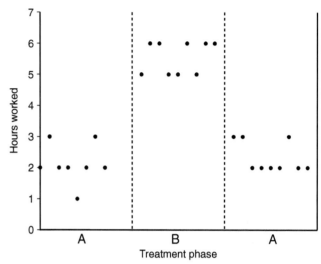

FIGURE 22-7 ■ Traditional A–B–A type *N*-of-1 design with phases of: **A**: multiple baseline, **B**: Intervention.

can vary along the expertise scale depending on whether an efficacy to effectiveness approach is preferred.

CLINICAL RESEARCH TO TEST TREATMENT EFFECTS: *N*-OF-1 TRIAL DESIGNS

As has been described above, RCTs require large samples, sometimes require challenging analyses, can be costly in terms of time and money, and the results are not directly transferable to making decisions regarding individual patients. RCTs will, on occasion, also present ethical dilemmas for clinicians, where it is not ethically sound to randomly allocate patients into treatment arms that are expected to be inferior (e.g. control or 'sham' groups). Finally, trials require the generalization of the results of a group (with variable results) to an individual.

N-of-1 or single-subject design (Fig. 22-7) provides an option to experimentally evaluate interventions in patients with chronic conditions by randomly allocating treatment and comparing standardized outcome measures. In traditional *N*-of-1 studies, a multiple baseline period is followed by random allocation of treatment options. Internal and external validity are strengthened with the addition of extra phases (e.g. A–B–A or A–B–A–C designs), consistent findings across several patients or consistency across environmental contexts. Where treatment is multimodal, one must avoid altering other aspects of care or co-intervention. *N*-of-1 trials work best when

John is a 35-year-old labourer whose primary job duties involve lifting and carrying over uneven terrain at jobsites. He has presented to physiotherapy for problems related to low back pain which are preventing him from working a full day. His primary goal is to resume full work duties and hours. As the physiotherapist, you have decided the best treatment for John's low back pain is a combination of manual mobilization for the lumbar spine, complemented with an exercise programme to improve stability and strength around the core, and the use of a hot pack or TENS for pain management. Currently he is only able to perform his regular job duties for an average of 2 hours per day before being limited by pain. This is down from a normal workload of 8 hours per day.

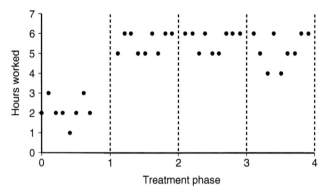

FIGURE 22-8 ■ *N*-of-1 sequential withdrawal design with phases of: **(0–1)** multiple baseline; **(1–2)** manual therapy, exercise and TENS; **(2–3)** manual therapy and exercise; **(3–4)** exercise only.

comparing two treatment alternatives and when return to a stable baseline occurs with removal of treatment (i.e. short washout). For example, comparing two different orthoses (splints) for carpometacarpal arthritis might provide an evidence-based answer as to which option will work best for a specific patient. However, in some cases it is unclear if all elements in a multimodal treatment programme are needed, as illustrated in Box 22-1. The treatment decision in Box 22-1 is to offer a combination of manual therapy, exercise and use of self-administered heating packs for pain management to improve number of hours worked at full job duties. The clinician may opt to conduct an *N*-of-1 study to evaluate treatment effectiveness in this case. Figure 22-7 shows the traditional approach using an A–B–A design, with each phase lasting 1 week. A positive treatment effect is indicated by the increase in John's average hours of full work duties with treatment and decay upon removal of treatment. While sound, there are two rather large pragmatic issues with this design and its interpretation. The first is on the surface it appears as though John may require manual therapy, exercise and hot pack in perpetuity. The second is, by virtue of conducting this study, the clinician has withdrawn a clearly effective treatment and reduced the patient's ability to work for at least 1 week, counter to most ethical practice guidelines.

The *withdrawal N-of-1 design* may be a better option for evaluating elements of multimodal programmes.[17] This is an extension of the *N*-of-1 design intended specifically for reversible conditions that require multimodal therapies. In a withdrawal design, the full set of therapies is offered once a stable baseline is established. Assuming effectiveness has been established, *one* aspect of the therapy is removed and another phase of repeated outcomes is collected. If the condition worsens again, that aspect of therapy can be re-introduced for another phase, and then a different aspect can be withdrawn. If removal of one aspect does not worsen the condition, the clinician may decide to subsequently remove a second aspect, and so on, until the gains can be maintained with the least amount of intervention. Figure 22-8 is our hypothetical patient John who comes to the clinic only able to work

an average of 2 hours per day at full duties. The intervention approach including manual therapy, exercise and TENS rapidly leads to improvement in his worked hours, up to 5.5 hours per day. In the next phase, the TENS is dropped, and gains are maintained with manual therapy and exercise. In the final phase, the manual therapy piece is withdrawn and a slight regression is seen with exercise alone.

Important consideration needs to be given to the order of withdrawal and the threshold for a satisfactory outcome. More burdensome interventions are often the most logical to withdraw first unless theoretical rationale suggests otherwise. The threshold for a satisfactory outcome may be based on existing literature (e.g. clinically important difference) or on the patient's individual goals. This is another advantage of this design. Using our hypothetical example, a slight regression in worked hours was noted in the final phase (exercise alone), down to 5 from 5.5 hours per day. Decisions regarding ongoing intervention can now be made using the data as a key information source; is an additional half hour of worked hours per day worth the time and cost burden of clinic visits for manual therapy treatments, or are the stakeholders content at 5 hours per day and exercises that can be performed at home?

CONCLUSION

Understanding alternative design when the usual parallel group design is not feasible will facilitate the choice of the most appropriate design for a given disorder–treatment–outcome situation. Each design may help to minimize systematic error such as selection bias, performance bias and detection bias. A traditional parallel group design is simple to understand but may be difficult to recruit for due to the placebo-controlled arm. Factorial designs require fewer patients and will answer two or more questions as well as their interaction, and thus save time. The cross-over trial design allows patients to receive both treatments in a pre-specified sequence and allows patients to act as their own control but assumes a stable disease or an absence of treatment-period interaction. The diamond design allows for an assessment of a delayed start of treatment however at the start of the second phase the patients are no longer comparable. The randomized withdrawal design reduces the time on a placebo since only the responders and those without adverse events are randomized. It however will overestimate the treatment effect. Expertise-based trial designs ensures therapists perform only the procedure where they are expert, provide a 'fair' comparison of the two treatment options, and enhances the participation of clinicians. Finally, for rare disorders, the *N*-of-1 trials design aims to assess the effect of more than one treatment in one person and patients are more likely to adhere to the treatment. Just like cross-over designs, *N*-of-1 requires a stable chronic disease. Thus innovative methodology will help answer specialized questions and address specific concerns such as engagement of physiotherapists in trial participation and encourage patient recruitment.

REFERENCES

1. Chalmer I. Unbiased, relevant, and reliable assessments in health care: Important progress during the past century, but plenty of scope for doing better. BMJ 1998;317:1167–8.
2. Bull JP. The historical development of clinical therapeutic trials. J Chronic Dis 1959;10:218–48.
3. Lilienfeld AM. Ceteris paribus: The evolution of the clinical trial. Bull History Medicine 1982;56:1–18.
4. Gross A, Kay TM, Paquin JP, et al. Exercises for mechanical neck disorders. Cochrane Database of Systematic Reviews 2015, Issue 1. Art. No.: CD004250. doi:10.1002/14651858.CD004250.pub5.
5. Miller J, Gross AR, Kay T, et al. Manual therapy with exercise for neck pain. Cochrane Database Syst Rev 2014;(in press).
6. Carlesso LC, MacDermid JC, Santaguida P. Standardization of adverse event terminology and reporting in orthopaedic physical therapy: Application to the cervical spine. J Orthop Sports Phys Ther 2010;40(8):455–63.
7. Cleland JA, Childs JD, Whitman JM. Psychometric properties of the Neck Disability Index and Numeric Pain Rating Scale in patients with mechanical neck pain. Arch Phys Med Rehabil 2008;89:69–74.
8. MacDermid JC, Miller J, Côté P, et al. Use of outcome measures in managing neck pain: an international multidisciplinary survey. The Open Orthop J 2013;7:506–20.
9. MacDermid JC, Ghobrial M, Quirion K, et al. Validation of a new test that assesses the functional performance of the upper extremity and neck (FIT-HaNSA) in patients with shoulder pathology. BMC Musculoskelet Disord 2007;8:42.
10. Pierrynowski MR, Gross AR, Miles M, et al. Reliability of the long-range power-law correlations obtained from bilateral stride intervals in asymptomatic volunteers whilst treadmill walking. Gait Posture 2005;22(1):46–50.
11. van Uum SH, Sauve B, Fraser LA, et al. Elevated content of cortisol in hair of paitents with severe chronic pain: a novel biomarker for stress. Stress 2008;Nov 11(6):483–8.
12. Gross AR, Langevin P, Andres C, et al. Manipulation or mobilization for neck pain. Cochrane Database Syst Rev 2014;(in press).
13. Patel KC, Gross AR, Graham N, et al. Massage for mechanical neck disorders. Cochrane Database Syst Rev 2012, Issue 9. Art. No.: CD004871. doi:10.1002/14651858.CD004871.pub4.
14. Helewa A, Goldsmith CH, Lee P, et al. Occupational therapy home service on patients with rheumatoid arthritis. Lancet 1991;337(8755):1453–6.
15. Helewa A, Goldsmith CH, Smythe HA, et al. Exercise and sleeping neck support on patients with chronic neck pain: A randomized clinical trial. J Rheumatol 2007;34(1):151–8.
16. Devereaux PJ, Bhandari M, Clarke M, et al. Need for expertise based randomised controlled trials. BMJ 2005;330(7482):88.
17. Rusch FR, Kazdin AE. Toward a methodology of withdrawal designs for the assessment of response maintenance. J Appl Behav Anal 1981;14(2):131–40.

RESEARCH APPROACHES TO MUSCULOSKELETAL PHYSIOTHERAPY

CHAPTER OUTLINE

NICOLA PETTY AND HUBERT VAN GRIENSVEN'S INTRODUCTION

Musculoskeletal (MSK) physiotherapy is a complex intervention delivered within a context of human and very often physical interaction. Practitioners deliver a service to people within a political, social and medical context. Consequently, a physiotherapy researcher is faced with a host of interdependent aspects that may be investigated, such as the clinical effects of a controlled intervention, the interaction between therapist and patient, the way patients experience their condition, or the political context of health care. The choice of research focus will suggest the type of data that need to be collected, the methods that may be used and the overall methodological approach that best suits the research. The predominantly quantitative focus of current MSK physiotherapy literature may have created the illusion that there is only one research approach.[1] This chapter series aims to broaden the options for the researching clinician by providing a brief overview of available methodological choices.

In developing a research question, researchers need to familiarize themselves with existing literature in the field to consider what is known, and what is unknown and needs to be investigated. Next, they may consider whether a subject requires a deductive or inductive approach. In the former the researcher formulates a hypothesis and then designs the research to either support or disprove it, usually on a statistical basis.[2] However, if not enough is known about a subject to generate a feasible hypothesis, an inductive approach may be needed, which involves generating theory from observation, interviewing, etc.[3]

The focus of the study may suggest the type of data required. If statistics are involved for instance, to compare the effect sizes of two treatments, the data are numerical and the research is quantitative in nature. Quantitative researchers try to be as objective as possible and to minimize the influence of anything other than predetermined controlled variables [see Chapter 23.1]. While this approach answers particular questions very well, not all practice can be reduced to numbers. A qualitative study may be needed where understanding of people is sought and therefore data consist of verbal and non-verbal communication, for example [see Chapter 23.2]. Finally, complex or new topics may benefit from a combination of qualitative and quantitative data in mixed methods research [see Chapter 23.3]. Each of these three approaches comes with certain assumptions about the nature of reality (ontology) and what can be known (epistemology).

The research approach and data type usually suggest the research method. Method refers to specific instruments and techniques of data collection, such as qualitative interviews, surveys or measurement of strain or angle. It also includes methods of data analysis such as statistical comparison and thematic analysis of interview data. Methods of data collection are not inextricably linked with specific approaches. For instance, questionnaires may be used to establish participants' opinions by asking multiple-choice questions, thus generating quantitative data. Conversely, the inclusion of free text sections in a questionnaire generates qualitative data.

The next three chapters discuss quantitative, qualitative and mixed methods research. Each chapter outlines the underlying theory of the approach as well as the methodologies, methods and potential questions. The concluding chapter lists a few recommended texts for readers who require more detailed information about specific research approaches.

REFERENCES

1. Petty NJ, Stew G, Thomson OP. Ready for a paradigm shift? Part 1: introducing the philosophy of qualitative research. Man Ther 2012;17(4):267–74.
2. Bowling A. Research Methods in Health – Investigating Health and Health Services. Maidenhead: Open University; 2009.
3. Teddlie C, Tashakkori A. Foundations of Mixed Methods Research. Integrating Quantitative and Qualitative Approaches in the Social and Behavioral Sciences. Thousand Oaks, CA: Sage; 2009. p. 26–7.

CHAPTER 23.1 ■ QUANTITATIVE RESEARCH

Lieven Danneels

WHAT IS QUANTITATIVE RESEARCH?

Quantitative research methods have been the foundation for traditional biomedical research for a long time.[1] The goal of quantitative research is to answer research questions or to test hypotheses.[2] Quantitative methods examine the effects of specified circumstances on an outcome of interest in ways that can be expressed numerically.[3] Thus, quantitative research deals with measurable characteristics, named parameters, variables or factors, and uses statistics to deduct conclusions.[4,5] Quantitative research aims to determine the relationship between one thing (an independent variable) and another (a dependent or outcome variable) in a population.

METHODOLOGY AND METHODS

Quantitative research designs can be descriptive/observational, experimental or quasi-experimental.

Descriptive/observational studies allow for associations between variables to be investigated. In these studies, the subjects are observed without otherwise intervening, thus a participant's exposure and outcome status are observed with no influence from the researcher. However, the evidence they provide is not strong enough to establish a causal link. Several types of studies can be classified as descriptive studies:

- *A case or a case series study* is the simplest form. A case study reports data on only one subject. Descriptive studies of a few cases are called a case series.
- *Cross-sectional studies* analyse variables of interest in a sample of subjects once, and the relationships between them are determined. A cross-sectional study examines a characteristic and an outcome in the same individuals at the same point in time.
- *A cohort study* is a study that follows over time a group of similar individuals (cohorts) who differ with respect to certain factors under study, to determine how these affect outcome. A cohort study can be either prospective or retrospective. The feature that distinguishes a prospective from a retrospective cohort is simply and solely whether the outcome of interest has occurred at the time the investigator initiates the study. *The prospective cohort study* is important for research on the aetiology of diseases and disorders. Therefore, the individuals are not randomly allocated to the groups. The study starts with the identification of the population and the exposure status (exposed/not exposed groups) and follows them (over time) for the development of disease. *Retrospective cohort studies* use existing data collected in the past to identify the population and the exposure status (exposed/not exposed groups) and determines at present the (development) status of disease. They use information that has usually been collected for reasons other than research, such as administrative data and medical records.

- *Case-control studies* compare cases with controls. Individuals who have the outcome of interest (cases) are compared to individuals who do not have the outcome of interest (controls) by looking back in time to identify the existence of possible causal factors. Case-control studies have a *retrospective* character, because they focus on conditions in the past that might have caused subjects to become cases rather than controls.

Besides the abovementioned group, there are the *experimental studies*, which are also referred to as *intervention studies*. This approach provides the best evidence about cause and effect. Instead of just observing the subjects, an independent variable (e.g. the therapeutic intervention) is manipulated to determine the effects on the dependent variables (i.e. the outcome). In an experiment, an effort is made to identify and impose control over all other variables except one. Further distinction can be made between an active and an attribute independent variable. The active independent variable is a manipulated variable, which is controlled within a specified period of time during the study (e.g. group A receives therapy X and group B is undergoing therapy Y). The attribute independent variable (e.g. ethnicity) is a measure of characteristics of the person and not study-dependent.[3,6] Experimental studies, also referred to as *longitudinal or repeated measures studies*, can be subdivided into several types.

- A *time series* is the simplest experiment. One or more measurements are taken on all subjects before and after a treatment. A major problem with a time series is to determine the changes seen as being the effect from nothing else but the treatment.
- A *crossover design* might be a solution to this problem. The subjects are given two treatments: one being the real treatment, the other a control or reference treatment. Half of the subjects receive the real treatment first and the other half the control first. After a period of time, sufficient to allow a treatment to effect to wash out, the treatments are crossed over. Multiple crossover designs involving several treatments are also possible. A problem with such a study design is that a long-term follow-up is not possible.
- A *controlled trial*, with a control group and an experimental group, is to be used if the researcher wants to evaluate long-term effects, or when the treatment effect is unlikely to be washed out between measurements. All subjects are measured but only half of them, the experimental group, receive the treatment. All subjects are then measured again and the change in the experimental group is compared with the change in the control group.
- The *randomized controlled trial* is believed to be the 'gold standard' to test the effectiveness of an intervention. Individuals who do not have the outcome of interest are randomly allocated to receive the intervention (the experimental group), or standard of care or conventional treatment (the comparison group), or no intervention (the control group) and are followed forward in time to determine whether they experience the outcome of interest.
- In a *single-blind controlled trial*, the subjects are blind to the identity of the treatment. In a *double-blind controlled trial*, both the subject and the researcher do not know what treatment the subjects receive until all measurements are taken.

Likewise, the *quasi-experimental research* attempts to establish cause–effect relationships among the variables. In a quasi-experimental research approach, there is again a manipulated independent variable, but the participants are not randomly allocated to a group. In a strong quasi-experimental design the participants are already in a few similar intact groups, but the treatment is randomly assigned. In a moderate strong quasi-experimental design, the participants are again in intact groups, but the treatment cannot be randomly appointed. And in a weak quasi-experimental design the participants assign themselves to a group by choosing to participate in the intervention or in the control group.[6–10]

FINDINGS

Statistics are a major tool in quantitative research. They allow the researcher to sample a portion of the population and to use probability to decide whether the findings from the sample are likely to apply to the entire population.[10] Statistical methods can be used to assess relationships between the variables measured.[3] Interpretation of the results should be done carefully. Significant findings may not reflect clinically important outcomes[10] and findings might be clinically relevant although not statistically significant.

SUMMARY

Quantitative research provides important tools to answer research questions that can be formulated as hypotheses. It should be noted, however, that quantitative research cannot answer all types of questions. In health care, a recognized error is the attribution of the properties which apply collectively to a group, to an individual. The critical need is to understand where generality ends and individuality begins, and that requires merging the two types of knowledge: quantitative and qualitative research are complementary.[1,3] The fundamental differences lie in the content of the research question to be answered.[4]

REFERENCES

1. Runciman WB. Qualitative versus quantitative research – balancing cost, yield and feasibility. Qual Saf Health Care 2002;11(2):146–7.
2. Vogelsang J. Quantitative research versus quality assurance, quality improvement, total quality management, and continuous quality improvement. J Perianesth Nurs 1999;14(2):78–81.
3. Lakshman M, Sinha L, Biswas M, et al. Quantitative vs qualitative research methods. Indian J Paediatr 2000;67(5):369–77.
4. Bergsjo P. Qualitative and quantitative research – is there a gap, or only verbal disagreement? Acta Obstet Gynecol Scand 1999;78(7):559–62.
5. Castillo-Page L, Bodilly S, Bunton SA. AM last page. Understanding qualitative and quantitative research paradigms in academic medicine. Acad Med 2012;87(3):386.
6. Enarson DA, Kennedy SM, Miller DL. Choosing a research study design and selcting a population study. Int J Tuberc Lung Dis 2004;8(9):1151–6.
7. Key Elements of a Research Proposal Quantitative Design, <http://www.bcps.org/offices/lis/researchcourse/develop_quantitative.html>; [accessed on April 25th 2014].
8. Hopkins WG. Quantitative Reserch Design Sportscience 4(1), <sportsci.org/jour/0001/wghdesign.html>; 2000.
9. Morgan GA, Gliner JA, Harmon RJ. Quantitative research approaches. J Am Acad Child Adolesc Psychiatry 1999;38(12):1595–7.
10. Dowrick AS, Tornetta P, Obremskey WT, et al. Practical research methods for orthopaedic surgeons. J Bone Joint Surg Am 2012;94(4):368–74.

CHAPTER 23.2 ■ QUALITATIVE RESEARCH

Nicola Petty

WHAT IS QUALITATIVE RESEARCH?

Qualitative research may be described as 'a form of social enquiry that focuses on the way people interpret and make sense of their experiences and the world in which they live'.[1] Qualitative research is sometimes referred to as naturalistic enquiry,[2] which aims to understand the social reality, such as behaviours, perspectives and experiences of individuals, groups and cultures.

ONTOLOGICAL AND EPISTEMOLOGICAL ASSUMPTIONS

The potential for a researcher to understand the views of an individual, group or culture is not straightforward. Reflecting on our everyday lives and our ability to understand others (and ourselves for that matter) highlight the challenges faced by qualitative researchers. The views of an individual may be considered subjective and constructed by the individual, and in this situation the researcher seeks knowledge about the meaning that the individual holds; this view would equate with the ontological position of idealism or relativism.[3] Qualitative researchers make explicit their ontological assumptions about the nature of the reality under investigation and these can lie on a continuum from realism to idealism (or relativism).[4] Closely related to the nature of what is being studied (ontology), is what can be known about what is being studied (epistemology). A researcher may, for example, consider that an individual creates meaning through engagement with others (an epistemological stance of social constructionism) or that an individual constructs meaning in their minds (an epistemological position of constructivism).[3] Qualitative researchers make explicit their epistemological assumptions about what can be known about that reality; these can lie on a continuum from positivism to interpretivism (or subjectivism).[4] Whatever ontological and epistemological positions are adopted, qualitative researchers seek to ensure these positions are congruent with the methodology and methods used to explore a given topic.

METHODOLOGY AND METHODS

There are a number of qualitative research methodologies available and these include case study, grounded theory, ethnography, phenomenology, narrative enquiry, evaluation research, action and participatory action research, discourse analysis, hermeneutics and feminism. Each methodology comes with its own set of processes and procedures as well as underlying ontological and epistemological assumptions. An example of a qualitative piece of research in MSK physiotherapy may serve to highlight some of the concepts considered so far in this chapter. The focus of the research was to explore the learning transition of physiotherapists following a Master's course in MSK physiotherapy.[5] It was assumed that the learning process was predominantly through social exchange with others (social constructionism). In relation to methodology, a constructivist (as opposed to objectivist) grounded theory approach[6] was chosen, as its assumptions were compatible with social constructionism. It was assumed that individuals would have unique learning transitions and so individual interviews (not focus groups) were used to collect data. The ontological and epistemological position of the researcher acts as an overarching paradigm to the study and influences decision making throughout the research process, from early inception to final write up.

In qualitative research the focus is on the views of people, their perceptions, meanings and interpretations of a phenomenon within a particular context. The individual or groups and the context are explored in all its complexity and it is assumed that there are multiple constructed views of reality with the participants' history, culture, setting, time and place shaping the phenomenon being explored. Researchers thus seek to understand (describe and explain) these individual meanings. This is done as far as possible in their natural setting as the context is considered part of the phenomenon and the process of gathering data can, of itself, influence participants.

There is an acknowledgement of the subjectivity of the researcher in qualitative research. The researcher's history, culture, setting, time, place, etc. will influence all aspects of a research study and in particular data collection and analysis. The researcher is the primary instrument of data collection, bringing their subjective self to the research and requires them to adopt a critically reflective and reflexive stance.[7] Researchers try to examine and understand the perceptions, actions and situations from the participant's point of view. This can be challenging when conducting research in one's own professional setting and may require an extended length of time to make what is familiar appear strange. The researcher collaborates interdependently with participants who are integral to the study and in some situations, particularly in participatory action research, may act as co-researchers. The quality of the researcher–participant relationship is thus of critical concern in qualitative research.

Data can come from multiple sources such as observation, interviews, documents, field notes and personal reflections to develop understanding of individuals in their context. Data, which are mostly in the form of words, have primacy. Data collection and analysis proceed together. Analysis and interpretation occur from the beginning of the study and are built from the data inductively, from the specific to the general. No initial hypothesis is developed at the start of the study; rather, tentative working propositions are developed (analysis) from initial data collection that is then modified in subsequent data collection. This iterative cycle of data collection and analysis continues until there are robust propositions to conclude the study. Detailed ('thick') description of the data and context aim to uncover the meanings of participants' experiences and actions, which can provide theoretical and analytical description and interpretation and in some cases, theory development. Study findings portray situated understandings that are reflective of the participants' perceptions; findings are therefore reported with a significant number of quotations from participants.

FINDINGS

Qualitative research can gain insight into the world of individuals, groups and/or cultures. Commonalities and patterns may be identified across individuals. In some cases an explanation of a social process may be developed. Thick description aims to allow the reader to put themselves into the situation of the participants and gain empathic and experiential understanding.[1] The social world and meanings held by individuals and groups will change over time, thus findings are temporary and uncertain. Theoretical (rather than statistical) generalizations are developed that may be transferable to other settings. The quality of the research is assessed though trustworthiness; this umbrella term includes credibility (findings ring true), transferability (of findings to other situations), dependability of the study procedures and confirmability that the findings relate to the data.[8] Strategies are put in place during the research study to address each of these aspects.

WHEN MIGHT YOU USE QUALITATIVE RESEARCH?

Qualitative research would, for example, enable exploration of patient-centred care, understanding the

perspective of the patient or practitioner and the values that underpin their behaviour and motivation.

Within MSK physiotherapy qualitative research questions could include:
- what is it like to live with chronic low back pain or neck pain?
- what triggers a person to seek physiotherapy?
- how do MSK physiotherapists decide to refer a patient on for further investigations?
- how do MSK physiotherapists develop expertise?
- what do patients expect from MSK physiotherapists?
- what is the nature of the patient–therapist relationship?

SUMMARY

The theoretical foundations of qualitative research are compatible with, and appropriate for, investigation of contemporary MSK practice. Each of the qualitative methodologies provides a particular perspective to understand the behaviour, perspective and experience of patients and practitioners that help inform practice.

REFERENCES

1. Holloway I. Basic Concepts for Qualitative Research. Oxford: Blackwell; 1997.
2. Lincoln YS, Guba EG. Naturalistic Inquiry. Beverly Hills: Sage; 1985.
3. Blaikie N. Approaches to Social Enquiry. Cambridge: Polity; 1993.
4. Savin-Baden M, Major C. Qualitative Research, the Essential Guide to Theory and Practice. London: Routledge; 2013.
5. Petty NJ. Towards Clinical Expertise: Learning Transitions Of Neuromusculoskeletal Physiotherapists. University of Brighton: Unpublished DPT thesis; 2009.
6. Charmaz K. Constructing Grounded Theory. A Practical Guide Through Qualitative Analysis. London: Sage; 2006.
7. Finlay L, Gough B. Reflexivity. A Practical Guide for Researchers in Health and Social Sciences. Oxford: Blackwell Science; 2003.
8. Erlandson DA, Harris EL, Skipper BL, et al. Doing Naturalistic Inquiry, A Guide to Methods. Newbury Park: Sage; 1993.

CHAPTER 23.3 ■ MIXED METHODS RESEARCH

Hubert van Griensven

WHAT IS MIXED METHODS RESEARCH?

Traditionally most research has been done from either a quantitative perspective based on hypothesis and deduction, or an interpretative and usually inductive qualitative perspective. Mixed methods research (MMR) utilizes both and may be defined/described as 'the type of research in which a researcher or team of researchers combines elements of qualitative and quantitative research approaches (e.g. use of qualitative and quantitative viewpoints, data collection, analysis, inference techniques) for the broad purposes of breadth and depth of understanding and corroboration'.[1] The choice of methods and the way in which they are combined is driven by the research

question.[2-4] Researchers may formulate at least one qualitative and one quantitative question[5] and should ensure that all research questions are open-ended and non-directional.[3]

In MMR both qualitative and quantitative data are integrated or connected in the overall study. All of the study's strands must be an essential part of the study, be investigated with rigour and analysed fully.[1] Their role and mutual relationship need to be considered throughout the design, execution and reporting of the entire study,[10] even when one element of the study receives more emphasis.[5] For example, the use of a patient questionnaire in a quantitative investigation of a drug or other treatment does not constitute MMR, because the data are rarely subjected to full qualitative analysis and are typically represented numerically.

WHEN MIGHT YOU USE MIXED METHODS RESEARCH?

Rationales for undertaking MMR include the engagement and recruitment of participants, the development and testing of a research instrument, the investigation of interventions and the enhancement of a study's significance.[7] MMR offers the potential to be both inductive and deductive, incorporate more views and provide stronger inferences compared with single method studies.[5] Some MMR researchers have utilized MMR specifically to address issues of social justice.[8,9]

METHODOLOGY AND METHODS

Only key design options for MMR studies will be discussed here, although many others are possible. A sequential study may be undertaken when one type of data is needed for the development of a subsequent study phase.[10] For instance, a large survey may be used to identify the most appropriate topics and participants for subsequent interviews, or a focus group may be used to generate a theory that is then tested with statistical methods. Alternatively, a researcher may decide to investigate qualitative and quantitative aspects of a phenomenon in parallel.[10] Other design possibilities include embedding one type of investigation within another[10] or the statistical analysis of agreement between codings of qualitative interview data.[11]

In addition to the best design for their study, researchers need to consider at which stage or stages mixing of qualitative and quantitative aspects will take place.[10] Both must be considered at the design stage and throughout the study.[6] In a sequential study, mixing takes place as data are collected. Mixing during data analysis may be done through triangulation or conversion of the results for direct comparison,[12] elaboration of one arm on the other,[12] or the use of a dialectic approach, which invites dialogue about paradoxical and conflicting results.[13] Alternatively, the arms of a study may be conducted and analysed separately, with mixing not taking place until the interpretation phase. Finally, mixing takes place at every stage of the research process in the *fully integrated design*.[5]

DIFFICULTIES ASSOCIATED WITH MIXED METHODS RESEARCH

Although MMR is an exciting field of research, it is not without its difficulties and controversies. Researchers who wish to truly integrate the findings of qualitative and quantitative methods must have a firm grasp of both.[14] MMR may therefore be problematic to researchers who have a background in only one approach or are new to research,[15] although changes in the way research methods are taught are likely to change this.[16] That said, even for competent researchers MMR can be more time-consuming and more costly than single method research.[15] Those with limited resources should therefore consider focusing their research question so that it can be answered using a single method.[2] This is especially pertinent because the level of unpredictability increases with the number of research methods, and more complex research does not necessarily yield more complete answers.[17] In a sequential MMR study the initial phase may yield results that do not support the second phase as anticipated, while a parallel design can produce findings which contradict each other.[6,18] Although unexpected findings have the potential to generate greater insight[15] or a dialogue about the multiplicity of viewpoints,[13] they may also be disruptive. For example, the criteria for validity or rigour set out at the design stage may not be appropriate for the actual findings.[2] Applications to commissioning bodies and ethics panels may therefore have to be revised significantly or completely.

A further difficulty is the exact way in which qualitative and quantitative findings should be combined, which is the subject of discussion among MMR scholars.[1,4,19] Even in sequential MMR studies where analysis and interpretation of one phase are completed before starting the next, integration of the findings remains essential. Direct comparison of data may require the transformation of at least one set of data, for instance by *qualitizing* quantitative data or vice versa,[3] which is likely to raise objections from mono-method researchers of either persuasion. Mixed methods researchers may find themselves under pressure to discuss only the part of their study that is acceptable to a particular audience when writing up or presenting their findings.[14]

SUMMARY

MMR involves the combination and integration of qualitative and quantitative data and research methods. As a consequence, it offers the possibility of investigations with greater scope and depth than mono-method research approaches. However, MMR adds its own complications and considerations to those associated with each method used, so it should only be considered if the research question cannot be answered by a quantitative or qualitative method alone.

CONCLUSION

This chapter has provided a brief overview of three research approaches to enable the reader to make an informed choice when planning a research study. The choice for a specific methodology is driven by the research question, which has to be considered carefully. For further reading, the following texts are recommended:

Quantitative Research

Bowling A 2009 Research methods in health – investigating health and health services. 3 ed. Maidenhead: Open University

Hicks C 2009 Research Methods for Clinical Therapists: Applied Project Design and Analysis. 2 ed. Edinburgh: Churchill Livingstone

Qualitative Research

Braun V, Clarke V 2013 Successful qualitative research, a practical guide for beginners. Los Angeles: Sage

Savin-Baden M, Major C 2013 Qualitative research, the essential guide to theory and practice. London: Routledge

Silverman D 2013 A very short, fairly interesting and reasonably cheap book about qualitative research. Los Angeles: Sage

Mixed Methods Research

Creswell J, Plano-Clark V 2011 Designing and conducting mixed methods research. 2 ed. Thousand Oaks, CA: Sage

Teddlie C, Tashakkori A 2009 Foundations of mixed methods research. Integrating quantitative and qualitative approaches in the social and behavioral sciences. Thousand Oaks, CA: Sage

REFERENCES

1. Johnson R, Onwuegbuzie A, Turner L. Toward a definition of mixed methods research. J Mixed Methods Res 2007;1(2):112–33.
2. Bryman A. Paradigm peace and the implications for quality. Int J Soc Res Methodol 2006;9(2):111–26.
3. Onwuegbuzie A, Leech N. Linking research questions to mixed methods data analysis procedures. Qual Rep 2006;11(3):474–98.
4. Greene J. Is mixed methods social inquiry a distinctive methodology? J Mixed Methods Res 2008;2(1):7–22.
5. Teddlie C, Tashakkori A. Foundations of Mixed Methods Research. Integrating Quantitative and Qualitative Approaches in the Social and Behavioral Sciences. Thousand Oaks, CA: Sage; 2009.
6. Brannen J. Mixing methods: the entry of qualitative and quantitative approaches into the research process. Int J Soc Res Methodol 2005;8(3):173–84.
7. Collins K, Onwuegbuzie A, Sutton I. A model incorporating the rationale and purpose for conducting mixed-methods research in special education and beyond. Learn Disabil: Contemp J 2006;4(1):67–100.
8. Mertens D. Transformative paradigm. Mixed methods and social justice. J Mixed Methods Res 2007;1(3):212–25.
9. Mertens D. Emerging advances in mixed methods: addressing social justice. J Mixed Methods Res 2013;7(3):215–18.
10. Creswell J, Plano-Clark V. Designing and Conducting Mixed Methods Research. 2nd ed. Thousand Oaks, CA: Sage; 2011. p. 66–96.
11. Castro F, Kellison J, Boyd S, et al. A methodology for conducting integrative mixed methods research and data analyses. J Mixed Methods Res 2010;4(4):342–60.
12. Greene J, Caracelli V, Graham W. Toward a conceptual framework for mixed-method evaluation designs. Educ Eval Policy Anal 1989;11(3):255–74.
13. Greene J. Mixed Methods in Social Enquiry. San Francisco: Wiley; 2007. p. 69.
14. Bryman A. Barriers to integrating quantitative and qualitative research. J Mixed Methods Res 2007;1(1):8–22.
15. Johnson R, Onwuegbuzie A. Mixed methods research: a research paradigm whose time has come. Educ Res 2004;33(7):14–26.
16. Hesse-Biber S, Johnson R. Coming at things differently: future directions of possible engagement with mixed methods research. J Mixed Methods Res 2013;7(2):103–9.
17. Bergman M. The good, the bad, and the ugly in mixed methods research and design. J Mixed Methods Res 2011;5(4):271–5.
18. Morgan D. Practical strategies for combining qualitative and quantitative methods: applications to health research. Qual Health Res 1998;8(3):362–76.
19. Tashakkori A, Teddlie C. Putting the human back in 'human research methodology': the researcher in mixed methods research. J Mixed Methods Res 2010;4(4):271–7.

CHAPTER 24

STANDARDIZED DATA COLLECTION, AUDIT AND CLINICAL PROFILING

Ann Moore

INTRODUCTION

As can be seen from other chapters in this section of the text, there are many different approaches to research that are relevant and essential to underpin musculoskeletal physiotherapy. One of the key elements of most research approaches is the inclusion of robust data that can underpin the study's findings, for example demographic data, clinical data, service delivery data, historical data and objective clinical data, which can be used often to explain why particular approaches to care have particular effects on a particular profile of patients. These data can also be used for clinical profiling and to inform clinical audit activities.

In addition there are various ways in which data collection and appropriate use of data can contribute to the care of patients, the quality of service delivery, marketing of services, production of business cases, and quality enhancement of the provision of services, together with cost-effectiveness calculations, outcomes of care, improvement of patient experiences and patient satisfaction and also job satisfaction of those involved in the data collection and interpretation of the data.

In research terms standardized data collection can help to rigorously profile research participants for inclusion, or for consideration for inclusion, in aspects of a research study. It can also enable further explanation of findings of studies focusing on profiling participants and how they have reacted to different types of interventions included in the study concerned. In addition, standardized data collection can help to further develop understandings of qualitative findings, for example what patient profiles appear to impact on their experiences and perhaps their expectations of certain techniques/approaches. One can only carry out such analyses of data if the data have been collected robustly and rigorously with no room for ambiguity. This chapter explores the concept of standardized data collection and the mechanisms for developing standardized data collection tools.

CONTEXT

Research, as defined broadly by Bailey[1] is 'any activity which increases knowledge'. Standardized data collection is a mechanism by which musculoskeletal clinicians can increase the knowledge of the work they undertake, the profiles of patients that they treat, the clinical approaches that they are taking, and how and when treatment takes place, as well as a range of other possible knowledge area developments.

The author, with a number of colleagues, has worked on the development of a range of standardized data collection tools for use in musculoskeletal physiotherapy since the mid-1990s and has published a master class on this topic area that describes the development processes in detail and also documents its historical development.[2] In this paper we defined a standardized data collection tool as:

'an agreed instrument which enables data concerning patients, therapists and/or healthcare settings and approaches to be collected unambiguously by a range of practitioners in a number of different settings'.[2]

The definition asserts that this would allow data to be shared and understood by practitioners working in the same organization, as well as across multiple organizations countrywide or potentially worldwide. The important things to note here are that if a tool is needed, then in order for it to work effectively or for clinicians to use the tool effectively, the tool must be developed in a robust and rigorous way which, in itself, requires some research activity. In addition, a process has to be in place for piloting the tool, and adapting the tool based on feedback from pilot studies. This process will be discussed in the rest of this chapter.

If data are being shared then of course the data collected must be anonymized to protect the identity of individual patients and ethics approval for the activity must be gained. Data collected can include aspects of patients' demographics, service delivery, process and type of care, referral pathways, clinical findings, outcomes of care, costs of care, profile of care providers, content of care and factors that may have influenced care and the outcome of care.

The reason that standardized data collection is important is that all health agendas and policies across the world are focusing on the quality issues relating to innovative, effective and efficient services that meet health-care needs. As economic growth continues to be slow in many countries and health-care costs often represent the largest proportion of government expenditure, hospital staffs are increasingly being required to provide good-quality information to commissioners of health care to support their service. This could relate to value for money, demonstrably high-quality patient outcomes and also in widening access and providing choice in health-care provision. In this context standardized data collection can help with the following:

- Sourcing evidence to demonstrate improved quality of care and improvement of services.
- Benchmarking outcomes against other similar and perhaps competitive service providers.
- Monitoring the productivity of the workforce.
- Delivering high-quality evidence-based services and auditing impact of services.
- Being able to match resources with projected health needs.
- Setting appropriate staffing levels in all areas of service delivery.
- Providing data concerning service delivery and outcomes to all stakeholders.
- Auditing clinical services against standards.
- Providing evidence on which commissioning decisions can be based.
- Facilitating patient profiling, especially if combined with screening tools and validated and reliable patient-recorded outcome measures.
- Identifying meaningful research questions for the profession/speciality.

It is well recognized that good-quality data are the foundation of good-quality information and that when decision makers use information well, services improve.[3] People who make decisions include patients and users of services who can chose particular hospitals/practices, clinicians and treatment approaches, professionals who exercise judgement on treatments and approaches, managers who prioritize service delivery and politicians who allocate resources for health care.[3]

The Audit Commission[3] defined good-quality data as the statistics, facts, numbers and records that can be organized and analysed into information that answers a specific need. Six characteristics of good-quality data were published by the Audit Commission[4] in a report Voluntary Data, Quality Standards:

- Accuracy – data need to be accurate for their intended purpose.
- Validity – data need to be recorded and used in compliance with relevant requirements.
- Reliability – data need to reflect stable and consistent data collection processes across collection points and over time.
- Timelines – data should be captured as quickly as possible after the event or activity and must be available for use within a reasonable time period.
- Relevance – data captured should be relevant to the purposes for which they are used.
- Completeness – data requirements need to be clearly specified based on information needs.[4]

For many years then, the concept of standardized data collection has been in growth and utilized in many areas of health practice, and there is substantial agreement that quality data collection is inextricably linked to quality improvement.[5] Standardized data collection has also been used in various health specialities, including tropical medicine,[6] sports medicine,[7,8] neurological physiotherapy[9] and cardiopulmonary settings.[10]

In relation to musculoskeletal physiotherapy settings the author has been involved in standardized data collection developments and applications since 1994, working with NHS hospital trusts in the United Kingdom and with private practitioners via PhysioFirst, the private physiotherapy practitioner organization in the UK, and also with osteopaths in the United Kingdom via the General Osteopathic Council. This work has led to a number of publications that detail the work[2,11,12] and other reports published on line.

There is no doubt that data emanating from practice need to be recorded in a systematic and accessible way. It is important that the reasons why data are needed and what purpose the data will serve, as well as a detailed plan of what data are to be collected and how, is created.[13] Data can be used for both clinical and research purposes (i.e. it can be used to identify research questions relevant to practice, to categorize/profile patients using diagnostic information, to provide descriptive/demographic data [e.g. age, height, weight, psychosocial circumstances, etc.]).

The information may be used to predict the patient outcome in the future, determine the suitability of particular interventions for particular patient profiles, inform the dosage and frequency of interventions, classify patients into profiling groups and indicate possible relationships between two or more factors across a range of patients with similar characteristics. The data/information can also be used to detect changes in patient profiles (diagnostic or personal) which can help further understanding and give more details of the patient's situation and enable comparison of patients to take place.

The data collection methods, however, can also focus heavily on service delivery if required, for example the number of treatments needed, the expertise available/needed, costs of treatments, quality of the patient experience, and a range of other possibilities depending on the need for the data collection which have been identified. The data collected can be qualitative or quantitative, again depending on the need and relevance of the data, and data collection tools to answer particular questions may already be available.

DEVELOPMENT OF A STANDARDIZED DATA COLLECTION TOOL

The methods most commonly used in the development of a standardized data collection tool are consensus methods. This involves bringing an expert team, or identifying an expert team that can work at a distance, relevant to the topic area (i.e. experts in musculoskeletal physiotherapy, in health delivery policy, users of musculoskeletal services, etc.). In this context the expert team identifies and agrees why a standardized collection tool is needed and necessary and what it is hoped it will achieve.

There are two consensus methods that can be utilized for this process. Firstly, there is the Delphi process and secondly, the nominal group technique.[14]

THE DELPHI PROCESS

The Delphi process or technique was developed by Dalkey and Helmer in 1963[15] and also discussed by

Linstone and Turoff.[16] It is a technique commonly used to achieve consensus opinion on certain topic areas and has been used in studies, particularly those looking at developing research priorities.[17,18] The Delphi technique is designed to achieve group communication via questions online or in paper copy and, eventually, consensus with regard to specific issues, for example research priority setting[17] (i.e. to seek out information which may generate a consensus on the majority of a respondent group).

The Delphi process includes a panel of 'experts'[19] to take part in up to four iterations/rounds of a questionnaire-type approach. In the Delphi process the panel of experts is set up together with a Delphi team of collators. The expert panel receives postal, email or web-based questionnaires on the research question or area of interest. Examples of sample questions include: what should be included in a standardized data collection tool for musculoskeletal physiotherapy to highlight the quality of patient care and service delivery? What topic areas should be included in the tool? Why should they be included? It is usual for each participant to be asked to give a rationale for the inclusion of certain topic areas.

The completed questionnaires are then sent back to the collation team to analyse and collate the responses, and then another more structured questionnaire, including the entire panel's views, is again sent out to the expert panel members for completion. In this round the participants are usually asked to rank topics in order of agreement or importance. The expert panel members send back their comments and the second round results are collated and analysed; further rounds continue until consensus is reached. Usually four rounds are sufficient. Although the Delphi process allows participants to be anonymous, it does not enable further discussion and therefore it may detract from individuals' understanding of issues that are held by other members of the expert panel. However, it has advantages where an international perspective is needed and the group cannot be brought together.

NOMINAL GROUP TECHNIQUE

The most common method used as a consensus methodology is a nominal group technique. This technique was first described by Delbecq and Van de Ven in 1971.[20] They described it as a method to facilitate effective group decision making in social psychological research.[20] Their process is clearly explained in a further paper.[21] Usually a nominal group would consist of five to ten participants. The nominal group technique is often considered a mixed-methods approach as it can utilize qualitative and quantitative methods.

The purpose of the group is to firstly identify why the data are needed and then to generate ideas for topics to be included in the data collection and eventually to decide how the data collection topics will be populated; for example, if one is collecting data concerning whiplash what classification system for whiplash will be utilized to capture the severity/mechanisms of the whiplash injury? This can be quite a complex process and the group needs to be well controlled during early discussions. The

nominal group needs to include representatives of all stakeholders in the standardized data collection tool. There could be more than one nominal group, but the outcome of each group discussion needs to be shared and discussed so that members of all groups understand the concern and/or the priorities of the different groups.

Process of Standardized Data Collection Development Utilizing a Nominal Group Technique

- The organizer should carry out a literature search to see if any standardized data collection tools are available and relevant.
- Preliminary work with several experts will be needed to identify appropriate discussion points/questions.
- A group or groups of experts need to be developed depending on the area in question, to come together for a discussion.
- Groups of patients, as well as clinicians, managers, other health professionals can be involved depending on the topic area.
- The individuals involved must have appropriate expertise and experience and interest in the topic area.
- Groups will normally meet for approximately two hours and the facilitator should be an expert on the discussion topic or be a credible non-expert.[20]

A Nominal Group Technique Protocol as an Example

- Introductions and explanation of purpose and procedure (5 to 10 minutes).
- Silent generation of ideas by all members of the group who write their thoughts down without discussion with others (10 minutes).
- Sharing of all participants' ideas and facilitator records all the ideas and comments. In addition, participants should write down any new ideas that arise as a result of these discussions (15 to 30 minutes).
- The group discussion then takes place. Participants seek more explanation/details of any ideas that are not clear to them and the facilitator controls the discussion, but allows all participants the opportunity to speak and feed in ideas (30 to 45 minutes).
- Voting and ranking process then takes place, prioritizing and confirming recorded ideas in relation to the initial question.
- At this point immediate results are available to all participants and the meeting concludes.[22]

With the development of a standardized data collection tool, several meetings will often be necessary to cover the complexities of the situation and the discussions around it. For an overall example of the procedure, see Moore et al.[2]

The findings from the nominal group technique are rarely the finishing point, hence the process shown below. The detailed discussion of the topics to be included and how the answers are to be recorded is complex, but agreement/consensus will mean that ambiguity of the standardized data collection will be low, at the first pilot (see Fig. 24-1)

Details and characteristics of consensus methods including the Delphi process and nominal group techniques have been published by Fink et al.,[23] as well as Jones and Hunter;[14] the Delphi technique has more recently been discussed in detail by Hsu and Sandford.[24]

It is useful to note that a manual of operation and completion and use of the tool for all participants is found to be very useful. To date, Moore et al.[2] have undertaken nine projects, developed nine standardized data collection tools that include a general tool for low back pain,

cervical spine dysfunction, whiplash, exercise prescription, over-60s, shoulder dysfunction, knee dysfunction and sports injuries. These tools have often been used in Snapshot surveys due to their length. A short-form standardized data collection tool is now being developed for daily and routine use in private practice.

Standardized data collection tools can be used in paper copy, electronically via data sticks, or web-based data storage, but obviously if data are being shared then it must be anonymized. Usually data systems can be easily modified to keep such data confidential and in an anonymized fashion.

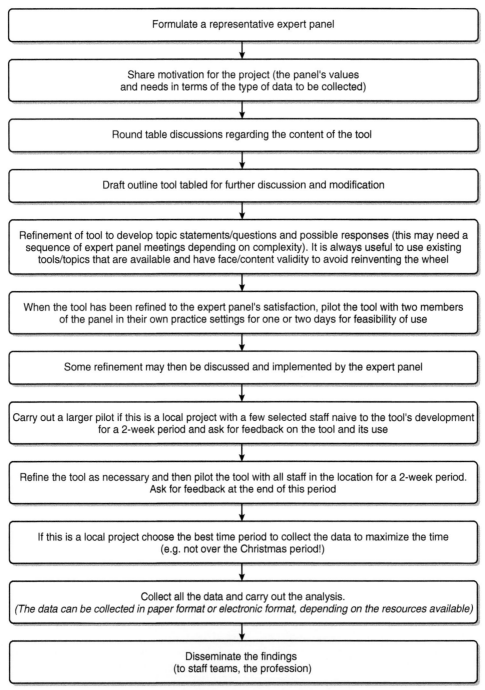

FIGURE 24-1 ■ Flow chart depicting the developmental process.

There are advantages of standardized data collection for patients, practitioner therapists, managers for practices and for the musculoskeletal speciality. If data can be collected across regions, countries, or even across the world using the same format, it provides very powerful information. In addition to the positive benefits of standardized data collection already described, the data collected can be utilized to set standards for clinical audit purposes.

Clinical audit has been defined as systematically looking at procedures used for diagnosis, care and treatment, examining how associated resources are used and investigating the effect care has on the outcome and quality of life for the patient.[25]

The use of data from research and standardized data collection and evaluation of service delivery and outcomes has been emphasized by authors including Øvretveit[26] as being an important area for development in clinical practice in the setting of standards which can then be audited. Clinical audits of course are founded on the need to monitor and improve quality of care and the audit cycle largely focuses on the structure, process and outcomes of treatment. Standardized data collection tools can, when necessary, be focused on deriving data much needed to inform standard setting in clinical environments. The importance of well-informed and timely standard setting cannot be underestimated and the results of a well-constructed quality audit of clinical activities and outcomes can be extremely powerful.

Together with detailed clinical subjective and objective data and the use of validated and reliable outcome measures, standardized data can be utilized to develop patient clinical profiles that may be very helpful in the development of treatment strategies and in formulating clinical research questions. The data can also be a powerful tool to influence commissioners of health services.

There are, however, some barriers to the use of standardized data collection tools. In a paper by Russek et al.,[27] attitudes were highlighted that may impact on standardized data collection tool use. Firstly, there is the inconvenience of collecting data in terms of the time taken. Secondly, the necessity to ensure appropriate training takes place with regard to the standardized data collection methods, so that large and high-quality databases can be constructed, i.e. training is needed in the operational definition and data collection procedures and it is of course highly relevant that computerized patient documentation systems can streamline data collection and increase clinicians' efficiency. The notion of the inconvenience of data collection, however, can be quickly rationalized with individuals if overall data produced is shared and discussed with them in an informative and constructive way. This often enables individuals who may be sceptical about the need for data collection to be brought up to speed with the impact that relevant data may have on a wide range of stakeholders including patients, carers, managers, commissioners and other health professionals.

REFERENCES

1. Bailey DM. Research for the Health Professional: A Practical Guide. Philadelphia: FA Davis Company; 1991.
2. Moore AP, Bryant E, Oliver G. Masterclass – development and use of standardised data collection tools to support and inform musculoskeletal practice. Man Ther 2012;17(6):489–96.
3. Audit Commission. In the Know: Using Information to Make Better Decisions – A Discussion Paper. Audit Commission Publications; 2008.
4. Audit Commission. Voluntary Data – Quality Standards. Audit Commission Publications; 2007.
5. Needham DM, Sinopoli DJ, Dinglas VD, et al. Improving data quality control in quality improvement projects. Int J Qual Health Care 2009;21(2):145–50.
6. Taylor T, Olola C, Valim C, et al. Standardised data collection for multi-centre clinical studies of severe malaria in African children: establishing the SMAC network. Transcr R Soc Trop Med Hyg 2006;100(7):615–22.
7. Finch CF, Valuri G, Ozanne-Smith J. Injury surveillance during medical coverage of sporting events – development and testing of a standardised data collection form. J Sci Med Sport 1999;2(1):42–56.
8. Fuller CW, Ekstrand J, Junge A, et al. Consensus statement on injury definitions and data collection procedures in studies of football (soccer) injuries. Br J Sports Med 2006;40(3):193–201.
9. Crow JL, Harmeling BC. Development of a consensus and evidence-based standardised clinical assessment and record form for neurological inpatients: the Neuro dataset. Physiotherapy 2002;88(1):33–46.
10. Jones P, Harding G, Wiklund I, et al. Improving the process and outcome of care in COPD: development of a standardised assessment tool. Prim Care Respir J 2009;18(3):208–15.
11. Fawkes C, Leach CMJ, Mathias S, et al. Development of a data collection tool to profile osteopathic practice: use of a nominal group technique to enhance clinician involvement. Man Ther 2014;19(2):119–24.
12. Fawkes C, Leach CMJ, Mathias S, et al. A profile of osteopathic care in private practices in the United Kingdom: a national pilot using standardised data collection. Man Ther 2014;19(2):125–30.
13. Wade DT. Editorial. Assessment, measurement and data collection tools. Clin Rehabil 2004;18:233–7.
14. Jones J, Hunter D. Consensus methods for medical and health services research. Br Med J 1995;331(7001):376–80.
15. Dalkey NC, Helmer O. An experimental application of the Delphi method to the use of experts. Manage Sci 1963;9(3):458–67.
16. Linstone HA, Turoff M. The Delphi Method: Technique and Applications. Massachussetts: Addison-Wesley Publishing Company.; 1975.
17. Rushton A, Moore A. International identification of research priorities for postgraduate theses in musculoskeletal physiotherapy using a modified Delphi technique. Man Ther 2010;15(2):142–8.
18. Rankin G, Rushton A, Olver P, et al. Chartered Society of Physiotherapy's identification of national research priorities for physiotherapy using a modified Delphi technique. Physiotherapy 2012;98(3):260–72.
19. Dalkey NC. An experimental study of group opinion. Futures 1969;1(5):408–26.
20. Delbecq AL, Van de Ven AH. A group process model for problem identification and program planning. Appl Behav Sci 1971;7:466–91.
21. Delbecq AL, Van de Ven AH, Gustafson DH. Group Techniques for Program Planning: A Guide to Nominal and Delphi Process. Glenview Illinois: Scott, Foresman & Company; 1975.
22. Potter M, Gordon S, Hamer P. The nominal group technique: a useful consensus methodology in physiotherapy research. N Z J Physiother 2004;32(3):126–30.
23. Fink A, Kosecoff J, Chassin M, et al. Consensus methods: characteristics and guidelines for use. Am J Public Health 1984;74:979–83.
24. Hsu CC, Sandford BA. The delphi technique: making sense of consensus. Practical Assessment, Research and Evaluation 2007;12(10):1–8.
25. Department of Health. Clinical Audit: Meeting and Improving Standards in Health Care. London: HMSO; 1993.
26. Øvretveit J. Evaluating Health Interventions. Milton Keynes: Open University Press; 1998.
27. Russek L, Wooden M, Ekedahl S, et al. Attitudes toward standardised data collection. Phys Ther 1997;77(7):714–29.

CHAPTER 25

IMPLEMENTATION RESEARCH

Simon French • Sally Green •
Rachelle Buchbinder • Jeremy Grimshaw

INTRODUCTION

The availability of high-quality research evidence is not sufficient to ensure high-quality health care is delivered, and the translation of research evidence into practice is difficult and complex. Implementation research, or translational research, explores the most effective ways to integrate research evidence into clinical practice and health policy. This chapter focuses on relevant research methods exploring the process of improving the implementation of research findings into physiotherapy practice. The use of theory, and theoretical frameworks, in implementation research is also discussed, including their use in the process of developing implementation interventions designed to change clinical practice.

WHAT IS THE PROBLEM?

Many people receiving health care are not receiving the best possible care through a failure of their health-care providers to incorporate up-to-date research evidence into clinical practice. Researchers continuously produce new findings that can contribute to effective and efficient health care as long as this research is implemented into practice. A common mechanism for synthesizing and disseminating high-quality research-supported information to clinicians is in the form of a clinical practice guideline. Guideline recommendations have the potential to improve the quality and safety of health care, but only with effective dissemination and uptake into clinical practice. In many clinical areas this does not occur and there is a gap between actual clinical practice and recommended, evidence-based practice.[1]

Evidence–practice gaps exist where there is variability between best recommended practice and actual clinical practice. There are numerous examples of evidence–practice gaps in different clinical settings, in different countries and for different clinical conditions, both in diagnosis and treatment,[2–12] resulting in some patients receiving care that is inappropriate, unnecessary or even harmful.[1] For example, an Australian study determined the percentage of health-care encounters at which care was in line with evidence-based or consensus-based guidelines.[3] Overall, Australian patients in the study received appropriate care at an average of 57% of eligible encounters during 2009 and 2010, and for people with low back pain or osteoarthritis, the percentage of encounters with appropriate care were 72% and 43%, respectively.

Timely implementation of evidence into clinical practice ensures that people who require health care receive the most contemporary, effective and safest care. However, in many cases, research findings do not result in a change in clinical practice or health-care policy. Using musculoskeletal health care as an example, in many cases diagnostic tests are not being used appropriately (e.g. too few bone density scans for osteoporosis diagnosis,[13] or too many plain X-rays for low back pain[14,15]) and interventions with established effectiveness are not being used in practice (e.g. too few people with hip fracture receive osteoporosis treatment to prevent further fracture[16]). Also, interventions are being used before there is established evidence to support them, and in some instances, being used despite research demonstrating they are ineffective and/or harmful (e.g. vertebroplasty for vertebral compression fractures,[17,18] opioid prescription for low back pain[19] and arthroscopy for osteoarthritis of the knee[20]).

Physiotherapists generally hold favourable attitudes towards evidence-based practice.[21–23] However, these positive attitudes alone do not guarantee best possible patient care informed by the latest research. Many health-care workers, including physiotherapists, base clinical decisions on potentially outdated knowledge obtained during their physiotherapy education, or on personal experience, rather than being informed by findings from up-to-date research.[21,24–27]

The process of implementing research evidence into an individual clinician's practice and subsequent improvement of patient health outcomes can be a long and complex one.[2] Much emphasis is placed on dissemination of research evidence, for example by making clinical practice guidelines available, or presentation at educational meetings. But ensuring clinician awareness of the evidence is only the beginning of the process and other aspects of translation into practice have received less attention. In busy clinical environments clinicians must not only remember the evidence, but also actively decide to vary their practice when relevant to an individual patient. In addition, if the evidence is contrary to the clinician's preconceived ideas and opinions, this may limit acceptance and uptake of the new information.[28] Even if the evidence is applicable to the clinician's setting and it is accepted, they may not have the appropriate skills, training or equipment to be able to implement the evidence. Finally, the evidence also needs to be acceptable and feasible to patients, and patient benefit relies upon adherence to the agreed course of action.[2]

WHAT IS IMPLEMENTATION RESEARCH?

To date, little is known about the best way to promote the uptake of research evidence into clinical practice. Implementation research aims to evaluate the most effective and efficient means of achieving this. Implementation research is a field of health service research that explores the development, delivery and evaluation of strategies and methods to implement research evidence into practice.[29] Implementation research can study any aspect of implementing evidence into practice, including exploring the factors affecting implementation, the processes of implementation, and the results of implementation.[30] Implementation researchers focus on understanding and influencing the process of uptake of evidence into practice by applying and developing theories on why health-care providers and policy makers do what they do, and on how to improve their performance through facilitating the use of evidence in their decision making.[31]

The practice of, and research about, improving the uptake of evidence into health-care practice and policy is relatively new. Reflecting this, there are inconsistencies in the literature about the best term to use to describe this field.[32] To add to the confusion, some of these terms have attempted to capture the entire process of research to practice or policy, some parts of the process, and some terms have been used interchangeably.[33] Some of the more common terms used in the literature include implementation research, knowledge translation research, translational research, research translation, research utilization, quality improvement research, knowledge transfer and exchange, and dissemination and implementation research. In this chapter we will use the term 'implementation research'.

Advances in implementation research have the potential to improve patient care. Implementation research is required to provide rigorous methods for improving the uptake of evidence into clinical practice so patients receive the best care. However, there exists a 'poverty of research' to inform decisions about how to improve the delivery of health care and there is great opportunity and scope to conduct research to improve the uptake of evidence into clinical practice.[12]

WHAT ARE THE TYPES OF IMPLEMENTATION RESEARCH?

A wide range of qualitative and quantitative research methods can be used in implementation research. Implementation research can be classified into three categories: descriptive, evaluative and methodological implementation research. Table 25-1 provides simple examples of the different types of implementation research that fall within these three categories.

Descriptive implementation research is investigation conducted to describe current practice. This typically includes observational research, using qualitative or quantitative methods, to determine what is occurring in practice and to attempt to understand why practitioners conduct practice in this way. This research explores whether an evidence–practice gap exists, and if so, the extent of this gap and the likely reasons for the gap.

Evaluative implementation research is the conduct of effectiveness studies of interventions that aim to improve the uptake of research into clinical practice. Evaluative implementation research generates substantive knowledge about how to implement research into practice. This typically includes quantitative study designs to test the effects of an intervention, such as uncontrolled or controlled before-and-after studies, interrupted time series studies, non-randomized controlled clinical trials and individual participant or cluster randomized controlled trials.[34,35] Of these, the randomized controlled

---

TABLE 25-1 Different Implementation Research Categories with Examples

Aim	Implementation Research Category	Examples
Describing practice	Descriptive	Demonstrating the extent to which clinicians practice according to recommendations of an evidence-based clinical practice guideline (CPG), e.g. a survey shows high rate of X-ray use for acute low back pain (LBP)
Understanding practice: barriers and enablers analysis	Descriptive	Determining reasons why clinicians do, and do not, practice in accordance with the CPG, e.g. focus groups with clinicians find that they feel pressure from patients to order an X-ray
Evaluation studies	Evaluative	Randomized controlled trial of an intervention to change health-care providers' behaviour, e.g. randomize clinicians to receive negotiation skills or not, then measure X-ray referral rates between groups
Implementation intervention design	Methodological	Using theoretical exploration and modelling to develop an intervention to overcome barriers to practicing in accordance with the CPGs, e.g. modelling suggests providing clinicians with negotiation skills will assist them when patients with acute LBP demand an X-ray
Assessing intervention fidelity	Methodological	Strategies to ensure that an intervention is delivered as planned and an evaluation of this, e.g. document how many clinicians receive negotiation skills training, and evaluating the content of the training
Methods development	Methodological	Research across all the different categories, contributing to the methods of each, e.g. the development of techniques to analyse cluster randomized controlled trials evaluating implementation strategies

trial is the most methodologically robust of the evaluative implementation research designs. The other designs have greater risk of bias, but may be appropriate in certain situations, such as when a randomized controlled trial is not feasible or ethical to conduct.

Methodological implementation research is a study conducted into the different methodological components of the implementation process. This category of research flows from, and informs, the conduct of both descriptive and evaluative implementation research. The study designs utilized for this research are varied, and will typically include qualitative and mixed-methods research. As implementation research is a relatively new field it requires foundational research to build the science, developing and testing hypotheses about why health professionals, patients and health organizations do what they do and how to improve their performance in clinical practice.[12]

WHICH INTERVENTIONS HELP TO CHANGE CLINICAL PRACTICE?

A systematic review published in 2010 synthesized all studies of knowledge translation strategies in allied health, including physiotherapy.[36] Only nine published studies involving physiotherapists could be found. The authors concluded that equivocal results, low methodological quality and outcome-reporting bias did not allow them to recommend one particular knowledge translation strategy over another to improve allied health practice. Although there are few studies specifically targeting physiotherapists, evidence from systematic reviews of other professionals might be useful because their findings are likely to be transferrable.

Complex interventions designed to increase the uptake of evidence into clinical practice can be termed *implementation interventions*. Implementation interventions have been extensively evaluated and the results synthesized in a number of systematic reviews.[37–40] Grimshaw and colleagues summarized the findings of 235 studies evaluating implementation interventions designed to improve the uptake of clinical practice guidelines.[41] The most common interventions evaluated included reminders, dissemination of educational materials, audit and feedback, educational outreach, patient-directed interventions and multifaceted interventions consisting of a combination of these strategies. Overall, the majority of the studies reported that the implementation interventions evaluated resulted in modest to moderate improvements in care. However, the improvements varied both within and across interventions. Despite the large number of previous implementation studies, there is currently no strong basis for selecting a particular implementation intervention to overcome a particular implementation problem.

The Cochrane Effective Practice and Organisation of Care (EPOC) Review Group publishes *Cochrane Systematic Reviews* of interventions designed to improve health-care delivery and health-care systems (http://epoc.cochrane.org/). EPOC reviews include continuing education, quality assurance, informatics, financial, organizational and regulatory interventions.[42] EPOC has developed a taxonomy of implementation interventions that describes interventions used to improve clinical practice. Table 25-2 lists some of these interventions and gives some examples relevant to the physiotherapy profession.

HOW ARE INTERVENTIONS DEVELOPED THAT AIM TO INCREASE IMPLEMENTATION OF RESEARCH?

Complex interventions, which are interventions made up of a number of components, are typically employed in studies aiming to implement evidence into clinical practice. Development of complex interventions for implementation research requires careful planning to ensure that the intervention specifically targets what requires change. Given the high proportion of trials of complex interventions in this area that do not show which interventions are effective in which situations, and the need to improve practice in line with evidence, researchers should provide a strong rationale for the development of their interventions.[44] This will ensure that the theoretical basis and feasibility of the intervention have been established prior to embarking upon a costly implementation project.

The science of developing complex interventions to change practitioner behaviour is at an early stage of development.[12] Only a minority of trials of complex implementation interventions have published details about how and why the intervention tested was developed.[41,45] Details of the theoretical basis, delivery and measures of the process of care targeted by these interventions are often lacking, making it difficult to know what exactly has been evaluated and how to replicate the intervention in other settings.

Pharmaceutical interventions are evaluated in randomized controlled trials only after there is a strong rationale for their use, based on empirical evidence of their mechanism of effect in animals and from modelling studies.[46] Pre-clinical studies then aim to elucidate the mechanism of effect in humans by measuring surrogate outcomes. In other words, it takes many years and much preliminary research before a drug is tested in definitive trials. The same principle could apply for interventions designed to change clinical practice; however, the need for change in practice is urgent and we cannot afford to wait many years using a pharmaceutical model of development. More explicit consideration of barriers to change and mechanisms of action of potential implementation interventions, underpinned by a theory or rationale that attempts to explain how and why the intervention may effect change, would likely enhance the field.

Implementation of evidence into practice often requires behaviour change. This behaviour change may be required at the general population or patient level, at the clinician level or health-care practice level (including non-clinical staff), at a regional health-care level or at a policy level. Behaviour change is complex and there are many recommendations and approaches in the literature

TABLE 25-2 **Examples of Interventions Designed to Change Health Professional Clinical Behaviour**

Type of Intervention	Subgroups	Examples
Professional interventions	Distribution of educational materials	Distribution of clinical practice guidelines via mass mailings
	Educational meetings	Clinicians participating in conferences
	Educational outreach visits	Use of a trained person who meets with a clinician in their practice settings to give information with the intent of changing the clinician's practice
	Local opinion leaders	Use of providers nominated by their clinician colleagues as 'educationally influential'
	Audit and feedback	A summary provided to a clinician of their clinical health-care performance over a specified period of time
	Reminders	Patient- or encounter-specific information, provided verbally, on paper or on a computer screen, which is designed or intended to prompt a clinician to recall information
	Marketing	Survey of health-care providers to identify barriers to change and subsequent design of an intervention that addresses identified barriers
	Mass media	Targeting the general population about best practice management of a particular health condition via the media (including television, radio, newspapers, social media, etc.)
Financial interventions	Provider interventions	A new fee-for-service is introduced into a clinical practice
Organizational interventions	Revision of professional roles	Use of allied health assistants
	Clinical multidisciplinary teams	Creation of a new team of health professionals to include different clinical disciplines
	Case management	A new coordination of assessment, treatment and arrangement for referrals for specific clinician groups
	Changes in medical records systems	Changing from paper to computerized records
Regulatory interventions	Changes in medical liability	Expanded scope of practice

Adapted from the Cochrane Effective Practice and Organisation of Care Group intervention taxonomy.[43]

proposing one way or another, or multiple approaches, to achieve sustained behaviour change.[47]

Various conceptual and theoretical frameworks are available when considering the development of implementation interventions to improve the uptake of research into clinical practice.[33,48–54] A systematic scoping review in 2010 identified 33 frameworks designed for use by researchers to guide research dissemination activities.[51] However, there is no specific guidance available to choose one framework over another for a specific clinical situation or for a specific evidence–practice gap.

One suggested approach, developed by the authors of this chapter, is to use a series of questions in a streamlined approach moving directly from identified theoretical domains relevant to the implementation problem to behaviour change techniques.[44] Figure 25-1 outlines the four steps of this framework. By answering these questions, researchers, practitioners or policy makers, wishing to develop implementation interventions to overcome evidence–practice gaps, can utilize a systematic theoretically informed method to develop implementation interventions.

The approach outlined in Figure 25-1 involves examining a potential evidence–practice gap and, if it is present, developing a means to overcome this gap. The first step is to systematically identify the evidence–practice gap itself. This involves determining high-quality evidence,

Step 1: Who needs to do what differently?

Action: Systematically identify the evidence–practice gap

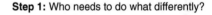

Step 2: Using a theoretical framework, which barriers and enablers need to be addressed?

Action: Systematically identify the barriers and enablers to change

Step 3: Which intervention components could overcome the modifiable barriers and enhance the enablers?

Actions: Select evidence-based behaviour change techniques that address barriers and enablers; combine techniques into a deliverable intervention; and test the intervention feasibility and acceptability

Step 4: How will we measure behaviour change?

Action: Evaluate the intervention using an appropriate research design

FIGURE 25-1 ■ A conceptual framework designed to guide researchers, practitioners and decision-makers to systematically develop implementation interventions.[44]

in the form of a systematic review and/or clinical practice guideline, which suggests a particular health-care practice should or should not be undertaken. Then clinical practice needs to be examined to determine the extent to which this practice is, or is not, occurring. For example, United Kingdom (UK) National Institute of Health and Clinical Excellence (NICE) guidelines for osteoarthritis made treatment recommendations based on high-quality evidence.[55] However, a survey of physiotherapists showed that while some of the guideline's recommendations including recommending exercise, undertaking patient education and encouragement of patient self-management were generally undertaken by physiotherapists, physiotherapists continued to use treatment modalities that the guidelines did not endorse.[56]

The next step is to systematically identify the barriers and enablers to clinical practice behaviour change. Using this information, evidence-based behaviour change techniques can be selected to address these barriers and enablers. Behaviour change techniques can then be combined into a deliverable intervention, and this intervention should be tested for feasibility and acceptability. Importantly, consideration of system factors is also required to ensure that there is general system support for any proposed clinician behaviour change. For example, efforts to change general population and clinician behaviour in response to a mass media campaign for back pain was much more successful in Australia in comparison to other countries, in part explained by the coexistence of supportive legislation and health policy that supported that change.[57] Finally, the intervention should be evaluated using an appropriate research design.

DOES THEORY HAVE A ROLE IN COMPLEX INTERVENTION DEVELOPMENT?

A possible explanation for the disappointing effects demonstrated to date for many complex interventions designed to change health professional behaviour is the use of inadequate methods for their development,[58] and a lack of consideration of the 'whole system'.[59] Without appropriate rationale to underpin their design, interventions may not be ideally suited to the context in which they are delivered or to the behaviour they are attempting to change, nor designed to overcome the barriers to change. The lack of an explicit process for development means that previous evaluations of complex interventions have provided little information on determining how or why they were either effective or ineffective, and there is little opportunity to determine the potential factors that may have modified the effects. Without information on this process it is also difficult for others to be informed about the application of the intervention to another setting or context. There is growing evidence in the literature suggesting that the design of complex implementation interventions requires a more systematic approach with a strong rationale for the chosen design and explicit reporting of the intervention development process.[60–62]

One proposed option to achieve this is to use behavioural theory, or behaviour change theory, to underpin the design of complex interventions aimed at implementing evidence into clinical practice.[46,63–65]

Theory can explain how different events relate to one another and may predict how these phenomena will relate under different conditions.[66] Proponents of the use of theory in the design of implementation interventions argue that theories have the potential to provide understanding of how societies work, how organizations operate and why people behave in certain ways.[67] Behaviour change scientists propose that the development of theoretical models for predicting when health-care professionals are likely to respond to different interventions would provide a framework for effective implementation.[64] This premise is built on an understanding that the uptake of evidence into practice depends on human behaviour, and so interventions aiming to change clinical practice may be improved by drawing on theories of human behaviour that have been extensively developed and tested for use in changing the health behaviour of individuals.[68,69]

Explaining and changing a health-care professional's practice behaviour could be informed by the use of theory.[70] However, to date implementation intervention development appears to be largely based on simple, mostly unstated, models of human behaviour, or commonly when it is reported that an intervention has been theory-based, a systematic process has not been followed.[47] In the Grimshaw and colleagues systematic review discussed earlier,[41] only 27% of included studies used theory and/or psychological constructs, and when theory was reported as used it was often not explained how the theory explicitly informed the design of the intervention.[45] There is a growing body of evidence demonstrating that interventions based on theory may be more effective in changing behaviour than those that are not.[65]

Currently, our understanding of factors that influence health-care professional clinical practice and optimal approaches to modify their behaviour in line with research evidence is incomplete. Research into the uptake of evidence into practice using a theoretical base to support the choice and development of interventions is yet to be widely applied and tested. Consequently, the interpretation of study results of the evaluations of these interventions into health-care practice is limited.[46] This has led to calls for more research into implementation interventions that are based on specific theories of behaviour change.[47,63,71–73] However, a significant challenge to using theories is choosing an appropriate theory for the context in which the change is required.

HOW BEST SHOULD THEORY BE USED IN IMPLEMENTATION RESEARCH?

Multiple theories and frameworks of individual and organizational behaviour change exist, and often these theories have conceptually overlapping constructs.[71,74,75] Only a few of these theories have been tested in robust research in health-care settings. There is currently no systematic basis for determining which among the various theories available predicts behaviour or behaviour change most precisely,[76] or which is best suited to underpin implementation research.[69,71]

Using a broadly based theoretical framework for behaviour change, rather than a single theory, may allow a more comprehensive examination of potential barriers and enablers, and possible mechanisms linking them to the target clinical behaviour. The Theoretical Domains Framework is a broad-based, comprehensive, framework for designing implementation interventions offering a broad coverage of potential change pathways;[77,78] however, other theoretical frameworks, or specific theories, could be used.

It is unlikely that there will be one theory (and one implementation intervention) that will apply equally well to every setting and every intervention.[79] The complex interaction of barriers and facilitators to change may influence the success of an intervention designed to implement evidence into practice. An understanding of these barriers and facilitators is considered an essential step in developing an effective implementation intervention.[71] A theory that can attempt to explain these barriers and facilitators could be used to develop a theory-based intervention for implementation research.

For example, in their study of 45 physiotherapists in various settings in Sweden, who participated in 11 focus group interviews, Dannapfel and colleagues used Self-Determination Theory to understand physiotherapists' use of research evidence in practice.[24,25] By using a theoretical framework in their qualitative analysis, they were able to systematically make recommendations about how to improve the use of evidence in physiotherapy practice, including the potential to tailor educational programmes to better account for differences in motivation among physiotherapists, using physiotherapists as change agents and creating favourable conditions to encourage autonomous motivation by way of feelings of competence, autonomy and a sense of relatedness.

CONCLUSION

Translation of research evidence into practice is complex and does not happen automatically. Well-designed implementation interventions are required to improve clinical practice, but currently there is limited research in physiotherapy settings to guide the choice of effective interventions to improve practice. The design and evaluation of implementation interventions aiming to improve the uptake of research into physiotherapy practice should be informed by theory and science.

REFERENCES

1. Grimshaw JM, Eccles MP, Lavis JN, et al. Knowledge translation of research findings. Implement Sci 2012;7(1):50.
2. Glasziou P, Haynes B. The paths from research to improved health outcomes. Evid Based Med 2005;10(1):4–7.
3. Runciman WB, Hunt TD, Hannaford NA, et al. CareTrack: assessing the appropriateness of health care delivery in Australia. Med J Aust 2012;197(2):100–5.
4. Davis D, Evans M, Jadad A, et al. The case for knowledge translation: shortening the journey from evidence to effect. BMJ 2003;327(7405):33–5.
5. Schuster MA, McGlynn EA, Brook RH. How good is the quality of health care in the United States? Milbank Q 1998;76(4):517–63, 509. Review.
6. McGlynn EA, Asch SM, Adams J, et al. The quality of health care delivered to adults in the United States. N Engl J Med 2003; 348(26):2635–45.
7. Leatherman S, Sutherland K. Quality of care in the NHS of England. BMJ 2004;328(7445):E288–90.
8. Schoen C, Davis K, How SK, et al. U.S. health system performance: a national scorecard. Health Aff (Millwood) 2006;25(6):w457–75.
9. Seddon ME, Marshall MN, Campbell SM, et al. Systematic review of studies of quality of clinical care in general practice in the UK, Australia and New Zealand. Qual Health Care 2001;10(3):152–8.
10. Steel N, Bachmann M, Maisey S, et al. Self reported receipt of care consistent with 32 quality indicators: national population survey of adults aged 50 or more in England. BMJ 2008;337:a957.
11. Bodenheimer T. The American health care system – the movement for improved quality in health care. N Engl J Med 1999; 340(6):488–92.
12. Grol R, Berwick DM, Wensing M. On the trail of quality and safety in health care. BMJ 2008;336(7635):74–6.
13. Elliot-Gibson V, Bogoch ER, Jamal SA, et al. Practice patterns in the diagnosis and treatment of osteoporosis after a fragility fracture: a systematic review. Osteoporos Int 2004;15(10):767–78.
14. Gandjour A, Telzerow A, Lauterbach KW. European comparison of costs and quality in the treatment of acute back pain. Spine 2005;30(8):969–75.
15. Walker BF, French SD, Page MJ, et al. Management of people with acute low-back pain: a survey of Australian chiropractors. Chiropr Man Therap 2011;19(1):29.
16. Majumdar SR. Recent trends in osteoporosis treatment after hip fracture: improving but wholly inadequate. J Rheumatol 2008; 35(2):190–2.
17. Buchbinder R, Osborne RH, Ebeling PR, et al. A randomized trial of vertebroplasty for painful osteoporotic vertebral fractures. N Engl J Med 2009;361(6):557–68.
18. Kallmes DF, Jarvik JG, Osborne RH, et al. Clinical utility of vertebroplasty: elevating the evidence. Radiology 2010;255(3):675–80.
19. Mafi JN, McCarthy EP, Davis RB, et al. Worsening trends in the management and treatment of back pain. JAMA Internal Medicine 2013;173(17):1573–81.
20. Bohensky MA, Sundararajan V, Andrianopoulos N, et al. Trends in elective knee arthroscopies in a population-based cohort, 2000–2009. Med J Aust 2012;197(7):399–403.
21. Heiwe S, Kajermo KN, Tyni-Lenne R, et al. Evidence-based practice: attitudes, knowledge and behaviour among allied health care professionals. Int J Qual Health Care 2011;23(2):198–209.
22. Nilsagård Y, Lohse G. Evidence-based physiotherapy: a survey of knowledge, behaviour, attitudes and prerequisites. Adv Physiother 2010;12(4):179–86.
23. Jette DU, Bacon K, Batty C, et al. Evidence-based practice: beliefs, attitudes, knowledge, and behaviors of physical therapists. Phys Ther 2003;83(9):786–805.
24. Dannapfel P, Peolsson A, Nilsen P. What supports physiotherapists' use of research in clinical practice? A qualitative study in Sweden. Implement Sci 2013;8:31.
25. Dannapfel P, Peolsson A, Stahl C, et al. Applying self-determination theory for improved understanding of physiotherapists' rationale for using research in clinical practice: a qualitative study in Sweden. Physiother Theory Pract 2014;30(1):20–8.
26. Filbay SR, Hayes K, Holland AE. Physiotherapy for patients following coronary artery bypass graft (CABG) surgery: limited uptake of evidence into practice. Physiother Theory Pract 2012;28(3):178–87.
27. Li LC, Bombardier C. Physical therapy management of low back pain: an exploratory survey of therapist approaches. Phys Ther 2001;81(4):1018–28.
28. Festinger L. A Theory of Cognitive Dissonance. Stanford, CA: Stanford University Press; 1957.
29. Eccles M, Mittman B. Welcome to Implementation Science. Implement Sci 2006;1(1):1.
30. Peters DH, Adam T, Alonge O, et al. Implementation research: what it is and how to do it. BMJ 2013;347:f6753.

31. Rubenstein LV, Pugh J. Strategies for promoting organizational and practice change by advancing implementation research. J Gen Intern Med 2006;21(Suppl. 2):S58–64.

32. Rabin BA, Brownson RC, Haire-Joshu D, et al. A glossary for dissemination and implementation research in health. J Public Health Manag Pract 2008;14(2):117–23.

33. Graham ID, Logan J, Harrison MB, et al. Lost in knowledge translation: time for a map? J Contin Educ Health Prof 2006;26(1):13–24.

34. Eccles M, Grimshaw J, Campbell M, et al. Research designs for studies evaluating the effectiveness of change and improvement strategies. Qual Saf Health Care 2003;12(1):47–52.

35. Grimshaw J, Campbell M, Eccles M, et al. Experimental and quasi-experimental designs for evaluating guideline implementation strategies. Fam Pract 2000;17(Suppl. 1):S11–16.

36. Scott SD, Albrecht L, O'Leary K, et al. Systematic review of knowledge translation strategies in the allied health professions. Implement Sci 2012;7:70.

37. NHS. Getting evidence into practice. Eff Health Care 1999;5(1).

38. Oxman AD, Thomson MA, Davis DA, et al. No magic bullets: a systematic review of 102 trials of interventions to improve professional practice. CMAJ 1995;153(10):1423–31.

39. Bero LA, Grilli R, Grimshaw JM, et al. Closing the gap between research and practice: an overview of systematic reviews of interventions to promote the implementation of research findings. The Cochrane Effective Practice and Organization of Care Review Group. BMJ 1998;317(7156):465–8.

40. Davis DA, Taylor-Vaisey A. Translating guidelines into practice. A systematic review of theoretic concepts, practical experience and research evidence in the adoption of clinical practice guidelines. CMAJ 1997;157(4):408–16.

41. Grimshaw JM, Thomas RE, MacLennan G, et al. Effectiveness and efficiency of guideline dissemination and implementation strategies. Health Technol Assess 2004;8(6):iii–iv, 1–72.

42. Grimshaw J, Shepperd S, Pantoja T, et al. Cochrane Effective Practice and Organisation of Care Group. About The Cochrane Collaboration (Cochrane Review Groups (CRGs) 2013(4) Art. No.: EPOC.

43. Cochrane Effective Practice and Organisation of Care Group (EPOC). Data collection checklist, section 2. 2007. Available from: <http://www.epoc.cochrane.org/>; [Accessed 13 January, 2015.].

44. French SD, Green SE, O'Connor DA, et al. Developing theory-informed behaviour change interventions to implement evidence into practice: a systematic approach using the Theoretical Domains Framework. Implement Sci 2012;7(1):38.

45. Davies P, Walker AE, Grimshaw JM. A systematic review of the use of theory in the design of guideline dissemination and implementation strategies and interpretation of the results of rigorous evaluations. Implement Sci 2010;5:14.

46. Eccles M, Grimshaw J, Walker A, et al. Changing the behavior of healthcare professionals: the use of theory in promoting the uptake of research findings. J Clin Epidemiol 2005;58(2):107–12.

47. Michie S. Designing and implementing behaviour change interventions to improve population health. J Health Serv Res Policy 2008;13(Suppl. 3):64–9.

48. Craig P, Dieppe P, Macintyre S, et al. Developing and evaluating complex interventions: the new Medical Research Council guidance. BMJ 2008;337:a1655.

49. Campbell M, Fitzpatrick R, Haines A, et al. Framework for design and evaluation of complex interventions to improve health. BMJ 2000;321(7262):694–6.

50. Bartholomew LK, Parcel GS, Kok G. Intervention mapping: a process for developing theory- and evidence-based health education programs. Health Educ Behav 1998;25(5):545–63.

51. Wilson PM, Petticrew M, Calnan MW, et al. Disseminating research findings: what should researchers do? A systematic scoping review of conceptual frameworks. Implement Sci 2010;5:91.

52. Estabrooks CA, Thompson DS, Lovely JJ, et al. A guide to knowledge translation theory. J Contin Educ Health Prof 2006; 26(1):25–36.

53. Damschroder LJ, Aron DC, Keith RE, et al. Fostering implementation of health services research findings into practice: a consolidated framework for advancing implementation science. Implement Sci 2009;4:50.

54. Zidarov D, Thomas A, Poissant L. Knowledge translation in physical therapy: from theory to practice. Disabil Rehabil 2013;35(18):1571–7.

55. National Institute for Health and Clinical Excellence (NICE). Osteoarthritis: the care and management of osteoarthritis in adults. NICE Clin Guide 2008;59.

56. Walsh NE, Hurley MV. Evidence based guidelines and current practice for physiotherapy management of knee osteoarthritis. Musculoskeletal Care 2009;7(1):45–56.

57. Gross DP, Deshpande S, Werner EL, et al. Fostering change in back pain beliefs and behaviors: when public education is not enough. Spine J 2012;12(11):979–88.

58. van Bokhoven MA, Kok G, van der Weijden T. Designing a quality improvement intervention: a systematic approach. Qual Saf Health Care 2003;12(3):215–20.

59. Loisel P, Buchbinder R, Hazard R, et al. Prevention of work disability due to musculoskeletal disorders: the challenge of implementing evidence. J Occup Rehabil 2005;15(4):507–24.

60. Des Jarlais DC, Lyles C, Crepaz N. Improving the reporting quality of nonrandomized evaluations of behavioral and public health interventions: the TREND statement. Am J Public Health 2004;94(3):361–6.

61. Baker EA, Brennan Ramirez LK, Claus JM, et al. Translating and disseminating research- and practice-based criteria to support evidence-based intervention planning. J Public Health Manag Pract 2008;14(2):124–30.

62. Boutron I, Moher D, Altman DG, et al. Extending the CONSORT statement to randomized trials of nonpharmacologic treatment: explanation and elaboration. Ann Intern Med 2008;148(4): 295–309.

63. ICEBeRG (The Improved Clinical Effectiveness through Behavioural Research Group). Designing theoretically-informed implementation interventions. Implement Sci 2006;1:4.

64. Sanson-Fisher RW, Grimshaw JM, Eccles MP. The science of changing providers' behaviour: the missing link in evidence-based practice. Med J Aust 2004;180(5):205–6.

65. Marteau T, Dieppe P, Foy R, et al. Behavioural medicine: changing our behaviour. BMJ 2006;332(7539):437–8.

66. Bem S, Looren de Jong H. Theoretical Issues in Psychology: An Introduction. 2nd ed. London; Thousand Oaks, California: Sage; 2006.

67. Reeves S, Albert M, Kuper A, et al. Why use theories in qualitative research? BMJ 2008;337:a949.

68. Armitage CJ, Conner M. Social cognition models and health behaviour: a structured review. Psychol Health 2000;15(2):173–89.

69. Lippke S, Ziegelmann JP. Theory-based health behavior change: developing, testing, and applying theories for evidence-based interventions. Appl Psychol 2008;57(4):698–716.

70. Sales A, Smith J, Curran G, et al. Models, strategies, and tools. Theory in implementing evidence-based findings into health care practice. J Gen Intern Med 2006;21(Suppl. 2):S43–9.

71. Grol RP, Bosch MC, Hulscher ME, et al. Planning and studying improvement in patient care: the use of theoretical perspectives. Milbank Q 2007;85(1):93–138.

72. Greenhalgh T, Robert G, Macfarlane F, et al. Diffusion of innovations in service organizations: systematic review and recommendations. Milbank Q 2004;82(4):581–629.

73. Thompson DS, Estabrooks CA, Scott-Findlay S, et al. Interventions aimed at increasing research use in nursing: a systematic review. Implement Sci 2007;2:15.

74. Ferlie EB, Shortell SM. Improving the quality of health care in the United Kingdom and the United States: a framework for change. Milbank Q 2001;79(2):281–315.

75. Ashford A. Behavioural Change in Professional Practice: Supporting the Development of Effective Implementation Strategies Report No 88. Newcastle upon Tyne: Centre for Health Services Research; 1998.

76. Noar SM, Zimmerman RS. Health Behavior Theory and cumulative knowledge regarding health behaviors: are we moving in the right direction? Health Educ Res 2005;20(3):275–90.

77. Michie S, Johnston M, Abraham C, et al. Making psychological theory useful for implementing evidence based practice: a consensus approach. Qual Saf Health Care 2005;14(1):26–33.

78. Cane J, O'Connor D, Michie S. Validation of the theoretical domains framework for use in behaviour change and implementation research. Implement Sci 2012;7(1):37.

79. Grimshaw J, Eccles M, Tetroe J. Implementing clinical guidelines: current evidence and future implications. J Contin Educ Health Prof 2004;24(Suppl. 1):S31–7.

PART **III**

ADVANCES IN CLINICAL SCIENCE AND PRACTICE

PRINCIPLES OF MANAGEMENT

One of the key characteristics of modern musculoskeletal physiotherapy is the use of multimodal approaches to the management of musculoskeletal disorders reflecting their biopsychosocial dimensions. This section on principles of management presents some of the main features and systems to be considered in modern musculoskeletal physiotherapy management.

Approaches to assessment and management of musculoskeletal disorders have become more complex and multifaceted over the years. In the first instance, the way clinicians may make decisions in terms of approach to assessment and choice of management methods can be based on a range of models (e.g. clinical reasoning, subgrouping, clinical prediction rules, clinical guidelines and evidence-based practice). A chapter discussing these models for management prescription has been included to contextualize these approaches to assist the clinician appraise them in respect of their own clinical practice.

Good communication is fundamental for every successful therapeutic relationship. Thus it was considered important to reflect on several aspects of communication including the use of language, the communication of risk and approaches to patient education to highlight the importance of the awareness of communication styles and approaches in providing patient-focused care.

There are many features for the clinician to consider when assessing and treating individuals with musculoskeletal disorders. Pain management is usually a priority for the patient. Pain is a multifaceted entity from biological and individual perspectives and to reflect this, the pain experience, physical interventions for pain management and educational approaches are overviewed. In addition, a further chapter considers cognitive and behavioural influences on physiotherapy practice with strategies which clinicians may use to help their patients in their daily practice.

The advances in knowledge of the very familiar areas for the musculoskeletal physiotherapist, namely in the articular, neuromuscular and nervous systems are featured. Chapters have been dedicated to the areas of manipulative therapy management, the management of the nervous system, the very large area of therapeutic exercise where re-education of motor control, strength and endurance are considered as well as management of the sensorimotor system in terms of proprioception and postural control. A chapter also considers adjuvant pain management strategies that are used by physiotherapists (electrophysical agents, acupuncture/dry needling, taping), realizing the importance to have as much dampening of pain as possible to facilitate rehabilitative exercises.

In summary, this section focuses on the fundamental principles involved in musculoskeletal physiotherapy and their rationales to inform delivery of quality care for patients.

CHAPTER 26

CLINICAL REASONING AND MODELS FOR CLINICAL MANAGEMENT

Peter Kent • Jan Hartvigsen

Clinical reasoning is the foundation for rational patient care in musculoskeletal and other health conditions. It includes the ability to think critically, to weigh different types of knowledge and evidence, and to reflect upon how a clinical conclusion has been reached, for example, about diagnosis and treatment.[1] In this chapter we discuss different clinical reasoning models used in musculoskeletal health care, including the roles of clinical guidelines, clinical prediction rules, stepped care, adaptive care, clinically important subgroups and stratified care.

EVIDENCE-BASED CLINICAL REASONING

Whether you are managing patients with similar clinical presentations in roughly the same way according to a predefined system, or whether you are more adaptive in customizing management strategies for patients based on their individual needs and presentation, you are using a clinical reasoning model. While models can vary greatly in their flexibility and content, the interpretive matrix that clinicians apply to each and every patient encounter is by definition a clinical reasoning model – whether they are conscious of it or not.

Currently, evidence-based practice is the dominant clinical reasoning model. This is in contrast to models focused on traditions or beliefs, such as opinion-based models promoted by people teaching particular treatment techniques, location-based models based on local traditions, or authority-based models that are based on opinions of respected and experienced clinicians.[2-5] This fundamental shift in clinical decision-making is primarily the result of the explosion in research activity over the last 30 years, but also the growing demand for clinical accountability from funders and the medico-legal system, and more recently, a recognition of the importance of patients in shared decision-making.[6-8] So, in addition to traditions and clinician judgement, contemporary clinical reasoning also embraces the contribution of evidence and patient input.[3]

In an evidence-based health-care environment, clinicians need to be able to read, appraise and apply scientific evidence to prognosis, diagnosis and the treatment of individual patients. This is because evidence-based clinical reasoning and life-long learning practices have become core competences required for clinicians to be able to adapt to changing standards of good clinical practice. In musculoskeletal care, this poses particular challenges, as the evidence base is incomplete. Therefore, clinicians need to adjust to a changing body of knowledge that responds to the publication of new research findings. This has proven to be difficult because the education of musculoskeletal clinicians such as physiotherapists, chiropractors and osteopaths has traditionally been grounded in profession-specific traditions and belief systems, and not in dynamic, evidence-based, clinical problem solving.[9,10] Consequently, modern musculoskeletal clinicians, in addition to their clinical skills, ideally are capable of appraising different types of scientific studies.

Observational studies inform us about the incidence, prevalence, course, prognosis and risk of health conditions, while intervention studies inform us about the effect of treatments or other interventions. The synthesis of evidence in systematic reviews and meta-analyses summarizes results of multiple comparable studies within a field of interest (Fig. 26-1). Because more tightly designed studies provide more trustworthy results, they carry greater scientific weight. Therefore knowledge and skills in the appraisal of scientific literature enable clinicians to make rational and evidence-based decisions about diagnostic procedures, therapeutic efficacy, prognosis and clinical impact.[11-15] However, in musculoskeletal care, as many areas of clinical interventions and management are under-researched, clinical reasoning is mostly informed by evidence that is patchy and imperfect.

BOX 26-1 Key Points

- Clinical reasoning is inherent in solving clinical problems, making a diagnosis or prognosis and formulating a clinical management plan
- Evidence-based practice involves clinical reasoning that includes best-available scientific evidence, clinician experience and patient preference
- Scientific evidence in musculoskeletal care is greater than ever before, but still quite incomplete
- Good clinical reasoning models allow for new knowledge to change clinical practice

---

SOURCES OF EVIDENCE

Information on recent evidence is available from a range of sources including electronic databases such as PubMed (www.ncbi.nlm.nih.gov/pubmed) – the world's largest free search engine of published peer-reviewed literature – and Trip Database (www.tripdatabase.com) – a broader database indexing and providing links to peer-reviewed

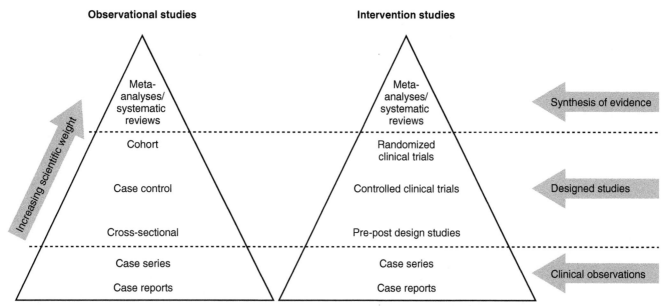

Observational studies **Intervention studies**

Increasing scientific weight

Observational studies	Intervention studies	
Meta-analyses/ systematic reviews	Meta-analyses/ systematic reviews	Synthesis of evidence
Cohort	Randomized clinical trials	
Case control	Controlled clinical trials	Designed studies
Cross-sectional	Pre-post design studies	
Case series	Case series	Clinical observations
Case reports	Case reports	

FIGURE 26-1 ■ Hierarchy of evidence for observational/epidemiological studies and intervention studies. Designed studies and syntheses of the evidence carry increasing scientific weight and are therefore shown higher up in the pyramids.

scientific papers plus clinical guidelines, reports, patient information material and opinion statements. These and other resources can be used to inform best practice based on scientific evidence (e.g. clinical guidelines, systematic reviews, clinical trials, prediction rules, case series, case studies). In contrast, other sources are more experiential, such as, using a patient's response to clinical tests and initial response to treatment to guide subsequent treatment decisions, and drawing on clinicians' previous experience.

Different types of research findings provide different types of evidence and have different uses in clinical decision-making (Table 26-1 and Fig. 26-1). Summaries of evidence from multiple studies are communicated in systematic reviews and meta-analyses. Clinical guidelines are based on systematic reviews of the literature but usually also take into account local circumstances regarding feasibility, side effects and costs. Systematic reviews and meta-analyses generally convey greater certainty than individual studies, but clinicians still need to assess the generalizability of these findings to their particular clinical setting and the demographic characteristics of their patients.

TABLE 26-1	Sources of Evidence to Inform Clinical Reasoning
Source	**Definitions**
Original (primary) research	Individual diagnostic, therapeutic, prognostic or clinical impact studies that provide varying levels of evidence (clinical trials, cohort studies, case series, case studies)
Clinical prediction rules	Clinically useful rules for the selection of diagnostic procedures, clinical assessment techniques and treatment, or for estimating prognosis
Systematic reviews/ meta-analyses	Syntheses of original research on a single topic, that are designed to give the most precise estimate of (a) how good a diagnostic procedure is; (b) how effective a specific treatment is; or (c) how prognostic a clinical feature is
Clinical guidelines	Overviews that aim to synthesize best-available evidence into clinically interpretable principles and procedures

INDUCTIVE AND DEDUCTIVE CLINICAL REASONING

When using inductive reasoning, we develop generalizations from specific observations, whereas in deductive reasoning, we develop specific hypotheses from general principles.[16,17] Clinical reasoning includes both inductive reasoning and deductive reasoning, with deductive reasoning being the mainstay of patient management. For example, a clinician who remembers evidence that some patients with lumbar disc lesions respond well to directional preference-based exercises and then decides that the best treatment for a specific patient would be such

exercises, he/she is using deductive reasoning – from the general to the specific. Deductive reasoning is inherent in almost all physiotherapy management of musculoskeletal conditions, because working from general principles to concrete decisions about specific patients is at the core of clinical practice.

Some deductive-based clinical reasoning models allow for repeated recalibration of the management plan based on monitoring a patient's response to treatment. Examples of these are stepped care models and adaptive care models.

Stepped Care and Adaptive Care

Stepped care is where the intensity, complexity and costs of care are 'stepped up' based on the complexity of a patient's presentation or response to initial care.[18–20] The principle is to commence care with 'first-line' low-intensity, low-cost diagnosis and treatment and only progress to more intense, complex and costly management strategies in those patients who do not improve adequately or present with obvious reasons for more costly and intense diagnostic procedures and/ or therapy. Therefore, individualized stepped care is a time-dependent strategy that Tiemens and Von Korff[21] describe as being based on three assumptions: (a) different levels of care are required for different people; (b) a monitoring of outcomes is often required to determine the right level of care for individual patients; and (c) health system effectiveness and cost efficiency can be improved by progressing patients from lower to higher levels of care based on their outcomes. In principle, stepped care may apply both within the range of management/treatment options that an individual clinician can self-administer, and also to the range of options available for co-management of patients with musculoskeletal conditions. For example, a patient with recurrent patellar dislocation might initially be commenced on a progressive exercise and taping programme. However, a monitoring of their adherence, treatment response and outcomes may subsequently indicate that use of a patellar brace, modification of functional/sports activities and referral for an opinion from a sports medicine physician or orthopaedic surgeon would be useful next steps. In the management of musculoskeletal conditions, care is often progressed on the basis of patient response to treatment rather than diagnosis alone.

Adaptive care is a closely related strategy for individualizing patient care that uses decision rules to guide whether, how and when to alter clinical management.[22] The main distinction between stepped care and adaptive care is that the latter uses more formalized clinical guidelines to specify the way in which care should be tailored for individual patients. Adaptive care strategies are also called adaptive interventions and dynamic treatment regimens.[23]

CLINICAL PREDICTION RULES

Clinical prediction rules are often simple, memorable rules for selecting clinical assessment techniques or treatment.

An example of a prediction rule for the selection of a clinical assessment technique is the Ottowa Knee Rule, which is a rule designed to help clinicians determine whether an X-ray is required in patients who have an acute knee injury.[24] This prediction rule states that an X-ray is required only in patients who have one or more of the following: age 55 years or older, tenderness at the head of the fibula, isolated tenderness of the patella, an inability to flex to 90°, or an inability to bear weight (unable to take four steps) both immediately after the injury and also in the clinic. This prediction rule was designed and validated for use in hospital emergency departments. In an initial validation study of 1096 adults in two hospitals, the rule had a sensitivity of 1.0 (95% CI 0.94 to 1.0) for identifying clinically important fractures, and the probability of fracture, when the decision rule was negative, was 0% (95% CI, 0% to 0.4%).[24] This rule is designed to be extremely sensitive – to not miss any clinically important fractures – and yet in this study the rule would have reduced the rate of unnecessary X-ray referrals by 28%. Replication in external validation studies is a very important step in the development of clinical prediction rules, and near-identical results for the Ottowa Knee Rule were obtained in a subsequent study of 3907 patients in four hospitals.[25] Also important in the assessment of clinical prediction rules are impact analysis studies[26] that examine whether such rules work in non-experimental conditions in routine clinical care settings (prediction rule practicality and acceptance).

An example of a clinical prediction rule for treatment selection in patients with acute non-specific low back pain is Flynn's Manipulation Prediction Rule.[27] Initial results indicated that patients who were positive on this prediction rule were more likely to benefit from spinal manipulation and range of movement exercises than from a low-stress aerobic and lumbar spine strengthening programme.[28] Patients were 'rule positive' if they met any four out of these five criteria: symptom duration of less than 16 days; no symptoms distal to the knee; score less than 19 on a fear-avoidance measure; at least one hypomobile lumbar segment; and at least one hip with more than 35° of internal rotation. Overall at 1-week follow-up in this clinical trial, 44% of participants improved with the manipulation (defined as a 50% or more improvement in their baseline activity limitation scores). However, 92% who were rule positive improved with the manipulation (positive likelihood ratio = 13.2) versus only 7% who were rule negative (negative likelihood ratio = 0.1). These results are promising, as this simple prediction rule appears to identify subgroups of people for whom manipulation is, or is not, effective. However, similar to the Ottawa Knee Rule, there is a need for independent external validation studies that test this rule using the same treatments and determine whether it is generalizable to, and feasible for use in, other clinical settings.

Classifying patients in diagnosis or treatment can go beyond simple clinical prediction rules and may involve more complex classification systems. An example is Classification-Based Cognitive Functional Therapy for people with chronic non-specific low back pain.[29] This targeted treatment approach contains a comprehensive decision-making algorithm that classifies patients based on the assessment of multiple health domains (physical impairment, pain, activity limitation, functional loss, psychological adaptation). A recent randomized controlled trial showed clinically important improvements in outcomes for people with chronic non-specific low back pain treated with this approach when compared with current best practice manual therapy and exercise.[30] Over the 12-month follow-up period, the group of patients treated with this approach had more than twice the improvement in pain and activity limitation than those receiving the control treatment. This is also an example of a physiotherapy management approach for which components have been systematically validated,[31] including its reproducibility,[32,33] prior to its clinical efficacy being examined in a clinical trial.

TECHNOLOGY AND PAPER-BASED AIDES FOR CLINICAL REASONING

Technology-based assistance for clinical reasoning involves the use of phone/tablet applications and computer algorithms embedded in electronic patient record systems and clinical care databases (Table 26-2). Using

TABLE 26-2	Features of Technology-Assisted and Paper-Based Aids for Clinical Reasoning
Definitions	**Strengths/Weaknesses**
Technology Assisted – Computer-Based Questionnaires or Algorithms	
Phone/tablet applications, or functions embedded in electronic patient records/clinical information systems	Strengths: • Automated scoring • May be more sensitive and patient-specific than paper-based systems, as they can be compared with large normative datasets • May provide novel or more precise information, or may automatically synthesize information from disparate sources • Easy storage and retrieval of information • May include skip logic to reduce questionnaire length • Can include multiple languages Weaknesses: • Require technology literacy • Need to be integrated into the clinical encounter in ways that do not excessively interrupt the workflow and clinician/patient engagement • Require ongoing expert IT support
Paper-Based Questionnaires or Algorithms	
Printed questionnaires or printed scoring algorithms, such as nomograms*	Strengths: • Easy to complete • Do not require technology literacy Weaknesses: • Require manual scoring and therefore the scoring method needs to be simple and time-efficient • Harder to store information • May provide less sophisticated information

*A nomogram is a visual method for predicting a patient's score on an unobserved or unmeasured clinical feature, when their score on related clinical features is known.

these technologies, clinicians are provided with value-adding information that they can choose whether to include in their clinical reasoning. This information is not intended to replace the role of individual clinicians taking responsibility for clinical decision-making about individual patients because only the clinician sees the patient in his or her entirety and there is always a need for clinical decisions to be adaptive and responsive to individual circumstances. One example of a computer algorithm designed to inform musculoskeletal clinical reasoning is an electronic nomogram that classifies the gait characteristics of children with spastic diplegia which can also be used for monitoring their gait outcomes.[34] Using three simple clinical measures as inputs – leg length in metres, stride length in metres and cadence in steps per minute – the computer algorithm characterizes and compares the child's neuromuscular function and classifies it into one of five characteristic patterns. The principle is that changes in cluster membership provide an objective measure of improvement in the child's neuromuscular function, using measures obtained with only simple clinical equipment: a stopwatch, tape measure, and talcum powder.

Another example of web-based computer algorithms designed to inform clinical reasoning is the Focus On Therapeutic Outcomes system (FOTO Inc. Knoxville, TN, USA). On the basis of standardized, validated baseline questions that are answered by the patient, the system calculates, for a range of musculoskeletal conditions, the patient's baseline functional status and predicted functional status taking into account such factors as age, episode duration, severity and co-morbidities, based on a large normative dataset. The clinician can then (a) base clinical decisions on the predicted change in functional status, predicted outcome, and predicted number of patient visits to achieve that outcome, which are based on the collective performance of other physiotherapists; and (b) measure and document actual functional status at the time of discharge from care. This allows for benchmarking of performance against a risk-adjusted average for similar patients, by effectiveness (functional outcome), by efficiency (number of visits) and by patient satisfaction.

An example of a paper-based questionnaire or algorithm is the STarT Back Tool.[35] The STarT Back Tool is a simple nine-item questionnaire that classifies patients with non-specific low back pain into one of three care streams. This classification is based on an estimate of each patient's risk of a poor outcome (low risk; medium risk; high risk) plus an estimate of the complexity of his or her presentation, that results in an estimate of the complexity of intervention that is likely to be required (minimal intervention/reassurance; manual therapy and exercise; manual therapy, exercise and psychologically informed physiotherapy). In a recent clinical trial, STarT Back Tool classification-based treatment showed modest improvements in patient outcomes and overall treatment costs (primarily by reducing unnecessary treatments for low-risk patients), compared with usual GP/physiotherapy care.[36] Noteworthy in this approach is that clinicians retain considerable flexibility in their choice of treatment for the medium-risk and high-risk subgroups.

STRATIFIED HEALTH CARE AND TREATMENT EFFECT MODIFICATION

Stratified health care is similar to stepped care and adaptive care models in that they all seek to match the right treatment to the right patient at the right time. Sometimes these concepts co-exist or overlap in the same setting. However, stratified health care in its pure form is designed for decision making about care pathways during the initial clinical encounter, rather than relying on a time-dependent response to treatment.

Stratified care targets treatment to patient subgroups based on characteristic patient profiles, such as their prognostic risk, the suspected underlying causal mechanisms of their health condition or their likely response to a particular treatment.[37] The idea of stratified health care is popular because it is seen as a method: (a) to tailor treatment to specific, sometimes biologically or psychologically distinct, individuals; (b) to maximize treatment response, reduce harm or both, and; (c) to rescue treatment that fails to show an overall effect by identifying subgroup(s) for whom it is effective.[38]

Stratified care is closely related to the concept of treatment effect modification, which confusingly is also sometimes called treatment effect moderation and treatment effect subgrouping. Research into treatment effect modification seeks to identify patients with distinct clinical profiles (phenotypes) who respond best to particular treatment.[37] It is based on the concept that not all patients respond to the same extent to a given treatment and the recognition that research methods exist to identify such patient phenotypes. This is also seen as a means to perform research that more closely mimics current clinical practice and the hope that research targeting clinically important subgroups will result in the demonstration of larger treatment effects.

Treatment effect modification research is more technically and procedurally demanding than traditional two-group clinical trials,[39] and although the appropriate methods vary depending on the specific research question being asked,[40] these methods are now well defined.[39,41-44] Given the current research interest in treatment effect modification, the goal is that in the medium term, robust evidence of treatment effect modification will become available that assists musculoskeletal clinicians in their clinical reasoning.

Clinical reasoning models can include both stratified care and treatment effect modification.[37] For example, a stratified care model, such as the STarT Back Tool, may identify preferred care pathways for patients based on their prognostic profile (low risk, medium risk, high risk

of poor outcome). However, within a care pathway, such as for the high-risk group, targeted treatment decisions can be informed by knowledge of treatment effect modification, that is, identifying which high-risk patients are likely to respond to a particular available treatment and which patients are better suited to different treatment methods. In addition, response to treatment in a given stratified care pathway may determine subsequent steps that merge the stratified and stepped care approaches.

Another concept with similar wording to treatment effect modification is treatment effect mediation and, although these concepts are often confused, they are quite different (Table 26-3). While treatment effect modification aims at matching the individual patient to the best treatment, treatment effect mediation is a method for testing theories about causal links between a treatment and an outcome[45] and so it seeks to understand how and why – and not if – a treatment works or does not work. A hypothetical mediational analysis might test whether the effect of a treatment (such as stabilization exercises for people with whiplash) on an outcome (such as activity limitation) occurs via a change in some modifiable intermediate variable (such as reduced fear of movement). If this were the case, then the effect of the treatment might be increased by also deliberately treating the intermediate variable. In musculoskeletal research, mediation analysis is becoming more common as it has the capacity to inform the design and delivery of more effective interventions.[46] Again, the goal is that in the medium term, robust evidence of effect mediation will become available to assist musculoskeletal clinicians in optimizing treatment effects.

THE CHALLENGE OF MAKING CLINICAL REASONING MODELS RELEVANT TO THE CARE OF INDIVIDUAL PATIENTS

The clinical reasoning models that we have discussed above attempt to integrate or provide best-available evidence to clinicians in forms that are accessible, understandable and useful in reducing uncertainty at the time of the clinical encounter. One of the challenges in providing this evidence is to extend findings from the group or subgroup level and make them as accurate as possible at the individual patient level. One way in which researchers are working on this challenge is by exploring the use of Bayesian statistical methods to create clinical reasoning tools.[47] Bayesian methods have a number of advantages that hold the promise of their being more adaptive and patient-specific than previous methods.[48,49] For example,

TABLE 26-3	**Treatment Effect Modification and Effect Mediation – How Are They Different?**	
Treatment effect modification	The identification of symptoms or signs that indicate a patient's likely response to a specific treatment	This information is often the basis for a clinical prediction rule
Treatment effect mediation	A method to identify factors that are causally linked to treatment response	This information helps with understanding the mechanisms by which a treatment is effective, how it could be more effective, or why it is ineffective

they are able to incorporate and respond to clinical information that may only emerge during an episode of care (such as initial response to treatment and the results of subsequent tests), and are therefore better able to model the dynamic temporal nature of a clinical trajectory. They are also able to model the causal relationships underlying that trajectory. As they are based on probability, Bayesian models typically result in outputs that clinicians find intuitive to understand, such as 'this patient has a 73% probability of improving by a clinically important amount by 6 weeks if he or she receives this treatment regimen'.

BOX 26-2 | **Key Points**

- Deductive reasoning is the mainstay of patient management because working from general principles to concrete decisions about specific patients is at the core of clinical practice
- Deductive-based clinical reasoning models, such as stepped care and adaptive care models, incorporate the repeated monitoring of a patient's response to treatment as a means to regularly calibrate the management plan
- Other models of clinical reasoning are based on identifying clinically important subgroups of patients by way of clusters of their symptoms and signs. Some of these models involve clinical prediction rules and classification systems, and are based on technology assistance or paper-based questionnaires and algorithms
- Stratified health care and the concept of treatment effect modification are based on a recognition that not all patients respond to the same extent to a given treatment

---

THE BIOPSYCHOSOCIAL MODEL – WHY DEALING WITH THE PHYSICAL IS OFTEN NOT ENOUGH

Currently, the dominant conceptual framework in musculoskeletal disorders is the biopsychosocial model put forward by, among others, Gordon Waddell in the mid-1980s.[50,51] This model suggests that taking a purely biomedical perspective may limit one's understanding of musculoskeletal disorders. This is because for many individuals the fundamental problem is not their experience of pain, which can often be temporary, but rather their own and society's views and responses to their pain.[52] Yet the concept of a 'diagnosable disease' is still central to most clinical reasoning in musculoskeletal health care, as diagnosis and staging of the condition identify the involved abnormal body function plus its pathological cause, and, at least theoretically, indicate appropriate treatment and prognosis. However, there is now good evidence showing that in musculoskeletal health, psychological factors (such as fear-avoidance beliefs, anxiety, depression, poor coping strategies, poor self-efficacy and pre-existing somatization) are important predictors of poor outcomes, and play significant roles in the transition from acute to persistent pain and disability.[53-56] In fact, often these are more strongly associated with outcome than biomedical factors. Similarly, social factors (social arrangements, health and disability structures and local cultural beliefs) have been shown to influence outcomes,

such as disability, beyond the factors operating at the level of individuals.[52,57-60]

One example of a physiotherapy clinical reasoning method that follows the biomedical model is the Mechanical Diagnosis and Therapy approach to the management of spinal pain.[61] This popular assessment approach[62] classifies patients into treatment subgroups using validated diagnostic procedures.[63,64] Although this approach classifies patients on the basis of their physical impairment and pain characteristics rather than patho-anatomical diagnosis, it nonetheless is based on the biomedical model to the extent that it does not incorporate psychological and social factors. A more recent physiotherapy clinical reasoning model – Classification-Based Cognitive Functional Therapy – does incorporate psychosocial factors because in addition to considering physical impairment and pain, this classification system clusters patients into subgroups based on cognitive constructs (negative back pain beliefs, fear, hypervigilance, anxiety, low mood), lifestyle behaviours (activity avoidance, poor pacing) and maladaptive movement (loss of movement awareness, protective and avoidance behaviours).[29,65]

Despite emerging evidence that embracing the biopsychosocial model may be more effective,[30,36] and the intuitive appeal of managing the 'whole person' in musculoskeletal patient care, there is evidence that many clinicians, including physiotherapists, frequently do not assess the psychosocial aspects of their patients[66] and are often uncomfortable addressing these aspects.[67,68] Many do not feel they possess adequate skills or training to deal effectively with psychosocial obstacles to recovery.[67,69] Perhaps this is because clinical education and culture have historically been too biomedically focused[70] and have largely failed to adopt the biopsychosocial model.[52] In response to this, a more psychologically informed practice[71] has recently been promoted and the model of the psychologically informed physiotherapist[72] has been implemented in some settings, such as in the training of physiotherapists to manage high-risk patients under the STarT Back Tool model. This can be seen as a 'middle way' between traditional biomedically focused physiotherapy and cognitive-behavioural therapy[71] because this training equips physiotherapists with skills to recognize and influence modifiable psychological risk factors for the development of unnecessary pain-associated disability.

BOX 26-3 | **Key Points**

- Much current management of musculoskeletal disorders is centred around a biological or biomedical paradigm
- The biopsychosocial model encourages clinicians to include in their clinical reasoning their patient's psychological and social barriers to recovery
- In musculoskeletal care, some of these psychosocial barriers are believed to be modifiable
- Many clinicians currently do not assess these aspects and feel inadequately trained or uncomfortable to address them
- Recent developments in clinical education have led to the model of the psychologically informed physiotherapist

FUTURE DIRECTIONS FOR CLINICAL REASONING AND MANAGEMENT

The volume of clinical and epidemiological research in musculoskeletal health is increasing and it is changing the face of musculoskeletal health care and the role of physiotherapists and other health-care providers. The principles behind clinical reasoning will remain, but clinicians will face new evidence that will challenge their beliefs and routines and require the development of new practice patterns. For example, clinicians are likely to be expected to systematically screen patients for risk of chronicity using psychological and social instruments, in addition to the physical clinical examination, in order to make evidence-based, biopsychosocially informed, decisions about prognosis and therapy. Stepped diagnosis and care that reserves expensive testing and therapy for patients with clear indications and evidence of benefit, and care stratified according to predefined criteria will gradually be implemented with the emergence of new evidence and the desire for more cost-effective health care. Wearable, discrete and affordable devices to monitor activity and motion will become common so that physiotherapists and other clinicians can capture information in real time about the activities of patients and thereby improve compliance with prescribed exercises (Actigraph, Pensacola, USA; actigraphcorp.com). Also, motion sensing and analysis technology to assist the assessment of movement, movement patterns, posture and work practices will extend physiotherapists' capacity to evaluate patients in the clinic and in their daily functional activity, and these data – whether from occupational, rehabilitation, sport, recreation or daily living settings – will require new forms of clinical reasoning (dorsaVi Ltd, Melbourne, Australia; www.dorsavi.com).

Importantly, patients will be informed and will expect to participate in decisions about their own care management.[6-8] Information technology will be a useful vehicle for disseminating evidence to both patients and clinicians, and interactive platforms for informed decision-making based on the presentation and circumstances of individual patients will become common. High-quality evidence and ready access to care are fundamental components in modern societies. However, good clinical reasoning from well-educated clinicians will remain the foundation for good health care.

REFERENCES

1. Anderson KJ. Factors Affecting the Development of Undergraduate Medical Students' Clinical Reasoning Ability. PhD Thesis, The University of Adelaide; 2006.
2. Sackett D, Richardson W, Rosenberg W, et al. Evidence-Based Medicine: How to Practice & Teach EBM. 1st ed. Edinburgh: Churchill Livingstone; 1998.
3. Sackett DL, Rosenberg WM, Gray JA, et al. Evidence based medicine: what it is and what it isn't. BMJ 1996;312(7023):71–2.
4. Hoffmann T, Bennett S, Del Mar C. Evidence-Based Practice Across the Health Professions. Australia: Elsevier; 2009.
5. Isaacs D, Fitzgerald D. Seven alternatives to evidence based medicine. BMJ 1999;319:1618.
6. Trede F, Higgs J. Collaborative decision making. In: Higgs JJM, Loftus S, Christensen N, editors. Chapter 4 in Clinical Reasoning in the Health Professions. Elsevier Health Sciences; 2008. p. 520.
7. Edwards A, Elwyn G. Shared Decision Making in Health Care: Achieving Evidence-Based Patient Choice. Shared Decision Making in Health Care. 2nd ed. Oxford UK: Oxford University Press; 2009.
8. Informed Medical Decisions Foundation. 2013. From: <http://www.informedmedicaldecisions.org>; [retrieved 31 December 2013].
9. Parsons S, Harding G, Breen A, et al. Will shared decision making between patients with chronic musculoskeletal pain and physiotherapists, osteopaths and chiropractors improve patient care? Fam Pract 2012;29(2):203–12.
10. Foster NE, Hartvigsen J, Croft PR. Taking responsibility for the early assessment and treatment of patients with musculoskeletal pain: a review and critical analysis. Arthritis Res Ther 2012;14(1):205.
11. Guyatt GH, Oxman AD, Kunz R, et al. Rating quality of evidence and strength of recommendations: going from evidence to recommendations. BMJ 2008;336(7652):1049–51.
12. Guyatt GH, Oxman AD, Kunz R, et al. Rating quality of evidence and strength of recommendations: incorporating considerations of resources use into grading recommendations. BMJ 2008; 336(7654):1170–3.
13. Guyatt GH, Oxman AD, Vist G, et al. Rating quality of evidence and strength of recommendations GRADE: an emerging consensus on rating quality of evidence and strength of recommendations. BMJ 2008;336:924–6.
14. Schünemann HJ, Oxman AD, Brozek J, et al. Grading quality of evidence and strength of recommendations for diagnostic tests and strategies. BMJ 2008;336(7653):1106–10.
15. Jaeschke R, Guyatt GH, Dellinger P, et al. Use of GRADE grid to reach decisions on clinical practice guidelines when consensus is elusive. BMJ 2008;337:a744.
16. Edwards I, Jones M, Carr J, et al. Clinical reasoning strategies in physical therapy. Phys Ther 2004;84:312–30.
17. Pottier P, Hardouin JB, Hodges BD, et al. Exploring how students think: a new method combining think-aloud and concept mapping protocols. Med Educ 2010;44(9):926–35.
18. Hartvigsen J, Natvig B, Ferreira M. Is it all about a pain in the back? Best Pract Res Clin Rheumatol 2013;27:613–23.
19. Roos E, Juhl C. Osteoarthritis 2012 year in review: rehabilitation and outcomes. Osteoarthr Cartil 2012;20:1477–83.
20. Von Korff KM, Moore JC. Stepped care for back pain: activating approaches for primary care. Ann Intern Med 2001;134:911–17.
21. Von Korff M, Tiemens B. Individualized stepped care of chronic illness. West J Med 2000;172(2):133–7.
22. Amirall D, Compton SN, Gunlicks-Stoessel M, et al. Designing a pilot sequential multiple assignment randomized trial for developing an adaptive treatment strategy. Stat Med 2012;31:1887–902.
23. Murphy SA. Optimal dynamic treatment regimes. J R Stat Soc Series B 2003;65:331–55.
24. Stiell IG, Greenberg GH, Wells GA, et al. Prospective validation of a decision rule for use of radiography in acute knee injury. JAMA 1996;275:611–15.
25. Stiell IG, Wells GA, Hoag RH, et al. Implementation of the Ottawa Knee Rule for the use of radiography in acute knee injuries. JAMA 1997;278:2075–9.
26. Moons KG, Royston P, Vergouwe Y, et al. Prognosis and prognostic research: what, why and how? BMJ 2009;338:b375.
27. Flynn T, Fritz JW, Whitman M, et al. A clinical prediction rule for classifying patients with low back pain who demonstrate short-term improvement with spinal manipulation. Spine 2002;27(24): 2835–43.
28. Childs JD, Fritz JM, Flynn TW, et al. A clinical prediction rule to identify patients with low back pain most likely to benefit from spinal manipulation: a validation study. Ann Intern Med 2004; 141(12):920–8.
29. O'Sullivan P. Diagnosis and classification of chronic low backpain disorders: maladaptive movement and motor control impairments as underlying mechanism. Man Ther 2005;10:242–55.
30. Vibe Fersum K, O'Sullivan P, Skouen JS, et al. Efficacy of classification-based cognitive functional therapy in patients with non-specific chronic low back pain: a randomized controlled trial. Eur J Pain 2012;17(6):916–28.
31. Dankaerts W, O'Sullivan P. The validity of O'Sullivan's classification system (CS) for a sub-group of NS-CLBP with motor control impairment (MCI): overview of a series of studies and review of the literature. Man Ther 2011;16(1):9–14.

32. Dankaerts W, O'Sullivan PB, Straker LM, et al. The inter-examiner reliability of a classification method for non-specific chronic low back pain patients with motor control impairment. Man Ther 2006;11(1):28–39.

33. Fersum KV, O'Sullivan PB, Kvåle A, et al. Inter-examiner reliability of a classification system for patients with non-specific low back pain. Man Ther 2009;14(5):555–61.

34. Vaughan CL, O'Malley MJ. A gait nomogram used with fuzzy clustering to monitor functional status of children and young adults with cerebral palsy. Dev Med Child Neurol 2005;47(6):377–83.

35. Hill JC, Dunn KM, Lewis M, et al. A primary care back pain screening tool: identifying patient subgroups for initial treatment. Arthritis Rheum 2008;59(5):632–41.

36. Hill JC, Whitehurst DG, Lewis M, et al. Comparison of stratified primary care management for low back pain with current best practice (STarT Back): a randomised controlled trial. Lancet 2011;378(9802):1560–71.

37. Foster NE, Hill JC, O'Sullivan P, et al. Stratified models of care. Best Pract Res Clin Rheumatol 2013;27:649–61.

38. Hingorani AD, Windt DA, Riley RD, et al. Prognosis research strategy (PROGRESS) 4: Stratified medicine research. BMJ 2013;346:e5793.

39. Hancock M, Herbert R, Maher CG. A guide to interpretation of studies investigating subgroups of responders to physical therapy interventions. Phys Ther 2009;89(7):698–704.

40. Kent P, Hancock M, Petersen DH, et al. Choosing appropriate study designs for particular questions about treatment subgroups. J Man Manip Ther 2010;18(3):147–52.

41. Kent P, Keating JL, Leboeuf-Yde C. Research methods for subgrouping low back pain. BMC Res Meth 2010;10:62. doi:10.1186/1471-2288-10-62.

42. Rothwell P. Subgroup analysis in randomised controlled trials: importance, indications, and interpretation. Lancet 2005;365(9454):176–86.

43. Royston P, Moons KG, Altman DG, et al. Prognosis and prognostic research: developing a prognostic model. BMJ 2009;338:b604.

44. Altman DG, Vergouwe Y, Royston P, et al. Prognosis and prognostic research: validating a prognostic model. BMJ 2009;338:b605.

45. Mansell G, Kent P, Kamper S. Why and how back pain interventions work: what can we do to find out? Best Pract Res Clin Rheumatol 2013;27(5):685–97.

46. van der Windt DA, Dunn KM. Preface. Best Pract Res Clin Rheumatol 2013;27:571–3.

47. van Gerven MA, Taal BG, Lucas PJ. Dynamic Bayesian networks as prognostic models for clinical patient management. J Biomed Inform 2008;41:515–29.

48. Verduijn M, Peek N, Rosseel PM, et al. Prognostic Bayesian networks I: Rationale, learning procedure and clinical use. J Biomed Inform 2007;40:609–18.

49. Verduijn M, Rosseel PM, Peek N, et al. Prognostic Bayesian networks II: an application in the domain of cardiac surgery. J Biomed Inform 2007;40:619–30.

50. Waddell G. A new clinical model for the treatment of low-back pain. Spine 1987;12(7):632–44.

51. Waddell G. Preventing incapacity in people with musculoskeletal disorders. BMJ 2006;77–78:55–69.

52. Pincus T, Kent P, Bronfort G, et al. Twenty-five years with the biopsychosocial model of low back pain – is it time to celebrate? A report from the Odense Forum XII. Spine 2013;38(14):2118–23.

53. Gatchel RJ, Peng YB, Peters ML, et al. The biopsychosocial approach to chronic pain: scientific advances and future directions. Psychol Bull 2007;133:581–624.

54. Mallen CD, Thomas E, Belcher J, et al. Point-of-care prognosis for common musculoskeletal pain in older adults. JAMA Intern Med 2013;173(12):1119–25.

55. Pincus T, Burton A, Vogel S, et al. A systematic review of psychological factors as predictors of chronicity/disability in prospective cohorts of low back pain. Spine 2002;27(5):E109–20.

56. Nicholas MK, Linton SJ, Watson PJ, et al. Early identification and management of psychological risk factors ('yellow flags') in patients with low back pain: a reappraisal. Phys Ther 2011;91:737–53.

57. Anema JR, Schellart AJM, Cassidy JD, et al. Can cross country differences in return-to-work after chronic occupational back pain be explained? An exploratory analysis on disability policies in a six country cohort study. J Occup Rehabil 2009;19:419–26.

58. Fransen M, Woodward M, Norton R, et al. Risk factors associated with the transition from acute to chronic occupational back pain. Spine 2002;27(1):92–8.

59. Lippel K, Lötters F. Public insurance systems: A comparison of cause-based and disability-based income support systems. In: Loisel PaA JR, editor. Handbook of Work Disability: Prevention and Management. New York: Springer Science+Business Media; 2013.

60. Loisel P, Buchbinder R, Hazard R, et al. Prevention of work disability due to musculoskeletal disorders: the challenge of implementing evidence. J Occup Rehabil 2005;15:507–24.

61. McKenzie R, May S. Lumbar Spine, Mechanical Diagnosis and Therapy. 2nd ed. Waikanae, New Zealand: Spinal Publications Ltd; 2003.

62. Battié MC, Cherkin DC, Dunn R, et al. Managing low back pain: attitudes and treatment preferences of physical therapists. Phys Ther 1994;74(3):219–26.

63. Donelson R, Aprill C, Medcalf R, et al. A prospective study of centralization of lumbar and referred pain: a predictor of symptomatic discs and annular competence. Spine 1997;22(10):1115–22.

64. Long A, Donelson R, Fung T. Does it matter which exercise? A randomized control trial of exercise for low back pain. Spine 2004;29(23):2593–602.

65. O'Sullivan PB. Lumbar segmental 'instability': clinical presentation and specific stabilizing exercise management. Man Ther 2000;5(1):2–12.

66. Kent P, Keating JL, Taylor NF. Primary care clinicians use variable methods to assess acute nonspecific low back pain and usually focus on impairments. Man Ther 2009;14:88–100.

67. Sanders T, Foster NE, Bishop A, et al. Biopsychosocial care and the physiotherapy encounter: physiotherapists' accounts of back pain consultations. BMC Musculoskelet Disord 2013;14:65. doi:10.1186/471-2474-14-65.

68. Shaw WS, Pransky G, Winters T, et al. Does the presence of psychosocial 'yellow flags' alter patient-provider communication for work-related, acute low back pain? J Occup Environ Med 2009;51:1032–40.

69. Savage R, Armstrong D. Effect of a general practitioner's consulting style on patients' satisfaction: a controlled study. BMJ 1990;301(6758):968–70.

70. Shepard KF. Thirty-eighth Mary McMillan Lecture: are you waving or drowning? Phys Ther 2007;87:1543–54.

71. Main CJ, George SZ. Psychologically informed practice for management of low back pain: future directions in practice and research. Phys Ther 2011;91:820–4.

72. Craik RL. A convincing case – for the psychologically informed physical therapist. Phys Ther 2011;91(5):606–8.

CHAPTER 27

COMMUNICATING WITH PATIENTS

EDITOR'S INTRODUCTION

One of the key elements of a successful patient–
therapist relationship is personal one-to-one
communication. In the absence of good-quality
communication, patients' satisfaction can be
reduced and patients' expectations may not be
achieved. In addition, the opportunity for mutual
understanding between the patient and the
clinician may be lost. Intelligence in the use of
language in the therapeutic setting is vital in
maintaining an empathetic and trusting
relationship which contributes to successful
treatment outcomes.

Frequently, patients need to be informed
about possible risks, for example the risk that
may occur as a result of proposed high-velocity
thrust manipulative procedures to the cervical
region. This enables them to make an informed
choice about the treatment that they receive.
One of the key areas highlighted by
musculoskeletal physiotherapists, as part of a
multimodal approach to treatment, is education.
A person-centred approach to communication
and how educational strategies and concepts
are articulated by the physiotherapist are vital in
ensuring that the pedagogic (educational)
element of a multimodal approach is appropriate
and effective. Thus this chapter focuses on these
three important components: the use of
language in the clinical setting, the
communication of relative risk of treatments and
patient education.

CHAPTER 27.1 ■ PATIENT-FOCUSED PRACTICE AND COMMUNICATION: USE OF COMMUNICATION IN THE CLINICAL SETTING

Ruth Parry

INTRODUCTION

Substantial evidence shows that the content and style of
clinicians' communication influence patient outcomes
including: attendance at subsequent appointments,
adherence with prescribed activities, symptom resolution, functional outcomes and reported satisfaction.[1,2]
The evidence indicates that effective communication
entails treating the patient as an active participant,
in-depth discussion of their problem(s), providing opportunities to ask questions, offering positive feedback and
emotional support, giving clear instructions and endeav-
ouring to reach common ground about the nature of the
problem and what needs to be done.[1-3] While these
insights are helpful, practitioners need to know precisely
how to go about 'treating patients as active participants',
'reaching common ground' and so on. Fortunately, a
growing body of research is providing explicit descriptions of practices through which we can implement these
kinds of communication.

In this section I consider evidence from this growing
body of research. This research uses the conversation
analytic approach, which entails systematically analysing
recordings of naturally occurring interactions to identify
and describe the structure and functioning of communication behaviours.[4-8] First, I will outline features of communication that one needs to grasp in order to analyse
one's own communication and that of patients and colleagues (Box 27-1). Then I describe the structure and
functioning of some specific practices relevant for working
with patients. In doing so, I provide a brief introduction
to conversation analytic findings and make recommendations for further reading.

BOX 27-1	Some Key Features of Communication

- The details of communication matter: meaning is built not just by what is said, but how and when it is said
- Communication is sequentially structured
- Any particular communicative task or action can be done in a variety of ways, and these have different consequences
- Each of our communicative 'moves' does several things at the same time
- Communication is more than information exchange: through communication we build relationships and identity – who we are to one another

BOX 27-2	Strategies by Which Practitioners Can Work to Build Common Ground

- Asking patients about their views and understandings
- Encouraging them to respond
- Designing what you say in relation to what the patient says
- Stepwise building of agreement
- 'You tell me first' sequences
- Online commentary about your examination findings
- Explaining reasons
- Making positive and specific recommendations before making any negative recommendations

SOME KEY FEATURES OF COMMUNICATION

Firstly, we should notice that not only what we say, but how and when we say it is important: details are highly significant for meaning-making.[9] These details include wording, pauses, intonation, gesture, gaze and so on. To illustrate: consider all the different ways you can pronounce words such as 'Oh' or 'Yeah', and notice how vastly their meanings differ depending on how you say them and at what conversational juncture you say them.

Secondly, communication is structured in sequences – think of greetings, or the question and response series during initial patient assessments. Therefore, when we think about communication, we should think of it sequentially, i.e. in terms how what we do shapes what the patient can and does say, and how this in turn shapes what we can and do say.

Thirdly, any particular communication task or activity can be done in multiple ways. For instance, we can seek information from another person via a quizzical look, by repeating what they have said in a puzzled tone of voice, or by asking indirect or direct questions.[10] Each different way of attempting a communication task will have different consequences for what the other person does and says, and for how they perceive you. Some communication tasks that are frequent in physiotherapy have been studied in great detail, for instance, different ways of seeking patients' views,[11-13] ways in which patients convey their views,[14] and different ways of making treatment recommendations.[15-17] This research helps illuminate how different ways of doing things have different consequences; for instance, how different question formats more or less strongly encourage in-depth or 'on-topic' responses.[13]

Fourthly, it is important to recognize that communication is the fundamental means by which we do things with one another, and furthermore that every communicative action does more than one thing at once. When I ask a patient to do a movement I not only request her physical efforts, but also convey that this is what therapy is and that I have therapeutic knowledge and skills. When the patient responds with a movement, they not only perform the action, they also convey things like cooperation and effort.[18] Communication is the key means by which we convey who we are to one another (trustworthy therapist, cooperative patient, etc.), make sense of one another's actions, wishes and perspectives; and build and maintain relationships with one another.

SOME SPECIFIC PRACTICES FOR BUILDING TOWARDS COMMON GROUND

Inevitably, therapists and patients will have different perspectives and understandings on physiotherapy-related matters. As noted, the research evidence suggests it is important that practitioners at least try to build common ground about treatment activities, recommendations and decisions, and about the rationale underpinning them. Box 27-2 lists some relevant strategies, and I describe them below.

Pursuing Patients' Contributions, and Designing What You Say in Relation to Their Contributions

Perhaps the simplest strategy for reaching common ground is asking questions, and – if you do not get the answer you need – asking again, or asking somewhat differently. Once a patient has responded, building common ground entails designing what you say in relation to their response.

Stepwise Building of Agreement

This practice can be particularly useful where there are some obstacles to building common ground. An illustrative example can be found in Box 27-3, a transcript of part of a physiotherapy session involving a patient who is receiving inpatient rehabilitation after acute stroke. The focus of the fairly lengthy session has been on sitting balance.

Analysis of some features I don't examine here can be found elsewhere.[19] Notice that as the episode begins, a difference between the patient's and therapist's positions becomes evident (L1–18). The therapist 'pursues' the patient's response and the patient resists, culminating in voicing a reason why he cannot answer (L18). At this point, the therapist begins building agreement in a

BOX 27-3	Transcribed Episode from Physiotherapy Illustrating Stepwise Building of Agreement

Parry_S4Ph9PaUT1/2.55 (simplified)

1	T	Have you 'ad <u>enough?</u>
2		(0.3)
3	P	No I'm not bothered ((*flat tone*)) (0.2) 's up to you en<u>tire</u>ly
4		(0.3)
5	T	No it's not (0.2) doesn' matter to us (it's up to) you
6	P	Mm
7		(1.0)
8	P	Oh. Think you (.) Think you ach<u>iev</u>ed something?
9	T	D'you think you achieved something?
10		(1.0)
11	P	Not up to me it's up to you (.) teacher
12	T	hh uh huh the teacher ((*patient and therapist are smiling*))
13	T	N<u>o</u>
14		(0.3)
15	T	It's what <u>you</u> want. <u>you</u> gotta get better ['aven't] you
16	P	[ahh ((*quietly*))]
17	T	[yeah?]
18	P	[No] but I can – I don't know what's better.
19	T	Al<u>right</u>. Well to be able to sit was your first <u>goal</u>
20	P	Ye[s]
21	T	[an]d you achieved it
22	P	Yes
23	T	So you have achieved something
24	P	(I've) achieved something yes.
25	T	Yeah.
26		(0.5)
27	P	Mm
28	T	Very good
29		(0.2)
30	T	Uhm, still sometimes Joe, you're you <u>are</u> falling this way?
31	P	Yes I know, ((*The next minute or two are not included in this transcript. During them, the therapist, and to a degree the patient talk about future treatment plans and what needs to be worked on. Then the therapist refers back to the higher level of assistance the patient needed in order to sit up earlier during the treatment session*))
32	T	… but we don't need three ((*meaning no longer needing three people to help him stay sitting up*))
33	P	Mm, ahm
34	T	So you must be better
35	P	Must be better hu hum
36	T	Try and keep yer … ((*instructions follow as the patient is assisted to get dressed*))

T = therapist
P = patient
<u>Underline</u> = emphasized word or syllable
[talk]
[talk] = overlapping talk
(0.x) = gap of silence of more than a tenth of a second
((*text*)) = supplementary descriptive information

stepwise manner. First, she cites a goal that it seems the patient had agreed to at the start of the session (L19). That is, she raises something about which she can reasonably expect agreement, and this proves to be the case (L20). The therapist then builds another 'step', it too results in agreement (L21,22) and then another (L23,24). A minute or so later, we see the same patterning: the therapist raises something about which she can predict the patient will agree, and she keeps building upon this,

coming to a conclusion (L34) that directly refers back to the patient's claim not to know 'what's better' (L18). Thus, common ground appears to be reached.

By the way, you may have noticed that I am being rather tentative about whether common ground is 'really' reached. In line with conversation analytic practice, I take the position that we cannot KNOW, we can only INFER what someone actually feels or thinks – what is inside someone's head. This is the case whether we are communicating with one another, or analysing that communication.

'You Tell Me First' Sequences

The 'perspective display', or 'you tell me first' sequence, has been documented in contexts where clinicians deliver bad news.[20-22] In musculoskeletal physiotherapy, this might be informing a footballer that they have severe damage to a ligament and need surgery, or explaining to someone hoping for a quick fix for their low back pain that they need a lengthy pain management and cognitive behavioural therapy programme. In these sequences, the clinician seeks the view of the person consulting them before they deliver any specific news, then the clinician goes on to deliver the news in ways that are fitted to the patient's perspective.[20-24] This practice has particular advantages when there is a chance the recipient of the news may disagree with and/or be highly distressed by it. It allows us to shape our news delivery to the patient's own understandings and perspectives, and to accomplish news delivery in a 'cautious', relatively gentle manner.

Online Commentary About Your Examination Findings

Another practice found to be effective in building common ground with patients – and in forestalling disagreements – is online commentary.[25-27] This entails the clinician providing the patient with information – 'commentary' – about what she is seeing and finding on physical examination. This paves the way towards common ground about what is (or is not) wrong, and thus what should be done about it. In terms of physiotherapy, one might consider deploying online commentary when examining a patient who in your clinical judgement has incorrect assumptions about their condition. For instance, commentary indicating 'no problem' or 'non-serious problem' may be helpful for building common ground with a patient who thinks a damaged joint is stopping them from various activities, whereas examination shows the absence of any serious damage.

Explaining Reasons for Treatments and Recommendations

Explaining reasons seems an obvious means of working towards common ground. However, in everyday life, people only provide reasons when they suspect that others might understand their actions as surprising or problematic. People also tend not to ask others to explain their reasons ('Why are you doing that?') because doing so can be interpreted as showing a lack of trust and respect. Thus 'social' pressures tend to work against providing reasons in everyday life and, indeed, in physiotherapy.[28] Nevertheless, some therapists manage to 'opportunistically' squeeze in talk about reasons. In particular, when a patient directly or indirectly refers to their physical limitations, besides giving some kind of reassurance and/or sympathy, some therapists go further by 'tacking on' explanations about how therapy activities can manage or alleviate these physical limitations.[28]

Make Positive, Specific Recommendations First

Conversation analytic research in primary care medicine has described how recommendations can be negatively or positively formulated and has found that positive, specific recommendations are more likely to be accepted.[15] Negative recommendations include 'You don't need antibiotics' or, to give a more physiotherapeutic example, 'You need to stop playing football for 4 weeks'. The research indicated that if a practitioner's first recommendation is a negative one, this is much more likely to be met with resistance and arguments than when their first recommendation is a positive and specific one, for example, 'I think the best thing to do at this point would be to elevate your head at night, have plenty of fluids to drink'. In our physiotherapy example, the therapist might want to first describe specific interventions (e.g. ultrasound, joint mobilization) and a specific home exercise programme, BEFORE recommending the patient stops playing football. While we cannot be certain that someone who has agreed to something will actually comply, it seems sensible nevertheless to make our recommendations maximally likely to be met with agreement.

Readers are directed towards other research on ways of working towards common ground and providing patients with opportunities to be active participants.[12,29-33]

CONCLUDING REMARKS

I have only been able to scratch the surface of the vast and important body of evidence about the structure and functioning of communication practices. Furthermore, there are some highly relevant areas of communication (body movement, facial expression, touch) that are still not well researched. On a more positive note, a key message is that when reflecting on and developing one's own and other's communication skills, it is helpful to be aware that there are always different ways – different communication practices – by which one can attempt any particular activity. Few if any will always be the right thing to do, or always the wrong thing to do. Rather, it is best to consider communication practices as having an array of pros and cons; trying to be conscious and analytical about these is a good way of developing one's own practice. Finally, it is important to be very clear that good communication takes time: time for staff training, development, support and reflection, and – very importantly – sufficient contact time with patients themselves.[34]

REFERENCES

1. Stewart M. Effective physician-patient communication and health outcomes: a review. Can Med Assoc J 1995;152(9):1423–33.
2. Brown J, Stewart M, Ryan BL. Outcomes of patient-provider interaction. In: Thompson T, Dorsey A, Miller K, et al., editors. Handbook of Health Communication. Mahwah NJ.: Lawrence Erlbaum Associates; 2003. p. 141–61.
3. Hall AM, Ferreira PH, Maher CG, et al. The influence of the therapist-patient relationship on treatment outcome in physical rehabilitation: a systematic review. Phys Ther 2010; 90(8):1099–110.

4. Clayman SE, Gill VT. Conversation analysis. In: Hardy M, Bryman A, editors. Handbook of Data Analysis. Beverly Hills: Sage; 2004. p. 589–606.

5. Heritage J. Conversation analysis and institutional talk: analysing data. In: Silverman D, editor. Qualitative Research: Theory, Method and Practice. London: Sage; 2004. p. 222–45.

6. Heritage J, Clayman S. Talk in Action: Interactions, Identities, and Institutions. Chichester: Wiley-Blackwell; 2010.

7. Parry R. Video-based conversation analysis. In: Bourgeault I, DeVries R, Dingwall R, editors. Sage Handbook of Qualitative Methods in Health Research. London: Sage; 2010. p. 373–96.

8. Sidnell J, Stivers T. The Handbook of Conversation Analysis. Malden MA: Wiley-Blackwell; 2013.

9. Sidnell J. Conversation Analysis. Chichester: Wiley-Blackwell; 2010.

10. ten Have P. Talk and institution: a reconsideration of the 'Asymmetry' of doctor-patient interaction. In: Boden D, Zimmerman DH, editors. Talk and Social Structure. Cambridge: Polity Press; 1991. p. 138–63.

11. Heritage J, Robinson J, Elliott MN, et al. Reducing patients' unmet concerns in primary care: the difference one word can make. J Gen Intern Med 2007;22(10):1429–33.

12. Heritage J. Questioning in medicine. In: Freed A, Ehrlich S, editors. Why do you Ask?': The Function of Questions in Institutional Discourse. Oxford: Oxford University Press; 2009. p. 42–68.

13. Parry R, Land V, Seymour J. How to communicate with patients about future illness progression and end of life: a systematic review. BMJ Support Palliati Care 2014. mjspcare-2014-000649. Published Online First: 24 October 2014; doi:10.1136/bmjspcare-2014-000649.

14. Gill VT, Pomerantz A, Denvir P. Pre-emptive resistance: patients' participation in diagnostic sense-making activities. Sociol Health Illn 2010;32(1):1–20.

15. Stivers T. Non-antibiotic treatment recommendations: delivery formats and implications for patient resistance. Soc Sci Med 2005;60:949–64.

16. Clark SJ, Hudak PL. When surgeons advise against surgery. Res Lang Soc Interac 2011;44(4):385–412.

17. Toerien M, Shaw R, Duncan R, et al. Offering patients choices: a pilot study of interactions in the seizure clinic. Epilepsy Behav 2011;20:312–20.

18. Parry RH. The interactional management of patients' physical incompetence: a conversation analytic study of physiotherapy interactions. Sociol Health Illn 2004;26(7):976–1007.

19. Parry RH. Communication Between Stroke Patients and Physiotherapists, PhD Thesis, University of Nottingham. British library reference DXN054515. 2002. EThOS ID 247132 http://ethos.bl.uk/OrderDetails.do?did=1&uin=uk.bl.ethos.247132. Copy available from the author.

20. Maynard DW. Bearing bad news in clinical settings. In: Dervin B, editor. Progress in Communication Sciences. New Jersey: Ablex; 1991a. p. 143–72.

21. Maynard DW. The perspective-display series and the delivery and receipt of diagnostic news. In: Boden D, Zimmerman D, editors. Talk and Social Structure. Cambridge: Polity Press; 1991b. p. 164–94.

22. Maynard DW. How to tell patients bad news: the strategy of 'forecasting. Cleve Clin J Med 1997;64(4):181–2.

23. Maynard DW. On clinicians co-implicating recipients' perspective in the delivery of diagnostic news. In: Drew P, Heritage J, editors. Talk At Work. Cambridge: Cambridge University Press; 1992. p. 331–58.

24. Lutfey K, Maynard DW. Bad news in Oncology: how physician and patient talk about death and dying without using those words. Soc Psychol Q 1998;61(4):321–41.

25. Heritage J, Stivers T. Online commentary in acute medical visits: a method of shaping patient expectations. Soc Sci Med 1999;49: 1501–17.

26. Mangione-Smith R, Stivers T, Elliott M, et al. Online commentary during the physical examination: a communication tool for avoiding inappropriate antibiotic prescribing? Soc Sci Med 2003;56:313–20.

27. Heritage J, Elliott MN, Stivers T, et al. Reducing inappropriate antibiotics prescribing: the role of online commentary on physical examination findings. Patient Educ Couns 2010;81(1):119–25.

28. Parry R. Practitioners' accounts for treatment actions and recommendations in physiotherapy: when do they occur, how are they structured, what do they do? Sociol Health Illn 2009;31(6):835–53.

29. Stivers T, Heritage J. Breaking the sequential mold: answering 'more than the question' during comprehensive history taking. Text 2001;21(1/2):151–85.

30. Collins S, Drew P, Watt I, et al. 'Unilateral' and 'bilateral' practitioner approaches in decision-making about treatment. Soc Sci Med 2005;61:2611–27.

31. Boyd E, Heritage J. Taking the patient's medical history: questioning during comprehensive history taking. In: Heritage J, Maynard D, editors. Communication in Medical Care: Interactions Between Primary Care Physicians and Patients. Cambridge: Cambridge University Press; 2006. p. 151–84.

32. Robinson J, Heritage J. Physicians' opening questions and patients' satisfaction. Patient Educ Couns 2006;60(3):279–85.

33. Peräkylä A, Ruusuvuori J, Lindfors P. What is patient participation: Reflections arising from the study of general practice, homeopathy and psychoanalysis. In: Collins S, Britten N, Ruusuvuori J, et al., editors. Patient Participation in Health Care Consultations. Maidenhead: Open University Press/McGraw-Hill Education; 2007.

34. Parry R. Communication and compassion need time and support: insights from end of life care. Int J Ther Rehabil 2013;20(10): 478–9.

CHAPTER 27.2 ■ PATIENT EDUCATION: A COLLABORATIVE APPROACH

Lynne Caladine • Jane Morris

Patient education is a relatively new development and can be traced from the early 1970s.[1] Since that time there has been an increasing emphasis on the concept of patient-centred care,[2] with increased patient involvement in decision making about their own health and promotion of self-care.[3] During this period there has also been significant growth in information technology, including the development of the internet, giving opportunities for wide access to medical information and advice. Patient education forms part of the role of a wide range of health professional groups but has developed at different rates. It is also a separate discipline in some countries (e.g. the USA).

The term 'patient education' and other terms such as 'health education' and 'health promotion' are often used interchangeably, which may lead to some confusion. Patient education has been defined as 'a planned systematic, sequential, and logical process of teaching and learning provided to patients and clients in all clinical settings'.[4] The same author considered patient education to include health education which 'concentrates mostly on wellness, prevention and health promotion'.[4]

Physiotherapists and other health professionals have a variety of roles, including that of educator. In this role they support the learning experiences of peers, colleagues and students as well as patients and their carers. Key aspects of the educator role in relation to the learner have been identified as facilitator, assessor and evaluator.[5] Despite being a demanding role it is an aspect for which there is often very little formal preparation or recognition. In a recent study physiotherapists acknowledged their educator role and reported that a high percentage (more than 50%) of their interactions with patients included educational activities.[6,7] These communications might include explanations, instructions (verbal or written), teaching exercises and assessing understanding. The author also suggested that the terms (e.g. verbs and metaphors) used when discussing aspects of patient education may give some insight into educational/pedagogic approaches likely to be adopted by individual therapists.[6,7] The expert therapists in a study in the USA were distinguished by:

> 'a patient-centred approach to care characterised by patient empowerment through education ... with an emphasis on problem solving and cultivation of a patient-practitioner relationship'.[8]

More recently this was reinforced by another author

> 'education that is tailored to the individual or to a group is perhaps the most important component of the expertise of the contemporary physical therapist to effect health behaviour change along with the individual's motivation to effect such change'.[9]

Despite this recognition, education related to students as learners has received more attention than education of patients in the literature over recent years. However, there is a substantial literature base across health professional contexts that uses patient education as a treatment intervention in research studies. In such studies 'patient education' is often used as a generic category to be compared against a treatment intervention of interest to the researchers. It is worth noting that there is wide variation in the operational definition of patient education in such studies and seldom consideration of the related educational approaches or methods (sometimes referred to as pedagogy).

In relation to student education there has been a marked shift in emphasis over the last two decades. 'Teacher-centred' approaches of the past, based on the belief that knowledge can be transmitted from one individual to another have given way to more 'student-centred' approaches which focus on the needs of the learner and change the teacher's role to one of facilitator of learning, helping people to learn. There are parallels that can be drawn between student-centred teaching and patient-centred care when patients are recognized as learners and the traditional, paternalistic, practitioner-centred approach to patient education is joined, if not replaced by, one in which the patient takes a more active part in self-care. In adopting a more patient-centred approach to patient education the principles of student-centred learning can be readily transferred and are listed below and then expanded upon:

1. Consider the characteristics of the learner (e.g. patient or carer).

2. Select approaches to facilitate the learning.
3. Assess the learning (i.e. check whether the patient understands and has learnt).
4. Evaluate your own practice as an educator through self-reflection, peer feedback or more formal feedback.

CONSIDER THE CHARACTERISTICS OF THE LEARNER (E.G. PATIENT OR CARER)

Several pertinent issues related to the individual learner are noted below.

What Are the Patient's Learning Needs?

By finding out what the patient already knows, relevant to their current condition, his or her learning needs can be identified and prior experience recognized. This may be achieved by the use of a modified learning agreement (or learning contract). The physiotherapist and the patient collaborate and contribute equally to this process. The format of the learning agreement need not be complex and could be based on those in wide use with students.

To give an example of how a modified learning agreement might be used, a possible case scenario (Table 27-1) for a recently retired 60-year-old male who has been diagnosed with osteoarthritis of the knee joint is presented below. He has had an active job as a project manager in the construction industry and is a keen golfer. His present condition is limiting his ability to pursue his hobby. He has good eyesight and hearing and no other disabilities.

The alternative name for a learning contract is a 'negotiated learning agreement' and the latter more accurately reflects their intended collaborative and constructive nature. More information about learning contracts may be accessed through various websites including http://www.learningace.com/doc/5825504/8fd61966eeb ed03ac44fb0a905b63823/learningcontracts/.

What Are the Learner's (Patient's) Personal Characteristics?

A wide range of personal characteristics may influence a patient's readiness or ability to learn. These may include age, cultural background, learning styles and preferences, and additional needs (including visual impairment, hearing impairment, dyslexia and ability to communicate effectively). How will you adapt your approach in response to these characteristics?

Many of the learners (patients) will be adults and an understanding of Knowles' ideas,[10] including his principles of adult learning, may help to guide the approaches to patient education that therapists choose to adopt.

Adult(s):
- are internally motivated and self-directed
- are goal-orientated
- need to see the relevance
- are practical
- like to be respected

TABLE 27-1 Possible Format for a Patient Education Learning Agreement

Patient's name:
Therapist's name:
Diagnosis: – Osteoarthritis R Knee joint
Date of learning agreement:
Date(s) of review:

What Do the Patient and Therapist Agree the Patient Needs to Learn?	How Will the Learning Be Achieved?	How Will the Learning Be Assessed?	Date by Which This Will Be Achieved
Basic anatomy of the knee joint	• Hand out with drawings of key structures • Use of anatomical model • Explanation by therapist	• Patient will self-assess • Therapist will check understanding through discussion	As appropriate (at next visit)
Basic pathology of the knee joint	• As above plus referral to website	• As above	• As above
Exercises to strengthen knee extensors and flexors	• Demonstration by therapist • Guidance and correction by therapist to help patient carry out the exercises • Hand out if appropriate • Written instructions on number and frequency of exercises	• Demonstration by patient • Assessment of muscle strength • Measurement of muscle bulk • Patient's reflective log	• As above
Exercises to improve mobility of the knee joint	• As above	• Demonstration by patient • Measurement of joint range	• As above

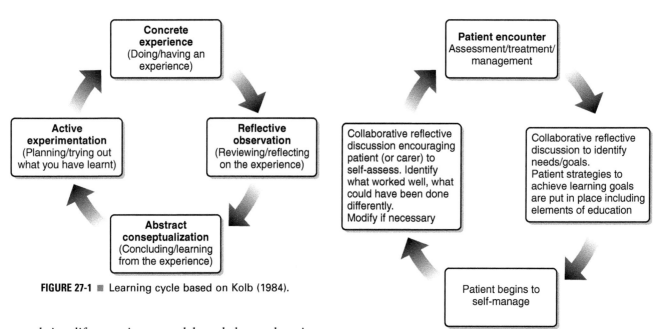

FIGURE 27-1 ■ Learning cycle based on Kolb (1984).

FIGURE 27-2 ■ Collaborative patient education learning cycle.

• bring life experiences and knowledge to learning experiences.

The vast array of past and continuing experience that learners can draw upon can form a basis for further learning based on Kolb's ideas[11] and his experiential learning cycle (Fig. 27-1). This may equally apply to the therapist developing their practice as an educator or be applied to the patient as a learner.

Figure 27-1 outlines Kolb's classic learning cycle in which experience is formalized as the basis for learning and builds upon previous knowledge through reflection. We suggest that a more collaborative version might be appropriate when helping patients and their carers to learn. Figure 27-2 identifies the phases of a collaborative patient education learning cycle.

SELECT APPROACHES TO FACILITATE THE LEARNING

Once the patients' learning needs have been established, learning outcomes can be identified. It is then necessary to decide how these outcomes can be achieved. Facilitation is about helping and enabling rather than telling and persuading. Once you have identified what needs to be learnt you may select from what Cross et al. referred to as a 'toolkit'.[5] They have identified ways in which

TABLE 27-2   Examples of Therapist-Centred and More Patient-Centred Approaches to Patient Education

Example of Type of Learning	Examples of Therapist-Centred/ Transmission Approach	Examples of Patient-Centred/Facilitatory Approach
Knowledge/information about a condition (e.g. low back pain)	Verbal explanation from therapist. Provision of information leaflet	1. Find out what the patient already knows about the condition. Use this as a base to suggest other sources of information (which might include leaflets) appropriate for their learning characteristics. Allow the opportunity for questions and discussion 2. Work with group of patients with similar learning needs and draw on their experiences. Your role is to facilitate discussion rather than provide all information. Consider principles of **peer learning** and **problem-based learning**
Practical skills (e.g. exercises for core stability)	Giving an information leaflet. Demonstration of a set of exercises	Use leaflet and demonstration if appropriate but observe, correct and help patient to adapt for own needs and learning characteristics Use anatomical models to aid explanation of rationale. Respond to questions by linking to current understanding Allow the opportunity for questions and progress difficulty of the exercises based on subsequent assessment and discussion with the patient
Use of equipment	Provision of instruction leaflet. Demonstration by therapist	Demonstrate use of the equipment; explain how it should be used; get the patient to try Use their self-assessment and your observations as a basis for correction Continue until performance is at a suitable standard Ask questions to ensure/support understanding
Health promotion	Provision of information sheet	Assess current level of understanding through observation/ questioning, identify learning needs Direct patient to website(s) and follow up If possible provide opportunity for group discussion facilitated by therapist

learning can be facilitated in the practice setting. As well as structuring learning, guidance is given on fostering collaboration and promoting empowerment. Dreeben[4] also addressed approaches to facilitate patient learning in a comprehensive way.

Some examples of ways in which patient learning may be facilitated are outlined in Table 27-2. These include 'traditional' therapist-centred approaches and more patient-centred strategies. A combination is likely to be most effective. Aim for a balance of providing information (transmission) to the patient and facilitating patient learning (helping people to learn). There may be times when it is appropriate to explain something verbally or give patients a well-constructed information leaflet, but it is also necessary to consider drawing on strategies that help patients to become more independent as learners in order to manage their condition. Group discussion is an example of how patients' prior knowledge and expertise of a condition can be used to help others (which may include the therapist) to learn. A recent master class by Sadlo[12] on the use of problem-based learning with students on placement in the practice learning environment contains some content which may be transferable to certain groups of patients as learners.

When directing patients to websites for information about their condition therapists will also need to ensure that they have a way of evaluating the quality of these sources. There are many guides available for critical appraisal of research articles but this site[13] includes consideration of websites.

ASSESS THE LEARNING

In the same way that student learning needs to be assessed in academic or clinical settings, therapists responsible for patient education also need to check whether the patient understands and has learnt. As a patient educator you may need to check understanding through questions, observation and exploration of how the patient has incorporated, for example, exercises and new information into functional activity. This will form a basis for deciding collaboratively with the patient how to proceed with the management of their condition or injury.

EVALUATE YOUR OWN PRACTICE AS AN EDUCATOR

When supporting student learning evaluating the educational episode is an important part of the cycle. Feedback obtained from the learner helps to guide the educator in making improvements to their strategies for the future. Suggestions are made below for how evaluation might be adapted for use with patients as learners.

- Seek verbal feedback from a patient or group of patients about an educational interaction or episode.
- Devise a simple form to gather written feedback about aspects of an educational episode.
- Be alert to occasions in your clinical practice which involve you as a 'teacher'. Take time to review individual educational patient interactions using a

reflective model such as that of Gibbs.[14] Use a recent example of patient education to try this. You might choose to talk this through with a trusted colleague. How might your patient education practice change in response to this reflection?

- Consider whether your teaching is based on a belief that knowledge can be transmitted between a teacher and a learner or whether you think of it as helping to facilitate learning. Thinking about the language you use when discussing your involvement in education with colleagues may be a guide. What sort of verbs and metaphors do you use? Use of terms such as 'giving', 'delivery', 'getting it through' might suggest that your ideas and approach to teaching are closer to transmission than facilitation. Whereas 'support', 'guiding', 'working with' when related to education may indicate a more collaborative, facilitatory and patient-centred approach.
- Note the way that your peers and colleagues talk about patient education (the terms and figures of speech they use – their discourse) and the approaches they adopt. Is there a link between their discourse and their approach? Do they predominantly follow a transmission or a facilitation model?

SUMMARY

Developments in patient education are driven by an increasing emphasis on more patient-centred approaches to care, self-management of health and financial imperatives. Parallels have been identified here between patients as learners and students as learners, noting that the principles of student-centred education may be applied with patients. Approaches to patient education which include collaboration and facilitation of learning may be more effective in some situations than traditional transmission-based approaches alone with their heavy reliance on the 'provision' of information. Therapists are encouraged to reflect on their own educational practice with patients.

REFERENCES

1. Hoving C, Visser A, Dolan Mullen P, et al. A history of patient education by health professionals in Europe and North America: from authority to shared decision making education. Patient Educ Couns 2010;78:275–81.
2. Mead N, Bower P. Patient-centredness: a conceptual framework and review of the empirical literature. Soc Sci Med 2000;51(7):1087–110.
3. Deccache A, Van Ballekom K. From patient compliance to empowerment and consumer's choice: evolution or regression? An overview of patient education in French speaking European countries. Patient Educ Couns 2010;78(3):282–7.
4. Dreeben O. Patient Education in Rehabilitation. Sudbury, MA: Jones & Bartlett; 2010.
5. Cross V, Moore A, Morris J, et al. The Practice-Based Educator – A Reflective Tool for CPD and Accreditation. Chichester: Wiley; 2006.
6. Caladine L. Physiotherapists' construction of their role in patient education. Doctoral thesis. University of Brighton; 2011.
7. Caladine L. Physiotherapists' construction of their role in patient education. Int J Practice-based Learn Health Soc Care 2013;1(1):37–49. doi:10.11120/pblh.2013.00005.
8. Resnik L, Jenssen GM. Using clinical outcomes to explore the theory of expert practice in physical therapy. Phys Ther 2003;83(12):1090–106.
9. Dean E. Physical therapy in the 21st century (Part 2): evidence-based practice within the context of evidence-informed practice. Physiother Theory Pract 2009;25(5–6):354–68.
10. Knowles M. The Adult Learner: A Neglected Species. 4th ed. Houston: Gulf Publishing; 1990.
11. Kolb D. Experiential Learning: Experience as the Source of Learning and Development. New Jersey: Prentice-Hall; 1984.
12. Sadlo G. Using problem-based learning during student placements to embed theory in practice. Int J Practice-based Learn Health Soc Care 2014;2(1):6–19. doi:10.11120/pblh.2014.00029.
13. Engle M. Evaluating web sites: criteria and tools. Online available from: <http://www.library.cornell.edu/olinuris/ref/research/webeval.html#context>; 2014 [May 2014].
14. Gibbs G. Learning by doing: A guide to teaching and learning methods. Oxford Centre for Staff and Learning Development, Oxford Polytechnic. Further Education Unit, London. <http://www2.glos.ac.uk/gdn/gibbs/ch4_3.htm#4.3.5>; 1988.

CHAPTER 27.3 ■ COMMUNICATING RISK

Roger Kerry

Risk is the probability that an event will give rise to harm.[1] As healthcare professionals, communicating risk is central to all our interactions. Risks associated with manual therapy might include rare and severe events (e.g. death, stroke), or common and mild ones (e.g. transient unwanted responses to treatment). Given these associations, we have a responsibility to consider and communicate risk as best we can. This section summarizes evidence on the best ways to communicate risk in order to optimize shared decision making.

Risk communication has become increasingly important with the publication of data and evidence-based practice. In contrast to traditional 'gut feelings' about risk, it is becoming possible to make data-informed judgements. Despite this numerical dimension, there is still uncertainty in understanding and communicating risk.[2] Paradoxically, communicating uncertain risk judgements using numerical ranges can worsen understanding, credibility, and perceptions of risk.[3] This section aims to provide some clarity and guidance on risk communication by focusing on three key areas: understanding risk; communication tools; and framing risk.

UNDERSTANDING RISK

Healthcare professionals are poor at understanding numbers.[2,4] Gigerenzer et al reported only 25% of subjects correctly identified 1 in 1000 as being the same as 0.1%, coining the phrase 'collective statistical illiteracy' in relation to health statistics users.[5] Education and numeracy levels have little impact on risk judgement or understanding.[6,7] Consensus on the best ways for health professionals to communicate risk is lacking.[8] These facts create barriers to communication, and can lead to aberrant use of research-generated data.[9] Regardless of this, a numerical interpretation of probability is an important aspect of the clinicians' understanding of risk. Risk communication should be inclusive of the numerical probability of an unwanted event happening, together with the effect of this on a patient; importance of the effect; and the context in which the risk might occur.[10]

'every representation of risk carries its own connotations and biases that may vary according to the individual's perspective concerning the way the world works'[11]

Understanding Probabilities

What does 5% mean? Is this the same as 0.05? Does 5 out of 100 mean the same thing as 50 out of 1000? Do the odds of 1:20–for say the same as 19:1–against? These are all mathematically valid expressions of the same data relating to probability judgement, but can and do *mean* different things. But what actually *is* a 5% risk? If I said you had a 5% chance of increased pain following intervention *X*, how do you interpret that? Does this mean you might be one of the 5 out of 100 people who will experience pain? Or that in every 100 patients I treat, 5 experience pain? Does it mean if you had 100 treatments, you would experience pain 5 times? Does it mean that in 5% of the time, people experience pain? Or that 5 out of every 100 manual therapists induce pain to all their patients? Is this 5% epistemological (i.e. it is already decided that you will have pain, but you just do not know it yet to the degree of 5%) or is it aleatory (i.e. a completely random notion to the degree of 5% that you will or will not experience pain)? These variables should be considered when communicating risk.

The first stage in effective communication is establishing the reference class to which the probability relates (e.g. time, location, person). In using population data for risk communication, most of the time the reference class will be historical (i.e. data from past events are used to inform the chance of the next event). Embedding a new individual event in data from a past population should carry some additional judgement, as new informative knowledge may be ignored. Spiegelhalter's report of pre-Obama odds on a black US President is a good example: $^{43}/_{43}$ of past US Presidents were white, indicating a statistical prediction of almost certainty of a 44th white President.[11]

Relative Versus Absolute Risk

Misinterpretations of absolute and relative risk contribute to data users' anxieties and misunderstandings.[12] Absolute risk (AR) can be the prevalence (or incidence), or indicate the absolute difference in risk between two groups. Relative risks (RR) – and their counterparts, odds ratios (OR) – are products of the division of AR in each group, to form a relative difference. RRs may help to make comparative judgements (e.g. 'this is riskier than that'). This way of communicating is encouraged in evidence-based medicine. However, RRs are more persuasive and make differences in risk appear larger than they are.[5] They are over-reported in lay-press and

research reports where authors want to exaggerate differences.[13]

'If the absolute risk is low, even if the relative risk is significantly increased to exposed individuals, the actual risk to exposed individuals will still be very low'[14]

A related statistic to absolute risk is number needed to harm (NNH). NNH is the inverse of the absolute risk difference. Although NNH might seem to hold informative content,[15] a recent Cochrane review concluded that this was poorly understood by patients and clinicians.[16] In summary both RR (including ORs) and NNH are poor means of communicating risk, and AR should be favoured.[4,17]

Probabilities Versus Natural Frequencies

So far we have considered risk expressed as some sort of probability. Alternatively, natural frequencies (NF) can be a clearer way of representing risk.[16,18] NFs are joint occurrences of two events (e.g. positive result on a clinical test and the presence of a condition). In terms of risk prediction, we may be familiar with probabilistic ideas of specificity, sensitivity, positive predictive value, etc. Although commonly used (e.g. these form the core of clinical predication rules), these statistics are a consistent source of confusion and error.[19-21] Reports have suggested that the human mind might be better evolved to understand risk in terms of NFs.[22,23] NFs are absolute frequencies arising from observed data. Risk representation using NFs avoids the complex statistics of probability expression, while maintaining the mathematical rigour and Bayesian logic necessary to calculate risk.

COMMUNICATION TOOLS

Stacey et al. found that use of decision aids can improve patients' knowledge and perception of risk, and improve shared decision making.[24] Such aids include visual representations of risk, and these have many desirable properties (e.g. reveal otherwise undetected data patterns, attract attention and evoke specific mathematical operations).[25] Specific types of aids are useful for specific types of risk (e.g. bar charts for group comparisons, line graphs for temporal interactions among risk factors, pie-charts for showing risk proportions, etc.).[26] Icon arrays are also used to display population proportions, and rare events can be demonstrated in magnified or circular images. Figures 27-3 and 27-4 shows examples of graphical images used for communicating common and rare events.

FRAMING RISK

The way risk is framed is considered important for effective communication.[1] Framing presents logically equivalent information in different ways. Generally, risks can be framed positively (gain-framed) or negatively (loss-framed). We might gain-frame the risk of stroke following manual therapy as 'you are very unlikely

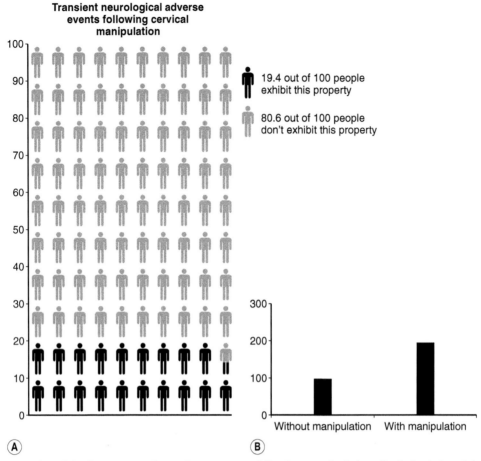

(A)   (B)

FIGURE 27-3 ■ Representing risk of common minor adverse events following manipulation. Pooled relative risk (RR) from meta-analysis,[27] RR = 1.96, or 194 events per 1000 with manipulation versus 99 per 1000 with no manipulation (control). (**A**) icon array pictorially representing absolute risk; (**B**) bar-graph demonstrating difference between the two groups.

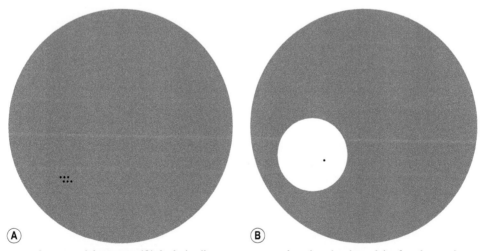

(A)   (B)

FIGURE 27-4 ■ Representing rare risk events. (**A**) A circle diagram representing the absolute risk of serious adverse event following manipulation. The grey circle represents 100 000 units, and the black dots represent the number of cases per 100 000. (**B**) From prevalence data on vertebrosbasilar insufficiency (VBI)[28] and diagnostic utility of a VBI test,[29] this graph shows a population of 100 000 (the large grey circle), the proportion who test positive on a VBI test (16 000: the white circle), and the proportion of people who will actually have VBI (1: the black dot).

to experience stroke following this intervention', or loss-frame it as 'this treatment could cause you to have a stroke'. Gain-framing can be more effective if the aim is preventative behaviour with an outcome of some certainty[30] (e.g. 'exercising more will reduce

cardiovascular risk' would be more effective than 'if you don't exercise, you will have an increased risk of cardiovascular disease'). However, loss-framing is generally more effective, and especially so when concerned with uncertain risks.[1]

- Data can help our naturally poor understanding of risk
- Probabilities should be considered in relation to a reference class
- Gain-framing can be effective for communicating risk related to preventative behaviour which has an outcome of at least some certainty
- Loss-frame is generally most effective, especially with uncertain risks
- Relative risk (including odds ratios) and numbers needed to harm should be avoided in preference to pure absolute risk expressions
- Natural frequencies are better understood than probabilistic interpretations of risk
- Visual representations of risk improve understanding
- Risk data ultimately need to be personalized and considered in the context of uncertainty

Personalizing Risk

Edwards et al. (2000) reported that risk estimates based on personal risk factors were most effective in improving patient outcomes.[31] A subsequent Cochrane review reported that compared to generalized numerical risk communication, personalized risk communication improved knowledge, perception and uptake of risk-reducing interventions.[32] Personalized risk may include attempts to identify a smaller sub-group akin to the individual patient, and/or consideration of the individual's own risk factors for an event. This dimension of risk communication contextualizes population data estimates within single patients' risk factors, together with their values and world-view.

Ultimately, despite the data, most risk estimates are communicated in the context of uncertainty. Data help inform decisions, but human nature and the complexity of the world make certainty impossible. This is an accepted difficult stance in risk communication.[33] Understanding uncertainty means accepting that risk communication is best done knowing that responses to risk depend on a patient's characteristics, values and experiences, and sociocultural worldviews.[11,33] This knowledge should be embraced, not ignored. Box 27-4 summarizes the key messages from this section.

REFERENCES

1. Edwards A, Elwyn G, Covey J, et al. Presenting risk information–a review of the effects of 'framing' and other manipulations on patient outcomes. J Health Commun 2001;6(1):61–82.
2. Gigerenzer G. How innumeracy can be exploited. In: Reckoning with Risk – Learning to Live with Uncertainty. London: Penguin Press; 2002. p. 201–10.
3. Longman T, Turner RM, King M, et al. The effects of communicating uncertainty in quantities health risk estimates. Patient Educ Cou 2012;89:252–9.
4. Ahmed H, Naik G, Willoughby H, et al. Communicating risk. Br Med J 2012;344:e3996.
5. Gigerenzer G, Gaissmaier W, Kurz-Milcke E. Helping doctors and patients make sense of health statistics. Psychol Sci Publ Int 2007;8:53–96.
6. Lipkus IM, Samsa G, Rimmer BK. General performance on a numeracy scale among highly educated samples. Med Decis Making 2001;21:37–44.
7. Gigerenzer G, Galesic M. Why do single event probabilities confuse patients. Br Med J 2012;344:e245.
8. Ghosh AK, Ghosh K. Translating evidence based information into effective risk communication: current challenges and opportunities. J Lab Clin Med 2005;145(4):171–80.
9. Moyer VA. What we don't know can hurt our patients: physician innumeracy and overuse of screening tests. Ann Intern Med 2012;156:392–3.
10. Edwards A. Risk communication. In: Edwards A, Elwyn G, editors. Shared Decision Making in Health Care: Achieving Evidence-Based Patient Choice. 2nd ed. Oxford: Oxford University Press; 2009. p. 135–42.
11. Speigelhalter DJ. Understanding uncertainty. Ann Fam Med 2008;6(3):196–7.
12. Mason D, Prevost AT, Sutton S. Perceptions of absolute versus relative differences between personal and comparison health risk. Health Psychol 2008;7(1):87–92.
13. should enforce transparent reporting in abstracts. Br Med J 2010;341:791–2.
14. Gordis L. Epidemiology. Philadelphia: Saunders; 2009. p. 102.
15. Sainani KL. Communicating risks clearly: absolute risk and numbers needed to treat. Am Acad Phys Med Rehabil 2012;4:220–2.
16. Akl EA, Oxman AD, Herrin J, et al. Using alternative statistical formats for presenting risks and risk reductions. Cochrane Database Syst Rev 2011;(3):CD006776.
17. Fagerlin A, Zikmund-Fisher BJ, Ubel PA. Helping patients decide: ten steps to better risk communication. J Natl Cancer Inst 2011;103:1436–43.
18. Gigerenzer G. What are natural frequencies? Br Med J 2011; 343:d6386.
19. Eddy DM. Probabilistic reasoning in clinical medicine: problems and opportunities. In: Kahneman D, Sloviv P, Tversky A, editors. Judgement under Uncertainty: Heuristics and Biases. Cambridge UK: Cambridge University Press; 1982. p. 249–67.
20. Cahan A, Gilon D, Manor O. Probabilistic reasoning and clinical decision-making: do doctors overestimate diagnostic probabilities? Q J Med 2003;96:763–9.
21. Ghosh AK, Ghosh K, Erwin PJ. Do medical students and physicians understand probability? Q J Med 2004;97:53–5.
22. Gigerenzer G, Huffage U. How to improve Bayesian reasoning without instruction: frequency formats. Psychol Rev 1996;102: 684–704.
23. Cosmides L, Tooby J. Are humans good intuitive statisticians after all? Rethinking some conclusions from the literature on judgement under uncertainty. Cognition 1996;58(1):1–73.
24. Stacey D, Bennett CL, Barry MJ, et al. Decision aids for people facing health treatment or screening decisions. Cochrane Database Syst Rev 2011;(1):CD001431.
25. Lipkus IM, Hollands J. The visual communication of risk. J Natl Cancer Inst 1999;25:149–63.
26. Lipkus IM. Numeric, verbal, and visual formats of conveying health risks: suggested best practices and future recommendations. Med Decis Making 2007;27(5):696–713.
27. Carlesso LC, Gross AR, Santaguida PL, et al. Adverse events associated with the use of cervical manipulation and mobilization for the treatment of neck pain in adults: a systematic review. Man Ther 2010;15(5):434–44.
28. Boyle E, Côté P, Grier AR. Examining vertebrobasilar artery stroke in two Canadian provinces. J Manipulative Physiol Ther 2009; 32:S194–200.
29. Hutting N, Verhagen AP, Vijverman V, et al. Diagnostic accuracy of premanipulative vertebrobasilar insufficiency tests: a systematic review. Man Ther 2013;18(3):177–82.
30. Fagerlin A, Peters E. Quantitative information. In: Fischhoff B, Brewer NT, Downs JS, editors. Communicating Risks and Benefits: An Evidence-Based User's Guide. Silver Spring, MD: US Department of Health and Human Services, Food and Drug Administration; 2011. p. 53–64.
31. Edwards A, Hood K, Matthews EJ, et al. The effectiveness of one-to-one risk communication interventions in health care: a systematic review. Med Decis Making 2000;20:290–7.
32. Edwards AG, Evans R, Dundon J. Personalised risk communication for informed decision making about taking screening tests. Cochrane Database Syst Rev 2006;(4):CD001865.
33. Politi MC, Han PK, Col NF. Communicating the uncertainty of harms and benefits of medical interventions. Med Decis Making 2007;27:681–95.

Pain Management Introduction

EDITOR'S INTRODUCTION

Pain is a multidimensional experience that has been defined as an unpleasant sensory and emotional experience associated with actual or potential tissue damage or described in terms of such damage (International Association for the Study of Pain). As the definition implies, pain not only involves the sensation (location, duration, intensity, quality) but also has an emotional component (unpleasantness). As a complex experience, pain can affect every dimension of a person's life including daily activities, work, family relationships and social interactions. Thus, successful treatment must use multiple approaches aimed at all dimensions of pain, including the sensory and emotional aspects. Physiotherapy management of a person with pain, therefore, involves multiple interventions that include education, exercise, manual therapy and modalities such as electrical and thermal agents. Along with these, understanding the individual patient's pain experience and context is critical to successful management. This chapter will address three areas in the very broad field of pain management by physiotherapists. The first section will discuss the patient's experience of pain and how this may impact on interactions with health professionals. Secondly, the current evidence base for the provision of education will be outlined and thirdly, the processes that may potentially underlie some commonly used physical interventions will be explored.

CHAPTER 28.1 ■ THE PATIENT'S PAIN EXPERIENCE

Hubert Van Griensven

Much of manual therapy rests on the assumption that pain results from nociception: increases and decreases in pain in response to positions, movements and manipulations are interpreted as indicators of the health of specific musculoskeletal and neural tissues. This *end-organ model* or *structure–pathology model* is powerful and persuasive but also has its limitations. Firstly, the central nervous system modifies sensory input, for instance when there is central sensitization, thus altering the relationship between stimulus and sensation (Chapter 2). Secondly, persistent pain is frequently not stimulus-dependent (Chapter 2), while much of the musculoskeletal examination is based on responses to stimuli. Finally, pain is ultimately an intensely subjective experience, which is intimately connected with personal meaning.

The subjective aspects of pain make it demand attention, interfere with some activities while driving others, and disrupt thought.[1] There are many pain scoring systems and questionnaires that can help the clinician to objectify the patient's pain experience.[2] However, patients with persistent pain find it difficult to quantify their pain and their own descriptions do not necessarily match formal tools for pain assessment.[3] Tools used to measure aspects of pain may therefore provide us with categorizations and outcome measures, but the wider pain assessment involves *empathy* or a sense of understanding the experience of another person in pain.[4] A clinician needs to be able to actively listen to the patient's story in order to be in a position to provide information and advice that is valued by the patient.[5,6]

This section discusses this subjective pain experience, drawing mostly on qualitative research (Chapter 23). Although it is acknowledged that an individual's pain is influenced by, for instance, age,[7] ethnicity,[8] religion[9] and gender,[10] the focus here is on personal experience.

COMING TO TERMS WITH PAIN AND DISABILITY

Most people who experience pain first try to find a resolution.[11] Unfortunately not all pain can be eliminated or even reduced, leading people with persistent pain to visit numerous health-care practitioners in search of a cure. A succession of failed treatments can eventually lead to the conclusion that there is no solution. This can be difficult to accept if clinicians do not provide a clear explanation for the pain.[12] Indeed, primary care research has found that patients only accept reassurance if it includes a positive explanation which covers all relevant factors.[13] Clinicians are therefore advised to find out what their patient's information needs are.[5] Explanations should help the patient make sense of not only the nociceptive origins of their pain, but also reasons for its persistence. Teaching pain mechanisms and how physical, psychological and circumstances may influence pain may play an important role in this.[14,15]

People with persistent pain find it difficult to maintain a sense of control, because long-term pain tends to fluctuate unpredictably.[12,16] This makes it difficult to plan activities and set goals, both in the shorter and longer term.[16] It also creates fear and uncertainty about life roles, both in the present and in the future.[17] It is therefore important for clinicians not to dismiss accounts of unpredictable and inconsistent pain patterns, but to believe their patients and listen. An understanding of the physiology and psychology of persistent pain, combined with a belief in what the patient reports, can aid in the provision of realistic and empathetic explanations. This can increase the patient's sense of control and ability to look beyond pain and suffering.

Clinicians are advised to check adherence to, and effectiveness of, any advice or treatment provided. Reasons for (non-)compliance can be deeply personal. For example, patients may not take prescribed medication because of side effects,[18] but also because some individuals with pain associate it with a lack of self-respect.[17] Non-compliance with any treatment may therefore warrant some careful and empathetic probing, in order to find strategies that suit the individual.

PERSONAL AND SOCIAL CHANGES IN RESPONSE TO PAIN

People with long-term pain have reported turning into a different person and experiencing a loss of 'self'.[19] Internally this may be associated with an experience of self-loathing, while externally it can lead to a hardening of attitudes towards others, a reduction in empathy and lashing out at friends and relatives.[19,20] These unpleasant aspects of their personality can be experienced as separate from the individual's old self.[19] This duality may extend to the way the body is experienced; although the body in general is not experienced consciously to a high degree, painful, numb or dysfunctional parts are.[17,21] As a consequence, these parts may be experienced as 'not me', while functioning and non-painful parts are identified as still

belonging to the individual.[21] The battle to maintain control therefore includes the internal battle to retain one's original self and body.[19,21] Bodywork approaches such as yoga, qigong, Feldenkrais or Rolfing, which aim to adjust overall wellbeing through adjustment of the body, may play a role in reintegrating a patient's experience of themselves.[22]

Externally, the battle for control includes a struggle to retain work, with the fear about the future a cause of anxiety and distress.[16,23,24] The unpredictability of pain can make it difficult to comply with the requirements of regular employment.[16,25] As a consequence of these and other changes, individuals with persistent pain are likely to experience a strong sense of loss, for instance of abilities, finances and identity.[24] Roles within the family also change, for instance when a parent is no longer able to pick up a child or have sex because of pain.[11] Although many pain sufferers experience a loss of hope, having a (pain) diagnosis and a supportive environment can help to counteract this.[24]

Several studies describe the development of social isolation. Individuals with pain who recognize their low mood and tendency at lash out at those around them, may feel forced to withdraw from interaction with others.[17,19] This withdrawal may be compounded by a fear of being judged by others,[19] a loss of physical ability and concentration[24] and feeling uneasy about having to rely on others.[17] Although many individuals with persistent pain feel a need to talk about their problems, this conflicts with fear that doing so will turn others away.[17] As a consequence, friendships and personal relationships are likely to change or end.[24] Visits to a familiar health-care practitioner over an extended period may therefore play a role in supporting patients with persistent pain, even if the treatments do not yield objective improvements.[24,26]

ADOPTING A ROLE IN THE HEALTH AND SOCIAL CARE SYSTEM

Individuals with persistent pain often go through numerous health-care appointments with long waits in between and repeated disappointments.[24] They experience poor communication and a lack of understanding of the patient's position on the part of medical professionals.[27] Pain sufferers have described how clinicians tend to lose interest once they realize that they are unable to provide an effective treatment for the pain, and may even make the patient feel as if they are to blame for their condition.[27]

Unsuccessful attempts at diagnosis and treatment can lead to individuals feeling stigmatized and written off by health-care practitioners.[23] In trying to get their complaint legitimized by the health profession, people with persistent pain have described how they feel under pressure to appear unwell, but not too unwell.[12,28] The resulting juggling act can increase feelings of helplessness and injustice[20] and may force them into a sick role.[12,20,27] The way patients present may therefore be influenced by previous consultations and what they think the clinician needs to see and hear. Building a relationship is therefore a key component of the consultation.[5]

Similar conflicting demands on the presentation of pain and other symptoms are experienced when dealing with the social security system. People with pain who are unable to work may wish to be viewed as normal people by the outside world,[17] but this can conflict with the need to demonstrate eligibility to receive compensation or benefits.[27] They are likely to feel under pressure to demonstrate that their pain is real, but this is difficult because pain itself is invisible and may not be consistent across different days.[16,20,23,24,27,29–31] As a consequence they encounter disbelief about why they are suffering, which in turn leads to frustration, anger, guilt and despair.[12,16]

CONCLUSION

Living with, and trying to cope with, ongoing pain can have a profound effect on the individual. This has been described in terms of loss or suspension of self, wellness, roles, employment and future.[11,32] This forces people with pain into different roles, not only in their personal lives but also when dealing with the health-care system. An understanding of subjective aspects of living and coping with pain can help clinicians to empathize and engage with their patients, and to find effective pain-management strategies for them as individuals.

Clinicians are advised to reflect on the fact that they are likely to come across as 'switching off' or 'turning away' to patients with persistent pain, and to examine how these patients make them feel. For example, they may feel helpless and useless, under pressure to see patients who are more responsive to physiotherapy, or angry because they are put in a position where their patient's problems do not match their expertise. Reflecting on these issues can lead to an improvement in the way a clinician relates to his or her patients with persistent pain. This process of introspection may be aided by the use of mindfulness techniques[33,34] and acknowledging one's vulnerabilities as a health-care practitioner.[35]

REFERENCES

1. Melzack R, Casey K. Sensory, motivational, and central control determinants of pain. In: Kenshalo D, editor. The Skin Senses. Springfield, Illinois: Charles C Thomas; 1968. p. 423–43.
2. Strong J, van Griensven H. Assessing pain. In: van Griensven H, Strong J, Unruh A, editors. Pain. A Textbook for Health Professionals. Edinburgh: Churchill Livingstone; 2013. p. 91–114.
3. De Souza L, Frank A. Subjective pain experience of people with chronic back pain. Physiother Res Int 2013;5(4):207–19.
4. Goubert L, Craig K, Vervoort T, et al. Facing others in pain: the effects of empathy. Pain 2005;118:285–8.
5. Main CJ, Buchbinder R, Porcheret M, et al. Addressing patient beliefs and expectations in the consultation. Best Pract Res Clin Rheumatol 2010;24(2):219–25.
6. Gask L, Usherwood T. ABC of psychological medicine. The consultation. Br Med J 2002;324:1567–9.
7. Gagliese L. Pain and aging: the emergence of a new subfield of pain research. J Pain 2009;10(4):343–53.
8. Edwards C, Fillingim R, Keefe F. Race, ethnicity and pain. Pain 2001;94:133–7.
9. Büssing A, Michalsen A, Balzat H, et al. Are spirituality and religiosity resources for patients with chronic pain conditions? Pain Med 2009;10(2):327–39.
10. Unruh A. Pain in women. Pain Res Manage 2008;13(3):199–200.
11. Nielsen M. The patient's voice. In: van Griensven H, Strong J, Unruh A, editors. Pain. A Textbook for Healthcare Practitioners. Edinburgh: Churchill Livingstone; 2013. p. 9–19.
12. Osborn M, Smith J. The personal experience of chronic benign lower back pain: an interpretative phenomenological analysis. Br J Health Psychol 1998;3:65–83.
13. Dowrick C, Ring A, Humphris G, et al. Normalisation of unexplained symptoms by general practitioners: a functional typology. Br J Gen Pract 2004;54:165–70.
14. Nijs J, van Wilgen C, Van Oosterwijck J, et al. How to explain central sensitisation to patients with 'unexplained' chronic musculoskeletal pain: practice guidelines. Man Ther 2012;16:413–18.
15. Moseley G. Unraveling the barriers to reconceptualization of the problem in chronic pain: the actual and perceived ability of patients and health professionals to understand the neurophysiology. J Pain 2003;4(4):184–9.
16. Corbett M, Foster N, Ong B. Living with low back pain – stories of hope and despair. Soc Sci Med 2007;65:1584–94.
17. Campbell C, Cramb G. 'Nobody likes a back bore' – exploring lay perspectives of chronic pain: revealing the hidden voices of nonservice users. Scand J Caring Sci 2008;22:383–90.
18. Smith M, Muralidharan A. Pain pharmacology and the pharmacological management of pain. In: van Griensven H, Strong J, Unruh A, editors. Pain. A Textbook for Health Professionals. Edinburgh: Churchill Livingstone; 2013. p. 159–80.
19. Smith J, Osborn M. Pain as an assault on the self: an interpretative phenomenological analysis of the psychological impacto of chronic benign low back pain. Psychol Health 2007;22(5):517–34.
20. McParland J, Eccleston C, Osborn M, et al. It's not fair: an interpretative phenomenological analysis of discourses of justice and fairness in chronic pain. Health 2010;15(5):459–74.
21. Osborn M, Smith J. Living with a body separate from the self. The experience of the body in chronic benign low back pain: an interpretative phenomenological analysis. Scand J Caring Sci 2006;20:216–22.
22. Maitland J. Spacious Body. Explorations in Somatic Ontology. Berkeley: North Atlantic Books; 1995.
23. Holloway I, Sofaer-Bennett B, Walker J. The stigmatisation of people with chronic back pain. Disabil Rehabil 2006;29(18):1456–64.
24. Walker J, Sofaer B, Holloway I. The experience of chronic low back pain: accounts of loss in those seeking help from pain clinics. Pain 2006;10:199–207.
25. Patel S, Greasley K, Watson P. Barriers to rehabilitation and return to work for unemployed chronic pain patients: a qualitative study. Eur J Pain 2007;11(8):831–40.
26. Pincus T, Vogel S, Breen A, et al. Persistent back pain – why do physical therapy clinicians continue treatment? A mixed methods study of chiropractors, osteopaths and physiotherapists. Eur J Pain 2006;10(1):67–76.
27. Walker J, Holloway I, Sofaer B. In the system: the lived experience of chronic back pain from the perspectives of those seeking help from pain clinics. Pain 1999;80:621–8.
28. Toye F, Barker K. 'Could I be imagining this?' – the dialectic struggles of people with persistent unexplained back pain. Disabil Rehabil 2010;32(21):1722–32.
29. Crowe M, Whitehead L, Gagan M, et al. Listening to the body and talking to myself – the impact of chronic lower back pain: a qualitative study. Int J Nurs Stud 2010;47:586–92.
30. Vroman K, Warner R, Chamberlain K. Now let me tell you in my own words: narratives of acute and chronic low back pain. Disabil Rehabil 2009;31(12):976–87.
31. Werner A, Widding Isaksen L, Malterud K. 'I'm not the kind of woman who complains of everything': illness stories on self and shame in women with chronic pain. Soc Sci Med 2004;59:1035–45.
32. Bunzli S, Watkins R, Smith A, et al. Lives on hold. A qualitative synthesis exploring the experience of chronic low back pain. Clin J Pain 2013;29(10):907–16.
33. Grabovac A, Lau M, Willett B. Mechanisms of mindfulness: a Buddhist psychological model. Mindfulness 2011;2(3):154–66.
34. Kabat-Zinn J. Full Catastrophe Living. How to Cope with Stress, Pain and Illness using Mindfulness Meditation. London: Piatkus; 1990.
35. Rowe L, Kidd M. First do no Harm. Being a Resilient Doctor in the 21st Century. Sydney: McGraw Hill; 2009.

CHAPTER 28.2 ■ EDUCATIONAL APPROACHES TO PAIN MANAGEMENT

James McAuley

Patient education is a cornerstone of contemporary health care; it is essential to the quality of care for chronic diseases and is important for the care of acute health conditions. Patient education improves outcomes for a range of health conditions including diabetes, asthma, chronic obstructive pulmonary disease, hypertension, cardiac disease, rheumatic disease and cancer.[1]

This section reviews the evidence for patient education for musculoskeletal conditions, with a focus on low back pain. The important role of patient education as the first-line management of musculoskeletal pain conditions is reflected in clinical practice guidelines.[2,3]

Broadly, patient education involves the provision of information by a health-care provider to a patient. This can range from advice or simple information on diagnosis, prognosis or treatment,[4] through to comprehensive education lasting several hours and across multiple occasions.[5]

The aim of patient education is to improve patient outcomes either as a single intervention or to add to the treatment effects of any other intervention that the patient is receiving. The goal is to move a patient from a passive recipient of health care to an active partner in the management of their health condition.

DELIVERY OF PATIENT EDUCATION

Education can be delivered verbally to individuals[6-9] or to groups of patients[10-12] via written materials such as leaflets or information booklets,[13-15] by material from the Internet including web pages,[16,17] social media/YouTube[18,19] and smartphone apps,[20-22] or by educational videos.[23,24] Education can also be delivered at a societal level and mass media campaigns have been developed to educate the public about pain,[25,26] most notably and successfully in Australia.[27] In clinical practice the delivery of patient education is usually verbal and/or written information provided to individual patients,[28] though information delivered through the Internet or smartphone apps is becoming increasingly common and important.[29]

Education for patients with musculoskeletal pain typically involves providing information on diagnosis,[30-32] prognosis[33] and management[34] of their condition. For a patient with a non-specific pain condition this information is intended to reassure the patient that their pain is not caused by a serious disease[32] and that increased activity and the resumption of normal activities is likely to speed up their recovery.[35] For patients with acute musculoskeletal pain, education also aims to increase the patient's expectations that their pain will resolve and that they will recover within a few weeks.[2,35,36]

CONTENT OF EDUCATION INTERVENTIONS FOR LOW BACK PAIN

Approaches to patient education for musculoskeletal disorders have mostly been developed for patients with low back pain. These approaches can be grouped into three broad categories: biomedical, biopsychosocial or pain neurophysiology education. Biomedical approaches to education focus on biomechanical properties of the spine and information is provided on ergonomics and advice on posture.[37] This type of education is most closely aligned with Back Schools,[38] developed in the late 1960s and early 1970s, and has been incorporated into multidisciplinary or functional restoration programmes.[39-41] Biopsychosocial approaches (including brief education) were developed in the late 1980s and early 1990s from the biopsychosocial model of back pain.[42] These educational approaches emphasize the importance of the relationship between thoughts and feelings to low back pain/disability[43] and advise patients to avoid bed rest[44] and that a gradual return to activity is likely to increase the rate of their recovery.[45,46] Much of the content of the biopsychosocial education can be found in the *Back Book*.[14] Pain neurophysiology education or pain biology education[47,48] was developed in the early 2000s and focuses on educating the patient about the neurophysiological mechanisms that underlie their pain.[5,49] This approach attempts to reconceptualize a patient's understanding of their pain by emphasizing that pain does not reflect the extent of tissue damage, but is rather a protective output produced by the brain when sensory information is evaluated as threatening, dangerous or harmful.[5,50]

THE EFFECTIVENESS OF PATIENT EDUCATION FOR LOW BACK PAIN

Much of the research on the effectiveness of patient education for musculoskeletal conditions has been conducted on patients with low back pain. The conclusions of systematic reviews of this research are summarized below. These conclusions broadly reflect those of education for other musculoskeletal conditions such as neck pain.[51,52] The effectiveness of educational interventions is usually determined by their effects on pain, disability and return to work. Findings and conclusions are typically made from comparing the educational approach to waitlist, placebo or usual care assessed at short term, when the effects are presumed to be largest.

Biomedical Education (Back Schools)

Five reviews have systematically reviewed the evidence for the effectiveness of biomedical education (Back

Schools).[10,12,53-55] Although Brox et al.[53] and Heymans et al.[12] found conflicting evidence, Turner[54] and Demoulin et al.[55] concluded that biomedical education is not effective at reducing either pain intensity or disability for patients with chronic low back pain. Brox et al.,[53] Demoulin et al.[55] and Turner[54] all concluded that for patients with chronic low back pain biomedical education does not reduce work absences, though Heymans et al.[10,12] found conflicting evidence. The quality of the evidence for these conclusions was typically low to moderate.[12]

Biopsychosocial Education (Advice/Brief Education)

There are four systematic reviews on the effect of biopsychosocial education for low back pain.[9,53,56,57] Advice or brief education does not reduce pain intensity for either acute,[9,53,56] subacute[9] or chronic low back pain patients.[9] Brox et al.[53] concluded that brief education is effective at reducing disability, whereas Engers et al.[9] and Shaheed et al.[56] concluded that it was not. Although Brox et al.[53] and Shaheed et al.[56] concluded that brief education was effective at reducing sick leave, Henrotin et al.[57] concluded a biopsychosocial booklet alone was insufficient to produce effects and Engers et al.[9] concluded that only education that lasted longer than 2.5 hours was effective, although there was no effect for patients with chronic low back pain. It should be noted that the quality of available evidence was 'very low', leading Shaheed et al.[56] to caution against conclusions that could be used to inform clinical management.

Pain Neurophysiology/Pain Biology Education

There is one systematic review on the effect of pain neurophysiology/pain biology education for chronic low back pain[58] and one of the effect of pain neurophysiology/pain biology education on chronic pain, with most included studies on low back pain.[59] Clarke et al.[58] and Louw et al.[59] concluded that pain neurophysiology education was effective at reducing pain intensity for patients with chronic low back pain or other chronic pain. Clarke et al.[58] found evidence that these effects become larger over time. Louw et al.[59] concluded that pain neurophysiology education decreased disability for patients with different chronic pain conditions whereas Clarke et al.[58] did not reach the same conclusion for patients with chronic low back pain. Neither of these reviews reported on sick leave/return to work. The quality of the evidence included in these reviews typically ranged from moderate- to high-quality studies,[59] providing some confidence in the conclusions.

The conclusions from systematic reviews provide conflicting evidence that biomedical and biopsychosocial education are effective at reducing pain and disability associated with low back pain. Even when effects are found, the size of the effect is often small and may not be clinically important. Larger and more robust effects are found for patients with chronic pain who are provided with pain neurophysiology education. Biomedical and biopsychosocial education are most consistently associated with reduced sick leave/increased return to work.

PATIENT EDUCATION AND MALADAPTIVE BELIEFS

Some authors have pointed out that as patient education is complex and aimed at changing behaviours, theoretical models are likely to provide a useful guide for their development or refinement.[9,60] Pain, disability and return to work are important outcomes that reflect patients' concerns[61] and are included in the core outcomes for research on low back pain.[62] Psychological theories suggest that underlying these outcomes are patient beliefs.[63] Patient beliefs can therefore be considered to be the primary targets of patient education, and changes in these beliefs are likely to lead to improved patient outcomes.

Inaccurate or unhelpful beliefs about low back pain are common in the general population[64-67] and are caused by poor or out-dated information.[68] For example, patients who have erroneous or unhelpful beliefs about pain are more likely to be distressed and worried about their condition, to report increased pain and disability and to seek inappropriate management.[60,63] For patients with low back pain the presence of these beliefs is a marker for increased risk of poor outcome and a slow recovery.[36]

Patient beliefs have been demonstrated to be stronger predictors of poor outcome than factors such as pain.[69] These beliefs are not only predictive of poor outcome,[70,71] but they are significant barriers to recovery.[63,72] Changes in these beliefs are associated with clinical improvements[73,74] and there is evidence that they underlie the development of chronic symptoms.[75] The causal relationships between beliefs and poor outcomes such as unhealthy behaviours, pain and disability are outlined in psychological theories such as the social cognition models including self-efficacy,[76,77] the theory of planned behaviour,[78] and the fear-avoidance model.[79-81]

When providing patient education, the aim of the health-care practitioner is to change unhelpful beliefs by providing accurate, evidenced-based information to reduce health anxiety or worries, increase confidence and make a patient an active participant in the management of their health (a patient-centred approach). Changing unhelpful beliefs to more adaptive beliefs is presumed to lead ultimately to decreased pain and disability.

Unfortunately, relatively few studies have tested whether education can effectively change maladaptive or unhelpful beliefs.[57] Those studies that have measured the effect of education on catastrophizing[6,82] and fear-avoidance beliefs[83] suggest that these beliefs may be difficult to change even with lengthy intervention (greater than 3 hours) heavily focused on psychosocial factors. It is therefore not known to what extent the conflicting evidence on the effectiveness of patient education provided by systematic reviews might be due to a failure to accurately target and change patient beliefs.[84]

COMMON BELIEFS TARGETED BY PATIENT EDUCATION

Education targets commonly held erroneous, faulty or maladaptive beliefs that patients may have about their pain and their condition.

Suitable targets for education are beliefs about pain that have been shown to be associated with poor outcome, including catastrophic pain beliefs (a belief that the pain has a serious cause, that the pain will persist and the condition will inevitably deteriorate), fear-avoidance beliefs (when pain is experienced physical activities should be avoided and rest should be taken) and self-efficacy beliefs (the confidence that a patient has the ability to achieve outcomes that are important and desirable).[60,63]

Research that shows that these beliefs are associated with poor outcomes such as pain and disability[70,71] was a major reason for the development of biopsychosocial education.[42] Pain neurophysiology education focuses on identifying and changing a belief that *hurt equals harm*.[49,85] A strong belief that the presence of pain is always associated with tissue damage is regarded by this approach as underpinning other maladaptive beliefs such as catastrophic and fear-avoidant beliefs.[48]

PAIN NEUROPHYSIOLOGY EDUCATION

In contrast to biomedical and biopsychosocial education there is evidence that pain neurophysiology education effectively targets and changes patients' beliefs. In particular, pain neurophysiology has been found to decrease pain-related catastrophizing in people with chronic or subacute pain.[47,86,87] A simple book using pain metaphors based on principles of the neurophysiology of pain has also been found to decrease catastrophizing in patients with chronic low back pain,[88] although written material provided to patients with fibromyalgia did not.[89] Investigations are underway to determine whether pain neurophysiology effectively targets and changes catastrophizing and self-efficacy in patients with acute low back pain and whether these effects are associated with pain and disability outcomes.[90]

REFERENCES

1. Lagger G, Pataky Z, Golay A. Efficacy of therapeutic patient education in chronic diseases and obesity. Patient Educ Couns 2010;79:283–6. doi:10.1016/j.pec.2010.03.015.
2. Koes BW, van Tulder M, Lin C-WC, et al. An updated overview of clinical guidelines for the management of non-specific low back pain in primary care. Eur Spine J 2010;19:2075–94. doi:10.1007/s00586-010-1502-y.
3. Dagenais S, Tricco AC, Haldeman S. Synthesis of recommendations for the assessment and management of low back pain from recent clinical practice guidelines. Spine J 2010;10:514–28. doi:10.1016/j.spinee.2010.03.032.
4. Henrotin YE, Cedraschi C, Duplan B, et al. Information and low back pain management: a systematic review. Spine 2006;31:E326–34. doi:10.1097/01.brs.0000217620.85893.32.
5. Nijs J, van Wilgen CP, Van Oosterwijck J, et al. How to explain central sensitization to patients with 'unexplained' chronic musculoskeletal pain: practice guidelines. Man Ther 2011;16:413–18. doi:10.1016/j.math.2011.04.005.
6. Pengel LHM, Refshauge KM, Maher CG, et al. Physiotherapist-directed exercise, advice, or both for subacute low back pain – A randomized trial. Ann Intern Med 2007;146:787–96.
7. Frost H, Lamb SE, Doll HA, et al. Randomised controlled trial of physiotherapy compared with advice for low back pain. BMJ 2004;329:708. doi:10.1136/bmj.38216.868808.7C.
8. Rantonen J, Vehtari A, Karppinen J, et al. Face-to-face information combined with a booklet versus a booklet alone for treatment of mild low-back pain: a randomized controlled trial. Scand J Work Environ Health 2013;40:156–66. doi:10.5271/sjweh.3398.
9. Engers A, Jellema P, Wensing M, et al. Individual patient education for low back pain. Cochrane Database Syst Rev 2008;CD004057, doi:10.1002/14651858.CD004057.pub3.
10. Heymans MW, van Tulder MW, Esmail R, et al. Back schools for nonspecific low back pain: a systematic review within the framework of the Cochrane Collaboration Back Review Group. Spine 2005;30:2153–63.
11. Cohen JE, Goel V, Frank JW, et al. Group education interventions for people with low back pain. An overview of the literature. Spine 1994;19:1214–22.
12. Heymans MW, van Tulder MW, Esmail R, et al. Back schools for non-specific low-back pain. Cochrane Database Syst Rev 2004;CD000261–CD000261, doi:10.1002/14651858.CD000261.pub2.
13. Udermann BE, Spratt KF, Donelson RG, et al. Can a patient educational book change behavior and reduce pain in chronic low back pain patients? Spine J 2004;4:425–35. doi:10.1016/j.spinee.2004.01.016.
14. Roland M, Dixon M. Randomized controlled trial of an educational booklet for patients presenting with back pain in general practice. J R Coll Gen Pract 1989;39:244–6.
15. Burton AK, Waddell G, Tillotson KM, et al. Information and advice to patients with back pain can have a positive effect. A randomized controlled trial of a novel educational booklet in primary care. Spine 1999;24:2484–91.
16. Hendrick PA, Ahmed OH, Bankier SS, et al. Manual therapy. Man Ther 2012;17:318–24. doi:10.1016/j.math.2012.02.019.
17. Washington TA, Fanciullo GJ, Sorensen JA, et al. Quality of chronic pain websites. Pain Med 2008;9:994–1000. doi:10.1111/j.1526-4637.2008.00419.x.
18. Fischer J, Geurts J, Valderrabano V, et al. Educational quality of youtube videos on knee arthrocentesis. JCR. J Clin Rheumatol 2013;19:373–6. doi:10.1097/RHU.0b013e3182a69fb2.
19. Stephen K, Cumming GP. Searching for pelvic floor muscle exercises on YouTube: what individuals may find and where this might fit with health service programmes to promote continence. Menopause Int 2012;18:110–15. doi:10.1258/mi.2012.012007.
20. Wallace LS, Dhingra LK. A systematic review of smartphone applications for chronic pain available for download in the United States. J Opioid Manag 2014;10:63–8. doi:10.5055/jom.2014.0193.
21. Reynoldson C, Stones C, Allsop M, et al. Assessing the quality and usability of smartphone apps for pain self-management. Pain Med 2014;15:898–909. doi:10.1111/pme.12327.
22. Rosser BA, Eccleston C. Smartphone applications for pain management. J Telemed Telecare 2011;17:308–12. doi:10.1258/jtt.2011.101102.
23. Oliveira AA, Gevirtz RR, Hubbard DD. A psycho-educational video used in the emergency department provides effective treatment for whiplash injuries. CORD Conf Proc 2006;31:1652–7. doi:10.1097/01.brs.0000224172.45828.e3.
24. Pozo-Cruz B, Parraca J, Pozo-Cruz J, et al. An occupational, internet-based intervention to prevent chronicity in subacute lower back pain: a randomised controlled trial. J Rehabil Med 2012;44:581–7. doi:10.2340/16501977-0988.
25. Gross DP, Russell AS, Ferrari R, et al. Evaluation of a Canadian back pain mass media campaign. Spine 2010;35:906–13. doi:10.1097/BRS.0b013e3181c91140.
26. Waddell G, O'Connor M, Boorman S, et al. Working Backs Scotland: a public and professional health education campaign for back pain. Spine 2007;32:2139–43. doi:10.1097/BRS.0b013e31814541bc.
27. Buchbinder R, Jolley D, Wyatt M. 2001 Volvo Award Winner in Clinical Studies: effects of a media campaign on back pain beliefs and its potential influence on management of low back pain in general practice. Spine 2001;26:2535–42.
28. Dupeyron A, Ribinik P, Gélis A, et al. Education in the management of low back pain. Literature review and recall of key

recommendations for practice. Ann Phys Rehabil Med 2011;54:319–35. doi:10.1016/j.rehab.2011.06.001.

29. Pellisé F, Sell P, EuroSpine Patient Line Task Force. Patient information and education with modern media: the Spine Society of Europe Patient Line. Eur Spine J 2009;18(Suppl. 3):395–401. doi:10.1007/s00586-009-0973-1.

30. Hancock MJ, Maher CG, Latimer J, et al. Systematic review of tests to identify the disc, SIJ or facet joint as the source of low back pain. Eur Spine J 2007;16:1539–50. doi:10.1007/s00586-007-0391-1.

31. Henschke N, Maher CG, Refshauge KM. A systematic review identifies five 'red flags' to screen for vertebral fracture in patients with low back pain. J Clin Epidemiol 2008;61:110–18. doi:10.1016/j.jclinepi.2007.04.013.

32. Henschke N, Maher CG, Refshauge KM, et al. Prevalence of and screening for serious spinal pathology in patients presenting to primary care settings with acute low back pain. Arthritis Rheum 2009;60:3072–80. doi:10.1002/art.24853.

33. da C Menezes Costa L, Maher CG, Hancock MJ, et al. The prognosis of acute and persistent low-back pain: a meta-analysis. Can Med Assoc J 2012;184:E613–24. doi:10.1503/cmaj.111271.

34. Koes BW, van Tulder MW, Thomas S. Diagnosis and treatment of low back pain. BMJ 2006;332:1430–4. doi:10.1136/bmj.332.7555.1430.

35. Hasenbring MI, Pincus T. Effective reassurance in primary care of low back pain. Clin J Pain 2014. doi:10.1097/AJP.0000000000000097; [Epub ahead of print].

36. Henschke N, Maher CG, Refshauge KM, et al. Prognosis in patients with recent onset low back pain in Australian primary care: inception cohort study. BMJ 2008;337:a171. doi:10.1136/bmj.a171.

37. Martin L. Back basics: general information for back school participants. Occup Med 1992;7:9–16.

38. Forssell MZ. The Swedish Back School. Physiotherapy 1980;66:112–14.

39. Bendix T, Bendix AF, Busch E, et al. Functional restoration in chronic low back pain. Scand J Med Sci Sports 1996;6:88–97.

40. Bendix T, Bendix A, Labriola M, et al. Functional restoration versus outpatient physical training in chronic low back pain: a randomized comparative study. Spine 2000;25:2494–500.

41. Poiraudeau S, Rannou F, Revel M. Functional restoration programs for low back pain: a systematic review. Ann Readapt Med Phys 2007;50:425–9, 419–24. doi:10.1016/j.annrmp.2007.04.009.

42. Waddell G. Biopsychosocial analysis of low back pain. Baillieres Clin Rheumatol 1992;6:523–57.

43. Waddell G, Main CJ, Morris EW, et al. Chronic low-back pain, psychologic distress, and illness behavior. Spine 1984;9:209–13.

44. Hagen KB, Jamtvedt G, Hilde G, et al. The updated cochrane review of bed rest for low back pain and sciatica. Spine 2005;30:542–6.

45. Dahm KT, Brurberg KG, Jamtvedt G, et al. Advice to rest in bed versus advice to stay active for acute low-back pain and sciatica (Review). Cochrane Database of Systematic Reviews 2010. doi:10.1002/14651858.CD007612.pub2.

46. Hagen EM, Eriksen HR, Ursin H. Does early intervention with a light mobilization program reduce long-term sick leave for low back pain? Spine 2000;25:1973–6.

47. Moseley GL, Nicholas MK, Hodges PW. A randomized controlled trial of intensive neurophysiology education in chronic low back pain. Clin J Pain 2004;20:324–30.

48. Moseley L. Unraveling the barriers to reconceptualization of the problem in chronic pain: the actual and perceived ability of patients and health professionals to understand the neurophysiology. J Pain 2003;4:184–9. doi:10.1016/S1526-5900(03)00488-7.

49. Butler DS, Moseley GL. Explain Pain, 2nd Edition. 2013. Noigroup Publications; Adelaide, pp. 133.

50. Moseley GL. A pain neuromatrix approach to patients with chronic pain. Man Ther 2003;8:130–40.

51. Haines T, Gross AR, Burnie S, et al. A Cochrane review of patient education for neck pain. Spine J 2009;9:859–71. doi:10.1016/j.spinee.2009.04.019.

52. Yu H, Côté P, Southerst D, et al. Does structured patient education improve the recovery and clinical outcomes of patients with neck pain? A systematic review from the Ontario Protocol for Traffic Injury Management (OPTIMa) Collaboration. Spine J 2014. pii: S1529-9430(14)00347-7. doi:10.1016/j.spinee.2014.03.039.

53. Brox JI, Storheim K, Grotle M, et al. Systematic review of back schools, brief education, and fear-avoidance training for chronic

54. Turner JA. Educational and behavioral interventions for back pain in primary care. Spine 1996;21:2851–7, discussion 2858–9.

55. Demoulin C, Marty M, Genevay S, et al. Effectiveness of preventive back educational interventions for low back pain: a critical review of randomized controlled clinical trials. Eur Spine J 2012;21:2520–30. doi:10.1007/s00586-012-2445-2.

56. Shaheed CA, Maher CG, Williams KA, et al. Critical Review. YJPAI 2014;15:2–15. doi:10.1016/j.jpain.2013.09.016.

57. Henrotin YE, Cedraschi C, Duplan B, et al. Information and low back pain management: a systematic review. Spine 2006;31:E326.

58. Clarke CL, Ryan CG, Martin DJ. Pain neurophysiology education for the management of individuals with chronic low back pain: a systematic review and meta-analysis. Man Ther 2011;16:544–9. doi:10.1016/j.math.2011.05.003.

59. Louw A, Diener I, Butler DS, et al. The effect of neuroscience education on pain, disability, anxiety, and stress in chronic musculoskeletal pain. Arch Phys Med Rehabil 2011;92:2041–56. doi:10.1016/j.apmr.2011.07.198.

60. Pincus T, McCracken LM. Psychological factors and treatment opportunities in low back pain. Best Pract Res Clin Rheumatol 2013;27:625–35. doi:10.1016/j.berh.2013.09.010.

61. Hush JM, Refshauge K, Sullivan G, et al. Recovery: what does this mean to patients with low back pain? Arthritis Rheum 2009;61:124–31. doi:10.1002/art.24162.

62. Dworkin RH, Turk DC, Farrar JT, et al. Core outcome measures for chronic pain clinical trials: IMMPACT recommendations. Pain 2005;113:9–19. doi:10.1016/j.pain.2004.09.012.

63. Main CJ, Foster N, Buchbinder R. How important are back pain beliefs and expectations for satisfactory recovery from back pain? Best Pract Res Clin Rheumatol 2010;24:205–17. doi:10.1016/j.berh.2009.12.012.

64. Bostick GP, Schopflocher D, Gross DP. Validity evidence for the back beliefs questionnaire in the general population. Eur J Pain 2013;17:1074–81. doi:10.1002/j.1532-2149.2012.00275.x.

65. Buer N, Linton SJ. Fear-avoidance beliefs and catastrophizing: occurrence and risk factor in back pain and ADL in the general population. Pain 2002;99:485–91.

66. Leeuw M, Houben RMA, Severeijns R, et al. Pain-related fear in low back pain: a prospective study in the general population. Eur J Pain 2012;11:256–66. doi:10.1016/j.ejpain.2006.02.009.

67. Ihlebæk C, Eriksen H. Are the 'myths' of low back pain alive in the general Norwegian population? Scand J Public Health 2003;31:395–8. doi:10.1080/14034940210165163.

68. Gross DP, Ferrari R, Russell AS, et al. A population-based survey of back pain beliefs in Canada. Spine 2006;31:2142–5. doi:10.1097/01.brs.0000231771.14965.e4.

69. Crombez G, Vlaeyen JW, Heuts PH, et al. Pain-related fear is more disabling than pain itself: evidence on the role of pain-related fear in chronic back pain disability. Pain 1999;80:329–39.

70. Wertli MM, Eugster R, Held U, et al. Catastrophizing-a prognostic factor for outcome in patients with low back pain: a systematic review. Spine J 2014;14(11):2639–57. pii: S1529-9430(14)00243-5. doi:10.1016/j.spinee.2014.03.003.

71. Wertli MM, Rasmussen-Barr E, Weiser S, et al. The role of fear avoidance beliefs as a prognostic factor for outcome in patients with nonspecific low back pain: a systematic review. Spine J 2014;14:816–36.e4. doi:10.1016/j.spinee.2013.09.036.

72. Pincus T, Vogel S, Burton AK, et al. Fear avoidance and prognosis in back pain: a systematic review and synthesis of current evidence. Arthritis Rheum 2006;54:3999–4010. doi:10.1002/art.22273.

73. Jensen MP, Turner JA, Romano JM. Changes in beliefs, catastrophizing, and coping are associated with improvement in multidisciplinary pain treatment. J Consult Clin Psychol 2001;69:655–62. doi:10.1037//0022-006X.69.4.655.

74. Mansell G, Kamper SJ, Kent P. Why and how back pain interventions work: what can we do to find out? Best Pract Res Clin Rheumatol 2013;27:685–97. doi:10.1016/j.berh.2013.10.001.

75. Costa LDCM, Maher CG, McAuley JH, et al. Self-efficacy is more important than fear of movement in mediating the relationship between pain and disability in chronic low back pain. Eur J Pain 2011;15:213–19. doi:10.1016/j.ejpain.2010.06.014.

76. Bandura A. Human agency in social cognitive theory. Am Psychol 1989;44:1175.

77. Bandura A. Social cognitive theory of self-regulation. Organ Behav Hum Decis Process 1991;50:248–87.
78. Armitage CJ, Conner M. Efficacy of the Theory of Planned Behaviour: a meta-analytic review. Br J Soc Psychol 2001;40:471–99.
79. Leeuw M, Goossens MEJB, Linton SJ, et al. The fear-avoidance model of musculoskeletal pain: current state of scientific evidence. J Behav Med 2006;30:77–94. doi:10.1007/s10865-006-9085-0.
80. Vlaeyen JW, Linton SJ. Fear-avoidance and its consequences in chronic musculoskeletal pain: a state of the art. Pain 2000;85:317–32.
81. Vlaeyen JWS, Linton SJ. Fear-avoidance model of chronic musculoskeletal pain: 12 years on. Pain 2012;153:1144–7. doi:10.1016/j.pain.2011.12.009.
82. Jellema P, van der Windt DAWM, van der Horst HE, et al. Should treatment of (sub)acute low back pain be aimed at psychosocial prognostic factors? Cluster randomised clinical trial in general practice. BMJ 2005;331:84. doi:10.1136/bmj.38495.686736.E0.
83. Hay E, Mullis R, Lewis M, et al. Comparison of physical treatments versus a brief pain-management programme for back pain in primary care: a randomised clinical trial in physiotherapy practice. Lancet 2005;365:2024–30. doi:10.1016/S0140-6736(05)66696-2.
84. Jellema P, van der Windt DAWM, van der Horst HE, et al. Why is a treatment aimed at psychosocial factors not effective in patients with (sub)acute low back pain? Pain 2005;118:350–9. doi:10.1016/j.pain.2005.09.002.
85. Moseley GL. Reconceptualising pain according to modern pain science. Phys Ther Rev 2007;12:169–78. doi:10.1179/108331907X223010.
86. Ryan CG, Gray HG, Newton M, et al. Pain biology education and exercise classes compared to pain biology education alone for individuals with chronic low back pain: a pilot randomised controlled trial. Man Ther 2010;15:382–7. doi:10.1016/j.math.2010.03.003.
87. Meeus M, Nijs J, Van Oosterwijck J, et al. Pain physiology education improves pain beliefs in patients with chronic fatigue syndrome compared with pacing and self-management education: a double-blind randomized controlled trial. Arch Phys Med Rehabil 2010;91:1153–9. doi:10.1016/j.apmr.2010.04.020.
88. Gallagher L, McAuley J, Moseley GL. A randomized-controlled trial of using a book of metaphors to reconceptualize pain and decrease catastrophizing in people with chronic pain. Clin J Pain 2013;29:20–5. doi:10.1097/AJP.0b013e3182465cf7.
89. van Ittersum MW, van Wilgen CP, Groothoff JW, et al. Is appreciation of written education about pain neurophysiology related to changes in illness perceptions and health status in patients with fibromyalgia? Patient Educ Couns 2010;85(2):269–74. doi:10.1016/j.pec.2010.09.006.
90. Traeger AC, Moseley GL, Hübscher M, et al. Pain education to prevent chronic low back pain: a study protocol for a randomised controlled trial. BMJ Open 2014;4:e005505. doi:10.1136/bmjopen-2014-005505.

CHAPTER 28.3 ■ PHYSICAL INTERVENTIONS OF PAIN MANAGEMENT AND POTENTIAL PROCESSES

Kathleen Sluka

EXERCISE

Exercise is a mainstay of physiotherapy interventions. For pain management, nearly all subjects will be prescribed an exercise programme to increase physical activity, increase strength and restore normal motion. There are numerous forms of exercise including stretching, strengthening, motor control, coordination, endurance and aerobic. Physiotherapists use a combination of different forms of exercise to individualize a programme to the person with pain.

Clinical Studies

Numerous studies show the effectiveness of exercise for a variety of pain conditions (Cochrane reviews) including chronic low back pain, neck pain, tendonitis, osteoarthritis, rheumatoid arthritis, fibromyalgia, myofascial pain and neuropathic pain.[1-12] Further exercise can reduce the number of recurrences of low back pain,[13] suggesting that regular exercise can reduce the chronicity of pain. Lastly, using a large-population database those who are regularly physically active are less likely to develop chronic musculoskeletal pain conditions than those who are sedentary.[14,15] Thus exercise and physical activity can reduce pain and disability, and improve function in people with a variety of painful conditions, can prevent the recurrence of pain and can prevent the development of chronic pain.

Dosing

Despite the strong evidence that exercise is effective, there are insufficient data to make recommendations regarding the frequency, duration and intensity of an effective exercise programme. Thus, future experiments need to determine optimal dosing parameters for development of an effective exercise programme. However, the type of exercise has been tested in a variety of pain conditions. In most instances for those with chronic pain, both strengthening and aerobic conditioning exercises are equally effective.[5,16,17] For example, in people with low back pain equivalent reductions in pain and disability and improvements in function and quality of life occurred when motor control exercises were compared with graded activity, or when motor control exercises were compared with general aerobic exercise.[5,18] Similarly, in fibromyalgia comparing muscle strengthening exercises to an aerobic exercise training programme produced similar reductions in pain and improvements in quality of life,[17] and in those with osteoarthritis aerobic exercise, strengthening exercises and aquatic exercises all reduce pain and improve function.[16] Additionally, complementary and alternative therapies that include exercise, such as yoga and tai chi, as well as lifestyle physical activity are also effective in people with a variety of pain conditions.[6,19-21] Thus, the type of exercise given for someone with chronic pain should be targeted towards patient preference and factors that improve compliance.

Basic Mechanisms

Although a significant amount of clinical literature supports the effectiveness of exercise for pain, few studies have addressed the underlying mechanisms. Early studies examined mechanisms in uninjured animals and humans. In animals, increases in withdrawal thresholds are observed in rats allowed free access to running wheels,[22] mice bred for high running wheel activity,[23] acute or long-term swimming[24,25] and after a strength training programme.[26]

Central Mechanisms

Endogenous opioids are produced in a wide range of tissue types, including the midbrain periaqueductal grey (PAG), rostral ventromedial medulla (RVM), spinal cord and muscle,[27,28] and are key players in exercise-induced analgesia. Further, serotonin is a major neurotransmitter found in endogenous inhibitory pathways including the PAG, RVM and spinal cord and plays a significant role in analgesia. In healthy human subjects there are increased serum levels of β-endorphin in response to aerobic exercise.[29-31] In animals without tissue injury, blockade of opioid receptors reduces analgesia produced by chronic running wheel activity and by strength training injury,[23,24] there is also reduced effectiveness of μ- and κ-opioid agonists in the PAG in the midbrain after chronic running wheel activity.[22,32-35] In animal models of pain, blockade of opioid receptors, systemically and in the brainstem, prevents the analgesia produced by regular aerobic exercise in neuropathic pain, chronic muscle pain and acetic-acid-induced pain.[24,36-39] In addition, there is an increased release of endogenous opioids in the PAG and RVM in response to aerobic exercise in animals with neuropathic pain.[36] On the other hand, blockade of peripheral opioid receptors has no effect on exercise-induced analgesia in animals with neuropathic pain.[36] In animals without tissue injury, aerobic exercise-induced analgesia is prevented by prior depletion of serotonin with p-chlorophenylalanine.[24] Thus these data support that exercise activates our central inhibitory pathways to produce analgesia through opioid and serotonergic mechanisms.

Central pathways not only inhibit pain, but can also facilitate and enhance pain behaviours. The RVM is a key nucleus in pain facilitation, and glutamate receptors mediate the facilitation. In animals, after induction of chronic muscle pain or exercise-induced pain, there is enhanced phosphorylation of the NR1 subunit of the NMDA receptor in the RVM,[40] suggestive of enhanced neuron activity in pain facilitation pathways. These increases in p-NR1 in the RVM are prevented by regular physical activity,[40] suggesting that regular exercise reduces central neuron sensitivity.

Peripheral Mechanisms

It is also possible that exercise has effects peripherally, reducing nociceptor activity or enhancing endogenous inhibitory neuromodulators. In animals with diabetic neuropathy, there is enhanced calcium current density for both low- (T-; LVA) and high-voltage activated activated calcium currents (N-, P/Q-, L-; HVA) in dorsal root ganglia neurons,[37] which is indicative of enhanced nociceptor activity. Aerobic exercise running reduced the enhanced current densities of HVA and LVA calcium channels, suggesting reductions in nociceptor activity and thus it is possible that regular exercise reduces pain hypersensitivity by normalization of enhanced ion channel activity of nociceptors.

Regular aerobic exercise in mice with muscle pain leads to increased expression of neurotrophin-3 mRNA and protein in the muscle tissue and follows the same time course as the analgesia.[41] Neurotrophin-3 is analgesic when injected or overexpressed in muscle,[42] and thus these data suggest exercise could increase NT-3 in muscle to reduce nociceptive activity and produce analgesia.

Additional Mechanisms

A recent study showed that the reduction of pain behaviours in an animal model of neuropathic pain was blocked by inhibition of adenosine receptors and enhanced by inhibition of adenosine degradation systemically,[39] and thus adenosine, either peripherally or centrally, could play a role in the analgesia produced by regular exercise.

TENS

Transcutaneous electrical nerve stimulation (TENS) is the application of electrical stimulation to the skin for pain relief. TENS is generally applied at low frequencies (<10 Hz) or high frequencies (>50 Hz), at varying intensities. These intensities include sensory threshold, strong sensory intensity, or intensities that produce motor contraction. Recent studies show that low and high frequencies produce analgesia through different mechanisms[43] and that greater intensities produce greater analgesia.[44] Electrodes can be placed to surround the site of pain, over a nerve or segmentally – not much research has been done to examine optimum electrode placement sites. TENS is a safe, non-invasive treatment with relatively few contraindications that can be either self-administered or administered by a therapist. TENS is typically used as an additional pain-management technique in a physical therapy management programme that includes education and exercise.

Clinical Studies

The clinical literature on TENS is controversial and recent reviews discuss potential reasons for this controversy related to design and quality of trials.[44,45] These reviews suggest that sub-optimal dosing, inappropriate outcome assessments and inadequate timing of outcomes assessments contribute to negative effects. Systematic reviews show significant reductions in pain in individuals post-operatively, those with osteoarthritis and those with peripheral neuropathy.[46-48] However, other systematic reviews similarly show TENS is ineffective or inconclusive for a variety of painful conditions including acute pain, osteoarthritis, low back pain and post-operative pain;[49-55] this effect may be dependent on dosing of TENS.[46,47]

TENS has also been shown in individuals with post-operative pain, osteoarthritis and fibromyalgia to reduce pain with movement, but not pain at rest,[56-58] suggesting that TENS is more effective for movement-related pain. TENS may be effective for other evoked pain like hyperalgesia and allodynia, in addition to movement pain. Indeed TENS reduces hyperalgesia in those with osteoarthritis and fibromyalgia, and allodynia in those with neuropathic pain.[56,59,60]

TENS produces its analgesic effect by activating opioid receptors (see Basic Science Mechanisms section for details) and as such it is important to understand potential pharmaceutical interactions. Low-frequency TENS activates mu-opioid receptors whereas high-frequency TENS activates delta-opioid receptors.[43] As opioids can produce analgesic tolerance, repeated daily use of TENS at the same frequency and intensity (dose) in healthy controls can also induce analgesic tolerance.[61] In addition, low-frequency TENS is less effective than high-frequency TENS in both people and animals that are opioid-tolerant.[62,63] Alternating frequencies between low and high, or increasing intensity daily delays analgesic tolerance in animal studies.[64,65] Thus, understanding mechanisms may assist in improving efficacy of treatment.

On the other hand, a cumulative effect of TENS (delivered two to five times per week) has been shown in individuals with chronic low back pain, osteoarthritis and neuropathic pain.[60,66-68] The reasons for this cumulative effect are not clear but may be secondary to increasing activity levels as a result of reduced movement pain. Alternatively, TENS could normalize pain physiology (i.e. reduce central sensitization or increase central inhibition). In support a recent study in individuals with fibromyalgia showed that TENS delivered to the neck or back increased pain thresholds outside the site of stimulation (leg) and increased central inhibition (central pain modulation).[56]

Dosing

It has become increasingly clear in the last decade that intensity of TENS is critically important to obtain a positive effect. Specifically, stimulation amplitude must be of sufficient strength to produce an analgesic response.[47,57,69,70] In healthy subjects, TENS delivered at a strong but comfortable intensity provided a significant analgesic effect, whereas TENS delivered at or below sensory threshold was ineffective.[69-71] Similarly, systematic reviews that consider dosing show that high intensities are associated with significant reductions in both post-operative and osteoarthritis pain while lower intensities are not effective.[46,47]

Basic Science Mechanisms

TENS activates a complex neuronal network to result in a reduction in pain. At frequencies and intensities used clinically, TENS activates large-diameter afferent fibres.[72,73] This afferent input is sent to the central nervous system to activate the descending inhibitory system to reduce hyperalgesia. Specifically, blockade of neuronal activity in the PAG, RVM and spinal cord inhibits the analgesic effects of TENS.[74-76]

In animals without tissue injury, both low- and high-frequency TENS reduce dorsal horn neuron activity.[77-81] In animals with peripheral inflammation or neuropathic pain, enhanced activity of dorsal horn neurons (i.e. central sensitization) to both noxious and innocuous stimuli is reduced by either high- or low-frequency TENS.[82-85] In parallel there is a reduction in both primary and secondary hyperalgesia by either low- or high-frequency TENS.[82-84,86-90]

In human subjects *high-frequency TENS* increases the concentration of β-endorphins in the bloodstream and cerebrospinal fluid, and methionine-enkephalin in the cerebrospinal fluid.[91,92] The reduction in hyperalgesia by high-frequency TENS is prevented by blockade of δ-opioid receptors in the RVM or spinal cord, or synaptic transmission in the ventrolateral PAG.[75,76,93] The reduction in hyperalgesia produced by high-frequency TENS is prevented by blockade of muscarinic receptors (M1, M3) in the spinal cord[94] – muscarinic receptors are implicated in opioid analgesia in the spinal cord. High-frequency TENS also enhances release of the inhibitory neurotransmitter GABA in the spinal cord dorsal horn and the TENS antihyperalgesia is reduced by blockade of GABA_A receptors in the spinal cord.[95] However, blockade of serotonin or noradrenergic receptors in the spinal cord has no effect on the reversal of hyperalgesia produced by high-frequency TENS.[96] Thus high-frequency TENS produces analgesia by activating endogenous inhibitory mechanisms in the central nervous system involving opioid, GABA and muscarinic receptors.

High-frequency TENS also reduces central neuron sensitization,[85] and release of the excitatory neurotransmitters glutamate and substance P in the spinal cord dorsal horn in animals with inflammation.[97,98] The reduction in glutamate is prevented by blockade of δ-opioid receptors. Thus, one consequence of activation of inhibitory pathways by TENS is to reduce excitation and consequent neuron sensitization in the spinal cord.

Peripherally, substance P, which is normally increased in injured animals, is reduced in dorsal root ganglia neurons by high-frequency TENS in animals injected with the inflammatory irritant, formalin.[97] In α-2a-adrenergic knockout mice, analgesia by high-frequency TENS does not occur.[99] Blockade of peripheral, but not spinal or supraspinal, α-2a receptors prevents the analgesia produced by TENS,[99] suggesting a role for peripheral α-2a-adrenergic in analgesia produced by TENS. Thus, some of the analgesic effects of TENS are mediated through actions on primary afferent fibres.

Low-frequency TENS reduces hyperalgesia after joint inflammation and this reduction is prevented by blockade of μ-opioid receptors in the spinal cord or the RVM, or synaptic transmission in the ventrolateral PAG.[93] The analgesia produced by low-frequency TENS is also reduced by blockade of GABA_A, serotonin 5-HT2A and

5-HT3 and muscarinic M1 and M3 receptors in the spinal cord.[94–96] Serotonin is released during low-frequency TENS in animals with joint inflammation.[100] Low-frequency TENS also reduces dorsal horn neuron sensitization in animals with inflammation.[85] Thus, these studies show that low-frequency TENS uses classical descending inhibitory pathways involving the PAG–RVM pathway activating opioid, GABA, serotonin and muscarinic receptors to reduce dorsal horn neuron activity and the consequent pain.

Low-frequency TENS also has effects on the peripheral nervous systems. Blockade of peripheral opioid receptors with naloxone at the site of application prevents the analgesic effects of low-frequency but not high-frequency TENS in an animal model of inflammatory pain.[101] The reduction in cold allodynia by low-frequency TENS is reduced by administration of systemic phentolamine to block α-adrenergic receptors.[83] In parallel, the antihyperalgesia produced by low-frequency TENS in animals with joint inflammation is reduced in α2a-noradrenergic receptor knockout mice, and prevented by peripheral blockade of α2-noradrenergic receptors (but not by spinal or supraspinal blockade).[99] Increases in blood flow occur with stronger low-frequency TENS at intensities that produce motor contraction (intensity greater than 25% above motor threshold).[102–106] Thus, peripheral effects of TENS may involve opioid receptors and changes in sympathetic activity utilizing local α2a-noradrenergic receptors.

MANUAL THERAPY

Manual therapy techniques may include traditional massage, soft tissue mobilization, joint mobilizations and manipulations, nerve or 'neural' mobilization procedures, joint stabilization exercises and self-mobilization exercises. Clinical evidence supports the use of massage and manipulations for a variety of pain conditions.[107–122]

Basic Science Mechanisms

The basic science mechanisms underlying massage have included evidence aimed at deciphering which central pathways are activated. In an animal model, 10 minutes of massage to the abdomen increases pain thresholds in a cumulative manner.[123] Following massage in this model there is an increase in the neuropeptide oxytocin in the plasma and PAG in response.[123] Blockade of oxytocin receptors, either systemically or in the PAG, reduces the analgesic effect of massage.[124] After delayed onset muscle soreness (DOMS) induced in otherwise healthy male subjects, 10 minutes of massage reduced excitatory signally at the level of the muscle (decreases in cytokines, heat shock protein phosphorylation and NFκB) and increased signalling proteins involved in tissue repair and metabolic control (MAP kinases, PGC-1).[125] Thus massage likely has local peripheral effects, as well as more systemic and central nervous system effects that either directly or indirectly reduce pain.

Joint manipulation and mobilization use similar multiple mechanisms to reduce pain that include effects peripherally at the site of application and in the central nervous system. Manipulation and mobilization clearly increase pain thresholds in healthy controls and increase pain-free range of motion of the upper limb tension test.[126–129] Peripherally, in healthy human subjects, manipulation produces a short-lived (10–30 seconds) decrease in motoneuron excitability.[130,131] However, these effects are longer lasting in people with low back pain – spinal manipulation increases the activity of the oblique abdominal muscle for several minutes and there is no effect in normal healthy controls.[132] In an animal model, a lumbar spinal thrust reduces activity of muscle spindle afferent fibres for several seconds[133] and decreases electromyographic activity in the paraspinal muscles for minutes.[134]

In addition, evidence suggests that joint mobilization activates central inhibitory mechanisms to reduce central excitability and have a more widespread effect. In healthy controls there is a decrease in temporal summation, which is a measure of central excitability, following spinal manipulation, suggesting central mechanisms may play a role.[135,136] In people with lateral epicondylalgia, joint mobilization of the cervical spine (grade III lateral glide of C5/6) increases pressure pain thresholds, pain-free range of motion for the upper limb tension test and pain-free grip force,[128] and in people with knee osteoarthritis application of joint mobilization to the knee increases pressure pain thresholds at the knee (i.e. primary hyperalgesia) and the heel (i.e. secondary hyperalgesia).[137] Similarly, in animal models of inflammatory pain, grade III mobilizations of the knee joint reduce hyperalgesia associated with inflammation of the knee or the ankle.[137–139] Further ankle joint mobilization in an animal model of neuropathic pain reduces the enhanced glial cell activity in the spinal cord,[146] further suggesting a reduction in central excitability. Thus, these data show that joint mobilizations not only have local effects but that the effects can be widespread, indicating reductions in central excitability.

Pharmacological studies in humans and animals have started to decipher potential mechanisms in the central nervous system underlying the analgesia produced by joint manipulation. The analgesia produced by joint manipulation and mobilization is not reversed by the opioid antagonist, naloxone, in human subjects[140–142] or in an animal model of mobilization-induced analgesia.[138] However, in an animal model of post-operative pain, blockade of opioids locally prevents the analgesia produced by mobilization.[143] The analgesia produced using grade III mobilization of the knee joint, in an animal model of ankle inflammation or post-operative pain, is prevented by spinal blockade of serotonin 5-HT1A and α-2 noradrenergic receptors.[138,144] However, blockade of GABA or opioid receptors spinally has no effect on the analgesia produced by mobilization.[138] In a post-operative pain animal model, blockade of adenosine-A1 and cannabinoid receptors CB1 and CB2 in the spinal cord prevents the effects of ankle joint mobilization.[144,145] These data suggest that joint mobilizations reduce pain through effects in the central nervous system by activating descending inhibitory pathways from the RVM and dorsolateral pontine tegmentum (DLPT) that are non-opioid.

REFERENCES

1. Bement MK. Exercise-induced hypoalgesia: an evidence-based review. In: Sluka KA, editor. Mechanisms and Management of Pain for the Physical Therapist. Seattle: IASP Press; 2009. p. 143–66.
2. Busch AJ, Barber KA, Overend TJ, et al. Exercise for treating fibromyalgia syndrome. Cochrane Database Syst Rev 2007; CD003786.
3. Chou R, Huffman LH. Nonpharmacologic therapies for acute and chronic low back pain: a review of the evidence for an American Pain Society/American College of Physicians clinical practice guideline. Ann Intern Med 2007;147:492–504.
4. Edmonds M, McGuire H, Price J. Exercise therapy for chronic fatigue syndrome. Cochrane Database Syst Rev 2004;CD003200.
5. Ferreira ML, Ferreira PH, Latimer J, et al. Comparison of general exercise, motor control exercise and spinal manipulative therapy for chronic low back pain: a randomized trial. Pain 2007;131 :31–7.
6. Fontaine KR, Conn L, Clauw DJ. Effects of lifestyle physical activity on perceived symptoms and physical function in adults with fibromyalgia: results of a randomized trial. Arthritis Res Ther 2010;12:R55.
7. Fransen M, McConnell S, Bell M. Therapeutic exercise for people with osteoarthritis of the hip or knee. A systematic review. J Rheumatol 2002;29:1737–45.
8. Hayden JA, van Tulder MW, Malmivaara A, et al. Exercise therapy for treatment of non-specific low back pain. Cochrane Database Syst Rev 2005;CD000335.
9. Kluding PM, Pasnoor M, Singh R, et al. The effect of exercise on neuropathic symptoms, nerve function, and cutaneous innervation in people with diabetic peripheral neuropathy. J Diabetes Complications 2012;26:424–8.
10. Lluch E, Arguisuelas MD, Coloma PS, et al. Effects of deep cervical flexor training on pressure pain thresholds over myofascial trigger points in patients with chronic neck pain. J Manipulative Physiol Ther 2013;36:604–11.
11. Munneke M, de JZ, Zwinderman AH, et al. Effect of a high-intensity weight-bearing exercise program on radiologic damage progression of the large joints in subgroups of patients with rheumatoid arthritis. Arthritis Rheum 2005;53:410–17.
12. Stegner AJ, Shields MR, Meyer JD, et al. Effects of acute and chronic physical activity on chronic pain conditions. In: Ekkekakis P, editor. Routledge Handbook of Physical Activity and Mental Health. London: Routledge; 2013. p. 387–99.
13. Choi BK, Verbeek JH, Tam WW, et al. Exercises for prevention of recurrences of low-back pain. Cochrane Database Syst Rev 2010;CD006555.
14. Landmark T, Romundstad PR, Borchgrevink PC, et al. Longitudinal associations between exercise and pain in the general population–the HUNT pain study. PLoS ONE 2013;8:e65279.
15. Landmark T, Romundstad P, Borchgrevink PC, et al. Associations between recreational exercise and chronic pain in the general population: evidence from the HUNT 3 study. Pain 2011; 152:2241–7.
16. Uthman OA, van der Windt DA, Jordan JL, et al. Exercise for lower limb osteoarthritis: systematic review incorporating trial sequential analysis and network meta-analysis. BMJ 2013;347: f5555.
17. Bircan C, Karasel SA, Akgun B, et al. Effects of muscle strengthening versus aerobic exercise program in fibromyalgia. Rheumatol Int 2008;28:527–32.
18. Macedo LG, Latimer J, Maher CG, et al. Effect of motor control exercises versus graded activity in patients with chronic nonspecific low back pain: a randomized controlled trial. Phys Ther 2012;92:363–77.
19. Busch AJ, Webber SC, Brachaniec M, et al. Exercise therapy for fibromyalgia. Curr Pain Headache Rep 2011;15:358–67.
20. Lauche R, Langhorst J, Dobos G, et al. A systematic review and meta-analysis of Tai Chi for osteoarthritis of the knee. Complement Ther Med 2013;21:396–406.
21. Holtzman S, Beggs RT. Yoga for chronic low back pain: a meta-analysis of randomized controlled trials. Pain Res Manag 2013;18:267–72.
22. Kanarek RB, Gerstein AV, Wildman RP, et al. Chronic running-wheel activity decreases sensitivity to morphine-induced analgesia in male and female rats. Pharmacol Biochem Behav 1998;61: 19–27.
23. Li G, Rhodes JS, Girard I, et al. Opioid-mediated pain sensitivity in mice bred for high voluntary wheel running. Physiol Behav 2004;83:515–24.
24. Mazzardo-Martins L, Martins DF, Marcon R, et al. High-intensity extended swimming exercise reduces pain-related behavior in mice: involvement of endogenous opioids and the serotonergic system. J Pain 2010;11:1393.
25. Blustein JE, McLaughlin M, Hoffman JR. Exercise effects stress-induced analgesia and spatial learning in rats. Physiol Behav 2006;89:582–6.
26. Galdino GS, Duarte ID, Perez AC. Participation of endogenous opioids in the antinociception induced by resistance exercise in rats. Braz J Med Biol Res 2010;43:906–9.
27. Denning GM, Ackermann LW, Barna TJ, et al. Proenkephalin expression and enkephalin release are widely observed in non-neuronal tissues. Peptides 2008;29:83–92.
28. Sluka KA. Central mechanisms involved in pain processing. In: Sluka KA, editor. Pain Mechanisms and Management for the Physical Therapist. Seattle: IASP Press; 2009. p. 41–72.
29. Colt EW, Wardlaw SL, Frantz AG. The effect of running on plasma beta-endorphin. Life Sci 1981;28:1637–40.
30. Rahkila P, Hakala E, Alen M, et al. Beta-endorphin and corticotropin release is dependent on a threshold intensity of running exercise in male endurance athletes. Life Sci 1988;43:551–8.
31. Rahkila P, Hakala E, Salminen K, et al. Response of plasma endorphins to running exercises in male and female endurance athletes. Med Sci Sports Exerc 1987;19:451–5.
32. Smith MA, Yancey DL. Sensitivity to the effects of opioids in rats with free access to exercise wheels: mu-opioid tolerance and physical dependence. Psychopharmacology (Berl) 2003;168:426–34.
33. D'Anci KE, Gerstein AV, Kanarek RB. Long-term voluntary access to running wheels decreases kappa-opioid antinociception. Pharmacol Biochem Behav 2000;66:343–6.
34. Mathes WF, Kanarek RB. Chronic running wheel activity attenuates the antinociceptive actions of morphine and morphine-6-glucouronide administration into the periaqueductal gray in rats. Pharmacol Biochem Behav 2006;83:578–84.
35. Mathes WF, Kanarek RB. Wheel running attenuates the antinociceptive properties of morphine and its metabolite, morphine-6-glucuronide, in rats. Physiol Behav 2001;74:245–51.
36. Stagg NJ, Mata HP, Ibrahim MM, et al. Regular exercise reverses sensory hypersensitivity in a rat neuropathic pain model: role of endogenous opioids. Anesthesiol 2011;114:940–8.
37. Shankarappa SA, Piedras-Renteria ES, Stubbs EB Jr. Forced-exercise delays neuropathic pain in experimental diabetes: effects on voltage-activated calcium channels. J Neurochem 2011; 118:224–36.
38. Bement MK, Sluka KA. Low-intensity exercise reverses chronic muscle pain in the rat in a naloxone-dependent manner. Arch Phys Med Rehabil 2005;86:1736–40.
39. Martins DF, Mazzardo-Martins L, Soldi F, et al. High-intensity swimming exercise reduces neuropathic pain in an animal model of complex regional pain syndrome type I: evidence for a role of the adenosinergic system. Neuroscience 2013;234:69–76.
40. Sluka KA, O'Donnell JM, Danielson J, et al. Regular physical activity prevents development of chronic pain and activation of central neurons. J Appl Physiol 2013;114:725–33.
41. Sharma NK, Ryals JM, Gajewski BJ, et al. Aerobic exercise alters analgesia and neurotrophin-3 synthesis in an animal model of chronic widespread pain. Phys Ther 2010;90:714–25.
42. Gandhi R, Ryals JM, Wright DE. Neurotrophin-3 reverses chronic mechanical hyperalgesia induced by intramuscular acid injection. J Neurosci 2004;24:9405–13.
43. Sluka KA, Walsh DM. Transcutaneous electrical nerve stimulation and interferential current. In: Sluka KA, editor. Mechanisms adn Management of Pain for the Physical Therapist. Seattle: IASP Press; 2009. p. 167–90.
44. Sluka KA, Marchand S, Bjordal JM, et al. What makes TENS work? Making sense of the clinical literature. Phys Ther 2013; 93:1397–402.
45. Bennett MI, Hughes N, Johnson MI. Methodological quality in randomised controlled trials of transcutaneous electric nerve stimulation for pain: low fidelity may explain negative findings. Pain 2011;152:1226–32.

46. Bjordal JM, Johnson MI, Lopes-Martins RA, et al. Short-term efficacy of physical interventions in osteoarthritic knee pain. A systematic review and meta-analysis of randomised placebo-controlled trials. BMC Musculoskelet Disord 2007;8:51.

47. Bjordal JM, Johnson MI, Ljunggreen AE. Transcutaneous electrical nerve stimulation (TENS) can reduce postoperative analgesic consumption. A meta-analysis with assessment of optimal treatment parameters for postoperative pain. Eur J Pain 2003;7:181–8.

48. Jin DM, Xu Y, Geng DF, et al. Effect of transcutaneous electrical nerve stimulation on symptomatic diabetic peripheral neuropathy: a meta-analysis of randomized controlled trials. Diabetes Res Clin Practice 2010;89:10–15.

49. Hurlow A, Bennett MI, Robb KA, et al. Transcutaneous electric nerve stimulation (TENS) for cancer pain in adults. Cochrane Database Syst Rev 2012;(3):CD006276.

50. Khadilkar A, Odebiyi DO, Brosseau L, et al. Transcutaneous electrical nerve stimulation (TENS) versus placebo for chronic low-back pain. Cochrane Database Syst Rev 2008;CD003008.

51. Kroeling P, Gross A, Goldsmith CH, et al. Electrotherapy for neck pain. Cochrane Database Syst Rev 2009;CD004251.

52. Nnoaham KE, Kumbang J. Transcutaneous electrical nerve stimulation (TENS) for chronic pain. Cochrane Database Syst Rev 2008;CD003222.

53. Rutjes AW, Nuesch E, Sterchi R, et al. Transcutaneous electrostimulation for osteoarthritis of the knee. Cochrane Database Syst Rev 2009;CD002823.

54. Walsh DM, Howe TE, Johnson MI, et al. Transcutaneous electrical nerve stimulation for acute pain (review). Cochrane Database Syst Rev 2009;CD006142.

55. Dowswell T, Bedwell C, Lavender T, et al. Transcutaneous electrical nerve stimulation (TENS) for pain relief in labour. Cochrane Database Syst Rev 2009;CD007214.

56. Dailey DL, Vance CGT, Liebano RE, et al. Transcutaneous Electrical Nerve Stimulation (TENS) reduces and improves function in people with fibromyalgia. J Pain 2012;12:23.

57. Rakel B, Frantz R. Effectiveness of transcutaneous electrical nerve stimulation on postoperative pain with movement. J Pain 2003;4:455–64.

58. Law PPW, Cheing GLY, Tsui AYY. Does transcutaneous electrical nerve stimulation improve the physical performance of people with knee osteoarthritis? J Clin Rheumatol 2004;10:295–9.

59. Vance CG, Rakel BA, Blodgett NP, et al. Effects of transcutaneous electrical nerve stimulation on pain, pain sensitivity, and function in people with knee osteoarthritis: a randomized controlled trial. Phys Ther 2012.

60. Cheing GL, Luk ML. Transcutaneous electrical nerve stimulation for neuropathic pain. J Hand Surg [Br] 2005;30:50–5.

61. Liebano R, Rakel B, Vance C, et al. An investigation of the development of analgesic tolerance to Transcutaneous Electrical Nerve Stimulation (TENS) in humans. Pain 2011;152:335–42.

62. Leonard G, Courtier C, Marchand S. Reduced analgesic effect of acupuncture-like TENS but not conventional TENS in opioid-treated patients. J Pain 2011;12:929–35.

63. Chandran P, Sluka KA. Development of opioid tolerance with repeated transcutaneous electrical nerve stimulation administration. Pain 2003;102:195–201.

64. Sato KL, Sanada LS, Rakel BA, et al. Increasing intensity of TENS prevents analgesic tolerance in rats. J Pain 2012;13:884–90.

65. DeSantana JM, Santana-Filho VJ, Sluka KA. Modulation between high- and low-frequency transcutaneous electric nerve stimulation delays the development of analgesic tolerance in arthritic rats. Arch Phys Med Rehabil 2008;89:754–60.

66. Facci LM, Nowotny JP, Tormen F, et al. Effects of transcutaneous electrical nerve stimulation (TENS) and interferential currents (IFC) in patients with nonspecific chronic low back pain: randomized clinical trial. Sao Paulo Med J 2011;129:206–16.

67. Marchand S, Charest J, Li J, et al. Is TENS purely a placebo effect? A controlled study on chronic low back pain. Pain 1993;54:99–106.

68. Law PP, Cheing GL. Optimal stimulation frequency of transcutaneous electrical nerve stimulation on people with knee osteoarthritis. J Rehabil Med 2004;36:220–5.

69. Rakel B, Cooper N, Adams HJ, et al. A new transient sham TENS device allows for investigator blinding while delivering a true placebo treatment. J Pain 2010;11:230–8.

70. Moran F, Leonard T, Hawthorne S, et al. Hypoalgesia in response to Transcutaneous Electrical Nerve Stimulation (TENS) depends on stimulation intensity. J Pain 2011;12:929–35.

71. Aarskog R, Johnson MI, Demmink JH, et al. Is mechanical pain threshold after transcutaneous electrical nerve stimulation (TENS) increased locally and unilaterally? A randomized placebo-controlled trial in healthy subjects. Physiother Res Int 2007;12:251–63.

72. Levin MF, Hui-Chan CW. Conventional and acupuncture-like transcutaneous electrical nerve stimulation excite similar afferent fibers. Arch Phys Med Rehabil 1993;74:54–60.

73. Radhakrishnan R, Sluka KA. Deep tissue afferents, but not cutaneous afferents, mediate TENS-induced antihyperalgesia. J Pain 2005;6:673–80.

74. Desantana JM, Sluka KA. Blockade of the ventrolateral PAG prevents the effects of TENS. Neuroscience 2009;163:1233–41.

75. Kalra A, Urban MO, Sluka KA. Blockade of opioid receptors in rostral ventral medulla prevents antihyperalgesia produced by transcutaneous electrical nerve stimulation (TENS). J Pharmacol Exp Ther 2001;298:257–63.

76. Sluka KA, Deacon M, Stibal A, et al. Spinal blockade of opioid receptors prevents the analgesia produced by TENS in arthritic rats. J Pharmacol Exp Ther 1999;289:840–6.

77. Lee KH, Chung JM, Willis WD. Inhibition of primate spinothalamic tract cells by TENS. J Neurosurg 1985;62:276–87.

78. Sjolund BH. Peripheral nerve stimulation suppression of C-fiber evoked flexion reflex in rats. Part 1: Parameters of continuous stimulation. J Neurosurg 1985;63:612–16.

79. Sjolund BH. Peripheral nerve stimulation suppression of C-fiber evoked flexion reflex in rats. Part 2. Parameters of low rat train stimulation of skin and muscle afferent nerves. J Neurosurg 1988;68:279–83.

80. Garrison DW, Foreman RD. Decreased activity of spontaneous and noxiously evoked dorsal horn cells during transcutaneous electrical nerve stimulation (TENS). Pain 1994;58:309–15.

81. Garrison DW, Foreman RD. Effects of prolonged transcutaneous electrical nerve stimulation (TENS) and variation of stimulation variables on dorsal horn cell activity. Europ J Phys Med Rehabil 1997;6:87–94.

82. Somers DL, Clemente FR. High-frequency transcutaneous electrical nerve stimulation alters thermal but not mechanical allodynia following chronic constriction injury of the rat sciatic nerve. Arch Phys Med Rehabil 1998;79:1370–6.

83. Nam TS, Choi Y, Yeon DS, et al. Differential antinociceptive effect of transcutaneous electrical stimulation on pain behavior sensitive or insensitive to phentolamine in neuropathic rats. Neurosci Lett 2001;301:17–20.

84. Leem JW, Park ES, Paik KS. Electrophysiological evidence for the antinociceptive effect of transcutaneous electrical nerve stimulation on mechanically evoked responsiveness of dorsal horn neurons in neuropathic rats. Neurosci Lett 1995;192:197–200.

85. Ma YT, Sluka KA. Reduction in inflammation-induced sensitization of dorsal horn neurons by transcutaneous electrical nerve stimulation in anesthetized rats. Exp Brain Res 2001;137:94–102.

86. Sluka KA, Bailey K, Bogush J, et al. Treatment with either high or low frequency TENS reduces the secondary hyperalgesia observed after injection of kaolin and carrageenan into the knee joint. Pain 1998;77:97–102.

87. Vance CG, Radhakrishnan R, Skyba DA, et al. Transcutaneous electrical nerve stimulation at both high and low frequencies reduces primary hyperalgesia in rats with joint inflammation in a time-dependent manner. Phys Ther 2007;87(1):44–51.

88. Ainsworth L, Budelier K, Clinesmith M, et al. Transcutaneous electrical nerve stimulation (TENS) reduces chronic hyperalgesia induced by muscle inflammation. Pain 2006;120:182–7.

89. Gopalkrishnan P, Sluka KA. Effect of varying frequency, intensity and pulse duration of TENS on primary hyperalgesia in inflamed rats. Arch Phys Med Rehabil 2000;81:984–90.

90. Resende MA, Sabino GG, Candido CRM, et al. Transcutaneous electrical stimulation (TENS) effects in experimental inflammatory edema and pain. Eur J Pharmacol 2004;504:217–22.

91. Salar G, Job I, Mingrino S, et al. Effect of transcutaneous electrotherapy on CSF β-endorphin content in patients without pain problems. Pain 1981;10:169–72.

92. Han JS, Chen XH, Sun SL, et al. Effect of low and high frequency TENS on met-enkephalin-arg-phe and dynorphin A immunoreactivity in human lumbar CSF. Pain 1991;47:295–8.

93. DeSantana JM, da Silva LF, De Resende MA, et al. Transcutaneous electrical nerve stimulation at both high and low frequencies activates ventrolateral periaqueductal grey to decrease mechanical hyperalgesia in arthritic rats. N S 2009;163:1233–41.

94. Radhakrishnan R, Sluka KA. Spinal muscarinic receptors are activated during low or high frequency TENS-induced antihyperalgesia in rats. Neuropharm 2003;45:1111–19.

95. Maeda Y, Lisi TL, Vance CG, et al. Releaes of GABA and activation of GABA$_A$ receptors in the spinal cord mediates the effects of TENS in rats. Brain Res 2007;1136:43–50.

96. Radhakrishnan R, King EW, Dickman J, et al. Blockade of spinal 5-HT receptor subtypes prevents low, but not high, frequency TENS-induced antihyperalgesia in rats. Pain 2003;105:205–13.

97. Rokugo T, Takeuchi T, Ito H. A histochemical study of substance P in the rat spinal cord: effect of transcutaneous electrical nerve stimulation. J Nippon Med Sch 2002;69:428–33.

98. Sluka KA, Vance CGT, Lisi TL. High-frequency, but not low-frequency, transcutaneous electrical nerve stimulation reduces aspartate and glutamate release in the spinal cord dorsal horn. J Neurochem 2005;95:1794–801.

99. King EW, Audette K, Athman GA, et al. Transcutaneous electrical nerve stimulation activates peripherally located alpha-2A adrenergic receptors. Pain 2005;115:364–73.

100. Sluka KA, Lisi TL, Westlund KN. Increased release of serotonin in the spinal cord during low, but not high, frequency TENS in rats with joint inflammation. Arch Phys Med Rehab 2006;87:1137–40.

101. Sabino GS, Santos CM, Francischi JN, et al. Release of endogenous opioids following transcutaneous electric nerve stimulation in an experimental model of acute inflammatory pain. J Pain 2008;9:157–63.

102. Sherry JE, Oehrlein KM, Hegge KS, et al. Effect of burst-mode transcutaneous electrical nerve stimulation on peripheral vascular resistence. Phys Ther 2001;81:1183–91.

103. Cramp FL, McCullough GR, Lowe AS, et al. Transcutaneous electric nerve stimulation: the effect of intensity on local and distal cutaneous blood flow and skin temperature in healthy subjects. Arch Phys Med Rehabil 2002;83:5–9.

104. Cramp AF, Gilsenan C, Lowe AS, et al. The effect of high- and low-frequency transcutaneous electrical nerve stimulation upon cutaneous blood flow and skin temperature in healthy subjects. Clin Physiol 2000;20:150–7.

105. Chen CC, Johnson MI, McDonough S, et al. The effect of transcutaneous electrical nerve stimulation on local and distal cutaneous blood flow following a prolonged heat stimulus in healthy subjects. Clin Physiol Funct Imaging 2007;27:154–61.

106. Sandberg ML, Sandberg MK, Dahl J. Blood flow changes in the trapezius muscle and overlying skin following transcutaneous electrical nerve stimulation. Phys Ther 2007;87:1047–55.

107. Patel KC, Gross A, Graham N, et al. Massage for mechanical neck disorders. Cochrane Database Syst Rev 2012;(9):CD004871.

108. Furlan AD, Imamura M, Dryden T, et al. Massage for low-back pain. Cochrane Database Syst Rev 2008;CD001928.

109. Furlan AD, Yazdi F, Tsertsvadze A, et al. A systematic review and meta-analysis of efficacy, cost-effectiveness, and safety of selected complementary and alternative medicine for neck and low-back pain. Evid Based Complement Alternat Med 2012;2012:953139.

110. Plews-Ogan M, Owens JE, Goodman M, et al. A pilot study evaluating mindfulness-based stress reduction and massage for the management of chronic pain. J Gen Intern Med 2005;20:1136–8.

111. Gross A, Miller J, D'Sylva J, et al. Manipulation or mobilisation for neck pain. Cochrane Database Syst Rev 2010;CD004249.

112. Rubinstein SM, Terwee CB, Assendelft WJ, et al. Spinal manipulative therapy for acute low-back pain. Cochrane Database Syst Rev 2012;(9):CD008880.

113. Rubinstein SM, van MM, Assendelft WJ, et al. Spinal manipulative therapy for chronic low-back pain. Cochrane Database Syst Rev 2011;CD008112.

114. Rubinstein SM, van MM, Assendelft WJ, et al. Spinal manipulative therapy for chronic low-back pain. Cochrane Database Syst Rev 2011;CD008112.

115. Delitto A, George SZ, Van Dillen LR, et al. Low back pain. J Orthop Sports Phys Ther 2012;42:A1–57.

116. Childs JD, Cleland JA, Elliott JM, et al. Neck pain: clinical practice guidelines linked to the International Classification of Functioning, Disability, and Health from the Orthopedic Section of the American Physical Therapy Association. J Orthop Sports Phys Ther 2008;38:A1–34.

117. Kelley MJ, Shaffer MA, Kuhn JE, et al. Shoulder pain and mobility deficits: adhesive capsulitis. J Orthop Sports Phys Ther 2013;43:A1–31.

118. Carcia CR, Martin RL, Houck J, et al. Achilles pain, stiffness, and muscle power deficits: achilles tendinitis. J Orthop Sports Phys Ther 2010;40:A1–26.

119. McPoil TG, Martin RL, Cornwall MW, et al. Heel pain–plantar fasciitis: clinical practice guildelines linked to the international classification of function, disability, and health from the orthopaedic section of the American Physical Therapy Association. J Orthop Sports Phys Ther 2008;38:A1–18.

120. Moss P, Sluka KA, Wright A. The initial effects of knee joint mobilisation on osteoarthritic hyperalgesia. Man Ther 2006;12:109–18.

121. Vicenzino B, Collins D, Wright A. The initial effects of a cervical spine manipulative physiotherapy treatment on the pain and dysfunction of lateral epicondylalgia. Pain 1996;68:69–74.

122. Vicenzino B, Paungmali A, Buratowski S, et al. Specific manipulative therapy treatment for chronic lateral epicondylalgia produces uniquely characteristic hypoalgesia. Man Ther 2001;6:205–12.

123. Lund I, Ge Y, Yu LC, et al. Repeated massage-like stimulation induces long-term effects on nociception: contribution of oxytocinergic mechanisms. Eur J Neurosci 2002;16:330–8.

124. Agren G, Lundeberg T, Uvnas-Moberg K, et al. The oxytocin antagonist 1-deamino-2-D-Tyr-(Oet)-4-Thr-8-Orn-oxytocin reverses the increase in the withdrawal response latency to thermal, but not mechanical nociceptive stimuli following oxytocin administration or massage-like stroking in rats. Neurosci Lett 1995;187:49–52.

125. Crane JD, Ogborn DI, Cupido C, et al. Massage therapy attenuates inflammatory signaling after exercise-induced muscle damage. Sci Transl Med 2012;4:119ra13.

126. George SZ, Bishop MD, Bialosky JE, et al. Immediate effects of spinal manipulation on thermal pain sensitivity: an experimental study. BMC Musculoskelet Disord 2006;7:68.

127. Bialosky JE, Bishop MD, Robinson ME, et al. The influence of expectation on spinal manipulation induced hypoalgesia: an experimental study in normal subjects. BMC Musculoskelet Disord 2008;9:19.

128. Vicenzino B, Gutschlag F, Collins D, et al. An investigation of the effects of spinal manual therapy on forequarter pressure and thermal pain thresholds and sympathetic nervous system activity in asymptomatic subjects In: Shacklock M (ed). Moving in on Pain, Butterworth Heinemann, Adelaide 1995.

129. Wright A, Vicenzino B. Cervical mobilisation techniques, sympathetic nervous system effects and their relationship to analgesia. In: Schacklock M, editor. Moving in on Pain. Adelaide: Butterworth Heinneman; 1995. p. 164–73.

130. Bulbulian R, Burke J, Dishman JD. Spinal reflex excitability changes after lumbar spine passive flexion mobilization. J Manipulative Physiol Ther 2002;25:526–32.

131. Dishman JD, Bulbulian R. Spinal reflex attenuation associated with spinal manipulation. Spine 2000;25:2519–24.

132. Ferreira ML, Ferreira PH, Latimer J, et al. Comparison of general exercise, motor control exercise and spinal manipulative therapy for chronic low back pain: a randomized trial. Pain 2007;131:31–7.

133. Sung PS, Kang YM, Pickar JG. Effect of spinal manipulation duration on low threshold mechanoreceptors in lumbar paraspinal muscles – A preliminary report. Spine 2005;30:115–22.

134. Pickar JG. Neurophysiological effects of spinal manipulation. Spine J 2002;2:357–71.

135. George SZ, Bishop MD, Bialosky JE, et al. Immediate effects of spinal manipulation on thermal pain sensitivity: an experimental study. BMC Musculoskelet Disord 2006;7:68.

136. Bialosky JE, Bishop MD, Robinson ME, et al. The influence of expectation on spinal manipulation induced hypoalgesia: an experimental study in normal subjects. BMC Musculoskelet Disord 2008;9:19.

137. Moss P, Sluka KA, Wright A. The initial effects of knee joint mobilisation on osteoarthritic hyperalgesia. Man Ther 2006; 12:109–18.

138. Skyba DA, Radhakrishnan R, Rohlwing JJ, et al. Joint manipulation reduces hyperalgesia by activation of monoamine receptors but not opioid or GABA receptors in the spinal cord. Pain 2003;106:159–68.

139. Sluka KA, Wright A. Knee joint mobilization reduces secondary mechanical hyperalgesia induced by capsaicin injection into the ankle joint. Europ J Pain 2001;5:81–7.

140. Zusman M, Edwards BC, Donaghy A. Investigation of a proposed mechanism for the relief of spinal pain with passive joitn movement. J Manual Med 1989;4:58–61.

141. Vicenzino B, O'Callahan J, Kermode F, et al. No influence of naloxone on the initial hypoalgesic effect of spinal manual therapy. In: Devor M, Rowbotham MC, Wiesenfeld-Hallin Z, editors. Proceedings from the 9th World Congress on Pain. Seattle: IASP Press; 2000. p. 1039–44.

142. Paungmali A, O'Leary S, Souvlis T, et al. Naloxone fails to antagonize initial hypoalgesic effect of a manual therapy treatment for lateral epicondylalgia. J Manipulative Physiol Ther 2004;27: 180–5.

143. Martins DF, Bobinski F, Mazzardo-Martins L, et al. Ankle joint mobilization decreases hypersensitivity by activation of peripheral opioid receptors in a mouse model of postoperative pain. Pain Med 2012;13:1049–58.

144. Martins DF, Mazzardo-Martins L, Cidral-Filho FJ, et al. Ankle joint mobilization affects postoperative pain through peripheral and central adenosine A1 receptors. Phys Ther 2013;93:401–12.

145. Martins DF, Mazzardo-Martins L, Cidral-Filho FJ, et al. Peripheral and spinal activation of cannabinoid receptors by joint mobilization alleviates postoperative pain in mice. N S 2013; 255:110–21.

146. Martins DF, Mazzardo-Martins L, Gadotti VM, et al. Ankle joint mobilization reduces axonotmesis-induced neuropathic pain and glial activation in the spinal cord and enhances nerve regeneration in rats. Pain 2011;152(11):2653–61.

CHAPTER 29

Spinal Manipulation

Christopher McCarthy • Joel Bialosky • Darren Rivett

INTRODUCTION

Spinal manipulation (SM) is a modality ubiquitous to most cultures, and possesses an evidence base that supports its use in contemporary musculoskeletal practice.[1] However, there are a number of issues regarding this ancient and modern practice that lead some health-care practitioners to take an adamant stance against the use of these techniques.[2,3] The debate regarding the use of manipulation in the modern musculoskeletal management of spinal dysfunction is fuelled by some crucial issues regarding the objectives of and evidence for SM. It may be that uncertainty regarding both the mechanisms and effectiveness of SM, coupled with uncertainty regarding the terminology being used to define SM are hampering the understanding of this approach to spinal dysfunction. It would appear that there is lack of clarity in the evidence base, resulting in differences in the relative importance placed on the techniques by differing manipulative professions. For example, British chiropractors will manipulate cervical spine patients 20 times more frequently than Irish physiotherapists.[4,5] If the understanding of the mechanisms, effectiveness and objectives of the technique were defined, presumably we would not see such marked professional differences in the utilization of SM techniques.

This chapter will endeavour to address these issues in three sections. The first section will consider some of the proposed aims and objectives of SM and suggest a definition of SM that reflects the biomechanical, neurophysiological and psychosocial mechanisms that will be discussed in the second section. In light of the evidence for clinical effectiveness, a discussion of some of the risks of SM and methods we may use to reduce risk will be discussed in Section 3 of this chapter.

DEFINING SPINAL MANIPULATION

When one considers the amount of scientific and lay literature on spinal manipulation, it is perhaps surprising to find no absolute consensus on the definition of manipulation. Typically the definition will make reference to some form of passive handling of the spine[6] or some reference to a low-amplitude highly accelerative thrusting movement applied to the passive patient.[7] In addition, there may be some reference to the point in passive range of movement where a technique is applied, varying from being at 'a restriction in range' to 'a range that extends slightly beyond the patient's physiological range of movement'.[6,7]

A commonly cited definition would take the form of 'a forced, passive movement of vertebral segments, carrying the elements of articulation beyond the usual range of movement to the limit of anatomic range'.[8] Clearly this form of definition details the mechanism of how one might apply a technique to the vertebral column but does not define what the technique is. This is not the typical format one expects when defining a therapeutic procedure. For example, another specific form of manual therapy, the Elpey manoeuvre,[9] is defined as 'a canalith repositioning manoeuvre to reposition otolithic debris from the semicircular ducts, to the utricle in benign paroxysmal positional vertigo'. It is not defined as 'four sequential movements of the neck performed in sitting and lying in paroxysmal positional vertigo'. An adequate definition carries some information regarding the objectives and mechanisms of the treatment, in the context of the dysfunction it is being utilized in. In light of the mechanisms discussed in this chapter we will offer a new definition of SM for the reader's consideration.

One method of developing a definition would be to undertake a review of SM techniques to identifying similarities and disparities in approach and thus define the key components of SM. A review of multidisciplinary textbooks,[10-13] reveal two common approaches to SM, which one might term 'direct contact gapping' and 'positional gapping'. Direct contact gapping techniques involve direct application of operator force on two adjacent vertebral segments, with force application in a direction that produces segmental motion leading to joint surface separation. The example in Figure 29-1 shows the right side of T5 is directed in a posterior–anterior and cephalad direction while the left side of T6 is simultaneously directed in a posterior–anterior and caudad direction.

In contrast, positional gapping is commonly applied in regions of the vertebral column, where it is difficult to directly contact both vertebrae and move them in the opposing directions simultaneously. For example, in the mid-lumbar and mid-cervical spines vertebral segments are positioned in starting positions that do not follow the normal coupled movements of the region (see Fig. 29-1). In these positions one segment can be stabilized while the other is moved away from it in a direction the patient cannot easily induce themselves.[14-16] Many authors[6,16,17] have suggested that the direction of motion produced results in separation of joint surfaces, in contrast to the typical translatory motions invoked by mobilization techniques that are aimed along facet joint planes (i.e. Nags

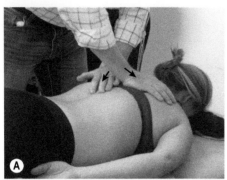
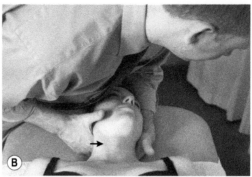

FIGURE 29-1 ■ **(A)** The direct gapping of T5 and T6 with little spinal position required but direct contact on adjacent vertebral segments and movement directed posterior–anteriorly (not along the plane of the facet joint). **(B)** The positioning of the vertebral segments in small degrees of extension, right lateral flexion and left rotation (not the natural coupling of these movements) with movement being induced at a plane perpendicular to the plane of the right zygapophyseal joint, unlike mobilizations following the facet joint surface plane.

and Snags).[18] Thus motion that results in joint surface separation or gapping could be considered to be a defining feature of manipulation, distinguishing the technique from segmental mobilizations that do not aim to produce surface separation.

The neurophysiological mechanisms for why this phenomenon might contribute to pain relief and return to function will be discussed in depth in Section 2 (Neurophysiological effects); however, there are a number of theoretical perspectives on the effects of manipulation that may have led to some of the disparity in perceived objectives of SM. With differing anticipated effects of a technique, come differing approaches to application of SM. An SM technique in the hands of one clinician could appear very gentle and comfortable whereas a clinician with a differing objective could undertake an SM technique that may appear to be a vigorous, end-of-range stretch. Both clinicians would define their intervention as an SM technique; however, the objective, application and therefore effect of the technique could be very disparate. When evaluating the effect of SM, researchers need to be aware that while a group of intervening clinician may be undertaking SM techniques, not all clinicians will perform the techniques in the same manner and perceptions of the objectives of SM may differ.

OBJECTIVES OF SPINAL MANIPULATION (BIOMECHANICAL)

Stretching/Tearing Tissue?

One commonly perceived objective of SM is the production of a tensile stress sufficient to cause lengthening of tissue, or even 'tearing of adhesions'.[19] With this objective in mind, manipulation is typically undertaken towards the end of passive range and has the objective of producing movement that extends to the anatomical integrity of tissue. However, if one accepts that one of the key defining features of SM is to gap the joint surfaces it would seem unlikely that this objective will be met if the joint capsule has been tightened to the limit of extensibility. If anything you could argue that the joint surfaces are in a position where they are least likely to separate when

moved under extreme capsular tension.[6] Spinal manipulation techniques, applied with this objective tend to involve low-amplitude, high-velocity and high-force thrusts, in order to overcome the tension induced by the end-of-range positioning.[19,20]

In light of the viscoelastic properties of collagenous tissue there is a natural rebound to rapidly applied forces, meaning that at higher speeds more force is required to produce elongation than when forces are applied at slow speeds.[21] Thus while the objective of this type of approach to SM is lengthening of tissue, one is left to consider if this is an optimal method of stretching the vertebral columns of patients in pain. It is proposed that the surface separation, induced by SM, could break microscopic, intra-articular adhesions evident in immobilized facet joints;[17] however, these adhesions are not currently visible in vivo when imaged with the highest resolution MRI scanners, and thus we have no evidence to support the theory. Of course it is equally feasible that mobilization, not just SM, could break these adhesions. Thus, as the link between SM and lengthening tissue is not clear we will not include it within our definition of SM.

Inducing Cavitation Within the Joint?

Cavitation phenomenon is the formation and collapse of bubbles (cavities) within the synovial fluid of spinal joints and has been observed during SM.[22-24] Surface separation, resulting in an increase in intra-articular volume, will drop intra-articular pressure. If pressures fall to a threshold level, 'vapour pressure' micro-clouds of bubbles will form within the synovial fluid.[15] The subsequent gaseous/fluid mix results in a transient period, where less force is required to induce movement.[25,26] This minor, transient effect lasts approximately 20–60 minutes.[22,24]

Cavitation phenomenon is well described in engineering fields as a phenomenon that is damaging to engines (associated with the rapid changes in fluid pressure in pistons) and this has led some authors to consider whether cavitation phenomenon is in itself damaging to the articular cartilage of the synovial joint.[27,28] However, cohort studies of metacarpophalangeal 'knuckle crackers' have revealed no increase in the odds of developing osteoarthritis in these joints.[29,30] One might extrapolate these

the dorsal horn of the spinal cord with a temporal summation protocol.[74,75] Subsequently, SM-related attenuation of temporal summation suggests a mechanism corresponding to modification of dorsal horn excitability.

A reflex link exists between the lumbar joint capsule and the paraspinal musculature.[76,77] The mechanical force from SM may stimulate this neuromuscular reflex response resulting in pain inhibition related to counter irritation[78] or proprioceptive input to the central nervous system.[79] Stimulation of this link is suggested by studies demonstrating afferent discharge in response to SM. For example, positive action potentials at the S1 nerve root have been recorded in response to SM in anaesthetized subjects undergoing spinal surgery.[80,81]

A lessening of the spinal motoneuron pool excitability is associated with SM. The Hoffman Reflex (H-reflex) is comparable to a monosynaptic stretch reflex; however, it utilizes electrical stimulation as the stimulus. A decrease in H-reflex has been observed following SM in the lumbar[40,82] and cervical spine.[83] Collectively, these findings suggest a brief inhibition of motoneuron pool excitability speculated to result from Ia afferents.[84] The characteristic hypoalgesia and decrease in muscle spasm frequently accompanying SM in the clinical setting may result from the related diminished afferent input to the spinal cord.

Potential Supraspinally Mediated Mechanisms

SM may directly influence the supraspinal structures to impart its clinical effect. Hypoalgesia accompanying SM is characterized by similar features as that observed in animal studies of direct stimulation of the periaqueductal grey leading to speculation of similar mechanisms.[85] More recently, changes in cortical excitability have been observed in response to SM in individuals with recurring neck pain as indicated by somatosensory evoked potentials[86,87] and transcranial magnetic stimulation.[88,89] Changes in cortical excitability as indicated by transcranial magnetic stimulation have also been observed in response to SM applied to the lumbar spine in healthy individuals.[90] Collectively, these studies suggest a supraspinally mediated effect of SM on nervous system excitability with potential implications for clinical outcomes. Imaging modalities are improving and offer the potential for more direct visualization of nervous system responses to SM. A recent study used functional magnetic resonance imaging to visualize changes in pain processing following SM. Ten healthy participants were imaged during a painful task prior to and immediately following SM directed to the thoracic spine. Changes in cerebral blood flow corresponding to changes in pain ratings were observed following the SM.[88]

Placebo is a psychological and biologically active process associated with a robust analgesic effect[91] and reflective of descending inhibitory mechanisms of pain inhibition.[92] Subsequently, placebo effects represent a supraspinally mediated mechanism of SM. Placebo mechanisms play a role in all interventions for pain. For example, pain medication is significantly more effective when patients are aware they are receiving it than treatment that is concealed.[93] Similarly, placebo

mechanisms are likely influential in the response to SM.[94] While not studied extensively in SM, placebo mechanisms are influential in other types of complementary and alternative medicine. For example, Kalauokalani et al.,[95] randomly assigned 135 individuals with chronic LBP to receive either acupuncture or massage. Group differences were not observed in clinical outcomes; however, participants with greater expectation for acupuncture and receiving acupuncture had significantly better outcomes than those with higher expectation for massage who received acupuncture and vice versa. Specific to SM, baseline expectations for improvement and to benefit from SM were associated with better clinical outcomes at 4 weeks in participants with neck pain receiving SM to the thoracic spine.[44] Additionally, attenuation of temporal summation in response to SM as has been observed in several studies[35,70–72] may be negated if participants expect more pain following the SM.[43]

SAFETY AND PRACTICAL ISSUES ASSOCIATED WITH SPINAL MANIPULATION

A number of systematic reviews of the randomized controlled trial literature have concluded that SM is effective in the reduction of spinal pain and is cost-effective[96–98] Despite this, there has been much controversy over many years regarding the risk of adverse events following the application of spinal manipulation, in particular cervical spine manipulation.[99] Risk estimates have focused on dissection injury to the vertebral artery leading to stroke, but vary widely from 1 in 163 000[100] manipulations to about 1 in 5 000 000.[101] Most estimates are inherently flawed as they have usually relied on retrospective methodologies, usually surveys of practitioners or searches of insurance or medical records. Recall bias, incomplete records and legal restrictions may limit the accuracy of the data relating to the number of adverse events, while the number of actual manipulations performed (the denominator) is generally an estimate extrapolated from a limited sample of practitioners. At best we can state that the risk of stroke following neck manipulation is unknown but that the actual incidence is likely very rare.[102] It is this rareness that makes it very difficult to conduct any sort of meaningful prospective study of serious complications, such as craniocervical arterial dissection and consequent stroke.

A recent systematic review[102] of adverse events related to manual therapy (including manipulation) reported that nearly half of all patients undergoing manual therapy will experience transient and minor adverse effects, typically increased pain and most commonly after the first treatment. No serious adverse events were found and it was concluded that the risk of such events was lower than from taking medication for the same condition.

Minimizing Risk in Applying Manipulation

To help avoid adverse events, manipulation should be applied using the same principles as for passive joint mobilization of the spine. That is, manipulation should be viewed simply as an extension or progression of mobilization, as Maitland et al.[103] and other clinical authorities have long advocated. Mobilization should be applied initially and its effects evaluated over the time period between consecutive treatment sessions. Manipulation should generally only be applied when mobilization has been progressed in vigour or grade, and when its effects are no longer satisfactory.

Further recommendations to promote the safe application of spinal manipulation are as follows.[104–107]

- Minimal force should be applied to any spinal structure. Low-amplitude and short lever thrust techniques are preferable.
- Spinal manipulation techniques should at all times feel comfortable to the patient. In applying cervical spine manipulation, placing the patient's head on a pillow in supine lying is often more comfortable to the patient than alternative positions. This position also allows the practitioner to better monitor the patient's facial expression and for any nystagmus.
- Neck manipulation techniques should not be performed at the end of range of overall cervical spine physiological movement, especially for extension and rotation. The head and cervical spine segments not included in the manipulation can be used to direct loads to the targeted segment, thus minimizing stress on the rest of the neck.[9]
- Positioning and briefly holding the patient in the pre-manipulative test position is advisable prior to thrusting to evaluate patient comfort and to feel for any protective muscle spasm or other concerning end-feel. In neck manipulation, enquiry should specifically be made about any dizziness in the pre-manipulative test position which may be indicative of vertebrobasilar insufficiency leading to cerebral ischaemia.
- Repeated manipulation within the same session or over a number of consecutive sessions should be avoided, owing to potential dangers of frequent, repeated manipulations and a lack of longer-term benefit.

The use of manipulation in the upper cervical spine is losing favour in manipulative physiotherapy because of the perceived increased risk in this region. In a survey of member organizations of the International Federation of Orthopaedic Manipulative Physical Therapists (IFOMPT) undertaken by Carlesso and Rivett in 2007,[108] eight member organizations (40%) reported that their members had decreased the use of manipulation in the upper cervical spine over the last decade. Thirteen member organizations (65%) further indicated that upper cervical spine manipulation techniques taught to practitioners in post-professional courses had been changed to limit the amount of rotation.

Clinical Reasoning and Patient Selection

Clinical reasoning refers to the thinking skills underpinning clinical practice. It is clear from the literature that many documented adverse events following the application of spinal manipulation could have been easily avoided if better clinical reasoning had been exercised by the practitioner.[104] With patients for whom spinal manipulation is contemplated, it is critically important that the patient history is used to establish and test reasoning hypotheses related to the potential for adverse events. The practitioner should aim during the patient history to make the best judgement on the likelihood of the presence of serious pathology and contraindications to spinal manipulation based on available information.

Contraindications to spinal manipulation include the following:[109]

- upper motoneuron lesion
- spinal cord compromise
- multi-level spinal nerve/nerve root compromise (cervical spine)
- deteriorating neurological status
- intense, unremitting, non-mechanical pain
- constant night pain (stopping patient from falling asleep)
- recent trauma to relevant region, especially the head and neck
- craniovertebral ligament instability
- vertebrobasilar insufficiency or internal carotid artery pathology.

The clinician should also exercise caution before applying manipulation in the presence of the following:[109]

- cervical spine anatomical anomaly
- congenital collagenous condition (e.g. Down syndrome)
- connective tissue disease
- currently or recently active cancer
- first episode of spinal pain before age 18 or after 55
- hypermobility syndrome
- inflammatory joint disease (e.g. rheumatoid arthritis, ankylosing spondylitis)
- local infection
- osteoporosis
- prolonged use of steroid medication
- recent or frequent manipulation
- systemic illness
- throat infection (cervical spine).

It is important that the clinician is aware that craniocervical arterial dissection may mimic musculoskeletal dysfunction in the early stage of its pathological progression as headache or neck pain may be the presenting symptom.[104,110,111] Indeed a patient experiencing pain from a dissecting artery may well seek manipulative therapy for the relief of their pain.[13] A high index of suspicion is particularly advisable in cases of severe, acute-onset neck or head pain described as 'unlike any other'.[111,112] To this end, it is therefore also important to recognize potential risk factors for arterial dissection because unless there are explicit signs or symptoms of neurovascular compromise (e.g. hemianopia, dysarthria) evident in the recent history or on examination, no individual or isolated clinical feature or clinical test has adequate clinical utility to detect the patient who will stroke following cervical spine manipulation.

The following factors have been proposed to increase the risk of craniocervical arterial pathology:[110–113]

- anticoagulant medication
- blood clotting disorders or changes in blood properties such as hyperhomocysteinaemia

- cardiovascular disease, especially a previous cerebrovascular accident or transient ischaemic attack
- diabetes mellitus
- history of smoking
- hypercholesterolaemia
- hyperlipidaemia
- hypertension
- immediately post-partum
- migraine-type headache
- past history of trauma to the cervical spine or head, or craniocervical arteries
- recent infection.

The physical examination generally provides minimal additional information related to the safe application of manipulation as most clinical tests have limited validity. Clearly if the physical examination elicits signs that are consistent with a mechanical joint presentation, then manual therapy (including manipulation) may be indicated in the absence of any contraindications or precautions ascertained in the patient interview or detected on testing.

Provocative positional testing for vertebrobasilar insufficiency has long been recommended in practice prior to cervical spine manipulation. Such testing is intended to provide a challenge to the vascular supply to the brain, and the provocation of signs or symptoms of cerebrovascular ischaemia during or immediately after testing is interpreted as a positive test result. Sustained end-range rotation has been advocated and has been proposed as the most provocative and valid test.[114,115] The sustained pre-manipulative test position has also been advocated.[115] However, the predictive ability of any of these positional tests to identify patients at risk of manipulative stroke is questionable and at best they can be considered a test of the adequacy of the collateral circulation in the presence of compromised contralateral vertebral artery flow.[116]

More recently, Kerry and Taylor[117] have advocated that a raft of physical tests of the cardiovascular status of an individual be undertaken pre-manipulatively, including blood pressure measurement, palpation of the carotid artery and examination of the cranial nerves. Biologically it is plausible that some of these tests may assist in detecting a patient presenting with a dissection in progress. However, there are no data demonstrating an ability of any of these cardiovascular tests, either individually or in combination, to predict the patient at risk of a craniocervical arterial dissection subsequent to neck manipulation. In fact, hypertension and most other general cardiovascular risk factors (such as smoking) have been shown as unlikely to be significant risk factors for craniocervical arterial dissection.[112]

It is important that the clinician refer the patient for immediate medical investigation when their clinical suspicion of progressive arterial dissection or other serious pathology is supported by reasoned historical features and clinical examination findings.

International Context

There are many different types of manipulative technique utilized across the world and between professions.

Interestingly, recent research into blood flow to the brain with two contrasting types of cervical spine manipulative technique found no significant differences with either technique, suggesting the type of manipulation employed may be less important than careful patient selection.[118]

There are also substantial jurisdictional differences in educational standards in spinal manipulation, as well as in regulatory restrictions to practice manipulation. To help address this, the IFOMPT member organizations have collectively endorsed an 'International Framework for Examination of the Cervical Region for Potential of Cervical Arterial Dysfunction Prior to Orthopaedic Manual Therapy Intervention'.[109] The framework is designed to provide guidance to practitioners in the assessment of the cervical spine region for the potential of cervical artery dysfunction in advance of planned manual therapy interventions, particularly neck manipulation.

CONCLUSION – DEFINITION OF SPINAL MANIPULATION

In light of the material we have presented in this chapter, we have proposed a definition of spinal manipulation that reflects our current understanding of the technique. It accepts the limitations of the evidence base in the field and thus our incomplete understanding of SM's mechanisms. It reflects our understanding of the mechanical, neurophysiological and psychological effects of SM.

Spinal manipulation is the application of rapid movement to vertebral segments producing joint surface separation, transient sensory afferent input and reduction in perception of pain. Joint surface separation will commonly result in intra-articular cavitation that, in turn, is commonly accompanied with an audible pop. Post-manipulation reductions in pain perception are influenced by supraspinal mechanisms including expectation of benefit.

REFERENCES

1. Livingston MC. The mystery and history of spinal manipulation. Can Fam Physician 1981;27(2):300–2.
2. Ernst E. Spinal manipulation: its safety is uncertain. CMAJ 2002;166(1):40–1.
3. Ernst E. Spinal manipulation: are the benefits worth the risks? Expert Rev Neurother 2007;7(11):1451–2.
4. Hurley L, Yardley K, Gross AR, et al. A survey to examine attitudes and patterns of practice of physiotherapists who perform cervical spine manipulation. Man Ther 2002;7(1):10–18.
5. Thiel H, Bolton J. Estimate of the number of treatment visits involving cervical spine manipulation by members of the British and Scottish Chiropractic association over a one year period. Clin Chiro 2004;7:163–7.
6. Evans DW. Why do spinal manipulation techniques take the form they do? Towards a general model of spinal manipulation. Man Ther 2010;15(3):212–19.
7. Moore A. Systematic review of spinal manipulation: including different techniques. J R Soc Med 2006;99(6):278–9.
8. Mosby's Medical Dictionary. 8th ed. Edinburgh: Elsevier; 2009.
9. Syed I, Ahmed W, Selvadurai D. Dix-Hallpike and Epley manoeuvres. Br J Hosp Med (Lond) 2012;73(10):C149–51.
10. Hartman L. Handbook of Osteopathic Technique. 3rd ed. London: Cengage Learning; 1996.

11. Gibbons P, Tehan P. Manipulation of the Spine, Thorax and Pelvis: An Osteopathic Perspective. 3rd ed. Elsevier Health Sciences; 2009.

12. Bergmann TF, Peterson D. Chiropractic Technique: Principles and Procedures. 3rd ed. New York: Elsevier Health Sciences; 2010.

13. McCarthy CJ. Combined Movement Theory; Rational Mobilisation and Manipulation of the Vertebral Column. Edinburgh: Elsevier Health Sciences; 2010.

14. Haas M. The physics of spinal manipulation. Part III. Some characteristics of adjusting that facilitate joint distraction. J Manipulative Physiol Ther 1990;13(6):305–8.

15. Haas M. The physics of spinal manipulation. Part IV. A theoretical consideration of the physician impact force and energy requirements needed to produce synovial joint cavitation. J Manipulative Physiol Ther 1990;13(7):378–83.

16. Herzog W. The biomechanics of spinal manipulation. J Bodyw Mov Ther 2010;14(3):280–6.

17. Cramer GD, Cambron J, Cantu JA, et al. Magnetic resonance imaging zygapophyseal joint space changes (gapping) in low back pain patients following spinal manipulation and side-posture positioning: a randomized controlled mechanisms trial with blinding. J Manipulative Physiol Ther 2013;36(4):203–17.

18. Exelby L. The Mulligan concept: its application in the management of spinal conditions. Man Ther 2002;7(2):64–70.

19. Forand D, Drover J, Suleman Z, et al. The forces applied by female and male chiropractors during thoracic spinal manipulation. J Manipulative Physiol Ther 2004;27(1):49–56.

20. Herzog W. The physics of spinal manipulation. J Manipulative Physiol Ther 1992;15(6):402–5.

21. Lopez-Garcia MD, Beebe DJ, Crone WC. Young's modulus of collagen at slow displacement rates. Biomed Mater Eng 2010; 20(6):361–9.

22. Cramer GD, Ross K, Pocius J, et al. Evaluating the relationship among cavitation, zygapophyseal joint gapping, and spinal manipulation: an exploratory case series. J Manipulative Physiol Ther 2011;34(1):2–14.

23. Ross JK, Bereznick DE, McGill SM. Determining cavitation location during lumbar and thoracic spinal manipulation: is spinal manipulation accurate and specific? Spine 2004;29(13): 1452–7.

24. Evans DW, Breen AC. A biomechanical model for mechanically efficient cavitation production during spinal manipulation: prethrust position and the neutral zone. J Manipulative Physiol Ther 2006;29(1):72–82.

25. Miller T, Smiley JT. Cavitation sounds during spinal manipulative treatments. J Manipulative Physiol Ther 1994;17(4):268–70.

26. Reggars JW. The therapeutic benefit of the audible release associated with spinal manipulative therapy. A critical review of the literature. Australas Chiropr Osteopathy 1998;7(2):80–5.

27. Ernst E. Does spinal manipulation have specific treatment effects? Fam Pract 2000;17(6):554–6.

28. Ernst E. Adverse effects of spinal manipulation: a systematic review. J R Soc Med 2007;100(7):330–8.

29. Castellanos J, Axelrod D. Effect of habitual knuckle cracking on hand function. Ann Rheum Dis 1990;49(5):308–9.

30. Deweber K, Olszewski M, Ortolano R. Knuckle cracking and hand osteoarthritis. J Am Board Fam Med 2011;24(2):169–74.

31. Reggars JW. The manipulative crack. Frequency analysis. Australas Chiropr Osteopathy 1996;5(2):39–44.

32. Dunning J, Mourad F, Barbero M, et al. Bilateral and multiple cavitation sounds during upper cervical thrust manipulation. BMC Musculoskelet Disord 2013;14:24.

33. Flynn T, Fritz J, Whitman J, et al. A clinical prediction rule for classifying patients with low back pain who demonstrate short-term improvement with spinal manipulation. Spine 2002;27(24): 2835–43.

34. Cleland JA, Flynn TW, Childs JD, et al. The audible pop from thoracic spine thrust manipulation and its relation to short-term outcomes in patients with neck pain. J Man Manip Ther 2007; 15(3):143–54.

35. Bishop MD, Beneciuk JM, George SZ. Immediate reduction in temporal sensory summation after thoracic spinal manipulation. Spine 2011;11(5):440–6.

36. Sillevis R, Cleland J, Hellman M, et al. Immediate effects of a thoracic spine thrust manipulation on the autonomic nervous system: a randomized clinical trial. J Man Manip Ther 2010; 18(4):181–90.

37. Sillevis R, Cleland J. Immediate effects of the audible pop from a thoracic spine thrust manipulation on the autonomic nervous system and pain: a secondary analysis of a randomized clinical trial. J Manipulative Physiol Ther 2011;34(1):37–45.

38. Herzog W. The physics of spinal manipulation: work-energy and impulse-momentum principles. J Manipulative Physiol Ther 1993;16(1):51–4.

39. Reggars JW. Recording techniques and analysis of the articular crack. A critical review of the literature. Australas Chiropr Osteopathy 1996;5(3):86–92.

40. Dishman JD, Weber KA, Corbin RL, et al. Understanding inhibitory mechanisms of lumbar spinal manipulation using H-reflex and F-wave responses: a methodological approach. J Neurosci Methods 2012;210(2):169–77.

41. Bialosky JE, Bishop MD, Robinson ME, et al. The relationship of the audible pop to hypoalgesia associated with high-velocity, low-amplitude thrust manipulation: a secondary analysis of an experimental study in pain-free participants. J Manipulative Physiol Ther 2010;33(2):117–24.

42. Teodorczyk-Injeyan JA, Injeyan HS, Ruegg R. Spinal manipulative therapy reduces inflammatory cytokines but not substance P production in normal subjects. J Manipulative Physiol Ther 2006;29(1):14–21.

43. Bialosky JE, Bishop MD, Robinson ME, et al. The influence of expectation on spinal manipulation induced hypoalgesia: an experimental study in normal subjects. BMC Musculoskelet Disord 2008;9:19.

44. Bishop MD, Mintken PE, Bialosky JE, et al. Patient expectations of benefit from interventions for neck pain and resulting influence on outcomes. J Orthop Sports Phys Ther 2013;43(7): 457–65.

45. Suter E, McMorland G, Herzog W. Short-term effects of spinal manipulation on H-reflex amplitude in healthy and symptomatic subjects. J Manipulative Physiol Ther 2005;28(9):667–72.

46. Dishman JD, Dougherty PE, Burke JR. Evaluation of the effect of postural perturbation on motoneuronal activity following various methods of lumbar spinal manipulation. Spine J 2005; 5(6):650–9.

47. Dishman JD, Greco DS, Burke JR. Motor-evoked potentials recorded from lumbar erector spinae muscles: a study of corticospinal excitability changes associated with spinal manipulation. J Manipulative Physiol Ther 2008;31(4):258–70.

48. Snodgrass SJ, Rhodes HR. Cervical spine posteroanterior stiffness differs with neck position. J Electromyogr Kinesiol 2012;22(6): 829–34.

49. Dishman JD, Bulbulian R. Comparison of effects of spinal manipulation and massage on motoneuron excitability. Electromyogr Clin Neurophysiol 2001;41(2):97–106.

50. Evans DW, Lucas N. What is 'manipulation'? A reappraisal. Man Ther 2010;15(3):286–91.

51. Evans DW. Mechanisms and effects of spinal high-velocity, low-amplitude thrust manipulation: previous theories. J Manipulative Physiol Ther 2002;25(4):251–62.

52. Triano JJ. Biomechanics of spinal manipulative therapy. Spine J 2001;1(2):121–9.

53. Abbott JH, Flynn TW, Fritz JM, et al. Manual physical assessment of spinal segmental motion: intent and validity. Man Ther 2009;14(1):36–44.

54. van Trijffel E, Oostendorp RA, Lindeboom R, et al. Perceptions and use of passive intervertebral motion assessment of the spine: a survey among physiotherapists specializing in manual therapy. Man Ther 2009;14(3):243–51.

55. van Trijffel E, Anderegg Q, Bossuyt PM, et al. Inter-examiner reliability of passive assessment of intervertebral motion in the cervical and lumbar spine: a systematic review. Man Ther 2005; 10(4):256–69.

56. Hollerwoger D. Methodological quality and outcomes of studies addressing manual cervical spine examinations: a review. Man Ther 2006;11(2):93–8.

57. Seffinger MA, Najm WI, Mishra SI, et al. Reliability of spinal palpation for diagnosis of back and neck pain: a systematic review of the literature. Spine 2004;29(19):E413–25.

58. Beneck GJ, Kulig K, Landel RF, et al. The relationship between lumbar segmental motion and pain response produced by a

posterior-to-anterior force in persons with nonspecific low back pain. J Orthop Sports Phys Ther 2005;35(4):203–9.

59. Landel R, Kulig K, Fredericson M, et al. Intertester reliability and validity of motion assessments during lumbar spine accessory motion testing. Phys Ther 2008;88(1):43–9.

60. Haas M, Groupp E, Panzer D, et al. Efficacy of cervical endplay assessment as an indicator for spinal manipulation. Spine 2003; 28(11):1091–6.

61. Herzog W, Kats M, Symons B. The effective forces transmitted by high-speed, low-amplitude thoracic manipulation. Spine 2001;26(19):2105–10.

62. Gal J, Herzog W, Kawchuk G, et al. Movements of vertebrae during manipulative thrusts to unembalmed human cadavers. J Manipulative Physiol Ther 1997;20(1):30–40.

63. Cramer GD, Ross JK, Raju PK, et al. Distribution of cavitations as identified with accelerometry during lumbar spinal manipulation. J Manipulative Physiol Ther 2011;34(9):572–83.

64. Tullberg T, Blomberg S, Branth B, et al. Manipulation does not alter the position of the sacroiliac joint. A roentgen stereophotogrammetric analysis. Spine 1998;23(10):1124–8.

65. Cleland JA, Fritz JM, Kulig K, et al. Comparison of the effectiveness of three manual physical therapy techniques in a subgroup of patients with low back pain who satisfy a clinical prediction rule: a randomized clinical trial. Spine 2009;34(25): 2720–9.

66. Kent P, Marks D, Pearson W, et al. Does clinician treatment choice improve the outcomes of manual therapy for nonspecific low back pain? A metaanalysis. J Manipulative Physiol Ther 2005;28(5):312–22.

67. Bialosky JE, Bishop MD, Price DD, et al. The mechanisms of manual therapy in the treatment of musculoskeletal pain: a comprehensive model. Man Ther 2009;14:531–8.

68. Degenhardt BF, Darmani NA, Johnson JC, et al. Role of osteopathic manipulative treatment in altering pain biomarkers: a pilot study. J Am Osteopath Assoc 2007;107(9):387–400.

69. McPartland JM, Giuffrida A, King J, et al. Cannabimimetic effects of osteopathic manipulative treatment. J Am Osteopath Assoc 2005;105(6):283–91.

70. George SZ, Bishop MD, Bialosky JE, et al. Immediate effects of spinal manipulation on thermal pain sensitivity: an experimental study. BMC Musculoskelet Disord 2006;7:68.

71. Bialosky JE, Bishop MD, Robinson ME, et al. Spinal manipulative therapy has an immediate effect on thermal pain sensitivity in people with low back pain: a randomized controlled trial. Phys Ther 2009;89(12):1292–303.

72. Bialosky JE, George SZ, Horn ME, et al. Spinal manipulative therapy specific changes in pain sensitivity in individuals with low back pain. J Pain 2014;15(2):136–48.

73. Price DD, Staud R, Robinson ME, et al. Enhanced temporal summation of second pain and its central modulation in fibromyalgia patients. Pain 2002;99(1–2):49–59.

74. Cuellar JM, Dutton RC, Antognini JF, et al. Differential effects of halothane and isoflurane on lumbar dorsal horn neuronal windup and excitability. Br J Anaesth 2005;94(5): 617–25.

75. Guan Y, Borzan J, Meyer RA, et al. Windup in dorsal horn neurons is modulated by endogenous spinal mu-opioid mechanisms. J Neurosci 2006;26(16):4298–307.

76. Licciardone JC, Kearns CM, Hodge LM, et al. Associations of cytokine concentrations with key osteopathic lesions and clinical outcomes in patients with nonspecific chronic low back pain: results from the OSTEOPATHIC Trial. J Am Osteopath Assoc 2012;112(9):596–605.

77. Solomonow M, Zhou BH, Harris M, et al. The ligamentomuscular stabilizing system of the spine. Spine 1998;23(23): 2552–62.

78. Boal RW, Gillette RG. Central neuronal plasticity, low back pain and spinal manipulative therapy. J Manipulative Physiol Ther 2004;27(5):314–26.

79. Pickar JG, Wheeler JD. Response of muscle proprioceptors to spinal manipulative-like loads in the anesthetized cat. J Manipulative Physiol Ther 2001;24(1):2–11.

80. Colloca CJ, Keller TS, Gunzburg R. Neuromechanical characterization of in vivo lumbar spinal manipulation. Part II. Neurophysiological response. J Manipulative Physiol Ther 2003;26(9): 579–91.

81. Colloca CJ, Keller TS, Gunzburg R, et al. Neurophysiologic response to intraoperative lumbosacral spinal manipulation. J Manipulative Physiol Ther 2000;23(7):447–57.

82. Dishman JD, Bulbulian R. Spinal reflex attenuation associated with spinal manipulation. Spine 2000;25(19):2519–24.

83. Dishman JD, Burke J. Spinal reflex excitability changes after cervical and lumbar spinal manipulation: a comparative study. Spine J 2003;3(3):204–12.

84. Dishman JD, Cunningham BM, Burke J. Comparison of tibial nerve H-reflex excitability after cervical and lumbar spine manipulation. J Manipulative Physiol Ther 2002;25(5):318–25.

85. Wright A. Hypoalgesia post-manipulative therapy: a review of a potential neurophysiological mechanism. Man Ther 1995;1(1): 11–16.

86. Taylor HH, Murphy B. Altered central integration of dual somatosensory input after cervical spine manipulation. J Manipulative Physiol Ther 2010;33(3):178–88.

87. Haavik-Taylor H, Murphy B. Cervical spine manipulation alters sensorimotor integration: a somatosensory evoked potential study. Clin Neurophysiol 2007;118(2):391–402.

88. Daligadu J, Haavik H, Yielder PC, et al. Alterations in cortical and cerebellar motor processing in subclinical neck pain patients following spinal manipulation. J Manipulative Physiol Ther 2013; 36(8):527–37.

89. Taylor HH, Murphy B. Altered sensorimotor integration with cervical spine manipulation. J Manipulative Physiol Ther 2008; 31(2):115–26.

90. Fryer G, Pearce AJ. The effect of lumbosacral manipulation on corticospinal and spinal reflex excitability on asymptomatic participants. J Manipulative Physiol Ther 2012;35(2):86–93.

91. Vase L, Petersen GL, Riley JL III, et al. Factors contributing to large analgesic effects in placebo mechanism studies conducted between 2002 and 2007. Pain 2009;145(1–2):36–44.

92. Price DD, Craggs J, Verne GN, et al. Placebo analgesia is accompanied by large reductions in pain-related brain activity in irritable bowel syndrome patients. Pain 2007;127(1–2):63–72.

93. Colloca L, Lopiano L, Lanotte M, et al. Overt versus covert treatment for pain, anxiety, and Parkinson's disease. Lancet Neurol 2004;3(11):679–84.

94. Bialosky JE, Bishop MD, George SZ, et al. Placebo response to manual therapy: something out of nothing? J Man Manip Ther 2011;19(1):11–19.

95. Kalauokalani D, Cherkin DC, Sherman KJ, et al. Lessons from a trial of acupuncture and massage for low back pain: patient expectations and treatment effects. Spine 2001;26(13):1418–24.

96. Michaleff ZA, Lin CW, Maher CG, et al. Spinal manipulation epidemiology: systematic review of cost effectiveness studies. J Electromyogr Kinesiol 2012;22(5):655–62.

97. Carroll LJ, Cassidy JD, Peloso PM, et al. Methods for the best evidence synthesis on neck pain and its associated disorders: the Bone and Joint Decade 2000–2010 Task Force on Neck Pain and Its Associated Disorders. J Manipulative Physiol Ther 2009; 32(2 Suppl.):S39–45.

98. Scholten-Peeters GG, Thoomes E, Konings S, et al. Is manipulative therapy more effective than sham manipulation in adults: a systematic review and meta-analysis. Chiropr Man Therap 2013;21(1):34.

99. Wand BM, Heine PJ, O'Connell NE. Should we abandon cervical spine manipulation for mechanical neck pain? Yes. Br Med J 2012;344:e3679.

100. Rivett DA, Reid D. Risk of stroke for cervical spine manipulation in New Zealand. N Z J Physiother 1998;26(2):14–17.

101. Hurwitz EL, Aker PD, Adams AH, et al. Manipulation and mobilization of the cervical spine. A systematic review of the literature. Spine 1996;21:1746–59.

102. Carnes D, Mars TS, Mullinger B, et al. Adverse events and manual therapy: a systematic review. Man Ther 2010;15(4): 355–63.

103. Maitland GD, Hengeveld E, Banks K, et al. Maitland's Vertebral Manipulation. 6th ed. London: Butterworths; 2000.

104. Rivett DA. Adverse effects of cervical manipulative therapy. In: Boyling JD, Jull GA, editors. Grieve's Modern Manual Therapy of the Vertebral Column. 3rd ed. Edinburgh: Churchill Livingstone; 2004. p. 533–49.

105. Childs JD, Flynn TW, Fritz JM, et al. Screening for vertebrobasilar insufficiency in patients with neck pain: manual therapy

decision-making in the presence of uncertainty. J Orthop Sports Phys Ther 2005;35(5):300–6.

106. Rushton A, Rivett D, Flynn T, et al. International framework for examination of the cervical region for potential of Cervical Arterial Dysfunction prior to Orthopaedic Manual Therapy intervention. Man Ther 2014;19(3):222–8.

107. Hing WA, Reid DA, Monaghan M. Manipulation of the cervical spine. Man Ther 2003;8(1):2–9.

108. Carlesso L, Rivett D. Manipulative practice in the cervical spine: a survey of IFOMPT member countries. JMMT 2011;19(2):66–70.

109. Rushton A, Rivett D, Carlesso L, et al. International Framework for Examination of the Cervical Region for Potential of Cervical Arterial Dysfunction Prior to Orthopaedic Manual Therapy Intervention. Auckland: International Federation of Orthopaedic Manipulative Physical Therapists; 2012.

110. Kerry R, Taylor AJ, Mitchell JM, et al. Cervical arterial dysfunction and manual therapy: a critical literature review to inform professional practice. Man Ther 2008;13(4):278–88.

111. Taylor AJ, Kerry R. A 'system based' approach to risk assessment of the cervical spine prior to manual therapy. Int J Ost Med 2010;13:85–93.

112. Thomas LC, Rivett DA, Attia JR, et al. Risk factors and clinical features of craniocervical arterial dissection. Man Ther 2011;16(4):351–6.

113. Arnold M, Bousser MG. Carotid and vertebral dissection. Practical Neurology 2005;5:100–9.

114. Mitchell J, Keene D, Dyson C, et al. Is cervical spine rotation, as used in the standard vertebrobasilar insufficiency test, associated with a measureable change in intracranial vertebral artery blood flow? Man Ther 2004;9(4):220–7.

115. Rivett DA, Shirley D, Magarey M, et al. Clinical Guidelines for Assessing Vertebrobasilar Insufficiency in the Management of Cervical Spine Disorders. Melbourne: Australian Physiotherapy Association; 2006.

116. McLeod LR, Thomas L, Osmotherly P, et al. The effect of end-range cervical rotation on vertebral and internal carotid arterial blood flow and cerebral inflow. Man Ther 2014 Nov 29. pii: S1356-689X(14)00233-1. doi: 10.1016/j.math.2014.11.012. [Epub ahead of print].

117. Kerry R, Taylor AJ. Cervical arterial dysfunction assessment and manual therapy. Man Ther 2006;11(4):243–53.

118. Thomas L, Rivett D, Levi C. The effect of selected manual therapy interventions for mechanical neck pain on vertebral and internal carotid arterial blood flow and cerebral inflow. Phys Ther 2013;93(11):1563–74.

CHAPTER 30

NEURODYNAMIC MANAGEMENT OF THE PERIPHERAL NERVOUS SYSTEM

Michel Coppieters • Robert Nee

INTRODUCTION

Recent surveys among musculoskeletal physiotherapists reveal that neurodynamic techniques are frequently part of a multimodal treatment approach to patients with compression neuropathies, such as cervical radiculopathy[1,2] and carpal tunnel syndrome (CTS).[3] To our knowledge, no survey datum exists that documents practice patterns for other compression neuropathies, such as cubital or tarsal tunnel syndrome, or sural nerve pathology. In this chapter we will discuss the use of neurodynamic tests as diagnostic tests, different neurodynamic treatment options and some clinical reasoning considerations behind their application, what pathophysiological processes may be influenced with treatment and an overview of the evidence from clinical studies. We will end this chapter with some final considerations regarding neurodynamics.

NEURODYNAMIC TESTS

Neurodynamic tests try to determine whether a patient's symptoms are related to increased nerve mechanosensitivity by using specific combinations of spine and limb movements that apply mechanical forces to a part of the nervous system (Fig. 30-1).[4–6] Biomechanical data show that joint movements involved in neurodynamic tests increase nerve strain, sliding and compression.[7–12] Neurodynamic tests also apply mechanical forces to non-neural tissues.[4,5] When central pain mechanisms are not the primary reason for a patient's pain experience, a positive neurodynamic test response could be related to neural or non-neural tissue sensitivity. A neurodynamic test response is thought to be related to neural tissue sensitivity when it changes with movement of a distant body part that further loads or unloads the nervous system (e.g. releasing neck flexion reduces a sensory response in the posterior thigh during the slump test). Analysing a neurodynamic test response by moving a distant body part is termed structural differentiation.[4,5,13]

Using structural differentiation to analyse neural tissue responses is supported by biomechanical and experimental pain model data. When a joint movement is performed at the end of a neurodynamic test, the biomechanical effects spread along the entire nerve.[9,14,15]

The spread of biomechanical effects along the nerve provides a credible explanation for why moving a distant body part can change sensory responses provoked at the end of a neurodynamic test. Experimental pain induced by injecting hypertonic saline into the thenar or calf muscles is not changed by applying structural differentiation manoeuvres associated with the median nerve, straight leg raise (SLR), or slump tests, respectively.[16,17] This indicates that neurodynamic tests can potentially be used to distinguish pain related to muscle irritation from pain related to increased nerve mechanosensitivity.[9]

Most asymptomatic individuals (≥80%) report sensory responses at the end of range of neurodynamic tests that change with structural differentiation.[9,18–20] Common descriptors include stretching, aching, pain, burning and tingling.[9,18–20] These data suggest that asymptomatic individuals have a certain level of nerve mechanosensitivity. The variety of sensory responses reported by asymptomatic individuals means it is important to specify the type of sensory response that qualifies as a 'positive' neurodynamic test in symptomatic populations. To be confident that a neurodynamic test is most likely identifying a patient with increased nerve mechanosensitivity, the test needs to reproduce at least part of the patient's symptoms and the symptoms should change with structural differentiation.[9]

Resistance to movement and range of motion (ROM) have also been proposed as criteria to define a 'positive' neurodynamic test.[4,5] Inter-examiner reliability for measuring elbow extension at the onset of resistance during the neurodynamic test for the median nerve is low.[9] Studies on detecting the onset of resistance during the SLR and slump tests have only reported intra-examiner reliability.[21,22] Poor inter-examiner reliability suggests that the onset of resistance is unlikely to be sensitive enough to be a useful criterion for defining a 'positive' neurodynamic test.[9]

Neurodynamic test ROM can be quantified by measuring the joint angle at pain onset or pain tolerance (e.g. elbow extension for the median nerve neurodynamic test, knee extension for the slump test). Neurodynamic test ROM is highly variable in asymptomatic and symptomatic individuals.[9,22–25] There is also considerable overlap in neurodynamic test ROM between asymptomatic and symptomatic individuals, and between the involved and uninvolved limbs of symptomatic individuals.[9,23] Neurodynamic test ROM variability and overlap make it unlikely that an absolute ROM cut-off can be found that

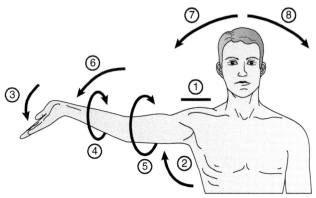

FIGURE 30-1 ■ End position of the base neurodynamic test for the median nerve. The components and sequence for this base test are: *1–2*, shoulder abduction to ~90–100°, while shoulder girdle elevation is prevented; *3*, wrist extension; *4*, forearm supination; *5*, shoulder external rotation; and *6*, elbow extension. Ipsilateral (*7*) or contralateral (*8*) lateroflexion of the mid and lower cervical spine are common manoeuvres to assist in structural differentiation if a patient's symptoms are (at least partially) reproduced in the distal upper quadrant. Wrist movements are commonly used to structurally differentiate if symptoms are elicited in the proximal upper quadrant. Base neurodynamic tests can be modified to suit individual patients. The upper limb neurodynamic tests for the median, ulnar and radial nerve, the slump and side-lying slump (femoral nerve) test and straight leg raise test are considered base neurodynamic tests.

accurately discriminates symptomatic from asymptomatic individuals.

Looking for a certain deficit in neurodynamic test ROM in the involved limb compared to the uninvolved limb (limb asymmetry) is another method for using ROM to define a 'positive' neurodynamic test. Asymptomatic individuals typically show a 5–10° difference between limbs in ROM for the median nerve[26–29] and SLR[25] tests. However, we are not aware of any data showing that a certain amount of limb asymmetry in neurodynamic test ROM can discriminate symptomatic from asymptomatic individuals. Consequently, at this stage it is unlikely that ROM can be a useful criterion for defining a 'positive' neurodynamic test.[9] Based on information available at this time, a 'positive' neurodynamic test should at least partly reproduce the patient's symptoms and the symptoms should change with structural differentiation.[9] This definition of a 'positive' neurodynamic test is reliable when applied to symptomatic populations.[23,30,31]

When electrodiagnostic tests are used as the reference standard to determine the diagnostic accuracy of neurodynamic tests, data suggest that the neurodynamic test for the median nerve can help diagnose cervical radiculopathy,[32] but not CTS.[33–35] However, care is required when interpreting these findings because of the limitations of using electrodiagnostic tests as the reference standard. Increased nerve mechanosensitivity can be present in cervical radiculopathy and CTS even when standard electrodiagnostic tests are normal.[36,37] This means that patients with peripheral neuropathic pain who have increased nerve mechanosensitivity rather than conduction loss will often be incorrectly classified by the reference standard as not having peripheral neuropathic pain. Potential misclassification of patients who have

peripheral neuropathic pain will bias the estimates of the diagnostic performance of neurodynamic tests.[38]

Studies investigating the ability of the SLR and slump tests to detect lumbar radicular pain have used electrodiagnostic testing, or surgical or imaging evidence of lumbar disc herniation as the reference standard. When using these reference standards, the diagnostic performance of the SLR is relatively poor.[39,40] Positive responses to a crossed SLR (a relatively uncommon clinical finding) or the slump test may help confirm the presence of lumbar radicular pain related to lumbar disc herniation.[39,41] Again, potential limitations in the reference standards require caution when interpreting these results. A surgical reference standard limits the generalizability of diagnostic performance findings because it narrows the spectrum of patients who can be included in the study and may alter the prevalence of the target condition.[39,42] Lastly, there is not necessarily a strong correlation between imaging findings and the presence or absence of lumbar radicular pain.[40,43] Therefore, similar to electrodiagnostic reference standards, imaging reference standards may misclassify patients and bias estimates of the diagnostic performance of neurodynamic tests.[38]

The difficulty in investigating the diagnostic performance of neurodynamic tests is that there is no agreed upon reference standard for establishing that an individual patient has increased nerve mechanosensitivity.[44] This means there is a mismatch between the intent of neurodynamic tests (identifying increased nerve mechanosensitivity) and the various reference standards that have been used in published research. Until a reference standard for increased nerve mechanosensitivity can be agreed upon, using neurodynamic tests for diagnostic purposes is primarily based on lower evidence from biomechanical and experimental pain model data described previously.

Another issue related to neurodynamic testing is the concept of sequencing. Standardized sequences for applying the movements involved in different neurodynamic tests have been described, yet clinicians have always been encouraged to change the order of movement to match an individual patient's presentation.[4,5,45] Neurodynamic test sequencing is partly based on the belief that different orders of movement can apply different levels of strain to a particular nerve segment at the end of a neurodynamic test.[5] However, cadaveric data have shown that, when joints are moved through similar ranges of motion, nerve strain at the end of the test does not change with different orders of movement.[10,46] However, when different neurodynamic test sequences are applied clinically, joints likely move through different ranges of motion. Potential differences between sequences in ranges of joint motion may be more likely to affect nerve biomechanics at the end of a neurodynamic test than any specific effects from the order of movement.[46]

We are not aware of any published or recent studies that have explored whether different sequences can improve the diagnostic performance of a neurodynamic test. Regardless of any potential impact on diagnostic performance, neurodynamic test sequencing may still have value clinically. A joint movement is not likely to reach a full ROM when performed in the later stages of a neurodynamic test.[47] This knowledge can help the clinician modify a neurodynamic test when examining a patient with a sensitive or stiff body part. Using a patient with a highly sensitive or stiff shoulder as an example, the best approach to neurodynamic testing for the median nerve might be to use a distal-to-proximal sequence where shoulder abduction would be the last movement. This sequence would apply less mechanical load to the non-neural tissues in the shoulder but would still apply adequate nerve strain and nerve compression to provoke sensitized neural tissues. Different neurodynamic test sequences may also help with structural differentiation. For example, in a patient who has plantar heel pain, it may be useful to modify the SLR so that ankle dorsiflexion and eversion are performed before hip flexion. Ankle dorsiflexion and eversion apply strain to the plantar fascia and tibial and plantar nerves simultaneously.[14] Subsequent hip flexion does not change strain on the plantar fascia but increases strain on the tibial and plantar nerves.[14] This modified test sequence could make it easier for the clinician to determine whether there is a nerve-related component to the patient's plantar heel pain.

NEURODYNAMIC MANAGEMENT

Neurodynamic techniques can be categorized as techniques that aim to either mobilize the nervous system itself, or mobilize the structures that surround it. Sliding and tensioning techniques mobilize the nervous system,[5,48] whereas a cervical contralateral lateral glide technique[49] is an example of a common technique that mobilizes the structures surrounding the nervous system. Whether it is indicated to mobilize the nervous system or its surrounding structures will depend on many factors, such as which pain mechanisms are in operation, the history, severity and 'irritability' of the condition, stages of tissue healing, associated pathologies, signs and symptoms and results from technical investigations.

Sliding and Tensioning Techniques

When clinicians first conceptualized the idea of mobilizing the nervous system as a treatment approach, techniques were implemented that resembled neurodynamic tests or parts thereof. These days, these techniques are referred to as tensioning techniques. Nerve gliding is obtained by moving one or several joints in such a manner that the nerve bed is elongated and, as a consequence, strain in the nervous system increases. Adjacent or more remote joints may also be positioned to further increase the load on the nervous system. Although very few adverse events were reported in the literature, clinicians quickly realized that these techniques were sometimes too aggressive. Clinicians therefore developed the concept of sliding techniques.

In a sliding technique, at least two joints are moved simultaneously, either actively or passively, in such a manner that one movement counterbalances the increase in nerve strain caused by another movement.[5] The clinical assumption is that – compared to tensioning techniques – sliding techniques are associated with much larger excursions of the nervous system relative to surrounding structures, but without the potentially large

increases in nerve strain.[5] These clinical assumptions were confirmed in a series of cadaveric[48,50] and in vivo studies[51] in the upper quarter (Fig. 30-2). When the same joints were moved through the same ranges of motion, with comparable start and end positions, the strain was substantially lower and the excursion of the nerve relative to surrounding structures was approximately 2.5[48,50] to 5[51] times larger for a sliding technique (Fig. 30-2). In contrast, a study in the lower limb reported much smaller differences.[52] Although the sliding technique still resulted in a significantly larger excursion of the sciatic nerve, it is questionable whether the observed mean difference of 0.6 mm is clinically meaningful. Because start and end positions varied significantly in this study,[52] we believe the results should be interpreted cautiously, especially because another in vivo study for the sciatic nerve that used identical start and end positions revealed large differences in excursion between the sliding and tensioning techniques (Fig. 30-3).[53]

Although sliding and tensioning techniques result in very different biomechanical effects on the nervous system, it is important to emphasize that one type of technique is not always superior to the other.[48] Sliding techniques are less vigorous and may be more appropriate in more irritable conditions; tensioning techniques may have a place in the later stages or in more sport-specific rehabilitation. To date, there is virtually no comparative clinical research to guide technique choices. Sound clinical reasoning, and perhaps erring on the side of caution, remains of cardinal importance.

Mobilization of Surrounding Structures

The cervical contralateral lateral glide technique (Fig. 30-4) was first described by Elvey as a treatment technique for neuropathic disorders.[49] The immediate effects of the technique have been investigated in several conditions, including nerve-related neck and/or arm pain[54,55] and musculoskeletal conditions, such as lateral epicondylalgia[56] and chronic whiplash-associated disorders.[57] To our knowledge, the technique has invariably demonstrated positive immediate effects across different conditions.[54-57] The equivalent technique for the lumbar spine – a segmental lumbar lateral flexion contralateral to the painful side – has also shown positive effects when administered to patients with peripheral nerve sensitization.[58]

Treating the Neural Container

Unhealthy neighbouring tissues or postural changes are likely important contributing factors in the development and maintenance of peripheral neuropathic pain states, and may require attention. Although important, this is beyond the scope of this chapter.

INDICATIONS AND CONTRAINDICATIONS

Elvey[4] proposed a set of specific signs that should be present, in addition to a patient interview suggestive of peripheral neuropathic pain, to support the hypothesis of

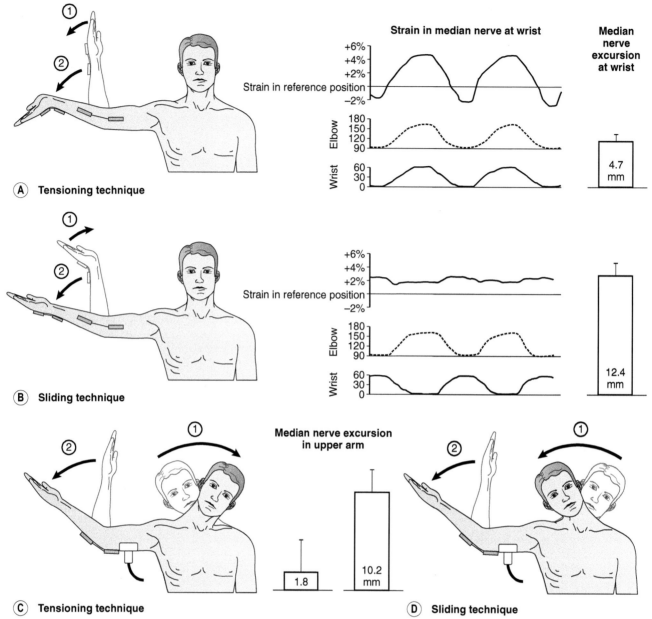

FIGURE 30-2 ■ Example of a tensioning technique and corresponding sliding technique for the median nerve at the wrist (**A,B**)[47,49] and the upper arm (**C,D**).[50] For the tensioning techniques, both depicted movements (1 and 2) increase the length of the nerve bedding. For the sliding techniques, the movement that elongates the length of the nerve bedding (2) is counterbalanced by another movement that reduces the length of the nerve bedding (1). The waveform diagrams in (A) and (B) represent the strain in the median nerve at the wrist (top waveform), and the range of motion of the elbow (middle waveform) and wrist (lower waveform) for two consecutive repetitions of the technique. For the elbow, 180° represents full extension. Clear differences in peak strain can be seen. The bar diagrams (A–D) demonstrate the large differences in excursion of the median nerve (in mm) relative to surrounding structures between the sliding and tensioning techniques.

a 'neurogenic disorder' for which physiotherapy management could be considered. These criteria were: (a) an active movement dysfunction that is related to non-compliance of a specific nerve; (b) a passive movement dysfunction that correlates with the active dysfunction; (c) a positive neurodynamic test; (d) an abnormal response to nerve palpation; (e) signs of a musculoskeletal dysfunction that would indicate that the cause of the neurogenic disorder would be responsive to physiotherapy; and (f) a protective posture that shortens the anatomical course of the affected nerve. Although the value of these criteria

has never been investigated directly, the criteria have been used as inclusion criteria in several clinical trials.[54,58,59] Furthermore, research has now identified which elements of the patient interview may be suggestive of neuropathic pain.[60,61] Various questionnaires may yield valuable information as well in this respect (e.g. S-LANNS,[62] DN4[63]). Several papers have investigated nerve palpation.[31,44,64,65] However, considering our current understanding of pathophysiological processes, if the entrapment site cannot be palpated directly or indirectly, we do not know whether abnormal responses to palpation can routinely be elicited at other points along the affected peripheral nerve. A protective posture may also not always be present, especially if the neuropathy is associated with minimal pain. The criterion regarding the presence of a musculoskeletal disorder is a good reminder that many of these criteria and neuropathic pain can be present following sinister space-occupying lesions or systemic diseases for which neurodynamic exercises are either contraindicated or for which we currently have no evidence. The criteria may have merit because they remind clinicians of potentially useful items to look out for before implementing neurodynamic techniques.

INFLUENCES ON PATHOBIOLOGICAL PROCESSES

Until recently,[48] we could only largely speculate on what pathophysiological changes could potentially be influenced with neurodynamics. Although there is still much to discover and much is still speculative, there are now at least some preliminary data on possible working mechanisms of neurodynamic techniques. Most of these studies have either been conducted in patients with CTS or in animal models. Because of the high prevalence of CTS in the general population (3.8%),[66] CTS is often used as a possible model for compression neuropathies in general.

Normalization of Impaired Nerve Movement

The majority of investigations demonstrated that patients with a compression neuropathy, such as CTS, have reduced longitudinal[67-69] and transverse[70-72] nerve movement compared to healthy controls. Due to the cross-sectional nature of these studies, it is still unclear whether altered nerve biomechanics is a consequence of the pathophysiological processes of a neuropathy, or possibly a predisposing factor for the development of a neuropathy. Recent unpublished work revealed that experimentally increasing carpal tunnel pressure to

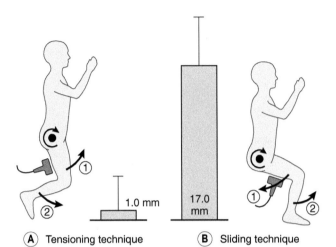

FIGURE 30-3 ■ Example of a tensioning technique and corresponding sliding technique for the sciatic and tibial nerve. **(A)** For the tensioning technique, both hip flexion (*1*) and knee extension (*2*) increase the length of the nerve bedding. **(B)** For the sliding technique, knee extension (*2*) which elongates the nerve bedding is counterbalanced by hip extension (*1*) which reduces the length of the nerve bedding. The bar diagrams demonstrate the large difference in excursion of the sciatic nerve (in mm) in the posterior thigh between the two techniques.[53] The location of the measurements is indicated with the ultrasound transducer.

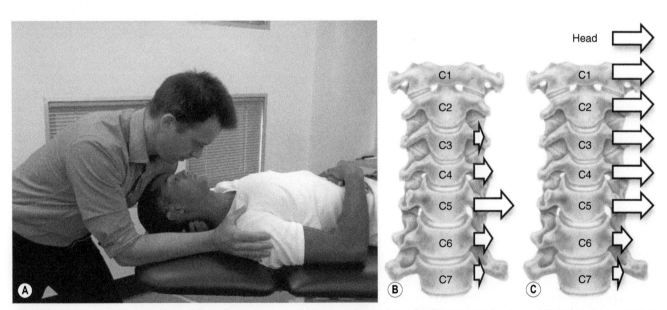

FIGURE 30-4 ■ A cervical contralateral lateral glide technique for (for example) the C5–C6 segment (i.e. to mobilize the structures that surround the C6 spinal nerve), can be performed in various ways. **(A)** The patient's head rests in neutral on the plinth while the therapist aims to translate C5 relative to C6, away from the affected side. **(B)** Because the technique is typically performed without fixation of adjacent spinal levels, the translation will also occur at neighbouring segments. **(C)** Alternatively, all spinal levels superior to the C6 nerve root can be translated together to the contralateral side. The patient's head then rests against the abdomen of the therapist, who shifts his/her trunk slightly to the contralateral side (not shown). When possible, the techniques are typically performed with the affected arm in a position that preloads the affected peripheral nerve.

similar and even higher levels than typically observed in patients with CTS did not influence longitudinal or transverse nerve movement.[73] Also, longitudinal excursion of the median nerve does not change following carpal tunnel release surgery.[74,75] These findings indicate that an acute increase or decrease in pressure does not alter nerve excursion. If a prolonged increase in pressure would, however, result in alterations in connective tissues, perhaps there is a place for interventions that aim to normalize nerve movement and restore the homoeostasis in and around the neuropathy. To the authors' knowledge, there are no studies yet to support this.

It has also been suggested that early mobilization may limit adhesions and scar formation following surgical release in patients with neuropathies.[76] A recent Cochrane review, however, indicated that there is currently no evidence available for or against post-operative rehabilitation following CTS surgery.[77] Two studies investigated the effect of early mobilization following ulnar nerve transposition for cubital tunnel syndrome.[78,79] Early mobilization resulted in substantially less contractures (4% versus 52%)[78] and a quicker return to work (1 month versus 2.75 months[79] or in half the time[78]).

Evacuation of Intraneural Oedema

Following nerve compression, impaired intraneural blood flow can lead to localized hypoxia, oedema, inflammation and fibrosis.[80] In many circumstances, symptoms such as paraesthesia or even numbness caused by reduced blood supply to a peripheral nerve due to temporary compression are easily reversible with movement or a change in posture. If pressure cannot be alleviated and hypoxia persists, the endothelial cells of the capillaries inside the peripheral nerve may break down, resulting in intraneural oedema.[81] Considering the absence of a lymphatic drainage system within the bundles of axons in a peripheral nerve,[82] evacuation of this oedema is more difficult, potentially resulting in an increase in intraneural pressure and possibly a mini-compartment syndrome within the nerve fascicles.[82] This is an ideal environment for fibroblasts to proliferate and form scar tissue, resulting in the fibrotic stage.[83] A recent MRI study revealed a reduction in intraneural oedema following neurodynamic exercises in patients with CTS, compared to a wait-and-see approach.[84] It is worthwhile noting that although the nerve was inflamed and swollen, mobilization exercises for the median nerve did not aggravate symptoms, suggesting that when applied skilfully, neurodynamic exercises can be performed safely, without significant adverse events. In fact, the reduction in nerve swelling was associated with an improvement in symptoms and function.[84] Perhaps movement-based interventions, such as neurodynamics, can play an important role in this oedematous stage, helping to prevent progression to the less reversible stage of nerve fibrosis. Also worthwhile noting is that splinting resulted in a similar reduction in intraneural oedema.[84] Although we believe there might be a place for the use of a splint in CTS and perhaps partial immobilization in other neuropathies (if limited in time and as part of a broader biologically plausible management approach), movement is likely to have additional benefits that splinting is unlikely to have. Some of these issues are discussed elsewhere in this chapter.

Reduction of Extraneural Oedema and Pressure

Carpal tunnel pressure is elevated in patients with CTS, and this elevated pressure is considered an important mechanism in CTS.[85,86] There is only preliminary evidence from a small randomized trial that suggests that neurodynamic exercises can reduce carpal tunnel pressure in a subgroup (around 50%) of patients with CTS.[87] Considering the invasive nature of carpal tunnel pressure measurements,[88] only a small sample of patients and only immediate effects have been studied. If neurodynamic exercises are capable of reducing extraneural pressure affecting a nerve and its functions, this reduction in pressure may also have a positive impact on intraneural blood flow and axonal transport. These two processes are considered vital for the integrity of the peripheral nervous system.[81,83,89,90]

Dispersal of Inflammatory Mediators

In a key paper, Dilley et al.[90] demonstrated that an inflamed nerve becomes extremely sensitive to mild compression or elongation, whereas the conduction velocity through the inflamed region may remain largely unaffected. Ectopic action potentials were generated mid-axon at the inflamed nerve region following mild mechanical provocation. At the demyelinated and inflamed nerve site, ion channel up-regulation and proliferation occurred resulting in the establishment of an abnormal or ectopic impulse-generating site, which can be triggered by elements of the inflammatory soup.[91] Song et al.[92] delivered inflammatory mediators around the L5 dorsal root ganglion in rodents to create a neuropathic pain state and investigated the effect of spinal mobilization. When compared to no intervention, mobilization resulted in reduced hyperexcitability of the dorsal root ganglion neurons, along with a reduction in severity and duration of thermal and mechanical hyperalgesia.[92] The authors concluded that mobilization resulted in faster elimination of the inflammation and excitability of the inflamed dorsal root ganglion neurons by improving blood supply and nutrition to the affected dorsal root ganglion.

Influence on the Neuro-Immune Response

Besides local inflammation and demyelination at the compression site,[83] animal models of (severe) nerve lesions revealed immune inflammatory responses in the corresponding ipsilateral dorsal root ganglia and dorsal horn of the spinal cord, but also in higher centres in the central nervous system, and even in the dorsal horn and dorsal root ganglia contralateral to the side of the nerve lesion.[93] These might be important mechanisms for the development of widespread pain and mirror pains that occur like mirror images on both sides of the body.[94,95]

Less severe nerve compression models, resulting in substantially less axonal loss at the compression site, also revealed inflammatory changes and glia cell activation in the dorsal root ganglia and spinal cord.[96] Santos et al.[97] investigated the effect of neural mobilization in rats with a sciatic nerve lesion. Compared to rats with a nerve lesion but no intervention, non-operated rats and sham-operated rats, the group that received neurodynamic mobilizations demonstrated a substantial decrease in nerve growth factor concentration and in glia cell activation in the corresponding dorsal root ganglia and spinal cord. Both nerve growth factor and glia cell activation are considered important players in neuropathic pain.[91,98,99] These changes were associated with pain reversal (hyperalgesia, allodynia and thermal sensitivity).[97] Further research is certainly required, but these findings suggest that movement-based interventions like neurodynamics may have positive effects on the neuro-inflammatory responses associated with the occurrence of widespread pain.

Facilitation of Descending Modulation

The initial analgesic effects following various forms of manual therapy have frequently been linked to the activation of the descending pain inhibitory system projecting from the periaqueductal grey region in the mid-brain to the spinal cord.[100–103] Temporal summation is considered a measure of dorsal horn excitability. Compared to a sham intervention, neurodynamic techniques resulted in a reduction of temporal summation in patients with CTS, suggesting reduced dorsal horn excitability, possibly due to activation of the descending inhibitory system.[104] An animal study revealed that neurodynamic techniques following a sciatic nerve injury modulate the expression of endogenous opioids in the periaqueductal grey region.[105] Furthermore, the injured animals that received neurodynamic mobilizations showed improved locomotion and muscle force compared to injured animals that did not receive treatment. These data support the view that neurodynamic exercises facilitate pain relief via endogenous analgesic modulation.

CLINICAL TRIAL EVIDENCE

Relatively few clinical trials have measured neurodynamic treatment effects. Lumbar and cervical radicular pain, CTS, cubital tunnel syndrome and tarsal tunnel syndrome have been the peripheral neuropathic pain conditions studied in these trials.

Patients with lumbar radicular pain do better when SLR or slump 'tensioning' techniques are added to a programme of lumbar mobilization and exercise.[106–108] Lumbar radicular pain was defined as reproduction of symptoms with SLR or slump testing, no neurological signs and no centralization of symptoms with repeated movements. Standardized mean differences (reported or calculated from reported data) for pain (0.65–1.42) and self-reported disability (0.75–1.96) after a 3-week intervention (six visits) favoured neurodynamic treatment. These standardized mean differences represent

'moderate' (≥0.6 but <1.2) to 'large' (≥1.2 but <2.0) treatment effects.[109] In contrast to these favourable results for non-operative management of lumbar radicular pain, one clinical trial suggests that neurodynamic treatment may not be helpful after lumbar surgery.[110]

Patients who have cervical radicular pain do better with neurodynamic treatment than advice to remain active.[111] Cervical radicular pain was defined as reproduction of symptoms with median nerve neurodynamic testing and less than two abnormal neurological signs at the same nerve root level. Neurodynamic treatment involved brief education, manual therapy with contralateral cervical lateral glide and shoulder girdle oscillation techniques, and a home programme of nerve gliding exercises for the cervical nerve roots and median nerve.[49,112] Standardized mean differences for pain (0.7–0.9) and self-reported function (0.6–0.9) showed 'moderate' treatment effects favouring neurodynamic treatment at a 3- to 4-week follow-up.[111] A previous clinical trial reported similar effect sizes that were not statistically significant because of a relatively small sample size.[59,113]

According to the published trials, neurodynamic treatment effects are less favourable for patients who have peripheral neuropathic pain conditions affecting the upper or lower limb. Although neurodynamic treatment appears to be better than no treatment for patients with CTS, it is not superior to other interventions (e.g. carpal bone mobilization, splinting).[114] Furthermore, adding neurodynamic techniques to other interventions such as splinting and tendon gliding exercises does not improve outcomes.[114] These findings are consistent regardless of whether neurodynamic techniques involve the entire upper limb or focus on moving only the wrist and hand. Despite these findings, it has been suggested that additional high-quality research on the efficacy of conservative interventions for CTS such as neurodynamic treatment is needed.[114] This additional research should blind participants to interventions where possible, blind outcome assessors and measure short-term and long-term outcomes, including the need for surgery.[114]

Based on the available evidence, neurodynamic treatment may not be beneficial for patients who have cubital tunnel syndrome. One randomized clinical trial showed that adding nerve gliding exercises to education on the pathomechanics of cubital tunnel syndrome and advice to avoid aggravating activities did not improve 6-month outcomes in patients who had mild to moderate symptoms.[115] However, nearly 30% of participants were lost to follow-up and were not included in the statistical analysis, which may have impacted the results.

It also appears from one small clinical trial that adding neurodynamic treatment to conservative management of tarsal tunnel syndrome may not be very helpful.[116] Conservative management involved ice, gastrocnemius stretching, lower extremity strengthening, shoe inserts for patients who had low medial arches or pronation deformities, and bandaging for patients who had ankle oedema. Neurodynamic treatment involved a slump 'tensioning' technique. Significantly fewer participants who received neurodynamic treatment still had a positive Tinel sign at the tibial nerve below the medial malleolus after the 6-week intervention (risk difference calculated from reported data = 0.54, 95% confidence interval 0.31–0.93). However, there were no differences between groups in pain, combined talocrural and subtalar joint ROM, foot muscle strength or the number of participants whose symptoms were provoked with the ankle dorsiflexion and eversion test for the tibial nerve.

Researchers have consistently been encouraged to identify characteristics that predict whether patients will respond to an intervention.[117,118] Schäfer et al.[58] and Nee et al.[119] provided preliminary data on characteristics that may help identify patients with lumbar or cervical radicular pain who are likely to improve with neurodynamic treatment. Patients who have physical signs of increased nerve mechanosensitivity (e.g. reproduction of symptoms with neurodynamic testing and a change in these symptoms with structural differentiation, increased sensitivity to nerve palpation), no neurological signs and an absence of neuropathic pain qualities (i.e. clinician-administered or self-report version of the Leeds Assessment of Neuropathic Symptoms and Signs score <12) are likely to improve with neurodynamic treatment.[58,119] For patients who have cervical radicular pain, older age and smaller deficits in median nerve neurodynamic test ROM in the involved limb relative to the uninvolved limb are also associated with improvement.[119] Further research is needed to determine whether these characteristics identify patients who do well regardless of the intervention (prognostic factors) or patients who respond better to neurodynamic treatment than to alternative treatments (treatment effect modifiers).[120,121]

FINAL CONSIDERATIONS

The number of studies investigating various aspects of neurodynamics has grown substantially over recent decades. There remain concerns however about the low quality of evidence due to the small number of clinical trials and/or relatively high risk of bias of studies. The interventions that are evaluated in clinical trials are often poorly described,[122] and this also applies to trials in neurodynamics. These factors make it difficult to provide strong recommendations for the management of peripheral neuropathic pain. More high-quality research is required.

Clinical research in neurodynamics, and neuropathies in general, is hampered by the absence of a gold standard or universally accepted criteria to diagnose any neuropathy.[123–125] Our understanding of the pathophysiology of compression neuropathies evolves rapidly. Unfortunately, taking nerve biopsies is rarely possible and the most commonly used animal models create more severe nerve lesions with much more damage[126] than the neuropathies we typically encounter in physiotherapy practices.

It is good to be aware that we treat many syndromes with neurodynamic techniques (e.g. carpal, cubital and tarsal tunnel *syndrome*, thoracic outlet *syndrome*, supinator and pronator teres *syndrome*). Most of these syndromes are still heavily debated, even CTS. Syndromes describe a collection of signs and symptoms that may not have a single identifiable pathogenesis. We have argued

previously that for the same syndrome (e.g. CTS), the dominant pathomechanism may be very different in different patients.[127] In some it may be localized at the entrapment site, but in others the dominant pain mechanism may be located in the dorsal root ganglia, spinal cord or brain. It is then to be expected that patients with the same syndrome but different pathomechanisms may respond differently in clinical trials to a more or less set intervention, be it neurodynamics, other forms of conservative management, or surgery. This may also explain the discrepancy that sometimes seems to exist between more physiological research findings with smaller and perhaps more uniform samples of patients in more controlled environments (this certainly also applies to animal studies), compared to large-scale clinical trials with long-term follow-up. In clinical practice, we want every patient to improve, but numbers needed to treat are rarely close to one. Identification of responders and non-responders remains important.

Discussing the potential effects of various interventions should not overshadow the importance of the quality of the patient–clinician relationship. Data suggest that a stronger therapeutic alliance between the patient and clinician is associated with better outcomes for patients who have musculoskeletal[128,129] or peripheral neuropathic pain.[130,131] Understanding the patient's perspective about the pain experience and the impact of any associated psychosocial issues, providing clear explanations to the patient (including a diagnosis where appropriate), and involving the patient in the decision-making process are examples of factors that can strengthen the patient–clinician relationship.[132,133]

There is an increased awareness of the role of the central nervous system in persistent pain states.[91,98,134,135] Patient perspectives have undoubtedly improved thanks to this. On the other hand, recent findings from respected research groups have reminded us that abnormal primary afferent input may also remain critical for maintaining pain in peripheral neuropathies[136] and phantom limb pain,[137] and that addressing this abnormal input can lead to drastic improvements.[137] As pointed out in this chapter, perhaps neurodynamics (and other movement-based interventions) can contribute to address both peripheral and central mechanisms in patients with persistent neuropathic pain states.

REFERENCES

1. Coppieters M, Nee RJ, Jull G, et al. How do you and your colleagues treat cervical radiculopathy? A nationwide survey of MPA members. In APA Conference New Moves. Melbourne, Australia: 2013.
2. Coppieters MW. The body and the brain. Current concepts in rehabilitation of neuropathic pain. 4th International Congress on Neuropathic Pain. IASP NeuPSIG; Toronto, Canada; 2013.
3. Coppieters M, Soon BT. Non-invasive management of carpal tunnel syndrome. A national practice survey among Australian hand therapists. In: APA Physiotherapy Conference, Brisbane, Australia; 2011.
4. Elvey RL. Physical evaluation of the peripheral nervous system in disorders of pain and dysfunction. J Hand Ther 1997;10(2):122–9.
5. Butler DS. The Sensitive Nervous System. 1st ed. Unley, S. Aust.: Noigroup Publications; 2000.
6. Smart K, Blake C, Staines A, et al. Clinical indicators of 'nociceptive', 'peripheral neuropathic' and 'central' mechanisms of

musculoskeletal pain. A Delphi survey of expert clinicians. Man Ther 2010;15:80–7.

7. Breig A, Troup J. Biomechanical considerations in the straight-leg-raising test: cadaveric and clinical studies of the effects of medial hip rotation. Spine 1979;4(3):242–50.

8. Gilbert K, Brismee J, Collins D, et al. 2006 Young Investigator Award Winner: lumbosacral nerve root displacement and strain. Part 2. A comparison of 2 straight leg conditions in unembalmed cadavers. Spine 2007;32(14):1521–5.

9. Nee RJ, Jull GA, Vicenzino B, et al. The validity of upper-limb neurodynamic tests for detecting peripheral neuropathic pain. J Orthop Sports Phys Ther 2012;42(5):413–24.

10. Boyd BS, Topp KS, Coppieters MW. Impact of movement sequencing on sciatic and tibial nerve strain and excursion during the straight leg raise test in embalmed cadavers. J Orthop Sports Phys Ther 2013;43(6):398–403.

11. Rade M, Kononen M, Vanninen R, et al. 2014 Young Investigator Award Winner: in vivo magnetic resonance imaging measurement of spinal cord displacement in the thoracolumbar region of asymptomatic subjects. Part 1: straight leg raise test. Spine 2014; 39(16):1288–93.

12. Ridehalgh C, Moore A, Hough A. Normative sciatic nerve excursion during a modified straight leg raise test. Man Ther 2014;19: 59–64.

13. Hall TM, Elvey RL. Nerve trunk pain: physical diagnosis and treatment. Man Ther 1999;4(2):63–73.

14. Coppieters MW, Alshami AM, Babri AS, et al. Strain and excursion of the sciatic, tibial, and plantar nerves during a modified straight leg raising test. J Orthop Res 2006;24(9):1883–9.

15. Alshami AM, Babri AS, Souvlis T, et al. Strain in the tibial and plantar nerves with foot and ankle movements and the influence of adjacent joint positions. J Appl Biomech 2008;24(4):368–76.

16. Coppieters MW, Kurz K, Mortensen TE, et al. The impact of neurodynamic testing on the perception of experimentally induced muscle pain. Man Ther 2005;10(1):52–60.

17. Coppieters MW, Alshami AM, Hodges PW. An experimental pain model to investigate the specificity of the neurodynamic test for the median nerve in the differential diagnosis of hand symptoms. Arch Phys Med Rehabil 2006;87(10):1412–17.

18. Walsh J, Flatley M, Johnston N, et al. Slump test: sensory responses in asymptomatic subjects. J Man Manipulative Ther 2007;15(4):231–8.

19. Lai W, Shih Y, Lin P, et al. Normal neurodynamic responses to the femoral slump test. Man Ther 2012;17:126–32.

20. Martinez M, Cubas C, Girbes E. Ulnar nerve neurodynamic test: study of the normal sensory response in asymptomatic individuals. J Orthop Sports Phys Ther 2014;44:450–6.

21. Hall T, Zusman M, Elvey R. Adverse mechanical tension in the nervous system? Analysis of straight leg raise. Man Ther 1998; 3(3):140–6.

22. Herrington L, Bendix K, Cornwell C, et al. What is the normal response to structural differentiation within the slump and straight leg raise tests? Man Ther 2008;13(4):289–94.

23. Walsh J, Hall T. Agreement and correlation between the straight leg raise and slump tests in subjects with leg pain. J Manipulative Physiol Ther 2009;32:184–92.

24. Johnson E, Chiarello C. The slump test: the effects of head and lower extremity position on knee extension. J Orthop Sports Phys Ther 1997;26(6):310–17.

25. Boyd B, Villa P. Normal inter-limb differences during the straight leg raise neurodynamic test: a cross sectional study. BMC Musculoskelet Disord 2012;13:245.

26. Covill L, Petersen S. Upper extremity neurodynamic tests: range of motion asymmetry may not indicate impairment. Physiother Theory Pract 2011;28:535–41.

27. Boyd B. Common interlimb asymmetries and neurogenic responses during upper limb neurodynamic testing: implications for test interpretation. J Hand Ther 2012;25:56–64.

28. Van Hoof T, Vangestel C, Shacklock M, et al. Asymmetry of ULNT1 elbow extension range-of-motion in a healthy population: consequences for clinical practice and research. Phys Ther Sport 2012;13:141–9.

29. Stalioraitis V, Robinson K, Hall T. Side-to-side range of movement variability in variants of the median and radial neurodynamic test sequences in asymptomatic people. Man Ther 2014;19: 338–42.

30. Philip K, Lew P, Matyas T. The inter-therapist reliability of the slump test. Aust J Physiother 1989;35:89–94.

31. Schmid AB, Brunner F, Luomajoki H, et al. Reliability of clinical tests to evaluate nerve function and mechanosensitivity of the upper limb peripheral nervous system. BMC Musculoskelet Disord 2009;10:11.

32. Wainner R, Fritz J, Irrgang J, et al. Reliability and diagnostic accuracy of the clinical examination and patient self-report measures for cervical radiculopathy. Spine 2003;28(1):52–62.

33. Wainner R, Fritz J, Irrgang J, et al. Development of a clinical prediction rule for the diagnosis of carpal tunnel syndrome. Arch Phys Med Rehabil 2005;86:609–18.

34. Vanti C, Bonfiglioli R, Calabrese M, et al. Upper limb neurodynamic test 1 and symptoms reproduction in carpal tunnel syndrome. A validity study. Man Ther 2011;16:258–63.

35. Vanti C, Bonfiglioli R, Calabrese M, et al. Relationship between interpretation and accuracy of the upper limb neurodynamic test 1 in carpal tunnel syndrome. J Manipulative Physiol Ther 2012; 35:54–63.

36. Slipman C, Plastaras C, Palmitier R, et al. Symptom provocation of fluoroscopically guided cervical nerve root stimulation: are dynatomal maps identical to dermatomal maps? Spine 1998; 23(20):2235–42.

37. Witt J, Hentz J, Stevens J. Carpal tunnel syndrome with normal nerve conduction studies. Muscle Nerve 2004;29:515–22.

38. Reitsma J, Rutjes A, Khan K, et al. A review of solutions for diagnostic accuracy studies with an imperfect or missing reference standard. J Clin Epidemiol 2009;62:797–806.

39. van der Windt D, Simons E, Riphagen I, et al. Physical examination for lumbar radiculopathy due to disc herniation in patients with low back pain. Cochrane Database Syst Rev 2010;(2): CD007430.

40. Scaia V, Baxter D, Cook C. The pain provocation-based straight leg raise test for diagnosis of lumbar disc herniation, lumbar radiculopathy, and/or sciatica: a systematic review of clinical utility. J Back Musculoskeletal Rehabil 2012;25:215–23.

41. Majlesi J, Togay H, Unalan H, et al. The sensitivity and specificity of the slump and the straight leg raising tests in patients with lumbar disc herniation. J Clin Rheumatol 2008;14:87–91.

42. Fritz J, Wainner R. Examining diagnostic tests: an evidence-based perspective. Phys Ther 2001;81(9):1546–64.

43. Beith I, Kemp A, Kenyon J, et al. Identifying neuropathic back and leg pain: a cross-sectional study. Pain 2011;152: 1511–16.

44. Walsh J, Hall T. Reliability, validity and diagnostic accuracy of palpation of the sciatic, tibial and common peroneal nerves in the examination of low back related leg pain. Man Ther 2009; 14(6):623–9.

45. Maitland G. Negative disc exploration: positive canal signs. Aust J Physiother 1979;25(3):129–34.

46. Nee RJ, Yang CH, Liang CC, et al. Impact of order of movement on nerve strain and longitudinal excursion: a biomechanical study with implications for neurodynamic test sequencing. Man Ther 2010;15(4):376–81.

47. Coppieters MW, Van de Velde M, Stappaerts KH. Positioning in anesthesiology: toward a better understanding of stretch-induced perioperative neuropathies. Anesthesiology 2002;97(1):75–81.

48. Coppieters MW, Butler DS. Do 'sliders' slide and 'tensioners' tension? An analysis of neurodynamic techniques and considerations regarding their application. Man Ther 2008;13(3): 213–21.

49. Elvey R. Treatment of arm pain associated with abnormal brachial plexus tension. Aust J Physiother 1986;32:225–30.

50. Coppieters MW, Alshami AM. Longitudinal excursion and strain in the median nerve during novel nerve gliding exercises for carpal tunnel syndrome. J Orthop Res 2007;25(7):972–80.

51. Coppieters MW, Hough AD, Dilley A. Different nerve-gliding exercises induce different magnitudes of median nerve longitudinal excursion: an in vivo study using dynamic ultrasound imaging. J Orthop Sports Phys Ther 2009;39(3):164–71.

52. Ellis RF, Hing WA, McNair PJ. Comparison of longitudinal sciatic nerve movement with different mobilization exercises: an in vivo study utilizing ultrasound imaging. J Orthop Sports Phys Ther 2012;42(8):667–75.

53. Coppieters MW, Andersen LS, Johansen R, et al. Excursion of the sciatic nerve during nerve mobilization exercises. An in vivo

cross-sectional study using dynamic ultrasound imaging. J Orthop Sports Phys Ther (in press).

54. Coppieters MW, Stappaerts KH, Wouters LL, et al. The immediate effects of a cervical lateral glide treatment technique in patients with neurogenic cervicobrachial pain. J Orthop Sports Phys Ther 2003;33(7):369–78.

55. Coppieters MW, Stappaerts KH, Wouters LL, et al. Aberrant protective force generation during neural provocation testing and the effect of treatment in patients with neurogenic cervicobrachial pain. J Manipulative Physiol Ther 2003;26(2):99–106.

56. Vicenzino B, Collins D, Wright A. The initial effects of a cervical spine manipulative physiotherapy treatment on the pain and dysfunction of lateral epicondylalgia. Pain 1996;68(1):69–74.

57. Sterling M, Pedler A, Chan C, et al. Cervical lateral glide increases nociceptive flexion reflex threshold but not pressure or thermal pain thresholds in chronic whiplash associated disorders: a pilot randomised controlled trial. Man Ther 2010;15(2):149–53.

58. Schäfer A, Hall T, Muller G, et al. Outcomes differ between subgroups of patients with low back and leg pain following neural manual therapy: a prospective cohort study. Eur Spine J 2011;20:482–90.

59. Allison GT, Nagy BM, Hall T. A randomized clinical trial of manual therapy for cervico-brachial pain syndrome – a pilot study. Man Ther 2002;7(2):95–102.

60. Smart KM, Blake C, Staines A, et al. The discriminative validity of 'nociceptive,' 'peripheral neuropathic,' and 'central sensitization' as mechanisms-based classifications of musculoskeletal pain. Clin J Pain 2011;27(8):655–63.

61. Smart KM, Blake C, Staines A, et al. Mechanisms-based classifications of musculoskeletal pain: part 2 of 3: symptoms and signs of peripheral neuropathic pain in patients with low back (+/– leg) pain. Man Ther 2012;17(4):345–51.

62. Bennett MI, Smith BH, Torrance N, et al. The S-LANSS score for identifying pain of predominantly neuropathic origin: validation for use in clinical and postal research. J Pain 2005;6(3):149–58.

63. Bouhassira D, Attal N, Alchaar H, et al. Comparison of pain syndromes associated with nervous or somatic lesions and development of a new neuropathic pain diagnostic questionnaire (DN4). Pain 2005;114(1–2):29–36.

64. Fernandez-de-Las-Penas C, Coppieters MW, Cuadrado ML, et al. Patients with chronic tension-type headache demonstrate increased mechano-sensitivity of the supra-orbital nerve. Headache 2008;48(4):570–7.

65. Hall T, Quintner J. Responses to mechanical stimulation of the upper limb in painful cervical radiculopathy. Aust J Physiother 1996;42(4):277–85.

66. Atroshi I, Gummesson C, Johnsson R, et al. Prevalence of carpal tunnel syndrome in a general population. JAMA 1999;282(2):153–8.

67. Hough AD, Moore AP, Jones MP. Reduced longitudinal excursion of the median nerve in carpal tunnel syndrome. Arch Phys Med Rehabil 2007;88(5):569–76.

68. Korstanje JW, Scheltens-De Boer M, Blok JH, et al. Ultrasonographic assessment of longitudinal median nerve and hand flexor tendon dynamics in carpal tunnel syndrome. Muscle Nerve 2012;45(5):721–9.

69. Valls-Sole J, Alvarez R, Nunez M. Limited longitudinal sliding of the median nerve in patients with carpal tunnel syndrome. Muscle Nerve 1995;18(7):761–7.

70. Allmann KH, Horch R, Uhl M, et al. MR imaging of the carpal tunnel. Eur J Radiol 1997;25(2):141–5.

71. Erel E, Dilley A, Greening J, et al. Longitudinal sliding of the median nerve in patients with carpal tunnel syndrome. J Hand Surg [Br] 2003;28(5):439–43.

72. Nakamichi K, Tachibana S. Restricted motion of the median nerve in carpal tunnel syndrome. J Hand Surg [Br] 1995;20(4):460–4.

73. Coppieters MW. Physiotherapy management of nerve-related neck and arm pain. In: Second Brazilian Conference of Manipulative and Musculoskeletal Physiotherapy (II COBRAFIMM) 2012. Sao Paulo, Brazil.

74. Tuzuner S, Inceoglu S, Bilen FE. Median nerve excursion in response to wrist movement after endoscopic and open carpal tunnel release. J Hand Surg [Am] 2008;33(7):1063–8.

75. Tuzuner S, Ozkaynak S, Acikbas C, et al. Median nerve excursion during endoscopic carpal tunnel release. Neurosurgery 2004;54(5):1155–60, discussion 1160–1.

76. Millesi H, Zoch G, Reihsner R. Mechanical properties of peripheral nerves. Clin Orthop Relat Res 1995;314:76–83.

77. Peters S, Page MJ, Coppieters MW, et al. Rehabilitation following carpal tunnel release. Cochrane Database Syst Rev 2013;(6):CD004158.

78. Warwick L, Seradge H. Early versus late range of motion following cubital tunnel surgery. J Hand Ther 1995;8(4):245–8.

79. Weirich SD, Gelberman RH, Best SA, et al. Rehabilitation after subcutaneous transposition of the ulnar nerve: immediate versus delayed mobilization. J Shoulder Elbow Surg 1998;7(3):244–9.

80. Sunderland S. The nerve lesion in the carpal tunnel syndrome. J Neurol Neurosurg Psychiatry 1976;39(7):615–26.

81. Rempel DM, Diao E. Entrapment neuropathies: pathophysiology and pathogenesis. J Electromyogr Kinesiol 2004;14(1):71–5.

82. Lundborg G, Myers R, Powell H. Nerve compression injury and increased endoneurial fluid pressure: a 'miniature compartment syndrome'. J Neurol Neurosurg Psychiatry 1983;46(12):1119–24.

83. Mackinnon SE. Pathophysiology of nerve compression. Hand Clin 2002;18(2):231–41.

84. Schmid AB, Elliott JM, Strudwick MW, et al. Effect of splinting and exercise on intraneural edema of the median nerve in carpal tunnel syndrome – an MRI study to reveal therapeutic mechanisms. J Orthop Res 2012;30(8):1343–50.

85. Chen SJ, Lin HS, Hsieh CH. Carpal tunnel pressure is correlated with electrophysiological parameters but not the 3 month surgical outcome. J Clin Neurosci 2013;20(2):272–7.

86. Diao E, Shao F, Liebenberg E, et al. Carpal tunnel pressure alters median nerve function in a dose-dependent manner: a rabbit model for carpal tunnel syndrome. J Orthop Res 2005;23(1):218–23.

87. Coppieters MW. Physiotherapy management of nerve-related neck and arm pain. In: Second Brazilian conference of manipulative and musculoskeletal physiotherapy (II COBRAFIMM). Sao Paulo, Brazil: 2012.

88. Coppieters MW, Schmid AB, Kubler PA, et al. Description, reliability and validity of a novel method to measure carpal tunnel pressure in patients with carpal tunnel syndrome. Man Ther 2012;17(6):589–92.

89. Bisby MA. Functions of retrograde axonal transport. Fed Proc 1982;41(7):2307–11.

90. Dilley A, Bove GM. Disruption of axoplasmic transport induces mechanical sensitivity in intact rat C-fibre nociceptor axons. J Physiol 2008;586(2):593–604.

91. Costigan M, Scholz J, Woolf CJ. Neuropathic pain: a maladaptive response of the nervous system to damage. Annu Rev Neurosci 2009;32:1–32.

92. Song XJ, Gan Q, Cao JL, et al. Spinal manipulation reduces pain and hyperalgesia after lumbar intervertebral foramen inflammation in the rat. J Manipulative Physiol Ther 2006;29(1):5–13.

93. Cheng CF, Cheng JK, Chen CY, et al. Mirror-image pain is mediated by nerve growth factor produced from tumor necrosis factor alpha-activated satellite glia after peripheral nerve injury. Pain 2014;155(5):906–20.

94. Milligan ED, Twining C, Chacur M, et al. Spinal glia and proinflammatory cytokines mediate mirror-image neuropathic pain in rats. J Neurosci 2003;23(3):1026–40.

95. Konopka KH, Harbers M, Houghton A, et al. Bilateral sensory abnormalities in patients with unilateral neuropathic pain; a quantitative sensory testing (QST) study. PLoS ONE 2012;7(5):e37524.

96. Schmid AB, Coppieters MW, Ruitenberg MJ, et al. Local and remote immune-mediated inflammation after mild peripheral nerve compression in rats. J Neuropathol Exp Neurol 2013;72(7):662–80.

97. Santos FM, Silva JT, Giardini AC, et al. Neural mobilization reverses behavioral and cellular changes that characterize neuropathic pain in rats. Mol Pain 2012;8:57.

98. Latremoliere A, Woolf CJ. Central sensitization: a generator of pain hypersensitivity by central neural plasticity. J Pain 2009;10(9):895–926.

99. Smith K. Neuroscience: settling the great glia debate. Nature 2010;468(7321):160–2.

100. Wright A. Hypoalgesia post-manipulative therapy: a review of a potential neurophysiological mechanism. Man Ther 1995; 1(1):11–16.

101. Sterling M, Jull G, Wright A. Cervical mobilisation: concurrent effects on pain, sympathetic nervous system activity and motor activity. Man Ther 2001;6(2):72–81.

102. Vicenzino B, Collins D, Benson H, et al. An investigation of the interrelationship between manipulative therapy-induced hypoalgesia and sympathoexcitation. J Manipulative Physiol Ther 1998;21(7):448–53.

103. O'Leary S, Falla D, Hodges PW, et al. Specific therapeutic exercise of the neck induces immediate local hypoalgesia. J Pain 2007;8(11):832–9.

104. Bialosky JE, Bishop MD, Price DD, et al. A randomized sham-controlled trial of a neurodynamic technique in the treatment of carpal tunnel syndrome. J Orthop Sports Phys Ther 2009;39(10): 709–23.

105. Santos FM, Grecco LH, Pereira MG, et al. The neural mobilization technique modulates the expression of endogenous opioids in the periaqueductal gray and improves muscle strength and mobility in rats with neuropathic pain. Behav Brain Funct 2014;10:19.

106. Adel S. Efficacy of neural mobilization in treatment of low back dysfunctions. J Am Sci 2011;7(4):566–73.

107. Cleland J, Childs J, Palmer J, et al. Slump stretching in the management of non-radicular low back pain: a pilot clinical trial. Man Ther 2006;11(4):279–86.

108. Nagrale A, Patil S, Gandhi R, et al. Effect of slump stretching versus lumbar mobilization with exercise in subjects with non-radicular low back pain: a randomized clinical trial. J Man Manipulative Ther 2012;20:35–42.

109. Hopkins W. A new view of statistics. 2011 Available from: <http://www.sportsci.org/resource/stats/index.html>; [cited 2011 December 7].

110. Scrimshaw S, Maher C. Randomized controlled trial of neural mobilization after spinal surgery. Spine 2001;26(24):2647–52.

111. Nee R, Vicenzino B, Jull G, et al. Neural tissue management provides immediate clinically relevant benefits without harmful effects for patients with nerve-related neck and arm pain: a randomised trial. J Physiother 2012;58:23–30.

112. Nee R, Vicenzino B, Jull G, et al. A novel protocol to develop a prediction model that identifies patients with nerve-related neck and arm pain who benefit from the early introduction of neural tissue management. Contemp Clin Trials 2011;32:760–70.

113. Gross A, Hoving J, Haines T, et al. A Cochrane review of manipulation and mobilization for mechanical neck disorders. Spine 2004;29(14):1541–8.

114. Page M, O'Connor D, Pitt V, et al. Exercise and mobilisation interventions for carpal tunnel syndrome (Review). Cochrane Database Syst Rev 2012;(6):Art. No.:CD009899.

115. Svernlov B, Larrson M, Rehn K, et al. Conservative treatment of the cubital tunnel syndrome. J Hand Surg 2009;34E:201–7.

116. Kavlak Y, Uygur F. Effects of nerve mobilization exercise as an adjunct to the conservative treatment for patients with tarsal tunnel syndrome. J Manipulative Physiol Ther 2011;34:441–8.

117. Foster N, Dziedzic K, van der Windt D, et al. Research priorities for non-pharmacological therapies for common musculoskeletal problems: nationally and internationally agreed recommendations. BMC Musculoskelet Disord 2009;10:3.

118. Goldstein M, Scalzitti D, Craik R, et al. The revised research agenda for physical therapy. Phys Ther 2011;91:165–74.

119. Nee R, Vicenzino B, Jull G, et al. Baseline characteristics of patients with nerve-related neck and arm pain predict the likely response to neural tissue management. J Orthop Sports Phys Ther 2013;43(6):379–91.

120. Hancock M, Herbert R, Maher C. A guide to interpretation of studies investigating subgroups of responders to physical therapy interventions. Phys Ther 2009;89(7):698–704.

121. Kent P, Keating J, Leboeuf-Yde C. Research methods for sub-grouping low back pain. BMC Med Res Methodol 2010;10:62.

122. Hoffmann TC, Glasziou PP, Boutron I, et al. Better reporting of interventions: template for intervention description and replication (TIDieR) checklist and guide. BMJ 2014;348:g1687.

123. Thoomes EJ, Scholten-Peeters GG, de Boer AJ, et al. Lack of uniform diagnostic criteria for cervical radiculopathy in conservative intervention studies: a systematic review. Eur Spine J 2012; 21(8):1459–70.

124. Genevay S, Atlas SJ, Katz JN. Variation in eligibility criteria from studies of radiculopathy due to a herniated disc and of neurogenic claudication due to lumbar spinal stenosis: a structured literature review. Spine (Phila Pa 1976) 2010;35(7):803–11.

125. Bland JD. Carpal tunnel syndrome. Curr Opin Neurol 2005; 18(5):581–5.

126. Hu P, Bembrick AL, Keay KA, et al. Immune cell involvement in dorsal root ganglia and spinal cord after chronic constriction or transection of the rat sciatic nerve. Brain Behav Immun 2007; 21(5):599–616.

127. Schmid AB, Nee RJ, Coppieters MW. Reappraising entrapment neuropathies–mechanisms, diagnosis and management. Man Ther 2013;18(6):449–57.

128. Hall A, Ferreira P, Maher C, et al. The influence of the therapist-patient relationship on treatment outcome in physical rehabilitation: a systematic review. Phys Ther 2010;90:1099–110.

129. Ferreira P, Ferreira M, Maher C, et al. The therapeutic alliance between clinicians and patients predicts outcome in chronic low back pain. Phys Ther 2013;93:470–8.

130. Ong B, Konstantinou K, Corbett M, et al. Patients' own accounts of sciatica. Spine 2011;36:1251–6.

131. Hopayian K, Notley C. A systematic review of low back pain and sciatica patients' expectations and experiences of health care. Spine J 2014;doi:10.1016/j.spinee.2014.02.029; (in press).

132. Pinto R, Ferreira M, Oliveira V, et al. Patient-centred communication is associated with positive therapeutic alliance: a systematic review. J Physiother 2012;58:77–87.

133. Peersman W, Rooms T, Bracke N, et al. Patients' priorities regarding outpatient physiotherapy care: a qualitative and quantitative study. Man Ther 2013;18:155–64.

134. Keefe FJ, Porter L, Somers T, et al. Psychosocial interventions for managing pain in older adults: outcomes and clinical implications. Br J Anaesth 2013;111(1):89–94.

135. Lee MC, Tracey I. Imaging pain: a potent means for investigating pain mechanisms in patients. Br J Anaesth 2013;111(1):64–72.

136. Haroutounian S, Nikolajsen L, Bendtsen TF, et al. Primary afferent input critical for maintaining spontaneous pain in peripheral neuropathy. Pain 2014;155(7):1272–9.

137. Vaso A, Adahan HM, Gjika A, et al. Peripheral nervous system origin of phantom limb pain. Pain 2014;155(7):1384–91.

CHAPTER 31

THERAPEUTIC EXERCISE

Deborah Falla • Rod Whiteley • Marco Cardinale • Paul Hodges

INTRODUCTION

This chapter aims to provide a framework to design exercise-based interventions to reach desired rehabilitation goals, be they improvements in neuromuscular control (muscle activation, movement strategy, alignment/posture and movement quality), strength, endurance, or some combination of these. This chapter focuses on motor control training and resistance training, but notes that exercise for other features may be relevant for a patient's presentation including range of motion, muscle length, sensory function and postural alignment.

PRINCIPLES OF MANAGEMENT

Clinical Prescription of Exercise

When working with an otherwise healthy patient, the physiotherapist must first conduct a needs analysis to define the desired exercise goal, prescribe the appropriate training parameters to achieve the goals and use validated measures to assess progress (Fig. 31-1). This chapter is arbitrarily divided into sections according to the desired outcomes of exercise, but it is necessary to remember that these outcomes are not mutually exclusive. Situations will often arise where multiple goals are important. For instance a person may initially require improvements in control of a movement, and once this is established move on to strength/endurance adaptation. A clear understanding of the parameters associated with exercise prescription will aid in this process. Accurate exercise prescription requires an understanding of an individual's existing function, along with a needs analysis regarding the functional requirements of his/her work/sport/daily activity (Fig. 31-1). It is then important to conduct an appropriate assessment to guide exercise prescription. Once this information is gathered, it is possible to define the training methodology, the specific means and exercises used, and the details of the programme in terms of its volume, intensity and progression. Finally, the continuous assessments to monitor progress and to ascertain the effectiveness of the therapeutic exercise programme to change the target features, represent fundamental milestones in the training programme in order to introduce adjustments and/or recalibrate the training contents to ensure the objectives are met.

Indications for Exercise

There is undoubtedly a link between pain and altered motor control. Disturbed motor control ultimately contributes to impaired motor output, which may include poor control/coordination, reduced strength, impaired endurance, diminished force steadiness or smoothness of movement, all of which are well documented in people with musculoskeletal pain (for a review see Chapter 6). The association between pain and motor control impairment is supported by the abundance of literature describing neuromuscular dysfunction in people across a range of musculoskeletal pain conditions, in addition to the numerous experimental pain studies confirming that pain may have an immediate and profound effect on motor control.[1-3] It is hypothesized that impaired motor function may contribute to the recurrence of musculoskeletal pain, further emphasizing the importance of early and effective exercise interventions. This has been particularly the case for spinal pain, where continuous motor impairments have been documented despite recovery from an acute episode and return to normal activity.[4-8] Ongoing deficits in motor control could lead to poor control of movement, abnormal loading, repeated microtrauma and eventually pain. Moreover, actual pain may not necessarily have to be present for motor control changes to persist. Factors such as fear of pain may have similar effects and may explain altered motor control in patients with pain when they are in remission.[9,10] Although there is no clear consensus on the cause–effect relationship between altered motor control and pain/injury, it is evident that pain/injury is associated with impaired motor function and thus training can be considered relevant in this context.

The importance of training as a component of rehabilitation is also supported by studies that show that a reduction in pain with treatment which excludes exercise (e.g. manipulative therapy as a sole treatment) is insufficient to enhance neuromuscular control in patients with musculoskeletal pain.[11-13] Guidance of an exercise programme depends on identifying features of motor output that are compromised in the patient, particularly those which underlie the deficit in performance of the patient's identified goal.

Assessment to Guide Exercise Prescription

Guidance of exercise relies on assessment of a range of potential targets including the quality of movement,

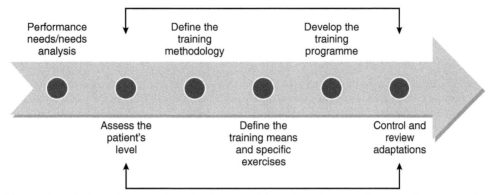

FIGURE 31-1 ■ A simple framework to develop an evidence-based approach to exercise prescription.

motor control, strength and endurance, and sensory function. The battery of tests used will depend on the patient's condition and the identified treatment goal. The following section outlines some of the general considerations when planning a patient's assessment to guide exercise prescription.

Assessment of Movement Quality

Movement quality refers to the kinematics of the performance of a movement, that is, the actual joint angles, velocities and variability associated with single bouts and repetitions of this movement pattern. Physiotherapists often consider that poor 'quality' of movement performance is related to excessive tissue loading and an individual's likelihood of injury (both past and present). Individuals generally present with some features of movement impairment (related to a function or a specific physiological movement direction), which is related to their presenting problem. Although a reference database of normative data may not be available for a complex functional task for comparison of an individual's performance, the physiotherapist will often examine a set of standardized movements such as shoulder abduction and flexion (for the upper limb) and a single leg squat, or walking (for the lower limb), and then extrapolate from the perceived quality of these movements to a clinical inference of the 'movement quality' in function. There is some evidence for the accuracy of this approach. For instance, in low back pain the quality (timing and amplitude) of pelvic motion during hip rotation provides reliable and meaningful information that guides exercise prescription.[14,15] Unfortunately, in many conditions such reliability is not evident. As an example, in assessment of the shoulder disorders, visual estimation of the quality of scapular movement associated with arm movements is considered clinically important. However, the accuracy of this visual estimation has poor inter-rater reliability and poor correlation to 'gold standard' examination of the tracking of implanted bone pins.[16] Acceptable reliability has been documented when the estimation is limited to classification as 'normal' versus either 'subtle' or 'obvious' dysfunction.[17] Similarly, clinical examination of the quality of a single leg squat is difficult, with good reliability only achieved for panel rating of video performance when ranked as 'good', 'fair', or 'poor'.[18]

Although there is some indication that tests of movement quality may provide information relevant for guidance of exercise prescription, the ability of such assessments to identify injury risk remains questionable.[19] Thus, it is important to keep in mind that the use of many assessments of movement quality is best restricted to guidance of exercise prescription.

Assessment of Motor Control

Pain and injury are commonly associated with changes in motor control and many clinical assessments have been developed to evaluate specific features of the control and coordination of muscle activation, posture and movement. The basic assumption is that features of the strategy of muscle activation, posture and movement may abnormally load the tissues and be responsible for at least part of the patient's symptoms. The specific assessments that are used depend on the clinical condition, the target task and the features of performance of the task that the clinician considers are a priority. In back and neck pain, specific assessments of muscle activation strategy, postures and movements have been developed. Methods such as observation, palpation and specific devices (e.g. air-filled cuff to quantify the quality of upper cervical flexion to assess the deep cervical flexor muscles; ultrasound imaging to measure the pattern of abdominal and back extensor muscle activation; photography to measure alignment of specific anatomical sites) are used to evaluate performance. Tests of motor control are diverse and the degree to which the validity and reliability have been assessed varies, with some tests evaluated extensively (e.g. voluntary activation of deep lumbar[20] and neck muscles[21–24]; dissociation of hip from spine motion[15]) and others not.

Assessment of Muscle Structure

Adequate muscle structure is essential to meet demands of motor output. Comprehensive assessment using imaging methods such us ultrasound/computed tomography/magnetic resonance imaging scans can provide the clinician with relevant information about muscle mass (cross-sectional area), structure, fatty infiltration and injury. These parameters will likely influence the motor output and have been identified as relevant for a range of conditions (e.g. muscle atrophy and fatty infiltration in back,[25] neck[26] and shoulder[27] pain).

Assessment of Strength Parameters

Comprehensive assessment of strength may consider a range of features including; peak force, rate of force development and rate of force relaxation. The use of instrumented devices to estimate muscle strength has gained increasing popularity over the last decade, especially with a more widespread clinical adoption of hand-held dynamometers. Typically, these devices only provide the peak force recorded by the load cell during a specific task, whereas more sophisticated dynamometers (such as isokinetic dynamometers or linear encoders, accelerometers and other isoinertial dynamometers) can calculate/measure the force (or torque when angular rotation is performed with an isokinetic dynamometer) produced at all angles of the range of motion, during different contractile activities (isometric, concentric or eccentric) and different velocities of contraction. Often, the maximum force generated in a specific task provides sufficient information for the clinician to detect differences between healthy and injured sides of an individual, or to screen for differences from normative data (as in the case of hamstrings to quadriceps[28] and shoulder internal to external rotation[29] strength ratios). In the context of a recovering injury, tracking progress on such force measures is a useful means of documenting response to treatment and the course of recovery. It is important to know that the information generated during such assessments is specific to the movement pattern used and the speed and modality of contraction. In the case of isometric actions, the value derived for a maximal voluntary contraction can only be extrapolated to a limited range of motion outside the angle used for testing. Assessment of strength parameters are used to identify the deficits to target with rehabilitation, to define the variables of a training intervention and to guide exercise intensity such as establishing the external load (as a percentage of maximum) to use in the rehabilitation programme. For instance, if the maximum force generated during elbow flexion is 120 N, this means the maximum load a patient can tolerate in that position is 12 kg. A 9.6 kg-load could be selected if the target intensity is 80% of the patient's maximal voluntary contraction.

Assessment of Muscle Fatigue

Muscle fatigue/endurance is important to consider clinically. The inability of a muscle to sustain force output will have consequences for maintenance of a function and could lead to poor control of movement. Traditionally, fatigue is quantified as time to task failure (when impossible to maintain a target force). Alternative measures can be used to quantify the processes that occur as the capacity of the muscle declines before task failure is reached (e.g. electromyography measures such as median frequency: see Chapter 17). Assessment of the fatigability of a muscle group could provide valuable information (if it is considered to be a relevant feature of the priority goal) when interpreting the target for exercise

prescription. Conventional assessment paradigms using isokinetic dynamometry provide limited validity for assessment of fatigue as the common algorithms simply consider performance decline from the first to last (typically five) repetition.[30] A better approach may be to derive the linear slope of the decline in work across the entire exercise test. Although a promising approach, this is unlikely to be implemented in clinical practice until this becomes a standard feature of the reporting software.[31]

Alternative measures of fatigue/endurance for clinical practice range from simple measures of time to task failure in standardized tasks (e.g. Biering Sorensen test to assess back extensor endurance), to comprehensive measurement of decline in median frequency of an electromyography recording using advanced clinical electromyography systems that provide this measure as an output. For a clinician it is important to consider which muscle/muscle group requires assessment and then determine from their available measurement tools how best to assess endurance to identify whether the feature should be targeted in the exercise programme.

Summary of Assessment

Assessment of the range of features of motor performance that the clinician considers to be relevant for the presentation of the patient (including motor control, endurance, strength/power capabilities) is of paramount importance to establish an optimal training programme, and is fundamental to assess progress of a patient. All relevant features of motor output need to be assessed to decide on the most appropriate intervention.

Specificity and Selectivity of Exercise

Clinical trials of patients with a range of musculoskeletal pain conditions report significant and clinically meaningful reductions in pain and disability for training programmes, including low-intensity training (often focused on precision and control) and high-intensity training (focused on strength and endurance effects). Thus, various training approaches require consideration for the individual patient and may be appropriate for the management of the patient's symptoms and presentation. An important consideration is that the neuromuscular and functional changes induced by the training paradigm are specific to the mode of exercise performed.[32,33] Depending on the training paradigm, the adaptations that transpire may involve distinct structural and functional changes in the periphery (e.g. enhanced muscle mass) and across the regions of the nervous system from the spinal cord to the motor cortex and other supraspinal centres.[32,34] Given that people with musculoskeletal pain present with an array of deficits of motor output ranging from subtle changes in coordination between muscles through to reduced maximal force capacity for a given muscle or muscle group (see Chapter 6), this knowledge implies that different forms of exercise will need to be considered and should be prescribed according to the neuromuscular impairments that are revealed by the clinical assessment of the patient.

The need for specificity in therapeutic exercise has been supported by a number of exercise trials in patients with musculoskeletal pain. For example, low-load motor control training, but not high-load resistance training of the neck/back, has been shown to be effective to enhance the activation of the deep cervical flexor muscles[35] or abdominal muscles,[36] restore the coordination between the deep and superficial flexors,[35,37] enhance the speed of deep muscle activation when challenged by a postural perturbation[35,36] and improve the patient's ability to maintain an upright posture of the cervical spine during prolonged sitting.[38] In contrast, resistance training of the neck muscles led to superior gains in cervical muscle strength, endurance and resistance to fatigue compared to a low-load motor control programme.[39,40] Likewise, resistance training targeted at atrophied muscles was required to ameliorate the long-standing atrophy and fatty infiltration in patients with chronic low back pain.[41] It is therefore established that in the presence of pain and/or dysfunction, specificity of training is an important concept to consider in the prescription of an exercise programme. Specificity of training should also be considered relative to the velocity of exercise, the position of the patient (joint angle) and the movement pattern during exercise.[42] Thus, if specific aspects of motor control are identified to be important features in a patient's presentation then it is likely that a 'specific' and targeted approach is required to achieve meaningful change.

Another issue that requires consideration is the potential for interaction between treatments in combined exercise approaches. Several studies have suggested that combining large volumes of endurance training with resistance exercise might impair the effectiveness of each modality. It is thought that endurance training has positive effects on endurance, but to the detriment of strength and power outcomes (and the reverse for strength training at the expense of endurance outcomes). Although the exact nature of this relationship is still debated with respect to its magnitude and the interaction for specific muscle groups of interest,[43,44] a strong molecular basis can explain why this might occur.[45]

Timing of Exercise

Changes in neuromuscular control appear early after the initial onset of pain or injury.[7,46] In addition, experimental pain studies confirm that pain has an immediate and profound effect on motor behaviour.[47,48] On this basis it has been suggested that exercise to address impairment of motor behaviour is commenced early within the rehabilitation programme.[49,50] Gentle and specific exercises have also been shown to provide immediate pain relief,[12,36,51] which further supports early inclusion of specific training for the management of musculoskeletal pain. Generally, it is considered important to address issues of motor control before loading the muscle to induce change in strength, endurance and structure.[41] Thus higher load resistance training typically follows later in the rehabilitation programme.[26,27]

Although the benefit of early rehabilitation of motor deficits has not been fully examined in clinical trials, it is assumed that early rehabilitation of motor function may also serve to prevent changes in muscle structural properties that have been documented in patients with chronic musculoskeletal pain (e.g. atrophy of selected muscles,[4,52] preferential atrophy of slow-twitch oxidative type-I fibres,[53,54] and fatty infiltration of muscle tissue[26,55]). For instance, the presence of fatty tissue infiltration of the neck extensor muscles, which is present in patients with moderate to severe pain following a whiplash injury, is not detected until 3 months after the injury[56] and changes in muscle fibre type in multifidus is not present until 6 months.[54] These observations suggest some of the structural changes may, at least in part, represent a secondary adaptation to altered motor control and may be potentially prevented by specific training interventions. In addition, it is hypothesized that early and effective training of motor control may help to prevent transition to chronicity and reduce the recurrence of symptoms.[57] Future studies are clearly warranted to confirm these hypotheses.

Variability in Response to Exercise

A multitude of neuromuscular adaptations have been documented in people with musculoskeletal pain with large variability noted between individual patients (see Chapter 6 for a review). Such variability in patient presentation may partly explain the variable symptomatic benefit experienced by patients from standardized exercise programmes; responses range from an excellent outcome to minimal benefit. An important determinant of symptomatic response to exercise is the degree of neuromuscular impairment before training. For example, in patients with low back pain, baseline transversus abdominis activation predicts those who respond best to specific motor control training.[13,58] Likewise, specific motor control exercise for the deep cervical flexor muscles is most effective at relieving pain in people with neck pain that demonstrate the poorest control of their deep muscles at baseline.[59] These findings further indicate that treatment outcome will likely be best when exercise is selected and tailored based on a precise assessment of a patients' neuromuscular control.

FORMS OF EXERCISE COMMONLY APPLIED TO MANAGE MUSCULOSKELETAL PAIN

A key aim of exercise programmes is to induce long-lasting changes in motor behaviour, either to restore correct motor patterns or to enhance other aspects of motor performance.[60] Optimization of motor output can be achieved with practice, reflecting the ability of the motor system to adapt and refine motor output towards higher efficiency. Numerous studies have confirmed that both muscle tissue and the neural control of muscle adapts in response to a variety of motor experiences, including motor control, strength and endurance training.[32,34,61-63] Moreover, these adaptations may persist despite the absence of continued training, which suggests the motor system is able to maintain these adaptations.[64] The following sections present two common forms of training applied for the rehabilitation of musculoskeletal conditions; namely motor control training and resistance (strength, endurance) training. The neuromuscular adaptations that occur with each form of training are reviewed and the general principles of each training approach presented.

Motor Control Training

Individuals with musculoskeletal pain present with deficits in motor control (e.g. coordination of muscles, posture and movement; reviewed in Chapter 6), which not only affect tissue loading, but also contribute to deficits in general features of motor output such as poor endurance and strength. Examples of motor control deficits that are commonly targeted with exercise are the compromised control of the deep spinal muscles that are frequently observed in people with back and neck pain. Among other features, compromised activation is characterized by delayed activation when the spine is perturbed (e.g. rapid arm movements are accompanied by delayed transversus abdominis and multifidus activation in back pain[65,66] and delayed longus colli and capitis[67] activation in neck pain), and reduced amplitude of activation across a range of functions.[68–73] Patients with musculoskeletal pain may also present with functional changes (reorganization) of the neuronal properties in the sensorimotor system. Exercise also targets neuroplastic changes in the nervous system. For instance, topography of the primary motor cortex representations of transversus abdominis[74] and the lumbar paraspinal[75] muscles, measured using transcranial magnetic stimulation, is modified in patients with recurrent episodes of low back pain. This is indicative of cortical reorganization and is related to behaviour features such as the activation of the muscle in association with arm movement.[74]

A critical issue for exercise prescription is that numerous studies have confirmed that many of the alterations in motor control of the spine cannot be ameliorated by strength or endurance training, or by general physical activity.[13,35–37] Thus, training approaches targeted at correction of the motor control faults and re-establishing normal motor strategies are an important aspect of the treatment of musculoskeletal pain.[76] The benefit of such training has been well documented for both low back pain and neck pain, and for some conditions of the limbs (e.g. training focused on rehabilitation of motor control of the knee in patellofemoral pain).[77] As a general recommendation it appears logical and consistent with many contemporary exercise approaches (e.g. Hodges et al.[50]) to correct aberrant features of motor control before loading the muscles to induce change in strength, endurance and muscle structure. Thus, the initial emphasis in prescription of an exercise programme should generally involve optimization of control, coordination and precision of movement.

Several training approaches that target restoration of features of motor control have been described, especially for the management of low back and neck pain.[49,50,78–81] Generally the objective is to address features of posture/alignment, movement and muscle activation strategies to achieve the goal of optimization of tissue loading and movement quality followed by progression into increasingly challenging situations towards full function[50] (Fig. 31-2). Most motor control training approaches encourage prescription of exercise that is tailored to the motor control deficits and functional demands that are identified for the individual patient based on findings of comprehensive assessment. Just like other forms of exercise management, motor control training cannot be applied in a uniform manner. Detailed assessment is essential to identify the features of motor control that are likely to

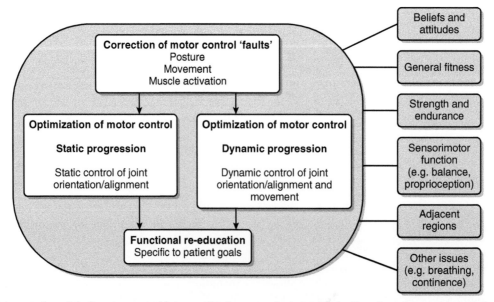

FIGURE 31-2 ■ Integrated model of motor control intervention for musculoskeletal pain disorders: An overview of the basic progression from initial goal of correction of faults in muscle activation, posture and movement to functional re-education and the intervening steps through static and dynamic training. On the right are additional issues that may be necessary to consider. (Adapted with permission from Hodges et al.[50])

be related to the patient's symptoms and the intervention is targeted to those features. As alluded to above, this must include assessment and subsequent intervention targeted at muscle activation, posture/alignment and movement.

In terms of muscle activation in spinal pain, considerable attention has been focused on evaluation and rehabilitation of the function of the deeper muscles of the lumbar and cervical spines.[16,17,21,27,28,81–83] Although changes in activation of the more superficial muscles must also be addressed, changes in activation of deeper muscles are commonly identified and often included as a component of the exercise programme. Considerable work has established that deficits in coordination of the deeper trunk muscles can be addressed by first encouraging the patient to learn the skill of voluntary activation of the muscles, repeated practice of this contraction, and then incorporation of the activation into dynamic and static functions.[35–38,49,50,79,84] In a similar manner, specific features of activation of superficial muscles, posture/alignment and movement are addressed by first using a range of clinical strategies to correct the 'fault' in motor control (e.g. feedback, instruction, manual guidance, etc.), followed by repetition and integration into function. Although less investigated, a similar motor control approach has/can be applied to other musculoskeletal conditions (e.g. lateral hip pain,[85] shoulder pain[82,86]).

The rationale for this approach is based on the principle of novel motor-skill training, which places emphasis on improved performance of selected (sub-optimal) components of function rather than the simple execution of a sequence of movements. This approach is consistent with accepted methods for training motor skills that involve initial cognitive attention to performance of task components, followed by repetition within changing environments and contexts to achieve more automatic activation.[87] It follows that this approach requires detailed assessment of motor deficits and then application of motor learning principles that are targeted to accurate modification of the relevant features of motor behaviour.[49,50] These include principles such as 'segmentation' (practice of individual components of a task before practice of the whole task), 'simplification' (practice with reduced demand to enable better-quality performance) and use of 'augmented feedback'.[50] The ability to target a specific component of movement requires greater skill and increased levels of attention and precision than contraction of all muscles (e.g. strength training) and several studies have shown that skill training achieves greater change in motor behaviour and motor cortex organization than these other types of muscle activation.[36,37,83]

Training Principles of Motor Control Training

Motor control training is typically commenced early within the rehabilitation programme. Ideally training should be performed in a pain-free manner in order to optimize success, since pain and the distraction associated with pain might interfere with the neuroplastic changes that would otherwise occur with motor-skill training.[88–90] Task repetitions should also be limited to ensure that factors such as fatigue are minimized. It is generally

considered that short sessions of high-quality practice are better than long sessions with deteriorating quality of performance. Rapid changes in cortical excitability are already apparent following short (10–15 minutes) intervals of motor control training[88] and extended within-session task repetitions may not facilitate additional gains in overall motor performance[91] or could be detrimental if performance quality is diminished. Cognitive effort is also known to significantly contribute to the extent of cortical neuroplastic changes associated with novel motor-skill acquisition,[92,93] thus the complexity of training should be slowly increased to encourage continued cognitive effort. The quality of training is critical to consider. For instance, improvements in the behaviour of activation of the transversus abdominis muscle in low back pain patients have been correlated to the quality of training and are associated with improvements in self-reported pain and function.[37]

As transfer to function is likely to be optimal when practice is performed as close to the function as possible,[94] progression to functional exercise is critical.[50] For instance, isolated motor control training of the deep cervical flexor muscles in people with chronic neck pain enhanced the activation of these muscles and reduced the necessary contribution of the superficial flexor muscles during performance of craniocervical flexion, but this did not transfer to reduced superficial neck muscle activity during a functional activity.[95] This highlights that training should be progressed to include specific training of problematic functional activities in order to optimize motor control in the tasks that the patient identifies as the priority functional goal.

Neuromuscular Adaptations

A key premise of motor control training is that the features of motor control that are targeted with the exercise approach are changed by the intervention and related to recovery. Besides a positive effect on pain and disability, specific motor control training has been shown to restore or reverse specific motor control impairments patients with in musculoskeletal pain. For instance, a single session of cognitive activation of transversus abdominis improves the timing of activation of this muscle during postural perturbations,[36] and this is further improved and maintained by repeated training.[63] Likewise, specific activation of deep cervical flexor muscles increases their activation during an isometric task,[35] improves the activation time when challenged by postural perturbations[35,59] and restores the directional specificity of neck muscle activity (which is normally observed in healthy individuals, but lost in many people with neck pain) during isometric contractions across a range of directions.[84] Activity of superficial trunk and neck muscles can also be reduced with specific motor control training,[35,37] even after a single session.[37,96] Interventions targeted at specific motor features also change posture,[38] movement[97] and sensory function.[98] Furthermore, motor cortex organization can be restored in association with improved pain and improved coordination of muscle activation in low back pain.[99] However, it should be noted that the specific features that need to be trained are individual-specific and treatment must be targeted to the changes identified in the individual patient.

Parameters of the muscle activation strategy at baseline are related to the responsiveness of an individual patient to a motor control intervention[13,58,59] and the degree of change in muscle activation is related to clinical improvement.[13,58,59,100] The weight of physiological evidence and evidence from high-quality clinical trials supports the relevance of exercise for motor control based on precise assessment to identify which features, if any, of posture/movement/muscle activation are considered relevant for the patient's presentation.[50]

Resistance Training

As highlighted earlier, musculoskeletal conditions are often accompanied by deficits in strength and endurance. Thus resistance training forms an important component of many rehabilitation programmes. Depending on the evaluation of the patient's capacity and their functional requirements, the intensity, frequency and duration of exercises are manipulated to optimize improvements in strength and/or endurance.

Strength training enhances maximum force production and maximal rate of force development,[101] which is accompanied by increased muscle cross-sectional area and fibre pennation angle.[102–104] Type II (phasic) muscle fibres preferentially hypertrophy with heavy resistance exercise.[105] Such structural alterations typically take several weeks to occur.[106] Changes in the myosin heavy chain isoforms,[103,107] Na^+–K^+ pump activity[108] and Ca^{2+} sensitivity[107,109] occur earlier than changes in the whole muscle morphology. Neural adaptations have also been observed following strength training which explain the disproportionate increase in muscle force compared to muscle size during the initial stages of training.[110] Early gains in strength have been attributed to a variety of mechanisms, including increased maximal motor unit discharge rates,[62,111] increased incidence of brief interspike intervals (doublets)[112] and decreased interspike interval variability.[113] Strength training also increases the tensile strength of tendons, ligaments and connective tissue in muscle.[114,115] This form of training usually involves lifting weights and/or using external resistances of moderate to high intensity. Prolonged programmes of resistance exercise produce muscle hypertrophy. Recent work also suggests that lifting relatively low-intensity loads to the point of task failure[116] or using blood flow restriction with low load[117] can induce a similar degree of hypertrophy to that obtained with heavy resistance exercise.

Endurance training programmes improve resistance to fatigue and are associated with reduced muscle fibre cross-sectional area, mitochondrial biogenesis and angiogenesis.[118–120] Transformation of muscle fibres from type IIB to type IIA is common with endurance training.[121] As observed for strength training, it has been shown that changes in the myosin heavy chain isoforms,[103,107] Na^+–K^+ pump activity[108] and Ca^{2+} sensitivity[107,109] occur earlier than changes in the whole muscle morphology following a period of endurance training. Metabolically, endurance training increases mitochondrial density and increases the use of lipids as a substrate.[120,122] These adaptations are accompanied by increased maximal oxygen uptake capacity.[122] Endurance training also leads to decreased motor unit interspike interval variability,[123] lower motor unit discharge rates[62] and a slower decline of motor unit conduction velocity during sustained contractions.[61]

Several studies have evaluated the effect of resistance training in patients with musculoskeletal complaints. Most show clinical benefit. A recent systematic review[124] confirmed that resistance training can increase muscle strength, reduce pain and improve functional ability in patients suffering from chronic low back pain, knee osteoarthritis, chronic tendinopathy and those under recovery after hip replacement surgery, especially for individuals presenting with loss of muscle strength and functional ability.

Intensity of Resistance Training

Force generation, or the peak force generated during a simple movement (e.g. knee extension, shoulder external rotation), has been well documented as an indicator for the strength abilities of a group of muscles in a given task. Such evaluation requires use of a dynamometer. It will likely be limited to an isometric task for a hand-held or fixed dynamometer, or through a single plane of movement for an isokinetic dynamometer with limited possibilities also achievable with isoinertial dynamometers. In practice, information from more complex multijoint movements is often of interest. In the occupational and sports setting this could be a lifting task that can be replicated using free weights. The maximum amount of weight able to be lifted by an individual for one repetition of a given exercise (but not two repetitions) is termed the 'one repetition maximum' (1 RM) for that person, for that exercise, on that day. In the field of weight training, this has become a commonly employed benchmark to estimate 'strength' of an individual for a given exercise. In a clinical setting, this is a useful technique to more accurately estimate the intensity of a given exercise for an individual.

Prescription of the intensity of the exercise is typically undertaken as a percentage of an individual's 1 RM. At the beginning of an exercise programme the percentage necessary to achieve training-induced adaptations in strength is low (30–40%) for sedentary, untrained individuals or very high (80–95%) for those already highly trained.[42] A typical training intensity would be between 60% and 70% of an RM for healthy but untrained adults.[42,125]

In practice, a patient may also perform a single exercise set to fatigue with the number of repetitions performed determined by the intensity. That is, if an individual performs a given exercise until fatigue, and completes 25 repetitions, then by definition this was a relatively low-intensity exercise (in spite of the fact that the individual will be fatigued at the end of the exercise). As the response to exercise is considered to be related to the intensity, it is useful to consult a table or formula to estimate the 1 RM from a fatiguing exercise and plan the appropriate resistance level for subsequent sessions.

Although regression equations are available that purport to predict the 1 RM of an individual from a submaximal test, the predictive abilities of such equations have variable accuracy and depend on the population and the exercise chosen with an error that ranges from <1% error (bench press) to 9–14% error (deadlift).[126] For clinical purposes, no single equation is clearly superior to another, and the differences in the predicted values could be relatively large if very low external loads are used (i.e. loads permitting more than ten repetitions) (as an example, see: Eston and Evans[127]).

Volume of Resistance Training

There has been substantial debate concerning the appropriate operational definition of training volume within the resistance exercise literature, making this parameter difficult to evaluate and replicate in research and/or provide practical guidelines for exercise prescription. One of the most widely accepted definitions for this variable is volume load, which takes into account the total number of repetitions performed and weight (kg) lifted (i.e. [repetitions (no.) × external load (kg)]. Through the use of volume load assignment, it is possible to manipulate the dosage of an exercise programme by altering (a) the number of sets performed per exercise, (b) the total number of exercises performed and/or (c) the loading parameters of exercise (i.e. the absolute intensity or the actual load lifted). The volume of exercise varies widely across training interventions depending on the main focus of the training prescription. For instance, several studies have demonstrated significant improvements in neck muscle strength in patients with chronic neck pain with application of different protocols and exercise volume. In the study by Falla et al.[39] patients with chronic neck pain trained using a head lift exercise and performed 12–15 repetitions with a weight that they could lift 12 times on the first training session (12 RM) and progressed to 15 repetitions over a 4-week period. For a further 2 weeks the patients performed three sets of 15 repetitions of the initial 12 RM load once per day. A significant improvement in neck muscle strength was also observed by Ylinen et al.,[128] yet this 12-day programme used Theraband® to train the neck flexor muscles and a single series of 15 repetitions directly forward, obliquely towards right and left, and directly backward were performed. The aim with this programme was to maintain the level of resistance at 80% of the participant's maximum isometric strength recorded at each visit. Rather than relying on a predefined volume of training, the volume of exercise should be determined based on the intended aim of training (e.g. a greater number of repetitions is more likely to enhance endurance than strength) and status of the patient so that the patient can perform the exercise without causing discomfort or reproduction of their symptoms.

Frequency and Duration of Resistance Training

The frequency of exercise to enhance strength and endurance also varies across training protocols. Although there are no firm rules, it is generally recommended that exercise can be performed more frequently (e.g. daily or even two to three times per day) in the early stages of training when the volume of exercise is relatively low.[42] As training progresses and the intensity and volume increase, the frequency of exercise is reduced.

The duration of training will also vary depending on the goals of exercise. For example, strength increase can occur with as little as 2 weeks of resistance training, but, if the aim is to increase muscle cross-sectional area then training must continue with high volume for at least 6–8 weeks.

Clinical Prescription of Resistance Training

When the aim of a training programme is to enhance strength, high loads are prescribed for a low number of repetitions, whereas a large number of repetitions at low intensity are used to enhance endurance. A key principle in resistance training is that of *overload*.[125,129] This principle states that a greater than normal stress or load on the body is required to induce training adaptation. As performance improves with training, the intensity or volume of exercise must increase to constantly place demand on the muscle/s. For endurance training, typically the duration of the contractions or the number of repetitions of the exercise are increased, whereas for strength training the amount of resistance is increased progressively.[42] Performance of too little exercise will fail to induce positive training adaptation, whereas prescription of excessive exercise can result in overtraining with associated decrements in performance, and possibly injury.[130] Regular, careful standardized assessment of capacity and adjustment of the exercise parameters is fundamental to optimal prescription of an individualized programme (Fig. 31-1).

Although systematic reviews confirm the efficacy of strength training in various musculoskeletal pain conditions, optimal exercise parameters have not been established.[124,131–133] For example, a recent systematic review examined the effects of resistance training for lateral epicondylosis/epicondylalgia.[131] Twelve studies were included (nine reporting on isotonic exercise, two isometric exercise and one isokinetic exercise). Exercise programme duration ranged from 4 to 52 weeks, and exercises were prescribed one to six times per day, with an average duration of 15 minutes per session, and three to 50 repetitions (average: 15), with one to four sets per session. Despite the variation in exercise dose and type, all studies reported substantial reduction in pain and improvement in grip strength. Thus, optimal exercise design and dosing is not defined. Research is necessary with systematic manipulation of intensity, volume, frequency and duration of exercise to determine the 'optimal dose' to enhance motor output and manage symptoms in patients with various musculoskeletal disorders.

A clearer understanding of dosage is available for design of a programme that is focused solely on strength gain. A meta-analysis[134] of dose–response relations in strength training (177 studies presenting 1803 effect sizes) suggested the response to exercise is dose-specific, non-linear and related to the baseline training status of the individual – higher gains are available for less absolute work in less trained individuals. For untrained individuals, maximal strength gains are elicited at a mean training intensity of 60% of 1 RM, 3 days per week, and with a mean training volume of four sets per muscle group. Recreationally trained non-athletes exhibit maximal strength gains with a mean training intensity of 80% of 1 RM, 2 days per week, and a mean volume of four sets. For athlete populations, maximal strength gains are elicited at a mean training intensity of 85% of 1 RM, 2 days per week, and with a mean training volume of eight sets per muscle group.[134] Thus for an untrained individual a large effect (effect size >2) could be achieved using 65% (of 1 RM) intensity, performed three times per week, three or four sets per session, whereas the same training parameters on an athlete will result in much smaller (effect size <0.5) gains. Thus, when setting goals for resistance training, not only the dose, but the training history of the individual must be considered to optimize the outcome.

SUMMARY AND CONCLUSION

Exercise has therapeutic effects for various musculoskeletal conditions. Evidence is accruing to support the role of exercise programmes that target motor control training and resistance training for their beneficial and profound effects on the neuromuscular system. The effectiveness of every exercise programme resides in the ability of the clinician to assess the status of the patient and prescribe the most appropriate exercise interventions to address the specific features of their presentation to achieve significant and durable improvements in clinical outcomes. Exercise is medicine, and as such it is important that the clinician develops and controls the effectiveness of the 'dosage' of its prescriptions (in terms of volume, intensity and exercise modalities). It is hoped that the framework provided in this chapter can be a guide to develop safe and effective exercise programmes.

REFERENCES

1. Hodges PW, Tucker K. Moving differently in pain: a new theory to explain the adaptation to pain. Pain 2011;152:S90–8.
2. Falla D, Farina D. Neural and muscular factors associated with motor impairment in neck pain. Curr Rheumatol Rep 2007; 9:497–502.
3. Graven-Nielsen T, Arendt-Nielsen L. Impact of clinical and experimental pain on muscle strength and activity. Curr Rheumatol Rep 2008;10:475–81.
4. Hides JA, Richardson CA, Jull GA. Multifidus muscle recovery is not automatic after resolution of acute, first-episode low back pain. Spine 1996;21(23):2763–9.
5. Falla D, Jull G, Edwards S, et al. Neuromuscular efficiency of the sternocleidomastoid and anterior scalene muscles in patients with chronic neck pain. Disabil Rehabil 2004;26(12):712–17.
6. Sterling M, Jull G, Vicenzino B, et al. Development of motor dysfunction following whiplash injury. Pain 2003;103:65–73.
7. Butler HL, Hubley-Kozey CL, Kozey JW. Changes in electromyographic activity of trunk muscles within the sub-acute phase for individuals deemed recovered from a low back injury. J Electromyogr Kinesiol 2013;23(2):369–77.
8. Moreside JM, Quirk DA, Hubley-Kozey CL. Temporal patterns of the trunk muscles remain altered in a low back-injured population despite subjective reports of recovery. Arch Phys Med Rehabil 2014;95:686–98.
9. Moseley G, Nicholas M, Hodges P. Does anticipation of back pain predispose to back trouble? Brain 2004;127:2339–47.
10. Tucker K, Larsson AK, Oknelid S, et al. Similar alteration of motor unit recruitment strategies during the anticipation and experience of pain. Pain 2012;153:636–43.
11. Jull G, Trott P, Potter H, et al. A randomized controlled trial of exercise and manipulative therapy for cervicogenic headache. Spine 2002;27(17):1835–43.
12. Lluch E, Schomacher J, Gizzi L, et al. Immediate effects of active cranio-cervical flexion exercise versus passive mobilisation of the upper cervical spine on pain and performance on the cranio-cervical flexion test. Man Ther 2014;19(1):25–31.
13. Ferreira P, Ferreira M, Maher C, et al. Changes in recruitment of transversus abdominis correlate with disability in people with chronic low back pain. Br J Sports Med 2009;55:153–69.
14. Hoffman SL, Johnson MB, Zou D, et al. Effect of classification-specific treatment on lumbopelvic motion during hip rotation in people with low back pain. Man Ther 2011;16:344–50.
15. Scholtes SA, Gombatto SP, Van Dillen LR. Differences in lumbopelvic motion between people with and people without low back pain during two lower limb movement tests. Clin Biomech 2009;24:7–12.
16. Bourne DA, Choo AM, Regan WD, et al. The placement of skin surface markers for non-invasive measurement of scapular kinematics affects accuracy and reliability. Ann Biomed Eng 2011;39: 777–85.
17. Myers JB, Oyama S, Hibberd EE. Scapular dysfunction in high school baseball players sustaining throwing-related upper extremity injury: a prospective study. J Shoulder Elbow Surg 2013;22: 1154–9.
18. Crossley KM, Zhang WJ, Schache AG, et al. Performance on the single-leg squat task indicates hip abductor muscle function. Am J Sports Med 2011;39:866–73.
19. Teyhen D, Bergeron MF, Deuster P, et al. Consortium for health and military performance and American College of Sports Medicine Summit: utility of functional movement assessment in identifying musculoskeletal injury risk. Curr Sports Med Rep 2014;13:52–63.
20. Pinto RZ, Ferreira PH, Ferreira M, et al. Reliability and discriminatory capacity of a clinical scale for assessing abdominal muscle coordination. J Manipulative Physiol Ther 2012;34:562–9.
21. Falla D, Campbell C, Fagan A, et al. Relationship between cranio-cervical flexion range of motion and pressure change during the cranio-cervical flexion test. Man Ther 2003;8(2):92–6.
22. Juul T, Langberg H, Enoch F, et al. The intra- and inter-rater reliability of five clinical muscle performance tests in patients with and without neck pain. BMC Musculoskelet Disord 2013;14:339.
23. O'Leary S, Falla D, Jull G. The relationship between superficial muscle activity during the cranio-cervical flexion test and clinical features in patients with chronic neck pain. Man Ther 2011; 16:452–5.
24. James G, Doe T. The craniocervical flexion test: intra-tester reliability in asymptomatic subjects. Physiother Res Int 2010;15: 144–9.
25. Hides JA, Stokes MJ, Saide M, et al. Evidence of lumbar multifidus muscle wasting ipsilateral to symptoms in patients with acute/subacute low back pain. Spine 1994;19(2):165–72.
26. Elliott J, Jull G, Noteboom JT, et al. Fatty infiltration in the cervical extensor muscles in persistent whiplash-associated disorders: a magnetic resonance imaging analysis. Spine 2006;31(22):847–55.
27. Beeler S, Ek ET, Gerber C. A comparative analysis of fatty infiltration and muscle atrophy in patients with chronic rotator cuff tears and suprascapular neuropathy. J Shoulder Elbow Surg 2013;22: 1537–46.
28. Croisier JL. Factors associated with recurrent hamstring injuries. Sports Med 2004;34:681–95.
29. Byram IR, Bushnell BD, Dugger K, et al. Preseason shoulder strength measurements in professional baseball pitchers: identifying players at risk for injury. Am J Sports Med 2010;38: 1375–82.
30. Pincivero DM, Lephart SM, Karunakara RA. Reliability and precision of isokinetic strength and muscular endurance for the quadriceps and hamstrings. Int J Sports Med 1997;18:113–17.
31. Maffiuletti NA, Bizzini M, Desbrosses K, et al. Reliability of knee extension and flexion measurements using the Con-Trex isokinetic dynamometer. Clin Physiol Funct Imaging 2007;27:346–53.

32. Adkins D, Boychuk J, Remple M, et al. Motor training induces experience-specific patterns of plasticity across motor cortex and spinal cord. J Appl Physiol 2006;101:1776–82.

33. Fluck M. Functional, structural and molecular plasticity of mammalian skeletal muscle in response to exercise stimuli. J Exp Biol 2006;209:2239–48.

34. Duchateau J, Semmler JG, Enoka RM. Training adaptations in the behavior of human motor units. J Appl Physiol 2006;101:1766–75.

35. Jull G, Falla D, Vicenzino B, et al. The effect of therapeutic exercise on activation of the deep cervical flexor muscles in people with chronic neck pain. Man Ther 2009;14:696–701.

36. Tsao H, Hodges PW. Immediate changes in feedforward postural adjustments following voluntary motor training. Exp Brain Res 2007;181:537–46.

37. Tsao H, Druitt TR, Schollum TM, et al. Motor training of the lumbar paraspinal muscles induces immediate changes in motor coordination in patients with recurrent low back pain. J Pain 2010;11(11):1120–8.

38. Falla D, Jull G, Russell T, et al. Effect of neck exercise on sitting posture in patients with chronic neck pain. Phys Ther 2007;87(4):408–17.

39. Falla D, Jull G, Hodges P, et al. An endurance-strength training regime is effective in reducing myoelectric manifestations of cervical flexor muscle fatigue in females with chronic neck pain. Clin Neurophysiol 2006;117:828–37.

40. O'Leary S, Jull G, Kim M, et al. Training mode-dependent changes in motor performance in neck pain. Arch Phys Med Rehabil 2012;93(7):1225–33.

41. Danneels LA, Vanderstraeten GG, Cambier DC, et al. Effects of three different training modalities on the cross sectional area of the lumbar multifidus muscle in patients with chronic low back pain. Br J Sports Med 2001;35:186–91.

42. Kisner C, Colby LA. Therapeutic Exercise: Foundations and Techniques. Philadelphia, USA: F.A. Davis Company; 2012.

43. Häkkinen K, Alen M, Kraemer WJ, et al. Neuromuscular adaptations during concurrent strength and endurance training versus strength training. Eur J Appl Physiol 2003;89:42–52.

44. Karavirta L, Häkkinen A, Sillanpää E, et al. Effects of combined endurance and strength training on muscle strength, power and hypertrophy in 40–67-year-old men. Scand J Med Sci Sports 2011;21:402–11.

45. Hawley JA. Molecular responses to strength and endurance training: are they incompatible? Appl Physiol Nutr Metab 2009;34:355–61.

46. Sterling M, Jull G, Vicenzino B, et al. Physical and psychological factors predict outcome following whiplash injury. Pain 2005;114:141–8.

47. Falla D, Arendt-Nielsen L, Farina D. Gender-specific adaptations of upper trapezius muscle activity to acute nociceptive stimulation. Pain 2008;138:217–25.

48. Muceli S, Falla D, Farina D. Reorganization of muscle synergies during multidirectional reaching in the horizontal plane with experimental muscle pain. J Neurophysiol 2014;111:1615–30.

49. Jull G, Sterling M, Falla D, et al. Whiplash, Headache and Neck Pain: Research Based Directions for Physical Therapies. Edinburgh: Elsevier, Churchill Livingstone; 2008.

50. Hodges P, Cholewicki J, van Dieen J. Spinal Control: The Rehabilitation of Back Pain. State of the Art and Science. Churchill Livingstone, Elsevier; 2013.

51. O'Leary S, Falla D, Hodges P, et al. Specific therapeutic exercise of the neck induces immediate local hypoalgesia. J Pain 2007;8:832–9.

52. Jull G, Amiri M, Bullock-Saxton J, et al. Cervical musculoskeletal impairment in frequent intermittent headache. Part 1: Subjects with single headaches. Cephalalgia 2007;27:793–802.

53. Uhlig Y, Weber BR, Grob D, et al. Fiber composition and fiber transformations in neck muscles of patients with dysfunction of the cervical spine. J Orthop Res 1995;13(2):240–9.

54. Hodges PW, James G, Blomster L, et al. Can pro-inflammatory cytokine gene expression explain multifidus muscle fiber changes after an intervertebral disc lesion? Spine 2014;In Press.

55. Alaranta H, Tallroth K, Soukka A, et al. Fat content of lumbar extensor muscles and low back disability: a radiographic and clinical comparison. J Spinal Disord 1993;6:137–40.

56. Elliott J, Pedler A, Kenardy J, et al. The temporal development of fatty infiltrates in the neck muscles following whiplash injury: an association with pain and posttraumatic stress. PLoS ONE 2011;6(6):e21194.

57. Hides JA, Jull GA, Richardson CA. Long-term effects of specific stabilizing exercises for first-episode low back pain. Spine 2001;26:243–8.

58. Unsgaard-Tøndel M, Lund Nilsen TI, Magnussen J, et al. Is activation of transversus abdominis and obliquus internus abdominis associated with long-term changes in chronic low back pain? A prospective study with 1-year follow-up. Br J Sports Med 2012;46:729–34.

59. Falla D, O'Leary S, Farina D, et al. The change in deep cervical flexor activity after training is associated with the degree of pain reduction in patients with chronic neck pain. Clin J Pain 2012;28(7):628–34.

60. Nielsen JB, Cohen LG. The Olympic brain. Does corticospinal plasticity play a role in acquisition of skills required for high-performance sports? J Physiol 2008;586:65–70.

61. Vila-Chã C, Falla D, Correia MV, et al. Adjustments in motor unit properties during fatiguing contractions after training. Med Sci Sports Exerc 2012;44:616–24.

62. Vila-Chã C, Falla D, Farina D. Motor unit behavior during submaximal contractions following six weeks of either endurance or strength training. J Appl Physiol (1985) 2010;109:1455–66.

63. Tsao H, Hodges PW. Persistence of improvements in postural strategies following motor control training in people with recurrent low back pain. J Electromyogr Kinesiol 2008;18:559–67.

64. Bawa P. Neural control of motor output: can training change it? Exerc Sport Sci Rev 2002;30:59–63.

65. Hodges PW, Richardson CA. Inefficient muscular stabilization of the lumbar spine associated with low back pain. A motor control evaluation of transversus abdominis. Spine 1996;21(22):2640–50.

66. MacDonald D, Moseley GL, Hodges PW. Why do some patients keep hurting their back? Evidence of ongoing back muscle dysfunction during remission from recurrent back pain. Pain 2009;142:183–8.

67. Falla D, Jull G, Hodges PW. Feedforward activity of the cervical flexor muscles during voluntary arm movements is delayed in chronic neck pain. Exp Brain Res 2004;157:43–8.

68. Falla D, Jull G, Hodges PW. Patients with neck pain demonstrate reduced electromyographic activity of the deep cervical flexor muscles during performance of the craniocervical flexion test. Spine 2004;29(19):2108–14.

69. Schomacher J, Boudreau S, Petzke F, et al. Localized pressure pain sensitivity is associated with lower activation of the semispinalis cervicis muscle in patients with chronic neck pain. Clin J Pain 2013;29:898–906.

70. Schomacher J, Farina D, Lindstroem R, et al. Chronic trauma-induced neck pain impairs the neural control of the deep semispinalis cervicis muscle. Clin Neurophysiol 2012;123(7):1403–8.

71. MacDonald D, Moseley G, Hodges P. People with recurrent low back pain respond differently to trunk loading despite remission from symptoms. Spine (Phila Pa 1976) 2010;35(7):818–24.

72. Ferreira PH, Ferreira ML, Hodges PW. Changes in recruitment of the abdominal muscles in people with low back pain: ultrasound measurement of muscle activity. Spine (Phila Pa 1976) 2004;29:2560–6.

73. O'Leary S, Cagnie B, Reeve A, et al. Is there altered activity of the extensor muscles in chronic mechanical neck pain? A functional magnetic resonance imaging study. Arch Phys Med Rehabil 2011;92(6):929–34.

74. Tsao H, Galea MP, Hodges PW. Reorganization of the motor cortex is associated with postural control deficits in recurrent low back pain. Brain 2008;131:2161–71.

75. Tsao H, Danneels L, Hodges PW. Smudging the motor brain in young adults with recurrent low back pain. Spine 2011;36:1721–7.

76. Boudreau SA, Farina D, Falla D. The role of motor learning and neuroplasticity in designing rehabilitation approaches for musculoskeletal pain disorders. Man Ther 2010;15(5):410–14.

77. Crossley KM, Bennell K, Green S, et al. Physical therapy for patellofemoral pain: a randomized, double-blinded, placebo-controlled trial. Am J Sports Med 2002;30:857–65.

78. Sahrmann S. Diagnosis and Treatment of Movement Impairment Syndromes. St Louis, MO: Mosby; 2002.

79. Richardson C, Hodges PW, Hides J. Therapeutic Exercise for Lumbopelvic Stabilization: A Motor Control Approach for the Treatment and Prevention of Low Back Pain. 2nd ed. Edinburgh: Churchill Livingstone; 2004.

80. McGill SM. Low Back Disorders: Evidence Based Prevention and Rehabilitation. Champaign, IL.: Human Kinetics; 2007.

81. O'Sullivan PB. Diagnosis and classification of chronic low back pain disorders: maladaptive movement and motor control impairments as underlying mechanism. Man Ther 2005;10:242–55.

82. Worsley P, Warner M, Mottram S, et al. Motor control retraining exercises for shoulder impingement: effects on function, muscle activation, and biomechanics in young adults. J Shoulder Elbow Surg 2013;22:e11–19.

83. Hall L, Tsao H, MacDonald D, et al. Immediate effects of co-contraction training on motor control of the trunk muscles in people with recurrent low back pain. J Electromyogr Kinesiol 2009;19:763–73.

84. Falla D, Lindstrøm R, Rechter L, et al. Effectiveness of an 8-week exercise programme on pain and specificity of neck muscle activity in patients with chronic neck pain: a randomized controlled study. Eur J Pain 2013;17:1517–28.

85. Grimaldi A. Assessing lateral stability of the hip and pelvis. Man Ther 2011;16:26–31.

86. Christiansen DH, Falla D, Frost P, et al. Physiotherapy after Subacromial Decompression Surgery: Development of An Exercise Intervention Submitted for Publication. 2014.

87. Fitts PM, Posner MI. Human Performance. USA: Wadsworth; 1967.

88. Boudreau S, Romaniello A, Wang K, et al. The effects of intra-oral pain on motor cortex neuroplasticity associated with short-term novel tongue-protrusion training in humans. Pain 2007;132:169–78.

89. Ferguson AR, Crown ED, Grau JW. Nociceptive plasticity inhibits adaptive learning in the spinal cord. Neuroscience 2006;141: 421–31.

90. Ingham D, Tucker KJ, Tsao H, et al. The effect of pain on training-induced plasticity of the corticomotor system. Eur J Pain 2011;15:1028–34.

91. Svensson P, Romaniello A, Arendt-Nielsen L, et al. Plasticity in corticomotor control of the human tongue musculature induced by tongue-task training. Exp Brain Res 2003;152:42–51.

92. Pascual-Leone A, Nguyet D, Cohen LG, et al. Modulation of muscle responses evoked by transcranial magnetic stimulation during the acquisition of new fine motor skills. J Neurophysiol 1995;74:1037–45.

93. Kleim JA, Barbay S, Cooper NR, et al. Motor learning-dependent synaptogenesis is localized to functionally reorganized motor cortex. Neurobiol Learn Memory 2002;77:63–77.

94. Shumway-Cook A, Woollacott M. Motor Control: Translating Research into Clinical Practice. Philadelphia, PA: Lippincott Williams & Wilkins; 2006.

95. Falla D, Jull G, Hodges P. Training the cervical muscles with prescribed motor tasks does not change muscle activation during a functional activity. Man Ther 2008;13:507–12.

96. Lluch E, Schomacher J, Gizzi L, et al. Immediate effects of active cranio-cervical flexion exercise versus passive mobilisation of the upper cervical spine on pain and performance on the cranio-cervical flexion test. Man Ther 2014;19:25–31.

97. Scholtes SA, Norton BJ, Lang CE, et al. The effect of within-session instruction on lumbopelvic motion during a lower limb movement in people with and people without low back pain. Man Ther 2010;15:496–501.

98. Jull G, Falla D, Treleaven J, et al. Retraining cervical joint position sense: The effect of two exercise regimes. J Orthop Res 2007; 25(3):404–12.

99. Tsao H, Galea MP, Hodges PW. Driving plasticity in the motor cortex in recurrent low back pain. Euro J Pain 2010;14:832–9.

100. Vasseljen O, Fladmark AM. Abdominal muscle contraction thickness and function after specific and general exercises: a randomized controlled trial in chronic low back pain patients. Man Ther 2010;15:482–9.

101. Aagaard P. Training-induced changes in neural function. Exerc Sport Sci Rev 2003;31:61–7.

102. Aagaard P, Andersen JL, Dyhre-Poulsen P, et al. A mechanism for increased contractile strength of human pennate muscle in response to strength training: changes in muscle architecture. J Physiol 2001;534:613–23.

103. Fitts RH. Effects of regular exercise training on skeletal muscle contractile function. Am J Phys Med Rehabil 2003;82:320–31.

104. Seynnes OR, de Boer M, Narici MV. Early skeletal muscle hypertrophy and architectural changes in response to high-intensity resistance training. J Appl Physiol 2007;102:368–73.

105. Kraemer WJ, Volek JS, Fleck SJ. Chronic musculoskeletal adaptations to resistance training. In: Roitman JL, editor. ACSM's Resource Manual for Guidelines for Exercise Testing and Prescription. 4th ed. Philadelphia: Lippincott Williams & Wilkins; 2001. p. 176.

106. Folland JP, Williams AG. The adaptations to strength training: morphological and neurological contributions to increased strength. Sports Med 2007;37:145–68.

107. Fluck M, Hoppeler H. Molecular basis of skeletal muscle plasticity – from gene to form and function. Rev Physiol Biochem Pharmacol 2003;146:159–216.

108. Green HJ, Barr DJ, Fowles JR, et al. Malleability of human skeletal muscle Na(+)-K(+)-ATPase pump with short-term training. J Appl Physiol 2004;97:143–8.

109. Green HJ, Ballantyne CS, MacDougall JD, et al. Adaptations in human muscle sarcoplasmic reticulum to prolonged submaximal training. J Appl Physiol 2003;94:2034–42.

110. Moritani T, deVries HA. Neural factors versus hypertrophy in the time course of muscle strength gain. Am J Phys Med 1979; 58:115–30.

111. Patten C, Kamen G, Rowland DM. Adaptations in maximal motor unit discharge rate to strength training in young and older adults. Muscle Nerve 2001;24:542–50.

112. Van Cutsem M, Duchateau J, Hainaut K. Changes in single motor unit behaviour contribute to the increase in contraction speed after dynamic training in humans. J Physiol 1998;513:295–305.

113. Griffin L, Painter PE, Wadhwa A, et al. Motor unit firing variability and synchronization during short-term light-load training in older adults. Exp Brain Res 2009;197:337–45.

114. Stone MH. Implications for connective tissue and bone alterations resulting from resistance exercise training. Med Sci Sports Exerc 1988;20:51–62.

115. Conroy BP, Earle RW, Beachle TR. Bone, muscle and connective tissue adaptations to physical activity. In: Essentials of Strength Training and Conditioning. Champaign, IL: Human Kinetics; 1994.

116. Mitchell CJ, Churchward-Venne TA, West DW, et al. Resistance exercise load does not determine training-mediated hypertrophic gains in young men. J Appl Physiol 2012;113:71–7.

117. Abe T, Loenneke JP, Fahs CA, et al. Exercise intensity and muscle hypertrophy in blood flow-restricted limbs and non-restricted muscles: a brief review. Clin Physiol Funct Imaging 2012; 32:247–52.

118. Baldwin KM, Haddad F. Effects of different activity and inactivity paradigms on myosin heavy chain gene expression in striated muscle. J Appl Physiol 2001;90:345–57.

119. Gibala MJ, Little JP, van Essen M, et al. Short-term sprint interval versus traditional endurance training: similar initial adaptations in human skeletal muscle and exercise performance. J Physiol 2006;575:901–11.

120. Hoppeler H, Fluck M. Plasticity of skeletal muscle mitochondria: structure and function. Med Sci Sports Exerc 2003;35:95–104.

121. Scott W, Stevens J, Binder-Macleod SA. Human skeletal muscle fiber type classifications. Phys Ther 2001;81:1810–16.

122. Wilmore JH, Costill DL, Kenney WL. Physiology Of Sport And Exercise. United Kingdom: Human Kinetics; 2008.

123. Cracraft JD. Effects of Exercise on Firing Patterns of Single Motor Units. Med Sci Sports Exerc 1975;7:86.

124. Kristensen J, Franklyn-Miller A. Resistance training in musculoskeletal rehabilitation: a systematic review. Br J Sports Med 2012;46:719–26.

125. Medicine ACoS. Position stand: progression models in resistance training for healthy adults. Med Sci Sports Exerc 2002;34: 364–80.

126. LeSuer DA, McCormick JH, Mayhew JL, et al. The accuracy of prediction equations for estimating 1-RM performance in the bench press, squat, and deadlift. J Strength Cond Res 2007; 11:211–13.

127. Eston R, Evans HJ. The validity of submaximal ratings of perceived exertion to predict one repetition maximum. J Sports Sci Med 2009;8:567–73.

128. Ylinen J, Takala EP, Nykanen M, et al. Active neck muscle training in the treatment of chronic neck pain in women: a randomized controlled trial. JAMA 2003;289(19):2509–16.

129. Hellebrandt F, Houtz SJ. Mechanisms of muscle training in man: experimental demonstration of the overload principle. Phys Ther Rev 1956;36:371.

130. Fry AC. The role of training intensity in resistance exercise, overtraining and overreaching. In: Kreider R, Fry A, O'Toole M, editors. Overtraining in Sport. Champaign, IL: Human Kinetics; 1998.

131. Raman J, MacDermid JC, Grewal R. Effectiveness of different methods of resistance exercises in lateral epicondylosis – a systematic review. J Hand Ther 2012;25:5–25.

132. Lange AK, Vanwanseele B, Fiatarone Singh MA. Strength training for treatment of osteoarthritis of the knee: a systematic review. Arthritis Rheum 2008;59:1488–94.

133. Taylor NF, Dodd KJ, Damiano DL. Progressive resistance exercise in physical therapy: a summary of systematic reviews. Phys Ther 2005;85:1208–23.

134. Peterson MD, Rhea MR, Alvar BA. Applications of the dose-response for muscular strength development: a review of meta-analytic efficacy and reliability for designing training prescription. J Strength Cond Res 2005;19:950–8.

MANAGEMENT OF THE SENSORIMOTOR SYSTEM

CHAPTER OUTLINE

CHAPTER 32.1 ■ THE CERVICAL REGION

Ulrik Röijezon • Julia Treleaven

The sensory and motor systems of the neck are vital for the perception, movement and stability of the head relative to the trunk, for eye and arm–hand functioning and for postural control. This section focuses on the somatosensory system of the cervical spine (i.e. cervical proprioception). The cervical proprioceptors are essential for the position and movement sense of the head and have abundant neurophysiological connections to the visual and vestibular organs and subsequent input to the sensorimotor control system. This has implications for head and eye movement control and postural control, as well as symptoms such as dizziness and visual complaints in people with neck pain disorders.

REPORTED COMPLAINTS AND IMPAIRMENTS

A large variety of complaints and motor control impairments presumed to be related to disturbed cervical somatosensory information and/or processing of this information have been reported in neck pain disorders, including cervical and upper extremity control as well as oculomotor and postural control.

Dizziness/unsteadiness and or light-headedness are common symptoms associated with neck pain, especially in those with chronic whiplash-associated disorder.[1–3] Loss of balance and actual falls occur but are less common.[3] In addition, light sensitivity, needing to concentrate to read and visual fatigue are the most prevalent visual complaints associated with neck pain.[4]

Impaired cervical movement control in neck pain includes reduced cervical position[1,3,5–7] and movement sense,[8–10] as well as reduced cervical force steadiness,[11] movement smoothness,[6,12,13] speed[14,15] and conjunct motions.[14,16] Impairments of upper limb kinematics documented in people with neck pain include reduced

position and movement sense of the shoulder,[17,18] elbow[17] and hand,[19] as well as reduced pointing acuity to a visual target.[20]

Oculomotor impairments include decreased smooth pursuit velocity gain, especially when the neck is in torsion, and altered velocity and latency of saccadic eye movements.[21–29] Moreover, changes in the activation of neck muscles during eye movements have been reported.[30]

Postural control is also known to be disturbed in people with neck pain. Several studies have reported increased sway in quite stance,[31–41] but impairments in more functional tasks (e.g. walking with head turns) have also been reported.[42]

Variations, however, are large between individuals with neck pain. While impairments have been reported in both non-traumatic (idiopathic) and trauma-induced neck pain disorders, some studies have reported no or only minor impairments. Several studies have reported more pronounced impairments in people following a whiplash injury and in individuals with dizziness.[3,9,26,32,40] The suggested pathophysiology underlying such impairments is illustrated in Figure 32-1.

OVERALL MANAGEMENT APPROACH

Assessment and treatment of altered cervical proprioception in the management of neck pain is as important as considering lower limb proprioceptive training following an ankle or knee injury. Sensorimotor disturbances in neck pain disorders are largely heterogeneous, and treatment therefore needs to be individually tailored and based on the patient's history and physical activities of daily living as well as findings from the clinical assessment.

Management should preferably include local neck treatment in combination with tailored sensorimotor exercises.[43] This combined approach will address the

Impact of somatosensory dysfunction in the cervical spine

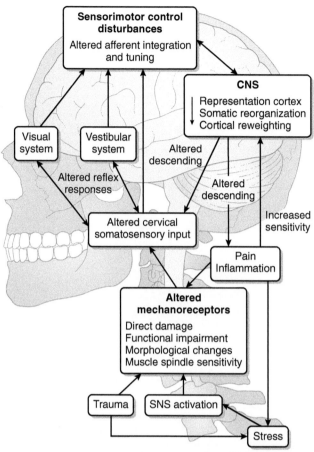

FIGURE 32-1 ■ The suggested pathophysiology of sensorimotor impairments associated with neck disorders. *CNS*, central nervous system; *SNS*, sympathetic nervous system.

local causes disturbing cervical afferent input and consider the important links between the cervical, vestibular and ocular systems and any secondary adaptive changes in sensorimotor control.

TAILORED LOCAL TREATMENT

Pain reduction, normalized range of motion and neuromuscular control, as well as adequate strength and endurance of the cervical spine, need to be addressed in neck pain disorders. This can be directed using traditional local treatment such as acupuncture, manual therapy and various training regimens. Specific traditional local treatments to the neck such as acupuncture, manual therapy and craniocervical flexion training have been shown to improve symptoms and dysfunctions related to disturbed cervical somatosensory information, including cervical position sense, dizziness and/or standing balance in patients with neck pain.[44-48] However, management of patients not responding sufficiently to traditional interventions should also include exercise regimens specifically targeting cervical proprioception and its relation to eye movement and postural control.

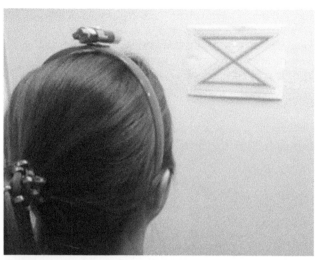

FIGURE 32-2 ■ Retraining cervical movement sense using a laser mounted on a headband. The patient traces patterns such as a zigzag placed 1 m from the laser.

TAILORED SENSORIMOTOR EXERCISE APPROACH BASED ON IMPAIRMENTS

The greatest deficits in sensorimotor tests have been measured in patients with whiplash complaining of dizziness,[3,27,40] but these deficits can be present in non-dizzy patients with idiopathic neck pain.[5,26,32] Although the causes of the disturbances are similar, an individual patient may present with dysfunction in either one or several aspects of sensorimotor control.[49]

Head Position and Movement Control

A low-cost method of mounting a laser pointer on a headband and directing the laser beam at a target, can be used to monitor both cervical position and movement sense.

Cervical Joint Position Error

The patient is seated and a target is placed to indicate the starting laser point (90 cm from wall). The patient, with eyes closed, performs at least three repetitions of an active neck movement and is asked to accurately return to the starting position. Errors, as little as 4.5° (equivalent to 7.1 cm with the patient seated 90 cm from the target) between the start and end position, can indicate a deficit in proprioception.[50,51] Joint position error can be retrained by practising relocating the head to a neutral position (guided by the laser beam).

Cervical Movement Sense

A laser mounted on a headband can also be used to allow the patient to trace patterns such as a zigzag (20 × 14 cm) placed 1 m from the laser (Fig. 32-2). Recently, pilot normative values (less than 25 seconds and seven times outside of a 5-mm radius) were suggested.[52] Cervical movement sense can be improved by practice of accurately tracing patterns using the laser. More sophisticated computerized assessment and treatment methods are commercially available[9] and a virtual reality device has been developed to measure and train velocity and accuracy of head movement.[15] Cervical movement acuity can also be trained using an unstable dynamic system such as controlling the movement of a ball on a plate mounted on the head.[53]

Oculomotor Control

Gaze Stability

In this test, the patient is requested to keep their eyes focused on a target while they actively move their head in rotation and flexion/extension. Inability to maintain focus, reduced or awkward cervical motion (less than 45°), reproduction of dizziness, blurring of vision or nausea are abnormal responses. Gaze stability can be practised by the patient by moving their head into directions of difficulty maintaining optimal movement and range of motion while fixating their gaze on the focus point.[54] Focusing on a point in a mirror may help initially. The patient or therapist can also passively move the trunk whilst the patient maintains focus.

Smooth Pursuit

The patient is requested to keep their head still while following, with the eyes, a moving target (20°/s through a visual angle of 40°). The test is repeated with the neck in torsion (head still but trunk rotated 45° to each side). Any decline in the smoothness of eye follow or an inability to keep up with the target with quick, catch-up eye movements, particularly when the target is crossing the midline, or symptom reproduction, in torsion compared to neutral is noted.[28] Smooth pursuit can be practised by following a laser pointer, moved backwards and forwards on a wall by the patient's hand (Fig. 32-3).

EYE–HEAD–TRUNK COORDINATION

Eye–Head Coordination

The patient moves the eyes first to a target which is then followed by head movement, ensuring that the eyes are kept focused on the target. The test is performed with movement in right and left rotation and flexion and extension of the neck. Often patients with neck pain are unable to keep the head still while the eyes move or they lose focus during the head movements.[54,55] Eye–head coordination can be practised with attention to correctly isolating eye and head movement.

Trunk–Head Coordination

The test is performed with the patient standing by asking them to hold the head still, eyes open, while rotating their trunk to the left and right. Patients with neck pain often have difficulty keeping their head still when their trunk is moving.[56] This can be practised with the patient using a mirror or laser to provide feedback for keeping the head stationary while turning the trunk (Fig. 32-4).

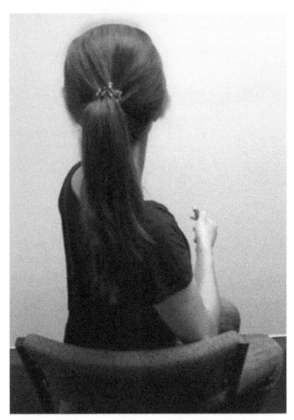

FIGURE 32-3 ■ Smooth pursuit eye movement practised by following a laser pointer, moved backwards and forwards on a wall by the patient's hand. The patient follows the laser with their eyes as accurately as they can, while keeping the head still. Here the patient is positioned in a neck torsion position to the left (head still while the trunk is rotated 45° to the right).

Postural Control

Inability to maintain stance for 30 seconds, large increases in sway, slower responses to correct or rigidity are considered abnormal responses in comfortable and narrow stance either on a firm or a soft foam surface with eyes open and closed. In younger patients, the same performance features can be evaluated in tandem and with single leg stance on a firm surface. Comparison of performance when the head is still and trunk rotated under the stationary head (biasing cervical proprioception) might be useful.[57] Dynamic tests such as the step test and the timed 10-m walk with head turns[42,58] can be used for elderly patients with neck pain and patients with neck pain complaining of dizziness, unsteadiness or loss of balance. The starting level for balance retraining will depend on which tests the patient failed or had difficulty with. Patients practise the exercise, gradually increasing stability time to 30 seconds.

General Recommendations, Progression of Treatment

It is recommended that exercises for each aspect of sensorimotor control should be performed two to five times per day. Temporary reproduction of dizziness or visual disturbances is acceptable; however, exacerbation of neck pain or headache is not. Decreasing the number

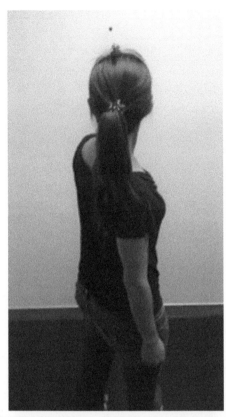

FIGURE 32-4 ■ Trunk head coordination practised with the patient using a laser pointer to provide feedback for keeping the head stationary while turning the trunk.

of repetitions or altering the patient position to a more supported position such as supine lying should prevent this. Progression can be achieved by increasing the duration, repetitions and the degree of difficulty of the task and by performing activities such as an oculomotor task simultaneously with a balance task. Exercises should be performed at a speed and range of movement and position that allows the patient to perform the task with precision and continuous correction. Exercises should also be performed in functional positions and contexts. Table 32-1 outlines some suggested exercises for each impairment and Table 32-2 outlines different ways to progress these exercises.

CONCLUSION

Assessment and management of altered cervical proprioception in people with neck pain is as important as considering lower limb proprioceptive retraining following a lower limb injury. Afferent information from the cervical receptors can be altered via a number of mechanisms and the findings of the assessment should direct and tailor the most appropriate management to the individual patient with a neck disorder. Management should include both local treatment to the neck in combination with tailored exercises to improve any deficits in cervical position and movement control, oculomotor control, eye–head–trunk coordination and postural control. This combined approach will address the local causes of altered

TABLE 32-1	**Examples of Exercises to Improve Sensorimotor Control in Neck Pain Disorders**
Activity	**Task**
Cervical joint position error	Relocate head back to neutral, eyes closed, laser on headband, check with eyes open Relocate trunk back to neutral, keep head still Relocate to predetermined positions in range (dots along wall), laser on headband, eyes closed, check eyes open
Cervical movement sense	Practice tracing intricate patterns on the wall with laser on headband and eyes open – increase speed, increase complexity of pattern
Balance	Eyes open then closed, firm then soft surface Different stances – comfortable, narrow, tandem, single leg Walking with head movements – rotation, flexion and extension of the neck whilst maintaining direction and velocity of gait Performing oculomotor or JPE, movement sense exercises whilst balance training
Eye follow	Eyes follow laser light moving backwards and forwards across a wall whilst sitting in a neutral neck position, then with the neck in torsion (move laser light with hand in lap), gradually increase speed and range of motion
Gaze stability	Maintain gaze as therapist moves the trunk or neck passively Maintain gaze as the patient actively moves their trunk or neck in all directions Change the focus point – e.g. spot to few words, business card Fix gaze, close eyes, move head and open eyes to check that they have maintained gaze (imaginary gaze) Change the background of the target – plain, stripes, checks
Eye–head coordination	Move eyes to focus on a point and then move head in the same direction. Return to neutral Move eyes to focus on a point in one direction and then move the head in the opposite direction Actively move head and eyes together Move head and eyes together whilst peripheral vision restricted (blackened sides of goggles) Move hand, arm, head and trunk following with the eyes with or without vision restricted
Trunk–head coordination	Passively hold head and actively move trunk left and right, and vice versa Keep head still, use focus point or laser for feedback, rotate trunk left and right Increase range and speed of movement

JPE, Joint position error

TABLE 32-2   **Variables That Can be Adjusted for Progression of Exercises**

Variable	Start	Progression	Further Progression	Applicable Exercise Task
Focus point	Dot	Word	Business card	Gaze stability, eye–head coordination
Background to focus point	Plain	Stripes	Checkerboard pattern	Gaze stability, eye–head coordination
Patient position	Supine	Sitting	Standing/walking	Gaze stability, JPE, eye follow
Neck position	Neutral	Torsion 30°	Torsion 45°	Eye follow, JPE, movement sense
Speed of movement	Slow	Medium	Fast	Eye follow, trunk–head coordination
Vision	Unrestricted	Peripheral restricted	Eyes closed	Gaze stability, eye–head coordination, balance
Range of motion	Small	Medium	Large	All
Duration of exercise	30 seconds	1–2 minutes	3–5 minutes	All
Frequency of exercise	2× day	3× day	5× day	All

JPE, Joint position error.

cervical afferent input and consider the important links between the cervical, vestibular and ocular systems and any secondary adaptive changes.

REFERENCES

1. Heikkila HV, Wenngren B-I. Cervicocephalic kinesthetic sensibility, active range of cervical motion, and oculomotor function in patients with whiplash injury. Arch Phys Med Rehabil 1998;799:1089.
2. Humphreys BK, Bolton J, Peterson C, et al. A cross-sectional study of the association between pain and disability in neck pain patients with dizziness of suspected cervical origin. J Whiplash Relat Disord 2003;1(2):63–73.
3. Treleaven J, Jull G, Sterling M. Dizziness and unsteadiness following whiplash injury: characteristic features and relationship with cervical joint position error. J Rehabil Med 2003;35(1):36–43.
4. Treleaven J, Takahashi H. Characteristics of visual disturbances reported by individuals with neck pain. Man Ther 2014; in press. <http://dx.doi.org/10.1016/j.math.2014.01.005>.
5. Kristjansson E, Dall'Alba P, Jull G. A study of five cervicocephalic relocation tests in three different subject groups. Clin Rehabil 2003;17(7):768–74.
6. Sjölander P, Michaelson P, Jaric S, et al. Sensorimotor disturbances in chronic neck pain – Range of motion, peak velocity, smoothness of movement, and repositioning acuity. Man Ther 2008;13(2):122–31.
7. Chen X, Treleaven J. The effect of neck torsion on joint position error in subjects with chronic neck pain. Man Ther 2013.
8. Kristjansson E, Hardardottir L, Asmundardottir M, et al. A new clinical test for cervicocephalic kinesthetic sensibility: 'The fly'. Arch Phys Med Rehabil 2004;85(3):490–5.
9. Kristjansson E, Oddsdottir GL. 'The Fly': a new clinical assessment and treatment method for deficits of movement control in the cervical spine reliability and validity. Spine 2010;35(23):E1298–305.
10. Woodhouse A, Liljeback P, Vasseljen O. Reduced head steadiness in whiplash compared with non-traumatic neck pain. J Rehabil Med 2010;42(1):35–41.
11. Woodhouse A, Stavdahl O, Vasseljen O. Irregular head movement patterns in whiplash patients during a trajectory task. Exp Brain Res 2010;201(2):261–70.
12. Grip H, Sundelin G, Gerdle B, et al. Cervical helical axis characteristics and its center of rotation during active head and upper arm movements-comparisons of whiplash-associated disorders, non-specific neck pain and asymptomatic individuals. J Biomech 2008;41(13):2799–805.
13. Sarig-Bahat H, Weiss PL, Laufer Y. The effect of neck pain on cervical kinematics, as assessed in a virtual environment. Arch Phys Med Rehabil 2010;91(12):1884–90.
14. Röijezon U, Djupsjöbacka M, Björklund M, et al. Kinematics of fast cervical rotations in persons with chronic neck pain: a cross-sectional and reliability study. BMC Musculoskelet Disord 2010;11.
15. Sarig Bahat H, Weiss PL, Laufer Y. The effect of neck pain on cervical kinematics, as assessed in a virtual environment. Arch Phys Med Rehabil 2010;91(12):1884–90.
16. Woodhouse A, Vasseljen O. Altered motor control patterns in whiplash and chronic neck pain. BMC Musculoskelet Disord 2008;9.
17. Knox JJ, Beilstein DJ, Charles SD, et al. Changes in head and neck position have a greater effect on elbow joint position sense in people with whiplash-associated disorders. Clin J Pain 2006;22(6):512–18.
18. Sandlund J, Djupsjöbacka M, Ryhed B, et al. Predictive and discriminative value of shoulder proprioception tests for patients with whiplash-associated disorders. J Rehabil Med 2006;38(1):44–9.
19. Huysmans MA, Hoozemans MJ, van der Beek AJ, et al. Position sense acuity of the upper extremity and tracking performance in subjects with non-specific neck and upper extremity pain and healthy controls. J Rehabil Med 2010;42(9):876–83.
20. Sandlund J, Röijezon U, Björklund M, et al. Acuity of goal-directed arm movements to visible targets in chronic neck pain. J Rehabil Med 2008;40(5):366–74.
21. Gimse R, Tjell C, Bjorgen IA, et al. Disturbed eye movements after whiplash due to injuries to the posture control system. J Clin Exp Neuropsychol 1996;18(2):178–86.
22. Hildingsson C, Wenngren B, Bring G, et al. Oculomotor problems after cervical spine injury. Acta Orthop Scand 1989;60(5):513–16.
23. Kelders WPA, Kleinrensink GJ, Van der Geest JN, et al. The cervico-ocular reflex is increased in whiplash injury patients. J Neurotrauma 2005;22(1):133–7.
24. Montfoort I, Kelders WPA, van der Geest JN, et al. Interaction between ocular stabilization reflexes in patients with whiplash injury. Invest Ophthalmol Vis Sci 2006;47(7):2881–4.
25. Storaci R, Manelli A, Schiavone N, et al. Whiplash injury and oculomotor dysfunctions: clinical-posturographic correlations. Eur Spine J 2006;15(12):1811–16.
26. Tjell C, Rosenhall U. Smooth pursuit neck torsion test: a specific test for cervical dizziness. Am J Otol 1998;19(1):76–81.
27. Tjell C, Tenenbaum A, Sandström S. Smooth pursuit neck torsion test – A specific test for whiplash associated disorders? J Whiplash Relat Disord 2003;1(2):9–24.
28. Treleaven J, Jull G, LowChoy N. Smooth pursuit neck torsion test in whiplash-associated disorders: relationship to self-reports of neck pain and disability, dizziness and anxiety. J Rehabil Med 2005;37(4):219–23.
29. Wenngren B, Pettersson K, Lowenhielm G, et al. Eye motiliy and auditory brainstem response dysfunction after whiplash injury. Acta Orthop Scand 2002;122(3):276–83.
30. Bexander CSM, Hodges PW. Cervico-ocular coordination during neck rotation is distorted in people with whiplash-associated disorders. Exp Brain Res 2012;217(1):67–77.
31. Alund M, Ledin T, Odkvist L, et al. Dynamic posturography among patients with common neck disorders. A study of 15 cases with suspected cervical vertigo. J Vestib Res 1993;3(4):383–9.
32. Field S, Treleaven J, Jull G. Standing balance: a comparison between idiopathic and whiplash-induced neck pain. Man Ther 2008;13(3):183–91.
33. Karlberg M, Magnusson M, Malmstrom EM, et al. Postural and symptomatic improvement after physiotherapy in patients with

dizziness of suspected cervical origin. Arch Phys Med Rehabil 1996;779:874–82.

34. Karlberg M, Persson L, Magnusson M. Impaired postural control in patients with cervico-brachial pain. Acta Otolaryngol Suppl 1995;440–2.

35. Madeleine P, Prietzel H, Svarrer H, et al. Quantitative posturography in altered sensory conditions: a way to assess balance instability in patients with chronic whiplash injury. Arch Phys Med Rehabil 2004;85(3):432–8.

36. Michaelson P, Michaelson M, Jaric S, et al. Vertical posture and head stability in patients with chronic neck. J Rehabil Med 2003;35(5):229–35.

37. Poole E, Treleaven J, Jull G. The influence of neck pain on balance and gait parameters in community dwelling elders. Man Ther 2008;13:317–24.

38. Röijezon U, Björklund M, Djupsjöbacka M. The slow and fast components of postural sway in chronic neck pain. Man Ther 2011;16(3):273–8.

39. Sjöström HJ, Allum J, Carpenter MG, et al. Trunk sway measures of postural stability during clinical balance tests in patients with chronic whiplash injury symptoms. Spine 2003;28(15):1725–34.

40. Treleaven J, Jull G, Low Choy N. Standing balance in persistent WAD – Comparison between subjects with and without dizziness. J Rehabil Med 2005;37(4):224–9.

41. Treleaven J, Jull G, Murison R, et al. Is the method of signal analysis and test selection important for measuring standing balance in chronic whiplash? Gait Posture 2005;21(4):395–402.

42. Stokell R, Lui A, Williams K, et al. Dynamic and functional balance tasks in those with persistent whiplash. Man Ther 2011;16:394–8.

43. Jull G, Sterling M, Falla D, et al. Whiplash, Headache and Neck Pain. London: Elsevier; 2008.

44. Fattori B, Borsari C, Vannucci G, et al. Acupuncture treatment for balance disorders following whiplash injury. Acupunct Electrother Res 1996;21(3–4):207–17.

45. Heikkila H, Johansson M, Wenngren BI. Effects of acupuncture, cervical manipulation and NSAID therapy on dizziness and impaired head repositioning of suspected cervical origin: a pilot study. Man Ther 2000;5(3):151–7.

46. Palmgren PJ, Sandström PJ, Lundqvist FJ, et al. Improvement after chiropractic care in cervicocephalic kinesthetic sensibility and subjective pain intensity in patients with nontraumatic chronic neck pain. J Manipulative Physiol Ther 2006;29(2):100–6.

47. Reid S, Rivett D, Katekar M, et al. Sustained natural apophyseal glides (SNAGs) are an effective treatment for cervicogenic dizziness. Man Ther 2008;13:357–66.

48. Jull G, Falla D, Treleaven J, et al. Retraining cervical joint position sense: the effect of two exercise regimes. J Orthop Res 2007;25(3):404–12.

49. Treleaven J, Jull G, LowChoy N. The relationship of cervical joint position error to balance and eye movement disturbances in persistent whiplash. Man Ther 2006;11(2):99–106.

50. Revel M, Andre-Deshays C, Minguet M. Cervicocephalic kinesthetic sensibility in patients with cervical pain. Arch Phys Med Rehabil 1991;72:288–91.

51. Roren A, Mayoux-Benhamou M, Fayad F, et al. Comparison of visual and ultrasound based techniques to measure head repositioning in healthy and neck-pain subjects. Man Ther 2008;14(3):270–7.

52. Pereira M, Beaudin C, Gurbans G, et al. Cervical movement sense: a proposed clinical tool. J Eval Clin Pract, Under Review.

53. Röijezon U, Björklund M, Bergenheim M, et al. A novel method for neck coordination exercise – a pilot study on persons with chronic non-specific neck pain. J Neuroengineering Rehabil 2008;5:doi:10.1186/743-0003-5-36.

54. Treleaven J, Jull G, Grip H. Head eye co-ordination and gaze stability in subjects with persistent whiplash associated disorders. Man Ther 2011;16(3):252–7.

55. Grip H, Jull G, Treleaven J. Head Eye Co-Ordination Using simultaneous measurement of eye in head and head in space movements: potential for use in subjects with a whiplash injury. J Clin Monit Comput 2009;23(1):31–40.

56. Treleaven J, Takasaki H, Grip H, editors. Trunk Had Co-Ordination in Neck Pain. Quebec Canada: IFOMPT IFOMPT; 2012.

57. Yu LJ, Stokell R, Treleaven J. The effect of neck torsion on postural stability in subjects with persistent whiplash. Man Ther 2011;16(4):339–43.

58. Herdman S. Vestibular Rehabilitation. Philadelphia Davis; 2000.

CHAPTER 32.2 ■ SENSORIMOTOR CONTROL OF LUMBAR SPINE ALIGNMENT

Jaap van Dieën • Idsart Kingma • Nienke Willigenburg • Henri Kiers

MOTOR CONTROL AND LOW BACK PAIN

Clinical guidelines advocate exercise to prevent chronic or recurrent low back pain (LBP)[1] and motor control training specifically appears to be a mainstay of treatment. The rationale for this is that inadequate motor control contributes to causation, recurrence and/or persistence of LBP. Inadequate motor control could indeed contribute to LBP, since the lumbar spine is inherently unstable[2] and, consequently, loss of control over spinal alignment might cause noxious tissue loading.[3,4] If this occurs repeatedly, it may cause 'wear-and-tear' of tissues, injury and inflammation. Conditions such as decreased segmental stiffness[3–6] due to injury or degeneration,[7,8] respiratory challenges,[9,10] dual tasking,[11] ligament creep after sustained trunk bending[12] and trunk muscle fatigue[14–17] increase the probability of a loss of control over lumbar alignment.

Athletes with reduced control over spinal motion after sudden perturbations have a higher chance of developing LBP.[17] Similarly, individuals with LBP from the general population display impaired control.[18–21] Whether this reflects a cause or a consequence of LBP, impaired control might contribute to recurrence or persistence of LBP.

Overall, the literature on changes in motor behaviour with LBP is rather inconsistent. Evidence for both increased and decreased muscle activity has been presented,[22] and for spinal alignment both hyper- and hypolordosis have been reported.[23–25] In addition, studies have reported increased variability in trunk movement,[26,27] but also reduced variability.[26,28] Part of this inconsistency could be due to competing effects of pain and associated impairments on one hand and secondary adaptations on the other hand. More specifically, decreased muscle activity and increased variability could be associated with pain-related inhibition and nociceptive interference with the control, while increased muscle activity and reduced variability could be consequences of so-called guarding behaviour. Guarding behaviour refers to a strategy of stiffening the spine by adapted muscle recruitment, possibly to compensate for a lack of control over spinal motion.[29] Such behaviour might prevent loss of control and consequent tissue irritation. However, in spite of the relatively low increase in muscle activation involved, this may come at the cost of increased muscle fatigue[30] and increased compression on the spine,[31-33] while reduced motor variability may cause more stereotypical loading patterns. The low variance in motor behaviour could also hamper behavioural flexibility and re-learning of trunk control.[34] Guarding behaviour, while primarily adaptive, might therefore in the long term contribute to persistence of pain.[22,35-37]

While a role of motor control impairments in causation and recurrence of LBP is plausible, current therapies aimed at enhancing motor control show only limited effect sizes.[38] This may indicate that motor control impairments are not the main problem in all patients with LBP, such that only a subgroup of patients will benefit from motor control training, or that the content of these interventions is sub-optimal. Therefore, more insight in to the nature of motor control impairments in LBP is needed. To this end, recent studies have focused on sensory feedback in spinal control and the implications of these studies will be discussed in the subsequent paragraphs.

SENSORIMOTOR CONTROL OF THE LUMBAR SPINE

The lumbar spine is controlled by means of intrinsic stiffness and damping resulting from spinal passive tissues and active trunk musculature. Intrinsic stiffness and damping can be enhanced by increasing co-activation of agonistic and antagonistic muscles. In addition, several feedback mechanisms contribute to spinal control.

The effect of visual feedback appears limited, both in the anteroposterior direction[39] and the mediolateral direction.[69] However, effects of visual manipulations on spinal control[40] and of closing the eyes when balancing on an unstable surface[41] indicate that, depending on the context, the contribution of visual feedback can be more pronounced. Vestibular feedback strongly affects spinal control, both in the anteroposterior[39] and in the mediolateral direction[40] and has an even greater effect in seated balancing on an unstable chair.[69] Tactile information, through contact with a stationary object with minimal force involved, whether at the hand or the trunk, reduces trunk sway[39] and contact with a moving object increases trunk sway.[69] Finally, proprioceptive feedback, specifically from muscle spindles in the paravertebral musculature, strongly affects trunk posture. This has been demonstrated by exciting muscle spindles through mechanical vibration, with bilateral stimulation leading to an illusion of trunk movement and compensatory responses in the anteroposterior direction[39,42] and unilateral stimulation leading to responses in the mediolateral direction.[69]

SENSORIMOTOR CONTROL IN LOW BACK PAIN

When sitting in a relaxed upright posture, individuals with LBP drift more from their starting position than healthy controls,[43] without a general preference for drift in a particular direction. This difference in drift disappears when subjects frequently observe an indication of their trunk orientation on a computer screen,[43] indicating that it is not a motor problem causing the reduced precision in maintaining a static trunk posture with LBP, but rather, a sensory problem – a problem in detecting slow drift. Basic neurophysiological studies have shown that pain may negatively affect proprioceptive information from muscle spindles[44] and the slow drift in thorax orientation observed was reminiscent of that seen in healthy subjects during stimulation of paraspinal muscle spindles.[39] Furthermore, in spite of inconsistent evidence,[45-51] proprioception appears affected at least in some patients with LBP.[52-62]

Combined, the above observations suggest that impaired sensorimotor control in patients with LBP may be due to a proprioceptive impairment. If so, the difference between patients and controls would be expected to decrease when muscle vibration is applied, since it would have more of an effect in controls than in patients. Although vibration negatively affects the precision of trunk control in both patients and controls, without such an interaction effect[43] a stronger response to paravertebral muscle vibration was observed in patients compared to controls when visual information was removed.[42]

Further evidence for a proprioceptive impairment in LBP was found when subjects were asked to perform a task which challenges control over lumbar spine movements.[63] When asked to make slow, spiral-like thorax movements tracking a target moving in the frontal and sagittal planes, subjects with LBP were less precise in tracking the target. When paravertebral muscle vibration was applied, performance of the healthy controls decreased to the level of the patients, while performance in patients was unaffected. Taken together, these results indicate that a proprioceptive impairment is present in LBP, which negatively affects trunk control when insufficiently compensated by other sensory modalities.

Proprioceptive impairments in spinal control may have effects on balance control. This could be relevant for recurrence and persistence of LBP, since recovery reactions after balance loss are associated with high trunk loading.[64,65]

To assess whether proprioceptive impairments in LBP affect balance control, LBP patients and controls were tested while sitting as still as possible on a chair mounted on a hemisphere, requiring the participants to use trunk movements to maintain balance. Muscle vibration induced a slight but similar deterioration of balance performance in both groups, whilst closing the eyes led to a large but again similar deterioration of balance performance in both groups.[41] Finally, the effects of LBP were small and inconsistent.[41,66-68] Effects of LBP and vibration in this task are thus quite subtle. In retrospect, this finding may not be that surprising. The main challenge in the task is to maintain a vertical orientation. Given the nature of this task, proprioceptive feedback does not provide information on the orientation relative to gravity – with the seat tilted one way and the thorax the other way a vertical orientation may still be present. In line with this, an experiment on healthy subjects showed that the effect of paravertebral muscle stimulation is substantially reduced when sitting on an unstable versus a stable chair, while the effects of visual and vestibular manipulations are strongly increased.[69]

While these data suggest that the proprioceptive impairments in LBP do not substantially affect the ability to control balance through trunk movement, LBP has been associated with adverse changes in balance control. LBP patients tend to make less use of trunk movements in control of standing balance, which renders them less effective in challenging conditions,[70,71] placing them at increased risk of falling.[72,73] Most likely this is a consequence of guarding behaviour that stiffens the spine.[70,71]

Studies on trunk control reviewed above assessed performance mostly in terms of thorax orientation. Visual, vestibular and tactile compensations for proprioceptive impairments are not likely to be as effective for controlling lumbar alignment as they are for thorax orientation, since lumbar alignment is only observable by means of proprioceptive information. Therefore, proprioceptive impairments may be even more important in relation to LBP than suggested by these measurements.

In conclusion, precision of trunk control in relatively simple, low-intensity tasks may be reduced in individuals with LBP. This appears to be due to a proprioceptive impairment rather than a motor impairment. Impaired proprioceptive feedback might also cause patients with LBP to adopt habitual sitting and standing postures towards either extreme of the range of motion. Adaptive, guarding behaviour may compensate for sensorimotor impairments. This may be positive, because of its initial benefits, or negative because of its long-term costs.

ASSESSMENT OF SENSORIMOTOR CONTROL IN LOW BACK PAIN

The effect of impaired proprioception on the quality of trunk control is context-dependent. Reduced precision of trunk control in LBP patients is not necessarily reflected in tasks that do not require maximum precision. In contrast, guarding behaviour may result in decreased movement variability compared to that in healthy controls. These are important considerations when diagnosing sensorimotor control impairment in LBP patients.

There is no accepted clinical test to assess lumbar proprioception. In research, it is usually measured by repositioning (i.e. the subject moves from neutral to a given pelvis or thorax inclination, moves back to neutral and subsequently is asked to move back again to what he or she assumes is the same posture).[45,47–50,52–56,58–61] Differences between this posture and the target posture are measured. Such a test requires minimal instrumentation, (e.g. an inclinometer or goniometer). The reliability of these measurements appears to be sufficient for individual assessment, provided that errors are averaged over six or more repeated trials.[60,74] However, the effects of memory and the fact that a conscious perception is tested could threaten the validity of this test. Moreover, normative data are not available. Alternatively, movement detection tests have been used,[46,57,62] but these require

expensive instrumentation. A promising approach, which needs further research, would be to test vibration effects on trunk control as described above.

MANAGEMENT OF SENSORIMOTOR CONTROL IN LBP

The results described above raise the question whether trunk proprioception can be improved via intervention. Spinal mobilization appears to have a small positive effect in this respect.[75] Balancing exercises, such as those using a 'Swiss ball', are popular and are often referred to as proprioceptive training. However, given the findings regarding sensory manipulations in balancing described above, it would seem that this is not appropriate. Perhaps these exercises teach patients to use vestibular and/or visual information more effectively, to enhance trunk control by compensating for a proprioceptive impairment. For cervical disorders, training repositioning, first under visual, augmented feedback, later without feedback, has been used with positive effects on proprioception.[76] In clinical practice, manually guided lumbar movement appears to be used to the same end. In addition, exposure to whole-body vibration did yield a short-term effect on trunk repositioning in healthy subjects.[77] However, these approaches have not been investigated in LBP. Other training modalities, such as those that focus on precise control like the tracking task described above, on isolated control of single trunk muscles[78,79] or on sensory discrimination[80,81] may have positive effects on proprioception.

Finally, the benefit of improving proprioception or the use of proprioceptive feedback on prevention of persistence and recurrence of LBP remains to be proven.

REFERENCES

1. Pillastrini P, Gardenghi I, Bonetti F, et al. An updated overview of clinical guidelines for chronic low back pain management in primary care. Joint Bone Spine 2012;79:176–85.
2. Crisco JJ, Panjabi MM. Euler stability of the human ligamentous spine. Part II Experiment. Clin Biomech (Bristol, Avon) 1992;7:27–32.
3. Panjabi MM. The stabilizing system of the spine. Part I. Function, dysfunction, adaptation, and enhancement. J Spinal Disord 1992;5:383–9, discussion 97.
4. Panjabi MM. The stabilizing system of the spine. Part II. Neutral zone and instability hypothesis. J Spinal Disord 1992;5:390–7.
5. Cholewicki J, Panjabi MM, Khachatryan A. Stabilizing function of trunk flexor-extensor muscles around a neutral spine posture. Spine 1997;22:2207–12.
6. van Dieën JH, Kingma I. Spine function and low back pain: interactions of passive and active tissues. In: Hodges PW, Cholewicki J, van Dieën JH, editors. Spinal Control: The Rehabilitation of Back Pain State of the Art and Science. 1st ed. Edinburgh: Churchill Livingstone; 2013. p. 41–58.
7. Quint U, Wilke HJ. Grading of degenerative disk disease and functional impairment: imaging versus patho-anatomical findings. Eur Spine J 2008;17:1705–13.
8. Zhao FD, Pollintine P, Hole BD, et al. Discogenic origins of spinal instability. Spine 2005;30:2621–30.
9. McGill SM, Sharratt MT, Seguin JP. Loads on spinal tissues during simultaneous lifting and ventilatory challenge. Appl Ergon 1995;38:1772–92.

10. Hodges PW, Heijnen I, Gandevia SC. Postural activity of the diaphragm is reduced in humans when respiratory demand increases. J Physiol 2001;37:99–1008.

11. Brereton LC, McGill SM. Effects of physical fatigue and cognitive challenges on the potential for low back injury. Hum Mov Sci 1999;18:839–57.

12. Sanchez-Zuriaga D, Adams MA, Dolan P. Is activation of the back muscles impaired by creep or muscle fatigue? Spine 2010;35:517–25.

13. van Dieen JH. Asymmetry of erector spinae muscle activity in twisted postures and consistency of muscle activation patterns across subjects. Spine (Phila Pa 1976) 1996;21:2651–61.

14. van Dieen JH, Luger T, van der Eb J. Effects of fatigue on trunk stability in elite gymnasts. Eur J Appl Physiol 2012;112:1307–13.

15. van Dieen JH, van der Burg P, Raaijmakers TA, et al. Effects of repetitive lifting on kinematics: inadequate anticipatory control or adaptive changes? J Mot Behav 1998;30:20–32.

16. Granata KP, Gottipati P. Fatigue influences the dynamic stability of the torso. Appl Ergon 2008;51:1258–71.

17. Cholewicki J, Silfies SP, Shah RA, et al. Delayed trunk muscle reflex responses increase the risk of low back injuries. Spine 2005;30:2614–20.

18. Alexiev AR. Some differences of the electromyographic erector spinae activity between normal subjects and low back pain patients during the generation of isometric trunk torque. Electromyogr Clin Neurophysiol 1994;34:495–9.

19. Magnusson ML, Aleksiev AR, Wilder DG, et al. Unexpected load and asymmetric posture as etiologic factors in low back pain. Eur Spine J 1996;5:23–35.

20. Radebold A, Cholewicki J, Panjabi MM, et al. Muscle response pattern to sudden trunk loading in healthy individuals and in patients with chronic low back pain. Spine 2000;25:947–54.

21. Reeves NP, Cholewicki J, Milner TE. Muscle reflex classification of low-back pain. J Electromyogr Kinesiol 2005;15:53–60.

22. van Dieen JH, Selen LP, Cholewicki J. Trunk muscle activation in low-back pain patients, an analysis of the literature. J Electromyogr Kinesiol 2003;13:333–51.

23. Evcik D, Yucel A. Lumbar lordosis in acute and chronic low back pain patients. Rheumatol Int 2003;23:163–5.

24. Harrison DD, Cailliet R, Janik TJ, et al. Elliptical modeling of the sagittal lumbar lordosis and segmental rotation angles as a method to discriminate between normal and low back subjects. J Spinal Disord 1998;11:430–9.

25. Dankaerts W, O'Sullivan P, Burnett A, et al. Differences in sitting postures are associated with nonspecific chronic low back pain disorders when patients are subclassified. Spine 2006;31:698–704.

26. Lamoth CJ, Meijer OG, Daffertshofer A, et al. Effects of chronic low back pain on trunk coordination and back muscle activity during walking: changes in motor control. Eur Spine J 2006;15:23–40.

27. Vogt L, Pfeifer K, Portscher M, et al. Influences of nonspecific low back pain on three-dimensional lumbar spine kinematics in locomotion. Spine 2001;26:1910–19.

28. van den Hoorn W, Bruijn SM, Meijer OG, et al. Mechanical coupling between transverse plane pelvis and thorax rotations during gait is higher in people with low back pain. J Biomech 2012;45:342–7.

29. van Dieen JH, Cholewicki J, Radebold A. Trunk muscle recruitment patterns in patients with low back pain enhance the stability of the lumbar spine. Spine (Phila Pa 1976) 2003;28:834–41.

30. van Dieen JH, Westebring-van der Putten EP, Kingma I, et al. Low-level activity of the trunk extensor muscles causes electromyographic manifestations of fatigue in absence of decreased oxygenation. J Electromyogr Kinesiol 2009;19:398–406.

31. Marras WS, Davis KG, Ferguson SA, et al. Spine loading characteristics of patients with low back pain compared with asymptomatic individuals. Spine 2001;26:2566–74.

32. Marras WS, Ferguson SA, Burr D, et al. Spine loading in patients with low back pain during asymmetric lifting exertions. Spine J 2004;4:64–75.

33. Healey EL, Fowler NE, Burden AM, et al. Raised paraspinal muscle activity reduces rate of stature recovery after loaded exercise in individuals with chronic low back pain. Arch Phys Med Rehabil 2005;86:710–15.

34. Moseley GL, Hodges PW. Reduced variability of postural strategy prevents normalization of motor changes induced by back pain: a risk factor for chronic trouble? Behav Neurosci 2006;120:474–6.

35. van Dieen JH, Moseley GL, Hodges PW. Motor control changes and low back pain: cause or effect? In: Hodges PW, Cholewicki J, van Dieen JH, editors. Spinal Control: The Rehabilitation of Back Pain State of the Art and Science. 1st ed. Edinburgh: Churchill Livingstone; 2013. p. 207–18.

36. van Dieen JH. Low-back pain and motor behavior: contingent adaptations, a common goal. In: 6th Interdisciplinary World Congress on Low Back and Pelvic Pain. Barcelona: 2007.

37. Hodges PW, Tucker K. Moving differently in pain: a new theory to explain the adaptation to pain. Pain 2011;152:S90–8.

38. Macedo LG, Maher CG, Latimer J, et al. Motor control exercise for persistent, nonspecific low back pain: a systematic review. Phys Ther 2009;89:9–25.

39. Maaswinkel E, Veeger HEJ, van Dieen JH. Interactions of touch feedback with muscle vibration and galvanic vestibular stimulation in the control of trunk posture. Gait Posture 2013.

40. Goodworth AD, Peterka RJ. Contribution of sensorimotor integration to spinal stabilization in humans. J Neurophysiol 2009;102:496–512.

41. Willigenburg NW, Kingma I, van Dieen JH. Center of pressure trajectories, trunk kinematics and trunk muscle activation during unstable sitting in low back pain patients. Gait Posture 2013;38:625–30.

42. Claeys K, Brumagne S, Dankaerts W, et al. Decreased variability in postural control strategies in young people with non-specific low back pain is associated with altered proprioceptive reweighting. Eur J Appl Physiol 2011;111:115–23.

43. Willigenburg NW, Kingma I, van Dieen JH. Precision control of an upright trunk posture in low back pain patients. Clin Biomech (Bristol, Avon) 2012;27:866–71.

44. Thunberg J, Ljubisavljevic M, Djupsjöbacka M, et al. Effects on the fusimotor-muscle spindle system induced by intramuscular injections of hypertonic saline. Exp Brain Res 2002;142:319–26.

45. Asell M, Sjölander P, Kerschbaumer H, et al. Are lumbar repositioning errors larger among patients with chronic low back pain compared with asymptomatic subjects? Arch Phys Med Rehabil 2006;87:1170–6.

46. Silfies SP, Cholewicki J, Reeves NP, et al. Lumbar position sense and the risk of low back injuries in college athletes: a prospective cohort study. BMC Musculoskelet Disord 2007;8.

47. Descarreaux M, Blouin JS, Teasdale N. Repositioning accuracy and movement parameters in low back pain subjects and healthy control subjects. Eur Spine J 2005;14:185–91.

48. Koumantakis GA, Winstanley J, Oldham JA. Thoracolumbar proprioception in individuals with and without low back pain: intra-tester reliability, clinical applicability, and validity. J Orthop Sports Phys Ther 2002;32:327–35.

49. Lam SSK, Jull G, Treleaven J. Lumbar spine kinesthesia in patients with low back pain. J Orthop Sports Phys Ther 1999;29:294–9.

50. Newcomer K, Laskowski ER, Yu B, et al. Repositioning error in low back pain. Comparing trunk repositioning error in subjects with chronic low back pain and control subjects. Spine 2000;25:245–50.

51. Hobbs AJ, Adams RD, Shirley D, et al. Comparison of lumbar proprioception as measured in unrestrained standing in individuals with disc replacement, with low back pain and without low back pain. J Orthop Sports Phys Ther 2010;40:439–46.

52. Brumagne S, Lysens R, Spaepen A. Lumbosacral position sense during pelvic tilting in men and women without low back pain: test development and reliability assessment. J Orthop Sports Phys Ther 1999;29:345–51.

53. Brumagne S, Cordo P, Lysens R, et al. The role of paraspinal muscle spindles in lumbosacral position sense in individuals with and without low back pain. Spine (Phila Pa 1976) 2000;25:989–94.

54. Newcomer KL, Laskowski ER, Yu B, et al. Differences in repositioning error among patients with low back pain compared with control subjects. Spine 2000;25:2488–93.

55. O'Sullivan PB, Burnett A, Floyd AN, et al. Lumbar repositioning deficit in a specific low back pain population. Spine 2003;28:1074–9.

56. Gill KP, Callaghan MJ. The measurement of lumbar proprioception in individuals with and without low back pain. Spine 1998;23:371–7.

57. Lee AS, Cholewicki J, Reeves NP, et al. Comparison of trunk proprioception between patients with low back pain and healthy controls. Arch Phys Med Rehabil 2010;91:1327–31.

58. Georgy E. Lumbar repositioning accuracy as a measure of proprioception in patients with back dysfunction and healthy controls. Asian Spine J 2011;5:201–7.

59. Astfalck RG, O'Sullivan PB, Smith AJ, et al. Lumbar spine repositioning sense in adolescents with and without non-specific chronic low back pain – an analysis based on sub-classification and spinal regions. Man Ther 2013;18:410–17.

60. Hidalgo B, Gobert F, Bragard D, et al. Effects of proprioceptive disruption on lumbar spine repositioning error in a trunk forward bending task. J Back Musculoskelet Rehabil 2013;26:381–7.

61. Olivier B, Stewart AV, McKinon W. Injury and lumbar reposition sense in cricket pace bowlers in neutral and pace bowling specific body positions. Spine J 2013.

62. Taimela S, Kankaanpaa M, Luoto S. The effect of lumbar fatigue on the ability to sense a change in lumbar position – A controlled study. Spine 1999;24:1322–7.

63. Willigenburg NW, Kingma I, Hoozemans MJ. van Dieen JH. Precision control of trunk movement in low back pain patients. Hum Mov Sci 2013;32:228–39.

64. van der Burg JC, Pijnappels M, van Dieen JH. Out-of-plane trunk movements and trunk muscle activity after a trip during walking. Exp Brain Res 2005;165:407–12.

65. Oddsson LIE, Persson T, Cresswell AG, et al. Interaction between voluntary and postural motor commands during perturbed lifting. Spine 1999;24:545–52.

66. Radebold A, Cholewicki J, Polzhofer GK, et al. Impaired postural control of the lumbar spine is associated with delayed muscle response times in patients with chronic idiopathic low back pain. Spine 2001;26:724–30.

67. van Dieen JH, Koppes LL, Twisk JW. Low back pain history and postural sway in unstable sitting. Spine (Phila Pa 1976) 2010;35:812–17.

68. Van Daele U, Hagman F, Truijen S, et al. Decrease in postural sway and trunk stiffness during cognitive dual-task in nonspecific chronic low back pain patients, performance compared to healthy control subjects. Spine (Phila Pa 1976) 2010;35:583–9.

69. Andreopoulou G, Maaswinkel E, Cofre Lizama LE, et al. Effects of support surface stability on feedback control of trunk posture. Exp Brain Res 2015;doi:10.1007/s00221-014-4185-5.

70. Mok NW, Brauer SG, Hodges PW. Hip strategy for balance control in quiet standing is reduced in people with low back pain. Spine (Phila Pa 1976) 2004;29:E107–12.

71. Mok NW, Brauer SG, Hodges PW. Changes in lumbar movement in people with low back pain are related to compromised balance. Spine (Phila Pa 1976) 2011;36:E45–52.

72. Lee WK, Kong KA, Park H. Effect of preexisting musculoskeletal diseases on the 1-year incidence of fall-related injuries. J Prev Med Public Health 2012;45:283–90.

73. Muraki S, Akune T, Oka H, et al. Prevalence of falls and the association with knee osteoarthritis and lumbar spondylosis as well as knee and lower back pain in Japanese men and women. Arthritis Care Res 2011;63:1425–31.

74. Allison GT, Fukushima S. Estimating three-dimensional spinal repositioning error: the impact of range, posture, and number of trials. Spine 2003;28:2510–16.

75. Learman KE, Myers JB, Lephart SM, et al. Effects of spinal manipulation on trunk proprioception in subjects with chronic low back pain during symptom remission. J Manipulative Physiol Ther 2009;32:118–26.

76. Jull G, Falla D, Treleaven J, et al. Retraining cervical joint position sense: the effect of two exercise regimes. J Orthop Res 2007;25:404–12.

77. Fontana TL, Richardson CA, Stanton WR. The effect of weight-bearing exercise with low frequency, whole body vibration on lumbosacral proprioception: a pilot study on normal subjects. Aust J Physiother 2005;51:259–63.

78. Tsao H, Hodges PW. Immediate changes in feedforward postural adjustments following voluntary motor training. Exp Brain Res 2007;181:537–46.

79. Tsao H, Hodges PW. Persistence of improvements in postural strategies following motor control training in people with recurrent low back pain. J Electromyogr Kinesiol 2008;18:559–67.

80. Wand BM, Abbaszadeh S, Smith AJ, et al. Acupuncture applied as a sensory discrimination training tool decreases movement-related pain in patients with chronic low back pain more than acupuncture alone: a randomised cross-over experiment. Br J Sports Med 2013;47:1085–9.

81. Luomajoki H, Moseley GL. Tactile acuity and lumbopelvic motor control in patients with back pain and healthy controls. Br J Sports Med 2011;45:437–40.

CHAPTER 32.3 ■ THE LOWER LIMB

Nicholas Clark • Scott Lephart

INTRODUCTION

Normal human movement depends on effective sensorimotor control. Sensorimotor control refers to central nervous system (CNS) regulation of joint stability, posture and movement,[1,2] operating on a 'sensory motor' basis where sensory input to the CNS is first required in order to generate effective motor output from the CNS.[3,4] Sensorimotor control is achieved by the sensorimotor system which includes all components involved in the acquisition of a sensory stimulus and its transmission to the CNS, the processing of that sensory stimulus within the CNS, and the resulting motor output from the CNS.[5] From a lower limb injury prevention and rehabilitation perspective, the sensorimotor system is predominantly employed for optimizing joint stability.[6–8] Joint stability refers to the ability of a joint to remain in or promptly return to proper alignment and functional position.[1] The primary role of sensorimotor control of joint stability is to activate muscle to stress-shield non-contractile tissues (bone,

cartilage, ligament, nerve) from potentially injurious tensile, compressive and torsional forces. In order to develop effective clinical management strategies for the sensorimotor system it is necessary to review the sensorimotor system and consider how it is affected by musculoskeletal injury. Findings from research will be presented and translated to the clinical context in a way that provides a sound scientific foundation for rational clinical interventions that beneficially affect lower limb sensorimotor control.

BRIEF REVIEW OF THE SENSORIMOTOR SYSTEM

The sensorimotor system is composed of sensory, processing (CNS), and motor components.[1,5] The sensory component refers to afferent pathways that include the sensory nerve ending, the sensory nerve fibre, the afferent synapses and interneurons and the ascending tracts; the processing component refers to

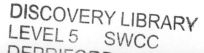

all elements within the CNS (spinal cord, brain stem and cerebral cortex); the motor component refers to efferent pathways that include an upper motor neuron, the efferent synapses and interneurons, the descending tracts, the lower motor neuron and the motor end plates.[1,5] The components of the sensorimotor system are integrated to control coordinated activation of the skeletal muscles (dynamic restraints) to optimize joint stability.[1,5] Appropriate sensorimotor control of joint stability and coordination of the dynamic restraints ultimately manifests with normal postural stability, kinematics and kinetics during human movement. Understanding the individual components of the sensorimotor system, and the way in which the components are configured and integrated, allows the clinician to plan interventions that are targeted at one or more components of the system.

THE SENSORY COMPONENT OF THE SENSORIMOTOR SYSTEM

The sensory component of the sensorimotor system includes the visual, vestibular, tactile, thermal, nociceptive and proprioceptive systems.[1] Of these, the proprioceptive system is most important with regard to joint stability, posture and movement.[1,3] Proprioception is composed of the senses of joint position (joint position sense), joint motion (kinaesthesia) and force (force sense).[1,9] Proprioception results from mechanoreceptor stimulation in the musculoskeletal tissues.[10,11] A mechanoreceptor is a specialized sensory nerve ending stimulated by mechanical deformation: mechanical deformation is converted into electrical signals that are transmitted to the CNS.[9,12] Mechanoreceptors in the non-contractile tissues of joints include Ruffini, Pacinian and Golgi endings.[13-20] Joint tissues, therefore, fulfil neurological as well as mechanical functions.[12,14] Mechanoreceptors in skeletal muscles include muscle spindles and Golgi tendon organs.[4,21,22] Different musculoskeletal tissues are thus innervated with different mechanoreceptor nerve endings. Joint and muscle mechanoreceptors have different functional properties due to different stimulus thresholds and adaptation characteristics and, consequently, different stimulation (intervention) techniques are needed (Table 32-3). Joint and muscle tissues can be targeted with a variety of manual and exercise therapy techniques to deliberately induce mechanoreceptor stimulation and proprioceptive feedback to the CNS. The clinician can, therefore, use specific intervention techniques to access the sensorimotor system to beneficially affect sensorimotor control of joint stability, posture and human movement.

EFFECTS OF INJURY ON THE SENSORIMOTOR SYSTEM

To administer effective interventions for the sensorimotor system it is important to know how the system can be affected by musculoskeletal injury. When the effects of musculoskeletal injury are recognized, effective interventions can then be selected for each component of the sensorimotor system. Lower limb joint injury frequently results in destruction of mechanoreceptors.[24,25] Loss of capsuloligamentous mechanoreceptors is consistently associated with impaired proprioception[26-29] and altered processing and organization of the somatosensory cortex.[30-32] Unilateral joint injury can manifest with an inability to fully activate peri-articular musculature.[33-35] Altered ipsilateral muscle activation patterns local to the injury site[36,37] and remote from the injury site[38] can be evident. Unilateral joint injury can manifest bilateral proprioceptive deficits[39,40] and inability to fully activate muscles contralateral to the injured side.[35,41,42] Pain can result in impaired proprioception,[43,44] muscle inhibition,[45,46] altered inter-muscular firing patterns[47,48] and reduced muscle strength.[45,49] Joint effusion is also associated with impaired proprioception[50] and muscle inhibition.[14,51,52] Since musculoskeletal injury affects all components of the sensorimotor system, it is not surprising that lower limb musculoskeletal injury, pain and effusion manifest with altered postural stability[53-55] and altered kinematics and kinetics during functional tasks.[51,56-58] Lower limb joint injury is not limited to the musculoskeletal system and, therefore, should also be considered a neurological problem. Unilateral joint injury can manifest ipsilateral motor dysfunction remote from the injury site. Furthermore, unilateral joint injury does not limit its effects to one side of the body but also extends its influence to the contralateral side. Because of the potentially widespread effects of apparently isolated joint injury, clinicians should extend management of the sensorimotor system beyond the local site and side of injury.

MANUAL THERAPY AND THE SENSORIMOTOR SYSTEM

This section will focus on lower limb joint manual therapy in the form of mobilizations and manipulations. Mobilizations and manipulations are passive movements of a patient's joint, performed by the clinician, and primarily used to improve joint mobility by reducing pain, mobilizing intracapsular fluid, and stretching capsuloligamentous tissues.[59-62] Pain neurons and proprioceptor neurons synapse in the dorsal horn of the spinal cord with shared ascending tracts that convey sensory information to supraspinal levels.[63] Stimulation of mechanoreceptor neurons activates an inhibitory interneuron that blocks the transmission of nociceptor impulses to higher CNS nuclei: this is the pain gate mechanism.[63,64] Manual therapy can use capsuloligamentous mechanoreceptor stimulation to block the inhibitory effects of pain on the sensorimotor system. Specific joint mobilization techniques are reported effective for immediately reducing knee and ankle pain.[65,66] Passive movement of peripheral joints causes intrasynovial fluid movement[67] and increased lymphatic drainage,[68,69] and both are desirable to decrease joint effusions. Manual therapy can be administered to facilitate clearance of excessive intrasynovial fluid, reverse effusion-induced inhibition of the sensorimotor system,

TABLE 32-3 Example Intervention Techniques to Stimulate Mechanoreceptors in Different Lower Limb Musculoskeletal and Cutaneous Tissues

Tissue	Mechanoreceptor Nerve Ending	Predominant Stimulation Type	Stimulation Threshold	Adaptation Characteristic	Proprioception Sub-Modality	Joint Manual Therapy Technique Examples	Taping/Bracing Technique Exercise	Active Examples Therapy Mode Examples
Capsule	Ruffini ending	Tension	Low	Slow	JPS/kinaesthesia	Sustained mobilization	–	Dynamic > static exercises
	Golgi ending	Tension	High	Slow	Kinaesthesia	Intermittent mobilizations	–	Dynamic exercises
Ligament	Ruffini ending	Tension	Low	Slow	JPS/kinaesthesia	Sustained mobilization	–	Dynamic > static exercises
	Pacinian ending	Tension/compression	Low	Fast	Kinaesthesia	Intermittent mobilizations	–	Dynamic exercises
	Golgi ending	Tension	High	Slow	Kinaesthesia	Intermittent mobilizations	–	Dynamic exercises
Meniscus/Labrum	Ruffini ending	Tension	Low	Slow	JPS/kinaesthesia	Sustained mobilization	–	Dynamic > static exercises
	Pacinian ending	Tension/compression	Low	Fast	Kinaesthesia	Intermittent mobilizations	–	Dynamic exercises
	Golgi ending	Tension	High	Slow	Kinaesthesia	Intermittent mobilizations	–	Dynamic exercises
Fat pad	Pacinian ending	Tension/compression	Low	Fast	Kinaesthesia	–	Fat pad taping	Dynamic exercises
Fascia	Pacinian ending	Tension/compression	Low	Fast	Kinaesthesia	–	Fascial taping	Dynamic exercises
Skin	Hair follicle receptor	Flutter, stroking	Low	Fast	–	–	EB/NS/Taping	–
	Merkel disc	Pressure/indentation	High	Slow	Kinaesthesia	–	EB/NS	–
	Meissner corpuscle	Flutter, stroking	Low	Fast	Kinaesthesia	–	EB/NS	–
	Ruffini ending	Skin tension	Low	Slow	JPS/kinaesthesia	–	Taping	Dynamic exercises
	Pacinian ending	Vibration	Low	Fast	Kinaesthesia	–	–	Dynamic exercises
Muscle	Spindle primary	Velocity of active length change	Low	Fast	Kinaesthesia	Intermittent mobilizations	–	Dynamic > static exercises
	Spindle secondary	Active length	Low	Fast	JPS/kinaesthesia	Intermittent mobilizations	–	Dynamic > static exercises
	Golgi Tendon Organ	Active tension	High	Slow	JPS/kinaesthesia/FS	–	–	Dynamic/static exercises

Mechanoreceptor information from references: 13–15, 18–20, 23.
JPS, Joint position sense; FS, force sense; EB, elastic bandage; NS, neoprene sleeve.

and promote reacquisition of normal lower limb biomechanics.

Capsuloligamentous tissue contains mechanoreceptor nerve endings and familiarity with sensorimotor system circuitry is useful for planning interventions to enhance proprioception. Feline knee studies have reported that low tensile forces in ligaments strongly stimulate gamma motor neurons and increase the sensitivity of the muscle spindle.[70-73] More recent studies in humans have described how tensile loads applied to the ankle ligaments elicit increased muscle spindle discharge in uninjured and injured athletes.[74] The range of forces applied by manual therapists during mobilizations and manipulations include the forces reported capable of stimulating ligament–muscle spindle circuitry.[75-77] Direct stimulation of capsuloligamentous mechanoreceptors and indirect stimulation of muscle spindles provides a pathway by which joint manual therapy can have an effect on proprioceptive feedback to the CNS. Authors have reported that lower quadrant joint mobilizations and manipulations are able to immediately enhance post-intervention proprioception.[78-80]

Proprioceptive information is transmitted to higher CNS centres by the ascending tracts in the spinal cord.[5,81] Stimulation of the knee ligaments and menisci results in increased electrical activity in the cerebral cortex.[82,83] This verifies the human brain can be directly accessed via sensory nerve endings in the periphery and, therefore, joint manual therapy can be used with the intent of stimulating the cerebral cortex. Interventions that stimulate the cerebral cortex are of importance because sensory information from cortical sensory nuclei is transmitted to the premotor and primary motor centres via transcortical axons and is important in modifying feedforward motor programmes and the learning of movement patterns.[84]

The components of the sensorimotor system are integrated to coordinate activation of skeletal muscle to optimize joint stability.[5] This requires reflex and voluntary activation of extrafusal muscle fibres.[1,85] A reflex is a stereotyped involuntary muscle response to a sensory stimulus.[10] Studies have described reflex activation of the hamstrings in response to mechanical stimulation of the anterior cruciate ligament,[86-88] reflex activation of the medial hamstrings and medial quadriceps in response to mechanical stimulation of the medial collateral ligament,[89,90] and reflex activation of the hamstrings in response to stimulation of the meniscus.[83] These studies indicate specific joint–muscle sensory-motor circuitry is hardwired into the human CNS. Sensory-motor circuitry mediates feedback activation of skeletal muscle to stress-shield non-contractile tissues: activation is specifically directed at muscles that are antagonists to the direction of joint motion and loading perceived by the CNS.

In the short term, lower quadrant joint mobilization and manipulation techniques have been shown to be capable of facilitating extrafusal muscle fibre activation and increasing muscle strength.[91-95] In the long term, stimulation of sensory-motor neurocircuitry via intermittent joint mobilizations (Fig. 32-5) is useful for beneficially affecting sensorimotor control of joint stability because repetitive activation of specific sensory-motor

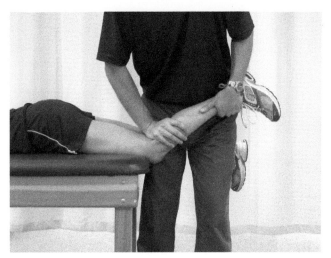

FIGURE 32-5 ■ Example of a knee accessory mobilization technique. (From Kaltenborn 1999.[60])

circuits results in long-term learning due to adaptation of neuron structure, increased effectiveness of synaptic transmission and modification of CNS somatotopic maps.[96,97]

Joint manual therapy has the potential to affect all components of the sensorimotor system. Because all components of the sensorimotor system can be affected by joint mobilizations and manipulations, there is the potential for joint manual therapy to have an immediate effect on the performance of functional tasks. Specific lower limb joint mobilizations have been shown to yield an immediate positive effect on postural stability and dynamic balance[98-100] and the kinematics of walking gait and drop-landing tasks.[101,102]

Joint manual therapy is capable of reducing pain and effusion, and positively affecting all components of the lower limb sensorimotor system. Because joint manual therapy can affect all components of the sensorimotor system, it is able to manifest an immediate beneficial effect in the performance of functional tasks. Joint manual therapy is, therefore, a clinically effective intervention that can be used to help patients prepare for more active rehabilitation in the form of exercise therapy sessions and the performance of functional movement patterns.

TAPING AND BRACING AND THE SENSORIMOTOR SYSTEM

This section will discuss the clinical use of athletic tape, elastic bandages and neoprene sleeves. The skin possesses three types of sensory nerve endings: thermoreceptors, nociceptors and mechanoreceptors.[9] Superficial cutaneous mechanoreceptors include hair follicle receptors, Merkel discs and Meissner corpuscles, while deeper subcutaneous tissue mechanoreceptors include Pacinian corpuscles and Ruffini endings.[4,9,23] Proprioception is predominantly the result of muscle and joint mechanoreceptor stimulation, although cutaneous mechanoreceptor stimulation also contributes to proprioception due to superficial tissue deformation during joint movement.[4,9]

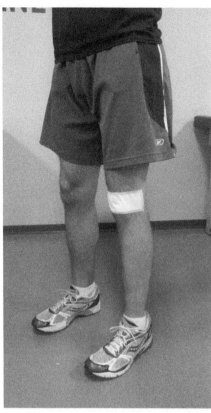

FIGURE 32-6 ■ Example of a knee taping technique. (From Callaghan et al. 2002.[111])

The application of athletic tape, elastic bandages or neoprene sleeves can immediately reduce the intensity of knee pain.[103–107] The application of athletic tape can also immediately enhance proprioception of the ankle[108–110] and knee,[111,112] as can wearing of elastic bandages and neoprene sleeves.[26,113,114] Furthermore, knee athletic tape and neoprene sleeves are able to modulate activity of the sensorimotor cortex,[115,116] and application of athletic tape has been reported to enhance lower limb muscle activation characteristics.[117–120] Stimulation of the skin, therefore, can be an important part of lower limb sensorimotor system rehabilitation.[121] Stimulation of the skin via athletic tape, elastic bandages and neoprene sleeves is capable of immediately reducing pain and beneficially affecting all components of the sensorimotor system. Lower limb taping (Fig. 32-6) and bracing is, therefore, a further potential intervention that clinicians can employ to help patients prepare for exercise therapy sessions and the performance of functional movement patterns.

EXERCISE THERAPY AND THE SENSORIMOTOR SYSTEM

Exercise therapy refers to repeated movements performed within structured and goal-directed exercise programmes. Repeated movements must be active versus passive in order to optimally and simultaneously stimulate all components of the sensorimotor system. The objective of exercise therapy is to integrate all components of the sensorimotor system and generate coordinated activity of the dynamic restraints to optimize joint stability.[8,11] Different training methods elicit different sensorimotor control training adaptations, and thorough exercise therapy for lower limb joint injuries must include several different types of exercise selected within a clinically reasoned and goal-directed process.[122–124]

The muscle spindle is the most potent mechanoreceptor which is always stimulated with active movements as a result of alpha-gamma co-activation.[4,10] The Golgi tendon organ is also a potent mechanoreceptor, being very sensitive to forces generated by active movements.[4,10] Any active exercise can, therefore, be considered proprioceptive training since it will generate a barrage of impulses from muscle mechanoreceptors.[122] Open kinetic chain and closed kinetic chain exercise generate proprioceptive feedback to the CNS,[125–127] although closed kinetic chain exercise results in better proprioception defined by less error in active joint repositioning tasks,[125,127] and full weight-bearing exercise enhances proprioceptive feedback more than partial weight-bearing exercise.[128] Long-term lower limb strength training,[129,130] balance training[131,132] and plyometric training[133] have all been reported to significantly improve active measures of proprioception.

Repeated use of the CNS is necessary to facilitate the neurological changes necessary for long-term learning of enhanced sensorimotor control programmes.[95,96] Activation of all components of the sensorimotor system is evident with the short-term active performance of repetitive goal-directed tasks.[134,135] Long-term strength and skill training stimulates spinal and cortical plastic adaptations that enhance both muscle performance characteristics and the execution of coordinated tasks.[136–138]

The sensorimotor system coordinates activation of skeletal muscle to optimize joint stability, posture and movement.[1,5] Goal-directed repeated movements result in learning new sensorimotor motor control programmes and enhanced functional properties of extrafusal muscle fibres,[95,96,139] which then manifest with changes in postural stability and the kinematics and kinetics of human movement. Strength training can enhance muscle performance characteristics, postural stability and the kinematics of walking.[140–142] Balance and perturbation training can enhance muscle activation patterns, muscle performance characteristics, postural stability, the kinematics of walking, and the kinematics and kinetics of landing tasks.[52,143–148] Plyometric training can alter muscle activation patterns, muscle performance characteristics, and the kinematics and kinetics of running and landing tasks.[147–151]

Exercise therapy integrates all components of the sensorimotor system to generate coordinated activity of skeletal muscle. Active exercises (Fig. 32-7) are the most effective intervention for stimulating all components of the sensorimotor system. A variety of exercise therapy training methods can positively affect proprioception, CNS processing, and the coordination of skeletal muscle activation. A selection of training methods is required to induce beneficial changes in lower limb muscle performance, joint stability, postural stability, kinematics and kinetics due to plastic adaptation in different parts of the sensorimotor system.

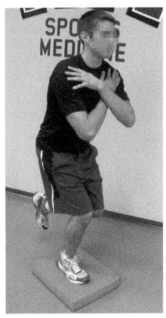

FIGURE 32-7 ■ Example of closed kinetic chain exercise technique on an unstable base-of-support.

SUMMARY

Normal human movement depends on effective sensorimotor control. Sensorimotor control is achieved by the sensorimotor system which includes sensory, processing and motor components. All components of the sensorimotor system are affected by lower limb joint injury. The effects of lower limb joint injury on the sensorimotor system can be widespread and extend far beyond the site and side of injury. Joint manual therapy, taping and bracing can all immediately reduce pain, stimulate the sensory (proprioception) and processing (CNS) components of the sensorimotor system, and enhance lower limb postural stability and kinematics during functional tasks. Joint manual therapy has also been reported to immediately stimulate motor function defined by increases in muscle strength. An integrated model for clinical management of the lower limb sensorimotor system, therefore, includes joint manual therapy, taping and bracing as effective interventions employed to help patients prepare for more active rehabilitation in the form of exercise therapy and the performance of functional movement patterns. Exercise therapy can then elicit long-term beneficial adaptations in all components of the sensorimotor system that manifest with measurable improvements in lower limb joint stability, postural stability, kinematics and kinetics.

REFERENCES

1. Riemann B, Lephart S. The sensorimotor system, part I: the physiologic basis of functional joint stability. J Athl Train 2002;37(1):71–9.
2. Shumway-Cook A, Woollacott M. Motor Control. Theory and Practical Applications. 2nd ed. Philadelphia: Lippincott; 2001.
3. Ghez C. The control of movement. In: Kandel E, Schwartz J, Jessell T, editors. Principles of Neural Science. 3rd ed. London: Prentice-Hall; 1991. p. 533–47.
4. Rothwell J. Control of Human Voluntary Movement. 2nd ed. London: Chapman Hall; 1994.
5. Lephart S, Riemann B, Fu F. Introduction to the sensorimotor system. In: Lephart S, Fu F, editors. Proprioception and Neuromuscular Control in Joint Stability. Illinois: Human Kinetics; 2000. p. xvii–xxiv.
6. Borsa P, Sauers E, Lephart S. Functional training for the restoration of dynamic stability in the PCL-injured knee. J Sport Rehabil 1999;8:362–78.
7. Lephart S, Pincivero D, Rozzi S. Proprioception of the ankle and knee. Sports Med 1998;25(3):149–55.
8. Swanik C, Lephart S, Giannantonio F, et al. Reestablishing proprioception and neuromuscular control in the ACL-injured athlete. J Sport Rehabil 1997;6:182–206.
9. Martin J, Jessell T. Modality coding in the somatic sensory system. In: Kandel E, Schwartz J, Jessell T, editors. Principles of Neural Science. 3rd ed. London: Prentice-Hall; 1991. p. 341–52.
10. Gordon J, Ghez C. Muscle receptors and spinal reflexes: the stretch reflex. In: Kandel E, Schwartz J, Jessell T, editors. Principles of Neural Science. 3rd ed. London: Prentice-Hall International; 1991. p. 564–80.
11. Lephart S, Pincivero D, Giraldo J, et al. The role of proprioception in the management and rehabilitation of athletic injuries. Am J Sports Med 1997;25(1):130–7.
12. Barrack R, Lund P, Skinner H. Knee joint proprioception revisited. J Sport Rehabil 1994;3(1):18–42.
13. Day B, Mackenzie W, Shim S, et al. The vascular and nerve supply of the human meniscus. Arthroscopy 1985;1(1):58–62.
14. Kennedy J, Alexander I, Hayes K. Nerve supply of the human knee and its functional importance. Am J Sports Med 1982;10(6):329–35.
15. Michelson J, Hutchins C. Mechanoreceptors in human ankle ligaments. J Bone Joint Surg Am 1995;77B(2):219.
16. Moraes M, Cavalcante M, Leite J, et al. Histomorphometric evaluation of mechanoreceptors and free nerve endings in human lateral ankle ligaments. Foot Ankle Int 2008;29(1):87–90.
17. Schutte M, Dabezies E, Zimny M, et al. Neural anatomy of the human anterior cruciate ligament. J Bone Joint Surg Am 1987;69A(2):243–7.
18. Moraes M, Cavalcante M, Leite J, et al. The characteristics of the mechanoreceptors of the hip with arthrosis. J Orthop Surg Res 2011;6:58.
19. Freeman M, Wyke B. The innervation of the knee joint. An anatomical and histological study in the cat. J Anat 1967;101(Pt 3):505–32.
20. Assimakopoulos A, Katonis P, Agapitos M, et al. The innervation of the human meniscus. Clin Orthop Relat Res 1992;275:232–6.
21. Kararizou E, Manta P, Kalfakis N, et al. Morphometric study of the human muscle spindle. Anal Quant Cytol Histol 2005;27(1):1–4.
22. Spiro A, Beilin R. Human muscle spindle histochemistry. Arch Neurol 1969;20(3):271–5.
23. Johansson R, Vallbo Å. Tactile sensory coding in the glabrous skin of the human hand. Trends Neurosci 1983;6:27–32.
24. Dhillon M, Bali K, Vasistha R. Immunohistological evaluation of proprioceptive potential of the residual stump of injured anterior cruciate ligaments (ACL). Int Orthop 2010;34(5):737–41.
25. Bali K, Dhillon M, Vasistha R, et al. Efficacy of immunohistological methods in detecting functionally viable mechanoreceptors in the remnant stumps of injured anterior cruciate ligaments and its clinical importance. Knee Surg Sports Traumatol Arthrosc 2012;20(1):75–80.
26. Borsa P, Lephart S, Irrgang J, et al. The effects of joint position and direction of joint motion on proprioceptive sensibility in anterior cruciate ligament-deficient athletes. Am J Sports Med 1997;25(3):336–40.
27. Lephart S, Kocher M, Fu F, et al. Proprioception following anterior cruciate ligament reconstruction. J Sport Rehabil 1992;1(3):188–98.
28. Safran M, Allen A, Lephart S, et al. Proprioception in the posterior cruciate ligament deficient knee. Knee Surg Sports Traumatol Arthrosc 1999;7(5):310–17.
29. Swanik C, Lephart S, Rubash H. Proprioception, kinesthesia, and balance after total knee arthroplasty with cruciate-retaining and

posterior stabilized prostheses. J Bone Joint Surg Am 2004; 86A(2):328–34.

30. Valeriani M, Restuccia D, Di Lazzaro V, et al. Central nervous system modifications in patients with lesion of the anterior cruciate ligament of the knee. Brain 1996;119: 1751–62.

31. Valeriani M, Restuccia D, Di Lazzaro V, et al. Clinical and neurophysiological abnormalities before and after reconstruction of the anterior cruciate ligament of the knee. Acta Neurol Scand 1999;99(5):303–7.

32. Kapreli E, Athanasopoulos S, Gliatis J, et al. Anterior cruciate ligament deficiency causes brain plasticity: a functional MRI study. Am J Sports Med 2009;37(12):2419–26.

33. Konishi Y, Fukubayashi T, Takeshita D. Possible mechanism of quadriceps femoris weakness in patients with ruptured anterior cruciate ligament. Med Sci Sports Exerc 2002;349: 1414–18.

34. Snyder-Mackler L, De Luca P, Williams P, et al. Reflex inhibition of the quadriceps femoris muscle after injury or reconstruction of the anterior cruciate ligament. J Bone Joint Surg Am 1994; 76A(4):555–60.

35. Chmielewski T, Stackhouse S, Axe M, et al. A prospective analysis of incidence and severity of quadriceps inhibition in a consecutive sample of 100 patients with complete acute anterior cruciate ligament rupture. J Orthop Res 2004;22(5):925–30.

36. De Mont R, Lephart S, Giraldo J, et al. Muscle preactivity of anterior cruciate ligament-deficient and -reconstructed females during functional activities. J Athl Train 1999;34(2): 115–20.

37. Swanik C, Lephart S, Giraldo J, et al. Reactive muscle firing of anterior cruciate ligament-injured females during functional activities. J Athl Train 1999;34(2):121–9.

38. Bullock-Saxton J. Local sensation changes and altered hip muscle function following severe ankle sprain. Phys Ther 1994;74(1): 17–28.

39. Roberts D, Fridén T, Stomberg A, et al. Bilateral proprioceptive defects in patients with a unilateral anterior cruciate ligament reconstruction: a comparison between patients and healthy individuals. J Orthop Res 2000;18(4):565–71.

40. Arockiaraj J, Korula R, Oommen A, et al. Proprioceptive changes in the contralateral knee joint following anterior cruciate injury. Bone Joint J 2013;95B(2):188–91.

41. Konishi Y, Konishi H, Fukubayashi T. Gamma loop dysfunction in quadriceps on the contralateral side in patients with ruptured ACL. Med Sci Sports Exerc 2003;35(6):897–900.

42. Urbach D, Nebelung W, Weiler H, et al. Bilateral deficit of voluntary quadriceps muscle activation after unilateral ACL tear. Med Sci Sports Exerc 1999;31(12):1691–6.

43. Matre D, Arendt-Neilsen L, Knardahl S. Effects of localization and intensity of experimental muscle pain on ankle joint proprioception. Eur J Pain 2002;6(4):245–60.

44. Rossi S, della Volpe R, Ginanneschi F, et al. Early somatosensory processing during tonic muscle pain in humans: relation to loss of proprioception and motor defensive strategies. Clin Neurophysiol 2003;114:1351–8.

45. Graven-Nielsen T, Lund H, Arendt-Neilsen L, et al. Inhibition of maximal voluntary contraction force by experimental muscle pain: a centrally mediated mechanism. Muscle Nerve 2002;26(5): 708–12.

46. Farina D, Arendt-Neilsen L, Merletti R, et al. Effect of experimental muscle pain on motor unit firing rate and conduction velocity. J Neurophysiol 2004;91(3):1250–9.

47. Graven-Nielsen T, Svensson P, Arendt-Neilsen L. Effects of experimental muscle pain on muscle activity and co-ordination during static and dynamic motor function. Electroencephalogr Clin Neurophysiol 1997;105(2):156–64.

48. Salomoni S, Ejaz A, Laursen A, et al. Variability of three-dimensional forces increase during experimental knee pain. Eur J Appl Physiol 2013;113(3):567–75.

49. Henriksen M, Rosager S, Aaboe J, et al. Experimental knee pain reduces muscle strength. J Pain 2011;12(4):460–7.

50. Baxendale R, Ferrell W. Disturbances of proprioception at the human knee resulting from acute joint distension. J Physiol 1987;392:60.

51. Palmieri-Smith R, Kreinbrink J, Ashton-Miller J, et al. Quadriceps inhibition induced by an experimental knee joint effusion affects knee joint mechanics during a single-legged drop landing. Am J Sports Med 2007;35(8):1269–75.

52. Stokes M, Young A. The contribution of reflex inhibition to arthrogenous muscle weakness. Clin Sci 1984;67(1):7–14.

53. Rozzi S, Lephart S, Sterner R, et al. Balance training for persons with functionally unstable ankles. J Orthop Sports Phys Ther 1999;29(8):478–86.

54. Lysholm M, Ledin T, Odkvist L, et al. Postural control – a comparison between patients with chronic anterior cruciate ligament insufficiency and healthy individuals. Scand J Med Sci Sports 1998;8(6):432–8.

55. Mohammadi F, Salavati M, Akhbari B, et al. Static and dynamic postural control in competitive athletes after anterior cruciate ligament reconstruction and controls. Knee Surg Sports Traumatol Arthrosc 2012;20(8):1603–10.

56. Fontboté C, Sell T, Laudner K, et al. Neuromuscular and biomechanical adaptations of patients with isolated deficiency of the posterior cruciate ligament. Am J Sports Med 2005;33(7): 982–9.

57. Seeley M, Park J, King D, et al. A novel experimental knee-pain model affects perceived pain and movement biomechanics. J Athl Train 2013;48(3):337–45.

58. Vairo G, Myers J, Sell T, et al. Neuromuscular and biomechanical landing performance subsequent to ipsilateral semitendinosus and gracilis autograft anterior cruciate ligament reconstruction. Knee Surg Sports Traumatol Arthrosc 2008;16(1):2–14.

59. Hengeveld E, Banks K, Maitland G, et al. Maitland's Peripheral Manipulation. Edinburgh: Butterworth-Heinemann; 2005.

60. Kaltenborn F. Manual Mobilizations of the Joints: The Kaltenborn Method of Joint Examination and Treatment. Oslo: Olaf Norlis Bokhandel; 1999.

61. Mulligan B. Manual Therapy: NAGs, SNAGs, MWMs. Minneapolis: Orthopaedic Physical Therapy Products; 2010.

62. Greenman P. Principles of Manual Medicine. Philadelphia: Lippincott; 2003.

63. Jessell T, Kelly D. Pain and analgesia. In: Kandel E, Schwartz J, Jessell T, editors. Principles of Neural Science. London: Prentice-Hall; 1991. p. 385–99.

64. Melzack R, Wall P. Pain mechanisms: a new theory. Science 1965;150(3699):971–9.

65. Yeo H, Wright A. Hypoalgesic effect of a passive accessory mobilisation technique in patients with lateral ankle pain. Man Ther 2011;16(4):373–7.

66. Moss P, Sluka K, Wright A. The initial effects of knee joint mobilization on osteoarthritic hyperalgesia. Man Ther 2007;12(2): 109–18.

67. Pedowitz R, Gershuni D, Crenshaw A, et al. Intraarticular pressure during continuous passive motion of the human knee. J Orthop Res 1989;7(4):530–7.

68. Ikomi F, Schmid-Schönbein G. Lymph pump mechanics in the rabbit hind leg. Am J Physiol 1996;271(1 Pt 2):H173–83.

69. McGeown J, McHale N, Thornbury K. The role of external compression and movement in lymph propulsion in the sheep hind limb. J Physiol 1987;387:83–93.

70. Sojka P, Johansson H, Sjölander P, et al. Fusimotor neurones can be reflexly influenced by activity in receptor afferents from the posterior cruciate ligament. Brain Res 1989;483(1):177–83.

71. Johansson H, Lorentzon R, Sjölander P, et al. The anterior cruciate ligament: a sensor acting on the γ-muscle-spindle systems of muscles around the knee joint. Neuro Orthop 1990;9(1):1–23.

72. Johansson H, Sjölander P, Sojka P. Activity in receptor afferents from the anterior cruciate ligament evokes reflex effects on fusimotor neurones. Neurosci Res 1990;8(1):54–9.

73. Sjölander P, Djupsjöbacka M, Johansson H, et al. Can receptors in the collateral ligaments contribute to knee joint stability and proprioception via effects on the fusimotor-muscle-spindle system? Neuro Orthop 1994;15(2):65–80.

74. Needle A, Charles BBS, Farquhar W, et al. Muscle spindle traffic in functionally unstable ankles during ligamentous stress. J Athl Train 2013;48(2):192–202.

75. Petty N, Maher C, Latimer J, et al. Manual examination of accessory movements – seeking R1. Man Ther 2002;7(1):39–43.

76. Venturini C, Penedo M, Peixoto G, et al. Study of the force applied during anteroposterior articular mobilization of the talus and its effect on the dorsiflexion range of motion. J Manipulative Physiol Ther 2007;30(8):593–7.

77. Silvernail J, Gill N, Teyhen D, et al. Biomechanical measures of knee joint mobilization. J Man Manip Ther 2011;19(3): 162–71.

78. Ju Y, Wang C, Cheng H. Effects of active fatiguing movement versus passive repetitive movement on knee proprioception. Clin Biomech (Bristol, Avon) 2010;25(7):708–12.

79. Vicenzino B, Jordan K, Brandjerporn M, et al. Mobilization with movement treatment of the ankle changes joint position sense in subjects with recurrent sprains: a preliminary report. J Orthop Sports Phys Ther 2005;35(5):A–21.

80. Learman K, Myers J, Lephart S, et al. Effects of spinal manipulation on trunk proprioception in subjects with chronic low back pain during symptom remission. J Manipulative Physiol Ther 2009;32(2):118–26.

81. Martin J, Jessell T. Anatomy of the somatic sensory system. In: Kandel E, Schwartz J, Jessell T, editors. Principles of Neural Science. 3rd ed. London: Prentice-Hall; 1991. p. 353–66.

82. Pitman M, Nainzadeh N, Menche D, et al. The intraoperative evaluation of the neurosensory function of the anterior cruciate ligament in humans using somatosensory evoked potentials. Arthroscopy 1992;8(4):442–7.

83. Saygi B, Yildirim Y, Berker N, et al. Evaluation of the neurosensory function of the medial meniscus in humans. Arthroscopy 2005;21(12):1468–72.

84. Saper C, Iversen S, Frackowiak R. Integration of sensory and motor function: the association areas of the cerebral cortex and the cognitive capabilities of the brain. In: Kandel E, Schwartz J, Jessell T, editors. Principles of Neural Science. 4th ed. New York: McGraw-Hill; 2000. p. 349–80.

85. Riemann B, Lephart S. The sensorimotor system, part II: the role of proprioception in motor control and functional joint stability. J Athl Train 2002;37(1):80–4.

86. Friemert B, Faist M, Spengler C, et al. Intraoperative direct mechanical stimulation of the anterior cruciate ligament elicits short-and medium-latency hamstring reflexes. J Neurophysiol 2005;94(6):3996–4001.

87. Huston L, Wojtys E. Neuromuscular performance characteristics in elite female athletes. Am J Sports Med 1996;24(4):427–36.

88. Beard D, Kyberd P, Fergusson C, et al. Proprioception after rupture of the anterior cruciate ligament. An objective indication of the need for surgery. J Bone Joint Surg Am 1993;75B(2):311–15.

89. Buchanan T, Kim A, Lloyd D. Selective muscle activation following rapid varus/valgus perturbations at the knee. Med Sci Sports Exerc 1996;28(7):870–6.

90. Dhaher Y, Tsoumanis A, Houle T, et al. Neuromuscular reflexes contribute to knee stiffness during valgus loading. J Neurophysiol 2005;93(5):2698–709.

91. Yerys S, Makofsky H, Byrd C, et al. Effect of mobilization of the anterior hip capsule on gluteus maximus strength. J Man Manip Ther 2002;10(4):218–24.

92. Makofsky H, Panicker S, Abbruzzese J, et al. Immediate effect of Grade IV inferior hip joint mobilization on hip abductor torque: a pilot study. J Man Manip Ther 2007;15(2):103–10.

93. Suter E, McMorland G, Herzog W, et al. Conservative lower back treatment reduces inhibition in knee-extensor muscles: a randomized controlled trial. J Manipulative Physiol Ther 2000;23(2): 76–80.

94. Suter E, McMorland G, Herzog W, et al. Decrease in quadriceps inhibition after sacroiliac joint manipulation in patients with anterior knee pain. J Manipulative Physiol Ther 1999;22(3):149–53.

95. Dishman J, Ball K, Burke J. Central motor excitability changes after spinal manipulation: a transcranial magnetic stimulation study. J Manipulative Physiol Ther 2002;25(1):1–9.

96. Ghez C. The cerebellum. In: Kandel E, Schwartz J, Jessell T, editors. Principles of Neural Science. 3rd ed. London: Prentice-Hall; 1991. p. 626–46.

97. Kandel E. Cellular mechanisms of learning and the biological basis of individuality. In: Kandel E, Schwartz J, Jessell T, editors. Principles of Neural Science. London: Prentice-Hall; 1991. p. 1009–31.

98. Vaillant J, Rouland A, Martigné P, et al. Massage and mobilization of the feet and ankles in elderly adults: effect on clinical balance performance. Man Ther 2009;14(6):661–4.

99. Ferreira G, Viero C, Silveira M, et al. Immediate effects of hip mobilization on pain and baropodometric variables – A case report. Man Ther 2013;18(6):628–31.

100. Wassinger C, Rockett A, Pitman L, et al. Acute effects of rearfoot manipulation on dynamic standing balance in healthy individuals. Man Ther 2013;(Accepted manuscript).

101. Delahunt E, Cusack K, Wilson L, et al. Joint mobilization acutely improves landing kinematics in chronic ankle instability. Med Sci Sports Exerc 2012;45(3):514–19.

102. Hunt M, Di Ciacca S, Jones I, et al. Effect of anterior tibiofemoral glides on knee extension during gait in patients with decreased range of motion after anterior cruciate ligament reconstruction. Physiother Can 2010;62(3):235–41.

103. Hinman R, Bennell K, Crossley K, et al. Immediate effects of adhesive tape on pain and disability in individuals with knee osteoarthritis. Rheumatology 2003;42(7):865–9.

104. Wilson T, Carter N, Thomas G. A multicenter, single-masked study of medial, neutral, and lateral patellar taping in individuals with patellofemoral pain syndrome. J Orthop Sports Phys Ther 2003;33(8):437–43.

105. Aminaka N, Gribble P. Patellar taping, patellofemoral pain syndrome, lower extremity kinematics, and dynamic postural control. J Athl Train 2008;43(1):21–8.

106. Bryk F, Jesus J, Fukuda T, et al. Immediate effect of the elastic knee sleeve use on individuals with osteoarthritis. Rev Bras Reumatol 2011;51(5):440–6.

107. Hassan B, Mockett S, Doherty M. Influence of elastic bandage on knee pain, proprioception, and postural sway in subjects with knee osteoarthritis. Ann Rheum Dis 2002;61(1):24–8.

108. Heit E, Lephart S, Rozzi S. The effect of ankle bracing and taping on joint position sense in the stable ankle. J Sport Rehabil 1996;5(3):206–13.

109. Simoneau G, Degner R, Kramper C, et al. Changes in ankle joint proprioception resulting from strips of athletic tape applied over the skin. J Athl Train 1997;32(2):141–7.

110. Jerosch J, Hoffstetter I, Bork H, et al. The influence of orthoses on the proprioception of the ankle joint. Knee Surg Sports Traumatol Arthrosc 1995;3(1):39–46.

111. Callaghan M, Selfe J, Bagley P, et al. The effects of patellar taping on knee joint proprioception. J Athl Train 2002;37(1):19–24.

112. Callaghan M, Selfe J, McHenry A, et al. Effects of patellar taping on knee joint proprioception in patients with patellofemoral pain syndrome. Man Ther 2008;13(3):192–9.

113. Barrett D, Cobb A, Bentley G. Joint proprioception in normal, osteoarthritic and replaced knees. J Bone Joint Surg Am 1991; 73B(1):53–6.

114. Jerosch J, Prymka M. Knee joint proprioception in normal volunteers and patients with anterior cruciate ligament tears, taking special account of the effect of a knee bandage. Arch Orthop Trauma Surg 1996;115(3–4):162–6.

115. Callaghan MJ, McKie S, Richardson P, et al. Effects of patellar taping on brain activity during knee joint proprioception tests using functional magnetic resonance imaging. Phys Ther 2012;92(6):821–30.

116. Thijs Y, Vingerhoets G, Pattyn E, et al. Does bracing influence brain activity during knee movement: an fMRI study. Knee Surg Sports Traumatol Arthrosc 2010;18(8):1145–9.

117. Karlsson J, Andreasson G. The effect of external ankle support in chronic lateral ankle joint instability. An electromyographic study. Am J Sports Med 1992;20(3):257–61.

118. Briem K, Eythörsdóttir H, Magnúsdóttir R, et al. Effects of kinesio tape compared with nonelastic sports tape and the untaped ankle during a sudden inversion perturbation in male athletes. J Orthop Sports Phys Ther 2011;41(5):328–85.

119. Chou E, Kim K, Baker A, et al. Lower leg neuromuscular changes following fibular reposition taping in individuals with chronic ankle instability. Man Ther 2013;18(4):316–20.

120. Csapo R, Herceg M, Alegre L, et al. Do kinaesthetic tapes affect plantarflexor muscle performance? J Sports Sci 2012;30(14): 1513–19.

121. Lewit K. Manipulative Therapy in Rehabilitation of the Locomotor System. Oxford: Butterworth Heinemann; 1999.

122. Clark N, Herrington L. The knee. In: Comfort P, Abrahamson E, editors. Sports Rehabilitation and Injury Prevention. Chichester: John Wiley; 2010. p. 407–63.

123. Clark N. Principles of injury rehabilitation. SportEx Medicine 2004;19:6–10.

124. Clark N. Functional rehabilitation of the lower limb. SportEx Medicine 2003;18:16–21.

125. Andersen S, Terwilliger D, Denegar C. Comparison of open versus closed kinetic chain test positions for measuring joint position sense. J Sport Rehabil 1995;4:165–71.

126. Benjaminse A, Sell T, Abt J, et al. Reliability and precision of hip proprioception methods in healthy individuals. Clin J Sport Med 2009;19(6):457–63.

127. Drouin J, Houglum P, Perrin D, et al. Weight-bearing and non-weight-bearing knee-joint reposition sense and functional performance. J Sport Rehabil 2003;12:54–66.

128. Bullock-Saxton J, Wong W, Hogan N. The influence of age on weight-bearing joint reposition sense of the knee. Exp Brain Res 2001;136(3):400–6.

129. Docherty C, Moore J, Arnold B. Effects of strength training on strength development and joint position sense in functionally unstable ankles. J Athl Train 1998;33(4):310–14.

130. Friemert B, Bach C, Schwarz W, et al. Benefits of active motion for joint position sense. Knee Surg Sports Traumatol Arthrosc 2006;14:564–70.

131. Eils E, Rosenbaum D. A multi-station proprioceptive exercise program in patients with ankle instability. Med Sci Sports Exerc 2001;33(12):1991–8.

132. Waddington G, Adams R, Jones A. Wobble board (ankle disc) training effects on the discrimination of inversion movements. Aust J Physiother 1999;45:95–101.

133. Waddington G, Seward H, Wrigley T, et al. Comparing wobble board and jump-landing training effects on knee and ankle movement discrimination. J Sci Med Sport 2000;3:449–59.

134. Lagerquist O, Mang C, Collins D. Changes in spinal but not cortical excitability following combined electrical stimulation of the tibial nerve and voluntary plantar-flexion. Exp Brain Res 2012;222(1–2):41–53.

135. Perez M, Lungholt B, Nyborg K, et al. Motor skill training induces changes in the excitability of the leg cortical area in healthy humans. Exp Brain Res 2004;159(2):197–205.

136. Jensen J, Marstrand P, Nielsen J. Motor skill training and strength training are associated with different plastic changes in the central nervous system. J Appl Physiol 2005;99(4):1558–68.

137. Adkins D, Boychuk J, Remple M, et al. Motor training induces experience-specific patterns of plasticity across motor cortex and spinal cord. J Appl Physiol 2006;101(6):1776–82.

138. Rosenkranz K, Kacar A, Rothwell J. Differential modulation of motor cortical plasticity and excitability in early and late phases of human motor learning. J Neurosci 2007;27(44):12058–66.

139. Flück M. Functional, structural and molecular plasticity of mammalian skeletal muscle in response to exercise stimuli. J Exp Biol 2006;209(12):2239–48.

140. Bruhn S, Kullmann N, Gollhofer A. The effects of a sensorimotor training and a strength training on postural stabilisation, maximum isometric contraction and jump performance. Int J Sports Med 2004;25(1):56–60.

141. Aagaard P, Simonsen E, Andersen J, et al. Increased rate of force development and neural drive of human skeletal muscle following resistance training. J Appl Physiol 2002;93(4):1318–26.

142. Snyder-Mackler L, Delitto A, Bailey S, et al. Strength of the quadriceps femoris muscle and functional recovery after reconstruction of the anterior cruciate ligament. A prospective, randomized clinical trial of electrical stimulation. J Bone Joint Surg Am 1995;77A(8):1166–73.

143. Chmielewski T, Hurd W, Rudolph K, et al. Perturbation training improves knee kinematics and reduces muscle co-contraction after complete unilateral anterior cruciate ligament rupture. Phys Ther 2005;85(8):740–9.

144. Gruber M, Gollhofer A. Impact of sensorimotor training on the rate of force development and neural activation. Eur J Appl Physiol 2004;92(1–2):98–105.

145. Hurd W, Chmielewski T, Snyder-Mackler L. Perturbation-enhanced neuromuscular training alters muscle activity in female athletes. Knee Surg Sports Traumatol Arthrosc 2006;14(1):60–9.

146. Heitkamp H, Horstmann T, Mayer F, et al. Gain in strength and muscular balance after balance training. Int J Sports Med 2001;22(4):285–90.

147. Myer G, Ford K, McLean S, et al. The effects of plyometric versus dynamic stabilization and balance training on lower extremity biomechanics. Am J Sports Med 2006;34(3):445–55.

148. Myer G, Ford K, Brent J, et al. The effects of plyometric vs. dynamic stabilization and balance training on power, balance, and landing force in female athletes. J Strength Cond Res 2006;20(2):345–53.

149. Lephart S, Abt J, Ferris C, et al. Neuromuscular and biomechanical characteristic changes in high school athletes: a plyometric versus basic resistance program. Br J Sports Med 2005;39(12):932–8.

150. Chimera N, Swanik K, Swanik C, et al. Effects of plyometric training on muscle-activation strategies and performance in female athletes. J Athl Train 2004;39(1):24–31.

151. Irmischer B, Harris C, Pfeiffer R, et al. Effects of a knee ligament injury prevention exercise program on impact forces in women. J Strength Cond Res 2004;18(4):703–7.

CHAPTER 33

CONSIDERATION OF COGNITIVE AND BEHAVIOURAL INFLUENCES ON PHYSIOTHERAPY PRACTICE

Justin Kenardy • Kim Bennell

Cognitive and behavioural factors may need to be considered in dealing with people with persistent/chronic musculoskeletal disorders. This chapter will provide a background to consideration of cognitive and behavioural influences in dealing with patients with persistent musculoskeletal disorders and how they may be managed in physiotherapy practice. It will also provide a practical guide to applying some important aspects of psychological care and behaviour change using cognitive and behavioural interventions. Rather than being separate and ancillary, cognitive and behaviour change will be described as an integral part of usual treatment. However, information will also be provided on management of significant psychological co-morbidity in this population when the problem falls outside the scope of physiotherapy practice. Understanding the context and function of cognitive and behavioural factors will provide the groundwork for the subsequent section on practical skills of relaxation, problem solving, coping skills training and graded activity.

UNDERSTANDING THE PROBLEM PRESENTATION

Chronic pain can have a complex presentation. A better understanding of the psychological factors that are part of chronic pain will assist the treating therapist in providing a better service for their patient. As pain transitions from acute to persistent, the patient will engage in thinking and behaviours that will be counterproductive and will contribute to ongoing distress and disability. These behaviours and thoughts will be influenced by people and environmental factors in their lives. The patient may change their work, either reducing their work capacity, requiring workplace and work role changes and concessions, or even ceasing work. These changes can often be a consequence of advice from healthcare providers, but can also come from the workplace directly or from family. Clearly these changes can have a stressful impact on the lives of patients, including financial stress. Successive interventions that are not effective in reducing the pain can often be demoralizing and lead to depression. Catastrophic thoughts may emerge that the pain will go on endlessly and that problems cannot be resolved. In addition, extended use of analgesic medications can have significant physical consequences that can also contribute to depression and anxiety. Activity levels will be reduced, sometimes on the basis of health care or other advice, and thoughts emerge that physical activity and pain associated with physical activity is harmful to recovery. The patient may avoid actions or situations out of fear that these might trigger or exacerbate pain. As activity is reduced depression can often develop, compounded by a reduction in physical fitness and increased fatigue and lethargy. In summary, these factors can occur individually and together, and they can interact with each other to create vicious cycles of physical factors, thinking and behaviour. This can be understood as the biopsychosocial model of chronic pain.[1]

The physiotherapist may choose to evaluate the person's presentation using this model through interview and careful assessment. The physiotherapist can also choose to use self-report tools as part of that assessment to assist in the formulation. Some examples of these are the Tampa Kinesiophobia Scale,[2] the Pain Self Efficacy Questionnaire,[3] the Pain Catastrophizing Scale,[4] and the Fear Avoidance Beliefs Questionnaire.[5]

PSYCHOLOGICAL CO-MORBIDITY AND WHAT TO DO ABOUT IT?

Patients who experience chronic illness may also experience a history of co-occurring psychological distress that may include mental illness. There is an increasing awareness among the general public and healthcare practitioners about mental illness. However in the context of a physical injury, it may well be overlooked as the focus is on physical rehabilitation and recovery. Mental illness is a relatively common occurrence in the population at large, with one in six people experiencing clinical depression and one in four experiencing clinical anxiety during their lives.[6] Adversity, including chronic illness and pain, can lead to the development of a mental illness, or exacerbate an existing one. Unfortunately there is a widely held and counterproductive view that the chronic pain itself is the psychological disorder.[7] This view should be avoided as much as possible unless the objective evidence is available to the contrary. Furthermore pain behaviours (e.g. fear of movement) and pain cognitions (e.g. pain catastrophizing) can occur with and without clinically significant distress, although distress is usually concomitant.

Both depression and anxiety have the potential to influence the patient's ongoing experience of pain and disability and their capacity to recover physically.[8,9] It should be stated that the presence of mental illness in the patient with chronic musculoskeletal pain should not necessarily prevent the progress of physical rehabilitation. Recognizing the psychological co-morbidity and understanding the impact on the chronic pain condition are essential to good patient management. Unfortunately recognition is not always easy. Patients may be reluctant to discuss their mental health with a physiotherapist whose focus is on the physical rehabilitation. In the patient's mind there may be a stigma associated with the mental illness. They may believe that the acknowledgement of a mental illness will 'discount' the validity of the physical disorder in the mind of the physiotherapist. The patient themselves may not even recognize their experience as a mental illness. Also, many of the symptoms of a mental illness will overlap with the presentation of a chronic musculoskeletal disorder (e.g. reduced activity) and increased weight, thereby complicating possible identification by the physiotherpist. Finally, the physiotherapist might be reluctant to address mental health issues within their treatment sessions through concerns about practicing outside their competance, or disenfranchising their patient. However, there are a number of simple and brief tools that can be given to patients that will help to identify mental illness if there is some concern that it might be present and impeding the effectiveness of physical rehabilitation. The Kessler Psychological Distress Scale (K10)[10] is a commonly used measure in general practice medicine to assess significant psychological distress. Its ten items can be completed quickly by the patient and has cut-points that provide an indication of clinically elevated anxiety and depression.[11] Alternatively the PHQ-4, derived from the PHQ-9 and GHQ-7[12] is a four-item screener that can detect possible clinical anxiety or depression (see www.phqscreeners.com). Either of these brief questionnaires could be administered if there was some concern by the physiotherapist about failure to progress in treatment. Referral for further assessment and care can then be negotiated with the patient.

SKILLS AND PROCEDURES OF COGNITIVE BEHAVIOURAL THERAPY RELEVANT TO PHYSIOTHERAPY PRACTICE

Stress, or distress, is common in injury and certainly present to some degree in most patients with chronic pain. There are a few simple skills that can be taught to patients that will help them to manage their stress.

Breathing Retraining and Body Scan Relaxation

Physiologically stress can manifest in increased body tension and arousal. A simple skill to manage that manifestation of stress is breathing retraining, using abdominal or diaphragmatic breathing. The rationale for the technique is that stress can change our breathing patterns, and that can lead to changes in our body's capacity to deal with stress and can create symptoms that can be stress-provoking in themselves such as shortness of breath and dizziness. Breathing retraining is designed to be used both on a regular basis to help reduce overall stress levels and at times where the patient might feel particularly stressed and overwhelmed. The physiotherapist can use the following script to help to teach the technique and should demonstrate the steps before observing the patient doing them.

'Find a quiet place and sit comfortably with your back straight. Put one hand on your diaphragm, between your belly button and the bottom of your ribcage, and the other hand on your upper chest. Close your eyes and breathe through your nose. Try to make the hand on your abdomen rise, while keeping the hand on your chest still. Exhale through your mouth, allowing your breath out and your abdominal muscles to contract. Count to three slowly as you inhale through your nose, pause and then count to three slowly as you exhale through your mouth. Continue breathing in. And out.'

The physiotherapist should provide encouragement and constructive feedback as it is sometimes difficult for the patient to perform the technique. While the technique should be able to be done in any position, it is sometimes easier for the patient to lie down to begin with, as this provides better feedback to the patient. Also some patients will attempt to breathe very deeply during the technique, this can be associated with light headedness and therefore can also be distressing. The depth of the breath should be guided by the simple rule that the technique is about the type of breathing rather than depth of breathing. Patients should be encouraged to breathe to a normal depth and use the diaphragm instead of the upper body.

A second technique can also be taught that focuses on breathing and body tension. The body scan is so called because the idea is to review the body for stress and tension and then undertake a brief muscular relaxation in combination with diaphragmatic breathing. The technique can be done at any time including before, during and after a treatment session. The steps are simple and the patient is taught to:

1. Undertake a self-evaluation of stress and tension using a ten-point scale.
2. Take a slow breath in, and then breathe out saying to 'relax' to yourself.
3. Begin to focus on sensations of relaxation within the body as you breathe out and allow sensations of heaviness and warmth to flow downwards through shoulders, arms and hands, stomach, legs and feet.
4. Remain as long as they wish in this state, relaxing more with each breath out.

The technique should be conducted once only or repeatedly, and can be performed in any position including standing. However, as with diaphragmatic breathing it may be easier if the patient starts in a lying position.

Problem Solving

Problem solving is a skill used to develop a plan to manage difficulties identified by the patient including overcoming barriers to self-management. It is a useful life skill that promotes self-efficacy through helping to improve a patient's capacity to overcome adversities. It should be said that the goal of problem solving is not to resolve the 'problem' of pain, which would be counterproductive and stressful,[13] but rather to develop solutions to specific life events and obstacles to recovery. The problem-solving approach should be modelled by the physiotherapist when a patient presents a difficulty as part of the therapy, for example finding time to complete an exercise. Problem solving is an iterative process with up to seven steps. The seven steps are:

1. **Identify the problem:** A problem that is solvable must be defined and it needs be broken down into separate and smaller components. Each component then becomes the focus of a problem-solving process.
2. **Explore the problem:** The aim is to better understand the scope of the problem, why it is relevant at this point in time, and in what ways it affects the patient.
3. **Set goals:** Problem solving implies that there is an end point to be achieved if the problem is resolved, this needs to be defined in order to understand possible solutions.
4. **Think of all possible solutions:** There are no bad ideas at this stage, creativity is encouraged. Consultation with others may be helpful.
5. **Select a possible solution:** Evaluate the generated solutions by asking how helpful, realistic, relevant, and manageable they are. Evaluate the pros and cons for each solution and ask whether the solution achieves the goals that are desired.
6. **Implement a possible solution:** Plan how and when the solution will be applied, and provide encouragement for attempting.
7. **Evaluate:** Was the solution effective? Did the solution achieve the personally relevant goals? Does another solution need to be sought?

If there is a need for further problem solving then the process should be repeated until a satisfactory endpoint is achieved.

Cognitive Coping Skills

Patients with chronic pain can experience a range of negative thoughts that will interfere with recovery. These thoughts can focus on the perceived negative consequences of pain, in particular where physical activity is avoided because of its believed deleterious effect on pain. To overcome these thoughts the patient may need to engage in a process of actively engaging in the avoided activities in a graded fashion. In order to assist in approaching these previously avoided activities it can be helpful for patients to substitute the negative and sometimes catastrophic thinking for thinking that will assist them in engaging in the approach behaviour, in continuing with the feared activity, and in reinforcing their new behaviour.

Hence the concept for the patient is that some thoughts work for them and others work against them. A first step is identifying unhelpful thoughts. This if followed by replacing these with more helpful coping statements. Unhelpful thoughts increase stress and avoidance and decrease use of helpful coping skills such as problem solving and relaxation. Examples of unhelpful thoughts are: 'This is too hard', 'I can't handle this' or 'I give up'. In contrast, helpful thoughts decrease stress and avoidance and increase use of helpful coping skills such as problem solving and relaxation. Examples of helpful thoughts are: 'I can handle this', 'This feeling will pass' or 'This is not dangerous'.

The physiotherapist can assist the patient identify unhelpful thoughts that increase stress and promote avoidance by using examples but then encouraging the patient to generate their own, especially by remembering what these might be from previous experience. The physiotherapist then assists the patient to generate their own cognitive coping statements. The use of examples helps to prompt the patient, but such thoughts always have greater valence when generated by the patient. A question that the therapist could ask is 'What could you say to yourself to increase your confidence and help yourself manage the situation?' The physiotherapist could practice a scenario with the patient where they might use these statements and then suggest that the patient record these statements on a card for use in situations outside of the treatment setting.

BEHAVIOURAL GRADED ACTIVITY APPROACHES

Graded exercise or activity encourages continued activity despite the presence of pain through the use of specific behavioural goals and systematic reinforcement for effort or achievement.[14] In a graded exercise approach, pain is not used to determine exercise or activity level. Instead, dosage is increased by preset quota in a time-contingent manner. A baseline exercise or activity level is first determined by having the patient perform a task until pain limits the patient's ability to perform the task. This level of exercise or activity provides the initial therapeutic quota. Subsequent sessions are based on this quota and if the patient reaches the quota, reinforcement is provided (e.g. verbal praise or some other reward). The quota is gradually increased across sessions. If the patient does not meet the quota, the therapist does not offer reinforcement and instead discusses the importance of continuing the activity and provides assistance for the patient to achieve the set goals.

Another graded activity approach is graded exposure. This approach can be useful for patients who have chronic pain and report high levels of fear of pain or injury and avoidance behaviours. It first involves patients identifying activities that they are highly fearful of performing because of their pain. Following this, a highly feared activity is incorporated into the rehabilitation programme first at a low level that elicits minimal fear and sequentially increased until the fear declines. A key aspect of graded exposures it that the exposure must also occur outside of the clinical setting.[14]

PROMOTING BEHAVIOUR CHANGE

A key part of many healthcare practices involve engaging with the patient to change their behaviours. A medical practitioner may prescribe a drug to control cholesterol with an implicit direction to the patient to adhere to the prescription. The patient must change their daily routine to incorporate the consistent and regular taking of the drug. Whether that occurs will depend on a multitude of factors, but an often overlooked yet key influence is the actions of the prescriber which will help or hinder the behaviour change. For a physiotherapist, a central part of patient recovery is providing advice on undertaking new behaviours such as strengthening exercises. It might be assumed that all patients are motivated by their desire to recover and that this is sufficient to ensure that they commence and maintain their changed behaviours. However this is a false assumption. As with the example of the medical practitioner prescribing a drug treatment, the beliefs, behaviours and communications of the physiotherapist will have a profound impact on the behaviours that are to be changed. In the case of a patient with a persistent musculoskeletal disorder, if the physiotherapist believes that the patient cannot or will not change their behaviours, these beliefs will implicitly impact on the physiotherapist's behaviours and communications, and therefore on their capacity to influence the patient to change their behaviour. If the physiotherapist provides complex instructions for the patient to undertake their new behaviours without checking for patient understanding of those instructions, it should come as no surprise that the patient is unable to complete the new behaviours. If, at the end of a treatment session, the physiotherapist gives the patient instruction on completing a series of regular exercises by the following session, and then fails to follow-up with a review of progress in the following session, there is less likelihood that the patient will continue with the exercise. Behaviour change is not about prescribing a set of new behaviours and expecting the prescription to be followed, it is an interactive and iterative process between the patient and the physiotherapist. The physiotherapist must see the patient as a collaborator in the process of change and the patient must be willing to hold the same view. The physiotherapist must understand and define what behaviour change is needed and the extent and circumstances of the change. The patient must share that understanding and be willing to accept, at least tentatively, that the behaviour change is what they will attempt. But there must also be an open process of collaborative negotiation about the behaviour to be changed in which the physiotherapist's expert knowledge and patient's needs and circumstances have equal value.

There are three main processes required to facilitate health behaviour change:[15] (a) assist the person to form a behavioural goal intention – this relates to whether a person has the required knowledge and sufficient motivation to form an intention to change; (b) help the person to convert that intention into action and maintenance; and (c) effective communication of information between the patient and the health professional. In essence, this can be simplified to several questions that the patient asks themselves: 'Do I know what to do?', 'Do I want to do it?' and 'Am I able to do it?'. From the clinician's perspective the question becomes: 'Are there techniques that can be applied to influence the patient's answers to these questions?'.

The first question, 'Does the patient know what to do?' relates to the effective communication of knowledge between the health practitioner and the patient. This relies on the 'therapeutic approach' taken by the clinician. A patient-centred approach where the patient's autonomy is respected and they are involved in collaborative decision making, is generally considered to be more effective than a 'traditional approach', where the patient is simply told what to do.[16,17] Once the patient knows what to do, the challenge for the clinician is to ensure that the patient is willing and able to act on their advice. Motivation (the desire to take action) and self-efficacy (the belief you can take action) are considered to be the two most important cognitive drivers of behaviour change.[18] The widely used model of stages of change[19] encapsulates these concepts. Readiness can be conceptualized as the resultant combined effect of thinking that it is important to take action, being somewhat confident of success and it being the right time to take action. Readiness can be influenced using interventions such as motivational interviewing (a collaborative conversation that seeks to identify, examine and resolve ambivalence about changing behaviour) and decisional balance (exploring the pros and cons of different choices). Once a patient has formed a goal intention, the clinician may need to assist them to engage in action and self-regulation leading to maintenance of behaviour change. It is recommended that the goal-setting and action-planning process should identify and address barriers to change and take into account strategies to identify when and how to act in a variety of situations.

INTEGRATING PSYCHOLOGICAL FACTORS IN TO CLINICAL PRACTICE

There are many challenges to integrating psychological perspectives within traditional physiotherapy clinical practice. Foster and Delitto[20] suggest a pyramid approach to this (Fig. 33-1). At the base of the pyramid are the common key psychological obstacles to recovery that are relatively easy to incorporate into physiotherapy practice, such as enhancing personal control and self-efficacy and reducing fear of movement in patients with pain. Identifying and addressing these factors is unlikely to require intensive additional education and skill development for physiotherapists. Moving up the pyramid are the psychological factors and intervention techniques that are likely to require more specialist training to identify and address, but that can and should be part of at least some physiotherapists' practice and skill set. At the top of the pyramid are the patients with psychological obstacles to recovery

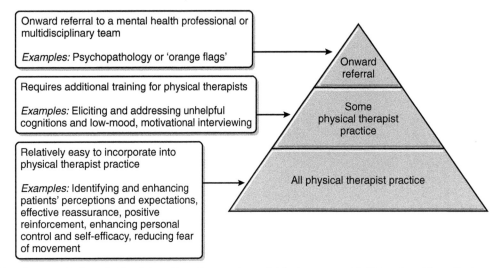

FIGURE 33-1 ■ A suggested model for integration: the psychosocial factors pyramid. (Reproduced from Foster and Delitto.[20])

that are most likely to require onward referral to mental health professionals.

Many physiotherapists feel ill-equipped to deal with psychological factors possibly because most training is biomedical in orientation with less attention paid to practical implementation of a biopsychosocial approach.[21] Certainly, incorporating higher-level psychological approaches into physiotherapy management of chronic conditions (Fig. 33-1, middle tier of the pyramid) requires additional training that can be extensive. For example, in a recent study investigating the effects of a physiotherapy-delivered integrated exercise and cognitive behavioural pain-coping skill training programme, physiotherapists underwent lengthy training in order to achieve a high degree of competence. This involved an initial 4-day group workshop followed by formal group mentoring and instruction, role-playing and performance feedback from a psychologist over the course of 3–6 months and continued throughout the study.[22] Interviews with the physiotherapists at the conclusion of the study found that they believed the extensive training to be critical to their ability to effectively deliver the intervention and to problem solve issues that arose (Boxes 33-1 and 33-2).[23] The fact that such extensive training is not feasible to implement widely in the real world, supports physiotherapy practice models whereby some practitioners gain the additional skills necessary to competently deliver higher-level psychological interventions.

CONCLUSION

Cognitive and behavioural factors often require consideration in people with persistent/chronic musculoskeletal disorders. Physiotherapists need to recognize and positively manage these factors as part of usual physiotherapy practice. They can use techniques such as relaxation, problem solving, coping skills training and graded activity, which are well within their scope of practice. However some patients may present with significant psychological co-morbidity which falls outside the scope of physiotherapy practice. It is important to recognize these

BOX 33-1

'[the workshop] was the tip of the iceberg … it set the groundwork or sort of gave us a taste of it, but then it was the weekly meetings we had with the psychologist that really concreted everything for us'

From Neilsen et al.[23]

BOX 33-2

'… because it's not a straightforward competency of just a performer's skill. It's a skill that has to adapt under the pressure of doing the interview. And that's a far more advanced skill than simply learning to be able to – I don't know – take a foot through a movement. If I learn that skill, then I've got that and I can go on. Whereas this sort of skill, I walk in and the client throws me a curve ball and I've got to adapt and make it all work.'

From Neilsen et al.[23]

patients and negotiate with them to gain appropriate psychological management. Such patients stand to gain better outcomes from multiprofessional management of the painful musculoskeletal condition.

REFERENCES

1. Gatchel RJ, Peng YB, Peters ML, et al. The biopsychosocial approach to chronic pain: scientific advances and future directions. Psychol Bull 2007;133:581–624.
2. Lundberg M, Styf J, Carlsson S. A psychometric evaluation of the tampa scale for kinesiophobia – from a physiotherapeutic perspective. Physiother Theory Pract 2004;20:121–33.
3. Nicholas MK. The pain self-efficacy questionnaire: taking pain into account. Eur J Pain 2007;11:153–63.
4. Sullivan MJL, Bishop SR, Pivik J. The pain catastrophizing scale: development and validation. Psychol Assess 1995;7(4):524–32.
5. Waddell G, Newton M, Henderson I, et al. A Fear-Avoidance Beliefs Questionnaire (FABQ) and the role of fear-avoidance beliefs in chronic low back pain and disability. Pain 1993;52:157–68.
6. Australian Bureau of Statistics. 2007 National Survey of Mental Health and Wellbeing: Summary of Results. Canberra: Australian Bureau of Statistics; 2008 Contract No.: 4326.0.

7. Crombez G, Beirens K, Van Damme S, et al. The unbearable lightness of somatisation: a systematic review of the concept of somatisation in empirical studies of pain. Pain 2009;145:31–5.

8. Surah A, Baranidharan G, Morley S. Chronic pain and depression. Cont Edu Anaesth Crit Care Pain 2014;14(2):85–9.

9. Liedl A, O'Donnell M, Creamer M, et al. Support for the mutual maintenance of pain and post-traumatic stress disorder symptoms. Psychol Med 2010;40:1215–23.

10. Kessler RC, Walters EE, Zaslavsky AM, et al. Screening for serious mental illness in the general population. Arch Gen Psychiatry 2003;60:184–9.

11. Andrews G, Slade T. Interpreting scores on the Kessler Psychological Distress Scale (K10). Aust N Z J Public Health 2001; 25:494–7.

12. Kroenke K, Spitzer RL, Williams JBW, et al. An ultra-brief screening scale for anxiety and depression: the PHQ-4. Psychosomatics 2009;50:613–21.

13. Eccleston C, Crombez G. Worry and chronic pain: a misdirected problem solving model. Pain 2007;132:233–6.

14. Michael KN, Steven ZG. Psychologically informed interventions for low back pain: an update for physical therapists. Phys Ther 2011;91:765–76.

15. Gale J, Skouteris H. Health coaching: facilitating health behaviour change for chronic condition prevention and self-management. In: Caltabiano M, Ricciardelli L, editors. Applied Topics in Health Psychology. Brisbane: John Wiley & Sons; 2012. p. 15–28.

16. Moller AC, Ryan RM, Deci EL. Self-determination theory and public policy: improving the quality of consumer decisions without using coercion. J Public Policy Mark 2006;25:104–16.

17. Wagner EH, Bennett SM, Austin BT, et al. Finding common ground: patient-centeredness and evidence-based chronic illness care. J Altern Complement Med 2005;11(Suppl.):S7–15.

18. Bandura A. Social cognitive theory: an agentic perspective. Annu Rev Psychol 2001;52:1–26.

19. Prochaska JO, DiClemente CC. The Transtheoretical Approach: Crossing Traditional Boundaries of Therapy. Homewood, Ill.: Dow Jones-Irwin; 1984.

20. Foster NE, Delitto A. Embedding psychosocial perspectives within clinical management of low back pain: integration of psychosocially informed management principles into physical therapist practice – challenges and opportunities. Phys Ther 2011;91:790–803.

21. Main CJ, George SZ. Psychologically informed practice for management of low back pain: future directions in practice and research. Phys Ther 2011;91(5):820–4. PubMed PMID: 21451091. [Epub 2011/04/01].

22. Bennell KL, Metcalf B, Egerton T, et al. A physiotherapist-delivered integrated exercise and pain coping skills training intervention for individuals with knee osteoarthritis: a randomised controlled trial protocol. BMC Musculoskelet Disord 2012; 13(1):129.

23. Nielsen M, Keefe FJ, Bennell K, et al. Physical therapist-delivered cognitive-behavioral therapy: a qualitative study of physical therapists' perceptions and experiences. Phys Ther 2014;94(2): 197–209.

ADJUNCT MODALITIES FOR PAIN

CHAPTER OUTLINE

EDITOR'S INTRODUCTION

The case for the integration of multimodalities in the management of complex musculoskeletal presentations is strong, as there is no panacea for musculoskeletal pain. It can be difficult to know what modality is the most 'effective/active' component within a programme of management, and thus what is the adjunct modality increasing effectiveness is equally difficult to establish. These treatment approaches, termed adjunct modalities, will undoubtedly continue to be crucial considerations in musculoskeletal management and will continue to attract similar levels of clinical and research interest as manual therapy and exercise.

In this chapter three internationally renowned experts in their respective fields have provided a summary of how electrophysical agents, acupuncture/dry needling and taping can facilitate the treatment of musculoskeletal pain. The potential is discussed for electrophysical agents to both address the underlying pathology of musculoskeletal pain presentations and relieve musculoskeletal pain as a distinct objective. Dry needling has become a popular modality and the theory underpinning needling is discussed in some detail, as are some issues regarding the evidence base for acupuncture. To complete a picture of the rationale for the use of taping within a programme of management for spinal pain has been described and some treatment examples are included.

CHAPTER 34.1   ■   ELECTROPHYSICAL AGENTS

Tim Watson

Electrophysical agents (EPAs, a term with greater accuracy and currency than the older term 'electrotherapy') have an established place as a component of therapy clinical practice, though their utilization appears to vary between professional groups, between countries and indeed within both of these. There is a substantial evidence to support their use but, for some clinical presentations, there appears to be a fundamental mismatch between the supportive evidence and current practice.

Historically, it is almost certainly the case that these 'modalities' were over-employed, with many, if not all, patients with a whole range of musculoskeletal presentations receiving some kind of electrotherapy. Given the current evidence base, the continued use of these interventions can be justified in some, but certainly not all, clinical circumstances. It is rarely, if ever, the case that

an EPA is most effectively employed in isolation. Transcutaneous electrical nerve stimulation (TENS) for example, may provide an effective and clinically useful method by which symptomatic pain relief can be achieved. Used in conjunction with a holistic treatment package, it can make a valuable contribution. Used alone, it will have an effect, evidenced and measurable, but it is unlikely to be optimal. It is the integration of manual therapy, exercise therapy, advice, education and, where appropriate, EPAs that is most likely to achieve optimal outcome.

In general, there has been a shift away from EPAs being delivered purely in the clinical environment. TENS was probably one of the first modalities provided as a 'home-based' treatment – the therapist teaching the patient how best to employ the machine, and the patient (or carer) being responsible for the day-to-day delivery. The machines were inexpensive and relatively easy to manage, making this a real-world possibility. Over time this approach has been adopted with other devices. There are now interferential therapy, neuromuscular electrical stimulation devices, therapy ultrasound, microcurrent and several others which can be delivered in this way.[1-6] Some clinics encourage patients to purchase their own machines while others lease, loan or rent to patients. That notwithstanding, the concept of home-based EPA treatment delivery is evidenced as being effective, and serves to 'free up' clinic time for those aspects of treatment which cannot be easily or effectively delivered by the patient at home.

In terms of potential uses in the musculoskeletal arena, there are two fundamental approaches that are employed for the use of EPAs. Firstly one can use the modality as a means to deal with the underlying pathology (e.g. to enhance repair of a damaged tissue). There are several modalities that are supported by the evidence base that can be used in this context such as ultrasound,[7-9] laser,[10,11] pulsed-shortwave therapy,[12,13] shockwave[14-16] and microcurrent.[5,17,18] Other modalities are sometimes also included in this group, for example radiofrequency applications that are similar to shortwave modalities but actually utilize electromagnetic energy delivered at slightly different frequencies[19,20] and magnetic-based therapies.[21-23] However, there is a need for more comprehensive clinical trial data before these can be confirmed as being supported by the evidence for this purpose, though such trials are currently underway, and the foundation studies (e.g. cell, animal) strongly suggest that they have this tissue repair capability.

The second, and equally valid approach would be to employ an EPA modality as a means to change the patient's perception of their pain without necessarily changing the underlying problem. EPA modalities in this group would most obviously include TENS;[24-26] interferential therapy;[27-29] various other forms of electrical stimulation[30,31] together with heat- and cold-based therapies,[32-37] and laser-based intervention.[38-41]

A detailed review of each of these modalities is clearly beyond the remit of this short overview. The essential/indicative references provided will provide a preliminary source of information for further evaluation.

Several reviews (Cochrane, systematic reviews and meta analyses) and clinical guidelines (e.g. NICE) have commonly drawn equivocal conclusions when these interventions have been considered. While not trying to defend the indefensible, one of the key issues is that these reviews tend not to consider treatment dose. Essentially, if five randomized controlled trial papers were shortlisted to the review, three demonstrating benefit whereas two do not, the common conclusion would be that there was insufficient supportive evidence. Taking into account the totality of the evidence base, there is strong support for a 'dose' dependency when using EPAs.[42] Strangely, dose-related issues do not often feature in the reviews. A detailed analysis of the effective and ineffective randomized controlled trials commonly reveals that the settings (dose) at which the EPA is delivered is key to a positive outcome. Several eminent authors[24,43-45] have explained

this phenomenon in considerable detail. If TENS, ultrasound or laser is applied at what is known to be a clinically effective dose, its use is supported by the evidence across the musculoskeletal physiotherapy range. If applied at an ineffective (or at least sub-optimal) dose, then it would be difficult to rationalize how a beneficial effect could be achieved, as would be the case with manual therapy, exercise, drug therapy or any other relevant intervention method.

In conclusion, various EPAs are evidenced as being effective when applied optimally and in line with best evidence. They can be used as a means to influence the underlying tissue problem (tissue damage, inflammation) or can be used as a means to change perception of pain or other disabling symptoms. One approach is not 'more valid' than another. They both have a potential value as a component of a therapeutic package of care, but none are evidenced as being optimal if used in isolation.

REFERENCES

1. Yik YI, Ismail KA, Hutson JM, et al. Home transcutaneous electrical stimulation to treat children with slow-transit constipation. J Pediatr Surg 2012;47(6):1285–90.
2. Bruce-Brand RA, Walls RJ, Ong JC, et al. Effects of home-based resistance training and neuromuscular electrical stimulation in knee osteoarthritis: a randomized controlled trial. BMC Musculoskelet Disord 2012;13:118.
3. Brown AS. At-home laser and light-based devices. Curr Probl Dermatol 2011;42:160–5.
4. Watanabe Y, Matsushita T, Bhandari M, et al. Ultrasound for fracture healing: current evidence. J Orthop Trauma 2010;24(Suppl. 1):S56–61.
5. Poltawski L, Johnson M, Watson T. Microcurrent therapy in the management of chronic tennis elbow: pilot studies to optimize parameters. Physiother Res Int 2012;17(3):157–66.
6. Persson AL, Lloyd-Pugh M, Sahlström J. Trained long-term TENS users with chronic non-malignant pain. A retrospective questionnaire study of TENS usage and patients' experiences. Phys Ther Rev 2010;15(4):294–301.
7. Watson T. Ultrasound in contemporary physiotherapy practice. Ultrasonics 2008;48:321–9.
8. Yildirim MA, Ones K, Celik EC. Comparision of ultrasound therapy of various durations in the treatment of subacromial impingement syndrome. J Phys Ther Sci 2013;25(9):1151–4.
9. Kinami Y, Noda T, Ozaki T. Efficacy of low-intensity pulsed ultrasound treatment for surgically managed fresh diaphyseal fractures of the lower extremity: multi-center retrospective cohort study. J Orthop Sci 2013;18(3):410–18.
10. Alayat MS, Elsodany AM, El Fiky AA. Efficacy of high and low level laser therapy in the treatment of Bell's palsy: a randomized double blind placebo-controlled trial. Lasers Med Sci 2014;29(1):335–42.
11. Sussmilch-Leitch SP, Collins NJ, Bialocerkowski AE, et al. Physical therapies for Achilles tendinopathy: systematic review and meta-analysis. J foot Ankle Res 2012;5(1):15.
12. Al Mandeel M, Watson T. Pulsed and continuous shortwave therapy. In: Watson T, editor. Electrotherapy: Evidence Based Practice. Edinburgh: Churchill Livingstone/Elsevier; 2008. p. 137–60.
13. Jan MH, Chai HM, Wang CL, et al. Effects of repetitive shortwave diathermy for reducing synovitis in patients with knee osteoarthritis: an ultrasonographic study. Phys Ther 2006;86(2):236–44.
14. Schmitz C, Csaszar NB, Rompe JD, et al. Treatment of chronic plantar fasciopathy with extracorporeal shock waves (review). J Orthop Surg 2013;8(1):31.
15. Reznik JE, Milanese S, Golledge J, et al. Extracorporeal shock wave therapy as a treatment for heterotopic ossification. Phys Ther Rev 2013;18(4):300–7.
16. Dizon JN, Gonzalez-Suarez C, Zamora MT, et al. Effectiveness of extracorporeal shock wave therapy in chronic plantar fasciitis: a meta-analysis. Am J Phys Med Rehabil 2013;92(7):606–20.

17. Poltawski L, Watson T. Bioelectricity and microcurrent therapy for tissue healing – a narrative review. Phys Ther Rev 2009;14(2):104–14.

18. Rockstroh G, Schleicher W, Krummenauer F. Effectiveness of microcurrent therapy as a constituent of post-hospital rehabilitative treatment in patients after total knee alloarthroplasty – a randomized clinical trial. Rehabilitation (Stuttg) 2010;49(3):173–9.

19. Guo L, Kubat NJ, Nelson TR, et al. Meta-analysis of clinical efficacy of pulsed radio frequency energy treatment. Ann Surg 2012;255(3):457–67.

20. Guo L, Kubat NJ, Isenberg RA. Pulsed radio frequency energy (PRFE) use in human medical applications. Electromagn Biol Med 2011;30(1):21–45.

21. Ueno S, Okano H. Static, Low-frequency and pulsed magnetic fields in biological systems. In: Lin JC, editor. Electromagnetic Fields in Biological Systems. CRC Press; 2012.

22. Assiotis A, Sachinis NP, Chalidis BE. Pulsed electromagnetic fields for the treatment of tibial delayed unions and nonunions a prospective clinical study and review of the literature. J Orthop Surg 2012;7(1):24.

23. Rosen AD. Studies on the effect of static magnetic fields on biological systems. PIERS Online 2010;6(2):133–6.

24. Sluka KA, Bjordal JM, Marchand S, et al. What makes transcutaneous electrical nerve stimulation work? making sense of the mixed results in the clinical literature. Phys Ther 2013;93(10):1397–402.

25. Johnson MI, Bjordal JM. Transcutaneous electrical nerve stimulation for the management of painful conditions: focus on neuropathic pain. Expert Rev Neurother 2011;11(5):735–53.

26. Johnson MI. Transcutaneous elecetrical nerve stimulation (TENS). In: Watson T, editor. Electrotherapy: Evidence Based Practice. Edinburgh: Elsevier/Churchill Livingstone; 2008. p. 253–96.

27. Rocha CS, Lanferdini FJ, Kolberg C, et al. Interferential therapy effect on mechanical pain threshold and isometric torque after delayed onset muscle soreness induction in human hamstrings. J Sports Sci 2012;30(8):733–42.

28. Gundog M, Atamaz F, Kanyilmaz S, et al. Interferential current therapy in patients with knee osteoarthritis: comparison of the effectiveness of different amplitude-modulated frequencies. Am J Phys Med Rehabil 2012;91(2):107–13.

29. Hurley DA, McDonough SM, Dempster M, et al. A randomized clinical trial of manipulative therapy and interferential therapy for acute low back pain. Spine 2004;29(20):2207–16.

30. Ediz L, Ceylan MF, Turktas U, et al. A randomized controlled trial of electrostimulation effects on effusion, swelling and pain recovery after anterior cruciate ligament reconstruction: a pilot study. Clin Rehabil 2012;26(5):413–22.

31. Lowry AM, Simopoulos TT. Spinal cord stimulation for the treatment of chronic knee pain following total knee replacement. Pain Physician 2010;13(3):251–6.

32. Thym DBM, Olmedija dAR, Dall'-Aqua JMG, et al. Evaluation of pain relief using a combination of TENS and cryotherapy. Kranken-Gymnastik 2005;57(5):894–901.

33. Ansari NN, Naghdi S, Naseri N, et al. Effect of therapeutic infrared in patients with non-specific low back pain: a pilot study. J Bodyw Mov Ther 2014;18(1):75–81.

34. Lewis SE, Holmes PS, Woby SR, et al. Short-term effect of superficial heat treatment on paraspinal muscle activity, stature recovery, and psychological factors in patients with chronic low back pain. Arch Phys Med Rehabil 2012;93(2):367–72.

35. Kettenmann B, Wille C, Lurie-Luke E, et al. Impact of continuous low level heatwrap therapy in acute low back pain patients: subjective and objective measurements. Clin J Pain 2007;23(8):663–8.

36. Chou R, Huffman LH. Nonpharmacologic therapies for acute and chronic low back pain: a review of the evidence for an American Pain Society/American College of Physicians clinical practice guideline. Ann Intern Med 2007;147(7):492–504.

37. Bleakley CM, Costello JT. Do thermal agents affect range of movement and mechanical properties in soft tissues? A systematic review. Arch Phys Med Rehabil 2013;94(1):149–63.

38. Al Rashoud AS, Abboud RJ, Wang W, et al. Efficacy of low-level laser therapy applied at acupuncture points in knee osteoarthritis: a randomised double-blind comparative trial. Physiotherapy 2014;100(3):242–8.

39. Maia ML, Bonjardim LR, Quintans Jde S, et al. Effect of low-level laser therapy on pain levels in patients with temporomandibular disorders: a systematic review. J Appl Oral Sci 2012;20(6):594–602.

40. Jovicic M, Konstantinovic L, Lazovic M, et al. Clinical and functional evaluation of patients with acute low back pain and radiculopathy treated with different energy doses of low level laser therapy. Vojnosanit Pregl 2012;69(8):656–62.

41. Jang H, Lee H. Meta-analysis of pain relief effects by laser irradiation on joint areas. Photomed Laser Surg 2012;30(8):405–17.

42. Watson T. Narrative review: key concepts with electrophysical agents. Phys Ther Rev 2010;15(4):351–9.

43. Bjordal JM, Lopes Martins RAB, Klovning A. Is quality control of Cochrane reviews in controversial areas sufficient? J Altern Complement Med 2006;12(2):181–3.

44. Bjordal JM, Lopes-Martins R, Johnson MI, et al. Inaccuracies in laser therapy meta-analysis for neck pain? J Physiother 2010;56(4):282.

45. Bjordal JM, Johnson MI, Lopes-Martins RA, et al. Short-term efficacy of physical interventions in osteoarthritic knee pain. A systematic review and meta-analysis of randomised placebo-controlled trials. BMC Musculoskelet Disord 2007;8(1):51.

CHAPTER 34.2 ■ ACUPUNCTURE/DRY NEEDLING

Panos Barlas

Acupuncture is a modality popular among physiotherapists as a safe and effective technique for the relief of pain. It was introduced to the physiotherapy profession in the early 1980s, and has steadily grown in popularity. It is estimated that over 10 000 physiotherapists in the UK alone have been trained in acupuncture and regularly use it for the treatment of musculoskeletal pain.

While acupuncture is an integral part of Traditional Chinese Medicine, recent scientific advances have deepened our understanding of the physiological mechanisms involved in sensory stimulation for the relief of pain and a number of other processes (e.g. healing). Furthermore, the traditional practice of acupuncture has evolved through the dissemination of acupuncture throughout the Western world and the influence of

modern, evidence-based, medical thinking. It is these developments that have shaped contemporary acupuncture to an amalgam of Traditional Chinese practices and modern needling techniques.

This short review will provide an overview of the main physiological effects of acupuncture and review its clinical efficacy on common musculoskeletal disorders, including a discussion on optimal stimulation parameters.

PHYSIOLOGICAL EFFECTS OF ACUPUNCTURE

Since the publication of Melzack and Wall's 'gate control theory' in 1965, and the subsequent development of transcutaneous electrical nerve stimulation (TENS), a considerable amount of research effort has been dedicated to the physiological mechanisms of analgesia through sensory stimulation. The historical coincidence of the publication of the 'gate control theory' (1965), the development of TENS (1967), the discovery of opiate-like substances in the cow's brain (1972) and the discovery of the opiate receptors (1975)[1] provided the necessary environment for the scientific establishment to accept that somatic stimulation is capable of stimulating endogenous pain-relieving mechanisms, which would explain the reported efficacy of traditional practices such as acupuncture and soft tissue techniques.

The following decades showed an explosion in acupuncture research that examined the physiological effects of such modalities (i.e. TENS, acupuncture and electroacupuncture) and their clinical efficacy.

The realization that Aδ and C fibres contribute to not only the generation and maintenance of pain, but also the stimulation of endogenous analgesic reflexes was perhaps the key to unlock the puzzle of the therapeutic effects of sensory stimulation modalities since they are designed to evoke stimuli capable of exciting such fibres.[2] Further research[3] showed the effects of somatosensory stimulation on the autonomic system, paving the way for further work in this area and explaining the effects of acupuncture on conditions such as migraine, infertility, etc.

The key points that emerge from this wealth of investigation are that acupuncture has peripheral, spinal (segmental) and supraspinal effects, and that these physiological responses to sensory stimulation (acupuncture) account for the analgesic, healing and mood effects observed after acupuncture treatment.[4] Full accounts of the complex events that take place after acupuncture stimulation are beyond the scope of this short review. An up-to-date account can be found in Zhang et al.[5]

Despite the abundance of scientific evidence on the physiological effects of acupuncture, the issue of its clinical efficacy remains perhaps one of the most hotly disputed subjects in the field of physical medicine. Proponents of acupuncture argue that traditional research methods employing double-blind, placebo-controlled designs fail to detect the full effect of complex therapies (such as acupuncture and exercise). Sceptics argue that acupuncture should provide a very robust set of evidence if it is to be included in the arsenal of the practitioner and should withstand the scrutiny of modern scientific investigation methods. Thankfully, the last decade has seen a significant amount of high-quality randomized clinical trials of acupuncture on a range of musculoskeletal conditions, which seem to overcome the methodological faults of earlier attempts. As such, the clinician can now make a reasoned, evidence-based decision as to whether acupuncture should feature in the rehabilitation programme of patients with musculoskeletal disorders and pain.

ACUPUNCTURE IN THE TREATMENT OF MUSCULOSKELETAL PAIN

The inclusion of acupuncture in the NICE guidelines for the management of low back pain[6] was perhaps the milestone for acupuncture since, for the first time, it was accepted by the medical establishment (in the United Kingdom) as a credible form of treatment for such a common condition. This recommendation was based on a range of clinical studies that showed acupuncture to be superior to the control intervention and placebo/sham interventions. Following this, a further review has demonstrated that the effect of acupuncture on chronic musculoskeletal pain is specific and significantly different to a sham procedure.[7] Earlier studies have also shown that acupuncture is an effective treatment for chronic knee pain,[8] and that this effect is dependent on a number of parameters, namely the number of treatments, the intensity and duration of stimulation as well as the repetition (treatment frequency) and the total number of treatments.[9] A similar recommendation was included in the NICE guidelines for the management of headache.[10] These recommendations were further validated in a later study that showed a positive correlation to the number of needles per session and the total number of treatments to successful treatment outcomes.[11]

Other popular applications of acupuncture include treatment of the hip, shoulder, elbow and neck pain. The evidence for the conditions needs further exploration and support from large clinical trials; nevertheless, they do point towards effectiveness of acupuncture as an adjunct to conventional treatment.[12,13] An interesting observation from the available trials is that acupuncture and sham acupuncture frequently outperform 'standard care' which may include a range of physiotherapy and manual medicine techniques.[14,15]

Acupuncture is also useful for the relief of myofascial pain and myofascial trigger points. It has been demonstrated that, when compared with other modalities, needling seems to be the most effective method for the deactivation of myofascial trigger points.[16] Frequently mentioned as 'dry needling' it is safe to say that there is no difference between the two modalities, other than the etymological one.

Despite the positive reports regarding the clinical efficacy of acupuncture on a range of conditions, closer examination of the literature reveals wide variation in practice and a lack of standardization of treatment parameters, namely number of needles, intensity and duration of stimulation and total number of treatments. As early as 2001, it was proposed that these parameters are crucial for the success to treatment,[17] and as a result of such observations, a consensus opinion for the reporting and designing clinical trials was proposed.[18] Perhaps more significantly the dose of acupuncture treatment has been discussed in relation to data from neurophysiological studies,[19] paving the way for a robust and science-based approach to designing effective clinical protocols.

Evident from these discussions is the fact that parameters such as intensity of stimulation, duration of treatment and frequency of treatment seem to be the determinants of treatment adequacy, moving away from the Traditional Chinese Medical model which places equal emphasis on point selection to the aforementioned variables.

Since the scientific validation of the mechanisms implicated in the analgesic effect of acupuncture, research has started to explore the effects of acupuncture in a number of other clinically relevant applications, namely its anti-inflammatory effects[20] and effects on mood[21,22] and the clinical efficacy of acupuncture on such conditions.[23,24] Such investigations further elaborate on the applications of sensory stimulation for the care of the patients with musculoskeletal pain, since depression and insomnia are common co-morbidities.[25,26]

Acupuncture has evolved in recent years to become a useful and effective tool in the arsenal of the musculoskeletal pain therapist. Frequently, its origins from Traditional Chinese Medicine create friction with an establishment whose point of reference is the Western medical model; however, as evidence for its physiological and clinical effects become available its acceptance as a valid, biologically plausible method of treatment is increasing. The biomedical model of clinical reasoning as evidenced from Western medical acupuncture seems to be the most promising development in the field of acupuncture or needling-based therapies in general.[27] The reports which show that the inclusion of acupuncture in a package of care for conditions prevalent in primary care such as back pain,[28] knee pain,[29] neck pain[30] and headache,[31] is a cost-effective measure, adds to the confidence of the therapist when choosing to include acupuncture in their treatment options.

The time has perhaps come to consider acupuncture (or dry needling) as a core skill in physiotherapy and advocate its inclusion to the core curriculum of physiotherapy education. Experience throughout the Western world has shown that physiotherapists are perhaps the best-suited practitioners to apply acupuncture since they have the scientific background, technical and clinical skills to effectively incorporate acupuncture in the care of their patients.

REFERENCES

1. Hughes J, Kosterlitz HW, Smith TW. The distribution of methionine-enkephalin and leucine-enkephalin in the brain and peripheral tissues. Br J Pharmacol 1997;120(4 Suppl.):428–36.
2. Sprenger C, Bingel U, Büchel C. Treating pain with pain: supraspinal mechanisms of endogenous analgesia elicited by heterotopic noxious conditioning stimulation. Pain 2011;152(2):428–39.
3. Sato A, Sato Y, Schmidt RF. The impact of somatosensory input on autonomic functions. Rev Physiol Biochem Pharmacol 1997;130(130):1–328.
4. Kawakita K, Gotoh K. Role of polymodal receptors in the acupuncture-mediated endogenous pain inhibitory systems. Prog Brain Res 1996;113:507–23.
5. Zhang ZJ, Wang XM, McAlonan GM. Neural acupuncture unit: a new concept for interpreting effects and mechanisms of acupuncture. Evid Based Complement Alternat Med 2012;2012:429412. doi:10.1155/2012/429412; [Epub 2012 Mar 8].
6. National Institute of Health and Clinical Excellence (NICE). Low back pain: early management of persistent low back pain. NICE Clin Guide 2009;88. <http://www.nice.org.uk/guidance/CG88>.
7. Vickers AJ, Cronin AM, Maschino AC, et al. Acupuncture Trialists' Collaboration. Acupuncture for chronic pain: individual patient data meta-analysis. Arch Intern Med 2012;172(19):1444–53.
8. White A, Foster NE, Cummings M, et al. Acupuncture treatment for chronic knee pain: a systematic review. Rheumatology (Oxford) 2007;46(3):384–90.
9. National Institute of Health and Clinical Excellence (NICE). Headaches: diagnosis and management of headaches in young people and adults. NICE Clin Guide 2012;150. <http://www.nice.org.uk/guidance/CG150>.
10. White A, Cummings M, Barlas P, et al. Defining an adequate dose of acupuncture using a neurophysiological approach–a narrative review of the literature. Acupunct Med 2008;26(2):111–20.
11. MacPherson H, Maschino AC, Lewith G, et al. Acupuncture Trialists' Collaboration. Characteristics of acupuncture treatment associated with outcome: an individual patient meta-analysis of 17,922 patients with chronic pain in randomised controlled trials. PLoS ONE 2013;8(10):e77438.
12. Green S, Buchbinder R, Hetrick S. Acupuncture for shoulder pain. Cochrane Database Syst Rev 2005;18(2):CD005319.
13. Trinh KV, Phillips SD, Ho E, et al. Acupuncture for the alleviation of lateral epicondyle pain: a systematic review. Rheumatology 2004;43(9):1085–90.
14. Stener-Victorin E, Kruse-Smidje C, Jung K. Comparison between electro-acupuncture and hydrotherapy, both in combination with patient education and patient education alone, on the symptomatic treatment of osteoarthritis of the hip. Clin J Pain 2004;20(3):179–85.
15. Witt CM, Jena S, Brinkhaus B, et al. Acupuncture for patients with chronic neck pain. Pain 2006;125(1-2):98–106. [Epub 2006 Jun 14].
16. Cummings TM, White AR. Needling therapies in the management of myofascial trigger point pain: a systematic review. Arch Phys Med Rehabil 2001;82(7):986–92.
17. Ezzo J, Hadhazy V, Birch S, et al. Acupuncture for osteoarthritis of the knee: a systematic review. Arhtritis Rheum 2001;44(4):819–25.
18. MacPherson H, Altman DG, Hammershlag R, et al. Revised standarts for teporting interventions in clinical trials of acupuncture (STRICTA): extending the CONSORT statement. J Evid Based Med 2010;3(3):140–55.
19. White A, Cummings M, Barlas P, et al. Acupunct Med 2008;26(2):111–20.
20. Kavoussi B, Ross BE. The neuroimmune basis of anti-inflammatory acupuncture. Integr Cancer Ther 2007;6(3):251–7.
21. da Silva MA, Dorsher PT. Neuroanatomic and clinical correspondences: acupuncture and vagus nerve stimulation. J Altern Complement Med 2014;20(4):233–40.
22. Hui KK, Marina O, Liu J, et al. Acupuncture, the limbic system, and the anticorrelated networks of the brain. Auton Neurosci 2010;157(1-2):81–90.
23. Hopton A, Macpherson H, Keding A, et al. Acupuncture, counselling or usual care for depression and comorbid pain: secondary analysis of a randomised controlled trial. BMJ Open 2014;4(5):e004964. doi:10.1136/bmjopen-2014-004964.
24. Spence DW, Kayumov L, Chen A, et al. Acupuncture increases nocturnal melatonin secretion and reduces insomnia and anxiety: a preliminary report. J Neuropsychiatry Clin Neurosci 2004;16(1):19–28.
25. Lavigne GJ, Nashed A, Manzini C, et al. Does sleep differ among patients with common musculoskeletal pain disorders? Curr Rheumatol Rep 2011;13(6):535–42.
26. Gorevic PD. Osteoarthritis. A review of musculoskeletal aging and treatment issues in geriatric patients. Geriatrics 2004;59(8):28–32.
27. Kavoussi B. The untold story of acupuncture. FACT 2009;14(4):276–85.
28. Ratcliffe J, Thomas KJ, MacPherson H, et al. A randomised controlled trial of acupuncture care for persistent low back pain: cost effectiveness analysis. BMJ 2006;333(7569):626.
29. Whitehurst DG, Bryan S, Hay EM, et al. Cost-effectiveness of acupuncture care as an adjunct to exercise-based physical therapy for osteoarthritis of the knee. Phys Ther 2011;91(5):630–41.
30. Willich SN, Reinhold T, Selim D, et al. Cost-effectiveness of acupuncture treatment in patients with chronic neck pain. Pain 2006;125(1-2):107–13.
31. Wonderling D, Vickers AJ, Grieve R, et al. Cost effectiveness analysis of a randomised trial of acupuncture for chronic headache in primary care. BMJ 2004;328(7442):747.

CHAPTER 34.3 ■ THE USE OF TAPE IN MANAGING SPINAL PAIN

Jenny McConnell

Patients with musculoskeletal problems usually present to physiotherapists for the treatment of pain. Treatment for chronic conditions frequently has to be modified because the patient experiences increased pain during treatment. Modifying the treatment can impede the recovery of the patient. The practitioner therefore needs to employ strategies that will minimize the aggravation of symptoms and facilitate the rehabilitation of the patient. Appropriate taping of a painful area has been found to decrease pain, alter muscle activity, change joint range of motion, improve joint loading and provide support for the injured area.[1-5]

WHAT IS PAIN?

Pain has been defined as an unpleasant sensory or emotional experience associated with actual or potential tissue damage (nociception). Pain involves the patient's reaction to the nociception, so it is very much an individual experience with a learned component.[6] Pain can become memorized because pain mechanisms are not fixed or hard-wired, but are plastic or soft-wired.[7] Through neuroplasticity, hyperalgesia can be learned and unlearned, from both tissue-based and environmental afferent inputs.[7]

Musculoskeletal pain syndromes are seldom caused by isolated precipitating events, but are the consequences of habitual imbalances in the movement system. The one-off injury such as the torn anterior cruciate ligament, can and does occur, but more often than not, physiotherapists are dealing with more complex pain syndromes such as low back pain and patellofemoral pain, so the problem is often multifactorial and the cause of the pain may be remote from the site of the symptoms.

WHY ARE SOME INDIVIDUALS MORE SUSCEPTIBLE TO PAIN?

An individual's mechanics has a marked effect on their inherent stability and passive control and hence their propensity for experiencing pain. Panjabi described a stability model for the spine which involves passive structures (osseus, ligamentous, tendinous and capsular structures of the joint), active structures (muscles) and neural control (centrally and peripherally. This means that a joint can be passively unstable, but dynamically stable, as the muscles via the neural control subsystem can compensate for the lack of stability in the passive structures.[9]

The amount of load through the soft tissues or the frequency of the loading will also affect joint structures and may result in tissue failure, as an individual may breach his/her threshold and stray out of the zone of homoeostasis.[10] Dye contends that symptoms will not be present if an individual is operating inside his/her envelope of function, but as soon as a threshold is reached a complex biological cascade of trauma and repair will occur, which will be manifested clinically by pain and swelling. In this model there are four factors determining the size of an individual's envelope of function: (a) anatomical (e.g. involving the morphology, structural integrity and biomechanical characteristics of the tissue); (b) kinematic (e.g. the dynamic control of the joint involving proprioceptive sensory output, cerebral and cerebellar sequencing of motor units, spinal reflex mechanisms, muscle strength and motor control); (c) physiological (e.g. the genetically determined mechanisms responsible for the quality and rate of repair of damaged tissues; and (d) treatment (e.g. the type of rehabilitation or surgery received).

WHERE IS THE PAIN COMING FROM?

In the first instance, pain will come from increased sensitivity of structures in the vicinity of the problem which will be mostly soft-tissue-related. Many soft tissues such as ligaments and tendons have tensile properties but these properties are affected when the ligament or tendon is disrupted so the tissues respond adversely to stretch, whereas other soft tissues such as menisci and discs are designed to minimize compressive stress but when they are damaged compression increases the sensitivity of the structures. Adams[11] has introduced the concept of 'functional pathology', whereby back pain can arise because postural habits generate painful stress concentrations within innervated tissues, even though the stresses are not high enough to cause physical disruption.

A study by Solomonow and colleagues[12] examining the effect of creep after loaded spinal flexion in the in vivo feline found that creep developed in the tissues during the 20 minutes of static or cyclic flexion and did not fully recover over the 7 hours of following rest. Histological data from the supraspinous ligament showed a tenfold increase in neutrophil density in the ligament 2 hours into the recovery and a hundredfold increase 6 hours into the recovery from the 20 minutes of sustained and cyclic flexion, indicating an acute soft tissue inflammation. A neuromuscular disorder of a decreasing magnitude of reflexive EMG from the multifidus upon flexion and superimposed spasms developed during and after the static and cyclic flexion. The recovery period was characterized by an initial muscle hyperexcitability, a slowly increasing reflexive EMG and a delayed hyperexcitability. The authors concluded that sustained static or cyclic loading of the lumbar viscoelastic tissues caused microdamage in the collagen structure resulting in spasms in the multifidus and hyperexcitability early in recovery when the majority of the creep occurs. The micro-damage caused the time-dependent development of inflammation and the resultant spasms (i.e. initial and delayed hyperexcitabilities) represented the increased muscular forces applied across the intervertebral joints in an attempt to limit the range of motion and unload the viscoelastic tissues in order to prevent further damage and to promote healing. The authors felt that this may give insight into development of idiopathic low back pain.[12] Thus, in the acute low back situation, it may be possible for clinicians to minimize the protective spasm of the erector spinae by improving the stability of vulnerable lumbar segments using firm tape (Fig. 34-1).

Unloading painful structures by using a firm, non-elastic, rayon-based tape with a hypoallergenic tape underneath allows the patient to exercise and train in a pain-free manner, which enhances treatment outcomes and further improves compliance. The principle of unloading is based on the premise that inflamed soft tissue does not respond well to stretch.

Hypomobility, which is a lack of flexibility of joint structures, neural, fascial and muscle tissues, can increase the stress on other relatively more mobile structures. An example would be tight hamstrings affecting forward flexion, so the lumbar spine demonstrates relatively more flexibility; firm tape across the muscle, perpendicular to the fibres at the musculotendinous junction is effective in decreasing hamstring tightness, allowing the patient to stretch the area more effectively (Fig. 34-2).

Hypermobility/instability, which is a lack of passive and dynamic control, can compromise joint function. Tape can be used to improve stability by being applied parallel to the muscle fibres to facilitate muscle activity. For control post whiplash, tape can be used to provide stability and minimize excessive protective spasm, particularly from the upper trapezius and scalenes. (Fig. 34-3).

If the pain persists central sensitization occurs, where extrinsic factors can amplify the pain experience. Fear-avoidance has long been recognized as an important factor in the development of pain-related disability. Exposure to stress initiates the secretion of several

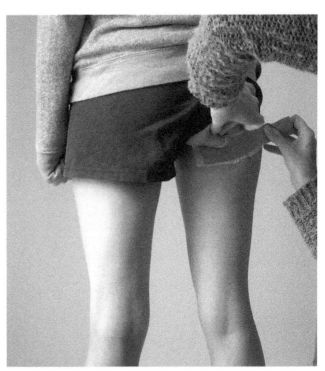

FIGURE 34-2 ■ Firmly tape across musculotendinous junction of hamstrings to help improve hamstring flexibility.

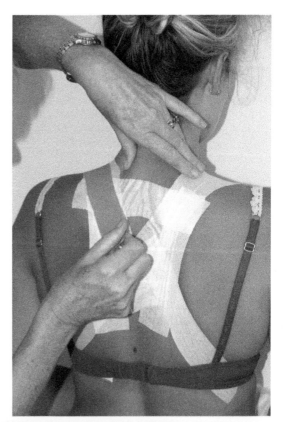

FIGURE 34-3 ■ Tape to facilitate stability post whiplash – unload the upper trapezius by lifting soft tissue towards neck and tape to support the scapular stabilizers.

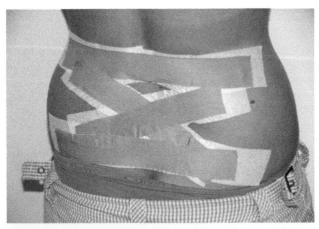

FIGURE 34-1 ■ Taping for acute low back pain. Tape towards the direction of pain with the horizontal strips, starting at the waist crease level. The diagonal strips start on the superior horizontal tape to the opposite buttock.

hormones as part of the survival mechanism, including corticosterone/cortisol, catecholamines, prolactin, oxytocin and renin. Such conditions are often referred to as 'stressors' and can be divided into three categories: (a) external conditions resulting in pain or discomfort; (b) internal homoeostatic disturbances; and (c) learned or associative responses to the perception of impending endangerment, pain or discomfort.[13] To test whether fear changes the motor control of the segment or whether the diminished motor control amplifies the fear of pain, pain has been induced in asymptomatic individuals in the lumbar spine. During anticipation of experimentally induced back pain, with repetitive arm movements there was decreased activity of the deep trunk muscles as well as a shift from biphasic to monophasic activation. Increased activity occurred in the superficial trunk muscles. These changes were similar to those observed in patients with recurrent back pain.[14] The implication is that if the patient is fearful about a movement causing pain, that alone will have a dramatic effect on muscle performance. It is important for clinicians to do whatever they have in their kitbag of treatment modalities to decrease pain so that the detrimental effects of pain and fear of pain can be reduced as soon as possible and muscle function can return to normal. Tape can be extremely successful in achieving this goal, particularly for controlling chronic low back and leg symptoms.[15] Using tape to unload inflamed tissues will decrease the pain and fear of pain, enabling the clinician to implement muscle-training strategies to provide a long-term control of symptoms for the patient.[15,16]

Chronic musculoskeletal conditions are managed, not cured. Taping should be used as an adjunct to treatment to decrease pain and improve control while normal mechanics are restored. The patient therefore needs to do something daily to ensure that the muscles stay working well and their symptoms do not recur. It is essential to improve the patient's awareness of the effects of uncontrolled sustained posture and to give them simple strategies so that they can cope with everyday life – how to stand, how to sit and how to get from sitting to standing, what type of mattress and pillow they need, what type of chair, position of arms on chairs, workstation advice, etc. They also need a home programme that uses minimal or no equipment, with a maximum of four exercises, taking no more than 5 minutes when on maintenance, otherwise they will not be compliant.

REFERENCES

1. Crossley K, Bennell K, Green S, et al. Physical therapy for patellofemoral pain: a randomized, double-blinded, placebo-controlled trial. Am J Sports Med 2002;30(6):857–65.
2. Derasari A, Brindle T, Alter K, et al. McConnell taping shifts the patella inferiorly in patients with patellofemoral pain: a dynamic magnetic resonance imaging study. Phys Ther 2010;90(3):411–19.
3. Gilleard W, McConnell J, Parsons D. The effect of patellar taping on the onset of vastus medialis obliquus and vastus lateralis muscle activity in persons with patellofemoral pain. Phys Ther 1998;78(1):25–32.
4. Kilbreath SL, Perkins S, Crosbie J, et al. Gluteal taping improves hip extension during stance phase of walking following stroke. Aust J Physiother 2006;52(1):53–6.
5. McConnell J, Donnelly CJ, Hamner S, et al. Effect of shoulder taping on maximum shoulder external and internal rotation range in uninjured and previously injured overhead athletes during a seated throw. J Orthop Res 2011;29(9):1406–11.
6. McConnell J, Donnelly CJ, Hamner S, et al. Is passive rotation shoulder range of motion indicative of active range of motion during throwing? PMR 2012;4(2):111–16.
7. Bogduk N. The anatomy and physiology of nociception. In: Crosbie J, McConnell J, editors. Key issues in Musculoskeletal Physiotherapy. Oxford: Butterworth-Heinemann; 1993.
8. Shacklock M. Central Pain Mechanisms: a new horizon in manual therapy. Aust J Physiother 1999;45(2):83–92.
9. Panjabi M. The stabilising system of the spine. Part I. J Spinal Disord 1992;5(4):383–9.
10. Dye S. The knee as a biologic transmission with an envelope of function: a theory. Clin Orthop 1996;325:10–18.
11. Adams MA. Biomechanics of back pain. Acupunct Med 2004;22(4):178–88.
12. Solomonow M, Baratta RV, Zhou BH, et al. Muscular dysfunction elicited by creep of lumbar viscoelastic tissue. J Electromyogr Kinesiol 2003;13(4):381–96.
13. Van de Kar LD, Blair ML. Forebrain pathways mediating stress-induced hormone secretion. Front Neuroendocrinol 1999;20(1):1–48.
14. Moseley GL, Nicholas MK, Hodges PW. Does anticipation of back pain predispose to back trouble? Brain 2004;127(Pt 10):2339–47.
15. McConnell J. Recalcitrant chronic low back and leg pain – a new theory and different approach to management. In: Karen B, editor. Manual Therapy in Masterclasses – The Vertebral Column. London: Churchill Livingstone; 2003.
16. McConnell J. Management of a difficult knee problem. Man Ther 2013;18(3):258–63.

CAUTIONS IN MUSCULOSKELETAL PRACTICE

EDITOR'S INTRODUCTION

Physiotherapists assessing, treating and providing guidance to people presenting with musculoskeletal conditions are, in many countries, primary contact practitioners who make autonomous decisions and provide the highest levels of care possible. Referrals for management may also come from other health professionals. Irrespective of the method of referral, physiotherapists must be accountable for their clinical practice. They must ensure that they remain vigilant to sinister conditions that may masquerade as musculoskeletal symptoms or that may be derived from non-musculoskeletal sources, such as the vascular system. They must also be aware of the possible side effects of medicines that may masquerade as musculoskeletal symptoms. It is highly relevant that one of the most common presenting symptoms of vascular pathology is pain, and that neoplasms may mimic the symptoms of musculoskeletal conditions. In addition, physiotherapists assessing musculoskeletal conditions, such as symptoms emanating from structures associated with cervical spine, must be aware of the value as well as the limitations of tests to implicate or

exclude instability in the upper cervical spine region as the source of symptoms. This highlights the importance of including a chapter discussing cautions in musculoskeletal practice. Chapter 35 brings together international experts in these fields of musculoskeletal practice to provide the reader with an essential overview of areas of concern that impact on clinical practice. Each subchapter provides invaluable information that will be indispensable to clinicians. Information includes methods of identifying sinister pathology and guidance on critical time frames required to respond to certain presenting symptoms. Guidance is provided to help identify clinical signs that may be associated with vascular impairment and methods of management. Finally a review of craniocervical ligament integrity assessment will provide important guidance for those using these tests to assess the stability of the upper cervical spine as well as part of pre-cervical spine manipulation screening. Chapter 35 is essential reading for all musculoskeletal physiotherapists, those newly qualified and those with considerable clinical experience.

CHAPTER 35.1 ■ MASQUERADERS

Susan Greenhalgh • James Selfe

INTRODUCTION

Musculoskeletal physiotherapists may be 'first contact' clinicians or receive referrals from other health specialities. It remains our duty of care to refer patients to an appropriate speciality in a timely manner if the presenting condition proves not to be musculoskeletal in origin. Although masqueraders of musculoskeletal conditions are rare in the general population, timely recognition of these presentations is essential. A key challenge for practitioners managing patients presenting to musculoskeletal services is that the source of symptoms is frequently extensive and may not originate from musculoskeletal tissues. The pathological mechanisms responsible for generating nociceptive signals may, particularly in the early stages of a non-musculoskeletal condition, present a confusing and indistinct clinical picture. For example serious pathology of the spine can initially masquerade as simple back pain (Box 35-1). The difficulties associated with early identification of serious causes of back pain are compounded by the sheer number of people suffering from low back pain and the variety and vagueness of symptoms articulated by the patients. It is also important to recognize that patients suffering with complex chronic pain states are not immune to other forms of pathology, and that musculoskeletal disorders may often coexist with other pathologies.

Masqueraders are usually related to a lesion of a system unrelated to the perceived site and nature of symptoms. The clinical severity of masqueraders covers a broad spectrum ranging from emergency life-threatening conditions (e.g. aortic aneurysm) through to minor disorders (e.g. carpal tunnel syndrome). Grieve first approached the subject of masqueraders in 1986 (p. 848),[4] he observed that: 'Neoplasms are sly surreptitious things, often masquerading as quite ordinary musculoskeletal syndromes'.

Those involved in musculoskeletal medicine work in an arena with some element of risk, with aspects of confusion and doubt occurring on a daily basis. Our clinical skills should guide us to reach a conclusion of greatest belief by considering the inherent likelihood of the cause (or causes) of a patient's pain and dysfunction. In order to do this accurately we must possess knowledge of the sometimes deceptive nature of symptoms referred from the viscera and from changes within metabolic systems (Fig. 35-1). In this short section it is impossible to discuss all the possible musculoskeletal masqueraders, or even to produce a comprehensive list. We have therefore chosen to focus on a small number of areas that are slightly more common and have important implications for musculoskeletal practitioners.

It is essential not to underestimate the power of sound anatomical knowledge in clinical reasoning. For example, anatomical knowledge clearly illustrates why a Pancoast tumour could produce symptoms in a C8/T1 distribution. Clinicians must also consider the wider holistic picture and actively listen to the patient's experiences (i.e. what makes symptoms worse, what improves the symptoms, when did it start, has anything else changed). The thoracic spine has a complex neural anatomy leading to difficulty in differentiating between visceral and somatic pain.[7] The close proximity of the intercostal nerves and the sympathetic plexus to the zygoapophyseal, costotransverse and costovertebral joints, disc and vertebral body account for referred band-like pain with any lesion compressing neural structures within this spinal complex. As with dermatomal distribution, there are discrepancies relating to the exact locations for some of these referred pains from viscera, which are often vague and ill-defined in nature. Figure 35-1 illustrates some of the less contentious areas. For more detailed information on this interesting subject see; *Topical Issues in Pain* 3e edited by Louis Gifford.[8]

CAUDA EQUINA SYNDROME

The estimated yearly incidence of cauda equina syndrome (CES) in England is 2 per 100 000.[9] It is a rare condition accounting for 2% of all herniated discs.

What is It?

CES occurs as a consequence of the loss of function of two or more of the 18 nerve roots that comprise the cauda equina.[10] CES is a potential emergency.[11,12] Consequently, it is mandatory that physiotherapists should routinely ask about bladder and bowel functions during the subjective examination.[3,13,14] Early diagnosis and surgical decompression are essential. Jalloh and Minhas[15] and Gleave and Macfarlane[16] suggest that spinal surgery within 48 hours of an individual developing sphincter dysfunction will optimize post-operative recovery. If left untreated, CES may lead to permanent loss of bowel and bladder control, sexual dysfunction or even paralysis.[17] Current evidence regarding the clinical presentation of CES demonstrates marked discrepancies related to its definition, with 17 different definitions of CES recorded.[11] Fraser et al.[11] have suggested that one or more of the

---

BOX 35-1	Definitions of Terms

Masquerader: A condition that 'appears in disguise or assumes a false appearance'
Red Herring:[1] Misleading biomedical or psychosocial factor that could deflect the course of accurate clinical reasoning
Red Flag:[2] Possible indicator of serious pathology
Serious pathology:[3] Fracture, cancer, infection, cauda equina syndrome, inflammatory disorder

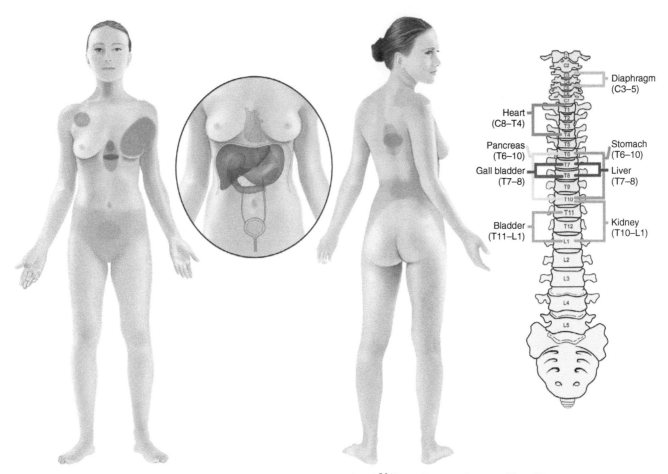

Diaphragm
(C3–5)

Heart
(C8–T4)

Pancreas
(T6–10)

Stomach
(T6–10)

Gall bladder
(T7–8)

Liver
(T7–8)

Bladder
(T11–L1)

Kidney
(T10–L1)

FIGURE 35-1 ■ Common sites of visceral pain referral.[5,6] For colour version see Plate 22.

following must be present in order to make a provisional diagnosis of CES: bladder and/or bowel dysfunction; reduced sensation in the saddle area; sexual dysfunction (Box 35-2).

Clinicians commonly consider CES as either incomplete (CES-I) or complete (CES-R).[19]

CES-I (48-Hour Emergency Window Open Where Surgery is Likely to be Helpful)

- Unilateral or bilateral sciatica may be present and increasing.
- Neurological deficit progressing.
- Unilateral or patchy perineal/perianal numbness.
- Anal sphincter tone may be reduced.
- Loss of desire to void, poor stream, strain to micturate but with sensation of full bladder.

CES-R (Emergency Window Passed Where Surgery is Less Likely to be Beneficial)

- May have no leg pain or may have unilateral/bilateral sciatica.
- May have unilateral or bilateral neurological deficit.
- Widespread perineal sensory deficit.
- No anal sphincter tone.
- Painless urinary retention with full bladder and overflow incontinence.

BOX 35-2	Sexual Dysfunction Associated with CES[18]

SEXUAL DYSFUNCTION

Vaginal anaesthesia and numbness
Incontinence during intercourse
Decreased intensity and/or inability to achieve orgasm
Inability to achieve erection
Inability to achieve ejaculation

- No bladder sensation or control.
- Faecal incontinence.

Important Issues

- Early diagnosis provides the best chance of optimal recovery.
- Diagnosis in early stages is not easy, yet is an orthopaedic/neurological emergency.
- To confound early diagnosis, the patient's experience of CES symptoms can be difficult for them to recognize or articulate.[20]
- It can be a highly litigious condition; damages on average can be £300000[17] because many cases are preventable.[20]

- Approximately 20% will have poor outcome (e.g. sexual dysfunction, self-catheterization, colostomy, psychosocial support).
- Potentially improved outcome if retention rather than incontinence present.
- Erectile dysfunction uncommon but a strong indicator of a poor prognosis.
- Early recognition is essential as decompression is preferably within 24–48 hours.

Gleave and Macfarlane[16] reported that the emergency surgical window is very small (48 hours) and they state that 'the die is cast at the time of the prolapse' depending on the speed of development and the severity of compression. This paper has been used subsequently to inform court decisions in the UK.[21] There is still debate surrounding the optimum point of surgical intervention with many authors suggesting that surgery should take place at the early stages of CES. This has been defined as unilateral or bilateral sensory/motor deficit in the lower extremities, prior to sphincter involvement.[22,23]

What Causes Confusion?

Variations in presentation may range from rapid onset of CES without previous history of back pain to acute bladder dysfunction with a history of back pain and sciatica, or even chronic backache and sciatica with gradual progression to CES.[9] In addition, a number of confounding factors may influence excretory organ dysfunction; these include medication (opioid salts; anticonvulsants; antidepressants), co-morbidity (prostate conditions; stress incontinence) or pain (acute or chronic).

Emerging Issues

The pattern of symptom progression in CES has not been defined.[22] Knowing that there appears to be no chronological pattern to symptoms developing may actually be clinically valuable. In 2013, in the UK a lengthy debate took place on the Chartered Society of Physiotherapy website (iCSP) relating to the definition of saddle anaesthesia. Part of the discussion involved the exact location of the saddle (bicycle versus horse). Personal communication with the CES UK Charity confirms that amongst their members, the anatomical area that would be in contact with a horse's saddle (including buttocks) is affected.

New Advances

A review of CES patient records has confirmed that these cases were regularly being missed in the early stages of symptom development.[20] A subsequent service improvement using an experience-based design model suggested that when suffering severe pain, bladder function was often not the main cause of a patient's concern.

For example the following quote was reported in sheer disbelief by the patient as she perceived the question was 'stupid'. 'I was crawling on the floor in agony when the ambulance man asked if me if I had any bladder problems?' This illustrates the importance of patients understanding the significance of Red Flag questions within the context of their suffering.

A CES guideline has recently been published by Gloucestershire Hospitals NHS (UK) that is designed to advance critical thinking skills and evidence-based management of CES.[24]

METASTATIC SPINAL CORD COMPRESSION

The guidelines for the physiotherapy management of low back pain[14] reported that there were 163 individual items that could be considered as Red Flags. Clearly this presents a major problem in terms of the practical and clinical utility of the current system of spinal Red Flags; none of the 163 items had been identified as being specific to metastatic spinal cord compression (MSCC).

The true incidence of MSCC is unknown; postmortem evidence indicates that it is present in 5–10% of patients with advanced cancer. In total, there are approximately 4000 new cases of MSCC reported in England and Wales per year.[25]

What is It?

MSCC is a well-recognized complication of cancer. The condition occurs when there is pathological vertebral body collapse or direct tumour growth causing compression of the spinal cord leading to irreversible neurological damage. In addition to the agonizing pain and spinal instability that the condition can cause; compression on the spinal cord can also lead to paraplegia or quadriplegia and double incontinence.[26]

Important Issues

- Frequently missed oncological emergency.[26]
- At diagnosis 82% of patients with MSCC are unable to walk or only able to do so with help.[26]
- Life expectancy significantly reduced once paraplegia has developed.[27]
- Those with established paraparesis and loss of bladder control by the time of treatment are unlikely to regain useful function.[28]
- The best outcome for MSCC in terms of function and prognosis depends on a high index of suspicion, early diagnosis, onward referral for urgent investigation ideally within 24 hours[25] and prompt treatment in order to prevent or limit neurological damage.
- Whole spinal scan required within 24 hours.[25]

What Causes Confusion?

MSCC may appear as simple mechanical back pain initially. Early detection and diagnosis of MSCC, before the development of neurological symptoms relies solely on the subjective history taking. This is extremely challenging when considering that on average patients present to a variety of non-specialist practitioners in a broad range of locations within three weeks of the onset of back pain.[26] Physical neurological examination is unremarkable until later stages in the disease process. Subjective leg symptoms may be vague: 'my legs feel odd and weak'.[29]

Emerging Issues

Studies have reported that around 25% of patients present with spinal cord compression as the first sign of malignancy with no previous diagnosis of primary cancer.[25] A combination of Red Flags increases suspicion, the more Red Flags the higher the risk and the greater the urgency.

TABLE 35-1	Musculoskeletal Side Effects of Medication[32-35]	
Musculoskeletal Side Effects: Signs and Symptoms	**Medication**
Mild aches, pains	Oral contraceptives (e.g. Microgynon)
	Statins (e.g. atorvastatin)
Muscle cramps	Diuretics (e.g. bendroflumethiazide)
	Calcium channel blockers (e.g. verapamil)
	Beta-agonists (e.g. salbutamol)
Proximal muscle weakness, atrophy	Oral corticosteroids (e.g. prednisolone)
	>10 mg daily dose, for at least 30 days
Severe pain, myopathy, malaise, fever, dark urine	Statins
	0.1–0.2% of patients in clinical trials have side effects
Osteoporosis, fracture	Oral corticosteroids
	Doses >5 mg daily lead to significant and rapid bone loss. A cumulative dose of >30 g associated with a high incidence of fracture 53%. Excessive risk of fracture disappears within 1 year of stopping therapy
Avascular necrosis	Corticosteroids
	5–40% of patients on long-term therapy
Tendinopathy, tendon rupture myopathy	Injected corticosteroids
	Oral corticosteroids
	Glucocorticoids have a direct catabolic effect on skeletal muscle tissue
Myalgia, arthralgia, arthritis, tendinitis	Quinalones (synthetic broad-spectrum antibiotics) (e.g. ciprofloxacin)
	World-wide incidence of side effects estimated as 15–20 per 100,000 patients treated
Bladder and bowel dysfunction	Opioid salts; constipation (e.g. tramadol, codeine)
	Anticonvulsants; urinary incontinence (e.g. gabapentin, pregabalin)
	Antidepressants; retention, sexual dysfunction (e.g. amitriptyline, nortriptyline)
Muscle cramp, muscle weakness	Thyroid hormones (e.g. levothyroxine sodium) at excessive dosage
Joint aches and pains (arthralgia)	Antithyroid drugs used to treat hyperthyroidism (e.g. carbimazole)

New Advances

A new eight-item tool aimed at helping clinicians to identify the early signs and symptoms of MSCC has been developed and produced in the form of a credit card.[30] The Greater Manchester and Cheshire Cancer Network (UK) brought together oncology expertise from the Regional Cancer Centre (Christie) and primary care musculoskeletal physiotherapy, to produce a user-friendly list of MSCC Red Flags for non-specialist front-line clinicians working in primary care settings.

Referred back pain that is multisegmental or band-like

Escalating pain which is poorly responsive to treatment (including medication)

Different character or site to previous symptoms

Funny feelings, odd sensations or heavy legs (multisegmental)

Lying flat increases back pain

Agonizing pain causing anguish and despair

Gait disturbance, unsteadiness, especially on stairs (not just a limp)

Sleep grossly disturbed due to pain being worse at night.

It is important to emphasize that established motor, sensory, bladder and bowel disturbances are considered to be late signs.

MEDICATION

In the UK, Chartered Physiotherapists have been performing injections since 1995; they were given supplementary prescribing rights in 2005 and independent prescribing rights in 2013.[31] Even if physiotherapy practice does not encompass these extended roles, knowledge of side effects of common medications which masquerade as musculoskeletal problems is useful in the clinical reasoning processes (Table 35-1). Medications can produce side effects, and it is essential for physiotherapists to be aware of these as they may include muscle pain, bladder and bowel dysfunction, osteoporosis, fractures and tendon ruptures. A large proportion of the structures within the musculoskeletal system have a high metabolic rate and blood flow. As a consequence the musculoskeletal system has a high exposure to circulating medications.[32] Within the clinical reasoning process the chronological sequence of symptoms is important. One of the main clues suggesting that the symptoms are caused by the medication is that the symptoms began after the medication was started and resolved once the medication had ceased.

REFERENCES

1. Sykes JB, editor. Concise Oxford Dictionary. 6th ed. Oxford: Clarendon Press.; 1978.
2. Greenhalgh S, Selfe J. Red Flags: A Guide to Identifying Serious Pathology of the Spine. Churchill Livingstone, Elsevier; 2006.
3. Clinical Standards Advisory Group. Report of a Clinical Standards Advisory Group on Back Pain. London: HMSO; 1994.
4. Grieve G. Modern Manual Therapy of the Vertebral Column. Edinburgh and New York: Churchill Livingstone; 1986.
5. Standring S, editor. Gray's Anatomy: the Anatomical Basis of Clinical Practice. 39th ed. Edinburgh: Elsevier Churchill Livingstone; 2005.

6. Ombregt L, Bisschop O, J ter Veer H. A System of Orthopaedic Medicine. 2nd ed. Elsevier Science Limited; 2003.

7. Boyling J, Jull G. Grieve's Modern Manual Therapy: The Vertebral Column. 3rd ed. Churchill Livingstone; 2005.

8. Gifford L, Thacker M. Complex regional pain syndrome: part 1. In: Gifford L, editor. Topical Issues in Pain 3. Sympathetic Nervous System and Pain. Pain Management. Clinical Effectiveness. Falmouth: CNS Press; 2002. p. 53–74.

9. Gitelman A, Hishmeh S, Morelli B, et al. Cauda equina syndrome: a comprehensive review. Am J Orthop 2008;37(11):556–62.

10. Woolsley R, Martin D. Spinal cord and cauda equina syndromes. In: Lin V, Cardenas D, Cutter N, et al., editors. Spinal Cord Medicine: Principles and Practice. New York Demos Medical Publishing; 2003.

11. Fraser S, Roberts L, Murphy E. Cauda equina syndrome: a literature review of its definition and clinical presentation. Arch Phys Med Rehabil 2009;90:1964–8.

12. Mestrum R, De Vooght P, Vanelderen P, et al. Cauda equina syndrome secondary to lumbar disc herniation: pitfalls in clinical pain management. Eur J Pain 2009;13:S138–9.

13. Royal College of General Practitioners. Clinical guidelines for the management of acute low back pain. [On line]. Available from: <http://www.rcgp.org.uk/clinspec/guidelines/backpain/index.asp>; 2001 [Accessed 14th November 2013].

14. The Chartered Society of Physiotherapy. Clinical guidelines for the effective physiotherapy management of persistent low back pain. [On line]. Available from: <http://corporate.csp.midev.rroom.net/director/libraryandpublications/publications.cfm?item_id=562CC348D28AC0F97B2AA357019A7C7C>; [Accessed 6 September 2010].

15. Jalloh I, Minhas P. Delays in the treatment of cauda equina syndrome due to its variable clinical features in patients presenting to the emergency department. Emerg Med J 2007;24(1):33–4.

16. Gleave JRW, Macfarlane R. Cauda equina syndrome: what is the relationship between timing of surgery and outcome? Br J Neurosurg 2002;16(3):325–8.

17. Markham DE. Cauda equina syndrome: diagnosis, delay and litigation risk. Curr Orthop 2004;18(1):58–62.

18. Shapiro S. Medical realities of cauda equina syndrome secondary to lumbar disc herniation. Spine 2000;25:348–52.

19. Gardner A, Gardner E, Morley T. Cauda equina syndrome: a review of the current clinical and medico-legal position. Eur Spine J 2011;20:690–7.

20. Anthony S. Cauda equina syndrome. UK Casebook 2003;20:9–13.

21. Oaks v Neininger, et al. [Online]. Available from: <http://www.bailii.org/ew/cases/EWHC/QB/2008/548.html>; [Accessed 15th July 2013].

22. Sun JC, Xu T, Chen KF, et al. Assessment of cauda equina syndrome progression pattern to improve diagnosis. Spine 2013; Spine publish ahead of print, doi:10.1097/BRS.0000000000000079.

23. Todd NV. Causes and outcomes of Cauda Equina Syndrome in medico-legal practice: a single neurosurgical experience of 40 consecutive cases. Br J Neurosurg 2011;25(4):503–8. [Epub 2011 Apr 22].

24. © GHNHSFT. Physiotherapy Guideline Cauda Equina Syndrome (CES) – Early Recognition v2 ISSUE DATE: v1 July 2012, v2 Apr 2013. [On line]. Available from: <www.esp-physio.co.uk>; 2013 [Accessed 14th November 2013].

25. National Institute for Health and Clinical Excellence (NICE). Metastatic Spinal Cord Compression: Diagnosis and Management of Patients at Risk of or with Metastatic Spinal Cord Compression. Clinical Guideline 75. 2008. [On line]. Available from: <www.nice.org.uk/Guidance/CG75>; [Accessed 14th November 2013].

26. Levack P, Graham J, Collie D, et al. Don't wait for a sensory level – listen to the symptoms: a prospective audit of the delays in diagnosis of malignant cord compression. Clin Oncol 2002;14:472–80.

27. Patchell RA, Tibbs PA, Regine WF. Direct decompressive surgical resection in the treatment of spinal cord compression caused by metastatic cancer: a randomised trial. Lancet 2005;266:643–8.

28. Christie Hospital NHS Foundation Trust. Spinal Cord Compression Guidelines. Manchester; 2008.

29. Greenhalgh S, Selfe J. A qualitative investigation of red flags for serious spinal pathology. Physiotherapy 2009;95:224–7.

30. Turnpenney J, Greenhalgh S, Richards L, et al. Developing an early alert system for metastatic spinal cord compression. Prim Health Care Res Dev 2013;1–7. [Epub ahead of print] [On line]. Available from: DOI: <http://dx.doi.org/10.1017/S1463423613000376>; [Accessed 14th November 2013].

31. Chartered Society of Physiotherapy. CSP History. [On line]. Available from: <http://www.csp.org.uk/about-csp/history/csp-history>; [Accessed 14th November 2013].

32. Randall C. Chapter 11. Musculoskeletal disorders; 293–325. In: Lee A, editor. Adverse Drug Reactions. 2nd ed. London: Pharmaceutical Press.; 2006.

33. BNF 65. March-September. BMA. Royal Pharmaceutical Society; 2013.

34. UPTODATE. Glucocorticoids. [On line]. Available from: <http://www.uptodate.com/contents/glucocorticoid-induced-myopathy?source=search_result&search=corticosteroids&selectedTitle=11%7E150>; [Accessed 14th November 2013].

35. Powell C, Chang C, Naguwa S, et al. Steroid induced osteonecrosis: an analysis of steroid dosing risk. Autoimmun Rev 2010;9:721–43.

CHAPTER 35.2 ■ HAEMODYNAMICS AND CLINICAL PRACTICE

Alan Taylor • Roger Kerry

INTRODUCTION

Altered haemodynamics is the forgotten Red Flag of manual therapy. While it is well understood in medicine that a failure to assess the vascular system could lead to dire consequences (limb loss, death) for patients, it seems manual therapists are less well versed in the art of vascular assessment. It is a sobering thought that most vascular pathologies, from deep vein thrombosis to stroke, have pain as their initial presenting feature – precisely the symptom for which patients may seek manual therapies.

This chapter highlights key advances in haemodynamic science that are relevant to the everyday practice of musculoskeletal physiotherapy.

The International Federation of Orthopaedic Manipulative Therapists (IFOMPT) produced a consensus document for cervical spine risk assessment,[1] which details a shift in thinking pertaining to manual therapy and vascular risk. This chapter provides an overview of this document for clinicians from a practical perspective, and goes on to consider how this change of practice may have implications when considering other anatomical regions.

The IFOMPT document recommends a number of evidence-informed changes to practice relating to cervical arterial dysfunction (CAD). Of note, the use of vertebral artery testing receives short thrift, in favour of a 'systems approach' based on existing reviews of the best of scientific evidence in the area.[2] This new model considers the whole vascular system, including knowledge of flow dysfunction, vessel mechanics and pertinent systemic pathologies. Clinicians are guided towards holistic assessment, incorporating general cardiovascular health and a consideration of pain as a symptom of arterial pathology, or impending events such as transient ischaemic attack or stroke.

The idea that cardiovascular status can inform judgement on the likelihood of a haemodynamic event, or predict such, is controversial in manual therapy.[3,4] However, these studies have over-focused on isolated pathologies, such as dissection events, and do not represent the range of presentations relevant to musculoskeletal therapists. Decades of data from medical literature leave little doubt that such a relationship exists.[2,5,6] The idea that pain is an early presenting feature of vascular dysfunction is clear.[7-9] The CAD model is well-aligned to the best of contemporary evidence regarding local vessel disease.[10-13] It utilizes the best of the medical data, demonstrating the relationship between mechanical vessel stress, fluid flow changes and disease formation.[14,15] It is suggested that an awareness of CAD is 'an important consideration as part of an orthopaedic manual therapy assessment'. Secondly, attention is drawn to the fact that, 'there are serious conditions which may mimic musculoskeletal dysfunction in the early stages of their pathological progression'.[1]

Clinicians should be aware that patients with potentially serious pathology (e.g. impending stroke) may attend for manual therapy treatment in the belief that they have a benign headache or migraine. Patterns of vascular pathologies are well known and should be central to clinical reasoning.[5]

An important subtle change in risk assessment has taken place. Attention is shifted away from specific structures, dysfunctions and tests, for example it is not a matter of 'is manipulation dangerous for the vertebral artery and should I do the vertebral artery test?'. The model gives consideration of all movements known to influence vessel mechanics (e.g. active and passive exercise and manual therapy techniques) in the context of the patient's haemodynamic status and with a background knowledge of a range of pathologies.

Subjective history taking requires clinicians to pay specific attention to known cardiovascular risk factors. This serves as a reminder for clinicians of the importance of detail, which should consider family history, as well as individual predilection towards cardiovascular disease. Haemodynamic principles are summarized in Box 35-3.

Of interest to clinicians is that more is now known about the subtle descriptors patients use which may alert therapists to the presence of underlying or impending vascular pathology. Table 35-2 presents typical subtle clinical presentation for CAD. Table 35-3 details the range of descriptors used for peripheral vascular pain.

Utilizing the evidence and knowledge of CAD and haemodynamic science, attempts may be made to develop

---

BOX 35-3 | **Principles of Clinical Reasoning as Illustrated by the IFOMPT Framework, Related to Haemodynamics**

- Haemodynamic science allows us to understand clinical aspects of vascular pathologies
- Vascular pathologies present in pre-ischaemic and ischaemic stages
- Pain is often an early (pre-ischaemic) symptom of vascular pathology; neurology is a late (ischaemic) presentation
- Vascular pathologies vary in nature and are not confined to dissection events
- Cardiovascular and hereditary risk factors predispose to a range of vascular pathologies
- Clinical tests currently used have poor diagnostic utility
- Reliance on any single clinical test is misleading, and physical findings should be considered in context with the subjective history

---

TABLE 35-2 **Clinical Presentations Related to CAD in Different Stages of the Pathologies**

Pre-Ischaemic		Ischaemic	
Vertebral Artery Pathology	Internal Carotid Artery Pathology	Vertebral Artery Pathology	Internal Carotid Artery Pathology
Ipsilateral posterior neck pain/occipital headache	Parietal, temporal headache; unilateral neck pain; jaw pain Horner's syndrome, pulsatile tinnitus Cranial nerve (CN) palsies (most commonly CN IX to XII) Less common local signs and symptoms include: ipsilateral carotid bruit, scalp tenderness, neck swelling, CN VI palsy, orbital pain and anhidrosis (facial dryness)	Hind-brain transient ischaemic attacks (dizziness, diplopia, dysarthria, dysphagia, drop attacks, nausea, nystagmus, facial numbness, ataxia, vomiting, hoarseness, loss of short-term memory, vagueness, hypotonia/limb weakness (arm or leg), anhidrosis (lack of facial sweating), hearing disturbances, malaise, perioral dysthesia, photophobia, papillary changes, clumsiness and agitation) Hind-brain stroke (e.g. Wallenberg's syndrome, locked-in syndrome)	Transient ischaemic attack Ischaemic stroke (usually middle cerebral artery territory) Retinal infarction Amaurosis fugax

Table 35-3 ■ **Descriptors Associated with Vascular Dysfunction in the Peripheral Regions**

| Sign/Symptom | Upper Limb | | Lower Limb | |
	Arterial Dysfunction	Venous Dysfunction	Arterial Dysfunction	Venous Dysfunction
Exercise-induced pain	☑	☑	☑	
Numbness/tingling	☑		☑	☑
Cold	☑	☑	☑	
Hot		☑		☑
Blue (back pressure of vein)		☑	☑	☑
Fatigue/weak	☑		☑	
Non-dermatomal pain	☑	☑	☑	☑
Cramp	☑	☑	☑	☑
Whitened skin/blanching	☑		☑	
Swelling		☑		☑
Subjective swelling (none seen)	☑	☑	☑	
Redness		☑		☑
Band of pain	☑		☑	
Throbbing/pulsatile	☑		☑	

(From detailed reviews of multiple case studies; case series; epidemiological studies; experimental studies; and clinical observations.)
Acknowledgments to Simon Meadows, Physiotherapist, for producing this table.

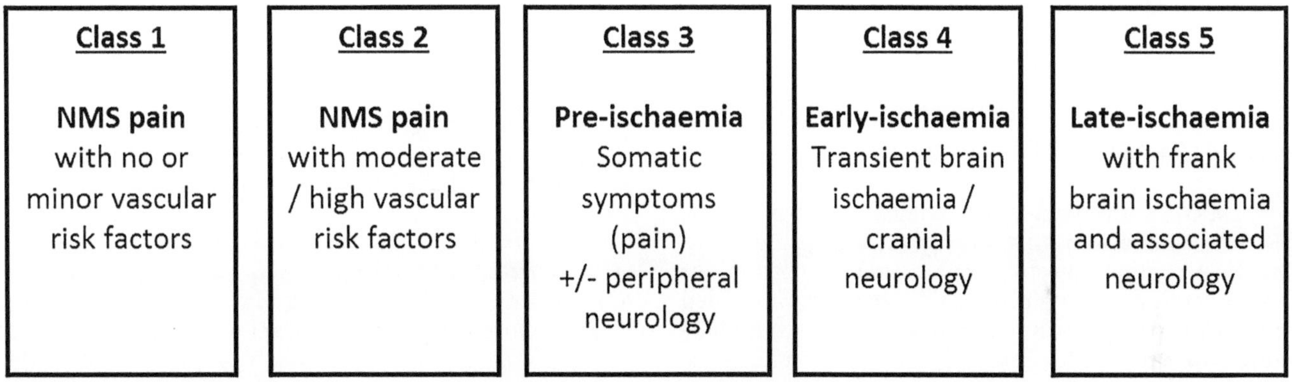

Class 1	Class 2	Class 3	Class 4	Class 5
NMS pain with no or minor vascular risk factors	**NMS pain** with moderate / high vascular risk factors	**Pre-ischaemia** Somatic symptoms (pain) +/- peripheral neurology	**Early-ischaemia** Transient brain ischaemia / cranial neurology	**Late-ischaemia** with frank brain ischaemia and associated neurology

FIGURE 35-2 ■ The Nottingham Cervical Arterial Dysfunction (nCAD) sub-classification system for profiling the haemodynamic status of a patient presenting with neck and/or head pain. Classes 3 to 5 represent patients presenting with haemodynamic pathology and medical referral should be considered. Disease progression is represented by the classification order (class 5 is advanced pathology). *NMS*, neuromusculoskeletal.

sub-classification systems to categorize patients. Figure 35-2 demonstrates a proposed system known as the Nottingham Cervical Arterial Dysfunction sub-classification (nCAD). The system categorizes patients first of all into whether they present with the potential of CAD (classes 1 and 2) or whether they present with signs and symptoms of actual CAD pathology (classes 3–5). This enables the clinician to make a decision on whether to continue with assessment or not, with a view to manual therapy treatment (classes 1 and 2), or to refer for medical assessment (classes 3–5).

The generic principles detailed in Box 35-3 may be distilled into a small number of clinical questions that the manual therapist can use to shape their evidence-informed reasoning. Box 35-4 summarizes these consideration.

BOX 35-4	Haemodynamic Considerations for Manual Therapists

1. What is the haemodynamic status of the patient?
2. Should manual therapy assessment proceed in the 'usual' way or be modified?
3. Are there haemodynamic considerations for treatment/management of the patient?

CASE STUDIES

In all musculoskeletal physiotherapy cases, regardless of proposed management strategies, a targeted subjective history should elucidate clues to potential underlying vascular pathology, or the need to explore this further using appropriate objective testing. Two short case scenarios, one involving a person with a cervical condition (Case Study 35-1) and one involving a person with a peripheral condition (Case Study 35-2), will follow which will illustrate key considerations.

CASE STUDY 35-1 MANUAL THERAPY-INDUCED TRANSIENT ISCHAEMIC ATTACK

A 75-year-old female with cervical spondylosis is referred for a 'flare up of neck pain' by her GP. She had a history of angina, heart disease and peripheral vascular disease (PVD) for which she was taking appropriate medications under the care of cardiac and vascular specialists.

CASE STUDY 35-2 DYNAMIC UPPER LIMB ARTERIAL OCCLUSION

An 18-year-old male competitive swimmer reported poor competitive performance associated with upper limb 'fatigue' and weakness when swimming (freestyle). The reported symptoms had been getting worse over the last 3 months and he and his mother were concerned that he may lose his place on the county team due to his deteriorating times/performance.

Case Study 1

The patient was examined by a domiciliary physiotherapist who took a subjective history (including the above detail). A routine objective examination revealed minor loss of cervical range globally. The therapist proceeded to treat the patient with longitudinal distraction mobilizations in sitting. Re-examination revealed mild gains (5°) in cervical rotation. At the follow-up visit the patient reported 'feeling funny' after the treatment, which was detailed further as 'feeling uncomfortable, light headed and woozy for a few hours'. This was ascribed to treatment soreness and manual therapy treatment continued. Variations of the same treatment continued for four sessions in total, with the 'treatment soreness' being reported after each session. Management was discontinued when the patient reported that her reaction to treatment was getting worse, 'post treatment arm and facial numbness/discomfort' and a report sent to the GP detailing the outcome.

At her routine visit to see her specialist she reported that her angina was stable, that her walking distance was the same, but that she had had some 'funny turns' following the visits of the domiciliary therapist. The vascular surgeon listened carefully to her description of events, palpated her carotid pulses and sent her for immediate ultrasound scans of her carotid arteries. She was found to have significant atherosclerotic stenosis bilaterally. She was listed for urgent carotid endarterectomy and made a full recovery. The surgeon's notes included the entry 'possible physiotherapy-induced transient ischaemic attacks'. Importantly, her neck pain cleared completely following the surgery.

Case Analysis

What Was the Haemodynamic Status of the Patient? The vascular status of the patient was known to the treating physiotherapist. The case notes detailed the vascular history and the drugs used to manage it. However, this knowledge did not appear to factor into the clinical reasoning. This patient would have reasonably been classified into class 3 or 4 on the nCAD system, indicating medical referral.

Should Manual Therapy Assessment Have Proceeded in the 'Usual' Way or Been Modified? There are strong indicators that further vascular assessment should have been undertaken. With the presenting vascular history there should have been a high index of suspicion for vascular pathology as it is well known that cardiac disease is associated with carotid disease.[16] Pulse palpation or auscultation may have revealed the abnormality.[17] Blood pressure examination may have been a pertinent aid to risk assessment prior to treatment.[18] Cranial nerve testing may have been performed at any stage, but particularly after the patient's report of an adverse response to treatment.

Were There Haemodynamic Considerations for Treatment/Management of the Patient? Where a patient details a range of vascular risk factors/events there is always a consideration for manual therapists to modify treatment. The belief that only manipulation is 'risky' is a dangerous fallacy; simple movement or exercise may have a haemodynamic effect that requires careful consideration, particularly in the presence of an adverse response to treatment. Empirically, it is known that normal physiological movements affected vessel mechanics.[18]

Clinical Reasoning Note

The therapist detailed all the vascular risk factors in the notes, but failed to raise an index of suspicion for concomitant carotid artery disease in a patient already under the care of the vascular team for heart disease, angina and peripheral vascular disease. When the patient reported an adverse response to the intervention, no further significant clinical reasoning took place and the patient was offered variations of a similar intervention until treatment was eventually halted. Furthermore, from a medico-legal perspective the surgeon's note relating to 'physiotherapy-induced transient ischaemic attacks' may have had deleterious effects, had a medico-legal case ensued. The patient's pain may have been associated with the carotid disease or 'carotidynia'.[19] Repeated movement of the head on neck might have been sufficient for microembolic events. Beyond the transient ischaemic attacks, no apparent neurology readily manifested itself during assessment. Clinicians should raise an index of suspicion for carotid disease in the presence of co-existing vascular disease and other cardiovascular risk factors[1] and modify examination accordingly.

Case Study 2

The patient was fit and healthy, taking no medications of any sort and had no history of trauma. The reported family history was unremarkable. Subjective history revealed an emphasis on upper limb fatigue/weakness and mild discomfort rather than pain. The symptoms were associated with swimming only (high-intensity training or competition) and did not manifest in normal activity.

Physical examination revealed glenohumeral joint instability and significant weakness of glenohumeral joint lateral rotation. The examination findings were reported to the patient and the mother by the therapist. The mother asked 'could this be circulatory? …because it only happens during exercise'. She was reassured by the therapist that this was unlikely, considering the patient's age and lack of vascular risk factors. However, the therapist suggested this would be checked at the next visit.

Case Analysis

What Was the Haemodynamic Status of the Patient? Because of the patient's age and activity levels, there appears to be no apparent traditional vascular risk factors. However, in certain populations the repetitive limb movement associated with that sport, together with mild anomalous body forms, may predispose vascular compromise.[20]

Should Manual Therapy Assessment Have Proceeded in the 'Usual' Way or Been Modified? Although subtle, there are sufficient historical indicators that would justify haemodynamic examination. At the follow-up visit, pulses and blood pressure were taken at rest and found to be entirely normal. Radial pulses were diminished in full glenohumeral joint flexion (compared to normal). Blood pressure readings were then performed in a temperate setting, with the person quiet and seated, with their arm outstretched and supported. This revealed the following results: left arm resting 124/82, elevated 80/62; right arm resting 118/78, elevated 76/60.

Were There Haemodynamic Considerations for Treatment/Management of the Patient? The patient was referred for further vascular testing and found to have restricted arterial flow in both upper limbs related to flexion/elevation. This was due to compression of the vessels by the humeral head. He was referred for intensive shoulder rehabilitation, with the goal of improving glenohumeral stability, to address the mechanical impingement of the artery. Importantly, positional blood pressure readings were used as a primary objective measure throughout the process. The patient returned to full competition 4 months later and achieved personal best times in all events after a period of re-conditioning.

Clinical Reasoning Note

Not all vascular problems are 'sinister' or require medical or surgical intervention. Some may respond to physiotherapy. It is the role of the clinician to modify examination and implement appropriate further testing in the light of findings. In this case, glenohumeral joint instability resulted in functional positional stenosis of the axillary artery, and the therapist's role was to identify the problem and then rehabilitate the underlying musculoskeletal cause, while monitoring key vascular markers.

CONCLUSION

Haemodynamic science has advanced substantially over the last decade. However, clinical practice has been slow to adapt. The IFOMPT risk assessment document for the cervical spine is an excellent example of how the evidence base should be used to inform clinical practice and reasoning. This chapter illustrates how clinicians can integrate that knowledge and apply it to real clinical situations. Above all it demonstrates how sound clinical reasoning allows for modification of physical examination and management for the benefit of the patient and the therapist. The fundamentals of simple vascular assessment together with a sound knowledge of haemodynamic principles and pathologies are an essential tool for the modern musculoskeletal therapist.

REFERENCES

1. Rushton A, Rivett D, Carlesso L, et al. International framework for examination of the cervical region for potential of cervical arterial dysfunction prior to orthopaedic manual therapy intervention. Man Ther 2013;pii:S1356-689X(13)00192-6. doi:10.1016/j.math.2013.11.005.
2. Taylor AJ, Kerry R. A 'system based' approach to risk assessment of the cervical spine prior to manual therapy. Int J Osteopath Med 2010;13:85–93.
3. Mitchell J. Vertebral artery atherosclerosis: a risk factor in the use of manipulative therapy? Physiother Res Int 2002;7:122–35.
4. Thomas LC, Rivett DA, Attia JR, et al. Risk factors and clinical presentation of craniocervical arterial dissection: a prospective study. BMC Musculoskelet Disord 2012;3;13:164. doi:10.1186/1471-2474-13-164.
5. Kerry R, Taylor AJ. Haemodynamics. In: McCarthy C, editor. Chapter 6 in: Combined Movement Theory. London: Elsevier; 2010. p. p79–99.
6. Romero JR, Wolf PA. Epidemiology of stroke: legacy of the framingham heart study. Glob Heart 2013;8(1):67–75.
7. Taylor AJ, George KP. Exercise induced leg pain in young athletes misdiagnosed as pain of musculoskeletal origin. Man Ther 2001;6(1):48–52.
8. Kerry R, Taylor AJ. Arterial pathology and cervicocranial pain – differential diagnosis for manual therapists and medical practitioners. Int Musculoskelet Med 2008;30(2):70–7.
9. Gottesman RF, Sharma P, Robinson KA. Clinical characteristics of symptomatic vertebral artery dissection: a systematic review. Neurologist 2012;18(5):245–54.
10. Engelter ST, Grond-Ginsbach C, Metso TM, et al. Cervical artery dissection: trauma and other potential mechanical trigger events. Neurology 2013;80(21):1950–7.
11. Lichy C, Metso A, Pezzini A, et al. Predictors of delayed stroke in patients with cervical artery dissection. Int J Stroke 2012;doi:10.1111/j.1747-4949.2012.00954.
12. Metso AJ, Metso TM, Debette S, et al. Gender and cervical artery dissection. Eur J Neurol 2012;19(4):594–602.
13. Debette S, Leys D. Cervical-artery dissections: predisposing factors, diagnosis, and outcome. Lancet Neurol 2009;8(7):668–78.
14. Cecchi E, Giglioli C, Valente S, et al. Role of hemodynamic shear stress in CV disease. Atherosclerosis 2011;214(2):249–56.

15. Anssari-Benam A, Korakianitis T. Atherosclerotic plaques: is endothelial shear stress the only factor? Med Hypotheses 2013;81(2):235–9.
16. Aboyans V, Lacroix P. Indications for carotid screening in patients with coronary artery disease. Presse Med 2009;38(6):977–86.
17. Cournot M, Boccalon H, Cambou JP, et al. Accuracy of the screening physical examination to identify subclinical atherosclerosis and peripheral arterial disease in asymptomatic subjects. J Vasc Surg 2007;46(6):1215–21.

18. Taylor AJ, Kerry R. Vascular profiling: Should manual therapists take blood pressure? Man Ther 2013;18(4):351–3.
19. Al-Obaidi SM, Asbeutah A, Al-Sayegh N, et al. To establish whether McKenzie lumbar flexion and extension mobility exercises performed in lying affect central as well as systemic hemodynamics: a crossover experimental study. Physiotherapy 2013;99(3):258–65.
20. Stanbro M, Gray BH, Kellicut DC. Carotidynia: revisiting an unfamiliar entity. Ann Vasc Surg 2011;25(8):1144–53.

CHAPTER 35.3 ■ PRE-MANIPULATIVE SCREENING FOR CRANIOCERVICAL LIGAMENT INTEGRITY

Peter Osmotherly

INTRODUCTION

Pre-manipulative screening to assess the integrity of the craniocervical junction is used to guide and alert clinicians who are considering manual treatments including end-range or high-velocity techniques to the upper cervical spine which, in the presence of hypermobility or instability, could result in adverse outcomes. The application of mechanical force in the presence of instability can result in catastrophic medical consequences[1] that may include motor incoordination,[2–4] disturbance of bladder or bowel control,[5–7] bilateral, hemilateral or quadrilateral paraesthesia or hypoaesthesia,[2,4,7–9] or even death from spinal cord compression or vascular injury secondary to excessive craniocervical range of rotation.[3,5,10]

Stability within the craniocervical complex is achieved by a complex interaction between the osseoligamentous and neuromuscular systems of this region.[11] Central to this interaction is the role of the ligaments that span the occipito-atlantoaxial complex,[12,13] particularly the transverse ligament of the atlas, the alar ligaments and the tectorial membrane.[14,15] Trauma, inflammatory disease or infection involving the craniocervical ligaments may result in injury or laxity to these structures. In conjunction with pertinent aspects of the patient history and physical examination, the performance of clinical screening tests developed to assess hypermobility or instability of the craniocervical ligaments is designed to inform the clinician to seek alternative management if appropriate, or to select treatment techniques with a lower risk of potential consequences in patients where ligamentous compromise may be suspected.[16]

SCREENING FOR CRANIOCERVICAL INSTABILITIES

The type and nature of symptoms associated with craniocervical instability are extremely diverse. One narrative literature review compiled 42 signs and symptoms associated with instability of the craniocervical region highlighting the considerable disagreement regarding the actual symptoms and signs exhibited by an individual with craniocervical ligament lesions.[16] A summary of the more commonly described signs and symptoms is given in Table 35-4. Many patients exhibit no symptoms at all, even in the presence of demonstrable instability.[4,19] In isolation, many of the described symptoms could be associated with other disorders of the cervical spine and cannot be considered indicative of craniocervical

TABLE 35-4 **Described Signs and Symptoms of Craniocervical Instability**

Symptoms	Signs
Bilateral or quadrilateral limb paraesthesia reproduced by active or passive movement[2,17,18]	Altered proprioception[2,7–9]
Buzzing in the ears/ tinnitus[18,19]	Altered sensation for vibration and deep pressure[2,7–9]
Dizziness[2,19,20]	Altered sphincter control (bladder/bowel)[5–7,14,22]
Facial pain or paraesthesia[18,19]	Pain within range of cervical motion[26–29]
Feeling of a lump in the throat[3,14,20,21]	Ataxia[2–4,14,22]
Hypoaesthesia of both hands or both feet[2]	Cardiac distress[2,30]
Metallic taste in the mouth[18]	Hyper-reflexia[7,8,14,17,31]
Nausea or vomiting[22]	Increased mobility on passive movement testing of the upper cervical spine[32]
Occipital numbness or paraesthesia[23]	Loss of cervical lordosis[26]
Paraesthesia of the lips reproduced by active or passive movement[24]	Nystagmus on head/ neck movement[8,14,19]
Popping in the ears[18]	Lingual deviation[2]
Retro-ocular pain[25]	Persistent, pain-free torticollis ('cock robin' position)[19,33]
Reflex swallowing or gagging[2]	Respiratory distress[2,30]
Upper cervical or suboccipital pain[3,19,26]	Syncope[14,17]
Pain on sudden movement of the head and neck[22]	
Vagal nerve symptoms e.g. chest and abdominal pain, tachycardia[10]	

instability on their own.[15,16,34] Currently, there is a lack of consensus as to any distinctive cluster of symptoms indicating the presence of clinical instability in this region.[4,16,35] The severity of symptoms has been reported to vary from vague discomfort to severe distress indicative of long tract compromise of the spinal cord.[17,36] Published clinical reports suggest that severe presentations are rare.[25,27,37–39] Many patients will tolerate marked instability without exhibiting neurological symptoms or signs, instead presenting with a wide variety of less severe symptoms. Furthermore, symptom severity often appears unrelated to the degree of pathological change present,[40,41] necessitating that assessment of instability occurs within a strong clinical reasoning framework.

A number of linear stress tests have been proposed to assess craniocervical ligament integrity. While descriptions of many of these tests may be found elsewhere,[9,14,15,42,43] the more commonly described linear stress tests used to assess this region are presented in Table 35-5 and discussed below.

Tests for Transverse Ligament Integrity

Sharp-Purser Test

Originally proposed as a clinical method of assessing spontaneous atlanto-axial dislocation in individuals with ankylosing spondylitis and rheumatoid arthritis, the Sharp-Purser test is commonly recommended to assess for integrity of the transverse ligament of the atlas. Interpretation of this test in its original form was that any sliding motion of the head when pressure was applied in a posterior direction indicated atlanto-axial instability.[2,14,22,39] Other descriptions of the interpretation of this test relate to symptom modification. As the test is proposed to relocate the odontoid process against the anterior arch of the atlas, it is considered that symptoms associated with this position may be relieved or ablated.[15,24,44–47] A 'clunk' on relocation of the atlas has also been interpreted as a positive finding.[15,22,24]

Exploration of the validity of this test has yielded sensitivity ranging from 43%[48] to 69%[39] and specificity from 77%[48] to 98%.[4] The higher estimate of specificity would suggest that the test, when positive, is potentially clinically useful in a rheumatoid arthritis population because of its low false-positive rate. However, estimates of both intra- and inter-observer reliability for the test are poor.[42,48] Assessments of the validity and reliability of this test have all been performed in non-traumatic populations, notably adults with rheumatoid arthritis and children with Down syndrome. While we may infer that the mechanism by which the test is proposed to be effective is the same, the applicability of the test to a traumatic population under conditions of acute pain and muscle spasm is not truly known.

Anterior Shear Test

Unlike the Sharp-Purser test, the anterior shear test is potentially a provocation test. For this reason, some authors have urged caution in its use, suggesting it should only be used in the presence of a negative Sharp-Purser

Table 35-5 Descriptions of Commonly Used Stress Tests to Assess Craniocervical Ligament Integrity

Test	Patient Position	Therapist Position	Action
Sharp-Purser test	Seated with neck relaxed in a semi-flexed position	Palm of one hand is placed on the patient's forehead Spinous process of the axis is gently fixed by a 'pinch grip' of thumb and fingertip of other hand	Using pressure of the palm on the patient's forehead, the occiput and atlas are translated posteriorly[15,26]
Anterior shear test	Supine lying with cervical spine neutrally positioned	Standing or seated at head of couch Both index fingers are placed posteriorly against the atlas and fingers III and IV resting against the occiput Axis is fixed by stabilization on the anterior aspect of the transverse processes by the clinician's thumbs	Gentle pressure is applied to the posterior arch of the atlas. The head and atlas move anteriorly as a unit while gravity fixes the lower portion of the cervical spine
Side-bending stress test	Sitting or supine	Spinous process and lamina of axis are stabilized by placing the thumb along one side of the neural arch and the index finger along the other, preventing both side-bending and rotation of the segment[14]	Slight compression is applied through the crown of the head to facilitate atlanto-occipital side-bending. Passive side-bending then applied using pressure through the patient's head[14,15,22,44] Test in upper cervical spine neutral, flexion and extension
Rotation stress test	Sitting or supine	Axis is stabilized around its lamina and spinous process using a lumbrical grip. The cranium is grasped with a wide hand span	Head rotated, the occiput taking the atlas segment with it, to the end of available range Test in upper cervical spine neutral, flexion and extension
Distraction test	Supine with head resting on a pillow	Therapist at the head of the plinth Fixate the axis around its neural arch with the lower hand Cup the occiput with the upper hand	Manual traction is then applied to the head Test in upper cervical spine neutral, flexion and extension

test.[14,22] No movement should be detected or symptoms produced on testing if the transverse ligament is normal.[14,15,17,22,45,47] An abnormal response occurs when the atlas glides forward on the axis, potentially allowing the dens to move into the space available for the spinal cord. In addition to movement, symptoms may be provoked or reproduced, including cardinal signs or a sensation of a 'lump in the throat'. A 'clunk' may indicate the atlas translating anteriorly on the axis.[14,15,22]

Although no data on the reliability or validity of this test have been published, the mechanism of the test has been demonstrated using magnetic resonance imaging to measure anterior displacement of the atlas against the axis in a normal population.[49]

Tests for Alar Ligament Integrity

Stress tests for integrity of the alar ligaments are based upon preventing the inherent coupling of rotation and lateral flexion in the occipito-atlantoaxial complex. Side-bending of the occiput on the atlas is accompanied by immediate ipsilateral rotation of the axis beneath the atlas. This rotation is proposed to result from tension generated in the alar ligaments.[50]

Side-Bending Stress Test

The side-bending stress test may be performed in sitting[44,47] or supine lying.[24] To account for variations in alar ligament orientation, testing is performed in three positions: (a) neutral posture of the upper cervical spine; (b) upper cervical flexion; and (c) upper cervical extension.[14,22] For a side-bending stress test to be considered positive for an alar ligament lesion, excessive movement in all three planes of testing should be evident.[15,22]

It has been proposed that testing in both directions is required to stress the alar ligament on one side.[22] It has been assumed that the occipital portion of the alar ligament contralaterally and the atlantal portion ipsilaterally will both be tensioned during side-bending. However, the importance of the atlantal portion of the alar ligament has recently been questioned,[51] suggesting that directing testing towards this component may be unnecessary.

Rotation Stress Test

The rotation stress test is regarded as primarily stressing the contralateral alar ligament. The test is described in both sitting[15,22] and supine lying[24] and no lateral flexion is permitted during the test. Similar to the side-bending stress test, the rotation test is repeated in positions of upper cervical spine neutral, flexion and extension, with laxity in all three positions necessary to establish a positive test finding.[15,22,24] Reports in standard textbooks of the amount of rotation that should be possible in the presence of intact alar ligaments has been inconsistent. While some rotation will occur during performance of the test, suggestions of the normal range of movement vary between 20° to 40°.[15,22,24,44,47] In the only study to quantify rotation occurring during this test, the maximum range measured using magnetic resonance imaging was 22°,[52] a finding consistent with the lower

published estimates. Cadaveric research has demonstrated a 30% increase in the range of contralateral rotation following unilateral alar ligament transection.[53] Therefore, it is possible that a person without alar ligament integrity may also have movement within these suggested ranges. This possibility presents difficulties in the interpretation of a test finding based upon range of rotation alone.

While the construct validity of both the side-bending and rotation stress tests have been demonstrated in a normal population using magnetic resonance imaging,[54] no examinations in any population of either the validity or reliability of these clinical tests in regard to detection of alar ligament lesions have been published. Investigations of this type remain unlikely in the absence of an accurate and reliable radiological gold standard for detecting and interpreting alar ligament injury.

Distraction Test for the Tectorial Membrane

Distraction testing is used to assess the integrity of the tectorial membrane because of its described role as a limiting factor in vertical translation.[55,56] The patient is positioned in supine lying with their head resting on a pillow. This is proposed to relax the upper cervical musculature[22] and to eliminate the stabilizing effect of ligamentum nuchae.[15] The test is performed in three positions with the upper cervical spine positioned in neutral, flexion where the tectorial membrane is tensioned as it passes over the tip of the dens and extension.[14,22,24]

Some movement on application of a distraction force is normal. A positive test response is considered to be excessive vertical translation when distraction is applied. Separation should not be greater than 1–2 mm.[22,24,47] There have been no examinations of the validity and reliability of this test published to date.

CONTROVERSIES IN CRANIOCERVICAL LIGAMENT TESTING

Testing for instability of the craniocervical region remains a controversial aspect of physiotherapy practice. While many authors have considered these tests to be a routine component of pre-manipulative screening for the upper cervical spine,[24,42,47] others have considered them to be provocative, potentially harmful and lacking validation.[2,7]

The predominant area of controversy regarding screening tests for this region pertains to their ability to discriminate individuals with lesions of the craniocervical ligaments from others in a neck pain population. While construct validity has been demonstrated for some of the clinical tests, little assessment of individuals with confirmed pathology of these ligaments has been undertaken. The impediment to completing this work at this time is technological. The consideration of magnetic resonance imaging being a 'gold standard' for the detection of lesions of the craniocervical ligaments has been seriously questioned due to the lack of reproducibility of interpretation of high-intensity signal changes within the cross-section of the ligaments and the consequent inability to determine pathological from normal ligaments.[57-59] Further investigation of highly reproducible methods to assess and measure ligament integrity is required before comparison of clinical tests against an acceptable reference standard may be undertaken.

The second major area of contention involves the use of tests where provocation of symptoms is required. This is particularly in regard to instability at the atlanto-axial joint. Given how rarely cardinal signs present in physiotherapy practice, rapid relocation of the atlanto-axial joint may be difficult when the clinician is working under the unfamiliar stress of a patient who may suddenly be demonstrating cardinal signs or gagging severely.[2] It is proposed that this may subject the transverse ligament to sustained stress and potentially further injury. Further, it is suggested that these tests have little practical application since patients with central nervous system signs should be appropriately referred for management elsewhere.[2] Certainly, the administration of tests to provoke cardinal signs is undesirable when there is any reasonable expectation that these symptoms may be present. However, it should be kept in mind that the tests described are screening tests designed to identify previously unidentified risk factors to manipulation in a largely unaffected population. As such, the tests are not intended to be diagnostic of craniocervical instability but rather highlight those individuals at greater risk of adverse outcome for whom other investigation and management may be instigated.

REFERENCES

1. Mathers KS, Schneider M, Timko M. Occult hypermobility of the craniocervical junction: a case report and review. J Orthop Sports Phys Ther 2011;41(6):444–57.
2. Meadows J. The Sharp-Purser test: a useful clinical tool or an exercise in futility and risk. J Man Manip Ther 1998;6(2):97–100.
3. Nguyen HV, Ludwig SC, Silber J, et al. Rheumatoid arthritis of the cervical spine. Spine J 2004;4:329–34.
4. Stevens JC, Cartlidge NEF, Saunders M, et al. Atlanto-axial subluxation and cervical myelopathy in rheumatoid arthritis. Q J Med 1971;40:391–408.
5. Meijers KAE, van Beusekom GT, Luyendijk W, et al. Dislocation of the cervical spine with cord compression in rheumatoid arthritis. J Bone Joint Surg 1974;56(B)(4):668–80.
6. Rahman N, Jamjoom ZA, Jamjoom A. Ruptured transvesre ligament: an injury that is often forgotten. Br J Neurosurg 2000;14(4):373–7.
7. Rana NA, Hancock DO, Taylor AR, et al. Atlanto-axial subluxation in rheumatoid arthritis. J Bone Joint Surg 1973;55-B(3):458–70.
8. Hensinger RN. Osseous anomalies of the craniovertebral junction. Spine 1986;11(4):323–33.
9. Mathews JA. Atlano-axial subluxation in rheumatoid arthritis. Ann Rheum Dis 1969;28:260–5.
10. Braaf M, Rosner S. Trauma of the cervical spine as a cause of chronic headache. J Trauma 1975;15(5):441–6.
11. Crisco JJI, Oda T, Panjabi MM, et al. Transections of the C1-C2 joint capsular ligaments in the cadaveric spine. Spine 1991;16(10S):S474–9.
12. Levine AM, Edwards CC. Traumatic lesions of the occipitoatlantoaxial complex. Clin Orthop Relat Res 1989;239:53–68.
13. Harris MB, Duval MJ, Davis JAJ, et al. Anatomical and roentgenographic features of atlantooccipital instability. J Spinal Disord 1993;6(1):5–10.
14. Aspinall W. Clinical testing for the craniovertebral hypermobility syndrome. J Orthop Sports Phys Ther 1990;12(2):47–54.
15. Pettman E. Stress tests of the craniovertebral joints. In: Boyling JD, Palastanga N, editors. Grieve's Modern Manual Therapy The Vertebral Column. 2nd ed. Edinburgh: Churchill Livingstone; 1994. p. 529–37.
16. Osmotherly PG, Rivett DA. Knowledge and use of craniovertebral instability testing by Australian physiotherapists. Man Ther 2011;16:357–63.
17. Meadows JTS. Orthopedic Differential Diagnosis in Physical Therapy. New York: McGraw-Hill; 1999.
18. Pettman E, editor. Subcranial Anatomy and Stress Testing the Anatomy. International Federation of Orthopaedic Manipulative Therapists 5th International Conference. Vail, Colorado; 1992.
19. Swinkels RAHM, Oostendorp RAB. Upper cervical instability: fact or fiction. J Manipulative Physiol Ther 1996;19(3):185–94.
20. Dvorak J, Hayek J, Zehnder R. CT-Functional diagnostics of the rotatory instability of the upper cervical spine. Part 2 An evaluation on healthy adults and patients with suspected instability. Spine 1987;12:726–31.
21. Coutts MB. Atlanto-epistropheal subluxations. Arch Surg 1934;29(2):297–311.
22. Beeton K. Instability in the upper cervical region; clinical presentation, radiological and clinical testing. Manipulative Physiother 1995;27(1):19–32.
23. Dugan M, Locke S, Gallagher J. Occipital neuralgia in adolescents and young adults. NEJM 1962;267:1166–72.
24. Hing W, Reid D. Cervical Spine Management. Pre-screening Requirement for New Zealand. New Zealand Manipulative Physiotherapists Association; 2004.
25. Derrick LJ, Chesworth BM. Post-motor vehicle accident alar ligament laxity. J Orthop Sports Phys Ther 1992;16(1):6–11.
26. Sharp J, Purser DW. Spontaneous atlanto-axial dislocation in ankylosing spondylitis and rheumatoid arthritis. Ann Rheum Dis 1961;20:47–77.
27. Niibayashi H. Atlantoaxial rotatory dislocation. Spine 1998;23(13):1494–6.
28. Hunter G. Non-traumatic displacement of the atlanto-axial joint. J Bone Joint Surg 1968;50-B(1):44–51.
29. Stauffer E. Subaxial injuries. Clin Orthop Relat Res 1989;239:30–9.
30. Akpinar G, Tekkok IH, Sumer M. Grisel's syndrome: a case of potentially lethal spinal cord injury in the adult. Br J Neurosurg 2002;16(6):592–6.
31. Floyd AS, Learmonth ID, Mody G, et al. Atlantoaxial instability and neurologic indicators in rheumatoid arthritis. Clin Orthop Relat Res 1989;241:177–82.
32. Kaale BR, Krakenes J, Albrektsen G, et al. Clinical assessment techniques for detecting ligament and membrane injuries in the upper cervical spine region – a comparison with MRI results. Man Ther 2008;13(5):397–403.
33. Parker DA, Selwyn P, Bradley PJ. Subluxation of the atlanto-axial joint. Br J Oral Maxillofac Surg 1985;23:275–8.
34. Rosa C, Alves M, Querios MV, et al. Neurologic involvement in patients with rheumatoid arthritis with atlatoaxial subluxation – a clinical and neuriphysiological study. J Rheumatol 1993;20:248–52.
35. Osmotherly PG, Rivett DA. Screening for craniovertebral instability; a new look at the evidence. Aust J Physiother 2005;51(4):S17.
36. Fielding JW, Griffin PP. Os odontoideum: an acquired lesion. J Bone Joint Surg 1974;56-A(1):187–90.
37. BenEliyahu DJ. Conservative management of posttraumatic cervical intersegmental hypermobility and anterior subluxation. J Manipulative Physiol Ther 1995;18(5):315–21.
38. Swinkels R, Beeton K, Alltree J. Pathogenesis of upper cervical instability. Man Ther 1996;1:127–32.
39. Uitvlugt G, Indenbaum S. Clinical assessment of atlantoaxial instability using the sharp-purser test. Arthritis Rheum 1988;31(7):918–22.
40. Castor WR, Miller JDR, Russell AS, et al. Computed tomography of the craniocervical junction in rheumatoid arthritis. J Comput Assist Tomogr 1983;7(1):31–6.
41. Grieve G. Common Vertebral Joint Problems. Edinburgh: Churchill Livingstone; 1981.
42. Cattrysse E, Swinkels RAHM, Oostendorp RAB, et al. Upper cervical instability: are clinical tests reliable? Man Ther 1997;2(2):91–7.
43. van der El A. Manuelle Diagnostiek. Rotterdam: Wervelkolom Manthel; 1992.
44. Gibbons P, Tehan P. Manipulation of the Spine, Thorax and Pelvis; An Osteopathic Perspective. Edinburgh: Churchill Livingstone; 2004.

45. Mintken PE, Metrick L, Flynn T. Upper cervical ligament testing in a patient with os odontoideum presenting with headaches. J Orthop Sports Phys Ther 2008;38(8):465–75.
46. Lincoln J. Clinical instability of the upper cervical spine. Man Ther 2000;5(1):41–6.
47. Westerhuis P. Cervical instability. In: von Piekartz HJM, editor. Craniofacial Pain Neuromusculoskeletal Assessment, Treatment and Management. Edinburgh: Butterworth Heinemann Elsevier; 2007. p. 119–47.
48. Forrester GA, Barlas P. Relaibility and validity of the sharp-purser test in the assessment of atlanto-axial instability in patients with rheumatoid arthritis. Physiotherapy 1999;85(7):376.
49. Osmotherly PG, Rivett DA, Rowe LJ. The anterior shear and distraction tests for craniocervical instability. An evaluation using magnetic resonance imaging. Man Ther 2012;17:416–21.
50. Dvorak J, Schneider E, Saldinger P, et al. Biomechanics of the craniocervical region: the alar and transverse ligaments. J Orthop Res 1988;6(3):452–61.
51. Osmotherly PG, Rivett DA, Mercer SR. Revisiting the clinical anatomy of the alar ligaments. Eur Spine J 2013;22(1):60–4.
52. Osmotherly PG, Rivett DA, Rowe LJ. Toward understanding normal craniocervical rotation occurring during the rotation stress test for the alar ligaments. Phys Ther 2013;93(7):986–92.
53. Dvorak J, Panjabi MM, Gerber M, et al. CT – functional diagnostics of the rotatory instability of upper cervical spine. 1. An experimental study on cadavers. Spine 1987;12(3):197–205.
54. Osmotherly PG, Rivett DA, Rowe LJ. Construct validity of clinical tests for alar ligament integrity: an evaluation using magnetic resonance imaging. Phys Ther 2012;92(5):718–25.
55. Werne S. Factors limiting the range of movement of the cranioverterbral joints. Acta Orthop Scand Suppl 1957;23(Pt 1):38–62.
56. White AAI, Panjabi MM. Clinical Biomechanics of the Spine. 2nd ed. Philadelphia: J.B. Lippincott Company; 1990.
57. Dullerud R, Gjertsen O, Server A. Magnetic resonance imaging of ligaments and membranes in the craniocervical junction in whiplash-associated injury and in healthy control subjects. Acta Radiol 2010;51:207–12.
58. Myran R, Kvistad KA, Nygaard OP, et al. Magnetic resonance imaging assessment of the alar ligaments in whiplash injuries. Spine 2008;33(18):2012–16.
59. Vetti N, Krakenes J, Damsgaard E, et al. Magnetic resonance imaging of the alar and transverse ligaments in acute whiplash-associated disorders 1 and 2. Spine 2011;36:E434–40.

THE BROADER SCOPE
OF MANAGEMENT

The personal and financial burden of musculoskeletal disorders is increasing worldwide, reflecting numerous factors (e.g. the ageing population, the recurrent and progressive nature of many musculoskeletal disorders and more sedentary lifestyles). Therefore, as well as conventional practitioner–patient encounters in the clinical setting, there is an increasingly broader scope to musculoskeletal physiotherapy in both the prevention and management of musculoskeletal pain to manage this global problem.

This section presents four key areas in this broader scope of patient management. The first is the concept and context of self-management that could arguably be a mandatory component of management for all patients, whether part of one-to-one patient/clinician encounters or when delivered more specifically to patient groups. The second explores the role of physiotherapy in lifestyle and health promotion in musculoskeletal conditions. This is another area where increased engagement is necessary. For people suffering musculoskeletal conditions, clinical outcomes may be improved if lifestyle and health promotion interventions for behaviours such as smoking, sub-optimal nutrition, unhealthy body mass, physical inactivity, low physical activity, sub-optimal sleep quality and quantity, and anxiety, depression and stress are included in patient management. The third chapter considers the important area of musculoskeletal health in the workplace. Here it is necessary to develop effective strategies for primary, secondary and tertiary prevention of work-related musculoskeletal disorders both to improve the workers' and management's outcomes. In the ideal world, prevention of musculoskeletal disorders would be the optimal management. No method or practice has yet achieved the ideal of prevention. Towards this ambition, the issue of musculoskeletal screening is discussed and an example of a musculoskeletal screening, testing and assessment model is presented.

Finally, over the last decade there has been a broader scope of management for physiotherapists. Advanced practice roles have developed internationally in response to increased demand and the need to provide high-quality cost-effective services. Musculoskeletal physiotherapists with appropriate knowledge and skills are ideally placed to take up these new opportunities. These roles include triage, referral for imaging and blood tests, listing for surgery, performing injections and independent prescribing. This chapter explores service models and evaluates their impact for patients as well as the health economy. It highlights professional issues associated with innovative practice and calls for further high-quality research to quantify the impact of these roles accurately as they continue to evolve.

CHAPTER 36

SUPPORTED SELF-MANAGEMENT AND AN OVERVIEW OF SELF-HELP

Ann Moore

INTRODUCTION

This chapter provides an overview of the context and definitions of self-management and self-help, and discusses the principles and theories underpinning successful self-management approaches. The perceptions of patients and clinicians of self-management and the implications of these perceptions for practice are also discussed with the main focus being on what patients' perspectives and expectations of self-management are.

CONTEXT AND DEFINITION

The concept of self-management has been around for many years in the field of health education. The term 'self-management' was first used in a text by Creer et al.[1] which focused on the rehabilitation of chronically ill children. Overall, however, there is a lack of clarity about the meaning of self-management from a range of stakeholder perspectives. Lorig and Holman[2] stressed that '*the issue of self-management is especially important for those with chronic disease, where only the patient can be responsible for his or her day to day care over the length of the illness, and for most of these people, self-management is a lifetime task*' (p. 1).[2] Lorig has much experience in the development of self-management programmes for patients with chronic disease, for example chronic arthritis. These programmes are often delivered for groups of patients and not necessarily on a one-to-one basis as is a common patient–clinician encounter in the musculoskeletal physiotherapy setting.[2]

The term self-management is often used in a similar context to 'self-help' and 'self-treatment'. The following definition of self-management by Gruman and Von Korff[3] is a helpful basis for this chapter:

> '*Self-management involves (the person with chronic disease) engaging in activities that protect and promote health, monitoring and managing symptoms and signs of illness, managing the impacts of illness on function, emotions and interpersonal relationships and adhering to treatment regimes*'.[3]

Barlow et al.[4] defined self-management as '*the individual's ability to manage the symptoms, treatment, physical and psychological consequences and lifestyle changes inherent in living with a chronic condition*' (p. 178).[4] Further, Richard and Shea[5] took the concept to a wider stance and contextualized self-management as '*the ability of the individual in conjunction with family, community and health care professionals to manage symptoms, treatments, lifestyles changes and psycho-social, cultural and spiritual consequences of health conditions*' (p. 261). This is in contrast to Richard and Shea's feelings about self-care which they contend '*broadly delineates the health lifestyle behaviours undertaken by individuals for optimal growth and development or the preventative strategies performed or maintain health*' (p. 261).[5]

Chronic disease across the world contributes to 60% of the global disease burden.[6] In terms of musculoskeletal physiotherapy, chronic low back pain, for example, has a high prevalence rate and is very costly in relation to health-care expenditure, the personal impact it has on patients, as well as the social and economic burden it places on society due to work absence and work loss.[7,8] Consequently, there is a strategic move by governments and health departments nationally and internationally to increase the focus on self-management in health services in order to reduce the impact of chronic diseases/disorders on society.[9,10] While health-service strategies are committed to reducing the burden of chronic disease on individuals and society in general, for some patients this may only be seen as a money-saving venture. In contrast, others may celebrate the move as the concept of self-management appears to support their own needs and desired personal direction.

PATIENT EDUCATION AND SELF-MANAGEMENT

For many decades, patient education has been one of the key elements of a multimodal approach to musculoskeletal patient care provided by musculoskeletal physiotherapists. Patient education is inextricably linked with self-management facilitation. Some authors, however, make the distinction between patient education and self-management education. Patient education has core components that are identifying, caring about and respecting patients' preferences, values, differences and expressed needs.[11] Self-management education, however, has been described as follows:

It should teach patients to:
- access the information they seek
- ensure they are proficient in carrying out medically related behaviours (e.g. insulin injections or using

an inhaler) and non-medically related behaviours (e.g. interacting with their doctor, exercising, etc.)
- enhance their levels of confidence (i.e. perceived self-efficacy) in their ability to engage with these behaviours
- ensure they are proficient in problem-solving.[12]

The interesting component of self-management is the understanding of the perceptions and expectations of self-management from both the patient's and the clinician's perspectives and how enmeshed or un-enmeshed they are at the first consultation. It is also important to note how these perceptions and expectations may change over time.

Self-care is distinguished from self-management as more broadly delineating healthy lifestyle behaviours undertaken by individuals for optimal growth and development, or the preventative strategies performed to promote or maintain health.[5] This is an important concept that should be considered by all musculoskeletal physiotherapists during each consultation. The concept relates to significant public health issues, for example, obesity, alcohol and drug abuse and lack of exercise.

Another two terms are linked to patient education and subsequently to patient self-management, namely self-efficacy and patient empowerment. Empowerment is an outcome of patient education as a result of which patients gain power, access to relevant resources to enable them to gain or take control over their lives.[13] Self-management education is an empowerment strategy in itself and enables patients to problem solve and make decisions about their condition and their approach to it. Self-efficacy, on the other hand, is related to patient education and is related to a person's belief or confidence in their ability to do something.[14] The two concepts are of course very much linked, as lack of self-confidence can significantly impact on self-management.

SELF-MANAGEMENT STRATEGIES

Lorig and Holman[2] identified five core self-management skills which need to be facilitated within a treatment self-management session. The five core self-management skills are:
- problem solving
- decision making
- resource utilization
- the forming of a patient/health-care provider partnership
- taking action.

Ewles and Simnett[15] made some useful suggestions as to how clinicians can help patients take more control of their health by:
- encouraging patients to make decisions
- encouraging patients to think things out for themselves
- respecting any unusual ideas that individuals may have about their health
- acceptance of individuals rather than judging them.

This means recognizing that the individual's knowledge and beliefs have emerged from their own life experiences, whereas the clinician's knowledge and beliefs have been modified and extended by their professional education and experience.

It is imperative to understand one's own (the physiotherapist's) knowledge, beliefs, values and standards, while also understanding the patient's beliefs, values and standards from their point of view and to recognize that you, the clinician, the patients and others you work with, may differ in knowledge, beliefs, values and standards. This will ensure that adequate communication occurs in the therapeutic workplace. It should be recognized that any differences do not imply that your views as a clinician are of greater worth than your patient's.[15] This is particularly relevant when considering the perceptions of self-management from both patients' and clinicians' perspectives. Some would agree, and some would not, with certain perspectives as illustrated by the work of Stenner et al.[16] The acknowledgement of differences in perspectives is vital in order to help the patient in their self-management journey.

EVIDENCE AND SELF-MANAGEMENT

In this section, some of the more recent evidence for self-management programmes will be presented. Butow and Sharpe[17] reviewed the research investigating the impact of communication on adherence to pain management strategies. Their conclusion was that although the treatment of chronic pain is challenging, good communication between health providers and patients can promote adherence and improve outcomes, and an intervention needs to be tailored to individuals' reasons for non-adherence. Du et al.[18] conducted a systematic review of 19 trials of self-management programmes for chronic musculoskeletal pain conditions. They concluded that self-management programmes have small to moderate effects on improving pain and disability in the long term but more research into self-management was needed, for example, on self-management for chronic low back pain. Since self-management as an approach is very complex and dependent on a range of factors, it is difficult to know from the review how tailored the self-management programmes included in the studies were to patient needs.

Schulman-Green et al.[19] studied processes of self-management in chronic illness. They highlighted the importance of health-care providers' ongoing communication with patients to explore their self-management preferences and how these may change over time. Their study was focused generally on chronic illness and disease and was not specific to chronic musculoskeletal conditions; however, the findings were broadly relevant to musculoskeletal patients and practitioners. They identified three categories of self-management processes and delineated the tasks and skills required for each:
- focusing on illness needs
- activating resources
- living with a chronic disease.

In a qualitative meta-synthesis of living with low back pain[20] it was found that professional and family support, self-efficacy, motivation, work conditions and exercise opportunities influenced the patient's pain experience.

This suggests that all need to be incorporated into self-management strategies in some way. Furthermore, a small qualitative study by Morris,[21] which explored patients' perspectives on self-management following a spinal rehabilitation programme, found a range of obstacles to continuing with exercise that included pain, time and family constraints. Some participants indicated that there were limitations to the extent to which their chronic low back pain would allow them to undertake certain activities and those activity limitations were perhaps inadvertently reinforced by physiotherapists in the rehabilitation sessions. Overall the study highlighted the need for very clear communication between the patient and their physiotherapist, and also the need for clinicians to have an understanding of patients' expectations and beliefs prior to engagement in a rehabilitation/self-management programme.[21]

In a qualitative study, Cooper et al.[22] explored patients' expectations of self-management of chronic low back pain. It appeared that self-management strategies that were largely focused on exercise were not always adopted by the patients/participants. There was a need for ongoing self-management support for patients following discharge to ensure that they more readily conformed to the exercises prescribed. Participants felt that physiotherapy had little influence on the management of chronic low back pain following discharge from treatment. Cooper et al.[22] concluded that self-management could be better facilitated and should include education on self-management, patient information and other aspects of patient education, as well as putting in place support for self-management via the telephone or by review appointments with the physiotherapist.

Sokunbi et al.[23] conducted a randomized controlled trial investigating the effects of stabilization exercises for patients with chronic low back pain. An extensive education programme was included in the study which was designed to facilitate self-management. It included video footage of the spine and its movements, the effects of certain positions on the spine and detailed descriptions of stabilization exercises. There were clear educational discussions with each participant on a one-to-one basis and many opportunities throughout the sessions for participants to ask questions and seek advice. The outcome of the patients' experiences of the programme was gathered using focus group interviews. Participants indicated that overall, they had found the whole process was enlightening and very positive, and that their confidence in relation to their problem had increased. The relationship that they had had with the lead researcher/clinician they felt was very open and their low back pain problems had reduced significantly. However, during the interviews it became very clear that the patients were not committed to carrying on with the management programme that they had received. They felt so much better that they wanted simply to get back to normal life and did not have the time to spend on the programme! This may indicate that the patient management programme may have lacked a key communication strategy which could help patients realize the need for ongoing self-management activities even when their pain has reduced or disappeared.[23]

Considering other delivery mediums, Zufferey and Schulz.[24] noted that patient-centred websites were useful in enhancing self-management of chronic low back pain. However, patient engagement appeared to depend on their stage of advancement in the self-management process. It seems that website information needs to be tailored to peoples' stage of self-management advancement. The authors identified and defined four types of self-management website users:

- *The selective user*: Experienced self-managers, who have a high level of awareness and experience of self-management of low back pain to good effect. Their expectation was to find tailored information on the website to further support their ongoing self-management.
- *The enthusiastic user*: Novices in self-management. They were aware that a medical cure for chronic low back pain did not exist and accepted that they had to be involved in their own care, but admitted that they did not know how to do it. They wanted the best way to deal with chronic low back pain from the website.
- *The magic user*: Passive self-managers who adhere to a traditional biomedical model of chronic low back pain, and were expecting that clinicians would find a cure/solution to their problem. They were mainly new to the problem of low back pain. This group expected the website to contain definitive solutions to the problem and, when not found, they became confused and felt discouraged.
- *The 'wait and see' user*: Latent self-managers where chronic low back pain was quite marginal and intermittent. They felt that they did not need to engage in long-term self-management.

Zufferey and Schulz.[24] concluded that information and support should be tailored to pave the way for people's stages of advancement. This indicates again the need for good communication between the clinician and the patient.

A systematic review and meta-analysis of the effectiveness of self-management of low back pain by Oliveira et al.[25] indicated that there is moderate quality evidence that self-management has a small effect on pain and disability in people with low back pain. They challenged the endorsement of self-management in treatment guidelines.[25] However, unless the approaches to self-management are clearly expressed and fully understood, it is difficult to make this challenge in a robust way.

Johnston et al.[26] provided a detailed approach to the use of self-management in facilitating workers with chronic musculoskeletal conditions to return to or remain in work. In particular, they highlighted the usefulness of the readiness to return to work scale.[27] They emphasized the need for detailed communication between the clinician and patient and the need for clinicians to ensure that they have the right skills to facilitate positive self-management behaviour in order to enable patients to return to work or stay in work. They presented a useful table of practical tips for the incorporation by clinicians of self-management into musculoskeletal practice.[26]

SELF-MANAGEMENT – PATIENTS' AND CLINICIANS' VIEWPOINTS

A recent study by our research team looked in detail at the perceptions of both patients (with chronic low back pain) and clinicians (from a variety of professions) of self-management. The work consisted of a detailed literature review (Defever et al., manuscript in preparation) and a series of focus groups involving patients and clinicians. Based on the findings, a further piece of research took place utilizing statements on self-management gleaned from the literature and from the focus group data. The study involved the use of Q-methodology[28] to explore patients' and health providers' viewpoints on the concept of self-management in the context of chronic low back pain[16] (Stenner et al. 2014, unpublished data). A set of 60 statements of opinion on self-management of chronic low back pain was developed (a 'Q set'). Subsequently, a wider group of stakeholders, which included 60 patients with chronic low back pain and 60 health-care practitioners, ranked the statements on a continuum from 'strongly agree' to 'strongly disagree' ('Q-sort'). The data were analysed by the research team which included clinicians, researchers and service users. What emerged from the data were four distinct viewpoints on self-management in chronic low back pain. The four viewpoints were:

- *'Changing myself'*: This viewpoint took a strong psychological approach, needing a lifestyle/mind-set change. This viewpoint was the largest perspective expressed mainly by health-care providers but also shared by some patients.
- *'Changing what I do'*: This was a strongly pragmatic approach to self-management guided by accurate information and practical strategies. This viewpoint was shared mostly by patients and some health-care practitioners.
- *'Not sure what to change'*: This viewpoint focused on managing medical uncertainty with a need for access to health-care resources and assistance. This was expressed mostly by patients and a few health-care providers.
- *'The others must change'*: This viewpoint was based on a concern with the stigmatic perception of being in chronic pain, with reliance on health-care providers to acknowledge and validate their problem. This viewpoint was only voiced by patients.

Overall, the study provided valuable insights into the diversity, complexity and tensions in and between viewpoints in relation to self-management in chronic low back pain. It shows that it is essential to address these issues and the resulting differences in expectations of care and self-management in order to establish more successful engagement in and accomplishment of effective self-management. Further research in education is needed both for those experiencing problems and those providing services to support the process of achieving effective and inclusive self-management in chronic low back pain, and most likely in a range of musculoskeletal conditions.

DISCUSSION

Clearly the philosophies, structures and processes associated with self-management are well grounded, but all those involved in facilitating self-management must be fully aware of these models and approaches, and develop strategies to incorporate them into routine day-to-day practice. In this context, the definitions of and approaches to empowerment and self-efficacy are very important.

Self-management should not be seen as a separate entity from an overall assessment and treatment strategy. There are a series of stages in a successful treatment pathway and self-management has to be part of these. Many stages of a successful treatment pathway depend on clear two-way communication between the clinician and the patient which was clearly articulated some years ago in a UK Department of Health document; *'the importance of patients may not always be appreciated by patients who feel talked at rather than listened to'*.[29] This led to the priority for more patient information, greater patient choice and more patient-centredness.[29]

The patient care continuum of Barr and Threlkeld[30] is a useful model in terms of the balance of patient/clinician partnership. The continuum has high control which is clinician-centred at one end of the spectrum and high control which is patient-centred at the other end of the continuum. Patient/clinician partnership is developed and comes to the fore throughout the treatment continuum. Early in treatment, there often needs to be a strong clinician-centred approach followed quickly by the development of a patient/clinician partnership. This then leads to patients' high control related to empowerment of self-efficacy and successful self-management strategies.

The importance of good-quality, effective and timely communication has been highlighted over the years. Richardson and Moran[31] suggest that good-quality communication can lead to patients' empowerment, advancement, enhancement of quality of care, improved patient satisfaction, improved health outcomes and modification of practice in response to patients' needs.[31] Some of the complexities of communication and its use in clinical practice are addressed in Chapter 27a.

Clinicians need to demonstrate good knowledge of the area, high-quality therapeutic skills, communication skills and also listening skills. Clinicians should offer high-quality tailored explanations, education and advice to patients, as well as clear guidance on the therapist's role. A consultative process within treatment sessions should be adopted. The facility of a flexible appointment system with 'SOS' appointment availability is important, particularly for patients who are at one end of the spectrum in their preparedness for self-management processes. Patients need to be facilitated to empower themselves. Self-efficacy needs to be facilitated in relation to behavioural change. It is important that clinicians give time to ensuring that these foci are addressed. This can present quite a challenge in some health services where, to become cost-effective, the numbers of treatments and treatment time available to patients is being reduced! Another challenge to self-management relates to the lack of, or low level of, pre-qualification training/education in patient education theories and practices. Post-registration, Masters level modules/courses are quite widely available but these are taken up only by a small percentage of clinicians. This is an important area for future development.

Fundamentally, successful self-management by patients is the result of patient-focused care in which the balance of the therapeutic partnership, consisting of trust, respect and understanding of patients' ideas, beliefs, knowledge and values, is in place, when patients are involved in decision making and also when patients' needs and expectations are shared and discussed and their expression of these is encouraged and facilitated. The issue for some clinicians working in some health service environments may be the time availability to engage with the patient at a personal level in order to explore their viewpoints on self-management and their learning needs in relation to resources, to help them decide on what approach to self-management would be best suited to their needs. This needs time which, well spent, could potentially be personally beneficial to the patient and cost effective for governments and health services if patients self-manage effectively and do not then need to receive or request further referrals for treatment. Having the opportunity for a review contact (i.e. SOS appointments) would lead to improved patient confidence in the support available to them and would also give clinicians insight to whether their approaches to self-management are being effective. The most important message from this chapter is the need for both the clinician and the patient to understand the range of perceptions of self-management that exist, and for clinicians to understand that the patient may be in a very different place along their perception of self-management according to their stage of advancement[24] which will alter their perception of self-management. If clinicians can understand this spectrum of perceptions of self-management and make time to explore the patients' position then this is likely to lead to an improved take up of a well-tailored self-management strategy.

Patient education skills play an important role in self-management, empowerment and self-efficacy. However, the term patient education is often used loosely in clinical practice so that clinicians very often take a didactic approach to education with little recognition of the patient's needs and learning styles. It is likely that more educational philosophies, principles and methods should be incorporated into health professionals' undergraduate and postgraduate curricula. The issue of patient education is discussed in Chapter 27b.

SUMMARY

This chapter has highlighted a number of issues relating to self-management. Firstly, there are a number of definitions associated with self-management and self-care which need to be clarified for the users. Secondly, there is a range of different interpretations and usages of the term self-management and self-care. Thirdly, there may not be a full understanding of the variety of viewpoints that might be held by all those involved in the self-management process. Unless detailed and clear communication can be held acknowledging that there may be differences in the perceptions of self-management, then self-management is unlikely to increase its effectiveness. Finally, it is important that all clinicians recognize that their perceptions, expectations and perspectives on self-management can vary considerably from those of their patients. It is extremely important that practitioners can spend time, at the initial meeting with their patients, to understand where they are coming from in terms of their perspectives on self-management and, indeed, on patient education.

REFERENCES

1. Creer T, Renne C, Christian W. Behavioral contributions to rehabilitation and childhood asthma. Rehabil Lit 1976;37:226–32.
2. Lorig KR, Holman HR. Self-management education: history, definition, outcomes, and mechanisms. Anns Behav Med 2003;26:1–7.
3. Gruman J, Von Korff M. Indexed Bibliography on Self-Management for People with Chronic Disease. Washington, DC: Center for Advancement in Health; 1996.
4. Barlow JH, Wright CC, Sheasby J, et al. Self-management approaches for people with chronic conditions: a review. Patient Educ Couns 2002;48:177–87.
5. Richard A, Shea K. Delineation of self-care and associated concepts. J Nurs Scholarsh 2011;43:255–64.
6. Murray CJL, Lopez AD, editors. The Global Burden of Disease: A Comprehensive Assessment of Mortality and Disability from Diseases, Injuries and Risk Factors in 1990 and Projected to 2020. Cambridge, MA: Harvard University Press on behalf of the World Health Organization and the World Bank; 1996.
7. Katz JN. Lumbar disc disorders and low-back pain: socioeconomic factors and consequences. J Bone Joint Surg Am 2006;88(Suppl. 2):21–4.
8. Johannes CB, Le TK, Zhou X, et al. The prevalence of chronic pain in United States adults: results of an internet-based survey. J Pain 2010;11:1230–9.
9. Department of Health. The Expert Patient: A New Approach to Chronic Disease Management for the 21st Century. London: Department of Health; 2001.
10. Department of Health. Self-Care – A Real Choice Self-Care Support: A Practical Option. London: Department of Health; 2005.
11. Barlow JH. How to use education as an intervention in osteoarthritis. In: Docherty M, Dougados M, editors. Osteoarthritis: Balliere's Best Practice and Research. London: Harcourt; Clinical Rheumatology, 15(4), 545–558; 2001.
12. World Health Organization. Preparing a Health Care Workforce for the 21st Century: The Challenge of Chronic Conditions. Geneva: WHO; 2005.
13. Lorig K. Self-management of chronic illness: a model for the future. Generations 1993;XVII(3):11–14.
14. Bandura A. Self-Efficacy: The Exercise of Control. New York: Freeman; 1977.
15. Ewles L, Simnett I. Promoting Health: A Practical Guide. 5th ed. Edinburgh: Ballière Tindall; 2003.
16. Stenner P, Cross V, McCrum CA, et al. Patient and healthcare provider viewpoints on the concepts of self-management in the context of chronic low back pain. Submitted for review in Social Science and Medicine (in review).
17. Butow P, Sharpe L. The impact of communication on adherence in pain management. Pain 2013;154:S101–7.
18. Du S, Yuan C, Xiao X, et al. Self-management programs for chronic musculoskeletal pain conditions: a systematic review and meta-analysis. Patient Educ Couns 2011;85:299–e310.
19. Schulman-Green D, Jaser S, Martin F, et al. Processes of self-management in chronic illness. J Nurs Scholarsh 2012;44:136–44.
20. Snelgrove S, Liossi C. Living with chronic low back pain: a metasynthesis of qualitative research. Chronic Illn 2013;9(4):283–301.

21. Morris AL. Patients' perspectives on self-management following a back rehabilitation programme. Musculoskeletal Care 2004;2(3):165–79.

22. Cooper K, Smith BH, Hancock E. Patients' perceptions of self-management of chronic low back pain: evidence for enhancing patient education and support. Physiotherapy 2009;95(1):43–50.

23. Sokunbi O, Cross V, Watt P, et al. A randomised controlled trial (RCT) on the effects of frequency of application of spinal stabilisation exercises on multifidus cross sectional area (MFCSA) in participants with chronic low back pain. Physiotherapy Singapore 2008;11(2):9–17.

24. Zufferey MC, Schulz PJ. Self-management of chronic low back pain: an exploration of the impact of a patient-centered website. Patient Educ Couns 2009;77(1):27–32.

25. Oliveira VC, Ferreira PH, Maher CG, et al. Effectiveness of self-management of low back pain: systematic review with meta-analysis. Arthritis Care & Research 2012;64(11):1739–48.

26. Johnston V, Jull G, Sheppard DM, et al. Applying principles of self-management to facilitate workers to return to or remain at work with a chronic musculoskeletal condition. Masterclass. Man Ther 2013;18(4):274–80.

27. Franche RL, Corbiere M, Lee H, et al. Readiness for Return-To-Work (RRTW) scale: development and validation of a self-report staging scale in lost-time claimants with musculoskeletal disorders. J Occup Rehabil 2007;17(3):450–72.

28. Stenner P, Stainton Rogers R. Q methodology and qualiquantology: the example of discriminating between emotions. In: Todd Z, Nerlich B, McKeown S, et al., editors. Mixing Methods in Psychology: The Integration of Qualitative and Quantitative Methods in Theory and Practice. Hove, UK: Psychology Press; 2004. p. 101–20.

29. Department of Health. The NHS Plan. London: Stationery Office; 2000.

30. Barr J, Threlkeld JA. Patient-practitioner collaboration in clinical decision-making. Physiother Res Int 2002;5:254–60.

31. Richardson KE, Moran S. Developing standards for patient information. Int J Health Care Qual Assur 1995;8(7):27–31.

CHAPTER 37

ROLE OF PHYSIOTHERAPY IN LIFESTYLE AND HEALTH PROMOTION IN MUSCULOSKELETAL CONDITIONS

Elizabeth Dean • Anne Söderlund

INTRODUCTION

There are two principal reasons why physiotherapists who specialize in musculoskeletal conditions, including treatment of spinal conditions, need to address risk factors for non-communicable diseases (NCDs) in their patients, which include ischaemic heart disease, smoking-related conditions, hypertension, stroke and cancer. Firstly, risk factors for back problems are comparable to those for NCDs (i.e. smoking, prolonged sitting, inactivity, being overweight, and depression and stress).[1,2] Secondly, contemporary physiotherapists focus on the comprehensive care of their patients consistent with the International Classification of Functioning, Disability and Health (ICF).[3] In this chapter, the authors translate evidence-based knowledge about the association between healthy living and musculoskeletal health that was synthesized in Chapter 11, to the musculoskeletal physiotherapy context. They first outline assessment and evaluation tools for lifestyle-related health practices and risk factors, and then strategies and interventions for health behaviour change that can be readily integrated into physiotherapists' practices. Attention to alcohol and drug abuse is beyond the scope of this chapter. Many of the behaviour change principles presented in this chapter may, however, be used to support change in these behaviours as well. Although other professionals may be primarily involved, the physiotherapist has a role in supporting and following their initiatives.

CLUSTERING OF UNHEALTHY LIFESTYLE-RELATED BEHAVIOURS AND RISKS

The clustering of commonalities among lifestyle-related NCDs, including chronic systemic low-grade inflammation[4] and contributing factors, have become a focus in the literature.[5-7] Understanding the role of the commonalities of these conditions provides valuable insight into best practices for their prevention, reversal and management.

PHYSIOTHERAPISTS AS HEALTH ADVOCATES

Motivating a patient to change health behaviour can appear daunting both to the physiotherapist and the patient. They both should be encouraged by the fact that healthy lifestyle practices and health benefits are dose-dependent.[8] Although strict dietary and activity changes do need to be instituted to reverse atherosclerosis,[8,9] high blood pressure,[10] type 2 diabetes mellitus[11] and reduce the growth of some tumors,[12] partial changes have substantial benefits.

HEALTH AND RISK ASSESSMENTS AND INTERVENTIONS

To comprehensively manage the needs of a person experiencing symptoms arising from the musculoskeletal system, the physiotherapist first needs to assess that person's health and lifestyle health practices. Based on these assessments, appropriate health education interventions may be negotiated between the physiotherapist and patient. Consistent with the ICF adopted by the World Confederation for Physical Therapy, a holistic approach is indicated with health as the base (see Chapter 11). Based on this perspective, physiotherapy assessment should include assessments of health, lifestyle-related health behaviours, lifestyle-related health risk, as well as any manifestations of lifestyle-related conditions (i.e. the signs and symptoms that constitute part of conventional physiotherapy management) (Box 37-1). The elements of these assessments are described below with the exception of the manifestations of lifestyle-related conditions, which is considered to be a fundamental physiotherapy practice whose resources can be found elsewhere.

Health Assessment

Health is a multifactorial construct, thus there is no single metric to quantify it. The ICF has provided guidance to clinicians to consider its multiple determinants

BOX 37-1	Tools for Assessing Health Status

GLOBAL HEALTH STATUS

> Short Form 12 and Short Form 36
> Health-related quality of life tools
> Life satisfaction tools

HEALTH-RELATED BEHAVIOUR ASSESSMENT/EVALUATION

> Health behaviours including smoking questionnaires (e.g. WISDOM and The WHY Test; and smoking abstinence self-efficacy questionnaire)
> Nutrition logs (in accordance with national food guidelines, e.g. Canada's Food Guide[13])
> Physical activity and exercise logs (in accordance with physical activity pyramid)
> Exercise self-efficacy assessment
> Sleep questionnaires
> Stress questionnaires

RISK FACTOR ASSESSMENT/EVALUATION FOR THE LIFESTYLE-RELATED CONDITIONS

> Ischaemic heart disease risk factor assessments (e.g. Grundy et al. 1999[14] and Harvard School of Public Health Disease Risk website[15])

ASSESSMENT/EVALUATION OF THE MANIFESTATIONS OF LIFESTYLE-RELATED CONDITIONS

> Established medical and surgical history taking
> Assessment and evaluation methods

and assess these and evaluate changes in them at its various levels (i.e. function and structure, activity and participation; see Chapter 11, Fig. 11-1).

Despite its limitations, self-report is typically how an individual's overall health and wellness are assessed. Functional status and independence are central to people's overall health and well-being, and these indices are reported to be singularly important within a social context (e.g. social participation, life satisfaction and health-related quality of life).

Assessment of Lifestyle-Related Health Behaviours

Lifestyle-related health behaviours are strongly associated with health status (see Chapter 11). Assessment of health behaviours (Fig. 37-1) enables the physiotherapist to identify the adequacy of the quality and quantity of these behaviours in terms of maximizing health (i.e. achieving the highest status possible at each level of the ICF and self-reported quality of life). They include the individual's status related to smoking, nutrition, body composition, activity and exercise, sleep, and anxiety, depression and stress. Assessment of lifestyle behaviours has some benefit over risk factor assessment for specific NCDs. The field of risk factor assessment is advancing rapidly with established tools being revised and new ones emerging. Thus tracking patients' risks over time or using these tools as outcome measures may be challenging. Basic lifestyle recommendations for maximal health (Box 37-2) are changing less quickly and dramatically than for risk factor assessment tools, therefore assessment

of lifestyle behaviours itself may be a superior focus than risk factor assessment.

Lifestyle-Related Health Risk Assessment

There are multiple health risk assessment tools. These typically focus on risk for a particular NCD (e.g. ischaemic heart disease, hypertension, stroke, type 2 diabetes mellitus and cancer). It is not feasible for the physiotherapist to administer all disease-specific risk assessment tools to every patient. Given there are common risks for these lifestyle-related conditions, assessment of risk factors for common lifestyle-related conditions however can yield important information. For example, the Canadian Diabetes Risk Questionnaire or CANRISK[17] has 12 items (Fig. 37-2). The questionnaire can be readily completed by the patient without the need for invasive procedures and blood tests, which some risk assessment tools require. CANRISK may be used to assess general lifestyle-related disease risk including type 2 diabetes mellitus. This tool has been expanded for use by Canadian pharmacists and this version also has utility for physiotherapists;[18] recommendations for specific interventions based on the individual's response are described. Other tools that are clinically applicable include cardiovascular disease risk[14] and stroke risk.[19] Also, a range of lifestyle-related risk factor tools can be accessed from the Harvard University School of Public Health website (e.g. heart disease, stroke, diabetes, cancer and osteoporosis).[15] Routine use of one of these tools, such as CANRISK, can provide a general assessment of lifestyle-related health and disease risk, and be used to evaluate change over time with health behaviour change intervention education and other physiotherapy or medical/surgical interventions. They also serve as effective patient education tools.

Multisystem Review

The multisystem review (Fig. 37-3) can be an effective way of identifying risk factors and the presence of chronic co-morbid conditions expediently, with the opportunity for more detailed questioning of the patient. Three levels of information can be gleaned that elucidate contributors to presenting musculoskeletal complaints, and insight into how these can be best managed. Firstly, the physiotherapist can identify lifestyle-related, non-musculoskeletal causes and conditions that contribute to a patient's musculoskeletal complaints; secondly, lifestyle-related non-musculoskeletal conditions that can be adversely affected by back complaints (e.g. a person with NCDs or their risk factors reducing activity level); and thirdly, insights into the 'best' strategies for managing patient's back pain including lifestyle behaviour change with traditional management, or alone.

Vital sign measurement has become an essential component of contemporary physiotherapy assessment. Heart rate and blood pressure are key indicators of physical health status and health risk.[20,21] These need to be recorded at the patient's initial visit and then as indicated.

Text continued on p. 371

Smoking
❑ Non-smoker   ❑ Life-long non-smoker

❑ Past smoker Amount: ❑ <½ pk/day   ❑ between ½ to 1 pk/day   ❑ between 1–2 pk/day   ❑ >2 pk/day

❑ I smoke.   Amount: ❑ >20 cigarettes/day   ❑ between 10 and 20 cigarettes/day   ❑ <10 cigarettes/day
                Duration: ❑ <5yr   ❑ 6–9 yr   ❑ 10–19 yr   ❑ >19 yr

If you smoke, what would help you to quit smoking?
    ❑ Counselling   ❑ Medication to help ❑ Knowledge of quitting methods   ❑ Will power   ❑ Support from a professional
    ❑ Fewer worries and stress   ❑ Other_____

If you don't smoke, are you exposed to the smoke of someone in your household or work place that smokes?
    ❑ No   ❑ Yes If yes, how much for how long_____

Plan: Smoking cessation

Diet and Nutrition
Body Composition

Weight (kg)_____   Height (m)_____   Body mass index (BMI (kg/m^2)_____   Waist girth (cm)_____
Hip girth_____   Waist–hip ratio (WHR)_____
Goal: WHR <85 cm for women and <90 cm for men

Plan: Achieve Recommended Food Guide Servings

Nutrition (example based on the Canada Food Guide [Health Canada[13]])

	Recommended Number of Food Guide Servings per Day*								
	Children			**Teens**		**Adults**			
	2–3	4–8	9–13	14–18 Years		19–50 Years		51+ Years	
	Girls and Boys			Female	Male	Female	Male	Female	Male
Vegetables and Fruit	4	5	6	7	8	7–8	8–10	7	7
Grain Products	3	4	6	6	7	6–7	8	6	7
Milk and Alternatives	2	2	3–4	3–4	3–4	2	2	3	3
Meat and Alternatives	1	1	1–2	2	3	2	3	2	3

*Serving Sizes for Each Food Group:

Vegetables and Fruit
125 mL (½ cup) fresh, frozen or canned vegetable or fruit or 100% juice
250 mL (1 cup) leafy raw vegetables or salad
1 piece of fruit

Grain Products
1 slice (35 g) bread or ½ bagel (45 g)
½ pita (35 g) or ½ tortilla (35 g)
125 mL (½ cup) cooked rice, pasta, or couscous
30 g cold cereal or 175 mL (¾ cup) hot cereal

Milk and Alternatives
250 mL (1 cup) milk or fortified soy beverage
175 g (¾ cup) yogurt
50 g (1½ oz.) cheese

Meat and Alternatives
75 g (2 ½ oz.)/125 mL (½ cup) cooked fish, shellfish, poultry or lean meat
175 mL (¾ cup) cooked beans
2 eggs
30 mL (2 Tbsp) peanut butter

FIGURE 37-1 ▩ Assessment of lifestyle-related health behaviours.

Physical Activity

Hours sitting with minimal activity in typical work day_____
Steps/day (measured by valid pedometer reading)_____
Weekly hours of structured exercise_____

During a week, how often do you accumulate at least 30 minutes of moderately intense physical activity a day. Circle the number of days that you achieve this?

0   1   2   3   4   5   6   7

0–2 days: design a walking plan
3–4 days: if not adding up to 150 minutes, introduce additional brisk walks and regular activity on another couple of days
5+ days: Goal met

Plan: Goal of at least 150 minutes of moderately intense activity a week (2008 Physical Activity Guidelines[14])

*Recommendation may need to be modified based on patient's disability and progressed accordingly under the physiotherapist's supervision
Strengthening exercise_____

Sleep

Hours sleep/typical night_____
Times up during a typical night_____
Feels restored in the morning (0 is not at all to 10 maximally restored)_____
Sleep Inventory (Coren 2009[15]) to assess sleep quality and sleep debt: Score:_____

Plan: Achieve optimal sleep between 7 and 10 hours depending on the individual

Stress

Self-rated daily stress 0 (none) to 10 (maximal, unbearable)_____
Stress triggers_____ Stress relievers_____
Psychological Stress Measure-9 (Lemyre et al 2009[16]) score:_____
Holmes-Rahe Stress Test[17] score:_____

Plan: Achieve manageable stress levels

FIGURE 37-1, cont'd

BOX 37-2	Guidelines on Nutrition and Physical Activity for Prevention of All-Cause Premature Mortality and Related Morbidity

ACHIEVE AND MAINTAIN A HEALTHY WEIGHT THROUGHOUT LIFE

Be as lean as possible throughout life without being underweight

Avoid excess weight gain at all ages. For those who are overweight or obese, losing even a small amount of weight has health benefits and is a good place to start

Get regular physical activity and limit intake of high-calorie foods and drinks as keys to help maintain a healthy weight

BE PHYSICALLY ACTIVE

Adults

Get at least 150 minutes of moderate intensity or 75 minutes of vigorous intensity activity each week (or a combination of these), preferably spread throughout the week

Children and Teens

Get at least 1 hour of moderate or vigorous intensity activity each day, with vigorous activity on at least 3 days each week

Limit sedentary behaviour such as sitting, lying down, watching TV and other forms of screen-based entertainment

Doing some physical activity above usual activities, no matter what one's level of activity, can have many health benefits

EAT A HEALTHY DIET, WITH AN EMPHASIS ON PLANT FOODS

Choose foods and drinks in amounts that help you get to and maintain a healthy weight

Limit how much processed meat and red meat you eat

Eat at least 2½ cups of vegetables and fruits each day

Choose whole grains instead of refined grain products

IF YOU DRINK ALCOHOL, LIMIT YOUR INTAKE

Drink no more than one drink per day for women or two per day for men

SOURCE: *McCullough et al, 2011; American Cancer Society. American Cancer Society guidelines on nutrition and physical activity for cancer prevention, <http://www.cancer.org/cancer/news/news/cancer-prevention-guidelines-also-helpful-against-other-diseases>.*[16]

THE **CANADIAN** DIABETES
RISK QUESTIONNAIRE

CANRISK

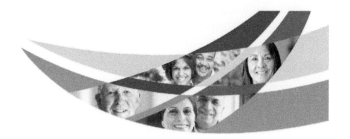

→ Are you at risk?

The following questions will help you to find out if you are at higher risk of having pre-diabetes or type 2 diabetes. Pre-diabetes is a condition where a person's blood sugar levels are higher than normal, but not high enough to be diagnosed as diabetes. You can have pre-diabetes or undiagnosed type 2 diabetes without having any obvious warning signs or symptoms.

Knowing your risk can help you make healthy choices now that will reduce your risk or even prevent you from developing diabetes.

Please answer the questions as honestly and completely as you can. If you wish, a friend or family member can help you to complete this form. The answers to these questions are completely confidential. Answer all questions. Enter your scores for each question in the box on the right-hand side and then add them up to calculate your total risk score.

This questionnaire is intended for adults aged 40 to 74 years.

→ AS YOU GET OLDER, YOUR RISK OF DEVELOPING DIABETES GOES UP.

		Score

1. **Select your age group:**
   - ○ 40-44 years — **0 points**
   - ○ 45-54 years — **7 points**
   - ○ 55-64 years — **13 points**
   - ○ 65-74 years — **15 points**

2. **Are you male or female?**
   - ○ Male — **6 points**
   - ○ Female — **0 points**

→ BODY SHAPE AND SIZE CAN AFFECT YOUR RISK OF DIABETES.

3. **How tall are you and how much do you weigh?**
   On the left-hand side of the BMI chart below, circle your height, then on the bottom of the chart circle your weight.
   Find the square on the chart where your height crosses with your weight, and note which shaded area you fall into.
   For example, if you were 5 feet 2 inches (or 157.5cm) and 163 pounds (or 74kg) you would fall in the LIGHT GREY area.

   Select your BMI group from the following choices:
   - ○ White (BMI less than 25) — **0 points**
   - ○ Light grey (BMI 25 to 29) — **4 points**
   - ○ Dark grey (BMI 30 to 34) — **9 points**
   - ○ Black (BMI 35 and over) — **14 points**

HEIGHT
feet/inches cm

6'4"	192.5	12 13 13 14 15 16 17 18 18 19 20 21 22 22 23 24 24 26 26 27 28 29 29 30 31 32 33 34
6'3"	190	12 13 14 15 16 16 17 18 19 20 20 21 22 23 24 24 25 26 27 28 29 29 30 31 32 33 34 34
6'2"	187.5	13 13 14 15 16 17 18 18 19 20 21 22 23 24 24 25 26 27 28 29 29 30 31 32 33 34 34 36
6'1"	185	13 14 15 15 16 17 18 19 20 21 22 22 23 24 25 26 27 28 29 29 30 31 32 33 34 34 36 37
6'0"	182.5	13 14 15 16 17 18 19 20 20 21 22 23 24 24 26 27 28 29 29 30 31 32 33 34 34 36 37 38
5'11"	180	14 15 15 16 17 18 19 20 21 22 23 24 24 26 27 27 28 29 30 31 32 33 34 34 36 37 38 39
5'10"	177.5	14 15 16 17 18 19 20 21 22 23 24 25 26 27 28 29 30 31 32 33 34 34 36 37 38 39 40
5'9"	175	14 15 16 17 18 19 20 21 22 23 24 25 26 27 28 29 30 31 32 33 34 34 36 37 38 39 40 41
5'8"	172.5	15 16 17 18 19 20 21 22 23 24 24 26 27 28 29 29 31 32 33 34 36 37 38 39 40 41 42
5'7"	170	15 16 17 18 19 20 21 22 24 24 26 27 28 29 31 32 33 34 34 36 37 38 39 40 41 42 43
5'6"	167.5	16 17 18 19 20 21 22 23 24 25 26 27 29 29 31 32 33 34 34 36 37 38 39 40 41 42 43 45
5'5"	165	16 17 18 19 21 22 23 24 24 26 27 28 29 30 32 33 34 34 36 37 38 39 40 42 43 44 45 46
5'4"	162.5	17 18 19 20 21 22 23 24 26 27 28 29 30 31 33 34 34 36 37 38 39 41 42 43 44 45 46 47
5'3"	160	17 18 20 21 22 23 24 25 27 28 29 30 31 32 34 36 37 38 39 41 42 43 44 45 46 48 49
5'2"	157.5	18 19 20 21 23 24 26 27 29 29 31 32 33 34 36 37 38 40 41 42 43 44 46 47 48 49 50
5'1"	155	18 20 21 22 23 24 26 27 28 29 31 32 33 34 36 37 38 40 41 42 43 45 46 47 48 50 51 52
5'0"	152.5	19 20 21 23 24 25 27 28 29 31 32 33 34 36 37 38 40 41 42 43 45 46 48 49 50 51 52 54
4'11"	150	20 21 22 24 24 26 28 29 30 32 33 34 36 37 38 40 41 42 44 45 46 48 49 50 52 53 54 56
4'10"	147.5	20 22 23 24 26 27 28 29 31 33 34 35 37 38 40 41 42 43 46 47 48 49 51 52 53 55 57 58
4'9"	145	21 22 24 25 27 28 29 31 32 35 37 38 39 41 42 44 45 47 48 49 51 52 54 55 57 58 59
4'8"	142.5	22 23 24 26 28 29 31 32 33 34 36 38 39 41 42 44 45 47 48 50 51 53 54 56 57 59 60 62

WEIGHT (kg)	44 47 50 53 56 59 62 65 68 71 74 77 80 83 86 89 92 95 98 101 104 107 110 113 116 119 122 125
WEIGHT (lbs)	97 103 110 117 123 130 136 143 150 156 163 169 176 183 189 196 202 209 216 222 229 235 242 249 255 262 268 275

4. **Using a tape measure, place it around your waist at the level of your belly button.**
   Measure after breathing out (do not hold your breath) and write your results on the line below.
   Then check the box that contains your measurement. (Note: this is not the same as the "waist size" on your pants).

   MEN – Waist circumference: ___ ___ ___ inches OR ___ ___ ___ cm
   - ○ Less than 94 cm or 37 inches — **0 points**
   - ○ Between 94-102 cm or 37-40 inches — **4 points**
   - ○ Over 102 cm or 40 inches — **6 points**

   WOMEN – Waist circumference: ___ ___ ___ inches OR ___ ___ ___ cm
   - ○ Less than 80 cm or 31.5 inches — **0 points**
   - ○ Between 80-88 cm or 31.5-35 inches — **4 points**
   - ○ Over 88 cm or 35 inches — **6 points**

Public Health Agency of Canada
Agence de la santé publique du Canada

Canada

FIGURE 37-2 ■ **Prototype of a lifestyle-related health risk assessment tool: CANRISK.** (Source: The Canadian Diabetes Risk Assessment Questionnaire. Public Health Agency of Canada; 2009. <http://www.diabetes.ca/documents/for-professionals/NBI-CANRISK.pdf>.[17]) (Source: © All rights reserved. Public Health Agency of Canada. Reproduced with permission from the Minister of Health, 2014.)

→ YOUR LEVEL OF PHYSICAL ACTIVITY AND WHAT YOU EAT CAN AFFECT YOUR RISK OF DEVELOPING DIABETES.

Score

5. **Do you usually do some physical activity such as brisk walking for at least 30 minutes each day?**
This activity can be done while at work or at home.
○ Yes   0 points
○ No   1 point

6. **How often do you eat vegetables or fruits?**
○ Every day   0 points
○ Not every day   2 points

→ HIGH BLOOD PRESSURE, HIGH BLOOD SUGAR, AND PREGNANCY-RELATED FACTORS ARE ASSOCIATED WITH DIABETES.

7. **Have you ever been told by a doctor or nurse that you have high blood pressure OR have you ever taken high blood pressure pills?**
○ Yes   4 points
○ No or don't know   0 points

8. **Have you ever been found to have a high blood sugar either from a blood test, during an illness, or during pregnancy?**
○ Yes   14 points
○ No or don't know   0 points

9. **Have you ever given birth to a large baby weighing 9 pounds (4.1 kg) or more?**
○ Yes   1 point
○ No, don't know, or not applicable   0 points

→ SOME TYPES OF DIABETES RUN IN FAMILIES.

10. **Have any of your blood relatives ever been diagnosed with diabetes?**
Check ALL that apply.
○ Mother   2 points
○ Father   2 points
○ Brothers/Sisters   2 points
○ Children   2 points
○ Other   0 points
○ No/don't know   0 points

Add your score.
Your combined score cannot be more than 8 points.
(2 points for each category, do not count multiple children or siblings twice).

11. **Please check off which of the following ethnic groups your biological (blood) parents belong to:**
MOTHER FATHER
○ ○ White (Caucasian)   0 points
○ ○ Aboriginal   3 points
○ ○ Black (Afro-Caribbean)   5 points
○ ○ East Asian (Chinese, Vietnamese, Filipino, Korean, etc.) 10 points
○ ○ South Asian (East Indian, Pakistani, Sri Lankan, etc.)   11 points
○ ○ Other non-white (Latin American, Arab, West Asian)   3 points

Choose only one score, the highest.
Do not add mother plus father scores together. (Your score cannot be more than 11 points for this section).

→ OTHER FACTORS ARE ALSO RELATED TO DEVELOPING DIABETES.

12. **What is the highest level of education that you have completed?**
○ Some high school or less   5 points
○ High school diploma   1 point
○ Some college or university   0 points
○ University or college degree   0 points

Total Score

Add up your points from questions 1 to 12

These risk scores are in no way a substitute for actual clinical diagnosis.
If you have any concerns, please consider discussing your results with a health care practitioner (eg. family doctor, nurse practitioner, pharmacist).

Lower than 21 → low risk	21-32 → moderate risk	33 and over → high risk
Your risk of having pre-diabetes or type 2 diabetes is fairly low, though it always pays to maintain a healthy lifestyle.	Based on your identified risk factors, your risk of having pre-diabetes or type 2 diabetes is moderate. You may wish to consult with a health care practitioner about your risk of developing diabetes.	Based on your identified risk factors, your risk of having pre-diabetes or type 2 diabetes is high. You may wish to consult with a health care practitioner to discuss getting your blood sugar tested.

Diabetes is a serious chronic disease and uncontrolled diabetes can lead to heart disease, kidney disease and other conditions.

While you can't change some factors such as, age, gender, family history, and ethno-cultural background, other risk factors for diabetes may respond to lifestyle changes. These include weight, physical activity, diet, and smoking.

If your BMI is 25 or higher, lowering your weight may help you reduce your risk of developing type 2 diabetes. Even a small change in body weight or physical activity can reduce your risk. Embrace a healthy balanced diet which emphasizes vegetables, fruit, and whole grains. Consult Canada's Food Guide for helpful suggestions. If you are not active, begin slowly and increase your activity gradually. Check with your doctor before beginning any exercise program.

If you smoke, it's never too late to quit. Every step you take to improve your health counts!

Thank you for completing the Canadian Diabetes Risk Questionnaire.

Public Health Agency of Canada, 2011

FIGURE 37-2, cont'd

Patient:_____   **Date:**_____

HISTORY

GENERAL	YES	NO	SYSTEMS REVIEW	YES	NO
Have you been examined and/or treated by a physician within the year?			**Hematologic or Blood-related Conditions** Do you:		
Are you taking any medication now? What? 1. 2. 3. 4.			29. Bleed a long time after an injury		
			30. Bruise easily		
			31. Have blood disorders, anemia, thin blood		
			Head, Ear, Eyes, Nose, and Throat Conditions Do you have:		
1. Have you been seriously ill? What?			32. Severe headaches		
2. Hospitalized?			33. Eye troubles		
3. Treated with x-ray, other for tumours What area(s)?			34. Frequent colds		
			35. Sinus trouble		
Have you had: 4. Major surgery? Type:			36. Frequent nosebleeds		
			37. Sore throats		
5. Blood transfusion			38. Ear aches		
SPECIFIC			**Cardiorespiratory Conditions**		
Have you had:			Do you have		
6. Rheumatic fever			39. High blood pressure		
7. Congenital heart disease			40. Shortness of breath		
8. Heart condition What?			41. Chest pains		
			42. Swollen ankles		
9. Stroke			43. Persistent cough		
10. Inflammatory rheumatism			44. Blood sputum produced by coughing		
11. Yellow jaundice			**Gastrointestinal Conditions** Have you had		
12. Tuberculosis			45. An ulcer		
13. Venereal disease			46. Recent change in appetite		
14. Liver damage			47. Foods you cannot eat		
15. Kidney condition			48. Difficulty in swallowing		
16. Diabetes			49. Frequent indigestion or vomiting		
17. Cancer			50. Feel thirsty much of the time		
18. Injury to face or jaws			51. Urinate more than 6 times per day		
19. Epilepsy			52. Kidney trouble		
20. Hepatitis			**Neuromuscular / Musculoskeletal Conditions**		
SENSITIVITY / ALLERGIES			53. Painful, swollen joints		
Have you had			54. Numb or prickling sensations on your skin		
21. Hives / skin rash			55. A history of broken bones		
22. Asthma, hay fever			56. A tendency to faint		
Have you had unusual reaction to any of the following medication 23. Dental anesthesia 24. Aspirin 25. Penicillin 26. Iodine 27. Sleeping pills 28. Other:			57. Fits or convulsions		
			Endocrine or Metabolic Conditions Do you		
			58. Get tired easily		
			59. Feel excessively nervous		
			60. Feel more discomfort in hot weather than other people		
			Hereditary Conditions		
For Women: Are you pregnant? How many months?			Do you have 61. A history of family disease What?		

Vital signs: Blood Pressure_____   Heart Rate_____   Respiratory Rate_____

FIGURE 37-3 ■ Multisystem Review.

Health Improvement Card

The World Health Professions Alliance published the Health Improvement Card[22] to provide a common tool for health professionals that could be readily used and implemented to address patients' lifestyle behaviours in terms of both basic lifestyle assessment and recommendations for health behaviour change. The World Health Professions Alliance also supports a practitioner NCD toolkit to further foster health promotion practice within the daily clinical context.[23]

The Health Improvement Card consists of two pages (Fig. 37-4). Page one outlines the patient's biometric information and includes lifestyle behaviours and some laboratory test results (cholesterol and blood sugar). Colour coding is used to indicate whether these are acceptable, caution is needed, or the patient is at high risk. Page two consists of colour-coded action items. Green signifies the lifestyle behaviour is within healthy limits and the person should continue accordingly. Yellow signifies warning and need for remediation, and red signifies risky health behaviour warranting priority attention by the patient and health practitioner. The Health Improvement Card provides a foundation for initiating a conversation with the patient about health behaviour change and realistic tangible targets. These targets are measurable and can be readily followed by the physiotherapist.

HEALTH BEHAVIOUR CHANGE INTERVENTIONS

A contemporary physiotherapy priority is to maximize health overall even in people living with chronic conditions. In addition, across health behaviour change initiatives, a primary goal is to avoid or reduce reliance on pharmacologic interventions as much as possible. The health psychology literature describes a range of strategies and interventions that can be incorporated into physiotherapy practice, to effect health behaviour change. Some established evidence-based interventions and related approaches are described below.

Interventions

Behaviour Modification

Physiotherapy-provided operant conditioning or behaviour modification has been a focus in multiple studies of chronic low back pain disability. In one recent systematic review, such intervention (described as a time-contingent, graduated increase in activity including goal setting and the education and reinforcement of positive pain behaviours with the ultimate aim of decreasing disability and increasing function) was considered efficacious in the treatment of low back pain.[24] Thus, physiotherapists may also consider operant conditioning for its additional effect on reducing long-term disability associated with chronic back pain. Another systematic review examined the use of behavioural strategies used by physiotherapists for the prevention of chronic low back pain.[25] The

investigators identified an operant treatment approach as a promising behavioural strategy to prevent chronic back pain, and one that can be readily integrated into ambulant physiotherapy practice.

Comparable to behavioural theories and models underlying lifestyle behaviour change in relation to patients with back problems, their applications have not been sufficiently studied. Their applications in relation to pain, its experience and remediation, may help inform best practice management of back pain. Although back pain was not a focus of a Cochrane review of weight loss strategies in people who were overweight or obese, weight loss was greatest when diet and exercise were combined with behaviour therapy.[26] Another review of the literature supported a behavioural approach to the management of acute whiplash-associated disorders.[27] Such behavioural approaches may be applicable to patients with whiplash and concurrent lifestyle-related conditions and by extension, those with thoracic and lumbar involvement. Study of the combined outcomes of physical and behavioural approaches in the management of spinal conditions is needed.

Cognitive Behaviour Therapy

Cognitive behaviour therapy (CBT) is an approach to behaviour change that focuses on the patient's emotional and behavioural responses as a vehicle for such change.[28] It is based on the assumption that emotional and behavioural responses are largely learned. The goal of therapy is for the patient to learn adaptive ways of responding emotionally and behaviourally to health problems, and to unlearn maladaptive responses. CBT is well suited for application to health behaviour change in the clinical setting. Intervention is focused, directed and brief, and often associated with rapid results. The therapeutic relationship needs to be empathetic and based on rapport. CBT enables the patient to accept a health or personal concern so that personal resources such as intelligence, knowledge and energy can be effectively harnessed to address it. CBT also uses elements of a Socratic method to enable patients to gain insight into their problems by posing questions to themselves and to the clinician. Overall, CBT has been promoted as a clinically useful evidence-based intervention to enable patients to better manage chronic back pain.[29]

Motivational Interviewing

Motivational interviewing (MI) has become a leading evidence-based interviewing strategy to enable patients to identify their health behaviour change needs and motivation. MI is a collaborative person-centred form of validating the patient's behaviours and guiding him or her to elicit and strengthen motivation for change.[30] A unique feature of MI is that it is 'evocative' in that it is designed to elicit the person's own motivation and commitment to change in a supportive, non-coercive manner. A patient's ambivalence about change is anticipated and MI strategies are designed to enable the patient to identify, examine and resolve any ambivalence. Examples of MI questions to identify the patient's 'positive motivation' to

HEALTH IMPROVEMENT CARD

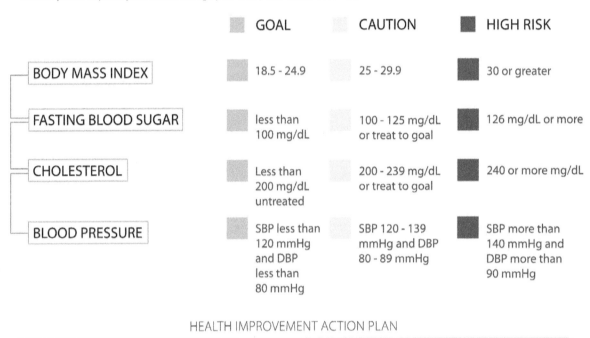

Male ( ) Female ( )

Age 20-34 ( ) 35-39 ( ) 40-44 ( ) 50-54 ( ) 55-59 ( ) 60-64 ( ) 65-69 ( ) 70-74 ( )

Height ( ) metres or feet   Weight ( ) kilograms or pounds

Waist circumference ( ) centimetres or inches

Body mass index = $\dfrac{\text{weight (kg)}}{\text{height (m) x height(m)}}$ ( ) kg/m²
(SI [metric] units)

OR

Body mass index = $\dfrac{\text{weight (lb)}}{\text{height (in) x height(in)}}$ x703   ( ) lb/in²
(Imperial/US customary units)

Biometrics scorecard

- helps you track measurable risk indicators which could over time damage your health, potentially leading to cancers, diabetes, respiratory diseases, heart disease, mental health problems and oral diseases.
- allows your health professional to help support you with information, advice, treatments (when indicated) and care
- enables you to improve your health through your own personalised action plan

	GOAL	CAUTION	HIGH RISK
BODY MASS INDEX	18.5 - 24.9	25 - 29.9	30 or greater
FASTING BLOOD SUGAR	less than 100 mg/dL	100 - 125 mg/dL or treat to goal	126 mg/dL or more
CHOLESTEROL	Less than 200 mg/dL untreated	200 - 239 mg/dL or treat to goal	240 or more mg/dL
BLOOD PRESSURE	SBP less than 120 mmHg and DBP less than 80 mmHg	SBP 120 - 139 mmHg and DBP 80 - 89 mmHg	SBP more than 140 mmHg and DBP more than 90 mmHg

HEALTH IMPROVEMENT ACTION PLAN

my commitment		my goal:
my action		
health professional action		target date:

For details, visit www.whpa.org   With the support of IFPMA

    World Confederation for Physical Therapy fdi⊂ FDI World Dental Federation WMA   IFPMA International Federation of Pharmaceutical Manufacturers & Associations

FIGURE 37-4 ■ Health Improvement Card. For colour version see Plates 23–24. (Source: Health Improvement Card. World Health Professions Alliance. Reprinted with permission. <http://www.ifpma.org/fileadmin/content/Publication/2011/ncd_Health-Improvement-Card_web-1.pdf>.[22])

Lifestyle scorecard

- helps you understand how you can improve your health by changing your lifestyle
- allows your health professional to help you improve your health and well-being
- enables you to own and personalise your health improvement action plan

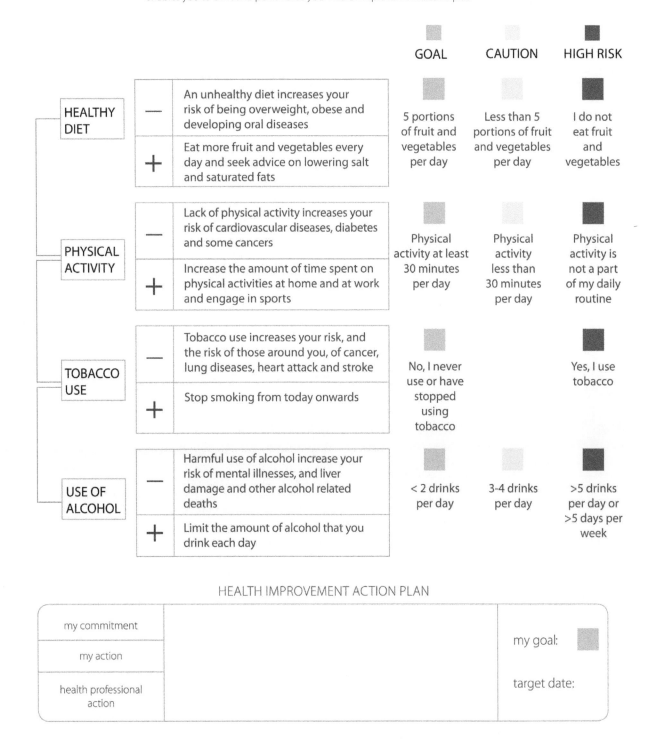

		GOAL	CAUTION	HIGH RISK
HEALTHY DIET	— An unhealthy diet increases your risk of being overweight, obese and developing oral diseases	5 portions of fruit and vegetables per day	Less than 5 portions of fruit and vegetables per day	I do not eat fruit and vegetables
	+ Eat more fruit and vegetables every day and seek advice on lowering salt and saturated fats			
PHYSICAL ACTIVITY	— Lack of physical activity increases your risk of cardiovascular diseases, diabetes and some cancers	Physical activity at least 30 minutes per day	Physical activity less than 30 minutes per day	Physical activity is not a part of my daily routine
	+ Increase the amount of time spent on physical activities at home and at work and engage in sports			
TOBACCO USE	— Tobacco use increases your risk, and the risk of those around you, of cancer, lung diseases, heart attack and stroke	No, I never use or have stopped using tobacco		Yes, I use tobacco
	+ Stop smoking from today onwards			
USE OF ALCOHOL	— Harmful use of alcohol increase your risk of mental illnesses, and liver damage and other alcohol related deaths	< 2 drinks per day	3-4 drinks per day	>5 drinks per day or >5 days per week
	+ Limit the amount of alcohol that you drink each day			

HEALTH IMPROVEMENT ACTION PLAN

my commitment		my goal:
my action		
health professional action		target date:

For details, visit www.whpa.org

With the support of IFPMA

FIGURE 37-4, cont'd

participate in health behaviour change and 'perceived barriers' to change, appear in Box 37-3.

Decision Balance Analysis

Decision balance analysis is based on principles associated with MI and CBT.[31,32] It is a strategy that enables the patient to identify and reflect on the pros and cons of changing a specific health behaviour and, as importantly, the pros and cons of not changing that behaviour. Completion of such a grid by the patient aims to increase his or her self-awareness of the facilitators to health behaviour change and to reduce the perceived barriers to such change. In addition, this information is useful to the physiotherapist in targeting health behaviour and health behaviour change strategies to the patient's needs.

The 5 As and the 5 Rs

At various points in their lives, patients are keen to address negative health behaviours such as quitting smoking, improving nutrition, losing weight, being less sedentary and more physically active, sleeping better and reducing stress. Their histories of health behaviour change attempts are important to identify in terms of

---

| BOX 37-3 | Motivational Interviewing: Examples of Questions and Their Interpretation; Implications for an Action Plan and Follow-Up |

QUESTION: Designed to elicit positive motivational statements from the patient about changing a given behaviour
'Pick a number from 1 to 10 (ten highest) that describes how motivated or interested you are in changing behaviour X?'
Follow-up probing question that would identify the degree to which the patient has no-to-low motivation
'Why did you not pick a lower number?'
QUESTION: Designed to identify the patient's barriers to making a given health behaviour change
'Pick a number from 1 to 10 (ten highest) that describes how confident you are in changing behaviour X?'
Follow-up probing question to identify factors that would indicate patient's increased confidence
'Why did you not pick a higher number?'

ACTION PLAN

• Summarize the patient's/client's responses for wanting and not wanting to change
• Prompt patient/client to come up with solutions
• Add other solutions that have worked for others (with patient's/client's permission)
• Systematic and agreed upon follow-up

FOLLOW-UP STRATEGY

• Set a follow-up date
• Clarify what the patient will do in terms of realistic expectations for changing behaviours
• What the practitioner will do
• Deliverables at follow-up

---

what has been tried, how many times and level of success. One barrier can be lack of systematic support and accountability to help sustain patient's efforts. With some modicum of interest by the patient in being supported for an attempt at behaviour change, the physiotherapist has an inroad. If the patient demonstrates readiness to change (Table 37-1) (i.e. is at the contemplative, preparation or action stages), the physiotherapist can initiative and/or support the patient with appropriate interventions or referral to other professionals with use of the 5 As endorsed by the World Health Organization.[33,34] The 5 As include Assess, Advise, Agree, Assist and Arrange. Their descriptions appear in Box 37-4. The 5 As constitutes a systematic sequential approach to effecting health behaviour change.

The physiotherapist needs to accept that a patient may be pre-contemplative and disinterested in considering change at this time. Given changing health behaviour is challenging and can appear formidable to a patient (e.g. one who smokes a pack of cigarettes a day or more to consider abstinence, or having to lose 25 kg), the 5 Rs can provide a systematic approach for the physiotherapist, to enable the patient to consider changing a health behaviour despite apparent lack of interest or motivation. The 5 Rs stand for Relevance, Resistance, Rewards, Roadblocks and Repetition.[36] These are also described in Box 37-4.

Finally, even if the patient is referred to one or more other health professionals, the physiotherapist has a role in continuing to follow the patient's progress in a manner that is as systematic as if that physiotherapist had initiated the behaviour change programme.

Other Behaviour Change Strategies

A physiotherapy clinic or department can take advantage of many resources available to health professionals to support health promotion. Ministries of Health in most countries, for example, circulate regular updated health bulletins, reports and information. User-friendly credible information is available on the Internet, available for clinic or department use, or to have the patient use at home as part of a take home assessment or health education strategy. The World Health Organization has identified key days of the year to promote specific health initiatives (e.g. May 31st is World No Tobacco Day). Resources are available for practitioners to promote such days in their settings. Disease/condition agencies and associations (e.g. heart, stroke, hypertension, diabetes and cancer) exist in most countries, and they too are eager to have their evidence-based resources fully used by patients, health professionals as well as the general public.

Engaging and informative clips are available in the form of 'edu-tainment' through Internet sites such as TED talks® and YouTube®. Although local professional associations need to preview these for quality and accuracy, some are well suited to being screened in waiting areas of clinics. A couple of evidence-based recommendations are Dean Ornish's healing through diet[37] and Dr. Mike's 23 and $\frac{1}{2}$ hours, on the effects of physical activity on health and disease prevention.[38]

TABLE 37-1 **Assessment of Readiness to Change Health Behaviour**

Circle a response to each question using the 'Y' or the 'N.'
Y = Yes, I meet my health objective on this question.
N = For each 'N' you circle, circle the readiness to change number that applies:
   1 = Not thinking about change at this time (pre-contemplative)
   2 = Thinking about change (contemplative)
   3 = Preparing to change (preparation)

Readiness to Change Checklist*	Response		Readiness to Change		
Do you exercise moderately intensely at least three times a week for 20 to 40 minutes?[†]	Y	N	1	2	3
Are you physically active during your average day (walk, walk briskly, take stairs)?	Y	N	1	2	3
Is your weight within normal range?	Y	N	1	2	3
Do you eat at least five servings of fruit and vegetables daily?	Y	N	1	2	3
Do you minimize the trans and saturated fats in your diet?	Y	N	1	2	3
Do you minimize highly refined carbohydrates in your diet (sugar and white flour)?	Y	N	1	2	3
Do you drink alcohol less often than five times a week?	Y	N	1	2	3
Are you a non-smoker?	Y	N	1	2	3
Are you generally relaxed during your day and do you feel in control?	Y	N	1	2	3

Modified from: *The Stages of Readiness to Change defined within the Transtheoretical Model of behaviour change (DiClemente and Prochaska, 1998)[35] is designed to help people adopt new health behaviours. Knowing where you are in the stages of readiness to change helps you to understand the steps you should take to move to subsequent stages to achieve lifelong sustainable health behaviours.*
*Behaviours that are consistent with healthy living. If patients give a No response to a question, then their readiness to change that behaviour is evaluated.
[†]Given patients vary with their capacity for exercise, the requirement for health should be adjusted.

BOX 37-4 **The 5 As and the 5 Rs**

Indication for the 5 As: The patient is ready to change health behaviour (i.e. either contemplating or preparing to change).
• **Ask** about the target health behaviour
• **Advise** to change the behaviour
• **Assess** willingness to attempt to change the behaviour
• **Assist** in changing the behaviour
• **Arrange** follow-up
Indication for the 5 Rs: The patient is not interested in changing a health behaviour at this time (i.e. at the pre-contemplative stage); the purpose is to maintain an open door for conversation should the patient become interested.
• Determine the **Relevance** of changing behaviour to patient
• Discuss the **Risks** of patient's continued deleterious behaviour
• Explore **Rewards** of changing behaviour
• Examine possible **Roadblocks** to changing behaviour
• Continue **Repetition** of the discussion

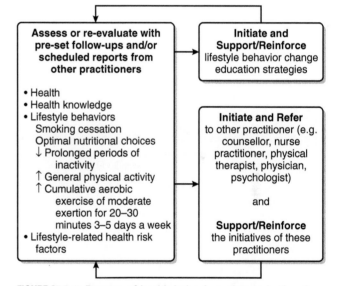

FIGURE 37-5 ■ Process of health behaviour change in the physiotherapy context. (Source: Adapted from Dean et al. 2012.[53])

Examples of Physiotherapy-Directed Health Behaviour Change Initiatives

The steps in the process for effecting lifestyle behaviour change with a patient are shown in Figure 37-5. This figure details the decision-making points for initiating health behaviour change or not; and whether to refer to another professional.

The key elements for assessing/evaluating and targeting strategies and interventions for modifying health behaviours are presented in Table 37-2. Comparable to physiotherapy assessment of a patient's musculoskeletal

complaints, baselines of lifestyle-related health behaviours as well as risk factors need to be assessed and addressed as indicated, in the interest of comprehensive patient care that is consistent with the ICF philosophy and goals.

Comparable to conventional assessments, self-reported assessments of smoking, basic nutrition, physical activity and structured exercise, sleep habits and stress are fundamental, despite the limitation of self-reported information. To maximize validity, patients are encouraged to record these behaviours as specifically and accurately as possible over a representative number of days. Quality baseline data are essential if the goals for health

TABLE 37-2   Examples of Evidence-Based Lifestyle-Related Assessment/Evaluation Tools and Strategies/Interventions for Health Behaviour Change Within an Orthopaedic Physiotherapy Context

SMOKING CESSATION

Assessment and Evaluation Tools

Smoking history and current practices (see Fig. 37-1 Smoking section)
The WHY test[39] (unvalidated) (helps to identify why the person smokes, i.e. stimulation, handling, pleasure, relaxation, habit, weight, image and social)

Strategies and Interventions

Brief advice (Bodner and Dean 2009;[40] Frerichs et al., 2012[41])
Referral to physician for potential pharmaceutical support and/or health psychologist/counsellor

OPTIMIZING NUTRITION AND HEALTHY WEIGHT

Assessment and Evaluation Tools

Detailed multi-day nutrition logs can be laborious and de-motivating, and may lack validity
Weight, height and body mass index
Waist–hip ratio (Zhu et al. 2002;[42] Janssen et al. 2004;[43] Yusuf et al. 2004;[44] Yusuf et al. 2005[45])
Use established and accepted food guides to establish a patient's typical consumption patterns related to servings of the basic food groups daily to identify gross excesses and deficits: servings of vegetables, fruit, whole grain, refined foods, dairy, animal protein (meat, poultry vs. fish sources), sweets
Added sweetener, salt, butter and oil
Food preparation: steam, bake and broil over frying and deep frying
Fast food meals per week
DETERMINE Your Nutritional Health Questionnaire (Morris et al. 2009[46])
Mini-Nutritional Assessment-SF (Morris et al. 2009[46])
Establish need for nutritionist intervention (beyond basic recommendations)

Strategies and Interventions

Implement basic nutrition education based on established guidelines (e.g. plant-based diets such as the Mediterranean diet)
Irrespective of body mass and waist–hip ratio, most patients can benefit from nutritional assessment and reinforcement of healthy food choices
Patients who are overweight and obese do require special consideration, however a healthy diet will help to modify body composition
Referral to dietician or nutritionist

MOTIVATING PATIENTS TO BE PHYSICALLY ACTIVE

Assessment and Evaluation Tools

International Physical Activity Questionnaire (IPAQ website[47]) (long and short versions in multiple languages that classify a person's general physical activity as low, medium, or high)
Pedometer to establish physical activity level, and whether is sedentary (<5000 step criterion) (Tudor-Locke et al. 2004[48])

Strategies and Interventions

Action planning worksheet (Rhodes et al. 2009[49])
Exercise barrier sheet (Rhodes et al. 2009[49])
Exercise enjoyment sheet (identifies suitable activities based on proximity, aesthetics and interest) (Rhodes et al. 2009[49])

OPTIMIZING SLEEP

Assessment and Evaluation Tools

Sleep inventory questionnaire (17 questions) (Coren 2009[50]) (helps to establish evidence for patient's sleep debt/deprivation and risk of related health problems)
Need to distinguish pathological disturbed sleep versus functionally/behaviourally disturbed sleep (if the former, may need to refer to sleep specialist and potential for sleep laboratory investigation)

Strategies and Interventions

Sleep is a physiological necessity but its quality and effectiveness to restore is highly behaviourally dependent
Sleep hygiene recommendations:
Regular hours
Quiet, no light (including electronic clock/TV lights), comfortable ventilated room
Avoid heavy meals, caffeine, alcohol within hours of bed

STRESS MANAGEMENT

Assessment and Evaluation Tools

Distinguish acute (daily hassle) type stress and chronic stress
Psychological Stress Measure-9 (nine questions) (Lemyre et al. 2009[51]) (evaluates short-term stress, past 4–5 days)
Holmes-Rahe Social Readjustment Stress Scale (Holmes-Rahe Stress Test[52]) (evaluates major life stressors over the past year and predicts health risks for the subsequent year)

Strategies and Interventions

Establish need for referral to other professionals
Methods based on principles of cognitive behavioural therapy and motivational interviewing

behaviour change are to be S.M.A.R.T. (i.e. Specific, Measurable, Attainable, Realistic and Timely). Such goal characteristics are necessary if effective change is to be demonstrated.

CONCLUSION

This chapter builds on the evidence and epidemiological base described in Chapter 11. It introduced physiotherapists involved in the management of people with musculoskeletal conditions to established assessment and evaluation tools, and theory- and evidence-based strategies and interventions to change their patients' lifestyle behaviours. Behaviours warranting assessment and potential intervention include smoking, sub-optimal nutrition, unhealthy body mass, regular prolonged periods of physical inactivity, low physical activity and exercise, sub-optimal sleep quality and quantity, and anxiety, depression and stress. Assessment tools and behavioural interventions are described that can be integrated into busy, resource-constrained physiotherapists' practices. With systematic attention to health behaviour change, physiotherapy outcomes related to musculoskeletal complaints including pain can be augmented as well as patients' general health and well-being improved. Both are priorities in contemporary physiotherapy practice.

REFERENCES

1. Huan HC, Chang HJ, Lin KC, et al. A closer examination of the interaction among risk factors for low back pain. Am J Health Promot 2014;28:372–9.
2. Melloh M, Elfering A, Stanton TR, et al. Low back pain risk factors associated with persistence, recurrence and delayed presentation. J Back Musculoskelet Rehabil 2014;27(3):281–9.
3. Sykes C, Myers B. Annual WHO Family of International Classifications Network Meeting: ICF Activities by the World Confederation for Physical Therapy and Its Member Organisations [Internet]. Seoul, Republic of Korea: World Confederation for Physical Therapy; 2009. Available from: <http://www.who.int/classifications/network/WHOFIC2009_D041p_Sykes.pdf>; [cited 2014 Feb 22].
4. Dean E, Gormsen Hansen R. Prescribing optimal nutrition and physical activity as 'first-line' interventions for best practice management of chronic low-grade inflammation associated with osteoarthritis: evidence synthesis. Arthritis 2012;2012:560634.
5. Buck D, Frosini F. Clustering of Unhealthy Behaviours Over Time: Implications for Policy and Practice [Internet]. London, UK: The King's Fund; 2012. Available from: <http://www.kingsfund.org.uk/sites/files/kf/field/field_publication_file/clustering-of-unhealthy-behaviours-over-time-aug-2012.pdf>; [cited 2014 Feb 21].
6. Schuit AJ, van Loon AJ, Tijhuis M, et al. Clustering of lifestyle risk factors in a general adult population. Prev Med 2002;35(3):219–24.
7. Spring B, Moller AC, Coons MJ. Multiple health behaviours: overview and implications. J Public Health 2012;34(Suppl. 1):i3–10.
8. Ornish D. Avoiding revascularization with lifestyle changes: the multicenter lifestyle demonstration project. Am J Cardiol 1998;82(10B):72T–76T.
9. Ornish D, Scherwitz LW, Billings JH, et al. Intensive lifestyle changes for reversal of coronary heart disease. JAMA 1998;280(23):2001.
10. Your Guide to Lowering Your Blood Pressure with DASH [Internet]. U.S Department of Health and Human Services; 2006. Available from: <http://www.nhlbi.nih.gov/health/public/heart/hbp/dash/new_dash.pdf>; [cited 2014 Feb 21].
11. Norris SL, Engelgau MM, Venkat Narayan KM. Effectiveness of self-management training in type 2 diabetes: a systematic review of randomized controlled trials. Diabetes Care 2001;24(3):561–87.
12. Ornish D, Weidner G, Fair WR, et al. Intensive lifestyle changes may affect the progression of prostate cancer. J Urol 2005;174(3):1065–9, discussion 1069–70.
13. Eating Well with Canada's Food Guide [Internet]. Ottawa, ON: Health Canada; 2007. Available from: <http://www.has.uwo.ca/hospitality/nutrition/pdf/foodguide.pdf>; [cited 2014 Feb 22].
14. Grundy SM, Pasternak R, Greenland P, et al. Assessment of cardiovascular risk by use of multiple-risk-factor assessment equations: a statement for healthcare professionals from the American Heart Association and the American College of Cardiology. Circulation 1999;100(13):1481–92.
15. Disease Risk Index [Internet]. Harvard School of Public Health; 2008. Available from: <http://www.diseaseriskindex.harvard.edu/update/>; [cited 2014 Feb 21].
16. 2008 Physical Activity Guidelines for Americans: Be Active, Healthy, and Happy [Internet]. U.S. Department of Health and Human Services; 2008. Available from: <http://www.health.gov/paguidelines/pdf/paguide.pdf>; [cited 2014 Feb 22].
17. The Canadian Diabetes Risk Assessment Questionnaire [Internet]. Public Health Agency of Canada; 2009. Available from: <http://www.diabetes.ca/documents/for-professionals/NBI-CANRISK.pdf>; [cited 2014 Feb 21].
18. Canrisk: The Canadian Diabetes Risk Questionnaire: User Guide for Pharmacists [Internet]. Public Health Agency of Canada. Available from: <http://www.pharmacists.ca/cpha-ca/assets/File/education-practice-resources/CanriskuserguideforpharmacistsEN.pdf>; [cited 2014 Feb 21].
19. Pearson TA, Blair SN, Daniels SR, et al. AHA guidelines for primary prevention of cardiovascular disease and stroke: 2002 update: Consensus Panel guide to comprehensive risk reduction for adult patients without coronary or other atherosclerotic vascular diseases. American Heart Association Science Advisory and Coordinating Committee. Circulation 2002;106(3):388–91.
20. Inoue T, Iseki K, Ohya Y. Heart rate as a possible therapeutic guide for the prevention of cardiovascular disease. Hypertens Res 2013;36(10):838–44.
21. Handler J. The importance of accurate blood pressure measurement. Perm J 2009;13(3):51–4.
22. Health Improvement Card [Internet]. World Health Professions Alliance; 2014. Available from: <http://www.ifpma.org/fileadmin/content/Publication/2011/ncd_Health-Improvement-Card_web-1.pdf>; [cited 2014 Feb 21].
23. Non Communicable Diseases: An Action Toolkit for Health Professionals, Patients and Public [Internet]. World Health Professions Alliance. Available from: <http://www.whpa.org/ncd_ActionToolkit_cover.pdf>; [cited 2014 Feb 21].
24. Bunzli S, Gillham D, Esterman A. Physiotherapy-provided operant conditioning in the management of low back pain disability: a systematic review. Physiother Res Int 2011;16(1):4–19.
25. Brunner E, De Herdt A, Minguet P, et al. Can cognitive behavioural therapy based strategies be integrated into physiotherapy for the prevention of chronic low back pain? A systematic review. Disabil Rehabil 2013;35(1):1–10.
26. Shaw K, O'Rourke P, Del Mar C, et al. Psychological interventions for overweight or obesity. Cochrane Database Syst Rev 2005;(2):CD003818.
27. Soderlund A, Sweden V. The role of educational and learning approaches in rehabilitation of whiplash associated disorders in lessening the transition to chronicity. Spine 2011;36(Suppl. 25):S280–5.
28. NACBT Online Headquarters [Internet]. National Association of Cognitive-Behavioral Therapists. 2010. Available from: <http://www.nacbt.org/whatiscbt.htm>; [cited 2014 Feb 21].
29. Gatchel RJ, Rollings KH. Evidence-informed management of chronic low back pain with cognitive behavioral therapy. Spine J 2008;8(1):40–4.
30. Rollnick S, Miller WL, Butler C. Motivational Interviewing in Health Care: Helping Patients Change Behavior (Applications of Motivational Interviewing). New York, NY: The Guilford Press; 2008.
31. Decisional balance worksheet [Internet]. Available from: <http://motivationalinterview.net/clinical/decisionalbalance.pdf>; [cited 2014 Feb 21].
32. Lipschitz JM, Fernandez AC, Larson HE, et al. Validation of decisional balance and self-efficacy measures for HPV vaccination in college women. Am J Health Promot 2013;27(5):299–307.

33. 5 A's behavior change model adapted for self-management support improvement [Internet]. 2002. Available from: <http://www.improvingchroniccare.org/downloads/3.5_5_as_behaviior_change_model.pdf>; [cited 2014 Feb 21].

34. Fiore MC, Jaen CR, Baker TB. A clinical practice guideline for treating tobacco use and dependence: 2008 Update. A U.S. Public Health Service report. Am J Prev Med 2008;35(2):158–76.

35. DiClemente CC, Prochaska JO. Toward a comprehensive, transtheoretical model of change: stages of change and addictive behaviors. In: Miller WR, Heather N, editors. Treating Addictive Behaviors. 2nd ed. New York, NY: Plenum Press; 1998. p. 3–24.

36. Newson RS, Lion R, Crawford RJ, et al. Behaviour change for better health: nutrition, hygiene and sustainability. BMC Public Health 2013;13(Suppl. 1):S1.

37. Dean Ornish: Healing through diet | Video on TED.com [Internet]. Ted Conferences; 2004. Available from: <http://www.ted.com/talks/dean_ornish_on_healing.html>; [cited 2014 Feb 21].

38. 23 and 1/2 hours: What is the single best thing we can do for our health? [Internet]. You Tube; 2011. Available from: <http://www.youtube.com/watch?v=aUaInS6HIGo>; [cited 2014 Feb 21].

39. The 'Why I Smoke' Test [Internet]. University of Virginia Health System. Available from: <http://uvahealth.com/patients-visitors-guide/smoke-free/smoke-free-pdfs/test.pdf>; [cited 2014 Feb 22].

40. Bodner ME, Dean E. Advice as a smoking cessation strategy: a systematic review and implications for physical therapy. Physiother Theory Pract 2009;25(5):369–407.

41. Frerichs W, Kaltenbacher E, van de Leur JP, et al. Can physical therapists counsel patients with lifestyle-related health conditions effectively? A systematic review and implications. Physiother Theory Pract 2012;28(8):571–87.

42. Zhu S, Wang Z, Heshka S, et al. Waist circumference and obesity-associated risk factors among whites in the third National Health and Nutrition Examination Survey: clinical action thresholds. Am J Clin Nutr 2002;76(4):743–9.

43. Jannsen I, Katzharzyk PT, Ross R. Waist circumference and not body mass index explains obesity-related health risk. Am J Clin Nutr 2004;79(3):379–84.

44. Yusuf S, Hawken S, Ounpuu S, et al. Effect of potentially modifiable risk factors associated with myocardial infarction in 52 countries (the INTERHEART study): case-control study. Lancet 2004;364(9438):937–52.

45. Yusuff S, Hawken S, Ôunpuu S, et al. Obesity and the risk of myocardial infarction in 27 000 participants from 52 countries: a case-control study. Lancet 2005;366(9497):1640–9.

46. Morris DM, Kitchin EM, Clark DE. Strategies for optimizing nutrition and weight reduction in physical therapy practice: the evidence. Physiother Theory Pract 2009;25(5–6):408–23.

47. International Physical Activity Questionnaire: IPAQ: short last 7 days self administered format. [Internet]. IPAQ website; 2001. Available from: <http://www.ipaq.ki.se/questionnaires/IPAQ_S7S_FINAL_MAY_01.pdf>; [cited 2014 Feb 22].

48. Tudor-Locke C, Bassett DR Jr. How many steps/day are enough? Preliminary pedometer indices for public health. Sports Med 2004;34(1):1–8.

49. Rhodes RE, Fiala B. Building motivation and sustainability into the prescription and recommendations for physical activity and exercise therapy: the evidence. Physiother Theory Pract 2009;25(5–6):424–41.

50. Coren S. Sleep health and its assessment and management in physical therapy practice: the evidence. Physiother Theory Pract 2009;25(5–6):442–51.

51. Lemyre L, Lalonde-Markon MP. Psychological stress measure (PM-9): integration of an evidence-based approach to assessment, monitoring, and evaluation of stress in physical therapy practice. Physiother Theory Pract 2009;25(5–6):453–62.

52. Holmes-Rahe Stress Test [Internet]. Fort Worth, TX: The American Institute of Stress. Available from: <http://www.stress.org/holmes-rahe-stress-inventory/>; [cited 2014 Feb 22].

53. Dean E, Li Z, Wong WP, et al. Cardiology best practice – effective health education meets biomedical advances: Reducing the ultimate knowledge translation gap. In: Lakshmanadoss U, editor. Novel Strategies in Ischemic Heart Disease. InTech Publishing; 2012. p. 301–18 [Online access].

CHAPTER 38

MUSCULOSKELETAL HEALTH IN THE WORKPLACE

Venerina Johnston • Leon Straker • Martin Mackey

INTRODUCTION

There is international consensus that work is generally good for health.[1] Maintenance of musculoskeletal health of the individual worker is a shared responsibility between the work organization and the worker. The organization has a responsibility to ensure the workplace and the way work is performed are safe and not detrimental to health and well-being. The worker has a responsibility to maintain their own health and ensure that work is practiced in the prescribed safe way. This symbiotic relationship between work organization and worker is confirmed in legislation in most developed countries. However, several features of modern society pose new challenges to this relationship – changes in workers themselves reflected in the ageing population and the increase in chronic diseases, and changes in the nature of work such as increases in precarious work and sedentary work. This chapter discusses contemporary approaches to assist the worker retain and regain musculoskeletal health within a constantly changing work environment.

Factors Threatening Worker Health

Population ageing is occurring globally due to a sustained reduction in fertility rates and a decline in mortality associated with improvements in health care and technology.[2] Ageing of the working population has significant social, economic and political implications for government, industry and the health professions.[3] For instance, in the future more mature-aged workers will need to remain active in the workforce beyond the current retirement age to meet workforce demands, and this is being encouraged by a range of legislative and social policy initiatives. There are several implications of an ageing workforce for workplace health and safety. Physical work capacity (impacted by changes in cardiovascular and musculoskeletal capacity) declines with increasing age, and after 50 years the deterioration is more marked.[4] If a worker's physical capacity cannot match the task demands, it could result in excessive fatigue, leading to a poor quality of work along with an increased risk of industrial accidents.[5] Older workers also tend to experience a higher rate of some work-related injuries (e.g. falls) than their younger counterparts.[6,7] Work injuries in mature-aged workers are more costly in terms of lost productivity partly due to the greater severity of injuries requiring longer recovery time.[8,9] In order to ensure the health and safety of older workers within the workplace, organizational practices will need to be adjusted, new technologies adopted and assistance given to help mature workers cope with work demands to ensure work ability is optimized in the face of increasing challenges to working life.[10-13] The physical changes with ageing need to be considered to enable workers to age productively.

The prevalence of some lifestyle risk factors for chronic disease is increasing, particularly physical inactivity and obesity across workers of all ages.[14] Asthma, cancer, cardiovascular disease, diabetes, arthritis, osteoporosis and other musculoskeletal conditions, including those associated with exposure to hazards in the workplace, are of particular concern.[14] These chronic diseases represent a major challenge for industry as they result in substantial absenteeism as well as presenteeism (reduced performance while at work).[14] In response to the growing impact of chronic disease on the health of workers and health-care systems, governments are currently implementing preventive strategies such as anti-smoking campaigns and lifestyle programmes to promote healthy eating choices and exercise participation including within the workplace.[15] With the majority of working-age people having one or more risk factors,[16] it is incumbent on health practitioners to assist workers to understand how these risk factors may impact on working life.

The nature of work is diversifying in many societies. Lifelong employment with a single organization in a single industry is becoming rarer, with more workers in precarious employment such as contract, temporary or part-time work. These work arrangements have been linked with negative health outcomes due to their associations with lower material well-being, adverse physical and psychosocial working conditions, less positive social contacts, and weaker support from supervisors and co-workers.[17,18] Concurrently, there is an increasing demand for greater flexibility in the location and timing of work. This is driven in part by portable technology, economic globalization and the desire of workers to combine family commitments and lifestyle interests while remaining in employment. Knowledge workers and those in information technology often have the option of working from home, whereas workers in the resource industry may utilize organization-sponsored 'fly-in fly-out' work arrangements. The changing nature of work requires clinicians to consider the current physical and psychosocial work environment and implement (often creative) strategies to increase the workers' knowledge and skills to ensure maintenance and/or improvement of musculoskeletal health.

There has also been an increase in sedentary work, with a shift in the proportion of workers employed in 'blue collar' industries to 'white collar' industries.[19] This increase in sedentary work is thought to be a significant contributor to the obesity epidemic facing many societies.[20] Even within traditionally physically demanding industries such as mining, forestry and agriculture, many tasks are now mechanized, creating sedentary jobs.[21] Some job tasks still remain that are physically demanding, such as hotel bed making, and there are other jobs that require only light physical exertion but are highly repetitive, such as electronics manufacturing. Thus there needs to be an awareness of the different types of work and current strategies to reverse the negative impact of sedentary work while maintaining employee musculoskeletal health. Such strategies include the use of adjustable sit–stand workstations in office environments[22] and initiatives to encourage increased physical activity in the workplace.[23]

What is a Work-Related Musculoskeletal Disorder?

Work-related musculoskeletal disorders (MSDs) are musculoskeletal conditions that may be caused, aggravated, accelerated or exacerbated by (non-accidental) work activities. They include disorders of inflammation, degeneration and physiological disruption of muscles, tendons, ligaments, nerves, synovia and cartilage of the limbs and/or trunk. MSDs are considered work-related when the work environment and performance of work contribute significantly to the condition but may be only one of a number of factors contributing to the causation of a multifactorial disease.[24,25] These entities are included in categories 353–355, 722–724 and 726–729 of the *International Classification of Diseases* (commonly referred to as ICD-9).[26] MSDs may include clinical syndromes such as tendon inflammations and related conditions (tenosynovitis, epicondylitis, bursitis), nerve compression disorders (carpal tunnel syndrome, sciatica) and osteoarthrosis, as well as conditions without clear diagnostic criteria such as myalgia, low back pain and other regional pain syndromes not attributable to known pathology. Body regions most commonly involved in prevalence order are the low back; hand, fingers and thumb; shoulder; and knee.[27,28] MSDs are associated with high costs to organizations in terms of absenteeism, lost productivity, and increased health-care, disability and worker's compensation costs. For example, workers' compensation claims for MSDs account for over 40% of the $57.5 billion annual expenditure of work-related injuries and diseases in Australia[29] and upto 1.6% of the gross domestic product of some European states.[30] MSDs are the most common cause of chronic severe pain and long-term physical disability, work limitations and unemployment.[31] They are often more severe than the average non-fatal

injury or illness.[24] As a result, there is increased recognition that the workplace is an ideal venue for health interventions and that work should be used not only for rehabilitation from injury but also to enhance and promote health.[32]

Health professionals such as physiotherapists who specialize in the preservation and improvement of movement for positive health and functional outcomes[33] have a key role to play in the prevention of work-related injuries[34–36] and in the prevention of work disability following a work-related injury or other pre-existing musculoskeletal health problem. While health professionals have traditionally focused mainly on management of symptoms related to MSDs, there is increasing awareness of their role in preventing subsequent disability (tertiary prevention) and also help prevent development of MSDs (primary and secondary prevention). The following presents a discussion of recent advances for the prevention and management of work-related MSDs.

PREVENTION

Prevention is often conceptualized in three stages: primary, secondary and tertiary. Primary prevention aims to avoid a health problem before it occurs; secondary prevention to minimize disability and recurrence in the early stages of a health problem; and tertiary prevention to reduce morbidity arising from a chronic health problem.[37] The definitions infer discreet phases, but taking the example of back or neck pain, the first episodes of spinal pain often occur during adolescence, prior to adult working life.[38,39] Similarly, the first experiences of disability associated with spinal pain often occur during adolescence.[40] For many MSDs there is a gradual onset and symptoms follow an episodic pattern.[38,41] Given these common life-course and episodic characteristics of many MSDs, the precise phase of prevention may not be clear for many MSDs' preventive activities. This chapter will discuss advances related to interventions aimed at primary prevention in the general workforce ('primary') and at those who have developed an MSD ('secondary' and 'tertiary').

Primary Prevention

The traditional intervention for primary prevention of spinal work-related MSDs was training in lifting technique. Several decades of research has provided evidence which questions the physical validity of recommended lifting techniques.[42–45] Further, high-quality intervention studies have been unable to demonstrate an improvement in MSD outcomes.[46] Systematic reviews have concluded that there is moderate evidence that training in manual handling techniques is *not* effective in preventing back pain.[47] This has prompted a change in approach to injury prevention – from changing the individual to meet the demands of the job (e.g. manual handling training) to a risk-management approach, creating a safe system of work. This approach is based on two models – an ergonomics human–technology systems model and a risk-management model.

Ergonomics Human–technology Systems Model

The ergonomics human–technology systems model is illustrated in Figure 38-1. Briefly, the model's focus is on the interaction between the human and the technology they are using to perform a task within a work environment, positioned within a broader organizational and societal context. It is becoming increasingly accepted in MSD management. Physical, psychological and social aspects of the interaction are important in the prevention of MSDs.[48] The aim of ergonomics is for the non-human aspects of the system to match the capabilities and limitations of the human. It is hypothesized that this will result in better health, satisfaction and productivity outcomes.

Risk-management Model

Figure 38-2 illustrates the risk-management model. Briefly, hazards within the work environment are identified and the risk for injury assessed. Measures to control the risks are identified and implemented and the impact of these changes is evaluated. Hazards are entities with the potential to cause harm (examples provided below). With respect to work-related MSDs these are commonly classified into hazards of physical aspects of work and hazards of psychosocial aspects of work. Risk, in contrast,

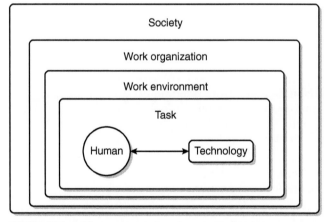

FIGURE 38-1 ■ The ergonomics human–technology systems model.

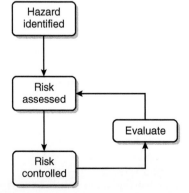

FIGURE 38-2 ■ The risk-management model.

is a product of the likelihood and consequences of harm being caused by the hazard. Likelihood is usually characterized as a probability, say a 1 in 5 chance each year of experiencing an MSD. Consequence is the outcome, which for MSDs would range from mild discomfort through to severe disability (more severe non-MSD consequences would include fatality).

Work-Related MSD Hazards. The main hazards identified as risks for MSDs are related to the different types of physical demands in work and psychosocial issues. Additional hazards are created by work organization factors (e.g. excessive work hours and shift systems) and work environment factors (e.g. high heat, inadequate lighting and arm or whole body vibration).

Physical hazards include individual technology and task aspects. Key physical hazards include:[49]
- Repetitive force – for example, repetitive gripping of bricks or using a nail gun to fix palings to a fence;
- Sustained force – for example, holding a plaster sheet while fixing it to a ceiling or supporting a patient limb during surgery;
- High force – for example, lifting a large container or cutting wire with pliers;
- Sudden force – for example, restraining an animal or catching a falling patient;
- Repetitive movement – for example cutting grape vines or typing;
- Awkward posture – for example, neck flexed and rotated to read document or arms reaching around an engine to adjust a bolt;
- Sustained posture – for example, continually standing on one leg or using a computer mouse.

Psychosocial hazards include individual task aspects in addition to broader job and organization aspects.[48] Key psychosocial hazards include:
- High mental workload – for example, excessive cognitive task demands where tasks have high perceptual demands with short time deadlines;
- Low control over work – for example, assembly line tasks where task pace is set by the conveyor belt;
- Low social support – for example, from work peers and supervisors.

There has been considerable debate about the level of evidence for work factors contributing to MSDs,[27,50,51] and therefore what the hazards are and what should be addressed in risk control measures. The continued debate about hazards is not surprising given the wide variety of work-related MSDs, the range of potential aetiological pathways, the cumulative nature and life-course of many MSDs and the difficulty in accurately assessing exposure to hazards and accurately defining MSD outcomes. However, a substantial body of evidence has now amassed that is convincing to most.[27,48,52]

Tools Available for Risk Management. A number of tools have been developed to assist practitioners assess the degree of risk associated with work. Often the relevant occupational safety and health authority will have produced guidelines, codes of practice or advice material which commonly include simple checklists (e.g. Safe Work Australia[49]). For more detailed assessments, there are a variety of tools to choose from. Macdonald and Evans[48] provide an accessible summary of tools available for assessment of posture (OWAS[53] and RULA[54]), loads (Health and Safety Executive[55], NIOSH lifting equation[56] and Liberty Mutual psychophysical tables[57]), repetition (Job Strain Index[58]), multiple physical hazards (ManTRA[59]), psychosocial hazards (Job Content Questionnaire[60]) and both physical and psychosocial hazards (Quick Exposure Check[61]).

Risk Control. Potential control options to reduce the risk of MSDs are often informed by the risks assessed. There is a recommended hierarchy of controls[62] where the strategy with the highest confidence for sustained success is to remove the hazard. An example would be a change in work processes to replace manual handling of bags of potatoes with forklift handling of pallets of potatoes. The second group of strategies recommended are based around engineering controls to control the hazard at its source. These do not rely on individual workers' behaviour. An example is the use of roller conveyors to eliminate the need to lift objects from the floor. The last group of strategies to deploy are administrative controls which rely on worker behaviour with protocols, training and the use of personal protective equipment. These administrative controls are the least reliable, and as stated earlier there is evidence that training in manual handling alone is not effective.

Evidence of the Efficacy of the Ergonomics/ Risk-Management Approach

In developed countries it is now very difficult to conduct controlled trials of the efficacy of ergonomics/risk-management approach as most work situations have already had some risk control measures implemented and ethics would not allow workers to be put at undue risk by reintroducing prior risks. Despite this challenge, a number of studies have demonstrated the efficacy of this approach. A randomized controlled trial tested this risk-management approach across 48 workplaces from three high-risk industry sectors in Queensland, Australia (food processing, aged care and construction related). The approach resulted in reduced risk based on occupational health and safety inspector audits.[63] Similarly, an intervention in 66 computer workers in Israel was able to show improvements in physical risk indicators and MSDs.[64]

Prevention of Work Disability – Secondary and Tertiary Prevention

The desired outcome of all primary prevention interventions in the workplace is an absence of injuries. However, the reality is that inevitably, some workers will sustain an MSD and that a small proportion will experience a chronic MSD. This section discusses the advances made for the secondary prevention of work disability immediately following an MSD and tertiary prevention of work disability for people with a chronic MSD. Inclusive of tertiary prevention, but not discussed further in this chapter, are vocational rehabilitation interventions that assist and support people who have an injury, disability

or health condition to find or keep a job when they are unable to return to their pre-injury occupation. These interventions include job capacity and functional capacity assessments to identify transferable skills and physical capacity for realistic vocational options.

There is consistent evidence that the longer a person is away from work, the longer it will take them to return to work and the likelihood of prolonged disability is increased.[65-67] Health professionals such as general practitioners and physiotherapists are intimately involved in the treatment of injured workers. The primary focus is often on relief of symptoms and restoration of function. Return to pre-injury work activities is the expected but often the secondary outcome of treatment. Increasingly, health-care practitioners are being encouraged and expected to take a more active role in the return to work (RTW) of the injured worker.[68-70] This is driven not only by the insurance authorities,[68] but also by the mounting evidence for the negative impact of worklessness.[71] For some practitioners, this may require a paradigm shift or, at least, clarification of the patient's treatment goals. RTW was once considered the end of the rehabilitation phase but complete recovery cannot always be assumed. There is evidence that for many workers the RTW was not sustained, with as many as two-thirds of workers experiencing a subsequent injury-related work absence.[72] Possible reasons are the recurrent nature of many MSDs, pressure from the organization to return sooner than ready or an organization's inability to modify the work environment. RTW is now recognized as a dynamic process, the success of which is dependent on the coordination of the various players in the process each with their own (sometimes competing) needs and demands.[73-76] This section will discuss three features of the advances made in the sphere of work disability prevention: adopting a systems approach to work disability prevention; looking beyond the physical symptoms; and the need to promote ability not disability in workers.

A Systems Approach to Work Disability Prevention

It is well-accepted that musculoskeletal conditions are best understood and managed according to a biopsychosocial model that includes biological, psychological and social dimensions.[77-81] Yet this model does not reflect the complexity of issues surrounding RTW after injury, which is influenced by a complex interaction of the individual and their health condition and the various stakeholders and systems (political, legislative, social, work environment, health care).[82] One model that reinforces the biopsychosocial perspective but also considers the various actors in the work disability prevention arena is that developed by Loisel et al.[82] This is an operational rather than an explanatory model to guide the management and understanding of the various systems on the disability process. The worker is at the centre of the recovery process and is exposed to the influence of four main systems (Fig. 38-3):

• their own personal resources to manage their condition and the impact on their life and family

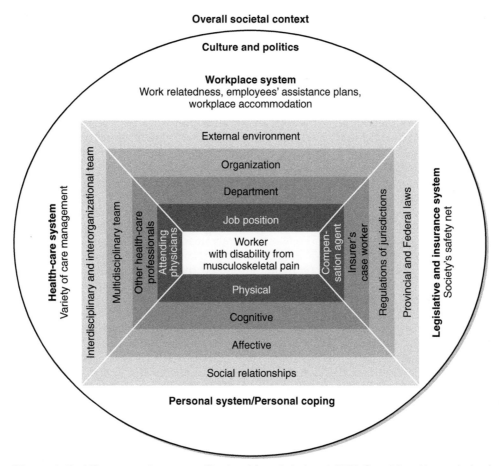

FIGURE 38-3 ■ The work disability prevention arena. (Reprinted from Loisel et al 2005. Copyright with permission from Springer.)

- the health-care system and various providers and their unique and overlapping roles
- the workplace system with its various policies and procedures to follow and
- the legislative and insurance system with the various actors and steps to follow.

By conceptualizing RTW as the result of an intricate interplay between various systems, it is necessary to accept that a transdisciplinary approach is required. This means that work optimization requires the involvement of professionals from various health disciplines such as medicine, occupational therapy, physiotherapy, nursing, psychology and ergonomics, as well as members of the organization such as human resource management, line manager, insurance and compensation systems. Thus, successful reintegration for work is a shared responsibility between the worker, health providers, the workplace and the insurance provider. The involvement of each stakeholder group from onset of injury is an important change in the way RTW is managed. Examples of system approaches include the 'Sherbrooke' model,[83] 'integrated care',[84] 'multifaceted' intervention,[85] coordinated and tailored work rehabilitation,[86] and the Return2Health programme.[87] Common to all these interventions is the active involvement of the worker and organization in addition to the health-care team.

The Sherbrooke model was developed and piloted by Loisel et al.[83] It consisted of a combined clinical rehabilitation and occupational intervention with the aim of returning workers with subacute back pain to their regular job. The clinical rehabilitation aspect involved a multidisciplinary approach whereas the occupational intervention included visits to the workplace by an occupational medicine physician, ergonomist, the injured worker, the supervisor, and management and union representatives. A participatory ergonomics[a] intervention was included to ensure that any work modifications or changes recommended would be feasible and acceptable to the organization that was at liberty to implement them or not. A 1-year follow-up revealed that the model was effective. Workers returned to pre-injury work 2.4 times faster than workers in usual care[88] and the model was cost effective in the long term for the insurer.[89] This Canadian intervention was replicated to suit the Dutch socioeconomic context by Anema et al.[90] and used for workers absent from work for 2–6 weeks due to non-specific low back pain. In comparison to usual care, workers returned to work sooner (77 versus 104 days) when participating in this active workplace intervention. The cost–benefit analyses showed that every £1 invested in integrated care

---

[a]Participatory ergonomics is defined as ergonomics with participation of the necessary actors in problem solving. A characteristic feature is the formation of an ergonomics team typically made up of employees or their representatives, managers, ergonomists, health and safety personnel, and research experts.

would return an estimated £26 with a net societal benefit of integrated care compared with usual care of £5744.[84]

Evidence of the success of multi-stakeholder interventions in countries without a workers' compensation insurance scheme is available from the UK and Denmark. In the UK, the Return2Health intervention was implemented to minimize the costs of long-term sickness absence and its adverse impact on health.[87] This intervention included representatives from the main stakeholders – human resource professionals, managers, employees and clinicians (occupational health physician, psychologist and physiotherapist). The focus of the intervention was restoration of function using a biopsychosocial approach, coordinated by a case manager. As a result of this intervention, the proportion of staff off work longer than 8 weeks decreased from 51.7% to 45.9% while increasing from 51.2% to 56.1% in the control group. Similarly, in Denmark workers receiving coordinated care by an interdisciplinary team had significantly fewer sickness absence hours than controls with savings of US$1366 per worker at 6-month review.[86]

In Australia, a multifaceted intervention was trialled that included early reporting, employee-centred case management by an experienced injury manager and removal of barriers to RTW through active involvement of the workplace. It resulted in a 40% reduction in the number of days on compensation and reduction in the average cost of claims by AUD$2329.[85]

These studies demonstrate that a systems approach to RTW after injury can result in benefits to the individual, the organization and the disability insurance scheme. This win–win approach is only possible when each stakeholder recognizes the differing perspective of each while sharing the ultimate goal of sustained RTW for the individual. The health-care provider can enhance this process by providing regular feedback regarding progress of the worker to the individual, insurer and organization to maintain or increase the stakeholders' levels of commitment and involvement and assist in the development of the RTW plan.

Beyond Physical Symptoms

The concept of Red Flags as signs of serious pathology is well engrained in a clinician's assessment of patients with musculoskeletal conditions. Less well known and assessed are the Yellow, Blue and Black Flags introduced to increase the focus on the psychological and workplace factors contributing to back disability after injury onset.[79] The flag concept has been extended for use in the secondary and tertiary prevention of disability after any musculoskeletal injuries, not only the back. Yellow Flags refer to those psychological features that may be considered normal but unhelpful reactions to pain such as the belief that pain implies damage; the Orange, less modifiable Flags are considered to be those conditions meeting the criteria for psychopathology (e.g. post-traumatic stress, major depression).[91] Blue Flags refer to the worker's (negative) perceptions about the workplace such as poor expectations for RTW, that work is stressful or harmful, and the workplace is unsupportive. Black Flags refer to the existing work conditions external to the individual

(e.g. high physical demands), interactions with the insurance system (e.g. access to treatment; questions of legitimacy) or the organization (e.g. availability of alternative duties) in which the injury is managed. The term 'procedural justice' refers to the worker's experience of the justice of the compensation process which has been linked with work absenteeism, high levels of stress and poorer long-term recovery.[92] Blue Flags may potentially be modifiable by therapeutic interventions whereas Black Flags require greater negotiation and often changes to the legislation or organizational policy and outside clinicians' influence.

In general, clinicians believe in the importance of assessing the psychosocial obstacles but may find management of these issues challenging.[93] There is preliminary evidence that few clinicians consider the work-relevant Blue Flags in their assessment.[94] Reasons offered include a lack of confidence in this area, not part of their professional role and the uncertainty in the assessment of these factors and interpretation of results. There are several tools available for use to assist in the assessment of psychosocial barriers to work. Yellow Flags are addressed in the Örebro Musculoskeletal Pain Questionnaire,[95] STarT Back Screening Tool[96] or the Fear Avoidance beliefs questionnaire.[97] For a comprehensive assessment of Blue Flags, the Obstacles to Return to Work Questionnaire[98] has been recommended, although its length may prohibit routine use in clinical practice.[99] Another option is to adopt the six-stage strategy recommended by Shaw et al.[69] as a means of incorporating workplace issues into usual clinical practice. Assessment of recovery expectations, one of the most consistent predictors of work disability and pain outcomes, can be assessed by the Return to Work Self-Efficacy Scale.[100] No one scale currently exists to measure all aspects of Black Flags; however, the physical demands of work may be assessed by a visit to the workplace or the Job Requirements and Physical Demands Scale.[101] Procedural justice may be assessed by the Perceived Justice of the Compensation Process Scale.[102]

With so many psychosocial factors implicated as important for the recovery from injury, the clinician may be at a loss to decide which to focus on as it is impossible to include all. A recent review by Laisné et al.[81] found strong evidence for two psychosocial constructs as predictors of work participation – recovery expectation and disability management systems such as availability of modified work or workplace accommodations. While psychosocial factors were once considered more relevant in the transition from acute to chronic state, this systematic review suggests that an integrated biopsychosocial approach early in the acute phase is important as many factors predate the injury or may have even contributed to the onset.

Much research has focused on low back pain as it is a common work-related MSD. Eight workplace factors are considered strong predictors of poor recovery from this injury: heavy physical demands at work, the inability to modify work, job stress, low social support from co-workers or supervisors, short job tenure, job dissatisfaction, poor expectation for return to work, and fear of re-injury.[69,103] Thus clinicians are advised to include assessment of these factors with either targeted questioning or the scales mentioned above in both the management of acute/subacute MSD and chronic MSD.

Promoting Ability Not Disability

There is evidence that workers who have sustained a work-related injury feel disempowered by the compensation process, experience difficulty navigating the social and procedural environment of RTW and are frustrated with the information imbalance between themselves, insurers and health-care providers. They are concerned about repercussions from disclosing their condition in the workplace, the perceived legitimacy of their injury and associated stigma with being injured.[104–108] Adopting a client-centred orientation and communication style may create an environment in which the worker feels comfortable discussing these concerns.[109] This opens discussions in which the clinician can help the worker identify and problem-solve their concerns about re-injury and their capacity to work, stigma and pressure from co-workers or supervisors to undertake more than they feel able. Techniques such as motivational interviewing,[87] problem solving[110] and goal setting with structured activity plans[111] have been successfully delivered by physiotherapists to benefit workers returning to work. These techniques motivate and empower the worker to self-manage obstacles to return to and remain at work and are particularly important for ongoing chronic MSD management. For practical tips on incorporating self-management strategies into practice when managing patients with a chronic musculoskeletal condition see Johnston et al.[112]

SUMMARY

Musculoskeletal health in the workplace is important for individuals, the work organizations and for society more broadly. Being able to work in a suitable job provides a very positive influence on a person's health and well-being. Clinicians have traditionally had a strong role in the management of MSDs and this role can be enhanced and extended to acknowledge and utilize the important influence of work in helping to prevent the development of MSDs and the disability related to them. Clinicians are ideally placed to be the conduit between the clinic and the workplace due to their proximity to the worker, their understanding of physical and psychosocial barriers to recovery and sustaining available ability, and their highly developed communication skills. However, to maximize their contribution to the musculoskeletal health of the working population, it is important for clinicians to stay abreast of the changes within society, such as the ageing population, and the work environment, such as the increase in precarious work. Evidence for the ergonomic/risk-management approach to injury prevention suggests that identifying and assessing the risks for injury is worthwhile with ample resources available to assist the clinician gain appropriate skills in this area. There is also evidence to support the systems approach for the prevention of work disability which

must consider all the stakeholders and RTW barriers. Clinicians are thus well placed to move 'beyond the clinic' to maximize the worker's opportunity to recover musculoskeletal health for a sustained return to work following an acute MSD or to remain at work with a chronic MSD.

REFERENCES

1. Dodu N. Is employment good for well-being? A literature review. J Occup Psychol Employ Disabil 2005;7:17–33.
2. World Health Organisation. Global Health and Aging. National Institute on Aging; National Institutes of Health; 2011 Contract No.: Contract No.: NIH Publication no. 11-7737.
3. NOHSC. Surveillance alert – OHS and the ageing workforce [Internet]. National Occupational Health and Safety Commission, Commonwealth of Australia; 2005.
4. Ilmarinen J. The ageing worker. J Occup Environ Med 2001;58: 546–52.
5. Shephard R. Age and physical work capacity. Exp Aging Res 1999; 25:331–43.
6. Kemmlert K, Lundholm L. Slips, trips and falls in different work groups – with reference to age and from a preventive perspective. Appl Ergon 2001;32:149–53.
7. Walton M. Graying, not falling. Occupa Health Saf 1999; 68:85–7.
8. Safe Work Australia. Australian work-related injury experience by sex and age 2009–10 [Internet]. Commonwealth of Australia. Available from: <http://www.safeworkaustralia.gov.au/>; 2012.
9. US Bureau of Labor Statistics. Non-fatal injuries and illnesses among older workers [Internet]. Available from: <http://www.bls.gov/>; 2009.
10. Gould R, Ilmarinen J, Järvisalo J, et al. Dimensions of work ability: results of the health 2000 survey. In: Helsinki: Finnish Centre for Pensions TSII, National Public Health Institute, editor. Finland: Finnish Institute of Occupational Health; 2008.
11. Ilmarinen J. The ageing workforce – challenges for occupational health. Occup Med 2006;56:362–4.
12. Ilmarinen J. Work ability – a comprehensive concept for occupational health research and prevention. Scand J Work Environ Health 2009;35:1–5.
13. Ilmarinen J, Rantanen J. Promotion of work ability during ageing. Am J Ind Med 1999;36:21–3.
14. Australian Institute of Health and Welfare. Chronic dsease and participation in work. In: Australian Institute of Health and Welfare, editor. Canberra: Australian Government; 2009.
15. Department of Health. Healthy workers initiative. Commonwealth of Australia. Available from: <www.healthyworkers.gov.au>; 2013 [updated 12.11.13; cited 2013 13.12.13.].
16. Australian Institute of Health and Welfare. Risk factors and participation in work. In: Australian Institute of Health and Welfare, editor. Canberra: Australian Government; 2010.
17. Quinlan M, Mayhew C, Bohle P. The global expansion of precarious employment, work disorganization, and consequences for occupational health: placing the debate in a comparative historical context. Int J Health Serv 2001;31:507–36.
18. Benach J, Muntaner C, Santana V. Employment Conditions and Health Inequalities Labor Markets and Welfare States: A Country Perspective. Barcelona: Final report to the WHO Commission on Social Determinants of Health: Employment Conditions Knowledge Network (EMCONET); 2007.
19. Straker L, Mathiassen SE. Increased physical work loads in modern work – a necessity for better health and performance? Ergonomics 2009;52:1215–21.
20. Mummery WK, Schofield GM, Steele R, et al. Occupational sitting time and overweight and obesity in australian workers. Am J Prev Med 2005;29:91.
21. Church TS, Thomas DM, Tudor-Locke C, et al. Trends over 5 decades in U.S. occupation-related physical activity and their associations with obesity. PLoS ONE 2011;6(5):e19657.
22. Alkhajah TA, Reeves MM, Eakin EG, et al. Sit–stand workstations: a pilot intervention to reduce office sitting time. Am J Prev Med 2012;43:298–303.

23. Conn VS, Hafdahl AR, Cooper PS, et al. Meta-analysis of workplace physical activity interventions. Am J Prev Med 2009;37:330–9.

24. Centers for Disease Control and Prevention C. Work-Related Musculoskeletal Disorders (Wmsd) Prevention. Atlanta, US: Centers for Disease Control and Prevention; 2013. Available from: <http://www.cdc.gov/workplacehealthpromotion/implementation/topics/disorders.html>; [cited 2013 23rd October.].

25. World Health Organization. Identification and Control of Work-Related Diseases: Report of a WHO Expert Committee. Geneva: World Health Organisation; 1985 Technical Report Series 714.

26. World Health Organisation W. World Health Classification: Manual of the International Statistical Classification of Diseases, Injuries, and Causes of Death. Geneva, Switzerland: World Health Organization; 1977.

27. Punnett L, Wegman DH. Work-related musculoskeletal disorders: the epidemiologic evidence and the debate. J Electromyogr Kinesiol 2004;14:13–23.

28. Safe Work Australia. Compendium of Workers' Compensation Statistics Australia 2010–11. Canberra: Commonwealth of Australia; 2013. p. 112; ISBN 978-1-74361-036-7 (Online PDF) ed.

29. Zheltoukhova K, Bevan S, Reich A. Fit for Work? Musculoskeletal Disorders and the Australian Labour Market. The Work Foundation, Part of Lancaster University; 2012.

30. European Agency for Safety and Health at Work. A European campaign on musculoskeletal disorders (en4): work-related musculoskeletal disorder-prevention report. In: Office for Official Publications of the European Communities, editor. Luxembourg: 2008.

31. Woolf AD, Vos T, March LM. How to measure the impact of musculoskeletal conditions. Best Pract Res Clin Rheumatol 2010;24:723–32.

32. Kuoppala J, Lamminpa L, Husman P. Work health promotion, job well-being, and sickness absences – a systematic review and meta-analysis. J Occup Environ Med 2008;50:1216–27.

33. World Confederation for Physical Therapy. Position Statement: Description of Physical Therapy. London: 2007.

34. Proper K, Koning M, van der Beek A, et al. The effectiveness of worksite physical activity programs on physical activity, physical fitness, and health. Clin J Sport Med 2003;13:106–17.

35. Verhagen AP, Karels C, Bierma-Zeinstra SMA, et al. Ergonomic and physiotherapeutic interventions for treating work-related complaints of the arm, neck or shoulder in adults. Cochrane Database Syst Rev 2006;(3):CD003471.

36. Verhagen AP, Karels C, Bierma-Zeinstra SMA, et al. Exercise proves effective in a systematic review of work-related complaints of the arm, neck, or shoulder. J Clin Epidemiol 2007;60:110–17.

37. Institute for Work & Health. At work, Issue 43. Toronto: Institute for Work & Health; 2006. Available from: <http://www.iwh.on.ca/system/files/at-work/at_work_43.pdf>; [cited January 2014.].

38. Dunn KM, Jordan KP, Mancl L, et al. Trajectories of pain in adolescents: a prospective cohort study. Pain 2011;152:66–73.

39. Rees C, Smith A, O'Sullivan P, et al. Back and neck pain are related to mental health problems in adolescence. BMC Public Health 2011;11:382.

40. O'Sullivan PB, Beales DJ, Smith AJ, et al. Low back pain in 17 year olds has substantial impact and represents an important public health disorder: a cross-sectional study. BMC Public Health 2012;12:100.

41. Axen I, Leboeuf-Yde C. Trajectories of low back pain. Best Pract Res Clin Rheumatol 2013;27:601–12.

42. Straker L. Evidence to support using squat, semi-squat and stoop techniques to lift low-lying objects. Int J Ind Ergon 2003;31:149–60.

43. Straker LM. A review of research on techniques for lifting low-lying objects: 1. Criteria for evaluation. Work 2002;19:9–18.

44. Straker LM. A review of research on techniques for lifting low-lying objects: 2. Evidence for a correct technique. Work 2003;20:83–96.

45. Van Dieen JH, Hoozemanns MJM, Toussaint HM. Stoop or squat: a review of biomechanical studies on lifting technique. Clin Biomech 1999;14:685–96.

46. Daltroy LH, Iversen MD, Larson MG, et al. A controlled trial of an educational program to prevent low back injuries. NEJM 1997;337:322–8.

47. Verbeek JH, Martimo KP, Karppinen J, et al. Manual material handling advice and assistive devices for preventing and treating back pain in workers. Cochrane Database Syst Rev 2011.

48. Macdonald W, Evans O. Research on the prevention of work-related musculoskeletal disorders. Stage 1 – literature review. In: Australian Safety and Compensation Council, editor. Canberra: Australian Government; 2006.

49. Safe Work Australia. Hazardous manual tasks code of practice. In: Australian Government, editor. Canberra: Australian Government; 2011.

50. da Costa BR, Vieira ER. Risk factors for work related musculoskeletal disorders: a systematic review of recent longitudinal studies. Am J Ind Med 2010;53:285–323.

51. Bernard B, Putz-Anderson V, Burt SE. Musculoskeletal Disorders and Workplace Factors: a Critical Review of Epidemiologic Evidence for Work-Related Musculoskeletal Disorders of the Neck, Upper Extremity and Low Back. Cincinatti: U.S. Department of Health and Human Services; 1997 Publication No. 97–141 Contract No.: July, 1997.

52. Xu Y-Y, Cheng ASK, Li-Tsang CWP. Prevalence and risk factors of work-related musculoskeletal disorders in the catering industry: a systematic review. Work 2013;44:107–16.

53. Kilbom A. Assessment of physical exposure in relation to work-related musculoskeletal disorders – what information can be obtained from systematic observations? Scand J Work Environ Health 1994;20:30–45.

54. McAtamney L, Corlett NE. Rula: a survey method for the investigation of work-related upper limb disorders. Appl Ergon 1993;24:91–9.

55. HSE HaSE. Manual handling assessment charts. In: Executive HaS, editor. UK: 2003.

56. Waters TR, Putz-Anderson V, Garg A, et al. Revised niosh equation for design and evaluation of manual lifting tasks. Ergonomics 1993;36:749–76.

57. Snook SH, Ciriello VM. The design of manual handling tasks: revised tables of maximum acceptable weights and forces. Ergonomics 1991;34:1197–213.

58. Moore JS, Garg A. The strain index: a proposed method to analyze jobs for risk of distal upper extremity disorders. Am Ind Hyg Assoc J 1995;56:443–58.

59. Burgess-Limerick R, Egeskov R, Straker L, et al. Manual tasks risk assessment tool (mantra) v2. 2004.

60. Karasek RA, Berisson C, Kawakami N, et al. The Job Content Questionnaire (JCQ): an instrument for internationally comparative assessments of psychosocial job characteristics. J Occup Health Psychol 1998;3:322–56.

61. Li G, Buckle P. Evaluating Change in Exposure to Risk for Musculoskeletal Disorders – A Practical Tool. London: Health and Safety Executive; 1999.

62. ILO-OSH. Guidelines on Occupational Safety and Health Management Systems. Geneva: International Labour Office; 2001.

63. Straker LM, Burgess-Limerick R, Pollock C, et al. A randomized and controlled trial of a participative ergonomics intervention to reduce injuries associated with manual tasks: physical risk and legislative compliance. Ergonomics 2004;47:166–88.

64. Levanon Y, Gefen A, Lerman Y, et al. Reducing musculoskeletal disorders among computer operators: comparison between ergonomics interventions at the workplace. Ergonomics 2012;55:1571–85.

65. Krause N, Dasinger L, Neuhauser F. Modified work and return to work: a review of the literature. J Occup Rehabil 1998;8:113–39.

66. Australian Institute for Social Research. The Role of the Workplace in Return to Work: Discussion Paper. WorkCover SA; 2008.

67. Watson PJ, Booker CK, Moores L, et al. Returning the chronically unemployed with low back pain to employment. Eur J Pain 2004;8:359–69.

68. Johnston V, Nielsen M, Corbiere M, et al. Experiences and perspectives of physical therapists managing patients covered by workers' compensation in Queensland, Australia. Phys Ther 2012;92:1306–15.

69. Shaw WS, Main CJ, Johnston V. Addressing occupational factors in the management of low back pain: implications for physical therapist practice. Phys Ther 2011;91:1–13.

70. Pincus T, Greenwood L, McHarg E. Advising people with back pain to take time off work: a survey examining the role of private musculoskeletal practitioners in the uk. Pain 2011;152:2813–18.

71. Australasian Faculty of Occupational & Environmental Medicine. Realising the Health Benefits of Work: A Position Statement. Sydney: The Royal Australasian College of Physicians; 2010.

72. Baldwin ML, Butler RJ. Upper extremity disorders in the workplace: costs and outcomes beyond the first return to work. J Occup Rehabil 2006;16:303–23.

73. Franche RL, Baril R, Shaw W, et al. Workplace-based return-to-work interventions: optimizing the role of stakeholders in implementation and research. J Occup Rehabil 2005;15:525–42.

74. Young AE, Roessler RT, wasiak R, et al. A developmental conceptualization of return towork. J Occup Rehabil 2005;15:557–68.

75. Kosny A, MacEachen E, Ferrier S, et al. The role of health care providers in long term and complicated workers' compensation claims. J Occup Rehabil 2011;21(4):582–90.

76. Wynne-Jones G, Buck R, Porteous C, et al. What happens to work if you're unwell? Beliefs and attitudes of managers and employees with musculoskeletal pain in a public sector setting. J Occup Rehabil 2011;21:31–42.

77. Engel GL. The need for a new medical model: a challenge for biomedicine. Science 1977;196:129–36.

78. Linton SJ. A review of psychological risk factors in back and neck pain. Spine 2000;25:1148–56.

79. Kendall NAS. Psychosocial approaches to the prevention of chronic pain: the low back paradigm. Baillieres Best Practice Res Clin Rheumatol 1999;13:545–54.

80. Pincus T, Burton AK, Vogel S, et al. A systematic review of psychological factors as predictors of chronicity/disability in prospective cohorts of low back pain. Spine 2002;27:E109–20.

81. Laisné F, Lecomte C, Corbière M. Biopsychosocial predictors of prognosis in musculoskeletal disorders: a systematic review of the literature. Disabil Rehabil 2012;34:355–82.

82. Loisel P, Buchbinder R, Hazard R, et al. Prevention of work disability due to musculoskeletal disorders: the challenge of implementing evidence. J Occup Rehabil 2005;15:507–24.

83. Loisel P, Durand P, Abenhaim L, et al. Management of occupational back pain: the Sherbrooke model. Results of a pilot and feasibility study. Occup Environ Med 1994;51:597–602.

84. Lambeek LC, Bosmans JE, Van Royen BJ, et al. Effect of integrated care for sick listed patients with chronic low back pain: economic evaluation alongside a randomised controlled trial. Br Med J 2010;341:c6414.

85. Iles RA, Wyatt M, Pranksy G. Multi-faceted case management: reducing compensation costs of musculoskeletal work injuries in Australia. J Occup Rehabil 2012;22:478–88.

86. Bultmann U, Sherson D, Olsen J, et al. Coordinated and tailored work rehabilitation: a randomized controlled trial with economic evaluation undertaken with workers on sick leave due to musculoskeletal disorders. J Occup Rehabil 2009;19:81–93.

87. Smedley J, Harris EC, Cox V, et al. Evaluation of a case management service to reduce sickness absence. Occup Med 2013;63:89–95.

88. Loisel P, Abenhaim L, Durand P, et al. A population-based, randomized clinical trial on back pain management. Spine 1997;22:2911–18.

89. Loisel P, Lemaire J, Poitras S, et al. Cost-benefit and cost-effectiveness analysis of a disability prevention model for back pain management: a six year follow up study. Occup Environ Med 2002;59:807–15.

90. Anema JR, Steenstra IA, Bongers PM, et al. Multidisciplinary rehabilitation for subacute low back pain: graded activity or workplace intervention or both? A randomized controlled trial. Spine 2007;32:291–8.

91. Nicholas M, Linton SJ, Watson PJ, et al. Early identification and management of psychological risk factors ('yellow flags') in patients with low back pain: a reappraisal. Phys Ther 2011;91:1–7.

92. Grant GM, O'Donnell ML, Spittal MJ, et al. Relationship between stressfulness of claiming for injury compensation and long-term recovery: a prospective cohort study. JAMA Psychiatry In press.

93. Sanders T, Foster NE, Bishop A, et al. Biopsychosocial care and the physiotherapy encounter: physiotherapists' accounts of back pain consultations. BMC Musculoskelet Disord 2013;14:65.

94. Gray H, Howe T. Physiotherapists' assessment and management of psychosocial factors (yellow and blue flags) in individuals with back pain. Phys Ther Rev 2013;18:379–94.

95. Linton SJ, Hallden K. Can we screen for problematic back pain? A screening questionnaire for predicting outcome in acute and subacute back pain. Clin J Pain 1998;14:209–15.

96. Hill JC, Dunn KM, Lewis M, et al. A primary care back pain screening tool: identifying patient subgroups for initial treatment. Arthritis Rheum 2008;59:632–41.

97. Waddell G, Newton M, Henderson I, et al. A fear-avoidance beliefs questionnaire (fabq) and the role of fear-avoidance beliefs in chronic low back pain and disability. Pain 1993;52:157–68.

98. Marhold C, Linton S, Melin L. Identification of obstacles for chronic pain patients to return to work: evaluation of a questionnaire. J Occup Rehabil 2002;12:65–75.

99. Gray H, Adefolarin AT, Howe TE. A systematic review of instruments for the assessment of work-related psychosocial factors (blue flags) in individuals with non-specific low back pain. Man Ther 2011;16:531–43.

100. Brouwer S, Franche RL, Hogg-Johnson S, et al. Return-to-work self-efficacy: development and validation of a scale in claimants with musculoskeletal disorders. J Occup Rehabil 2010;21:244–58.

101. Daniels C, Huang GD, Feuerstein M, et al. Self-report measure of low back-related biomechanical exposures: clinical validation. J Occup Rehabil 2005;15:113–28.

102. Franche R-L, Severin C, Lee H, et al. Perceived justice of compensation process for return-to-work: development and validation of a scale. Psychol Inj Law 2009;2:225–37.

103. Costa-Black KM, Loisel P, Anema JR, et al. Back pain and work. Best Pract Res Clin Rheumatol 2010;24:227–40.

104. Eggert S. Psychosocial factors affecting employees' abilities to return to work. AAOHN J 2010;58:51–5.

105. MacEachen E, Clarke J, Franche RL, et al. Systematic review of the qualitative literature on return to work after injury. Scand J Work Environ Health 2006;32:257–69.

106. Baril R, Clarke J, Friesen M, et al. Management of return-to-work programs for workers with musculoskeletal disorders: a qualitative study in three canadian provinces. Soc Sci Med 2003;57:2101–14.

107. Roberts-Yates C. The concerns and issues of injured workers in relation to claims/injury management and rehabilitation: the need for new operational frameworks. Disabil Rehabil 2003;25:898–907.

108. Young AE, Wasiak R, Phillips L, et al. Workers' perspectives on low back pain recurrence: 'it comes and goes and comes and goes, but it's always there'. Pain 2011;152:204–11.

109. Shaw WS, Chin EH, Nelson CC, et al. What circumstances prompt a workplace discussion in medical evaluations for back pain? J Occup Rehabil 2012;23(1):125–34.

110. van den Hout JH, Vlaeyen JWS, Heuts PH, et al. Secondary prevention of work-related disability in non-specific low back pain: does problem-solving therapy help? A randomized clinical trial. Clin J Pain 2003;19:87–96.

111. Sullivan MJL, Ward CL, Tripp D, et al. Secondary prevention of work disability: community-based psychosocial intervention for musculoskeletal disorders. J Occup Rehabil 2005;15:377–92.

112. Johnston V, Jull G, Sheppard DM, et al. Applying principles of self-management to facilitate workers to return to or remain at work with a chronic musculoskeletal condition. Man Ther 2013;18:274–80.

SCREENING

EDITOR'S INTRODUCTION

Screening in health care is used to identify potential risk factors for people without symptoms that, if left untreated, may lead to serious illness. Examples include assessment of blood pressure, monitoring blood glucose levels and bowel cancer screening programmes. The management of musculoskeletal conditions has not taken this approach and traditionally has involved assessment and management of symptoms as and when they present. The authors invited to contribute the two musculoskeletal screening chapters are international leaders in the field of musculoskeletal screening. These chapters explore the potential role of screening as a method to prevent musculoskeletal symptoms, as well as providing guidance when treating individuals with symptoms with a view of preventing or reducing recurrence. This is relevant as recurrence rates associated with musculoskeletal conditions are high, and the number one risk factor for musculoskeletal injury is previous injury. As such, attempts to reduce recurrence are warranted and welcome. The first subchapter deals mainly with athletic populations and identifies the independent predictors, risk factors and associated factors measured using field-expedient screening tests that have consistently been linked to future injury. The second subchapter presents a method and structure for undertaking musculoskeletal screening. Screening functional movement patterns, rather than single musculoskeletal variables, as predictors for injury is becoming increasingly popular and this is discussed in the two subchapters. The synthesis of these two subchapters will provide the reader with an understanding of the potential value for screening in musculoskeletal conditions. It will also highlight uncertainties and areas where our knowledge base with respect to screening for musculoskeletal conditions requires further research.

CHAPTER 39.1   ■   SCREENING FOR MUSCULOSKELETAL DISORDERS

Tania Pizzari • Carolyn Taylor

INTRODUCTION

Injury can detrimentally affect an athlete's performance, their team's success and, in extreme cases, curtail their career. Injuries may linger after the athlete has finished competing and result in long-term disability,[1,2] with an associated high cost for both the individual and society.[3] Screening of athletes for current injury and risk of future injury is common practice throughout the world in an attempt to reduce this injury burden. This screening is often called 'pre-participation examination' and is conducted by sports medicine personnel with the aim of identifying risk of illness, injury or sudden death in athletes.[4,5] Assessment prior to commencing organized sport is compulsory in some areas of the world (such as Italy and some parts of the United States of America)[6] and is also mandated by some sporting organizations.[2] However, in other places, this screening is voluntary (United Kingdom and Australia).[4,5] A pre-participation examination may have multiple components and include screening for cardiovascular, neurological, pulmonary, urogenital and musculoskeletal injury.[2,4,7,8] This chapter is concerned with musculoskeletal screening.

THE IMPORTANCE OF MUSCULOSKELETAL SCREENING

Although there are many reasons to conduct musculoskeletal screening, the most common are to identify current injuries or physical deficits due to previous injuries and to identify potentially modifiable intrinsic risk factors that may predispose the athlete to future injury.[4] Intrinsic risk factors may be present as a result of an inadequately rehabilitated previous injury[2] or be an inherent physical characteristic of that athlete, such as limited joint range of motion. The identification of modifiable risk factors may then allow counselling of athletes with sports-specific deficits and rehabilitation or prevention programmes to be implemented with the aim of reducing the risk of future injury.[7,9,10]

Other potential benefits of screening include building a professional rapport with the athlete, having first-hand knowledge of current and previous musculoskeletal injuries and physical deficits, educating athletes[4] and providing research data.

THE DIFFICULTIES OF SCREENING

The identification of potential risk factors for injury is an underdeveloped area of sports medicine research and there are few proven risk factors for injury.[2,6,8] In part this is because large, well-designed, cohort studies employing appropriate and generalizable outcome measures that screen uninjured athletes for potential risk factors and then follow them up for 1 to 2 years, without preventative intervention, are difficult to conduct.[9] Scientifically robust screening protocols based on evidence for the incidence of injury, the mechanism of injury and the established risk factors that utilize tests with predictive validity and reliability to identify those risk factors are required to conduct longitudinal cohort studies of value.

Research into musculoskeletal injury has predominantly yielded single variables as predictors of injury and these may vary depending on the requirements of the sport and the athlete characteristics. It is unrealistic to identify individual tests to predict every musculoskeletal injury in all athlete types and to conduct screening for each potential risk factor.[10,11] The multifactorial aetiology of most injuries means that a focus on single predictors neglects the inter-relationship between the intrinsic risk factors and extrinsic risks present at the moment of an inciting injury event.[12]

Musculoskeletal screening protocols are highly variable[4,6] and are often developed on an ad hoc basis based on practitioner preferences with no regard for the reliability or the predictive validity of the tests. Problems also arise when the musculoskeletal tests are conducted differently by different sports medicine personnel.[4] The field-expedience of screening protocols may also limit their use.

The time, cost, equipment and expertise required to conduct screening are an important consideration.[11,13]

Interpretation of screening outcomes is also complicated. No screening test is 100% accurate and therefore athletes may be falsely identified as having a positive or negative risk based on a test result. An athlete estimated to be at risk might then undertake unnecessary, costly and onerous steps in an attempt to minimize this risk.

RISK FACTORS AND INJURY

The identification of risk factors for injury using tests with predictive validity is an essential aspect of the musculoskeletal screening process. There are three different levels of 'risk factor': associated factors, risk factors and independent predictors. An associated factor is identified when a positive musculoskeletal test is associated with an injury in a cross-sectional cohort study.[14] A risk factor is where a musculoskeletal test is related to an injury in a prospective study using univariate or bivariate analysis.[15] An independent predictor is where the outcome of a musculoskeletal test has a significant contribution to an injury in a prospective study using a multivariate analysis, where all identified risk factors are included and where all other risk factors are controlled for.[16] A musculoskeletal test used to identify an independent predictor is said to have 'predictive validity', that is, the ability to predict future injury; however, a very limited number of independent predictors for injury in sport have been identified.[4]

While there are a small number of risk factors with predictive validity for injury risk, there are some with established links to injury risk. Table 39-1 outlines commonly used field-expedient screening tests with known reliability properties and some level of predictive validity.

There is a need for normative data for many of the tests used for musculoskeletal screening and a need to identify the threshold for abnormality.[63] It is important to establish what is normal and does not pose an increased injury risk, and what is an abnormal test result that could mean an increased risk of injury and allow for preventative strategies to be adopted. It should be noted that normative values and threshold might vary depending on the type and level of activity and the personal characteristics of the athlete.

Many non-modifiable risk factors such as age, gender, height, race, previous history, sport and climate, have been implicated in altering the risk of musculoskeletal injury.[64–67] The majority of such factors can be collated using a questionnaire and may be used together with screening tests to build a risk profile for an individual athlete.[11]

SCREENING AND PREVENTION

The assumption of screening is that the identification of risk factors and protective factors may then inform the development of preventative strategies. To date, however, there has been limited evidence that risk

TABLE 39-1 Commonly Used Field-Expedient Screening Tests: Independent Predictors, Risk Factors and Associated Factors with Injury

	Independent Predictors		
Test	**Intra-Rater Reliability**	**Inter-Rater Reliability**	**Predictive Validity**
Prone passive hip internal rotation	ICC >0.94 (95%CI range 0.68–0.97)[17–21]	ICC >0.30 (95%CI range 0.00–0.87)[19–21]	Reduced hip IR on ipsilateral leg independent predictor for lower limb/back injury in amateur cricket players.[22] Hip IR ≤ 30°: OR = 0.20 (0.06–0.073), $p = 0.045$, Hip IR = 31–40°: OR = 0.36 (0.12–1.11), $p = 0.045$
Modified Thomas test (quadriceps flexibility)	ICC >0.99[17] ICC = 0.69 (95%CI 0.29–0.88)[18]	ICC = 0.90 (95% CI 0.72–0.96)[18]	Reduced quadriceps flexibility (<50° of knee flexion) independent predictor of time to sustaining a hamstring injury. More flexible amateur Australian football players had a lower risk of sustaining a hamstring injury.[23] RR >51° knee flexion: RR = 0.3 (0.1–0.8), $p = 0.022$ Reduced hip flexibility (hip neutral/flexion) was an associated factor for sustaining a hamstring injury in professional Australian football players. RR = 1.47 (0.77–2.82)[15]
Hip muscle strength with HHD – hip adduction and abduction	ICC >0.77 (95% CI range 0.24–0.99)[24–28]	ICC >0.62 (95% CI range 0.19–0.97)[24,26,28–41]	Strength of adductor muscles independent predictor for groin injury in amateur soccer players.[32] Adjusted OR = 4.28 (1.38–14.0), $p = 0.02$ Hip adduction to hip abduction strength ratio a risk factor for groin injury (adductor strain) (p = 0.01) and independent predictor (p = 0.03) RR = 17:1 based on hip adduction strength less than 80% of abduction strength in professional ice hockey players[33]
Ankle dorsiflexion lunge	ICC >0.97 (95% CI range 0.92–0.99)[19,34,35]	ICC >0.96 (95% CI range 0.89–0.99)[19,34]	Reduced ankle dorsiflexion on contralateral leg an independent predictor for lower limb/back injury in amateur cricket players[22] Reduced ankle dorsiflexion (<10 cm) an independent predictor for hamstring injury in professional Australian football players[15] Reduced ankle dorsiflexion (≤12 cm) a risk factor for lower limb injury in amateur Australian football players[36]
Single leg balance	ICC = 0.88 (95%CI 0.76–0.94)[37]	ICC = 0.83 (95%CI 0.71–0.91)[37] Kappa = 0.90[38]	A positive SLB test independent predictor for ankle sprains in varsity and intercollegiate athletes, OR = 2.54 (1.02–6.03) $p < 0.05$[38]
Beighton score/ general hypermobility	% agreement = 69% Spearman rho = 0.86[39]	% agreement = 51% Spearman rho = 0.87[39]	Female amateur soccer players who had general joint laxity (Beighton score <4) were at great risk of any injury OR = 5.3 (2.0–13.5), $p < 0.001$. Joint laxity was an independent predictor of knee injury, OR = 5.0 (1.3–18.9), $p < 0.05$[40] Beighton score ≤5 a risk factor for traumatic leg injuries in female soccer players[41] Beighton score <4 a risk factor for any injury in male rugby players[42] General laxity (≥5 regions) a risk factor for non-contact ACL injury in both male and female military cadets[43]
Knee hyperextension (genu recurvatum)	ICC >0.88 (SEM = 1.8 degrees)[44]	ICC >0.48 (SEM = 2.9 degrees)[44] Kappa >0.85 (95% CI 0.64–1.06)[45]	Knee hyperextension an independent predictor for traumatic leg injuries in female soccer players, OR = 3.84 (1.51–9.79), $p = 0.005$[41] Knee hyperextension a risk factor for ACL injury in male American football players OR = 15.56 (3.61–138.32)[46]

TABLE 39-1	**Commonly Used Field-Expedient Screening Tests: Independent Predictors, Risk Factors and Associated Factors with Injury** (Continued)

	Risk Factors		
Test	**Intra-Rater Reliability**	**Inter-Rater Reliability**	**Predictive Validity**
Prone passive hip external rotation	ICC >0.88 (95% CI 0.54–0.96)[17,19]	ICC = 0.66 (95% CI 0.25–0.90)[19]	Restricted hip external rotation range of motion a risk factor for groin injury in amateur soccer players. OR = 1.53 (1.13–2.07) $p < 0.01$[32]
Supine passive hip internal rotation with hip at 90°	ICC >0.88 (95% CI 0.84–0.91)[21,47]	ICC >0.75 (95% CI 0.60–0.84)[21,48]	Restricted total hip rotation was a risk factor for groin injury. For each degree increase in hip rotation there was a 10% reduction in injury rate in professional Australian football players[49]
Supine passive hip external rotation with hip at 90°	ICC >0.91 (95%CI 0.93–0.96)[21,47]	ICC = 0.63 (95%CI 0.44–0.76)[21]	Restricted total hip rotation was a risk factor for groin injury. For each degree increase in hip rotation there was a 10% reduction in injury rate in professional Australian football players[49]
Adductor squeeze test	ICC >0.76 (95%CI range 0.61–0.97)[20,50–52]	ICC >0.77 (95%CI range 0.62–0.96)[20,51,52]	Hip adductor strength decreased 2 weeks preceding and during the onset of groin injury during in-season monitoring of junior elite Australian football players[53]
Single leg hamstring bridge test		ICC = 0.56 (95%CI 0.00–0.83)[19]	Amateur and semi-elite Australian football players who sustained right-sided hamstring strains had significantly lower preseason single leg bridge scores than uninjured players[54]
Biering-Sorenson test	ICC = 0.69 (95%CI 0.59–0.85)[55]	ICC >0.59 (95%CI 0.44–0.97)[55–60]	Extensor muscle endurance was a risk factor for serious low back pain at 36 months follow-up ($p = 0.01$), but not at 12 months follow-up ($p = 0.133$)[61] Risk factor for predicting first-time low back pain in 12-month follow-up period in men ($p = 0.029$), but not in women ($p = 0.34$)[62]
	Associated Factors		
Test	**Intra-Rater Reliability**	**Inter-Rater Reliability**	**Predictive Validity**
Supine active hip internal rotation	ICC = 0.83 (95%CI 0.57–0.94)[18]	ICC = 0.94 (95%CI 0.82–0.98)[18]	Reduced active hip internal rotation was associated with hamstring injury in professional Australian football players[15]

ACL, Anterior cruciate ligament; *CI*, Confidence interval; *HHD*, Hand-held dynamometer; *ICC*, Interclass correlation coefficient; *IR*, Internal rotation; *OR*, Odds ratio; *RR*, Relative risk; *SEM*, Standard error of measurement.

profiles can be altered with intervention[11] or that prevention programmes implemented to address risk factors reduce the risk of injury.[5] The cost benefit of screening must be questioned if it does not reduce the frequency and severity of musculoskeletal injury. Labelling an athlete 'at risk' without the ability to reduce injury may have a detrimental impact on an individual. Improving the quality of screening protocols may enhance the relationship between risk identification and injury prevention.

DEVELOPING A SCREENING TOOL

Ideally, a screening protocol should be highly relevant to a specific sport, and if a team sport, relevant to the individuals and their specific roles. The protocol should include reliable tests that are able to predict injuries and identify risk factors for those injuries. The tool should be simple, financially viable, easy to administer, take a

relatively short amount of time to conduct and not involve complicated tests or expensive equipment. The information should also follow the athlete as they progress through their career and move between teams.

Musculoskeletal screening has two components: a questionnaire and a physical examination.[7,68] Since one of the most consistent predictors of injury is previous injury,[15,65,67] the questionnaire should identify current and previous injuries. Caution needs to be adopted when relying on the information provided in the questionnaire as athletes' recall of injuries beyond the previous 12 months is poor.[69] Athletes may also be less inclined to disclose a complete injury history if they believe the outcome of a potential contract may depend on the extent of their previous injuries. The physical examination component of the musculoskeletal screen should include tests to identify physical deficits that may require further comprehensive assessment, and not to comprehensively assess every area of the athlete at that time.[13,68]

WHEN TO SCREEN

Musculoskeletal screening is conducted at various points in the season or the athlete's career. Screening may be prior to signing a contract, during the preseason, in-season or at the end of the season.[2,7] Preseason screening should be conducted at least 6 to 8 weeks prior to the commencement of the competition season to allow for further investigation and rehabilitation if problems are identified.[4] In-season screening monitors athletes during the season with the aim to identify risk factors that arise as a result of training and competition.[53] The end of season screening identifies issues that the athlete needs to work on during the off-season.

SCREENING FUNCTIONAL MOVEMENT PATTERNS

In response to the difficulties of screening to date, musculoskeletal evaluations have more recently shifted towards the identification of deficits in fundamental movement patterns.[10,11] The assumption that individuals who display poor movement patterns have an elevated risk of injury has been shown to be accurate in a number of studies.[70,71] Movement deficits are believed to limit performance and render the athlete susceptible to injury. The Lower Quarter Y Balance Test™ and the Functional Movement Screen™ are two examples of reliable, field-expedient screening protocols that use grading of movement to develop an injury risk profile for an athlete.[11] Assessment of movement patterns attempts to combine multiple potential risk factors of muscle strength, flexibility, range of motion, coordination, balance and proprioception into one test, and might better account for the multifactorial nature of injury. Screening is not sport-specific and allows the implementation of training programmes based around movement patterns rather than individual joints and muscles. This new generation of screening assessments shows promise; however, further research is required to establish the predictive validity of the tools across a range of populations, reliability across varying examiner levels and their ability to assist in the prevention of injury. The impracticalities of assessor training and equipment are also a consideration with the tools currently available. Care should also be taken to interpret the outcome of movement screening appropriately. The protocols are not diagnostic tools and simply highlight an increase in the risk of injury.

The move towards quantifying movement patterns as an indicator of injury risk signifies an important advancement in the sports medicine and injury prevention fields. The clinical evaluation of functional movement has been a part of clinical practice for many years but failed as a screening tool due to subjectivity and reduced reliability. The current movement screening tools attempt to objectively grade movement using explicit criteria. No doubt there will be continual evolution of fundamental movement pattern screening in years to come.

CLINICAL SCREENING

While this chapter has concentrated on screening for sport and exercise, future research may identify the value of screening people presenting to physiotherapists with a range of musculoskeletal conditions. Screening for general strength, endurance, range of motion and function might identify deficits in addition to the presenting musculoskeletal problem. Identifying and addressing these deficits may improve the rehabilitation outcomes and reduce future injury incidence.

For example, an elderly individual presenting with a fractured neck of humerus or massive inoperable rotator cuff tear who may normally have relied on both upper and lower limbs to stand up from a chair, or ascend stairs, would now have reduced function due to the inability to effectively use the upper limb. If rehabilitation concentrates on re-establishing upper limb function without using reliable, age- and function-specific screening to identify if the lower limbs have appropriate capacity to address the loss of upper limb contribution to these activities, it is arguable that clinical practice should be deemed as sub-standard. The value of screening across all musculoskeletal presentations, ages, co-morbidities and functional needs should be considered.

REFERENCES

1. Oiestad BE, Engebretsen L, Storheim K, et al. Knee osteoarthritis after anterior cruciate ligament injury. Am J Sports Med 2009;37(7):1434–43.
2. Tscholl PE, Dvorark J. Pre-competition orthopaedic assessment in elite athletes: experiences and general considerations from international football. Eur Musculoskel Rev 2011;6(4):260–4.
3. Dallinga JA, Benjaminse A, Lemmink KAPM. Which screening tools can predict injury to the lower extremities in team sports: a systematic review. Sports Med 2012;42(9):791–815.
4. Brukner P, White S, Shawdon A, et al. Screening of athletes: Australian experience. Clin J Sport Med 2004;14(3):169–77.
5. Carek PJ. Evidence-based preparticipation physical examination. In: MacAuley D, Best TM, editors. Evidence-Based Sports Medicine. 2nd ed. Carlton, Vic: Blackwell Publishing Asia; 2007. p. 18–35.
6. Wingfield K, Matheson GO, Meeuwisse WH. Preparticipation evaluation. Clin J Sport Med 2004;14(3):109–22.
7. Batt ME, Jaques R, Stone M. Preparticipation examination (screening): practical issues as determined by sport: a United Kingdom Perspective. Clin J Sport Med 2004;14(3):178–82.
8. Garrick JG. Preparticipation orthopedic screening evaluation. Clin J Sport Med 2004;14(3):123–6.
9. Finch CF. A new framework for research leading to sports injury prevention. J Sci Med Sport 2006;9(1–2):3–9.
10. Schneiders AG, Davidsson A, Horman E, et al. Functional movement screen normative values in a young, active population. Int J Sports Phys Ther 2011;6(2):75–82. [Epub 2011/06/30].
11. Lehr ME, Plisky PJ, Butler RJ, et al. Field-expedient screening and injury risk algorithm categories as predictors of noncontact lower extremity injury. Scand J Med Sci Sports 2013;23(4):e225–32. [Epub 2013/03/23].
12. Bartlett RBM. Sports biomechanics: reducing injury risk and improving sports performance. London; New York: Routledge; 2012.
13. Gomez JE, Landry GLB. Critical evaluation of the 2-minute orthopedic screening examination. Am J Dis Child 1993;147(10):1109–13.
14. Cowan SM, Schache AG, Brukner P, et al. Delayed onset of transversus abdominus in long-standing groin pain. Med Sci Sports Exerc 2004;36(12):2040–5.

15. Gabbe BJ, Bennell KL, Finch CF, et al. Predictors of hamstring injury at the elite level of Australian football. Scand J Med Sci Sports 2006;16(1):7–13.
16. Brotman DJ, Walker E, Lauer MS, et al. In search of fewer independent risk factors. Arch Intern Med 2005;165(2):138–45.
17. Bullock-Saxton J, Bullock M. Repeatability of muscle length measures around the hip. Physiother Can 1994;46(2):105.
18. Gabbe B, Bennell K, Wajswelner H, et al. Reliability of common lower extremity musculoskeletal screening tests. Phys Ther Sport 2004;5(2):90–7.
19. Dennis RJ, Finch CF, Elliott BC, et al. The reliability of musculoskeletal screening tests used in cricket. Phys Ther Sport 2008;9(1): 25–33. [Epub 2008/12/17].
20. Malliaras P, Hogan A, Nawrocki A, et al. Hip flexibility and strength measures: reliability and association with athletic groin pain. Br J Sports Med 2009;43(10):739–44. [Epub 2009/03/14].
21. Prather H, Harris-Hayes M, Hunt DM, et al. Reliability and agreement of hip range of motion and provocative physical examination tests in asymptomatic volunteers. PM R 2010;2(10):888–95. [Epub 2010/10/26].
22. Dennis RJ, Finch CF, McIntosh AS, et al. Use of field-based tests to identify risk factors for injury to fast bowlers in cricket. Br J Sports Med 2008;42(6):477–82. [Epub 2008/04/09].
23. Gabbe BJ, Finch CF, Bennell KL, et al. Risk factors for hamstring injuries in community level Australian football. Br J Sports Med 2005;39(2):106–10.
24. Kelln BM, McKeon PO, Gontkof LM, et al. Hand-held dynamometry: reliability of lower extremity muscle testing in healthy, physically active, young adults. J Sport Rehabil 2008;17(2):160–70. [Epub 2008/06/03].
25. Thorborg K, Petersen J, Magnusson SP, et al. Clinical assessment of hip strength using a hand-held dynamometer is reliable. Scand J Med Sci Sports 2010;20(3):493–501. [Epub 2009/06/30].
26. Krause DA, Schlagel SJ, Stember BM, et al. Influence of lever arm and stabilization on measures of hip abduction and adduction torque obtained by hand-held dynamometry. Arch Phys Med Rehabil 2007;88(1):37–42. [Epub 2007/01/09].
27. Phillips BA, Lo SK, Mastaglia FL. Muscle force measured using 'break' testing with a hand-held myometer in normal subjects aged 20 to 69 years. Arch Phys Med Rehabil 2000;81(5):653–61. [Epub 2000/05/12].
28. Scott DA, Bond EQ, Sisto SA, et al. The intra- and interrater reliability of hip muscle strength assessments using a handheld versus a portable dynamometer anchoring station. Arch Phys Med Rehabil 2004;85(4):598–603. [Epub 2004/04/15].
29. Katoh MYH. Comparison of reliability of isometric leg muscle strength measurements made using a hand-held dynamometer with and without a restraining belt. J Phys Ther Sci 2009;21(1): 37–42.
30. Thorborg K, Serner A, Petersen J, et al. Hip adduction and abduction strength profiles in elite soccer players: implications for clinical evaluation of hip adductor muscle recovery after injury. Am J Sports Med 2011;39(1):121–6. [Epub 2010/10/12].
31. Lu YM, Lin JH, Hsiao SF, et al. The relative and absolute reliability of leg muscle strength testing by a handheld dynamometer. J Strength Cond Res 2011;25(4):1065–71. [Epub 2010/09/15].
32. Engebretsen AH, Mykelurst G, Holme I, et al. Intrinsic risk factors for groin injuries among male soccer players: a prospective cohort study. Am J Sports Med 2010;38(10):2051–7.
33. Tyler T, Nicholas S, Campbell R, et al. The association of hip strength and flexibility with the incidence of adductor muscle strains in professional ice hockey players. Am J Sports Med 2001; 29(2):124–8.
34. Bennell KL, Talbot RC, Wajswelner H, et al. Intra-rater and interrater reliability of a weight-bearing lunge measure of ankle dorsiflexion. Aust J Physiother 1998;44(3):175–80. [Epub 2001/10/26].
35. Crossley KM, Thancanamootoo K, Metcalf BR, et al. Clinical features of patellar tendinopathy and their implications for rehabilitation. J Orthop Res 2007;25(9):1164–75. [Epub 2007/05/01].
36. Gabbe BJ, Finch CF, Wajswelner H, et al. Predictors of lower extremity injuries at the community level of Australian football. Clin J Sport Med 2004;14(2):56–63. [Epub 2004/03/12].
37. Finnoff JT, Peterson VJ, Hollman JH, et al. Intrarater and interrater reliability of the Balance Error Scoring System (BESS). PM R 2009;1(1):50–4. [Epub 2009/07/25].
38. Trojian TH, McKeag DB. Single leg balance test to identify risk of ankle sprains. Br J Sports Med 2006;40(7):610–13. [Epub 2006/05/12].
39. Boyle KL, Witt P, Riegger-Krugh C. Intrarater and interrater reliability of the Beighton and Horan joint mobility index. J Athl Train 2003;38(4):281–5. [Epub 2004/01/23].
40. Ostenberg A, Roos H. Injury risk factors in female European football. A prospective study of 123 players during one season. Scand J Med Sci Sports 2000;10(5):279–85. [Epub 2000/09/23].
41. Soderman K, Alfredson H, Pietila T, et al. Risk factors for leg injuries in female soccer players: a prospective investigation during one out-door season. Knee Surg Sports Traumatol Arthrosc 2001;9(5):313–21. [Epub 2001/10/31].
42. Stewart DR, Burden SB. Does generalised ligamentous laxity increase seasonal incidence of injuries in male first division club rugby players? Br J Sports Med 2004;38(4):457–60. [Epub 2004/07/27].
43. Uhorchak JM, Scoville CR, Williams GN, et al. Risk factors associated with noncontact injury of the anterior cruciate ligament: a prospective four-year evaluation of 859 West Point cadets. Am J Sports Med 2003;31(6):831–42. [Epub 2003/11/19].
44. Shultz SJ, Nguyen AD, Windley TC, et al. Intratester and intertester reliability of clinical measures of lower extremity anatomic characteristics: implications for multicenter studies. Clin J Sport Med 2006;16(2):155–61. [Epub 2006/04/11].
45. Juul-Kristensen B, Rogind H, Jensen DV, et al. Inter-examiner reproducibility of tests and criteria for generalized joint hypermobility and benign joint hypermobility syndrome. Rheumatology 2007;46(12):1835–41. [Epub 2007/11/17].
46. Nicholas JA. Injuries to knee ligaments: relationship to looseness and tightness in football players. JAMA 1970;212(13): 2236–9.
47. Nussbaumer S, Leunig M, Glatthorn JF, et al. Validity and test-retest reliability of manual goniometers for measuring passive hip range of motion in femoroacetabular impingement patients. BMC Musculoskelet Disord 2010;11:194. [Epub 2010/09/03].
48. Wyss TF, Clark JM, Weishaupt D, et al. Correlation between internal rotation and bony anatomy in the hip. Clin Orthop Relat Res 2007;460:152–8. [Epub 2007/02/10].
49. Verrall G, Slavotinek J, Barnes P, et al. Hip joint range of motion restriction precedes athletic chronic groin injury. J Sci Med Sport 2007;10(6):463–6.
50. Delahunt E, McEntee BL, Kennelly C, et al. Intrarater reliability of the adductor squeeze test in gaelic games athletes. J Athl Train 2011;46(3):241–5. [Epub 2011/06/15].
51. Fulcher ML, Hanna CM, Raina Elley C. Reliability of handheld dynamometry in assessment of hip strength in adult male football players. J Sci Med Sport 2010;13(1):80–4. [Epub 2009/04/21].
52. Mens JM, Vleeming A, Snijders CJ, et al. Reliability and validity of hip adduction strength to measure disease severity in posterior pelvic pain since pregnancy. Spine 2002;27(15):1674–9. [Epub 2002/08/07].
53. Crow JF, Pearce AJ, Veale JP, et al. Hip adductor muscle strength is reduced preceding and during the onset of groin pain in elite junior Australian football players. J Sci Med Sport 2010;13(2): 202–4.
54. Freckleton G, Cook J, Pizzari T. The predictive validity of a single leg bridge test for hamstring injuries in Australian Rules Football Players. Br J Sports Med 2013;[Epub 2013/08/07].
55. Lindell O, Eriksson L, Strender LE. The reliability of a 10-test package for patients with prolonged back and neck pain: could an examiner without formal medical education be used without loss of quality? A methodological study. BMC Musculoskelet Disord 2007;8:31. [Epub 2007/04/05].
56. Dedering A, Roos af Hjelmsater M, Elfving B, et al. Between-days reliability of subjective and objective assessments of back extensor muscle fatigue in subjects without lower-back pain. J Electromyogr Kinesiol 2000;10(3):151–8. [Epub 2000/05/20].
57. Latimer J, Maher CG, Refshauge K, et al. The reliability and validity of the Biering-Sorensen test in asymptomatic subjects and subjects reporting current or previous nonspecific low back pain. Spine 1999;24(20):2085–9. [Epub 1999/10/30].
58. Mannion AF, Dolan P. Electromyographic median frequency changes during isometric contraction of the back extensors to fatigue. Spine 1994;19(11):1223–9. [Epub 1994/06/01].

59. Moreland J, Finch E, Stratford P, et al. Interrater reliability of six tests of trunk muscle function and endurance. J Orthop Sports Phys Ther 1997;26(4):200–8. [Epub 1997/10/06].
60. Simmonds MJ, Olson SL, Jones S, et al. Psychometric characteristics and clinical usefulness of physical performance tests in patients with low back pain. Spine 1998;23(22):2412–21. [Epub 1998/12/04].
61. Adams MA, Mannion AF, Dolan P. Personal risk factors for first-time low back pain. Spine 1999;24(23):2497–505. [Epub 2000/01/08].
62. Biering-Sorensen F. Physical measurements as risk indicators for low-back trouble over a one-year period. Spine 1984;9(2):106–19.
63. Smith J, Laskowski ER. The preparticipation physical examination: Mayo Clinic experience with 2739 examinations. Mayo Clin Proc 1998;73(5):419–29. [Epub 1998/05/15].
64. Bahr R, Holme I. Risk factors for sports injuries – a methodological approach. Br J Sports Med 2003;37(5):384–92. [Epub 2003/09/30].
65. Freckleton G, Pizzari T. Risk factors for hamstring muscle strain injury in sport: a systematic review and meta-analysis. Br J Sports Med 2013;47(6):351–8. [Epub 2012/07/06].
66. Hrysomallis C. Injury incidence, risk factors and prevention in Australian rules football. Sports Med 2013;43(5):339–54. [Epub 2013/03/27].
67. Murphy DF, Connolly DA, Beynnon BD. Risk factors for lower extremity injury: a review of the literature. Br J Sports Med 2003; 37(1):13–29. [Epub 2003/01/28].
68. Gray J, Naylor R. BokSmart: musculoskeletal assessment form. 2009. <http://www.sarugby.co.za/boksmart/pdf/BokSmart%20-%20Musculoskeletal%20Assessment%20for%20Rugby%20Players.pdf>.
69. Gabbe BJ, Finch CF, Bennell KL, et al. How valid is a self reported 12 month sports injury history? Br J Sports Med 2003;37(6):545–7.
70. Kiesel K, Plisky PJ, Voight ML. Can serious injury in professional football be predicted by a preseason functional movement screen? N Am J Sports Phys Ther 2007;2(3):147–58. [Epub 2007/08/01].
71. Plisky PJ, Rauh MJ, Kaminski TW, et al. Star Excursion Balance Test as a predictor of lower extremity injury in high school basketball players. J Orthop Sports Phys Ther 2006;36(12):911–19. [Epub 2006/12/30].

CHAPTER 39.2 ■ WHAT IS OUR BASELINE FOR MOVEMENT? THE CLINICAL NEED FOR MOVEMENT SCREENING, TESTING AND ASSESSMENT

Gray Cook • Kyle Kiesel

INTRODUCTION

More than any other health-related problem in the United States, the cost of treating musculoskeletal disorders has risen to become the greatest financial burden.[1] Treatment associated with arthritis, back pain and other musculoskeletal dysfunction accounted for US$128 billion in 2012 as compared to US$116 billion for heart disease. Unlike approaches to other areas of health care that are often guided by agreed care guidelines, the treatment of musculoskeletal disorders continues to be dominated by varied patterns of practice and a lack of standardization.

The musculoskeletal system is unique among the other systems of the human body. Unlike other systems, the traditional approach in musculoskeletal medicine has been to wait for symptoms to appear before treatment is instigated.

In other systems, heath-care providers frequently screen for underlying abnormalities, using biomarkers of elevated risk and dysfunction as part of routine care to prevent more serious conditions from occurring. Examples include blood testing for elevated cholesterol and colonoscopy screening for bowel cancer. There has been no meaningful approach that has successfully followed this example for the musculoskeletal system.

MOVEMENT PATTERNS

Traditional models consider the musculoskeletal system as individual anatomical parts. Basic impairment measures such as isolated joint range of motion and muscle strength have not been shown to consistently correlate with functional outcomes such as return to previous level of activity or self-reported participation.[2] Additionally, these measures have been shown to be predictive of future injury in only small subgroups when considering specific patho-anatomical diagnosis such as hamstring strain[3] or anterior cruciate ligament tears.[4]

Fundamental movement patterns are seen as key milestones in human growth and development.[5] They are systematically used as developmental biomarkers for charting normal acquisition of motor development during the first 3 or 4 years of life. When these fundamental movement patterns are delayed or compromised, this information is used as a trigger to evaluate the systems involved with mobility and motor control. In this population, a compromised movement pattern provides an entry point for investigation as well as a baseline for the intervention progress.

Understanding that the measurement of individual parts may not yield desired results, some have described models that consider more comprehensive systems of analysis of human movement focused on the motor control aspect of the musculoskeletal system. Two such approaches are described by Janda and colleagues[6] and the movement systems approach described by Sahrmann.[7]

A key component of the Janda and Sahrmann models is that they consider patterns of movement, that is, how the parts work together to produce functional movement. While these approaches have provided alternative methods of assessment and management of musculoskeletal pain and dysfunction, there remains a need for standardization and the establishment of clinically measurable risk factors that can be utilized in preventative efforts.

Clinicians need to consider that symptom resolution and functional restoration require independent measurement tools to assess progress and should be used together to demonstrate successful rehabilitation and protection against future episodes. Outcomes data from the physical therapy literature related to two of the most commonly encountered diagnoses treated, low back pain and anterior cruciate ligament reconstruction, suggest somewhat disappointing results. Low back pain reoccurrence rates remain high, disability associated with low back pain remains common and at 41 months post-anterior cruciate ligament reconstruction only 63% of participants have returned to their previous level of function but 90% demonstrated normal impairment testing.[2,8] These are examples of less than desirable outcomes, and regardless of the rehabilitation approach or programme employed for a given musculoskeletal condition, there is arguably a need for standardized movement pattern screening, testing and assessment measures that may be applied across the many disciplines of musculoskeletal healthcare providers. In this new paradigm, where movement pattern screening, testing and assessment may complement each other, the clinician must understand that patients with the same musculoskeletal presentation will often have unique movement profiles. Because of these differences, the ideal treatment and preventative approaches, particularly from an exercise perspective, may vary based on the movement profile of the patient rather than the orthopaedic medical diagnosis.

FUNCTIONAL MOVEMENT SYSTEMS

The Functional Movement System (Fig. 39-1) is a series of movement-based measurement tools (screening, testing, assessment) that focus on biomarkers of movement quality. The system has been proposed to establish biomarkers within human movement patterns and to provide a standard operating procedure for screening, testing and assessment of movement pattern mobility and motor control limitations and asymmetry. In practice, the system is used to categorize risk and provides suggested corrective strategies. The system also offers higher levels of testing when asymmetry and motor control are considered competent with basic screening and to assist with risk assessment. Lastly, the system provides a movement pattern assessment model for the clinician, when treating a patient with known musculoskeletal pain, that separates asymptomatic and dysfunctional movement patterns from movement patterns that produce symptoms and may or may not be dysfunctional. Taken together, the functional movement systems provide a basic screening standard operating procedure, a measurement and testing standard operating procedure, and a diagnostic assessment standard operating procedure. Each has its own unique place in prevention and patient care from any entry point into the system from screening for prevention through to discharge at the completion of rehabilitation

The Functional Movement Screen – The Categorization and Predictive System

The Functional Movement Screen (FMS) is a reliable (ICC values ranging from 0.76–0.90 and Kappa values from 0.70–1.0)[9-15] screening tool created to rank movement patterns that are fundamental to normal function. The screen includes movements that require the basic mobility and motor control needed to complete a majority of fundamental movements utilized routinely by active individuals in daily function and sport. The FMS includes seven movements: overhead deep squat, hurdle step, in-line lunge, shoulder mobility, active straight leg raise, trunk stability push up and rotary stability. Each of these patterns is graded on a 0–3 ordinal scale where 0 represents pain with the movement, 1 represents dysfunctional movement, 2 represents acceptable movement

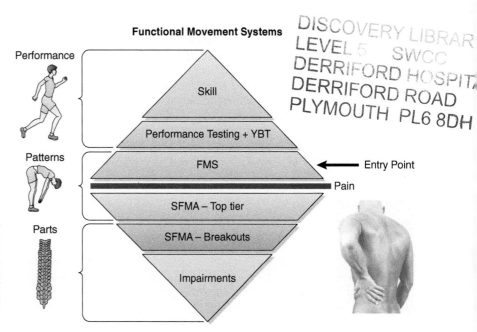

FIGURE 39-1 ■ A representation of the Functional Movement System showing the Functional Movement Screen as the entry point and pain being an indicator of moving up towards higher level testing or down towards the Selective Functional Movement Assessment for rehabilitation purposes. *FMS*, Functional Movement Screen; *SFMA*, Selective Functional Movement Assessment; *YBT*, Y Balance Test.

and 3 represents optimal movement. By screening these patterns, movement limitations and asymmetries are readily identified and measured. Basic movement pattern limitation and asymmetry are thought to reduce the effects of training and physical conditioning and recent data suggest these factors may be related to future injury. One goal of the FMS is to identify the asymptomatic population with movement pattern limitations or asymmetry so individualized correct exercise can be prescribed to normalize movement prior to an increase in physical training or activity or a competitive sports season. Research has linked low or asymmetrical scores on the FMS to injury risk in professional football players,[16,17] firefighters,[18,19] college athletes[20,21] and military personal.[22,23] Researchers have demonstrated that a standardized individual programme based on corrective exercise does improve dysfunctional movement and asymmetry as measured by the FMS.[24,25] The FMS is a screening tool and is designed for those individuals who do not have a known musculoskeletal injury or patients who are asymptomatic and as part of a standardized discharge programme when patients are returning to active, athletic, or tactical situations following rehabilitation.[26]

The Y Balance Tests – The Measurement System

The Y Balance Tests are clinically reliable[27,28] and serve as both clinical measurement tools and have demonstrated predictive validity related to injury risk in multiple populations including high school and college athletes.[29–31] They functionally represent the upper and lower quarters of the body and measure how the subject performs at their limits of stability. The test is scored on a continuous scale where the maximum amount of linear movement produced in each of the three reach directions is normalized by dividing by the subject's respective limb length. This provides a measurement that is a percentage of limb length; researchers have demonstrated that normative values on Y Balance Test performance vary based on gender, age and sport played.[32] The tests require moderate to advanced motor control and should be used in asymptomatic situations to accurately measure motor control abilities. The tests can also be used throughout the rehabilitation process and provide systematic feedback about the effectiveness of treatment, including therapeutic exercise, on motor control and movement pattern symmetry. Along with the FMS, the Y Balance Tests are also recommended as part of a standardized discharge protocol for patients returning to an active lifestyle after the rehabilitation programme has concluded to ensure that movement pattern risk factors have been appropriately managed.

The Selective Functional Movement Assessment – The Diagnostic System

The Selective Functional Movement Assessment (SFMA) is specifically designed for clinical situations where movement is complicated by symptoms (Fig. 39-2). The SFMA is a series of seven full-body movements including cervical patterns, shoulder patterns, multisegmental flexion, multisegmental extension, multisegmental rotation, single leg stance and the overhead deep squat, and is designed to assess fundamental patterns of movement in those with known musculoskeletal pain.[26]

The SFMA is a tool within the complete evaluation that complements the standard musculoskeletal examination in two distinct ways. Firstly, when the clinical assessment is initiated from the perspective of the movement pattern, the clinician has the opportunity to identify meaningful impairments that may be seemingly unrelated to the main musculoskeletal complaint, but contributing to the associated disability. This concept, known as regional interdependence, is a hallmark of the SFMA that guides the clinician to the most dysfunctional non-painful movement pattern that is then assessed in detail. Secondly, the SFMA is specifically designed to assist the clinician in the most effective therapeutic exercise choices targeting movement pattern restoration. Manual therapy, such as joint mobilization and manipulation and soft tissue treatments such as trigger point and myofascial releases and stretching, are techniques that may be considered to treat the impairment level of motor control; however, the musculoskeletal clinician must also consider strategies to restore motor control through developmental movement patterns and facilitation techniques.

Following the logic in the SFMA, the clinician separates painful patterns from non-painful patterns. Next, following a systematic approach, the dysfunctional patterns are broken down to identify the root cause of the dysfunction as primarily a mobility deficit or a stability/motor control deficit. The system accounts for managing multiple dysfunctional patterns simultaneously and with this knowledge a precise intervention may be prescribed to normalize the dysfunctional patterns from a motor control perspective. The SFMA is measured clinically as each of the seven patterns are categorized into one of the four following categories:

1. Functional and non-painful (FN)
2. Functional and painful (FP)
3. Dysfunctional and painful (DP)
4. Dysfunctional and non-painful (DN)

Simple criteria for each movement have been established, allowing the clinician to quickly determine if the movement is 'functional' which is defined as meeting the criteria as described. If one or more of the criteria are not met, the pattern is labelled as 'dysfunctional'. If pain is present during the movement it is considered painful, if not it is non-painful allowing for categorization in one of the four categories.

Once the seven major movement patterns have been categorized, the patterns that were scored as DNs are addressed first. By prioritizing DN patterns the clinician is able to address underlying dysfunction in the movement system that is not complicated by pain. Each DN pattern is broken down in detail to diagnose the cause of dysfunction as either a mobility problem or a stability/motor control problem. To achieve this diagnosis a systematic 'breakout examination' is applied in a logical manner. The breakout logic includes assessing movement in different conditions to determine the diagnosis. Firstly, the influence of the extremities on the movement is reduced (such as placing hands on hips during the

FIGURE 39-2 ■ The score sheet for each of the top-tier movements of the Selective Functional Movement Assessment. *DN*, Dysfunctional and non-painful; *DP*, Dysfunctional and painful; *FN*, Functional and non-painful; *FP*, Functional and painful; *L*, Left; *LRF*, Lateral rotation flexion; *MRE*, Medial rotation extension; *R*, Right; *SFMA*, Selective Functional Movement Assessment.

extension movement rather than overhead), next the movement is assessed in an unloaded condition, and finally active versus passive movement is considered. By applying these breakout principles to each dysfunctional pattern, a movement-orientated diagnosis is obtained. To capture the breakout logic in a systematic way and to be sure that no step is missed, the use of the breakout flow-charts is recommended. The flowcharts take the clinician through each step of the breakout logic in an efficient manner.

There are 15 total flowcharts that encompass the entire SFMA breakout system. Using multisegmental flexion (toe-touching pattern) as an example, we will describe how each part of the logic is applied to obtain a movement-orientated diagnosis. Firstly, to reduce the influence of one lower extremity on the pattern, the patient shifts their weight to bear the majority of their weight on one side and then repeats the forward bending movement. If the pattern can now be completed normally we have our first piece of information to help us with the diagnosis. Next, the movement is performed in the unloaded position (sit and reach movement). This is to say that the lower extremities are now unloaded and if

the movement can now be completed we have our second piece of information to help us with the diagnosis. For this example, let us assume that our patient does achieve a score of functional on the unloaded movement. This demonstrates that the patient has the requisite mobility to complete the pattern (adequate ankle dorsiflexion, hip flexion, posterior chain soft tissue mobility and adequate spinal flexion mobility) but was not able to coordinate the parts of the movement into a functional pattern.

This is the definition of a 'stability/motor control dysfunction' and is further broken down to determine the severity of the stability/motor control dysfunction by assessing functional rolling patterns. If, for example, the patient would have been unable to complete the unloaded toe-touching movement, the logic would have taken us to look at each part, that is, active leg raising, followed by passive if needed, then to hip flexion mobility and spinal mobility as indicated. This example provides the reader with the basic logic and process of how the SFMA structure allows for a movement diagnosis to be obtained, allowing for a targeted intervention to be applied. If the patient would have been diagnosed with a stability/motor control dysfunction for multisegmental flexion our intervention would need to be motor control re-training rather than mobility or stretching. If our diagnosis ends up as a mobility problem, either joint mobility dysfunction or a tissue extensibility dysfunction, then mobility techniques would be indicated prior to the re-establishment of motor control with appropriate exercise.

To simplify the process, we are simply looking for mobility problems first, and when they are present, they are treated accordingly prior to movement re-training. If mobility is considered acceptable, then the treatment can proceed to movement re-training. An important point here is that this can only be applied to patterns that are non-painful. When a pattern is complicated by pain, caution must be utilized, as it is not recommended to provide exercise re-training to a painful pattern because of the profound unpredictable effects of pain on motor control. The approach employed by the SFMA is based in fundamental movement logic and at the moment is based on experience and clinical observation. There are published reliability and validity studies referred to above indicating that movement patterns may be reliably measured and are related to injury risk when using the FMS and Y Balance Tests at the screening and testing levels. The SFMA is designed to manage patients from a movement perspective with known musculoskeletal pain but is not designed as a predictive tool. The system, including the FMS, Y Balance Tests and SFMA, is presented as a whole and recommended to be used together. There are reliability and validity data at the screening and testing levels which are recommended to be performed near discharge from the rehabilitation process. The reliability of the top-tier SFMA has been reported to be substantial to almost perfect with Kappa values from 0.72–0.83.[33] There are no SFMA specific validity data published to date.

CONCLUSION

Currently, when managing the musculoskeletal system our opportunity to intervene is largely driven by symptoms. Other medical specialties screen for biomarkers that may indicate the development and onset of more serious pathology. This may be a direction for musculoskeletal physiotherapy to evolve and build on the reliable and validated screens and tests that have been established. In addition, evidence is necessary to demonstrate that normalizing the screening and testing risk factors does indeed make a meaningful long-term difference to the patient's disability and may even prevent symptoms from starting. This evolution in musculoskeletal care moves us away from just assessing and treating pain originating from the musculoskeletal system. To move away from a pain-driven model we must become experts at screening, testing and assessing human movement patterns. We must define dysfunction and relate it to risk where applicable. Previous injury is the number one risk factor for a future injury, and if we become better at managing movement dysfunction we may influence future risk as well.

REFERENCES

1. Medical Expenditure Panel Survey. 2011. Available from: <http://meps.ahrq.gov/> [cited 2014].
2. Ardern CL, Taylor NF, Feller JA, et al. Return-to-sport outcomes at 2 to 7 years after anterior cruciate ligament reconstruction surgery. Am J Sports Med 2012;40(1):41–8.
3. Opar DA, Williams MD, Shield AJ. Hamstring strain injuries: factors that lead to injury and re-injury. Sports Med 2012;42(3):209–26.
4. Myer GD, Ford KR, Brent JL, et al. Differential neuromuscular training effects on ACL injury risk factors in 'high-risk' versus 'low-risk' athletes. BMC Musculoskelet Disord 2007;8:39.
5. Cech JDMS. Functional Movement Development. 3rd ed. St. Louis Missouri: Elsevaier; 2012.
6. Key J, Clift A, Condie F, et al. A model of movement dysfunction provides a classification system guiding diagnosis and therapeutic care in spinal pain and related musculoskeletal syndromes: a paradigm shift-Part 2. J Bodyw Mov Ther 2008;12(2):105–20.
7. Sahrmann SA. Diagnosis and Treatment of Movement Impairment Syndromes. St Louis, MO: Mosby; 2002.
8. Delitto A, George SZ, Van Dillen LR, et al. Low back pain. J Orthop Sports Phys Ther 2012;42(4):A1–57.
9. Minick KI, Kiesel KB, Burton L, et al. Interrater reliability of the functional movement screen. J Strength Cond Res 2010;24(2):479–86.
10. Teyhen DS, Shaffer SW, Lorenson CL, et al. The functional movement screen: a reliability study. J Orthop Sports Phys Ther 2012;42(6):530–9.
11. Gribble PA, Brigle J, Pietrosimone BG, et al. Intrarater reliability of the functional movement screen. J Strength Cond Res 2013;27(4):978–81.
12. Frohm A, Heijne A, Kowalski J, et al. A nine-test screening battery for athletes: a reliability study. Scand J Med Sci Sports 2012;22(3):306–15.
13. Onate JA, Dewey T, Kollock RO, et al. Real-time intersession and interrater reliability of the functional movement screen. J Strength Cond Res 2012;26(2):408–15.
14. Smith C, Chimera N, Wright N, et al. Interrater and intrarater reliability of the functional movement screen. J Strength Cond Res 2013;27(4):982–7.
15. Gulgin H, Hoogenboom B. The functional movement screening (fms)™: an inter-rater reliability study between raters of varied experience. JISPT 2014;9(1):14–20.
16. Kiesel K, Plisky PJ, Voight ML. Can serious injury in professional football be predicted by a preseason functional movement screen? N Am J Sports Phys Ther 2007;2(3):147–58.
17. Kiesel KB, Butler RJ, Plisky PJ. Limited and asymmetrical fundamental movement patterns predict injury in american football players. J Sport Rehabil 2013.
18. Butler RJ, Contreras M, Burton LC, et al. Modifiable risk factors predict injuries in firefighters during training academies. Work 2013;46(1):11–17.
19. Peate WF, Bates G, Lunda K, et al. Core strength: a new model for injury prediction and prevention. J Occup Med Toxicol 2007;2:3.
20. Chorba RS, Chorba DJ, Bouillon LE, et al. Use of a functional movement screening tool to determine injury risk in female collegiate athletes. N Am J Sports Phys Ther 2010;5(2):47–54.
21. Lehr ME, Plisky PJ, Butler RJ, et al. Field-expedient screening and injury risk algorithm categories as predictors of noncontact lower extremity injury. Scand J Med Sci Sports 2013.
22. Lisman P, O'Connor FG, Deuster PA, et al. Functional movement screen and aerobic fitness predict injuries in military training. Med Sci Sports Exerc 2013;45(4):636–43.
23. O'Connor FG, Deuster PA, Davis J, et al. Functional movement screening: predicting injuries in officer candidates. Med Sci Sports Exerc 2011.
24. Bodden JG, Needham RA, Chockalingam N. The effect of an intervention program on functional movement screen test scores in mixed martial arts athletes. J Strength Cond Res 2013.
25. Kiesel K, Plisky P, Butler R. Functional movement test scores improve following a standardized off-season intervention in professional football players. Scand J Med Sci Sports 2011;21(2):287–92.
26. Cook E. Movement. Aptos California: On Target Publishing; 2010.
27. Plisky PJ, Gorman PP, Butler RJ, et al. The reliability of an instrumented device for measuring components of the star excursion balance test. N Am J Sports Phys Ther 2009;4(2):92–9.

28. Westrick R, Miller J, Carow S, et al. Exploration of the y-balance test for assessment of upper quarter closed kinetic chain performance. Int J Sports Phys Ther 2012;7(2):139–47.

29. de Noronha M, Franca LC, Haupenthal A, et al. Intrinsic predictive factors for ankle sprain in active university students: a prospective study. Scand J Med Sci Sports 2012.

30. Plisky PJ, Rauh MJ, Kaminski TW, et al. Star Excursion Balance Test as a predictor of lower extremity injury in high school basketball players. J Orthop Sports Phys Ther 2006;36(12):911–19.

31. Butler RJ, Lehr ME, Fink ML, et al. Dynamic balance performance and noncontact lower extremity injury in college football players: an initial study. Sports health 2013;5(5):417–22.

32. Gorman PP, Butler RJ, Rauh MJ, et al. Differences in dynamic balance scores in one sport versus multiple sport high school athletes. Int J Sports Phys Ther 2012;7(2):148–53.

33. Glaws K, Juneau C, Becker L, et al. Intra- and Inter-rater Reliability of the Selective Functional Movement Assessment (SFMA). Int J of Sports Phys Ther 2014;9(2):195–207.

CHAPTER 40

ADVANCED ROLES IN MUSCULOSKELETAL PHYSIOTHERAPY

Jill Gamlin • Maree Raymer • Jeremy Lewis

INTRODUCTION

Innovative and cost-effective service models are sought to address the challenges of rising demand on health services and unsustainable growth in health expenditure. Health service redesign, in which physiotherapists take on an expanded role and level of responsibility in service provision for patients with musculoskeletal conditions, has been implemented in many countries, particularly in public sector services. This chapter will provide an overview of the development of advanced roles in musculoskeletal physiotherapy. Current models of practice and the evidence for the impact of these roles will also be presented, as will key current issues associated with advanced practice and the potential for future development.

BACKGROUND TO DEVELOPMENT OF ADVANCED ROLES

Advanced musculoskeletal physiotherapy roles were first developed in the military in the 1970s.[1,2] In the United Kingdom (UK), advanced practice roles began in the 1980s, as an innovative way to address long waiting times for rheumatology and orthopaedic clinics in secondary care services.[3,4] A combination of undergraduate and postgraduate education, autonomous practice, mentorship, vision and close collaboration with medical colleagues, enabled physiotherapists to undertake these roles. As examples of these service developments began to appear in the literature, these advanced roles developed and flourished across the UK and began to emerge and become embedded in health services in other countries.[5–18]

DRIVERS OF ADVANCED ROLE DEVELOPMENT

A range of factors have been associated with the development of advanced roles in musculoskeletal physiotherapy practice. These include unmet and unsustainable demand on health systems, which is contributed to by the growing burden of musculoskeletal conditions and related disability worldwide,[19] working patterns and workforce shortages,[20–23] professional interest from physiotherapists,[24–27] and emerging evidence relating to the impact of new service delivery models. Organizational and politically driven factors, such as the desire to reduce waiting times have been suggested as the dominant factor.[27]

In the UK, political directives such as the European Working Time Directive that restricted doctors working hours were a key driving factor.[20,21,23] Initial development of advanced practice roles related to local circumstances and local innovation; however, this was subsequently supported by Department of Health policy and governance arrangements and these roles have become a standard part of service delivery models.[28–31] Advanced roles have also developed in other countries, predominantly in public sector services. In Australia, the key driving factors have been similar to those in the UK, including unsustainable demand on public hospital services, resulting in extended waiting lists and unacceptable waiting times to access care.[16,18,32] In some Australian states a jurisdiction-wide approach has been taken, while in others, service developments have occurred at individual facilities. Advanced practice roles have also developed in response to medical workforce shortages. For example, Aiken[8] describes the development of a collaborative care model in Ontario, Canada, in which physiotherapists undertake an advanced role in hospital orthopaedic services to manage patients referred to hip and knee arthroplasty clinics.

The common feature in service redesign has been an aim to maximize the value of the knowledge and skills of experienced musculoskeletal physiotherapists and their contribution to streamlined pathways of care and improved outcomes for patients. Physiotherapists in advanced roles may now be found in diverse settings in many countries. The breadth and depth of work undertaken has evolved to include independent assessment, referral for imaging investigations and pathology tests, diagnosis as the first point of contact in the management pathway for patients referred for specialist medical opinion or those presenting to emergency care settings, case management and clinical consultancy and discharge decision making. In the UK advanced roles have developed to also include listing for surgery and additional therapeutic interventions such as injection therapy and ultrasound-guided injections for joints and soft tissues, hydro-distension for contracted frozen shoulders and, more recently, independent prescribing of medicines.

Musculoskeletal conditions are associated with high and increasing prevalence rates. They are one of the major causes of disability worldwide and the demands on services to provide timely and effective health care are predicted to increase.[19] Advanced roles that capitalize on the knowledge and skills of experienced musculoskeletal physiotherapists are expected to continue to develop to help meet this challenge.

DEFINITIONS

Initially, advanced roles were developed to address local needs and requirements. Ad hoc development has resulted in inconsistent terminology and definition of roles and a wide range of nomenclature exists to describe these positions. Titles include advanced physiotherapy practitioner, advanced practice physiotherapist, extended scope practitioners, orthopaedic physiotherapy practitioners, specialist physiotherapists, highly specialist physiotherapist, physiotherapy specialist, Norwegian manual therapist and consultant physiotherapist. This list is not exhaustive and in different countries different criteria must be met to attain these roles. This may vary from completing post graduate qualification(s), undertaking in-house education and training, demonstrating work-based competency or passing an examination defined by a national physiotherapy professional body. While titles will vary between organizations, jurisdictions and countries, the development of consistent definitions of advanced scope of practice roles would be beneficial to support progress in research and professional practice worldwide.

While separate descriptions of advanced or extended scope of practice exist,[33] perhaps what best defines these roles is that they require:

- post graduate education and training beyond initial qualification standards
- significant clinical experience
- location in an area of specialization and
- inclusion of activities and a level of work that may have previously been undertaken by medical or other health-care practitioners.

The degree of autonomy and accountability may vary between roles but, at the highest level, an individual practitioner may be totally responsible for the assessment, investigation, diagnosis and management of specific patient groups across an entire episode of care. The development of the consultant physiotherapist role in the UK, which combines 50% expert practice with dedicated time for research, teaching and service redesign, gives the opportunity for further expansion and evaluation of advanced roles. With many consultants participating in local and national advisory bodies, strategic influence may be exercised in shaping pathways of care around the needs of patients to achieve improved quality and better outcomes.

MODELS OF ADVANCED PRACTICE

Patients with musculoskeletal conditions are seen in a variety of subspecialty services in hospital settings, as well as in primary care services. Some examples of service settings in which advanced roles are found are discussed in the following sections.

Orthopaedics, Neurosurgery and Rheumatology in Hospital-Based Services

Referrals to an orthopaedic surgeon that are triaged as 'unlikely to require immediate surgical intervention' are directed to a physiotherapy-led service where the physiotherapist is responsible for providing a high level of diagnostic assessment and management planning.[27,34,35] In some services where the focus includes optimizing non-surgical management, the physiotherapist's role includes high-level consultancy and in some cases leadership of a multidisciplinary team.[32] Services may be targeted to manage patients with a broad range of musculoskeletal conditions, or to specific body regions (e.g. spine/shoulder/knee) or specific diagnoses (e.g. arthritis).[4,7,9–18,32]

Services have developed to manage an entire episode of care that may include initial assessment, referral for non-surgical management, monitoring of progression of the condition/disease, listing for surgery when required, pre-operative preparation and post-operative rehabilitation. There are also examples of physiotherapist-led fracture follow-up clinics,[36] post-operative review clinics[37] and the management of spinal pain referred to neurosurgical outpatient services.[38] Advanced roles in rheumatology have developed to include triage and the ongoing management of patients with inflammatory conditions.[3,39]

Emergency Departments

Advanced roles in emergency departments (EDs) involve independent assessment, referral for diagnostic tests, diagnosis, management and discharge of patients presenting with musculoskeletal conditions. Depending on their scope of practice and jurisdiction in which they work, ED roles may include independent interpretation of imaging findings and prescription and/or administration of medications.[40–45] In some ED services, physiotherapists also provide primary contact management of patients with uncomplicated fractures and dislocations.[45]

Primary Care Settings

Since the late 1990s, orthopaedic screening services have also been implemented in primary care settings in the UK.[46] In these services, physiotherapists provide assessment and management of patients who would otherwise be referred to hospital orthopaedic services for review by a consultant physician or surgeon. The development of services that bridge the gap between primary and secondary care was a major recommendation of the Musculoskeletal Services Framework developed for the United Kingdom National Health Service (NHS).[47] While multidisciplinary in nature, community assessment and treatment services specifically include physiotherapists working in an advanced role and are now in place in the majority of NHS Primary Care Trusts.[48] Orthopaedic physiotherapy screening in primary care is also being trialled in other jurisdictions.[5]

OTHER ASPECTS OF ADVANCED PRACTICE

Prescribing and administration of medicines for patients with musculoskeletal conditions is an example of an element of advanced practice that has been undertaken by physiotherapists across both hospital and primary care settings. While supplementary prescribing rights for physiotherapists have been in place in the UK since 2005, the granting of independent rights is aimed at improving access to care, convenience and choice for patients while maximizing the value of physiotherapy workforce resources within the NHS.[49,50] Physiotherapists in the UK are the first to be granted independent prescribing rights under legislation that came into effect in 2013.[49] Prescribing has also been part of advanced roles in other countries in particular circumstances and development of competency-based frameworks and nationally consistent pathways for non-medical prescribing are being explored.[1,2,51–53]

Physiotherapists in the UK have been performing injections for musculoskeletal conditions since the mid-1990s. This is another important area of advanced practice as it allows physiotherapists to embed these skills within an evidence-based package of care for individual patients with defined musculoskeletal conditions. This reduces the requirement for additional referrals and reduces waiting times.[54] More recently this practice has evolved further with increasing numbers of physiotherapists performing ultrasound-guided injections to target specific structures. Physiotherapists have also completed education programmes to be able to perform ultrasound-guided hydro-distension procedures for conditions such as contracted frozen shoulders. Audit evidence exists that demonstrates that patients with conditions such as frozen shoulder may be entirely managed (assessment, referral for imaging, ultrasound-guided corticosteroid and analgesic injections, hydro-distension injections and appropriate physiotherapy treatments together with advice and education) in a cost-effective manner with high levels of patient satisfaction, without the need for referral to other medical/health professionals.[54]

EVALUATION OF ADVANCED PRACTICE ROLES AND IMPACTS ON HEALTH SERVICES

Advanced roles in musculoskeletal physiotherapy have rapidly expanded in recent years, but the pace of change in response to significant service delivery challenges often means that robust evaluation of new roles and service models lags behind their uptake.[21] Current evidence regarding advanced musculoskeletal physiotherapy roles is briefly summarized in the following section.

Diagnostic Accuracy

Systematic reviews of studies conducted in orthopaedic and ED settings have concluded that physiotherapists in advanced roles are able to triage, diagnose musculoskeletal conditions and identify patients requiring surgery with comparable ability to that of orthopaedic consultants.[34,35]

Treatment Effectiveness

A systematic review of the impact of advanced roles in EDs reported high-level evidence of improved short-term clinical outcomes for patients managed by physiotherapists compared to routine ED care.[55] A subsequent randomized controlled trial concluded that patients managed by physiotherapists in advanced roles in EDs achieve equivalent outcomes compared to care provided by medical staff.[56]

A systematic review including studies in both ED and orthopaedic settings concluded that outcomes of care provided by physiotherapists in advanced roles may be as good as, or more beneficial than, usual care.[35] A pilot study by Comans et al.[32] also suggests that overall treatment effectiveness, as measured in quality adjusted life years (QALYs) gained, may be higher in physiotherapy-led orthopaedic service models than that achieved in traditional models of care. In addition, Chambers et al.[57] demonstrated that appropriately educated physiotherapists were as accurate as orthopaedic surgeons in performing landmark-guided subacromial bursal injections (67% accuracy in both groups), whereas orthopaedic registrars demonstrated lower accuracy (48%).

Patient Satisfaction/Experience

Patient satisfaction is the most commonly reported outcome in the evaluation of new allied health professional (AHP) roles and service models.[6] Kilner's systematic review identifies that there is high-level evidence of improved patient satisfaction for advanced ED physiotherapy services.[55] In their systematic review of advanced and extended roles, Desmeules et al.[35] included seven studies that evaluated patient satisfaction across a range of practice settings including ED, orthopaedics and rheumatology. Satisfaction levels with these services were high in all seven studies, with physiotherapy-led care resulting in significantly higher levels of satisfaction in three studies and equivalent levels of satisfaction to usual care in another three studies.

Process/Organizational Impacts

Reporting of process-related outcomes, such as waiting times, is also common and usually indicates reduced waiting times for patients.[6] Emergency and orthopaedic department waiting times are the subject of key health service performance targets internationally and the ability to impact on waiting times can be a key driver for service model reform. McClellan et al.[58] found that streaming patients appropriate to be seen by physiotherapists in advanced roles can reduce overall ED waiting times, a finding also supported by the review by Desmeules et al.[35]

In orthopaedic services, many observational and audit studies describe reduced waiting times. The systematic review by Stanhope et al.[34] identified two high-quality studies which reported reductions in orthopaedic waiting times associated with the introduction of advanced role physiotherapy services.

Health Economic Impacts

While many studies evaluate process measures and stakeholder satisfaction, relatively few analyse the economic impacts of new roles.[6] The results of early studies that included economic measures are mixed and hampered by methodological limitations, being criticized for lacking a comprehensive description of services provided, how resources were valued and information relevant to making a purchasing decision.[35]

A cost-effectiveness evaluation of a randomized controlled trial suggests that physiotherapy-led care in the ED is clinically equivalent, but may not be cost saving.[59] Another study has attempted to address the methodological issues associated with previous economic evaluations of advanced physiotherapy roles in orthopaedic settings.[32] In this study an economic (Markov) model was constructed in order to assess the costs, health outcomes, value for money and potential cost savings of a physiotherapy-led orthopaedic service in Queensland, Australia. The economic model was populated with retrospective, published, administrative and audit data and indicates the physiotherapy-led service could be considered to be highly cost effective and may be cost saving in some circumstances. It is expected that the Markov model proposed in this preliminary study could be modified to support robust economic evaluation of other advanced roles and services in the future.

Professional Issues

Changes to service provision require evaluation to ensure patients are receiving optimal care as well as to understand the clinical, financial and psychosocial impact on clinicians involved in the change. Collins et al.[60] found that nurses and allied health professionals in innovative roles in the UK generally experienced high levels of job satisfaction, which was related to increased freedom and autonomy in managing their own caseload and increased responsibility. They concluded that increased job satisfaction is likely to contribute to retention of experienced professionals within the NHS. Dawson and Ghazi[61] undertook a very small-scale qualitative study to explore the experience of physiotherapists in extended roles in orthopaedic services in the UK and concluded that although advanced roles can be stressful for the clinician, they are also very satisfying. It is evident, however, that the workforce and professional impacts of advanced roles, both on the clinician themselves and on other health professionals, have not been widely explored.

From a historic perspective the delivery of health care is constantly evolving, responding to new knowledge and demands. Advanced roles are best developed in environments where knowledge is shared within multidisciplinary teams, providing integrated evidence-based pathways that are patient-centred. This process works best when all involved in the provision of health care construct meaningful pathways, based on care delivered by the right practitioner, at the right time, in the right place and within a cost-effective delivery model.

While the current evidence base is promising in relation to the impacts of advanced roles, it is apparent that the evidence base lags behind the rate at which these services have been developed and implemented. Key criticisms of the majority of published studies include the small numbers of clinicians involved, single-centre designs, short-term follow-up periods, limited focus on patient-centred outcomes and little direct comparison of patient outcomes between physiotherapist-led and routine care.[6,34,35,62] There are also unanswered questions about cost effectiveness, impacts on the workforce and numerous education and training issues. Deficits in knowledge supporting these pathways need to be addressed with further research. Access to suitable education, training and mentorship to support individual development and longer-term service sustainability is fundamental to the continual evolution of advanced clinical practice roles.

The aims of these roles are to deliver seamless care to patients in a timely and cost-effective manner and support optimum use of the skills of the entire health workforce. It is conceivable that in the future physiotherapists may take on additional roles as health teams continue striving to streamline pathways of care. These new roles should be built upon the foundations of physiotherapists' existing scope of practice, knowledge and expertise and add measurable value to patient outcomes and experiences.

CONCLUSIONS AND RECOMMENDATIONS

Role and service innovations have become widespread in an attempt to address the almost universal burden of musculoskeletal conditions on health services. Since the inception of advanced practice roles, physiotherapists have pushed the boundaries of clinical practice in pursuit of providing seamless, evidence-based care pathways for patients, which maximize the value of the knowledge and skills of experienced musculoskeletal physiotherapists and other health professionals to the patient and health services. This development in health care has transformed service delivery in many ways. It aims to provide access to the right practitioner, at the right time in a cost-effective manner, while maintaining or improving the quality of care provided, together with improved outcomes and experiences for patients. Current evidence suggests a range of potential benefits for patients and health services. Care provided by physiotherapists in advanced roles may be as beneficial, or more beneficial, than traditional service models in terms of access to treatment, diagnostic accuracy and patient satisfaction, and result in more timely provision of care. However, the pace of development means there are persistent gaps in the evidence which indicate that further high-quality, methodologically sound research is required in order to explore fully the benefits and impacts of the introduction of these roles. International consensus on definitions of advanced practice will assist in progressing this research.

REFERENCES

1. James JJ, Stuart RB. Expanded role for the physical therapist. Screening musculoskeletal disorders. Phys Ther 1975;55(2):121–31. [Epub 1975/02/01].
2. Benson CJ, Schreck RC, Underwood FB, et al. The role of army physical therapists as nonphysician health care providers who prescribe certain medications: observations and experiences. Phys Ther 1995;75(5):380–6. [Epub 1995/05/01].
3. Langridge JC, Moran CJ. A comparison of two methods of managing patients suffering from rheumatoid arthritis. Physiotherapy 1984;70(3):109–13. [Epub 1984/03/01].
4. Byles S, Ling R. Orthopaedic out-patients: a fresh approach. Physiotherapy 1989;75(7):433–7.
5. Samsson K, Larsson ME. Physiotherapy screening of patients referred for orthopaedic consultation in primary healthcare – A randomised controlled trial. Man Ther 2013;[Epub 2013/11/20].
6. Comans TA, Clark MJ, Cartmill L, et al. How do allied health professionals evaluate new models of care? What are we measuring and why? J Healthc Qual 2011;33(4):19–28. [Epub 2011/07/08].
7. Dunlop B, McLaughlin L, Goldsmith C. Non-physician triage in patients with low back pain, sciatica and spinal stenosis. J Bone Joint Surg Br 2011;93-F(Suppl. IV):584.
8. Aiken A. Improved use of allied health professionals in the health care system: the case of the advanced practice physiotherapist in orthopedic care. World Hosp Health Serv 2012;48(1):28–30. [Epub 2012/09/29].
9. Aiken AB, Harrison MM, Atkinson M, et al. Easing the burden for joint replacement wait times: the role of the expanded practice physiotherapist. J Healthc Qual 2008;11(2):62–6. [Epub 2008/03/26].
10. Hockin J, Bannister G. The extended role of a physiotherapist in an out-patient orthopaedic clinic. Physiotherapy 1994;80(5):281–4.
11. Hourigan P, Weatherley C. The physiotherapist as an orthopaedic assistant in a back pain clinic. Physiotherapy 1995;81(9):546–8.
12. Weale AE, Bannister GC. Who should see orthopaedic outpatients – physiotherapists or surgeons? Ann R Coll Surg Engl 1995;77(2 Suppl.):71–3. [Epub 1995/03/01].
13. Daker-White G, Carr AJ, Harvey I, et al. A randomised controlled trial. Shifting boundaries of doctors and physiotherapists in orthopaedic outpatient departments. J Epidemiol Community Health 1999;53(10):643–50. [Epub 2000/01/05].
14. Hattam P. The effectiveness of orthopaedic triage by extended scope physiotherapists. Clinical Governance 2004;9(4):244–52.
15. Pearse EO, Maclean A, Ricketts DM. The extended scope physiotherapist in orthopaedic out-patients – an audit. Ann R Coll Surg Engl 2006;88(7):653–5. [Epub 2006/11/30].
16. Oldmeadow LB, Bedi HS, Burch HT, et al. Experienced physiotherapists as gatekeepers to hospital orthopaedic outpatient care. Med J Aust 2007;186(12):625–8. [Epub 2007/06/20].
17. Aiken AB, Atkinson M, Harrison MM, et al. Reducing hip and knee replacement wait times: an expanded role for physiotherapists in orthopedic surgical clinics. Healthc Q 2007;10(2):88–91, 6. [Epub 2007/05/12].
18. Blackburn MS, Cowan SM, Cary B, et al. Physiotherapy-led triage clinic for low back pain. Aust Health Rev 2009;33(4):663–70. [Epub 2010/02/20].
19. Vos T, Flaxman AD, Naghavi M, et al. Years lived with disability (YLDs) for 1160 sequelae of 289 diseases and injuries 1990–2010: a systematic analysis for the Global Burden of Disease Study 2010. Lancet 2012;380(9859):2163–96. [Epub 2012/12/19].
20. Pickersgill T. The European working time directive for doctors in training. BMJ 2001;323(7324):1266. [Epub 2001/12/04].
21. Kersten P, McPherson K, Lattimer V, et al. Physiotherapy extended scope of practice – who is doing what and why? Physiotherapy 2007;93(4):235–42.
22. Comeau P. Crisis in orthopedic care: surgeon and resource shortage. CMAJ 2004;171(3):223. [Epub 2004/08/04].
23. Suckley J. Core Clinical Competencies for Extended Scope Physiotherapists Working in Musculoskeletal Interface Clinics Based in Primary Care: A Delphi Consensus Study. Manchester, UK: College of Health and Social Care, School of Nursing, Midwifery and Social Work, University of Salford, UK; 2012. Available from: <http://usir.salford.ac.uk/26989/>; [cited 2013 12/8/13].
24. Durrell S. Expanding the scope of physiotherapy: clinical physiotherapy specialists in consultants' clinics. Man Ther 1996;1(4):210–13. [Epub 1996/09/01].
25. Li LC, Westby MD, Sutton E, et al. Canadian physiotherapists' views on certification, specialisation, extended role practice, and entry-level training in rheumatology. BMC Health Serv Res 2009;9:88. [Epub 2009/06/06].
26. Robertson VJ, Oldmeadow LB, Cromie JE, et al. Taking charge of change: a new career structure in physiotherapy. Aust J Physiother 2003;49(4):229–31. [Epub 2003/11/25].
27. ACT-Health. ACT Health 2008 Physiotherapy Extended Scope Practice: Phase 1 Final Report. Australian Capital Territory (ACT), Australia: ACT Government Health Directorate, ACT Government; 2008. Available from: <http://www.health.act.gov.au/professionals/allied-health/allied-health-projects>; [12/8/13].
28. Modernisation Agency Department of Health UK. 10 High Impact Changes for Service Improvement and Delivery. A Guide for NHS Managers. United Kingdom: UK Department of Health; 2004. Available from: <http://www.skane.se/Upload/Webbplatser/Utvecklingscentrum/dokument/10%20bra%20punkter%20NHS1.pdf>; [01/10/2013].
29. Department of Health UK. Freedom to Practice: Dispelling the Myths. London: United Kingdom UK Department of Health; 2003. Available from: <http://webarchive.nationalarchives.gov.uk/+/www.dh.gov.uk/en/Publicationsandstatistics/Publications/PublicationsPolicyAndGuidance/DH_4061524>; [01/12/2013].
30. Department of Health UK. Meeting the Challenge: A Strategy for the Allied Health Professionals. London: United Kingdom UK Department of Health; 2000. Available from: <http://webarchive.nationalarchives.gov.uk/+/www.dh.gov.uk/en/publicationsandstatistics/Publications/Publicationspolicyandguidance/DH_4025477>; [01/10/2010].
31. Department of Health UK. The NHS Plan – A Plan for Reform London. UK Department of Health; 2000. Available from: <http://webarchive.nationalarchives.gov.uk/+/www.dh.gov.uk/en/publicationsandstatistics/publications/publicationspolicyandguidance/dh_4002960>; [01/12/2010].
32. Comans T, O'Leary S, Raymer M, et al. Cost-effectiveness of a physiotherapist-led service for orthopaedic outpatients. J Health Serv Res Policy 2014;19(4):216–23.
33. Association AP. Positions Statement – Scope of Practice. Australia: Australian Physiotherapy Association; 2009. Available from: <http://www.physiotherapy.asn.au/DocumentsFolder/Advocacy_Position_Scope_of_Practice_2009.pdf>; [13/08/2013].
34. Stanhope J, Grimmer-Somers K, Milanese S, et al. Extended scope physiotherapy roles for orthopedic outpatients: an update systematic review of the literature. J Multidiscip Healthc 2012;5:37–45. [Epub 2012/02/24].
35. Desmeules F, Roy JS, MacDermid JC, et al. Advanced practice physiotherapy in patients with musculoskeletal disorders: a systematic review. BMC Musculoskelet Disord 2012;13:107. [Epub 2012/06/22].
36. Moloney A, Dolan M, Shinnick L, et al. A 6 month evaluation of a clinical specialist physiotherapist's role in a fracture clinic. Physiother Irl 2009;30(1):8–15.
37. Walton MJ, Walton JC, Bell M, et al. The effectiveness of physiotherapist-led arthroplasty follow-up clinics. Ann R Coll Surg Engl 2008;90(2):117–19. [Epub 2008/03/08].
38. Blackburn M, Cowan S, Cary B, et al. Physiotherapy-led triage for low back pain. Aust Health Rev 2009;33(4):663–70.
39. MacKay C, Veinot P, Badley EM. Characteristics of evolving models of care for arthritis: a key informant study. BMC Health Serv Res 2008;8:147. [Epub 2008/07/16].
40. Morris CD, Hawes SJ. The value of accident and emergency based physiotherapy services. J Accid Emerg Med 1996;13(2):111–13. [Epub 1996/03/01].
41. Jibuike OO, Paul-Taylor G, Maulvi S, et al. Management of soft tissue knee injuries in an accident and emergency department: the effect of the introduction of a physiotherapy practitioner. Emerg Med J 2003;20(1):37–9. [Epub 2003/01/21].
42. Bethel J. The role of the physiotherapist practitioner in emergency departments: a critical appraisal. Emerg Nurse 2005;13(2):26–31. [Epub 2005/05/26].

43. McClellan CM, Greenwood R, Benger JR. Effect of an extended scope physiotherapy service on patient satisfaction and the outcome of soft tissue injuries in an adult emergency department. Emerg Med J 2006;23(5):384–7. [Epub 2006/04/22].

44. Anaf S, Shepherd L. Physiotherapy as a clinical service in emergency departments: a narrative review. Physiotherapy 2007;93: 243–52.

45. Ball ST, Walton K, Hawes S. Do emergency department physiotherapy practitioners, emergency nurse practitioners and doctors investigate, treat and refer patients with closed musculoskeletal injuries differently? Emerg Med J 2007;24(3):185–8. [Epub 2007/03/14].

46. Hattam P, Smeatham A. Evaluation of an orthopaedic screening service in primary care. Clin Perform Qual Health Care 1999;7(3):121–4. [Epub 2000/06/10].

47. Department of Health UK. The Musculoskeletal Services Framework, a Joint Responsibility: Doing Things Differently. United Kingdom: UK Department of Health; 2006. Available from: <http://webarchive.nationalarchives.gov.uk/20130107105354/http://www.dh.gov.uk/en/Publicationsandstatistics/Publications/PublicationsPolicyAndGuidance/DH_4138413>; [23/10/2013].

48. Arthritis and Musculoskeletal Alliance (ARMA). The Musculoskeletal Map of England. United Kingdom: Arthritis and Musculoskeletal Alliance (ARMA); 2010. Available from: <http://arma.uk.net/wp-content/uploads/2014/10/England-Musculoskeletal-map-FINAL2.pdf>; [20/10/13].

49. Chartered Society of Physiotherapy. Independent Prescribing Gets legal Green Light. United Kingdom: Chartered Society of Physiotherapy; 2013. Available from: <http://www.csp.org.uk/news/2013/08/20/independent-prescribing-gets-legal-green-light>; [23/10/2013].

50. Department of Health-(UK). Allied health Professions Prescribing and Medicines Supply Mechanisms Scoping Project Report. United Kingdom: Department of Health (UK); 2009. Available from: <http://webarchive.nationalarchives.gov.uk/+/www.dh.gov.uk/en/Publicationsandstatistics/Publications/DH_103948>; [20/10/2013].

51. Department of Health Queensland. A Framework for Allied Health Professional Prescribing Trials within Queensland Health (Revised April 2013). Queensland, Australia: Queensland Department of Health; 2011. Available from: <http://www.health.qld.gov.au/ahwac/docs/min-taskforce/prescribefwork.pdf>; [21/11/2013] April 2013.

52. Morris J, Grimmer K. Non medical prescribing by physiotherapists: issues reported in the current evidence. Man Ther 2014;19(1):82–6.

53. Health Workforce Australia. Health Professionals Prescribing Pathway (HPPP) Project Final Report. Australia: Health Workforce Australia; 2013. Available from: <http://www.hwa.gov.au/sites/default/files/HWA%20HPPP%20final%20report_LR.pdf>; [21/11/2013].

54. O'Connaire E, Lewis JS. Arthrographic hydrodistension for frozen shoulder. A physiotherapy-led initiative in primary care. 2011. Available from: <http://www.health.org.uk/media_manager/public/75/programme_library_docs/Central%20London%20-%20Frozen%20Shoulder.pdf>.

55. Kilner E. What evidence is there that a physiotherapy service in the emergency department improves health outcomes? A systematic review. J Health Serv Res Policy 2011;16(1):51–8. [Epub 2010/12/28].

56. McClellan CM, Cramp F, Powell J, et al. A randomised trial comparing the clinical effectiveness of different emergency department healthcare professionals in soft tissue injury management. BMJ Open 2012;2(6):[Epub 2012/11/13].

57. Chambers I, Hide G, Bayliss N. An audit of accuracy and efficacy of injections for subacromial impingement comparing consultant, registrar and physiotherapist. J Bone Joint Surg Supp II Orthop Proc 2005;87-B(Suppl. II Orthopaedic Proceedings):160.

58. McClellan C, Cramp F, Powell J, et al. Extended scope physiotherapists in the emergency department: a literature review. Phys Ther Rev 2010;15:106–11.

59. McClellan CM, Cramp F, Powell J, et al. A randomised trial comparing the cost effectiveness of different emergency department healthcare professionals in soft tissue injury management. BMJ Open 2013;3(1):[Epub 2013/01/08].

60. Collins K, Jones ML, McDonnell A, et al. Do new roles contribute to job satisfaction and retention of staff in nursing and professions allied to medicine? J Nurs Manag 2000;8(1):3–12. [Epub 2000/10/03].

61. Dawson LJ, Ghazi F. The experience of physiotherapy extended scope practitioners in orthopaedic outpatient clinics. Physiotherapy 2004;90(4):210–16.

62. Cramp F. Systematic Review of Literature Evaluating Extended Scope of Practice and Advanced Practice Physiotherapy Provision within Musculoskeletal Healthcare. United Kingdom: Chartered Society of Physiotherapy; 2013. Available from: <http://www.esp-physio.co.uk/?page_id=43>; [23/10/2013].

PART **IV**

OVERVIEW OF CONTEMPORARY ISSUES IN PRACTICE

INTRODUCTION

The last 20 years in particular has seen an ever-growing body of research in the basic and applied clinical and behavioural sciences which has shaped and undoubtedly advanced musculoskeletal physiotherapy clinical practice. Clinicians, researchers and healthcare funders are seeking research-informed and evidence-based practices to offer to patients in their care. Despite considerable advances in knowledge of the basic and clinical sciences and advances in the art of clinical practice, we are not yet at a point where any one scientific or philosophical approach to management for a musculoskeletal disorder has the answers for all individuals. Nor is there strong evidence for the superiority of a particular treatment approach to the exclusion of all others. Thus this section has not attempted to present 'How to treat' monologues. Rather the aim of this section is to inform the clinician on contemporary issues in practice as well as the comprehensive practice of current musculoskeletal physiotherapy.

A somewhat eclectic approach has been taken in this section devoted to clinical practice so that the reader is broadly informed about the state of present-day practice, current thinking and research. In some chapters, as for example in the cervical spine, contemporary issues in the field have been chosen and discussed. In other regions, such as the thoracic spine and pelvis, there are quite different approaches to management internationally. Thus clinicians and researchers in the field have presented overviews of these different approaches, including their rationale and evidence base. There is now widespread recognition of the patient heterogeneity which is present within any 'diagnostic label'. A major field of clinical research in many conditions is addressing this problem of heterogeneity in patient presentation. Perhaps the field which is most advanced is subgrouping of low back pain patients to inform/direct therapeutic approaches. The chapter on low back pain has principally been devoted to the subgrouping approaches developed by physiotherapists. This is the first edition of *Grieve's Modern Musculoskeletal Physiotherapy* to include discussion on musculoskeletal disorders in the extremities. Chapters in this section present current research and practice across a scope of disorders in a particular region. For example, the chapter dealing with the knee discusses three prevalent presentations, acute knee injuries, anterior knee pain and knee osteoarthrosis, while the chapter on the shoulder covers the complexity of shoulder assessment and discusses a range of shoulder conditions including; rotator cuff tendinopathy, subacromial pain syndrome, shoulder instability, posterior shoulder tightness and frozen shoulder.

This section will hopefully inform and inspire clinicians and researchers towards better practice for patients with musculoskeletal disorders and provide motivation for further research and innovation to optimize their patients' quality of life.

CHAPTER 41

CERVICAL SPINE:

IDIOPATHIC NECK PAIN

Gwendolen Jull • Deborah Falla • Shaun O'Leary • Christopher McCarthy

The personal and societal burdens of mechanical neck pain of idiopathic origin are growing and likely reflect both contemporary occupational and lifestyle influences as well as the ageing population internationally.[1-6] The annual prevalence of neck pain is variably reported as between 30% and 50%.[7,8] The annual incidence of more bothersome or activity-limiting neck pain is up to 13% and is most common in the middle-aged population.[7,8] Neck pain is characteristically a recurrent disorder which underscores the burden of neck pain and its effects on quality of life. Episodes may occur over a lifetime with variable degrees of recovery between occurrences. Up to 85% of those who experience first episode neck pain will have a recurrence.[9] A Swedish multi-year cohort study found that only 11% of women and 14% of men reported recovery periods of at least 1 year duration.[7] In the USA, neck pain ranks fourth of the 30 diseases contributing to years lived with disability.[2] These statistics call for effective primary, secondary and tertiary interventions for people with mechanical neck pain to reduce both the personal and societal burdens.

Three distinct contemporary issues have been chosen for discussion in relation to mechanical neck pain towards more effective prevention and management:

1. patient profiling
2. training
3. cervical spine mobilization and manipulation.

PROFILING PATIENTS WITH MECHANICAL NECK PAIN

Patients with neck pain disorders are usually regarded within both medical diagnostic[10] and biopsychosocial models. The diagnostic label of mechanical neck pain is used for disorders where current imaging techniques fail to identify a relevant lesion in the cervical structures, onset is not related to a motor vehicle crash (for which the term whiplash-associated disorder is used), a cervical radiculopathy is not present and there is no evidence that neck pain comes from a non-musculoskeletal cause.[11] Over 80% of people with neck pain fall into the mechanical neck pain category. The potential problem with this one-dimensional term is that it can infer homogeneity in patient presentations. Likewise, the term biopsychosocial provides no indication of consideration of the relative contributions of biological, psychological and social features. The consequence is the potential for prescriptive and generic management approaches rather than patient-centred management that considers the requirements of the individual.

Patient presentations are variable. Biological, psychological and social features differ within and between domains and change at various time points within the course of a patient's recovery. This suggests that an optimal management approach is based on gaining a comprehensive profile of the individual patient which appreciates the diversity within, the relationships between and relative weighting of importance of the biological, psychological and social domains in the individual at initial and progressive time points. This is achieved through good communication and technical skills within a clinical reasoning process. Considerable research over the last two to three decades into mechanical neck pain across biological, psychological and social domains has revealed its many and varied features. This section illustrates some of this heterogeneity to support the position for multidimensional profiling of patients with mechanical neck pain as the basis for best practice management.

Biological Perspectives

Pain mechanisms are a primary consideration in diagnosis and management of patients with neck pain. They are variable between people and disorders. For instance, studies investigating primary and secondary mechanical hyperalgesia and thermal hyperalgesia have demonstrated that central sensitization (secondary hyperalgesia) may be present, but generally is a less dominant feature of mechanical neck pain when compared to whiplash-associated disorders.[12-14] Nevertheless, there are specific instances which vary from such a generalization. For instance, Chua et al.[15] demonstrated that a zygapophysial joint disorder was associated with primary hyperalgesia when it was a nociceptive source of a persistent neck pain disorder. Yet when the zygapophysial joint was a nociceptive source in patients with cervicogenic headache, it was also associated with secondary hyperalgesia and central sensitization.[15] Pain mechanisms need to be identified in the individual patient as they influence treatment delivery. The greater the sensory disturbances, the less any intervention (manual therapy or exercise) should be pain provocative in nature to avoid potential symptom aggravation.[16] Likewise, when there is evidence that nerve tissue mechanosensitivity is contributing to a patient's pain syndrome, whether cervicobrachial pain or cervicogenic headache,[17,18] a similar careful approach to management is in order.

The multidimensional and diverse responses to neck pain and pathology are also evident within the sensorimotor system. There is now clear evidence of a reorganization of cervical motor control strategies. These include altered coordination between deep and superficial neck muscles,[19–21] a loss of muscles' directional specificity[22] and increased co-activation of neck flexor and extensor muscles during functional tasks.[23,24] There are altered temporal features of muscle activity demonstrated by an increased latency between the onset of the deltoid muscle and onset of the neck muscles with rapid arm movement[25,26] and delayed activation of the neck muscles during full body perturbations.[27] People with neck pain display reduced strength and endurance at various contraction intensities and their neck muscles demonstrate increased fatigability.[28–30] Patients may present with altered joint position and/or movement sense and control, impaired balance and altered oculomotor control particularly when there are complaints of light-headedness or unsteadiness in association with neck pain and/or headache.[31–36] In summary, disturbances in sensorimotor function are a common feature of neck pain disorders but their presence and magnitude varies considerably between patients.[37] This exemplifies the necessity for individual profiling when prescribing patient-specific exercise programmes.

Psychological Perspectives

Pain is an individual sensory and emotional experience. The adoption of the biopsychosocial model spurred an increase in research into psychological features. Most research initially concerned low back pain and then interest was directed towards neck pain disorders. Whiplash-associated disorders have received the greatest attention, being compensable disorders with some unique psychological reactions (e.g. post-traumatic stress symptoms) identified.[38] Here the focus is on findings in persons with idiopathic mechanical neck pain.

Some level of anxiety and depression accompanies pain regardless of its source.[39] Various psychological features have been identified in association with the neck pain experience, including fear avoidance, somatization, catastrophization, poorer physical health and well-being,[40–43] as have behavioural factors such as illness beliefs, coping skills[44–46] and pain self-efficacy.[47] The moderating effect of various psychological features on the course of recovery of patients with mechanical neck pain has received attention.[42,45,48,49] A recent overview of systematic reviews on prognostic factors[50] found that there was limited evidence of significant associations, and thus very low confidence in the risk, between several psychological and behavioural features and recovery from mechanical neck pain. The features with more substantive evidence of moderate risk were a history of musculoskeletal disorders in other body regions and older age. This lack of evidence does not necessarily mean that psychological features have little role in the course of mechanical neck pain. Rather at this point in time there are too few studies or studies have produced conflicting results.

Studies of fear avoidance or fear of activity illustrate the conflicting results and lack of definitive evidence. They exemplify why multidimensional profiling is necessary, rather than making any generic assumptions for patients with mechanical neck pain. Some studies have found fear of activity to be a prognostic feature or a feature able to explain a reasonable proportion of the level of neck pain and disability.[40,42,51] In contrast, a study of health workers with neck pain found that fear avoidance was not a risk factor.[41] Other studies have found that fear of movement was more evident in patients in the acute state but not so evident in patients in the subacute phase or in patients with persistent disorders.[52–55] In most studies, the scores on the various questionnaires used to examine fear constructs (Fear-Avoidance Beliefs Questionnaire,[56] Tampa Scale for Kinesiophobia,[57] Pictorial Fear of Activity Scale-Cervical[58]) were either quite low or within normal range with few patients exhibiting high scores.[48,52–55] In view of such low scores, Cleland et al.[59] suggested that the experience of idiopathic, mechanical neck pain may not provoke the same level or type of fear as might the experience of low back pain. Thus it would seem that fear avoidance has some role in mechanical neck pain in the acute stage but may not have a substantial moderating effect on recovery for the majority of patients in the subacute or persistent stages of mechanical neck disorders.

Features other than fear-avoidance beliefs may contribute to a greater extent to persistent disability in patients with neck pain. Nevertheless it seems that psychological responses are not a major feature in most patients with mechanical neck pain. For instance, Verhagen et al.[49] studied patients with mechanical neck pain in primary care. They found that pain severity and catastrophizing modified treatment success, but catastrophizing scores were not high. Mercardo et al.[45] found that poor coping skills only predicted the 9% of their cohort ($n = 571$) with very disabling neck or back pain. More research is required to understand the incidence and role of psychological and behavioural features in mechanical neck pain. However, at this point in time, it would seem that they may have a substantive role in only the minority of patients, which emphasizes the need for individual profiling.

Social Perspectives

In considering social perspectives, extensive research has been undertaken into work-related neck pain. Generally, work absenteeism is not as great a problem for persons with neck disorders as it is in low back pain. Office or sedentary workers with mechanical neck pain in the main attend work (presenteeism) albeit their neck pain results in loss of productivity which is a problem in itself.[60] Several social features have been identified as moderating work-related mechanical neck pain. They include low supervisor support, high job demands, low co-worker support, poor job satisfaction and low job control as well as work features (occupation type, manual labour, sustain work postures, awkward work postures) and poor physical work environment.[6,61–65] A recent systematic review[65] concluded that the most consistent predictors of occupational neck pain were social factors of high job demands and low levels of supportive leadership and work features of sustained neck flexion and lifting in awkward postures. Psychological distress was not a risk factor, as was also determined by Walton et al.[50] Interestingly, a study of health-care workers did not find associations between high job strain, low supervisor support and neck pain,[41] which again emphasizes the need for individual and multidimensional profiling in assessment and management of the patient with mechanical neck pain.

It is artificial to consider physical, psychological or social features separately. As examples of how they may interact, Johnson et al.[66] found that high supervisor support, decision authority and skill discretion reduced the impact of several physical risk factors for neck pain in female office workers. Thompson et al.[43] determined that greater catastrophizing and lower pain vigilance and awareness together, moderated greater pain intensity and McLean et al.[47] found that pain self-efficacy mediated the relationship between neck pain and disability and upper limb disability. Thus, true to the biopsychosocial model, the different elements of the model may interact and have the potential to positively or negatively influence neck pain.

Patient Profiling in Clinical Practice

Mechanical neck pain needs to be considered from multidimensional perspectives in the context of the biopsychosocial model. As illustrated, each domain has multiple dimensions and the weighting of each domain can be very different between patients. An optimal management approach is based on gaining a comprehensive profile of the individual patient that appreciates the diversity and weights the biological, psychological and social aspects.

We propose that from the biological perspective, it is necessary to understand physiological pain mechanisms and identify sources of peripheral nociception in the articular, neural and muscle systems that might benefit from physical therapies. Likewise it is necessary to fully profile the functional status of these systems in the upper quadrant through the assessment of posture, local and regional cervical and thoracic motion, nerve tissue motion and neck and axio-scapular muscle function. Clinical assessment of kinaesthetic sense, balance and oculomotor control is relevant especially in patients with symptoms of light-headedness or unsteadiness in association with their neck pain.[67] Within a clinical reasoning framework the relationship between these sensorimotor impairments and the patient's pain and functional complaints as well as how the dysfunction in one system relates to or moderates function of another system must be understood to profile the patient and prescribe patient-specific multimodal management.

The research into psychosocial features of patients with mechanical neck pain of idiopathic origin indicates that in the majority of cases, psychological factors are likely to be a normal illness behaviour and often scores on psychological questionnaires are not high. This suggests that the weighting of this domain may be less than the biological domain for the majority of these patients.

The information from psychological questionnaires should be used constructively to inform the therapeutic approach, rather than be regarded as a negative prognostic feature.[68] As mentioned above, many of the psychological features are normal but unhelpful reactions to pain (Yellow Flags). For instance, fear of movement is a normal and understandable response when neck pain is in the acute stage. It directs management to include assurance and education about pain and movement along with interventions to reduce the pain and increase motion. Fear usually declines as pain resolves.[69] It would not be unusual for the patient to have some anxiety associated with a pain state. Good clinician–patient communication skills, empathy and education can assure the patient and help relieve the anxiety often associated with 'the unknown' about their pain or disorder. Likewise, it is important to understand patients from perspectives of coping skills, pain self-efficacy and perceived barriers to recovery. Clinicians may need to apply behavioural modification and health coaching skills to optimize recovery, particularly with regard to concordance to management strategies.

There will be some patients with neck pain who present with abnormally elevated scores on questionnaires for various psychological behaviours and beliefs or who demonstrate persisting abnormal illness behaviours, increasing the weighting of the psychological domain. The clinician should endeavour to understand why a person, for example is scoring highly on a catastrophization scale, and provide education and implement strategies that may assure or help relieve their distress within the management programme. If issues persist, however, referral to a clinician with appropriate advanced skills in behavioural modification or managing the patient in collaboration with an appropriately qualified practitioner such as a psychologist may be beneficial. It should be noted that scores from psychological questionnaires provide an indication of certain psychological symptoms, rather than a diagnosis. A diagnosis requires a clinical examination by a qualified practitioner such as a psychologist. The clinician should be alert to abnormally elevated scores on questionnaires. These may be an indicator of, for instance, severe psychological distress (which may or may not be associated with the neck disorder) or a true psychopathology such as depression. In such circumstances a timely referral to an appropriate health professional is required.

In instances of occupationally related neck pain in particular, the social domain will assume a greater weighting. There is considerable evidence for the association between work-related physical exposures and neck pain.[70] It is vital that any physical aspect of work that is a potential driver or moderator of the neck pain state is identified and rectified as much as is possible to gain long-term health benefits for the patient. Likewise, the clinician must gain an insight into the patient's work environment with the knowledge that, for example, low supervisor support, most likely in association with other features, can moderate the course of recovery and outcome. Negotiations with workplace personnel and knowledge of workplace legislation may help modify these effects to achieve desired outcomes.

Summary Statement

The biopsychosocial model emphasizes the interactions between different domains and stresses the importance of the interaction between domains in a patient's musculoskeletal pain state. There is no argument that mechanical neck pain is positioned well within the biopsychosocial model and no suggestion that patients present within only one domain of the model. Rather it is suggested that the weighting of the relative importance of biological, psychological and social domains varies between patients and that multidimensional profiling of patients is necessary to offer best practice patient-centred care.

TRAINING

Numerous studies support the prescription of exercise for the clinical management of mechanical neck pain.[67,71] In particular, exercise aimed at improving neuromuscular control of the cervical spine and shoulder girdle has shown the strongest evidence of effect of all conservative therapies for mechanical neck pain, particularly when combined with manual therapy.[72] The prescription of this form of exercise is justified by the numerous sensorimotor impairments that have been identified in mechanical neck pain including alterations in the timing and amplitude of activation of the neck and axio-scapular muscles during tasks of the cervical spine[20,22,25,73,74] and upper limb,[23,75,76] increased muscle fatigability,[28,77] physical changes in muscle size,[78] and fibre type composition.[79-81] Ultimately, these alterations contribute to impaired motor output which include deficiencies in contractile

strength and endurance,[82-84] force steadiness[30,73,85] and acuity of movement.[86,87]

Training for Pain Relief

Similar changes in perceived neck pain and disability have been observed for various exercise programmes ranging from low-load training to improve neuromuscular control and posture,[88] to high-load training to improve muscular strength and endurance.[89,90] Thus various training approaches may be appropriate for the management of pain. However, patients may respond to different exercise protocols depending on the stage of their disorder and their level of pain and disability.[71] For instance, gentle low-load exercise of the neck produces a superior immediate hypoalgesic effect compared to higher load exercise[91] (Fig. 41-1) and thus may be more appropriate in the initial stages of rehabilitation where the focus is on pain relief.

Training to Restore Neuromuscular Function

Therapeutic exercise of the neck has been shown to induce alterations in neck muscle behaviour in patients with mechanical neck pain including changes in the amplitude[88,92,93] and specificity[94] of neck muscle activity (Fig. 41-2), as well as timing of muscle activity during postural perturbations.[92] Changes in the physical structure of the neck muscles have also been demonstrated following neck exercise programmes including changes at the cellular level,[95] as well as improvements in strength and endurance.[90,92,93] Although these studies confirm that

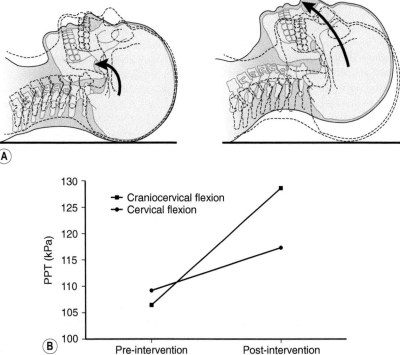

FIGURE 41-1 ■ **(A)** Patients with chronic neck pain were randomized into two training groups. The craniocervical flexion exercise involved a nodding movement of the head which remained in contact with the supporting surface. The flexion motion occurs predominantly about the upper cervical motion segments. In contrast in the cervical flexion exercise, the head is lifted off the supporting surface and flexion occurs predominantly about the lower cervical motion segments. **(B)** Change in pressure pain threshold recorded over the most symptomatic cervical motion segment immediately following one session (~3 minutes) of exercise. Note the significantly increased pressure pain threshold (reduced pain sensitivity) following the craniocervical flexion exercise only. (Reprinted with permission from O'Leary et al.[91])

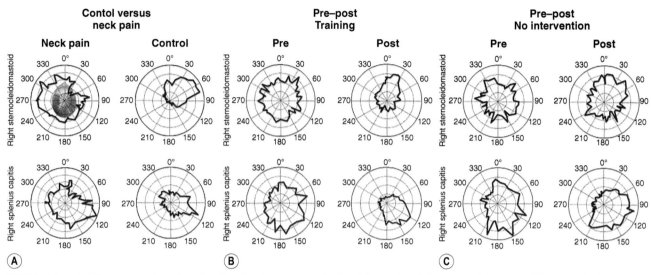

FIGURE 41-2 ■ **(A)** Representative directional activation curves obtained from the right sternocleidomastoid and splenius capitis muscles during a circular contraction performed at 15°N with change in force direction in the range 0–360°, for a control subject and a patient with chronic neck pain. The directional activation curve represents the modulation in intensity of muscle activity with the direction of force exertion. Note the defined activation of the sternocleidomastoid and splenius capitis for the control subject with minimal activity during the antagonist phase of the task. Conversely, the directional activation curves for the patient indicate more even activation levels of each muscle for all directions. **(B)** Representative directional activation curves for a patient with chronic neck pain performing the circular contraction at 15°N at baseline and at week 9, following an 8-week specific training intervention. Note that at baseline the patient shows undefined directional activation curves of their neck muscles largely due to co-activation of the neck muscles when acting as an antagonist, that is, activation of the sternocleidomastoid muscle during the extension phase of the contraction and activation of the splenius capitis during the flexion phase of the contraction. However, after training the patient from the exercise group displays more defined directional activation curves which more appropriately reflect the anatomical action of the muscle. **(C)** In contrast, no change in the directional activation curves was observed for a patient assigned to the control group (no intervention). (Reprinted with permission from Falla et al.[94])

motor function can be modified by exercise in mechanical neck pain, it is relevant to compare the specific changes achieved by different training interventions. In contrast to the similar effects on clinical symptoms, neuromuscular changes in response to training are specific to the mode of exercise performed. For example, low-load coordination training, but not high-load strength training, is effective in increasing the activation of the deep cervical flexor muscles in mechanical neck pain,[92] restoring the coordination between the deep and superficial flexors,[92] enhancing the speed of activation of the deep muscles when challenged by a postural perturbation[92] and improving the patient's ability to maintain an upright posture of the cervical spine during prolonged sitting.[96] In contrast, neck exercise programmes utilizing higher load endurance and strength protocols have shown superior gains in cervical muscle strength, endurance and resistance to fatigue compared to coordination training.[93,97] These clinical studies confirm basic studies in exercise physiology which show that specific neuronal[98] and muscle changes[99] are dependent on the primary behavioural demand of training undertaken.[98-101]

Differences in the change in neck muscle behaviour induced by exercise may even occur when the biomechanical demands of two exercises are similar. A reduction in superficial neck flexor muscle activity during a task of craniocervical flexion was observed in patients with mechanical neck pain after 10 weeks of low-load through-range craniocervical flexion (coordination) training, but not following isometric craniocervical flexion endurance training (despite biomechanical similarities between the

two exercise protocols) or active movement training (despite an emphasis on correct movement patterns during training)[93] (Fig. 41-3). As expected from earlier studies,[26,97] substantially greater gains in neck muscle endurance were acquired by the endurance training group compared to the other training groups.[93] Thus higher load resistance training can be introduced in the rehabilitation programme with the aim of inducing morphological adaptations in order to ameliorate endurance and strength of selected muscles and movements also known to be associated with mechanical neck pain.[82-84] Such exercises typically follow later in the rehabilitation programme, once more specific changes in motor control have been addressed.[67]

Transfer to Function

A primary focus of rehabilitation is retraining capacity to perform daily functional activities that are often work-related. Specific technique correction of functional activities is recommended as a means of normalizing muscle behaviour during problematic functional tasks[67] such as the correction of aberrant scapular orientation during typing.[75] Importantly, optimizing muscle control when training a functional task requires specific instruction and facilitation. For example, enhanced activation of the longus colli/longus capitis and lumbar multifidus muscles has been shown in patients with mechanical neck pain during a therapist-facilitated postural correction exercise compared to independent sitting correction.[102] What is unknown at this stage, however, is the degree to which

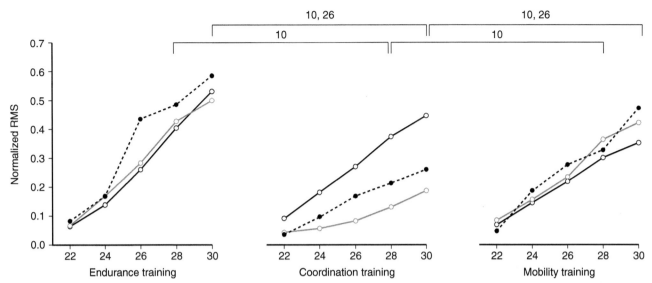

FIGURE 41-3 ■ EMG activity (normalized root mean square) of the sternocleidomastoid muscles during the progressive stages of the craniocervical flexion test (22–30) for all three training groups at baseline (open circles), and after 10 weeks (grey circles) and 26 weeks (black circles). The brackets denote significant between-group differences for a single stage of the craniocervical flexion test at 10 weeks (10) and/or 26 weeks (26). Note only the group who performed specific coordination training demonstrated a change in the coordination measure (reduced superficial muscle activity during the craniocervical flexion test) in response to training. (Reprinted with permission from O'Leary et al.[93])

specific changes in muscle control induced during formal exercise of muscle groups are transferred to the performance of functional tasks. While there is some initial evidence that specific neck exercise can alter postural orientation during functional tasks in sitting,[96,103] the degree of transference of muscle behaviour changes between specific exercise and functional activities is inconclusive. In the reverse scenario, there is some evidence that specific training of posture will improve neck muscle behaviour and reduce superficial neck flexor muscle activity during the craniocervical flexion task.[104] These studies collectively support clinical recommendations to include specific training of problematic functional activities to optimize patterns of muscle behaviour during rehabilitation.[67]

Variability in Response to Training

There is considerable variability in the extent of impairment in neuromuscular control of the cervical spine between individuals with mechanical neck pain.[23] This variability is partially related to the magnitude of the patient's neck pain intensity. For instance, augmented sternocleidomastoid and anterior scalene muscle activity during repetitive arm movements is greatest in patients reporting higher levels of pain and disability.[23] Furthermore, higher levels of pain are associated with greater delays in the activation of the deep cervical flexors during postural perturbations and lower amplitude of activation during isometric craniocervical flexion.[37] The variability of motor control impairments in patients with mechanical neck pain partly explains the variable symptomatic benefit experienced by patients from neck exercise programmes.[88,92] Recent work has shown that specific training of the deep cervical flexor muscles in patients with chronic neck pain reduces pain and increases the activation of these muscles, especially in patients with the least

activation of their deep cervical flexors prior to training (Fig. 41-4).[105] This study also demonstrated that the degree of improvement in motor control was associated with the extent of symptomatic improvement.[105] Thus although training is relevant to some degree for all patients with mechanical neck pain, the extent to which therapeutic exercise will benefit the patient from the point of view of pain will vary between individuals. These findings suggest that exercise interventions will be most effective when targeted to findings of a precise assessment of the patients' neuromuscular control and delivered within a multimodal context in which several modalities may be used to address the pain.

Exercise Dosage to Address Recurrence

Neck pain disorders are recurrent in nature.[9] Logically, good neuromuscular control would contribute substantially to primary prevention and especially to secondary and tertiary prevention towards decreasing recurrence rate and slowing disease progression. Impaired neuromuscular control does not necessarily automatically resolve following relief of pain,[88,106] which emphasizes the necessity for adequate rehabilitative exercise to restore normal muscle function (Fig. 41-5). At present, there is little specific knowledge of what 'dosage' of exercise is required to restore 'normal' cervical neuromuscular control and research is required to address this issue. Outcomes of exercise in clinical trials are usually presented as the average changes for the cohort in the measures of the muscle function under investigation. This may signify improvement but it does not tell if full rehabilitation of the impairment was achieved for any or all individuals in the cohort. It would be a step forward for outcome data to also be presented in terms of what percentage of the group returned to values within, for example, the 95% confidence intervals of a healthy

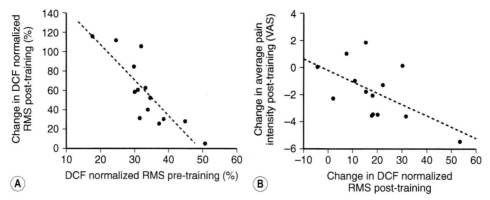

FIGURE 41-4 ■ **(A)** Scatter plot of pre-training normalized deep cervical flexor (*DCF*) electromyographic (*EMG*) amplitude (root mean square [*RMS*]) and the percentage change in DCF EMG amplitude values after 6 weeks of specific training of the DCF muscles in a group of patients with chronic neck pain. **(B)** Scatter plot of post-training normalized DCF EMG amplitude and change in average neck pain intensity rated on a visual analogue scale (VAS) post training. (Reprinted with permission from Falla et al.[105])

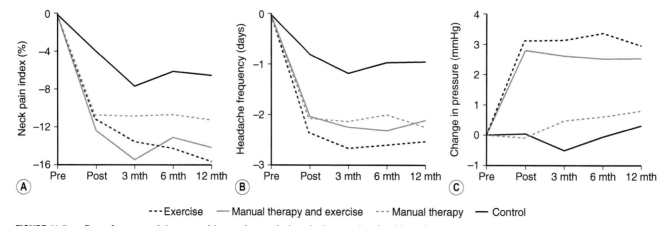

---Exercise   —— Manual therapy and exercise   --- Manual therapy   —— Control

FIGURE 41-5 ■ Data from participants with cervicogenic headache randomized into four groups: manual therapy, exercise, manual therapy combined with exercise, and a control (no intervention) group. Mean values for the **(A)** Northwick Park Neck Pain Questionnaire, **(B)** headache frequency and **(C)** change in pressure on the clinical test of craniocervical flexion recorded at baseline, in the week immediately after treatment (week 7) and 3, 6 and 12 months (mth) after the intervention. Note that although each intervention group demonstrated a reduction in neck pain intensity and headache frequency, only the groups that received specific muscle rehabilitation (exercise or manual therapy combined with exercise) improved their performance on the craniocervical flexion test (clinical test of deep cervical flexor muscle activation). (Reprinted with permission from Jull et al.[88])

population. This would start to provide insight and promote further research into dosage parameters (frequency, intensity and duration of training) required for 'normalization' of cervical muscle function. It would also inform on whether it is possible to 'normalize' muscle function in all persons after an episode of neck pain or whether in some, subclinical pathology may drive a level of dysfunction.[107] At present, the costs of health care are a primary consideration of governments and insurers around the world. If knowledge of dosage suggests that extended interventions are necessary to 'normalize' muscle function, the cost benefits of extended interventions would have to be clearly demonstrable for any translation in primary or secondary health-care protocols. These would include decreasing recurrence rates and lifetime costs of neck pain and increasing quality of life and productivity.

Summary

Exercise is a key element of any rehabilitation programme for patients with mechanical neck pain. Although various exercise protocols may have similar beneficial

effects on neck pain and disability, cervical motor adaptations to training are dependent on the specific behavioural demands of the training tasks. Changes in motor behaviour acquired with exercise have questionable transference to daily functional activities and exercise should incorporate training of cervical/shoulder girdle muscles as well as technique correction of problematic functional activities. The outcome of training will likely be best when exercise is tailored to the patient's presenting neuromuscular deficits. Further knowledge is required about appropriate dosage of exercise.

CERVICAL SPINE MOBILIZATION AND MANIPULATION

There is strong evidence supporting the benefits of manipulative therapy in the management of mechanical neck pain, albeit best when combined with exercise. Yet there is still uncertainty regarding the most appropriate application of this therapy particularly with regard to cervical manipulation. It is difficult to draw clear conclusions regarding the effectiveness of spinal manipulation compared to cervical mobilization for mechanical neck pain. The terminologies of mechanical neck pain and spinal manipulation are 'catch all' terms, which make precise estimates of effect difficult. Cervical mobilization refers to low-frequency, oscillatory or sustained passive movement typically aiming to encourage movement of intervertebral segments along the planes of their zygapophysial joints. Spinal manipulation as yet does not have a universally accepted definition (see Chapter 29). After a review of the mechanisms of the technique, a definition was proposed to facilitate discussion in the field. The definition suggested is as follows:

Spinal manipulation is the application of rapid movement to vertebral segments producing joint surface separation, transient sensory afferent input and reduction in perception of pain. Joint surface separation will commonly result in intra-articular cavitation, which in turn, is commonly accompanied with an audible pop. Post manipulation reductions in pain perception are influenced by supraspinal mechanisms including expectation of benefit.

Spinal manipulation is commonly undertaken to reduce patients' pain and impairment.[108] The spine is positioned in a manner such that when rapid passive movement is applied, gapping of spinal joint surfaces occurs.[109–111] As a consequence there may be transient alterations in spinal biomechanics,[111–113] pain perception[114–116] and muscle recruitment,[117–120] with the magnitude of effect being influenced by the patient's expectations and other psychological features.[121,122] In light of these observations it would seem likely that the utilization of manipulative therapy (mobilization or manipulation) could facilitate the effectiveness of exercise programmes, designed to regain cervical motor control. However, many questions remain regarding the specific technique selection. The uncertainty regarding the specific objectives of spinal manipulation and the complex interaction of its mechanisms suggest that more mixed-methods research is required before we fully understand the rationale behind selection, integration and application of this complex intervention.[123]

Controversy and clinician concern regarding the use of spinal manipulation in the cervical region is magnified by the small chance of serious neurovascular adverse events that have been reported to occur in response to cervical manipulation.[124,125] Research to establish the profile of patients who are most likely to benefit and have the lowest concomitant risk of serious adverse events, is in its infancy.[126,127] However, despite uncertainties within the literature one can have reasonable confidence in the assertion that neck pain is reduced with the utilization of spinal manipulation.[128,129] Associated with this are reductions in neck disability and health costs.[130,131] Spinal manipulation is both clinically and cost effective in the treatment of mechanical neck pain.

Specific Effectiveness of Cervical Spinal Manipulation

The use of spinal manipulation appears to be equally effective as the provision of a home exercise programme in acute[132] and chronic neck pain.[133] This is similar to its use with chronic low back pain.[134,135] Combining spinal manipulation with a neck exercise programme has been shown to be more effective than the provision of spinal manipulation alone.[136,137] The latest Cochrane Review comparing outcomes of manipulation versus mobilization of the neck concludes there is no difference in pain-relieving effect between the two passive modalities.[128] Data from Leaver et al.,[138] who compared the rate of pain reduction and recovery of function in acute mechanical neck pain, also showed equivalent outcomes for spinal manipulation and mobilization. Some authors have shown a greater reduction in pain with spinal manipulation compared to mobilization in the very short term, suggesting a greater transient analgesic effect of spinal manipulation.[139,140] However, the addition of spinal manipulation to a course of mobilization treatments does not appear to add any additional clinical benefit.[141] There is some debate regarding the effect of spinal manipulation on range of cervical movement. One review suggests there is some increase in range of movement with manipulation, compared to sham treatment,[113] while other authors demonstrate equal improvements in cervical range of movement when mobilization and manipulation treatments were compared.[112]

There has also been a discussion of the validity of the assumed need for localization of spinal manipulation techniques to particular symptomatic levels, as improvements in neck pain have been demonstrated with manipulation techniques applied to the thoracic spine.[142–144] In addition, the validity of the passive testing procedures used to identify symptomatic levels to which spinal manipulation techniques are targeted, is only moderate,[145] and the application of spinal manipulation techniques, targeted to symptomatic levels, provides equivocal pain relief compared to manipulation randomly applied to any level of the cervical spine.[146] However, one study showed superior short-term reduction in neck pain relief for those receiving cervical spinal manipulation compared to those who received thoracic spinal manipulation.[69] While there are clinical rationale for the benefit of spinal manipulation not specifically applied to cervical symptomatic levels (i.e. improved mobility to biomechanically dependent adjacent regions such as the thoracic spine), it would appear that the beneficial effect of non-specific spinal manipulation may be due to other factors. For example, the response also appears to be mediated by expectation of effect. Those expecting improvement have greater pain reduction.[147,148] Expectation of benefit is one of the predictive features of greater pain relief.[126] The therapeutic effects of spinal manipulation may also be widespread due to their known neurophysiological effects.

Neurophysiological Mechanisms of Spinal Manipulation

A number of studies have demonstrated spinal manipulation-induced hypoalgesia in accord with up-regulation of noradrenergic fight-or-flight system responses.[114] In spinal manipulation-induced hypoalgesia, the periaqueductal grey and rostro-ventromedial medullary centres of the brain stem are likely to be important components of the descending pain inhibition systems. These are distinct areas within the periaqueductal grey that mediate transmission of nociceptive information. Afferent stimulation of the dorsal periaqueductal grey elicits a fight-or-flight reaction, with sympatho-excitation leading to a modulation of pain that is effectively instantaneous.[149]

The potential for spinal manipulation to selectively inhibit C fibre afferent information has been highlighted in recent studies measuring the effect of spinal manipulation on the extent of dorsal horn wind up (or sensitization).[116,150] Aδ fibre information appears to be less influenced by spinal manipulation than that carried by C fibres, suggesting that the thresholds for the Aδ transportation of instantaneous, 'protective' pain is less influenced by manipulation. This may be explained by the fact that simple pain sensations, carried by Aδ fibres, appear to have less limbic and cortical moderation en route to the somatosensory cortex, with less need for interpretation of its value.[151] It has been suggested that spinal manipulation may rapidly adjust the maladaptive cortical integration of sensory afferent information,[152–154] induce a brief inhibition of the spinal motoneuron pool excitability[155–157] and facilitate the return of efficient motor control.[120,152–154]

Spinal manipulation may also inhibit pain by reducing inflammatory cytokines in treated tissues and systemically. For example, Teodorczyk-Injeyan et al.[158] assessed inflammatory cytokines in response to a single spinal manipulative thrust compared to a sham procedure and a control condition and showed a brief, systemic down-regulation of pro-inflammatory cytokines. The mechanisms of effect of spinal manipulation are clearly complex and interactive and thus an understanding of both its local biomechanical and wider neurophysiological effects is necessary so that treatment with spinal manipulation can be utilized effectively. Recently a thorough discussion and proposal of a mechanistic model of spinal manipulation was proposed by Bialosky and colleagues.[147] While complex, the model does provide the clinician with some guidance regarding the aims and objectives of spinal manipulation (see Chapter 29 for more detail).

Risks of Cervical Spinal Manipulation

Recently the International Federation of Orthopaedic Manipulative Physical Therapists, a subgroup of the World Congress of Physical Therapy, produced a document discussing the screening of patients prior to cervical manual therapy.[127] The document reflects the need to clinically reason the individual weighting of risk and benefit before selecting spinal manipulation, in light of the common minor adverse reactions to spinal manipulation (treatment soreness for 24 hours)[159,160] and the rare serious neurovascular adverse events associated with dissection of a cervical artery.[159] The reported risk of vertebral artery dissection associated with recent spinal manipulation is estimated to be in the order of 1.3 in 100 000 patients under the age of 45 (interestingly, not observed in the over-45-years age group).[161] Nevertheless, it is important to remember that this point estimate is not necessarily the individual patient's level of risk.

There are a number of cardiovascular[162] and connective tissue factors[127] that increase the chance of spontaneous arterial dissection. Thus specific 'screening' for these risk factors during the patient interview is recommended. Furthermore, it is recommended that the practitioner attempts to establish if the patient has a pre-existing arterial dissection. This is difficult as an arterial dissection may mimic common musculoskeletal presentations, with the typical referral pattern of pain with an arterial dissection reported in the neck and head.[163] Also, in the early stages of an arterial dissection, symptoms may be present while signs of brainstem ischaemia may not.[163] Thus, neurological examination (including cranial nerve examination) may be negative.[164] Pain of an unusual, throbbing, 'never experienced anything like it before' nature are features suggested to indicate the early non-ischaemic arterial dissection (see Chapter 35).[165,166]

Summary

In light of the equivocal effectiveness of spinal manipulation, when compared with mobilization techniques, the clinician has the option of choosing either. In some patients, likely to be those with an expectation that spinal manipulation will be effective, there may be a superior, short-term improvement in pain. However, there is evidence to suggest that in isolation, spinal manipulation is not superior to other manual or exercise approaches. Currently, we are unable to accurately predict those who should be offered the approach, beyond those who have an expectation that it will be beneficial. While the practical technique of spinal manipulation is targeted towards individual spinal joints, the specificity of effect is thought to be poor, with the influence of spinal manipulation on pain being systemic in nature. Widespread pain relief and improvement in spinal movement can follow the application of cervical spinal manipulation. How to best optimize these effects, and reduce the small risk of serious adverse events, requires further biomechanical, vascular and neurophysiological investigation.

REFERENCES

1. Farioli A, Mattioli S, Quaglieri A, et al. Musculoskeletal pain in Europe: the role of personal, occupational, and social risk factors. Scand J Work Environ Health 2014;40:36–46.
2. US Burden of Disease Collaborators. The state of US health, 1990–2010. Burden of diseases, injuries, and risk factors. JAMA 2013;310:597–608.
3. Son K, Cho N, Lim S, et al. Prevalence and risk factor of neck pain in elderly Korean community residents. J Korean Med Sci 2013;28:680–6.
4. Steinmetz A, Scheffer I, Esmer E, et al. Frequency, severity and predictors of playing-related musculoskeletal pain in professional orchestral musicians in Germany. Clin Rheumatol 2014;doi:10.1007/s10067-013-2470-5; [Epub ahead of print].
5. Long M, Bogossian F, Johnston V. The prevalence of work-related neck, shoulder, and upper back musculoskeletal disorders among midwives, nurses, and physicians: a systematic review. Workplace Health Saf 2013;61:223–9.
6. Carroll LJ, Hogg-Johnson S, Cote P, et al. Course and prognostic factors for neck pain in workers. Spine 2008; 33:S93–100.
7. Skillgate E, Magnusson C, Lundberg M, et al. The age- and sex-specific occurrence of bothersome neck pain in the general population – results from the Stockholm public health cohort. BMC Musculoskelet Disord 2012;13:185.

8. Hogg-Johnson S, van der Velde G, Carroll LJ, et al. The burden and determinants of neck pain in the general population – results of the bone and joint decade 2000–2010 task force on neck pain and its associated disorders. Spine 2008;33:S39–51.

9. Carroll L, Hogg-Johnson S, van der Velde G, et al. Course and prognostic factors for neck pain in the general population. Spine 2008;33:S75–82.

10. Gellhorn A, Katz J, Suri P. Osteoarthritis of the spine: the facet joints. Nat Rev Rheumatol 2013;9:216–24.

11. Acute Musculoskeletal Pain Guidelines Group Australia. Evidence Based Management of Acute Musculoskeletal Pain. Brisbane: Australian Academic Press; 2004.

12. Chien A, Sterling M. Sensory hypoaesthesia is a feature of chronic whiplash but not chronic idiopathic neck pain. Man Ther 2010; 15:48–53.

13. Johnston V, Jimmieson NL, Jull G, et al. Quantitative sensory measures distinguish office workers with varying levels of neck pain and disability. Pain 2008;137:257–65.

14. Scott D, Sterling M, Jull G. A psychophysical investigation of pain processing mechanisms in chronic neck pain. Clin J Pain 2005;21:175–81.

15. Chua N, van Suijlekom H, Vissers K, et al. Differences in sensory processing between chronic cervical zygapophysial joint pain patients with and without cervicogenic headache. Cephalalgia 2011;31:947–57.

16. Sterling M. A proposed new classification system for whiplash associated disorders – implications for assessment and management. Man Ther 2004;9:60–70.

17. Nee R, Vicenzino B, Jull G, et al. Neural tissue management provides immediate clinically relevant benefits without harmful effects for patients with nerve-related neck and arm pain: a randomised trial. J Physiother 2012;58:23–31.

18. Zito G, Jull G, Story I. Clinical tests of musculoskeletal dysfunction in the diagnosis of cervicogenic headache. Man Ther 2006;11:118–29.

19. Cagnie B, Dolphens M, Peeters I, et al. Use of muscle functional magnetic resonance imaging to compare cervical flexor activity between patients with whiplash-associated disorders and people who are healthy. Phys Ther 2010;90:1157–64.

20. Falla DL, Jull GA, Hodges PW. Patients with neck pain demonstrate reduced electromyographic activity of the deep cervical flexor muscles during performance of the craniocervical flexion test. Spine 2004;29:2108–14.

21. Jull G, Kristjansson E, Dall'Alba P. Impairment in the cervical flexors: a comparison of whiplash and insidious onset neck pain patients. Man Ther 2004;9:89–94.

22. Lindstrom R, Schomacher J, Farina D, et al. Association between neck muscle co-activation, pain, and strength in women with neck pain. Man Ther 2011;16:80–6.

23. Falla D, Bilenkij G, Jull G. Patients with chronic neck pain demonstrate altered patterns of muscle activation during performance of a functional upper limb task. Spine 2004;29:1436–40.

24. Johnston V, Jull G, Souvlis T, et al. Neck movement and muscle activity characteristics in office workers with neck pain. Spine 2008;33:555–63.

25. Falla D, Jull G, Hodges PW. Feedforward activity of the cervical flexor muscles during voluntary arm movements is delayed in chronic neck pain. Exp Brain Res 2004;157:43–8.

26. Jull G, Falla D, Vicenzino B, et al. The effect of therapeutic exercise on activation of the deep cervical flexor muscles in people with chronic neck pain. Man Ther 2009;14:696–701.

27. Boudreau S, Falla D. Chronic neck pain alters muscle activation patterns to sudden movements. Exp Brain Res 2014;232: 2011–20.

28. Falla D, Rainoldi A, Merletti R, et al. Myoelectric manifestations of sternocleidomastoid and anterior scalene muscle fatigue in chronic neck pain patients. Clin Neurophysiol 2003;114:488–95.

29. Edmondston S, Björnsdóttir G, Pálsson T, et al. Endurance and fatigue characteristics of the neck flexor and extensor muscles during isometric tests in patients with postural neck pain. Man Ther 2011;16:332–8.

30. O'Leary S, Jull G, Kim M, et al. Cranio-cervical flexor muscle impairment at maximal, moderate, and low loads is a feature of neck pain. Man Ther 2007;12:34–9.

31. Beinert K, Taube W. The effect of balance training on cervical sensorimotor function and neck pain. J Mot Behav 2013;45:271–8.

32. Woodhouse A, Vasseljen O. Altered motor control patterns in whiplash and chronic neck pain. BMC Musculoskelet Disord 2008;9:90.

33. Chen X, Treleaven J. The effect of neck torsion on joint position error in subjects with chronic neck pain. Man Ther 2013;18: 562–7.

34. Tjell C, Rosenhall U. Smooth pursuit neck torsion test: a specific test for cervical dizziness. Am J Otol 1998;19:76–81.

35. Yahia A, Ghroubi S, Jribi S, et al. Chronic neck pain and vertigo: is a true balance disorder present? Ann Phys Rehabil Med 2009;52:556–67.

36. Jørgensen M, Skotte J, Holtermann A, et al. Neck pain and postural balance among workers with high postural demands – a cross-sectional study. BMC Musculoskelet Disord 2011;12:176.

37. Falla D, O'Leary S, Farina D, et al. Association between intensity of pain and impairment in onset and activation of the deep cervical flexors in patients with persistent neck pain. Clin J Pain 2011;27:309–14.

38. Sterling M, Hendricks J, Kenardy J. Developmental trajectories of pain/disability and PTSD symptoms following a whiplash injury. Pain 2010;150:22–8.

39. Ligthart L, Gerrits M, Boomsma D, et al. Anxiety and depression are associated with migraine and pain in general: an investigation of the interrelationships. J Pain 2013;14:363–70.

40. Feleus A, van Dalen T, Bierma-Zeinstra1 S, et al. Kinesiophobia in patients with non-traumatic arm, neck and shoulder complaints: a prospective cohort study in general practice. BMC Musculoskelet Disord 2007;8:117.

41. Hoe V, Kelsall H, Urquhart D, et al. Risk factors for musculoskeletal symptoms of the neck or shoulder alone or neck and shoulder among hospital nurses. Occup Environ Med 2012;69: 198–204.

42. Karels C, Bierma-Zeinstra S, Burdorf A, et al. Social and psychological factors influenced the course of arm, neck and shoulder complaints. J Clin Epidem 2007;60:839–48.

43. Thompson D, Urmston M, Oldham J, et al. The association between cognitive factors, pain and disability in patients with idiopathic chronic neck pain. Disabil Rehabil 2010;32:1758–67.

44. Hurwitz E, Goldstein M, Morgenstern H, et al. The impact of psychosocial factors on neck pain and disability outcomes among primary care patients: results from the UCLA Neck Pain Study. Disabil Rehabil 2006;28:1319–29.

45. Mercado A, Carroll L, Cassidy J, et al. Passive coping is a risk factor for disabling neck or low back pain. Pain 2005;117:51–7.

46. Stenberg G, Fjellman-Wiklund A, Ahlgren C. 'I am afraid to make the damage worse' – fear of engaging in physical activity among patients with neck or back pain – a gender perspective. Scand J Caring Sci 2014;28:146–54.

47. McLean S, Klaber Moffett J, Sharp D, et al. An investigation to determine the association between neck pain and upper limb disability for patients with non-specific neck pain: a secondary analysis. Man Ther 2011;16:434–9.

48. Pool J, Ostelo R, Knol D, et al. Are psychological factors prognostic indicators of outcome in patients with sub-acute neck pain? Man Ther 2010;15:111–16.

49. Verhagen A, Karels C, Schellingerhout J, et al. Pain severity and catastrophising modify treatment success in neck pain patients in primary care. Man Ther 2010;15:267–72.

50. Walton D, Carroll L, Kasch H, et al. An overview of systematic reviews on prognostic factors in neck pain: results from the International Collaboration on Neck Pain (ICON) Project. Open Orthop J 2013;7:494–505.

51. Saavedra-Hernández M, Castro-Sánchez A, Cuesta-Vargas A, et al. The contribution of previous episodes of pain, pain intensity, physical impairment, and pain-related fear to disability in patients with chronic mechanical neck pain. Am J Phys Med Rehabil 2012;91:1070–6.

52. Äng BO. Impaired neck motor function and pronounced pain-related fear in helicopter pilots with neck pain – a clinical approach. J Electromyogr Kinesiol 2008;18:538–49.

53. Edmond S, Cutrone G, Werneke M, et al. Association between centralization and directional preference; and functional and pain outcomes in patients with neck pain. J Orthop Sports Phys Ther 2014;44:68–75.

54. Hanney W, Kolber M, George S, et al. Development of a preliminary clinical prediction rule to identify patients with neck pain that

may benefit from a standardized program of stretching and muscle performance exercise: a prospective cohort study. Int J Sports Phys Ther 2013;8:756–76.

55. Osborn W, Jull G. Patients with non-specific neck disorders commonly report upper limb disability. Man Ther 2013;18: 492–7.

56. Waddell G, Newton M, Henderson I, et al. Fear-Avoidance Beliefs Questionnaire (FABQ) and the role of fear-avoidance beliefs in chronic low back pain and disability. Pain 1993;52: 157–68.

57. Kori S, Miller R, Todd D. Kinisophobia: a new view of chronic pain behavior. Pain Manag 1990;Jan/Feb:35–43.

58. Turk D, Robinson J, Sherman J, et al. Assessing fear in patients with cervical pain: development and validation of the Pictorial Fear of Activity Scale-Cervical (PFActS-C). Pain 2008;139: 55–62.

59. Cleland JA, Fritz J, Childs J. Psychometric properties of the fear-avoidance beliefs questionnaire and Tampa scale of kinesiophobia in patients with neck pain. Am J Phys Med Rehabil 2008;87: 109–17.

60. Collins J, Baase C, Sharda C, et al. The assessment of chronic health conditions on work performance, absence, and total economic impact for employers. J Occup Environ Med 2005;47: 547–57.

61. Bugajska J, Zołnierczyk-Zreda D, Jędryka-Góral A, et al. Psychological factors at work and musculoskeletal disorders: a one year prospective study. Rheumatol Int 2013;33:2975–83.

62. Carroll L, Hogg-Johnson S, van der Velde G, et al. Course and prognostic factors for neck pain in the general population. Spine 2008;33:S75–82.

63. De Loose V, Burnotte F, Cagnie B, et al. Prevalence and risk factors of neck pain in military office workers. Mil Med 2008;173:474–9.

64. Larsman P, Kadefors R, Sandsjö L. Psychosocial work conditions, perceived stress, perceived muscular tension, and neck/shoulder symptoms among medical secretaries. Int Arch Occup Environ Health 2013;86:57–63.

65. Sterud T, Johannessen H, Tynes T. Work-related psychosocial and mechanical risk factors for neck/shoulder pain: a 3-year follow-up study of the general working population in Norway. Int Arch Occup Environ Health 2014;87:471–81.

66. Johnston V, Jull G, Souvlis T, et al. Interactive effects from self-reported physical and psychosocial factors in the workplace on neck pain and disability in female office workers. Ergonomics 2010;53:502–13.

67. Jull G, Sterling M, Falla D, et al. Whiplash, Headache and Neck Pain: Research Based Directions for Physical Therapies. Edinburgh: Elsevier UK; 2008.

68. Stewart J, Kempenaar L, Lauchlan D. Rethinking yellow flags. Man Ther 2011;16:196–8.

69. Puentedura E, Landers M, Cleland J, et al. Thoracic spine thrust manipulation versus cervical spine thrust manipulation in patients with acute neck pain: a randomized clinical trial. J Orthop Sports Phys Ther 2011;41:208–20.

70. Mayer J, Kraus T, Ochsmann E. Longitudinal evidence for the association between work-related physical exposures and neck and/or shoulder complaints: a systematic review. Int Arch Occup Environ Health 2012;85:587–603.

71. O'Leary S, Falla D, Elliott JM, et al. Muscle dysfunction in cervical spine pain: implications for assessment and management. J Orthop Sports Phys Ther 2009;39:324–33.

72. Gross AR, Goldsmith C, Hoving JL, et al. Conservative management of mechanical neck disorders: a systematic review. J Rheumat 2007;34:1083–102.

73. Falla D, Lindstrom R, Rechter L, et al. Effect of pain on the modulation in discharge rate of sternocleidomastoid motor units with force direction. Clin Neurophysiol 2010;121:744–53.

74. O'Leary S, Cagnie B, Reeve A, et al. Is there altered activity of the extensor muscles in chronic mechanical neck pain? A functional magnetic resonance imaging study. Arch Phys Med Rehabil 2011;92:929–34.

75. Wegner S, Jull G, O'Leary S, et al. The effect of a scapular postural correction strategy on trapezius activity in patients with neck pain. Man Ther 2010;15:562–6.

76. Zakharova-Luneva E, Jull G, Johnston V, et al. Altered trapezius muscle behavior in individuals with neck pain and clinical signs of scapular dysfunction. J Manipulative Physiol Ther 2012;35: 346–53.

77. Falla D, Farina D. Muscle fiber conduction velocity of the upper trapezius muscle during dynamic contraction of the upper limb in patients with chronic neck pain. Pain 2005;116: 138–45.

78. Elliott JM, Pedler AR, Jull GA, et al. Differential changes in muscle composition exist in traumatic and nontraumatic neck pain. Spine 2014;39:39–47.

79. Uhlig Y, Weber BR, Muntener DGM. Fiber composition and fiber transformations in neck muscles of patients with dysfunction of the cervical spine. J Orthop Res 1995;13:240–9.

80. Kadi F, Waling K, Ahlgren C, et al. Pathological mechanisms implicated in localized female trapezius myalgia. Pain 1998;78: 191–6.

81. Lindman R, Hagberg M, Angqvist KA, et al. Changes in muscle morphology in chronic trapezius myalgia. Scand J Work Environ Health 1991;17:347–55.

82. Falla D, Jull G, Edwards S, et al. Neuromuscular efficiency of the sternocleidomastoid and anterior scalene muscles in patients with neck pain. Disabil Rehabil 2004;26:712–17.

83. Jordan A, Mehlsen J, Ostergaard K. A comparison of physical characteristics between patients seeking treatment for neck pain and aged-matched healthy people. J Manipulative Physiol Ther 1997;20:468–75.

84. Watson DH, Trott PH. Cervical headache: an investigation of natural head posture and upper cervical flexor muscle performance. Cephalalgia 1993;13:272–84.

85. Muceli S, Farina D, Kirkesola G, et al. Force steadiness in women with neck pain and the effect of short term vibration. J Electromyogr Kinesiol 2011;21:283–90.

86. Kristjansson E, Dall'Alba P, Jull G. A study of five cervicocephalic relocation tests in three different subject groups. Clin Rehabil 2003;17:768–74.

87. Sjolander P, Michaelson P, Jaric S, et al. Sensorimotor disturbances in chronic neck pain – range of motion, peak velocity, smoothness of movement, and repositioning acuity. Man Ther 2008;13:122–31.

88. Jull G, Trott P, Potter H, et al. A randomised controlled trial of exercise and manipulative therapy for cervicogenic headache. Spine 2002;27:1835–43.

89. Andersen LL, Jorgensen MB, Blangsted AK, et al. A randomized controlled intervention trial to relieve and prevent neck/shoulder pain. Med Sci Sports Exerc 2008;40:983–90.

90. Ylinen J, Takala EP, Nykanen M, et al. Active neck muscle training in the treatment of chronic neck pain in women: a randomized controlled trial. JAMA 2003;289:2509–16.

91. O'Leary S, Falla D, Hodges P, et al. Specific therapeutic exercise of the neck induces immediate local hypoalgesia. J Pain 2007;8: 832–9.

92. Jull GA, Falla D, Vicenzino B, et al. The effect of therapeutic exercise on activation of the deep cervical flexor muscles in people with chronic neck pain. Man Ther 2009;14:696–701.

93. O'Leary S, Jull G, Kim M, et al. Training mode-dependent changes in motor performance in neck pain. Arch Phys Med Rehabil 2012;93:1225–33.

94. Falla D, Lindstrom R, Rechter L, et al. Effectiveness of an 8-week exercise programme on pain and specificity of neck muscle activity in patients with chronic neck pain: a randomized controlled study. Eur J Pain 2013;17:1517–28.

95. Mackey AL, Andersen LL, Frandsen U, et al. Strength training increases the size of the satellite cell pool in type I and II fibres of chronically painful trapezius muscle in females. J Physiol 2011; 589:5503–15.

96. Falla D, Jull G, Russell T, et al. Effect of neck exercise on sitting posture in patients with chronic neck pain. Phys Ther 2007;87: 408–17.

97. Falla D, Jull G, Hodges P, et al. An endurance-strength training regime is effective in reducing myoelectric manifestations of cervical flexor muscle fatigue in females with chronic neck pain. Clin Neurophysiol 2006;117:828–37.

98. Adkins DL, Boychuk J, Remple MS, et al. Motor training induces experience-specific patterns of plasticity across motor cortex and spinal cord. J Appl Physiol 2006;101:1776–82.

99. Coffey VG, Hawley JA. The molecular bases of training adaptation. Sports Med 2007;37:737–63.

100. Fluck M. Functional, structural and molecular plasticity of mammalian skeletal muscle in response to exercise stimuli. J Exp Biol 2006;209:2239–48.
101. Gabriel DA, Kamen G, Frost G. Neural adaptations to resistive exercise: mechanisms and recommendations for training practices. Sports Med 2006;36:133–49.
102. Falla D, O'Leary S, Fagan A, et al. Recruitment of the deep cervical flexor muscles during a postural correction exercise performed in sitting. Man Ther 2007;12:139–43.
103. Lee MH, Park SJ, Kim JS. Effects of neck exercise on high-school students' neck-shoulder posture. J Phys Ther Sci 2013;25:571–4.
104. Beer A, Treleaven J, Jull G. Can a functional postural exercise improve performance in the cranio-cervical flexion test?–a preliminary study. Man Ther 2012;17:219–24.
105. Falla D, O'Leary S, Farina D, et al. The change in deep cervical flexor activity after training is associated with the degree of pain reduction in patients with chronic neck pain. Clin J Pain 2012;28:628–34.
106. Sterling M, Jull G, Vicenzino B, et al. Development of motor dysfunction following whiplash injury. Pain 2003;103:65–73.
107. Lee H, Nicholson LL, Adams RD. Cervical range of motion associations with subclinical neck pain. Spine 2003;29:33–40.
108. Bialosky JE, Simon CB, Bishop MD, et al. Basis for spinal manipulative therapy: a physical therapist perspective. J Electromyogr Kinesiol 2012;22:643–7.
109. Cramer GD, Cambron J, Cantu JA, et al. Magnetic resonance imaging zygapophyseal joint space changes (gapping) in low back pain patients following spinal manipulation and side-posture positioning: a randomized controlled mechanisms trial with blinding. J Manipulative Physiol Ther 2013;36:203–17.
110. Evans DW, Breen AC. A biomechanical model for mechanically efficient cavitation production during spinal manipulation: pre-thrust position and the neutral zone. J Manipulative Physiol Ther 2006;29:72–82.
111. Herzog W. The biomechanics of spinal manipulation. J Bodyw Mov Ther 2010;14:280–6.
112. Cassidy JD, Lopes AA, Yong-Hing K. The immediate effect of manipulation versus mobilization on pain and range of motion in the cervical spine: a randomized controlled trial. J Manipulative Physiol Ther 1992;15:570–5.
113. Millan M, Leboeuf-Yde C, Budgell B, et al. The effect of spinal manipulative therapy on spinal range of motion: a systematic literature review. Chiropr Man Therap 2012;20:23.
114. Coronado RA, Gay CW, Bialosky JE, et al. Changes in pain sensitivity following spinal manipulation: a systematic review and meta-analysis. J Electromyogr Kinesiol 2012;22:752–67.
115. Fernandez-de-las-Penas C, Alonso-Blanco C, Cleland JA, et al. Changes in pressure pain thresholds over C5–C6 zygapophyseal joint after a cervicothoracic junction manipulation in healthy subjects. J Manipulative Physiol Ther 2008;31:332–7.
116. George SZ, Bishop MD, Bialosky JE, et al. Immediate effects of spinal manipulation on thermal pain sensitivity: an experimental study. BMC Musculoskelet Disord 2006;7:68.
117. Dishman JD, Bulbulian R. Comparison of effects of spinal manipulation and massage on motoneuron excitability. Electromyogr Clin Neurophysiol 2001;41:97–106.
118. Dunning J, Rushton A. The effects of cervical high-velocity low-amplitude thrust manipulation on resting electromyographic activity of the biceps brachii muscle. Man Ther 2009;14:508–13.
119. Fernandez-Carnero J, Fernandez-de-las-Penas C, Cleland JA. Immediate hypoalgesic and motor effects after a single cervical spine manipulation in subjects with lateral epicondylalgia. J Manipulative Physiol Ther 2008;31:675–81.
120. Haavik TH, Murphy B. The effects of spinal manipulation on central integration of dual somatosensory input observed after motor training: a crossover study. J Manipulative Physiol Ther 2010;33:261–72.
121. Bialosky JE, Bishop MD, George SZ, et al. Placebo response to manual therapy: something out of nothing? J Man Manip Ther 2011;19:11–19.
122. Bialosky JE, Bishop MD, Robinson ME, et al. The influence of expectation on spinal manipulation induced hypoalgesia: an experimental study in normal subjects. BMC Musculoskelet Disord 2008;9:19.
123. Dieppe P. Complex interventions. Musculoskelet Care 2004;2:180–6.
124. Cassidy JD, Boyle E, Cote P, et al. Risk of vertebrobasilar stroke and chiropractic care: results of a population-based case-control and case-crossover study. Spine 2008;33:S176–83.
125. Kerry R, Taylor AJ, Mitchell J, et al. Manual therapy and cervical arterial dysfunction, directions for the future: a clinical perspective. J Man Manip Ther 2008;16:39–48.
126. Puentedura EJ, Cleland JA, Landers MR, et al. Development of a clinical prediction rule to identify patients with neck pain likely to benefit from thrust joint manipulation to the cervical spine. J Orthop Sports Phys Ther 2012;42:577–92.
127. Rushton A, Rivett D, Carlesso L, et al. International framework for examination of the cervical region for potential of cervical arterial Dysfunction prior to orthopaedic manual therapy intervention. Man Ther 2014;19:222–8.
128. Gross A, Miller J, D'Sylva J, et al. Manipulation or mobilisation for neck pain: a Cochrane review. Man Ther 2010;15:315–33.
129. Millan M, Leboeuf-Yde C, Budgell B, et al. The effect of spinal manipulative therapy on experimentally induced pain: a systematic literature review. Chiropr Man Therap 2012;20:26.
130. Haldeman S, Carroll L, Cassidy JD, et al. The bone and joint decade 2000–2010 task force on neck pain and its associated disorders: executive summary. Spine 2008;33:S5–7.
131. Michaleff ZA, Lin CW, Maher CG, et al. Spinal manipulation epidemiology: systematic review of cost effectiveness studies. J Electromyogr Kinesiol 2012;22:655–62.
132. Bronfort G, Evans R, Anderson AV, et al. Spinal manipulation, medication, or home exercise with advice for acute and subacute neck pain: a randomized trial. Ann Intern Med 2012;156:1–10.
133. Martel J, Dugas C, Dubois JD, et al. A randomised controlled trial of preventive spinal manipulation with and without a home exercise program for patients with chronic neck pain. BMC Musculoskelet Disord 2011;12:41.
134. Bronfort G, Maiers MJ, Evans RL, et al. Supervised exercise, spinal manipulation, and home exercise for chronic low back pain: a randomized clinical trial. Spine J 2011;11:585–98.
135. Ernst E. Chiropractic spinal manipulation for neck pain: a systematic review. J Pain 2003;4:417–21.
136. Bronfort G, Evans R, Nelson B, et al. A randomized clinical trial of exercise and spinal manipulation for patients with chronic neck pain. Spine 2001;26:788–97.
137. Evans R, Bronfort G, Nelson B, et al. Two-year follow-up of a randomized clinical trial of spinal manipulation and two types of exercise for patients with chronic neck pain. Spine 2002;27:2383–9.
138. Leaver AM, Maher CG, Herbert RD, et al. A randomized controlled trial comparing manipulation with mobilization for recent onset neck pain. Arch Phys Med Rehabil 2010;91:1313–18.
139. Cassidy JD, Quon JA, LaFrance LJ, et al. The effect of manipulation on pain and range of motion in the cervical spine: a pilot study. J Manipulative Physiol Ther 1992;15:495–500.
140. Dunning JR, Cleland JA, Waldrop MA, et al. Upper cervical and upper thoracic thrust manipulation versus nonthrust mobilization in patients with mechanical neck pain: a multicenter randomized clinical trial. J Orthop Sports Phys Ther 2012;42:5–18.
141. Boyles RE, Walker MJ, Young BA, et al. The addition of cervical thrust manipulations to a manual physical therapy approach in patients treated for mechanical neck pain: a secondary analysis. J Orthop Sports Phys Ther 2010;40:133–40.
142. Cleland JA, Childs JD, McRae M, et al. Immediate effects of thoracic manipulation in patients with neck pain: a randomized clinical trial. Man Ther 2005;10:127–35.
143. Cross KM, Kuenze C, Grindstaff TL, et al. Thoracic spine thrust manipulation improves pain, range of motion, and self-reported function in patients with mechanical neck pain: a systematic review. J Orthop Sports Phys Ther 2011;41:633–42.
144. Krauss J, Creighton D, Ely JD. Podlewska-Ely J. The immediate effects of upper thoracic translatoric spinal manipulation on cervical pain and range of motion: a randomized clinical trial. J Man Manip Ther 2008;16:93–9.
145. Triano JJ, Budgell B, Bagnulo A, et al. Review of the methods used by Chiropractors to determine the site for applying manipulation. Chiropr Man Therap 2013;21:36.

146. Haas M, Groupp E, Panzer D, et al. Efficacy of cervical endplay assessment as an indicator for spinal manipulation. Spine 2003; 28:1091–6.

147. Bialosky JE, Bishop MD, Price DD, et al. The mechanisms of manual therapy in the treatment of musculoskeletal pain: a comprehensive model. Man Ther 2009;14:531–8.

148. Bishop MD, Mintken PE, Bialosky JE, et al. Patient expectations of benefit from interventions for neck pain and resulting influence on outcomes. J Orthop Sports Phys Ther 2013;43:457–65.

149. Wright A. Hypoalgesia post-manipulative therapy: a review of a potential neurophysiological mechanism. Man Ther 1995;1: 11–16.

150. Bialosky JE, Bishop MD, Robinson ME, et al. Spinal manipulative therapy has an immediate effect on thermal pain sensitivity in people with low back pain: a randomized controlled trial. Phys Ther 2009;89:1292–303.

151. Rolls ET. The functions of the orbitofrontal cortex. Brain Cogn 2004;55:11–29.

152. Dishman JD, Dougherty PE, Burke JR. Evaluation of the effect of postural perturbation on motoneuronal activity following various methods of lumbar spinal manipulation. Spine J 2005; 5:650–9.

153. Haavik H, Murphy B. The role of spinal manipulation in addressing disordered sensorimotor integration and altered motor control. J Electromyogr Kinesiol 2012;22:768–76.

154. Haavik-Taylor H, Murphy B. Cervical spine manipulation alters sensorimotor integration: a somatosensory evoked potential study. Clin Neurophysiol 2007;118:391–402.

155. Dishman JD, Ball KA, Burke J. Central motor excitability changes after spinal manipulation: a transcranial magnetic stimulation study. J Manipulative Physiol Ther 2002;25:1–9.

156. Dishman JD, Burke J. Spinal reflex excitability changes after cervical and lumbar spinal manipulation: a comparative study. Spine J 2003;3:204–12.

157. Dishman JD, Weber KA, Corbin RL, et al. Understanding inhibitory mechanisms of lumbar spinal manipulation using H-reflex and F-wave responses: a methodological approach. J Neurosci Methods 2012;210:169–77.

158. Teodorczyk-Injeyan JA, Injeyan HS, Ruegg R. Spinal manipulative therapy reduces inflammatory cytokines but not substance P production in normal subjects. J Manipulative Physiol Ther 2006;29:14–21.

159. Cagnie B, Vinck E, Beernaert A, et al. How common are side effects of spinal manipulation and can these side effects be predicted? Man Ther 2004;9:151–6.

160. Carnes D, Mars TS, Mullinger B, et al. Adverse events and manual therapy: a systematic review. Man Ther 2010;15:355–63.

161. Miley ML, Wellik KE, Wingerchuk DM, et al. Does cervical manipulative therapy cause vertebral artery dissection and stroke? Neurologist 2008;14:66–73.

162. Debette S, Leys D. Cervical-artery dissections: predisposing factors, diagnosis, and outcome. Lancet Neurol 2009;8:668–78.

163. Kerry R, Taylor AJ. Cervical arterial dysfunction: knowledge and reasoning for manual physical therapists. J Orthop Sports Phys Ther 2009;39:378–87.

164. Kerry R, Taylor AJ, Mitchell J, et al. Cervical arterial dysfunction and manual therapy: a critical literature review to inform professional practice. Man Ther 2008;13:278–88.

165. Kerry R, Taylor AJ. Cervical arterial dysfunction assessment and manual therapy. Man Ther 2006;11:243–53.

166. Taylor AJ, Kerry R. Neck pain and headache as a result of internal carotid artery dissection: implications for manual therapists. Man Ther 2005;10:73–7.

CHAPTER 42

WHIPLASH-ASSOCIATED DISORDERS

Michele Sterling • Tze Siong Ng • David Walton • Ashley Smith

INTRODUCTION

Whiplash-associated disorders (WAD) are a controversial condition associated with substantial personal and economic costs. Most individuals with WAD incur the injury as a result of a road traffic collision but the symptoms can arise from other traumatic events such as sporting incidents. Consistent international data indicate that up to 50% of those injured will not fully recover, with approximately 30% reporting ongoing moderate to severe pain and disability.[1] Mental health problems are also associated with the whiplash condition,[2] with disorders such as post-traumatic stress disorder, depression and anxiety being common.[3,4] The predominant symptom of WAD is neck pain, but headaches, arm pain, neck stiffness, dizziness and paraesthesia/anaesthesia in the upper quadrant are also frequently reported.

Whiplash is a controversial condition, most likely due to it being a compensable injury where a clinical diagnosis of tissue damage or lesion in the neck cannot usually be made.[5] Some still doubt the veracity of patients' complaints and deny it as a legitimate condition.[6] This is despite much research data in recent years demonstrating the presence of both physical and psychological manifestations including psychophysical indictors of augmented central nociceptive processing, movement loss, altered muscle recruitment patterns, morphological muscle changes, post-traumatic stress symptoms, psychological distress, fear of movement and pain catastrophizing amongst others.

It is not the aim of this chapter to discuss these changes and for interested readers, more in-depth detail of these factors and their implications for physiotherapy assessment and management of WAD is available elsewhere.[7] Rather, this chapter will focus on some current unresolved issues surrounding the whiplash condition; the research evidence base around these issues and their implications for the management of the whiplash condition. Specifically the chapter will discuss four main issues: (a) is there tissue damage in WAD and what is the clinical relevance of this?; (b) is WAD a culturally dependent condition?; (c) the clinical relevance of outcome prediction; and (d) what needs to be done in the area of treatment in order to improve health outcomes?

THE ROLE OF TISSUE DAMAGE IN WHIPLASH-ASSOCIATED DISORDERS

It is generally presumed that individuals sustain a peripheral injury to the neck following whiplash trauma,[5,8] despite conventional imaging usually not being able to detect such tissue damage.[9] Evidence for the presence of peripheral tissue damage stems from a combination of cadaveric dissection, animal and biomechanical studies, together with recent studies documenting the presence of inflammatory biomarkers in individuals with persistent moderate to severe symptoms.[10,11] However, the importance of patho-anatomical lesions and underlying sources of nociception is debatable in regard to their significance and relevance for the initiation and/or maintenance of whiplash pain. This section will summarize the mechanisms of injury and symptom production following whiplash injury, including tissue lesions that have been identified, and whether modulation of nociception arising from these lesions results in improved clinical outcomes.

Evidence Supporting the Presence of Tissue Damage

Mechanisms of whiplash injury have been demonstrated using high-speed cineradiography in human volunteers,[12] cadaveric experiments[13] and computer models.[14] Essentially, energy from the road traffic collision is transferred from the collision to the body, resulting in a cervical acceleration/deceleration motion, as the inertia of the head reacts to this energy.[15] These forces are non-physiological in nature[16] and could theoretically result in injury to various tissues in the cervical spine. Engineers have responded to results of these studies, by developing car seats to minimize the forces individuals are exposed to with whiplash trauma.[17,18] As a result, neck injury rates have reduced significantly.[19] Given that the injury rates have fallen in response to these lower forces, it can be presumed that injuries to neck tissues are associated with whiplash symptoms.

Supporting evidence for the presence of potential tissue damage identified in engineering studies can be found from post-mortem dissection studies of non-survivors of road traffic collisions who presumably have more serious injuries.[20-23] Multiple injuries have been demonstrated, including disruption to the facet joints, spinal ligaments, vertebral arteries, dorsal root ganglia and muscle tissue. Detection of these lesions has proven difficult, likely due to insensitivity of current radiological imaging techniques,[23,24] but has been demonstrated utilizing techniques such as cryomicrotomy (frozen sectioning and detailed microscopic investigation) where lesions involving the capsule, ligaments and discs can be detected.[25]

Clinical studies are also available to support the presence of tissue damage in chronic WAD. These studies have utilized diagnostic injections to provide a diagnosis of cervical facet joint pathology and have determined that the cervical facet joint is probably the most common tissue lesion contributing to chronic WAD symptoms.[26,27] Injuries to the cervical facet joint are proposed to arise from synovial fold impingement or capsular distension,[8] and facet joint capsules are rich with nociceptors.[28] In vivo animal experiments demonstrate a relationship between capsular distension and altered collagen fibre organization,[29] afferent fibre sensitization,[30,31] dorsal root ganglion sensitization and spinal cord metabolite changes,[32,33] and behavioural sensitivity (pain)[34] under experimental conditions similar to those observed in simulated whiplash.[35] A treatment for cervical facet joint dysfunction is available. Radiofrequency neurotomy (RFN) is a neuroablative technique directed at the medial branch of the dorsal rami of the cervical facet joints,[27] providing 7–14 months relief of pain,[36] together with resolution of psychological distress.[37] The procedure can successfully be repeated when pain returns.[36]

Thus convergent data from cadaveric, biomechanical and clinical studies indicate that tissue damage, in some form, is likely following whiplash injury.

The Relationship of Tissue Damage to the Clinical Presentation of Whiplash-Associated Disorders

The inability of current diagnostic imaging modalities to accurately detect tissue damage in individual patients following whiplash injury presents a dilemma. However, caution also needs to be applied when possible tissue damage is identified to determine if it is relevant to the patient's symptoms and whether effective treatment for such damage is available. Magnetic resonance imaging has demonstrated possible pathology of the cranioverte-bral ligaments[38–40] in people with whiplash. However, similar 'pathologic' changes in these ligaments were observed in asymptomatic, age- and gender-matched individuals and individuals with non-traumatic neck pain.[41] Moreover, even when detected by magnetic resonance imaging, correlation with clinical symptoms is questionable,[41] and outcomes did not differ significantly between those with high signal changes of the alar and transverse ligaments compared to those without these changes.[42]

Moreover, evidence suggests that nociception from the cervical facet joint contributes to other physiological and psychological manifestations of the whiplash condition. In a recent series of studies, individuals with chronic WAD (3–4 years post-road traffic collision) underwent RFN following successful response to diagnostic facet joint injections. Individuals were assessed on two occasions prior to undergoing the procedure (10 months apart) and then at 1 and 3 months post-procedure as well as at a subsequent time point upon the return of pain. Prior to receiving RFN, no changes were measured in any physical or psychological manifestations.[43] Following RFN, pain, disability and central hyperexcitability decreased (Fig. 42-1) with concomitant increases in neck range of movement[43] and reduced psychological distress

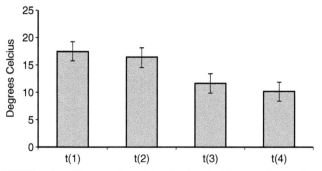

Cold Pain Thresholds vs. Time

FIGURE 42-1 ■ Changes in cold pain thresholds over time prior to and following radiofrequency neurotomy of the cervical facet joints. t(1), one month after initial preliminary cervical facet joint blockade; t(2), immediately prior to radiofrequency neurotomy of cervical facet joints; t(3), one month following radiofrequency neurotomy; t(4), three months following radiofrequency neurotomy.

and pain catastrophization.[44] These changes were evident within 1 month of receiving RFN and remained stable at 3 months. Physical measures returned to values similar to those of a healthy control cohort. No changes were observed in post-traumatic stress symptoms.[44] Upon return of pain, these findings reversed, with increased central hyperexcitability and deterioration of neck range of movement, pain catastrophizing and psychological distress.[45] Measures were not significantly different to those present prior to undergoing RFN.

Hence, these data indicate that neck tissue pathology contributes to the physical and psychological manifestations of chronic WAD. However, RFN did not result in complete resolution of pain and disability.[43] This is not surprising, as many factors are likely responsible for symptom persistence, including psychological factors, the social context of the patient,[46,47] compensation-related factors,[48] beliefs and expectations.[49]

Clinically, it is evident that individuals with chronic WAD presenting with a combination of physical and psychological manifestations may also have peripheral tissue pathology. Consideration for referral for diagnostic facet joint injection can be made in patients not responding to conservative physiotherapy treatment. These individuals may be identified by a positive response to each of the following clinical tests: extension–rotation test, segmental tenderness and provocation of familiar neck pain upon manual spinal examination.[50] Unfortunately, at the present time it is not possible to anaesthetize other cervical tissues in order to determine their role in whiplash symptoms. Until then, as in other conditions characterized by persistent pain, treatment directed at mechanisms and impairments underlying the disorder need to be addressed.[51]

Summary

Convergent evidence suggests that peripheral pathology is evident in individuals following whiplash injury. Lack of diagnostic imaging evidence does not preclude the presence of a lesion, with most evidence currently supporting cervical facet joint involvement. Successful treatment of a tissue lesion demonstrated significant improvements in physical and psychological manifestations, but future research needs to consider other lesions and treatment options.

IS WHIPLASH-ASSOCIATED DISORDER A CULTURALLY DEPENDENT CONDITION?

Chronic WAD has been proposed to be a culturally dependent condition. In Western countries such as Australia, Canada and the United Kingdom, the proportion of people who develop chronic WAD following a whiplash injury is as high as 50%.[1,52] The condition is purported to be less prevalent in countries such as Lithuania and Germany.[53-55] There has been little research on WAD in Asian countries but an early study reported the prevalence as being low in Singapore.[56] While there are no more recent data available for WAD, the prevalence of chronic pain in general would seem to be lower in Singapore ranging from 9–16%[57,58] compared to 19–50% in Australia.[59-61]

The prevalence of WAD may be affected by the compensation and social systems in each society. In the province of Saskatchewan in Canada, the incidence of WAD was 417 per 100 000 persons under a fault-based motor insurance system and decreased to 300 per 100 000 persons under a no-fault system.[48] The prevalence of chronic WAD in Brisbane, Australia, is believed to be higher than in Singapore.[56,62] Brisbane and Singapore both have a fault-based motor insurance system. Public health care is universal and the permanently disabled receive some form of social support in both cities. However, unemployment social benefits are provided in Brisbane while in Singapore there is an emphasis on employment benefits and unemployment benefits are not provided.[63] The culture and social systems may be factors which affect the cross-cultural prevalence of WAD.

The cross-cultural difference in prevalence of WAD could also be related to cultural differences in pain perception and psychological responses to pain.[64-66] In the United States, African-Americans with chronic neck and back pain have reported greater pain and disability when compared to Caucasians with similar conditions.[64,67] A systematic review revealed white patients generally exhibited higher pain thresholds and pain tolerances than African-American and Asian patients in studies that used experimental pain models to assess pain sensitivity,[68] and this may explain the greater levels of pain and disability in African-American patients with chronic pain conditions. Investigation of cultural responses to pain and injury in WAD is scant but recent investigation has been undertaken to directly compare chronic WAD in Singapore and Australia. The results of these recent studies are briefly described in this section.

Singapore is a multiracial Asian society comprising of three major ethnic groups: Chinese, Malay and Indian. Singaporean patients with chronic WAD demonstrated lowered cold and mechanical pain threshold as well as cold pain tolerance, when compared to healthy controls.[69]

This was consistent with findings of sensory hypersensitivity found in patients with chronic WAD in Australia, Europe, Canada and the United States of America.[43,70-72] A recent study found mechanical and thermal pain thresholds were not significantly different between white Australians and Asian Singaporeans with WAD when both groups were compared directly using the same research methodology (Ng et al., unpublished data). There were differences in cold pressor pain threshold and tolerance, with Singaporean patients demonstrating lower pain thresholds and tolerance than Australian patients with the cold pressor test. This was consistent with studies which reported higher cold pressor pain sensitivity in Asian than white patients.[68] Due to previous reports of lower WAD prevalence in Singapore, the findings that Singaporeans were more pain sensitive than Australians was not expected.

It is clear that various psychological factors including post-traumatic stress symptoms, pain catastrophizing and general distress amongst others are common in patients with WAD.[73] The lifetime prevalence of psychological disorders of post-traumatic stress disorder, anxiety and depression is higher in Western than Asian countries.[74-76] Psychological factors of post-traumatic stress disorder symptoms and depression have also been shown to be correlated with neck disability in patients with WAD.[77,78] The higher prevalence of psychological disorders in Western than Asian countries may have implications on the cross-cultural presentation of chronic WAD. A preliminary study that compared psychological factors between Australian and Singaporean patients with chronic WAD revealed no statistically significant difference in post-traumatic stress symptom severity, depression severity, self-efficacy, catastrophizing and fear-avoidance beliefs between both groups (Ng et al., unpublished data). However, Australian patients reported lower perceived injustice and held more positive illness perceptions. This is contrary to expectations of poorer psychological presentation in Australians given the previously reported greater prevalence of chronic WAD and chronic pain. The relatively few social benefits for Singaporean patients with WAD who may have difficulty seeking employment post injury could contribute to their higher level of perceived injustice and more negative illness perceptions. However, this cultural difference between Australians and Singaporeans did not reflect the higher prevalence of WAD in Brisbane.

The social–cognitive model suggests that expectations of health outcomes are shaped both by beliefs and the sociocultural context.[79] Another possible reason for the difference in WAD prevalence between various countries may be related to different beliefs and expectations about WAD and its recovery. There is strong evidence showing that health-care professionals' beliefs are known to influence both their clinical management as well as their patients' beliefs about their condition.[80,81] With respect to WAD, the beliefs and expectations of the injured person have been shown to predict health outcomes with studies in Canada and Sweden showing that patients with acute WAD who reported more pessimistic expectations of recovery had slower recovery[82] and higher disability levels 6 months post injury.[83] A comparison of physiotherapists' whiplash beliefs in Brisbane and Singapore found physiotherapists in both cities generally held beliefs that were positive and consistent with clinical practice guidelines for WAD. However, a higher proportion of physiotherapists in Singapore than Brisbane believed in a psychogenic origin of WAD and also believed in more positive recovery for a patient vignette depicting chronic WAD.[84] It is unclear whether this stronger belief in a psychogenic origin of chronic WAD and more positive expectation of long-term outcome of chronic WAD has any relationship with the prevalence of chronic WAD in Singapore.

A few studies have investigated expectations about WAD and its recovery on non-injured laypersons, namely employees from local utilities companies. The results indicate that Canadians hold more negative expectations than Lithuanian,[85] Greek,[86] and German people.[87] These studies suggest that in countries like Canada with a higher prevalence of chronic WAD, there is expectation of worse long-term outcomes. Using the whiplash beliefs questionnaire, a recent study compared whiplash beliefs in laypersons in Brisbane, Australia and Singapore. There is a presumably higher prevalence of chronic WAD in Brisbane than Singapore[36,62] but laypersons' expectations of recovery and beliefs about WAD in Brisbane and Singapore were generally similar and mostly positive.[88] The equivocal evidence suggests that laypersons' beliefs may not reflect the cross-cultural differences in prevalence of chronic WAD.

In summary, the proposal of chronic WAD being culturally dependent is debatable. In Brisbane and Singapore, which have similar fault-based motor insurance systems but different social benefits for the unemployed, patients with chronic WAD were largely similar in their physical and psychological presentation. Laypersons, and physiotherapists' whiplash beliefs in these two cities were also generally similar. The cultural differences in cold pressor pain sensitivity, perceived injustice and illness perceptions did not seem to reflect the higher prevalence of WAD in Brisbane. Further studies are needed to more accurately determine the current prevalence of chronic WAD in Asian countries. Nevertheless, the largely similar physical and psychological presentation of patients with chronic WAD in Brisbane and Singapore indicated that clinicians may treat patients with WAD similarly in different cultures, regardless of patients' country, ethnicity or jurisdiction. Clinicians in Asia may adopt the recommendations of clinical practice guidelines written for patients with WAD in Western populations.

THE CLINICAL RELEVANCE OF OUTCOME PREDICTION

The ability to establish a prognosis for clinical conditions is being increasingly recognized as a vital skill for clinicians. When the prognosis is favourable, clinicians may opt for less-intensive interventions, reassurance, advice and education. When the prognosis is unfavourable, the astute clinician will attempt to identify specific targets for intervention in an effort to mitigate the risk of poor outcome. Unlike many medical conditions, for the physiotherapist prognosis is rarely about survival of the patient. Rather, outcomes we most commonly consider important include pain or other symptoms, function and disability, work status (or role participation), and global satisfaction or well-being. Such outcomes pose a unique challenge for prognostic research, in that it is rare that they can be easily dichotomized as good/bad, alive/dead, recovered/not recovered, etc. The continuous nature of many clinical physiotherapy outcomes has forced researchers in the area into rather difficult and sometimes arbitrary decisions about the outcomes to be predicted, what constitutes a 'good' or 'bad' outcome, and what early variables can and should be captured that may predict them. WAD offers an interesting context from which to conduct such research, as chronic problems are relatively common,[1] gross structural lesions are often unable to explain the problems,[5] and it often occurs within a highly litigious medico-legal context that requires some degree of defensibility of complaints. This section will summarize the current state of evidence in the area of whiplash prognosis, will briefly describe some of the caveats and pitfalls of research in this area, and will offer some concrete suggestions for applying the current evidence in clinical practice.

Predisposed Does Not Mean Predestined

It is beyond the scope of this text to offer a comprehensive description of the characteristics of good prognostic research. Fortunately, such accounts can easily be found on the internet, including that of Kamper and colleagues,[89] and the statement of the 'strengthening the reporting of observational studies in epidemiology (STROBE)' group (http://www.strobe-statement.org). Briefly, there are key caveats of prognostic research of which clinicians must be aware in order to make prudent and judicious use of the evidence. Arguably the most important is an awareness of the nature of cause and effect. In 1965, Sir Austin Bradford-Hill offered nine criteria for causality that still hold relevance today.[90] The criteria are presented in Table 42-1. At best, purely observational prognostic research, where potential predictors are measured early and then analysed for their association with a later outcome, can only provide evidence for strength of association, temporality, possibly dose–response relationships, indirect or theoretical evidence for biologic plausibility, and then independent verification could offer consistency. Therefore, while good prospective 'prognostic' research can offer support for some of the *Bradford-Hill* criteria, it cannot support all of them. In practical terms this means that clinicians need to be willing to look critically at the evidence before them, and decide whether a variable reported in a research paper is in fact a causative factor.

As an example of the above comments, Hill and colleagues[91] conducted a large prospective study of 786 people with neck pain of varying cause and duration, following them for a period of 1 year to determine who continued to complain of neck pain for at least 1 day over the past month. Of the significant risk factors they identified, one was cycling. That is, those who indicated they cycle at least sometimes were at significantly greater risk

TABLE 42-1　**Criteria for Cause and Effect**

Criterion	Description
Strength of association	The magnitude of the association (e.g. correlation, effect size) should be strong enough to provide confidence that the cause and effect are in fact connected
Consistency of findings	The association should be consistent across different samples, contexts, designs and research groups
Specificity of the relationship	In current terms, this refers to the degree to which an association is real, and not influenced by confounders or other variables that may be related to both cause and effect but are actually driving the association. If the cause is associated with a specific set of effects (very specific symptoms for example, rather than a broad range of symptoms), this criterion is satisfied
Temporality	The cause MUST always occur before the effect
Dose–response relationship	In most cases, more (or less) of exposure to the cause should lead to more (or less) effect. Note however that in some conditions, the mere presence of the cause is enough to trigger the effect so this criterion is not inherently critical in all cases
Plausibility	The association between cause and effect should make sense. The burden of this criterion falls largely on the authors who should make the case for at least a theoretical connection between cause and effect
Coherence	Refers to a more general coherence of findings between large-scale population-based or epidemiological research and lab-based basic science research. In other words, if the relationship exists in the lab, does it also exist in the field? If it exists in the field, can it be reproduced in the laboratory?
Experimental evidence	In the current era of evidence-informed practice, this criterion seems almost superfluous, but as Bradford-Hill put it: 'Occasionally it is possible to appeal to experimental evidence'
Causation through analogy	A sort of 'pre-scientific' criterion which is probably the weakest of the bunch. Analogy and clinical observation form the basis of most scientific research, in that someone, somewhere, has observed and related the apparent association. An example here might be an observation that whiplash is a result of car accidents, but not all car accidents result in whiplash. Empirical scientific evidence is then required to clarify that relationship
Reversibility	Not part of Bradford-Hill's initial criteria, but a logical addition for conditions that are reversible. If the presence of a factor (e.g. high catastrophic thinking) is in fact a cause of an outcome (e.g. chronic pain-related disability), then removing the cause *should* reduce or abolish the effect

Adapted from Bradford-Hill (see text).[90]

(2.4 times greater) of belonging to the 'persistent pain' group than those who stated they never cycle. If cycling were in fact a cause of persistent neck pain, then clinicians should routinely recommend that their patients not cycle, and when a new patient enters their practice who states they even occasionally ride a bike, the clinician should immediately become concerned about the risk of long-term problems. But clearly (and encouragingly), this does not appear to be the case. The question then becomes: is cycling in fact a cause of chronic neck pain? Or could there be something else about those who cycle compared to those who never cycle that could explain this finding (a question of specificity)? Is it biologically reasonable? Are those who cycle *more* at greater risk than those who cycle *less* (dose–response)? If cyclists stopped cycling, would they be more likely to improve (reversibility)? Is it possible that this is a chance finding, a risk that increases with increasing comparisons performed? Is the outcome (at least 1 day of neck pain in the preceding month) of importance for your clinical population? All of these are questions that clinicians should consider before implementing such evidence into practice.

One additional important point to be made before moving to the summary of evidence is with respect to the title of this subsection: predisposed does not mean pre-destined. It is extremely rare that a predictor variable is able to perfectly classify all people into those that will develop chronic problems and those that will not. Even

newer and more complex risk algorithms that consider multiple factors average around 70–80% classification accuracy at best.[92,93] Many univariate analyses provide things like odds ratios or relative risk, which in most cases can be interpreted as the increase in odds that a person falls into the high-risk group, rather than any definitive dooming of the person to developing chronic pain. Finally, it potentially becomes a self-fulfilling prophecy when risk is ascribed to an individual if there's nothing to be done about it. Sex, age, educational attainment or socioeconomic status; these are all factors for which at least some evidence exists to suggest they may be useful to identify those at risk of a poor outcome. However, their clinical usefulness is questionable considering, at least as of today, there is nothing that can easily be done to address them.

With these caveats in mind, the next section provides a summary of the current evidence (updated to the end of 2012) for or against the prognostic factors that have been examined to date.

Summary of Current Evidence – What are Risk Factors, What are Not?

For the purposes of this chapter, and with space limitations in mind, only those factors for which the evidence provides adequately compelling evidence for or against their status as risk factors for a poor outcome exists, are discussed. An issue that has yet to be resolved in this field is the best definition and operationalization of a 'poor' outcome.[94] While this is problematic on many levels, meta-analytic procedures have so far not found a consistent difference in the predictive capacity of a variable based on the outcome it was predicting, as long as those outcomes were at least reasonably similar.[95,96] With this caveat in mind, Box 42-1 presents those prognostic variables for which the current balance of evidence provides the greatest confidence in their status as either predictors or non-predictors of a poor outcome. The box has been adapted from that of Walton and colleagues.[95,96] Of particular note, high neck pain intensity ('high' can be confidently considered as 6/10 or higher) is the most consistent predictor of a poor outcome, but as per a previous comment, may not be the most valuable clinical decision aid. High neck-related disability, most commonly assessed using the Neck Disability Index (NDI),[97] is likely most prognostic when neck-related disability is also the outcome being predicted. On balance, there is considerably greater evidence for the risk posed by strong psychological distress (catastrophizing, post-traumatic stress) than for physical or clinical signs such as range of motion or neck strength. Similarly, mechanisms of the event itself, including direction or speed of impact and seating position of the victim, appear to have little impact on the likelihood of a smooth recovery. However, caution must be observed when interpreting these findings: it is rare that a *valid, systematic approach* to evaluating clinical or diagnostic signs or parameters of the event has been employed in research, which leads to under-representation of such findings in systematic reviews. Evidence is slowly mounting that biological processes may well play an important role in the development of long-term problems despite the recent focus on psychosocial factors.[70,98,99] As clinical and observational evidence continues to mount, a true biopsychosocial understanding of the factors that drive the onset and maintenance of chronic post-WAD problems is likely to emerge.

Summary

The science of predicting the future is growing in the whiplash field, due largely to the recognition that chronic WAD is notoriously difficult to treat in the majority of cases. The balance of evidence currently suggests that high initial neck pain intensity, high self-reported disability, indicators of central hyperexcitability, and psychological distress are the strongest predictors of poor medium- to long-term outcome. The challenge for academics and clinicians is to unravel the meaning and mechanisms underlying these factors, and to identify additional areas in which intervention may mitigate the risk of chronicity. The field is still relatively young by most standards, and continues to struggle with inconsistent methods and operationalization of key variables. However, current evidence syntheses provide at least some guidance for clinicians hoping to identify the 'at risk' patient in their practice, and may offer useful windows through which to view the best targets for intervention.

THE TREATMENT OF WHIPLASH-ASSOCIATED DISORDERS

The most recent systematic reviews conclude that activity and/or exercise-based interventions are the most effective conservative treatments for acute and chronic WAD but that effects are modest and the relative effectiveness of various exercise regimens is not clear.[100,101] Since these reviews in 2010, further randomized controlled trials have been conducted and these demonstrate only small, if any, effects with physical rehabilitation approaches.

Acute Whiplash-Associated Disorders

In acute WAD, a recent randomized trial conducted in emergency departments of UK hospitals demonstrated that six sessions of physiotherapy (a multimodal approach of exercise, manual therapy) was only slightly more effective, but not cost effective, than a single session of advice from a physiotherapist.[102] However, only 45–50% of participants in either treatment group reported their condition as being 'much better' or 'better' at short- (4 months) and long-term follow-up (12 months) – a low recovery rate that is little different to the usual natural recovery following the injury.[4] In view of the physical and psychological factors shown to be present in acute WAD,[103] it could be surmised that a physiotherapy approach alone would not be sufficient to address these factors. For this reason another recent randomized controlled trial investigated if the early targeting of these factors would provide better outcomes than usual care.[104] Participants with acute WAD (≤4 weeks duration) were assessed using measures

---

BOX 42-1	Factors for Which the Current Balance of Evidence (to May 2012) Provides Confidence in Their Status as Either Risk Factors of a Poor Outcome, or as Having No Association with Outcome

STRONG OR MODERATE CONFIDENCE OF AN ASSOCIATION WITH A POOR OUTCOME

  High pain intensity
  High neck-related disability
  Post-traumatic stress symptoms at inception
  Catastrophizing
  Cold hyperalgesia/hypersensitivity

STRONG OR MODERATE CONFIDENCE IN NO ASSOCIATION WITH A POOR OUTCOME

  Angular deformity of the neck (scoliosis, flattened cervical lordosis)
  Impact direction
  Seating position
  Aware of impending collision
  Head-rest in place
  Older age
  Vehicle stationary when hit

Adapted from Walton et al.[95]

of pain, disability, sensory function and psychological factors including general distress and post-traumatic stress symptoms. Treatment was tailored to the findings of this baseline assessment and could range from a multimodal physiotherapy approach of advice, exercise and manual therapy for those with few signs of central hyperexcitability and psychological distress to an interdisciplinary intervention comprising medication (if pain levels were greater than moderate and signs of central hyperexcitability were present) and cognitive behavioural therapy delivered by a clinical psychologist (if scores on psychological questionnaires were above threshold). This pragmatic intervention approach was compared to usual care where the patient could pursue treatment as they normally would. Analysis revealed no significant differences in frequency of recovery (defined as Neck Disability Index <8%) between pragmatic and usual care groups at 6 months (OR 0.55, 95% CI 0.23 to 1.29) or 12 months (OR 0.65, 95% CI 0.28 to 1.47). There was no improvement in non-recovery rates at 6 months (64% for pragmatic care and 49% for usual care), indicating no advantage of the early interdisciplinary intervention.[104] Several possible reasons for these results were proposed. The design of the trial may have been too broad and not sensitive enough to detect changes in subgroups of patients, suggesting better outcomes would be achieved by specifically selecting patients at high risk of poor recovery. Additionally, 61% of participants in the trial found the medication (low-dose opioids and/or adjuvant agents) to be unacceptable due to side effects such as dizziness and drowsiness and did not comply with the prescribed dose,[104] indicating that more acceptable medications need to be evaluated. Compliance with attending sessions with the clinical psychologist was less than compliance with physiotherapy, perhaps indicating patient preference for physiotherapy.

The results of the above-mentioned trial should not mean that attempts to address and target potentially modifiable risk factors in the early injury stage be abandoned. There were, as outlined, several methodological issues that may have influenced the results. It is recognized that the risk factors for chronic pain development following whiplash injury are not necessary causally related, it still remains logical that further studies investigate the targeting of factors such as pain, central hyperexcitability, catastrophizing and post-traumatic stress symptoms. Such an approach has been explored in the area of low back pain where stratified care was provided to patients depending upon their risk of developing chronic pain and disability with results showing some promise.[105] Recently a clinical prediction rule including some of these factors was developed to identify both chronic moderate/severe disability and full recovery at 12 months post injury with good specificity and adequate sensitivity.[93] Whether or not the use of a stratified pathway of care for whiplash can improve recovery remains to be seen.

In addition to identifying patients at risk of poor recovery, an important aspect of such clinical prediction rules is also the identification of patients with good potential for recovery (low-risk patients). These patients will likely require less-intensive interventions and treatment comprising advice, assurance, together with simple exercises may be most effective for this group, although this proposal requires formal testing. Those patients at medium or high risk of poor recovery will likely need additional treatments to the basic advice/activity/exercise approach. This may include medication to target pain and nociceptive processes as well as methods to address early psychological responses to injury. As can be seen in a recent trial by Jull et al.,[104] this approach may not be straightforward. The participants of this trial not only found the side effects of medication unacceptable but also were less compliant with attendance to a clinical psychologist (46% of participants attended fewer than four of ten sessions) compared to attendance with the physiotherapist (12% attended fewer than four sessions over 10 weeks).[104] The reasons for non-compliance are not clear but the burden of attending numerous healthcare visits with different practitioners may have played a role. An alternative approach, currently being evaluated, is to train physiotherapists to deliver psychological interventions and to play more of a 'gatekeeper' role in the early assessment, risk stratification and triaging of patients with acute WAD. This approach has been investigated in mainly chronic conditions such as arthritis[106] as well as in acute low back pain[105] with results showing some early promise. This is not to say that patients with a diagnosed psychopathology such as depression or post-traumatic stress disorder should be managed by physiotherapists and of course, these patients will require referral to an appropriately trained professional.

Chronic Whiplash-Associated Disorders

The most recent systematic review of treatments for chronic WAD identified only 22 randomized trials that met the criteria for inclusion and only 12 were of good quality.[101] The authors concluded that exercise programmes are effective at relieving pain, although it does not appear that these gains are maintained over the long term.[101] It is also not clear if one form of exercise is more effective than another. Since this review further trials investigating exercise approaches for chronic WAD have been conducted and shown only small to modest effects of the interventions. In one trial, a specific motor and sensorimotor retraining programme for the cervical spine combined with manual therapy[107] resulted in just clinically relevant decreases in pain-related disability compared to usual care. Similar effects were demonstrated in another trial of graded functional exercise and advice compared to advice alone where small improvements in pain, bothersomeness and functional ability were found at short-term follow-up.[108] In a recent subsequent large randomized controlled trial,[109] these two forms of exercise were combined to a comprehensive exercise intervention that first focused on improving cervical motor and postural control before progressing to more functional higher load activities. Aerobic exercise was also performed by the participants throughout the 12-week treatment period. The results were disappointing with the comprehensive exercise programme being no more effective than advice in reducing pain (the primary outcome). At 14 weeks the treatment effect was 0.0 (95%

CI −0.7 to 0.7), 6 months 0.2 (−0.5 to 1.0) and at 12 months −0.1 (−0.8 to 0.6). Some of the effects on secondary outcomes were statistically significant but none were sufficiently large to be considered clinically worthwhile.

Two studies have investigated factors that may moderate the effects of predominantly exercise-based interventions. In an earlier trial, participants with both cold and mechanical hyperalgesia did not respond to a specific cervical muscle retraining as those without these features[107] but this analysis was performed post-hoc and the study was not powered to specifically detect any moderation effects. In the recent larger trial, the sample size was increased in order to be able to evaluate the possible moderation effects of factors such as measures of central hyperexcitability, post-traumatic stress symptoms, pain catastrophizing and symptom duration.[109] None of these factors were shown to moderate the effect of the exercise programme. So at present it remains unclear which patients will respond to exercise interventions.

In accordance with the biopsychosocial model of chronic pain, it may be expected that physical rehabilitation-only approaches for chronic WAD will not be sufficient. Few trials of interdisciplinary approaches have been conducted in a chronic WAD group and these approaches have been varied, from physiotherapists delivering psychological-type interventions in addition to physiotherapy to psychological interventions alone. In their systematic review, Teasell et al.[101] concluded that although the majority of studies suggest that interdisciplinary interventions are beneficial, it is difficult to formulate conclusions given the heterogeneity of the interventions. Since that review, additional trials have investigated psychological approaches for chronic WAD. Dunne and colleagues showed that trauma-focused cognitive behavioural therapy provided to individuals with chronic WAD and post-traumatic stress disorder led to decreased psychological symptoms of post-traumatic stress disorder, anxiety and depression, as well as decreased pain-related disability.[110] Although this was a small preliminary study, the results suggest that psychological interventions may be useful to improve not only psychological symptoms but also pain-related disability.

Future Directions

We are at cross-roads in the research and clinical management of acute and chronic WAD. The evidence is demonstrating that the usual 'traditional' treatment approaches that comprise predominantly of physical rehabilitation are offering only small effects. This is not to say that exercise-based interventions should not be provided to people with WAD as exercise and activity is important for their long-term general health. It may be that activity/exercise is combined with other treatments such as psychological approaches, educational approaches and medication. The optimal combination and dosage of such approaches will need to be determined. The results of the randomized controlled trials also indicate that some people respond to physical rehabilitation, but our ability to recognize these patients is lacking. Factors that

showed initial promise as moderators of treatment effectiveness[107] have not stood up to further scrutiny[109] and the investigation of additional or different factors requires thought.

With respect to acute WAD, an important goal of treatment should be to prevent the development of chronic pain and disability. The time period for this to be achieved appears to be short – within about 2–3 months of injury.[4] Physiotherapists play a vital role in this stage of the injury and as such may need to take a greater role in the overall care plan of the patient. This would mean having expertise in the assessment of risk factors and an understanding of when additional treatments such as medication and psychological interventions are required. While this has traditionally been the role of general practitioners, it is difficult to see how the busy structure of medical primary care will allow for the appropriate assessment of patients to first identify those at risk, develop a treatment plan, follow the patient's progress and modify treatment as necessary. Physiotherapists are well-placed to take on a coordination or 'gatekeeper' role in the management of WAD and research into health services models that include physiotherapists in such a role is also needed.

REFERENCES

1. Carroll L, Holm L, Hogg-Johnson S, et al. Course and prognostic factors for neck pain in whiplash-associated disorders (WAD). Results of the bone and joint decade 2000–2010 task force on neck pain and its associated disorders. Spine 2008;33:583–92.
2. Wilson S, Derrett S, Cameron I, et al. Prevalance of poor outcomes soon after injury and their association with the severity of injury. Inj Prev 2014;20(1):57–61.
3. Mayou R, Bryant B. Psychiatry of whiplash neck injury. Br J Psychiatry 2002;180:441–8.
4. Sterling M, Hendrikz J, Kenardy J. Developmental trajectories of pain/disability and PTSD symptoms following whiplash injury. Pain 2010;150:22–8.
5. Curatolo M, Bogduk N, Ivancic P, et al. The role of tissue damage in whiplash associated disorders. Spine 2011;36:S309–15.
6. Schiltenwolf M, Beckmann C. letter to the editor: whiplash disorder – is it a valid disease definition? Pain 2013;154(10):2235.
7. Sterling M. Physiotherapy management of whiplash associated disorders (WAD). J Physiother 2014;60(1):5–12.
8. Siegmund G, Winkelstein B, Ivancic P, et al. The anatomy and biomechanics of acute and chronic whiplash injury. Traffic Inj Prev 2009;10:101–12.
9. Haldeman S, Carroll L, Cassidy D, et al. The bone and joint decade 2000–2010 task force on neck pain and its associated disorders executive summary. Spine 2008;33:S5–7.
10. Linman C, Appel L, Fredrikson M, et al. Elevated (11C)-D-deprenyl uptake in chronic whiplash associated disorder suggests persistent musculoskeletal inflammation. PLoS ONE 2011;6: e19182.
11. Sterling M, Elliott J, Cabot P. The course of serum inflammatory biomarkers following whiplash injury and their relationship to sensory and muscle measures: a longitudinal cohort study. PLoS ONE 2013;8(10):e77903.
12. Kaneoka K, Ono K, Inami S, et al. Motional analysis of cervical vertebrae during whiplash loading. Spine 1999;24:763–70.
13. Panjabi M, Paerson A, Ito S, et al. Cervical spine curvature during simulated whiplash. Clin Biomech 2004;19:109.
14. Stemper B, Yoganandan N, Pintar F. Gender- and region-dependent local facet joint kinematics in rear impact: implications in whiplash injury. Spine 2004;29:1764–71.
15. McConnell W, Howard R, Guzman H, et al. Analysis of human test subject kinematic response to low velocity rear end impacts. SAE Tech Pap 1993;21–30.

16. Grauer J, Panjabi M, Cholewicki J, et al. Whiplash produces S-shaped curvatures of the neck with hyperextension at lower levels. Spine 1997;22:2489–94.

17. Jakobsson L, Lundell B, Norin H, et al. WHIPS–Volvo's Whiplash Protection Study. Acc Anal Prevent 2000;32:307–91.

18. Viano D, Olseon S. The effectiveness of active head restraint in preventing whiplash. J Trauma 2001;51:959–69.

19. Farmer C, Wells J, Lund A. Effects of head restraint and seat redesign on neck injury risk in rear-end crashes. J Spinal Disord 2003;4:251–63.

20. Jonsson H, Cesarini K, Sahlstedt B, et al. Findings and outcome in whiplash-type neck distortions. Spine 1994;19:2733–42.

21. Taylor J, Taylor M. Cervical spinal injuries: an autopsy study of 109 blunt injuries. J Musculoskeletal Pain 1996;4:61–79.

22. Taylor J, Twomey L. Acute injuries to cervical joints. Spine 1993;18:1115–22.

23. Uhrenholt L, Grunnet-Nilsson N, Hartvigsen J. Cervical spine lesions after road traffic accidents. a systematic review. Spine 2002;27:1934–41.

24. Davis S, Teresi L, Bradley W, et al. Cervical spine hyperextension injuries: MR findings. Radiology 1991;180:245–51.

25. Yoganandan N, Cusick J, Pintar F, et al. Whiplash injury determination with conventional spine imaging and cryomicrotomy. Spine 2001;26:2443–8.

26. Barnsley L, Lord S, Bogduk N. Comparative local anaesthetic blocks in the diagnosis of cervical zygapophyseal joint pain. Pain 1993;55:99–106.

27. Lord S, Barnsley L, Wallis B, et al. Chronic cervical zygapophysial joint pain after whiplash: a placebo-controlled prevalence study... including commentary by Derby R Jr. Spine 1996;21:1737–45.

28. McLain R. Mechanoreceptors endings in human cervical facet joints. Spine 1994;19:495–501.

29. Quinn K, Winkelstein B. Detection of altered collagen fiber alignment in the cervical facet capsule after whiplash-like joint retraction. Ann Biomed Eng 2011.

30. Lee K, Thinnes J, Gokhin D, et al. A novel rodent neck pain model of facet-mediated behavioral hypersensitivity: Implications for persistent pain and whiplash injury. J Neurotrauma 2004;137:151–9.

31. Quinn K, Winkelstein B. Cervical facet capsular ligament yield defines the threshold for injury and persistent joint-mediated neck pain. J Biomechanics 2007;40:2299–306.

32. Dong L, Odeleye A, Jordan-Sciutto K, et al. Painful facet joint injury induces neuronal stress activation in the DRG: implications for cellular mechanisms of pain. Neurosci Lett 2008;443:90–4.

33. Dong L, Winkelstein B. Simulated whiplash modulates expression of the glutamatergic system in the spinal cord suggesting spinal plasticity is associated with painful dynamic cervical facet loading. Neurotrauma 2011;27:163–74.

34. Winkelstein B, Santos D. An intact facet capsular ligament modulates behavioral sensitivity and spinal glial activation produced by cervical facet joint tension. Spine 2008;33:856–62.

35. Winkelstein BA, Nightingale RW, Richardson WJ, et al. The cervical facet capsule and its role in whiplsh injury. Spine 2000;25:1238–46.

36. McDonald G, Lord S, Bogduk N. Long-term follow-up of patients treated with cervical radiofrequency neurotomy for chronic neck pain. Neurosurgery 1991;45:61–7.

37. Wallis B, Lord S, Bogduk N. Resolution of psychological distress of whiplash patients following treatment by radiofrequency neurotomy: a randomised, double-blind, placebo controlled trial. Pain 1997;73:15–22.

38. Krakenes J, Kaale B. Magnetic resonance imaging assessment of craniovertebral ligaments and membranes after whiplash trauma. Spine 2006;31:2820–6.

39. Krakenes J, Kaale B, Moen G, et al. MRI assessment of the alar ligaments in the late stage of whiplash injury – a study of structural abnormalities and observer agreement. Neuroradiology 2002;44:617–24.

40. Krakenes J, Kaale B, Moen G, et al. MRI of the tectorial and posterior atlanto-occipital membranes in the late stage of whiplash injury. Neuroradiology 2003;44:637–44.

41. Myran R, Zwart J, Kvistad K, et al. Clinical characteristics, pain, and disability in relation to alar ligament MRI findings. Spine 2008;36:E862–7.

42. Vette N, Krakenes J, Eide G, et al. Are MRI high-signal changes of alar and transverse ligaments in acute whiplash injury related to outcome? BMC Musculoskelet Disord 2011;11.

43. Smith A, Jull G, Schneider G, et al. Cervical radiofrequency neurotomy reduces central hyperexcitability and improves neck movement in individuals with chronic whiplash. Pain Med 2014;15(1):128–41.

44. Smith A, Jull G, Schneider G, et al. Cervical radiofrequency neurotomy reduces psychological distress and pain catastrophization, but not post-traumatic stress in individuals with chronic WAD. Pain Res Manag 2013;18:e13.

45. Smith A, Jull G, Schneider G, et al. Modulation of cervical facet joint nociception and pain attenuates physical and psychological features of chronic whiplash: a prospective study. Pain Manage Res 2015;accepted.

46. Carroll L, Cassidy D, Cote P. The role of pain coping strategies in prognosis after whiplash injury: passive coping predicts slowed recovery. Pain 2006;124:18–26.

47. Sterling M, Jull G, Kenardy J. Physical and psychological predictors of outcome following whiplash injury maintain predictive capacity at long term follow-up. Pain 2006;122:102–8.

48. Cassidy JD, Carroll LJ, Cote P, et al. Effect of eliminating compensation for pain and suffering on the outcome of insurance claims for whiplash injury. N Engl J Med 2000;20:1179–213.

49. Bostick G, Ferrari R, Carroll L, et al. A population-based survey of beliefs about neck pain from whiplash injury, work-related neck pain, and work-related upper extremity pain. Europ J Pain 2009;13:300–4.

50. Schneider G, Jull G, Thomas K, et al. Derivation of a clinical decision guide in the diagnosis of cervical facet joint pain. Arch Phys Med Rehabil 2014;95:1695–701.

51. Jensen T, Baron R. Translation of symptoms and signs into mechanisms in neuropathic pain. Pain 2003;102:1–8.

52. Rebbeck T, Sindhausen D, Cameron I. A prospective cohort study of health outcomes following whiplash associated disorders in an Australian population. Inj Prev 2006;12:86–93.

53. Ferrari R, Pieschl S. An examination of coping styles and expectations for whiplash injury in Germany: comparison with Canadian data. Clin Rheumatol 2011;30:1209–14.

54. Obelieniene D, Schrader H, Bovim G, et al. Pain after whiplash: a prospective controlled inception cohort study. J Neurol Neurosurg Psychiatry 1999;66:279–93.

55. Richter M, Ferrari R, Otte D, et al. Correlation of findings, collision parameters and psychological factors in the outcome of whiplash associated disorders. J Neurol Neurosurg Psychiatry 2004;75.

56. Balla J. The late whiplash syndrome: a study of an illness in Australia and Singapore. Cult Med Psychiatry 1982;6:191–210.

57. Subramaniam M, Abdin E, Vaingankar J, et al. Impact of psychiatric disorders and chronic physical conditions on health-related quality of life: Singapore Mental Health Study. J Affect Disord 2013;147.

58. Yeo S. Pain prevalence in Singapore. Ann Acad Med Singapore 2009;38:937–42.

59. Blyth F, March L, Brnabic A, et al. Chronic pain in Australia: a prevalence study. Pain 2001;89:127–34.

60. Harstall C, Ospina M. How prevalent is chronic pain. Pain Clin Updates 2003;XI:1–4.

61. Henderson J, Harrison C, Britt H, et al. Prevalence, causes, severity, impact, and management of chronic pain in Australian general practice patients. Pain Med 2013;14:1346–61.

62. MAIC. Motor Accident Insurance Commission Annual Report 2009–10. Queensland Government 2010.

63. <www.mof.gov.sg/budget_2011/pd.html>; 2012. (Accessed May 2013.).

64. Campbell C, Edwards R. Ethnic differences in pain and pain management. Pain Manag 2012;2:219–30.

65. Lasch K. Culture and pain. Pain Clin Updates 2002;X.

66. Rahim-Williams B, Riley JL III, Herrera DG, et al. Ethnic identity predicts pain sensitivity in African Americans and Hispanics. Pain 2007;129:177–84.

67. Carey T, Freburger J, Holmes G, et al. Race, care seeking, and utilization for chronic back and neck pain: population perspectives. J Pain 2010;11:343–50.

68. Rahim-Williams B, Riley J, Williams A, et al. A quantitative review of ethnic group differences in experimental pain response:

do biology, psychology, and culture matter? Pain Med 2012; 13:522–40.

69. Ng T, Pedler A, Vicenzino B, et al. Less efficacious conditioned pain modulation and sensory hypersensitivity in chronic whiplash-associated disorders in Singapore. Clin J Pain 2014;30(5): 436–42.

70. Stone A, Vicenzino B, Lim E, et al. Measures of central hyperexcitability in chronic whiplash associated disorder – a systematic review and meta-analysis. Man Ther 2012;18:111–17.

71. Curatolo M, Petersen-Felix S, Arendt-Nielsen L, et al. Central hypersensitivity in chronic pain after whiplash injury. Clin J Pain 2001;17:306–15.

72. Elliott J, Sterling M, Noteboom T, et al. The clinical presentation of chronic whiplash and the relationship to findings of MRI fatty infiltrates in the cervical extensor musculature: a preliminary investigation. Eur Spine J 2009;18:1371–8.

73. Williamson E, Williams M, Gates S, et al. A systematic review of psychological factors and the development of late whiplash syndrome. Pain 2008;135:20–30.

74. Chen C, Wong J, Lee N, et al. The Shatin community mental health survey in Hong Kong. II. Major findings. Arch Gen Psychiatry 1993;50:125–33.

75. Chong S, Abdin E, Vaingankar J, et al. A population-based survey of mental disorders in Singapore. Ann Acad Med Singapore 2012;41:49–66.

76. Kenardy J, Dunne R. Traumatic injury and traumatic stress. Spine 2011;36:S233–7.

77. Merrick D, Stalnacke B. Five years post whiplash injury: symptoms and psychological factors in recovered versus non-recovered. BMC Res Notes 2010;3.

78. Sterling M, Hendrikz J, Kenardy J. Similar factors predict disability and PTSD trajectories following whiplash injury. Pain 2011;152:1272–8.

79. Janzen J, Silvius J, Jacobs S, et al. What is a health expectation? Developing a pragmatic conceptual model from psychological theory. Health Expect 2006;9:37–48.

80. Darlow B, Fullen B, Dean S, et al. The association between health care professional attitudes and beliefs and the attitudes and beliefs, clinical management, and outcomes of patients with low back pain: a systematic review. Eur J Pain 2012;16:3–17.

81. Parsons S, Harding G, Breen A, et al. The influence of patients' and primary care practitioners' beliefs and expectations about chronic musculoskeletal pain on the process of care: a systematic review of qualitative studies. Clin J Pain 2007;23:91–8.

82. Carroll L, Holm L, Ferrari R, et al. Recovery in whiplash-associated disorders: do you get what you expect. J Rheumatol 2009;36:1063–70.

83. Holm L, Carroll L, Cassidy D, et al. Expectations for recovery important in the prognosis of whiplash injuries. PLoS Med 2008;5:e105.

84. Ng T, Pedler A, Vicenzino B, et al. Physiotherapists' beliefs about whiplash injury: a cross-cultural comparison between Singapore and Queensland. Physiother Res Int 2014;in press.

85. Ferrari R, Obelieniene D, Russell A. A cross-cultural comparative study between Canada and Lithuania. Med Sci Monitor 2002;8.

86. Ferrari R, Constantoyannis C, Papadakis N. Laypersons' expectation of the sequelae of whiplash injury: a cross-cultural comparative study between Canada and Greece. Med Sci Monitor 2003;9:CR120–4.

87. Ferrari R, Lang C. A cross-cultural comparison between Canada and Germany of symptom expectation for whiplash injury. J Spinal Disord Tech 2005;18:92–7.

88. Ng T, Bostick G, Pedler A, et al. Laypersons' expectations of recovery and beliefs about whiplash injury: a cross-cultural comparison between Australians and Singaporeans. Eur J Pain 2013;17(8):1234–42.

89. Kamper S, Hancock M, Maher C. Optimal designs for prediction studies of whiplash. Spine 2011;36:s268–74.

90. Bradford Hill A. The environment and disease: association or causation? Proc Royal Soc Med 1965;58:6.

91. Hill J, Lewis A, Papageorgiou K, et al. Predicting persistent neck pain: a 1-year follow-up of a population cohort. Spine 2004;29:1648–54.

92. Kasch H, Kongsted A, Qerama E, et al. A new stratified risk assessment tool for whiplash injuries developed from a prospective observational study. BMJ Open 2013;3.

93. Ritchie C, Hendrikz J, Kenardy J, et al. Development and validation of a screening tool to identify both chronicity and recovery following whiplash injury. Pain 2013;154:2198–206.

94. Walton D. A review of the definitions of 'recovery' used in prognostic studies on whiplash using an ICF framework. Disabil Rehabil 2009;31:943–57.

95. Walton D, Macdermid J, Giorgianni A, et al. Risk factors for persistent problems following acute whiplash injury: update of a systematic review and meta-analysis. JOSPT 2013;43:31–42.

96. Walton D, Pretty J, MacDermid J, et al. Risk factors for persistent problems following whiplash injury: results of a systematic review and meta-analysis. JOSPT 2009;39:334–50.

97. Vernon H, Mior S. The neck disability index: a study of reliability and validity. J Manipulative Physiol Ther 1991;14:409–15.

98. Borstov A, Smith L, Diatchenko L, et al. Polymorphisms in the glucocorticoid receptor co-chaperone FKBP5 predict persistent musculoskeletal pain after traumatic stress exposure. Pain 2013;154:1419–26.

99. Elliott J, Pedler A, Kenardy J, et al. The temporal development of fatty infiltrates in the neck muscles following whiplash injury: an association with pain and posttraumatic stress. PLoS ONE 2011;6:e21194.

100. Teasell R, McClure J, Walton D, et al. A research synthesis of therapeutic interventions for whiplash-associated disorder (WAD): part 2 – interventions for acute WAD. Pain Res Manag 2010;15:295–304.

101. Teasell R, McClure J, Walton D, et al. A research synthesis of therapeutic interventions for WAD: part 4 – non invasive interventions for chronic WAD. Pain Res Manag 2010;15:313–22.

102. Lamb S, Gates S, Williams M, et al. Emergency department treatments and physiotherapy for acute whiplash: a pragmatic, two-step, randomised controlled trial. Lancet 2013;381:546–56.

103. Sterling M, Jull G, Vicenzino B, et al. Characterisation of acute whiplash associated disorders. Spine 2004;29:182–8.

104. Jull G, Kenardy J, Hendrikz J, et al. Management of acute whiplash: a randomized controlled trial of multidisciplinary stratified treatments. Pain 2013;154:1798–806.

105. Hill J, Whitehurst D, Lewis M, et al. Comparison of stratified primary care management for low back pain with current best practice (STarT Back): a randomised controlled trial. Lancet 2011;378:1560–71.

106. Hunt M, Keefe F, Bryant C, et al. A physiotherapist-delivered, combined exercise and pain coping skills training intervention for individuals with knee osteoarthritis: a pilot study. Knee 2013; 20:106–12.

107. Jull G, Sterling M, Kenardy J, et al. Does the presence of sensory hypersensitivity influence outcomes of physical rehabilitation for chronic whiplash? – A preliminary RCT. Pain 2007;129:28–34.

108. Stewart M, Maher C, Refshauge K, et al. Randomised controlled trial of exercise for chronic whiplash associated disorders. Pain 2007;128:59–68.

109. Michaleff Z, Maher C, Lin C, et al. Comprehensive physiotherapy exercise program or advice alone for chronic whiplash (PROMISE): a pragmatic randomised controlled trial. Lancet 2014;384: 133–41.

110. Dunne R, Kenardy J, Sterling M. A randomised controlled trial of cognitive behavioural therapy for the treatment of PTSD in the context of chronic whiplash. Clin J Pain 2012;28:755–65.

CHAPTER 43

Temporomandibular Disorders: Neuromusculoskeletal Assessment and Management

Harry von Piekartz

INTRODUCTION

Orofacial pain with headache is common in society. Its prevalence ranges from 8–15% for women and from 3–10% for men.[1,2] The American Academy of Orofacial Pain uses orofacial pain as a collective term for a number of dysfunctions and sensory complaints associated with the temporomandibular joint (TMJ), the masticatory muscles and associated structures.[3] It encompasses terms such as Costen syndrome, temporomandibular disorders (TMDs), craniomandibular disorders and mandibular dysfunction. This chapter focuses on TMDs. It presents a discussion of clinical patterns and possible contributing factors for different myogenic, arthrogenous and neurogenic TMDs and highlights aspects of assessment and management.

DO TEMPOROMANDIBULAR DISORDERS HAVE THEIR OWN ENTITY?

The diagnosis 'TMD' is based on signs and symptoms produced during movements of the mandible. Movement can affect both masticatory muscles and joint structures. Signs include changes in the range and quality of mandibular movements such as an opening shift (deviation) and TMJ sounds. Symptoms include headache, vertigo, tinnitus or swallowing impairments.[4] Clinical and research reports indicate that head and orofacial pain around the TMJ may or may not be related to TMJ neuromusculoskeletal dysfunctions.[5] TMD pain may overlap with other headaches types such as migraine, tension and cervicogenic headache. Glaros et al.[6] demonstrated that there were more complaints of headache in patients with TMD than without TMD, and Ballenberger et al.[1] suggest that migraine and tension-type headache could be risk factors for the development of TMD. Likewise a recent study concluded that cervicogenic headache was often associated with TMD pain with 44% of patients having clear TMD signs.[7,8] Thus there is evidence to support the involvement of TMD in orofacial and cervical pain and dysfunction, but there may be overlap with other headache types. It is important for the physiotherapist to assess the neuromusculoskeletal domain of the TMJ to determine its role and relevance to the individual patient's presenting orofacial complaint.

Figure 43-1 presents a modified flowchart (based on the second Research Diagnostic Criteria for Temporomandibular Disorders (RCD/TMD) classification) of the clinical diagnostic process. The RCD/TMD) classification is divided into three sub-classifications.[9,11] The neurogenic classification has been added to the original version by the author. AXIS I represents the physical disorders and AXIS II represents psychosocial factors such as altered mood, context and beliefs, which are particularly important in the chronic situation. AXIS III represents clinical considerations or contributing factors, which may maintain the patient's complaints. In 2013 the RCD/TMD Taxonomy was reviewed by different professional societies resulting in a proposed expanded TMD taxonomy; the Diagnosed Criteria of TMD (DC/TMD).[9,11] New recommendations include short and simple screenings instruments for Axis I and II focused on structural diagnosis with a more patient-centred approach. It is relevant to investigate the characteristics of myogenic, arthrogenic and neurogenic categories of TMDs.

Myogenic Temporomandibular Disorders

Muscle dysfunction is common in craniomandibular dyskinesia during orofacial activities such as chewing, swallowing, sucking, speaking and facial expression.[2] Pain from the masticatory system is difficult to localize. It is characterized by dull pressure, pulling sensations and feelings of stiffness.[12] It may be referred from other facial regions such as the teeth, eyes, sinuses and middle ear.[13] Myofascial TMD pain is often described as pain around the TMJ without reference to a particular pathophysiological mechanism.[14] TMD pain is related to a variety of biomedical, neurobiomedical and psychological/emotional factors.[14] Other sub-factors such as dental occlusion, hormones and stress may also be related to chronic TMD pain. Thus myofascial TMD pain is considered as a phenomenon related to multiple factors.[15,16]

Risk factors influencing muscle activity at rest include dental occlusion, neuroendocrine and genetic factors and parafunctional activities, but recent research has challenged some factors.

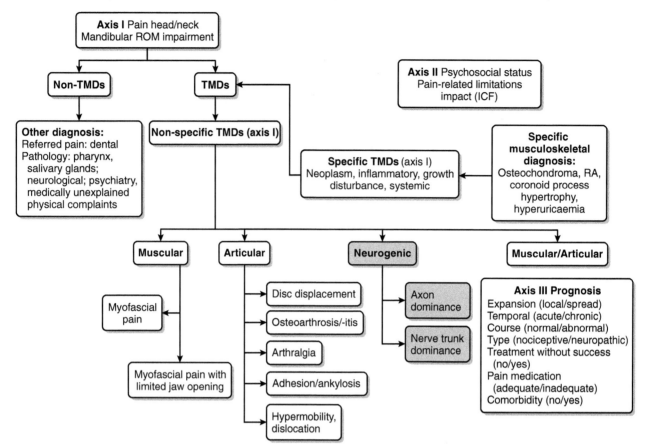

FIGURE 43-1 ■ A modified flowchart of the clinical diagnosis process during subjective and physical examination based on the revised RCD/TMD.[9,10] *ICF*, International Classification of Function; *RA*, Rheumatoid arthritis; *ROM*, Range of motion; *TMD*, Temporomandibular disorder.

Dental Occlusal Factors

It was assumed for decades that changes in dentition directly influence movement patterns, neuromuscular imbalance and masticatory pain.[17] Recent evidence refutes this view.[18] In a systematic review, Türp and Greene[16] concluded that occlusal factors were overestimated in models of myofascial TMD and pain. Nevertheless, questions about altered motor activity and pain during orofacial activity in relation to a history of occlusal interference are still included in the examination to determine any direct relationships.

Neuroendocrine and Genetic Factors

The incidence of TMD muscle pain is more prevalent in women than men. This may reflect the influence of female reproductive hormones on orofacial pain.[19] Oestrogen in particular has a strong influence on nerve growth factor and hence depolarization of nociceptors, which may play an important role in the genesis of TMD pain, allodynia and increased muscle activity.[20,21] This is even more important when genetic factors play a role such as enzyme polymorphism.[22]

Parafunctions

Parafunctional activities (abnormal oral habits) are not directly associated with TMD pain but there is some

evidence of their contribution to headache and orofacial pain.[23–25] The neurobiological relationship between parafunctions and myofascial pain is still debated.[23] Parafunctional habits seem to be associated with postural habits such as the forward head posture and bracing. The latter may cause TMD pain, headache and joint strain.[26] In assessment, different orofacial motor functions and habits may be noticed that might support the role of parafunctional activities. Motor control deficits may be observed in oral habits (chewing, nail biting), linguistic activities (speech, singing) or functions such as swallowing and sucking.

Parafunctional activities such as bruxism are characterized by clenching and grinding of the teeth during the night or day, and bracing or thrusting the mandible.[27] Terminologies such as bruxomania (grinding during the day) and bracing (diurnal teeth pressing without vertical teeth movement) are no longer distinguished because of their overlap and blurring of the underlying pathobiological mechanism.[27] Clinically, bruxism and bracing are related to different clinical patterns, which have to be distinguished as they require different (neuromusculoskeletal) management strategies.[28] Table 43-1 presents the different clinical patterns.

Increased Muscle Activity During Rest

Increased resting activity of the jaw muscles is found in orofacial pain patients,[29,30] but it is unclear if pain increases

TABLE 43-1	**Manifestation of Dominant Bruxism and Bracing Patterns**
Bruxism	**Bracing**
a.m. masticatory stiffness, symptoms	a.m. no masticatory stiffness, symptoms
Eases during the day	Increases during the day
Not really conscious of mechanism	Conscious of mechanism
Sleep disturbances (superficial sleep)	No sleep disturbances
Abrasion*	Less abrasion*
Unilateral muscular signs and symptoms	Bilateral muscular signs and symptoms
Restricted opening (muscular related)	Restricted opening (muscular related)

Note: Clinically, an overlap is often seen with one pattern being dominant.
*Abrasion: the loss of tooth structure by mechanical forces.
Modified after von Piekartz[28] and Lobbezoo et al.[27]

muscle activity or vice versa.[31] Factors such as changes of head position[1] neuropathic pain and local ischaemic changes in the muscle fibres may deregulate the motor end-plates. This might maintain a neural loop of sensory afferent information and consequently sustain abnormal motor and autonomic afferents. In turn this may result in myofascial trigger points.[31]

Arthrogenic Temporomandibular Disorders

Arthrogenic TMDs include disc displacements, arthralgia, hypermobility/dislocation, osteoarthrosis/itis adhesion and ankylosis.[3] The discussion in this chapter is limited to the non-specific arthrogenic disorders such as disc derangements, hypermobility, dislocation and arthralgia, which are commonly seen by physiotherapists.

Disc Displacements

Disc displacements or derangements are characterized by an abnormal condyle–disc relationship, which is classified into displacement with or without reduction or posterior displacement. The usual direction of displacement is anterior and anteriomedial.[10] The aetiology of disc displacements is not established. Anatomical research has shown that the capsule around the head of the mandibular and ligaments attaching the disc to the condyle are elongated. This allows increased movement of the disc, often found in disc displacements, trophic changes, impairment and osteoarthritis.[32,33]

The most common disc dysfunction is *disc displacement with reduction* (unstable relationship between the disc and condyle), characterized by a clicking or popping sound during mouth opening and closing (closing often produces less sound than opening). Opening of the mouth is slightly restricted with a shift usually towards the other side. The disc hurts or starts to click during correction of the mandible. In contrast, *disc displacement without reduction* is due to malposition (anterior position) of the disc in front of the condyle during habitual teeth contact.

It is characterized by restriction in mouth opening, pain, no clicking sounds but usually a history of clicking in the TMJ. If the disc displacement becomes chronic, mouth opening improves and active and end-range movements are less painful. Joint crepitation with (minor) inflammation may persist.[34–36]

It must be noted that approximately 33% of the general population have moderate to severe disc derangement[37,38] and there is no correlation between disc position and TMD pain.[39] Although disc displacements may, in the long-term, lead to degeneration, there is no correlation between degenerative changes and pain.[39,40] Imaging techniques are promoted as gold standard tests for assessment of disc–condyle position. However, they do not guarantee the correct diagnosis of the type of disc displacement.[41–43] Thus the clinician has to interpret the results of imaging in line with clinical diagnostic tests and ask the question: do the results fit?

Hypermobility and Dislocation

Hypermobility and dislocation are strongly related to disc instabilities. TMJ hypermobility is characterized by increased condylar anterior glide during mouth opening.[44] In dislocations the condyle is subluxed out of the fossa behind the crest of the articular eminence, which restricts mouth closure.[44,45] Hypermobility is often seen in (young) people with general hypermobility and/or after a (small) trauma to the mandible.[46] Functionally, neuromusculoskeletal contributing factors include reduced muscular control especially with excessive pterygoid muscle activity,[47] stiffness in the opposite TMJ, craniocervical posture changes[48] and occlusal interference. Orofacial functions such as chewing, talking and singing may be affected. During the assessment of the TMJ the clinician aims to identify possible contributing factors, which might maintain the hypermobility or (minor) dislocation.

Arthralgia

Arthralgic pain is not a single pathological entity. It is non-specific articular TMD (see Fig. 43-1) and is classified by clinical characteristics and clinical tests.[49] An arthralgia is diagnosed when pain is present around the ear, provoked by mandibular movements, which are restricted. Palpation of masticatory structures can provoke the familiar pain.[3] Pain mapping (structural diagnosis of TMJ pain by joint palpation and in combination with passive TMJ movements[50]) may help the clinician differentiate pain dominantly from a peripheral sensitized local structure or from a more central mechanism. This decision has important consequences for further assessment and treatment.

Neurogenic Temporomandibular Disorders

Neuropathic orofacial pain is classified in the RCD/TMD II as non-TMD and is sub-classified as episodic or continuous neuropathic pain with diagnoses such as trigeminal, laryngeal and glossopharyngeal neuralgia.[3] It is characterized by unpredictable episodic sharp, stabbing face pain with different triggers such as temperature changes, emotional and mechanical stress and hormone changes.[51] In the more peripheral part of the trigeminal nerve (distal to the trigeminal ganglion), spontaneous demyelination may occur after a traumatic event, such as teeth extractions, mandibular trauma, or long-term minor pressure on branches of the mandibular nerve (e.g. long-term pressure of the pterygoid muscle on the lingual branch). Trauma and pain onset may not be obviously linked. In many cases the aetiology is unknown.

An underestimated cause of head and orofacial pain may be neurogenic dysfunction where the signs and symptoms come from the nerve trunk and the mechanically or chemically sensitized nociceptors in the connective tissue sheaths of the nervous system (i.e. nervi nervorum).[52–54] For example, the trigeminal branches may be predisposed to nerve trunk pain by:

- Long-term minor pressure on the intracranial blood vessels in the pontine angle at the entry zone of the trigeminal nerve from craniocervical postures and movement.[55,56]
- Compression phenomena around the foramen rotundum and oval foramen (entry zone to the skull floor) during neck movements, particularly during lateral flexion.[57,58]
- Long-term pressure on the alveolar nerve by mandibular implants.[59]
- Intermittent compression, traction and friction on the mandibular nerve during mouth opening in patients with an anterior disc displacement. The mandibular nerve moves by an average distance of 4–5 mm towards the disc.[60]

A set of clinical diagnostic tests may support a hypothesis of peripheral neurogenic TMD pain. Table 43-2

presents a proposed classification of nerve dysfunction and pain caused by the axon or the nerve trunk compiled from literature and from patients presenting clinically.[61–64]

ASSESSMENT

Subjective Examination

A systematic subjective examination provides a hypothesis for the type of TMD, possible pain mechanisms, the patient's activity and participation level, as well as possible Yellow and Red Flags. It forms the basis for planning the physical examination.[65] The standardized taxonomy research diagnostic criteria for temporomandibular disorders (RCD/TMD) is recommended for research purposes as well as multidisciplinary practice.[66] For a detailed description of a subjective examination, the reader is referred to existing literature.[3,67,68]

Physical Examination

The physical examination of the TMJ includes observation and analysis of posture, assessment of active and passive movement as well as muscle testing, which includes an evaluation of endurance, strength and length and palpation for muscle tightness. This provides information on the general function of the masticatory system. It must be appreciated that the findings may not be directly related to the aetiology of the dysfunction and the clinician has to consider possible contributing/risk factors, which might support and maintain TMD pain.

TABLE 43-2 Proposed Features of Neurogenic Facial Dysfunction and Pain

Qualities	Axon Dominance	Nerve Trunk Dominance
Pathogenesis	Axonal destruction, emerging of AIGS	Trophic changes in connective tissue
Subjective Examination		
Pain description	Burning, itching, raw, electric	Dragging, dull, searing, aching/sore muscles, background pain
History	Spontaneous, first episode	Several small traumas in the same nerve region
Exacerbation	Stress, temperature changes, immunologic dysfunctions, tissue stretch	Moving and stretching, palpation
Relief	Rest	Rest and posture changes
Clinical Examination		
Nerve palpation	Delayed symptoms. Pain has a 'shooting' character	Slow increase and spread of symptoms during palpation
	No obvious nerve swelling	Obvious swelling of the nerve, less transverse movements possible
	Transverse movements possible	
Neurological examination (e.g. strength, reflexes, sensitivity)	Neurological signs evident in cranial nerve innervation	No neurological signs or rapid improvement after short trial of treatment of the nerve and its environment
Cranial neurodynamic tests	No obvious resistance. Pain behaviour/latent pain reaction possible	Resistant-pain behaviour during tests/sensitizing movement positive
	Protective spasm without pain during the test may persist	Protective spasm without pain during the test may persist
Electromyogram	Delayed or absence of conductivity	No obvious disturbance of conductivity

The Relationship between an Altered Posture of the Head and Temporomandibular Disorders

There is strong evidence for a neurophysiological, biomechanical and functional connection between the cervical spine and the TMJ.[68] Nevertheless, there is still debate regarding whether or not head posture is directly related to TMD and orofacial pain. Two reviews[68,69] found several studies reporting a relationship between head posture and the stomatognathic system; however, the evidence was inconclusive for the functional relationship between head posture, jaw posture and occlusion. On the other hand, a recent study found that different head postures, especially the forward head posture, changed mouth opening and decreased pressure pain thresholds over the TMJ and masticatory muscles.[70] Even though evidence at present is somewhat inconclusive, it is still recommended that the clinician assesses the influence of the individual patient's head posture on their condition. If changing head posture improves a patient's complaints, it may be reasoned that it has a role in the TMD pain or associated symptoms. Furthermore, a measure of posture can be used as an outcome measure to evaluate the effect of any head posture muscle control exercises. A simple, cheap and safe method to (re)assess the posture of the head is photometry. Van Niekerk[71] compared photometry and radiographic measures and found a good to moderate correlation between body angles and a moderate to good reliability for repeated photographs (intraclass correlation coefficient ranging from 0.78 to 0.99).

Measurement of Head Position

The craniocervical angle is the most common angle of interest. It is usually measured with photometry which has moderate to good validity when compared to radiographs.[68,72–74] The role of the craniocervical angle in headache and TMD is still controversial.[4,72–75] The head can also be forced into rotation about the sagittal plane, described as a posterior rotation of the cranium/head.[50] This is often observed in individuals who have a mouth-breathing pattern, in persons with an angle class II and those with an anterior atlas tilt position.[76] Including face reference points in measurement of the head position may provide indicators of anteroposterior or posterior rotation of the head.

A system for the measurement of head position has been proposed by Armijo-Olivo et al.[77] (Fig. 43-2):
- Eye–tragus–horizontal angle: the angle between a line connecting the midpoint of the lateral corner of the eye with the tragus of the ear and the horizontal line starting at the level of the tragus.
- Pogonion–tragus–C7 angle: the angle between a line connecting the pogonion (the most forward projecting point on the anterior surface of the chin) with the tragus and a line connecting the tragus to the C7 vertebra.
- Tragus–C7–shoulder angle: the angle formed by the intersection between the upper middle point of the shoulder with the C7 vertebra and the line connecting the tragus with the C7 vertebra.

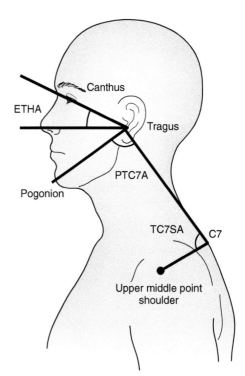

FIGURE 43-2 ■ Head posture measurements as proposed by Armijo-Olivo et al.[77] *ETHA*, Eye(Canthus)–Tragus–Horizontal Angle; *PTC7A*, Pogonion–Tragus–C7 Angle; *TC7SA*, Tragus–C7–Shoulder Angle

Armijo-Olivo et al.[77] found a clear difference between patients with TMD and healthy persons for the eye–tragus–horizontal angle and all measures showed excellent intra- and inter-rater reliability (intraclass correlation coefficient 0.996–0.998). Studies are in progress adding extra lines/angles to better depict forward head posture and posterior rotation of the head (upper cervical extension).[78] The challenge with these studies is the marked individual variability in postures which makes clear (clinical) significance between groups difficult to determine.

Clinical Diagnostic Testing of Temporomandibular Disorders

Quality of Clinical Tests

In general, results of single clinical tests have limited value due to large variations in values.[79] Clustering of relevant tests related to symptoms and multi-test scores (MTS) stand to increase the diagnostic value of clinical tests. For example, if TMJ 'noises' are provoked during active movements AND an additional test such as a static test is positive, then one can conclude that the applied MTS is positive. Table 43-3 presents the results of the inter-examiner reliability of MTS for most cardinal symptoms of TMD: pain, 'noise' and movement restriction.[49] It may be possible to confirm the hypothesized clinical pattern or diagnosis using clustered MTS and this will be the starting point for management.

The combination of symptoms and a clinical test, which has a moderate to high reliability (*k*-values >0.4),

TABLE 43-3 **Inter-Examiner Reliability for Multi-Test Scores (MTS) of Test Combinations for the Three Main Symptoms of Temporomandibular Disorders**

MTS Categories	Agreement %	K	Signs/Symptoms Present %
Pain			
During active movements	65	0.3	49
During additional tests (passive opening, joint play, compression static pain)	6	0.4	59
During function (active movements and/or additional tests)	89	0.7	69
During function and palpation	96	0.8	91
Noises			
During active movements	80	0.6	55
During additional tests	68	0.3	32
During function	77	0.5	60
Restriction of Movement			
During active movements	92	0.6	10
During active movements and/or joint play tests	75	0.4	29

K = Cohen's Kappa statistic in a TMD patient group (n = 79).
Modified after Steenks et al.[49]

assists the clinician to sub-classify the patient's presentation into arthrogenic, myogenic or neurogenic TMD. Steenks et al.[49] using a stepwise logistic regression, classified a sample of TMD patients (n = 160) by different tests and test combinations into myogenic (n = 69) and arthrogenic groups (n = 91).

Which Clinical Neuromusculoskeletal Tests Should be Chosen for Assessing Temporomandibular Disorders?

The aim of the examination is to sub-classify signs and symptoms of TMD pain to identify its source as more arthrogenic, myogenic or neurogenic. Physiological and accessory movements, together with structural differentiation, in general give a good overview of the cardinal signs which may be confirmed by additional tests.

Physiological and Accessory Movements. A combination of active and passive movements (mouth opening, laterotrusion, retrusion and protrusion) related to the MTS provides a sense of TMD and its sub-classifications. Accessory movements, as longitudinal caudal, cranial, medial and lateral transverse, anteroposterior, posteroanterior glides and variations (angulation and combinations) are used for testing peri- and intra-articular structures. Accessory movements contribute to a test battery, which can distinguish between the sub-classifications arthrogenic and myogenic, but the end-feel/stiffness, especially of the caudal longitudinal movement is not structure-specific.[80,81]

Structural Differentiation of Temporomandibular Disorder Pain Associated with Peripheral Nerve Sensitization. When there is clear (long-term) nociceptive pain in the TMJ area, structural differentiation by physiological and accessory movement might support sub-classifications of TMD. For example if the mandibular branch of the trigeminal nerve is involved, a combination of movements (craniocervical flexion, upper cervical lateroflexion, mouth opening (depression) and/ or contralateral laterotrusion of the mandible) are more sensitive than accessory movements to the ipsilateral mandibular head. Alternatively, the longitudinal caudal movement together with anteroposterior movement and laterotrusion may be stiff and locally painful on the symptomatic side. When palpation of the temporal muscle provokes the same pain and craniocervical flexion and lateroflexion do not change the pain, then the TMD may have myogenic characteristics.

Additional Tests

Muscle Testing. An indication of myogenic TMD is often obtained from the five physiological movements (active and/or passive) and static muscle tests.[82] In myogenic TMD, the typical pattern is that, in restricted mouth opening, overpressure beyond the active range results in more mouth opening (10–15 mm), mostly without noises, and restriction of laterotrusions or protrusion. Additional tests such as lengthening tests (a combination of physiological and accessory movement) and palpation of muscle tenderness or trigger points may support the hypothesis of myogenic TMD. It is appropriate to implement pressure pain threshold tests to gain another parameter of the patient's pain experiences. Pressure pain threshold tests can also be used to test for trigeminal or extratrigeminal sensitivity to support the classification of a TMD pain mechanism or for assessment of treatment effectiveness.[83,84] Recent studies indicate the presence of both local and widespread mechanical hypersensitivity in persons with TMD.[83–86]

Nervous System. A battery of quantitative sensory tests can be performed to suggest (cranial) nervous system involvement in pain mechanisms. Cranial neural tissue testing will inform on the function of nerves.

- *Quantitative sensory testing* includes the reaction to vibration, thermal, electrical, and mechanical stimuli.[87,88] Quantitative sensory testing is not a diagnostic test for a particular disease entity but a tool for helping in the mechanism-based diagnosis of pain.[89] Quantitative sensory testing has been used in the diagnosis of neurogenic TMD.[90–92]
- *Cranial neural tissue testing:* Assessment of cranial neural tissue consists of several modalities: conduction tests, palpation and neuromechanical sensitivity. Discussion will focus on the mandibular branch (V3) of the trigeminal nerve as this nerve innervates the temporomandibular region.
- *Conduction tests:* Tests include sensory features of discriminative touch, simple touch, pain, temperature, motor function and the mandibular jaw jerk or reflex. These tests may confirm a peripheral lesion or dysfunction of the mandibular branch.[93]
  - The mandibular jaw jerk (a small tap on the chin on a slightly opened mouth) is, in contrast to a spinal reflex, multisegmental in origin. It is altered in sensorimotor disturbances of the trigeminal nerve. It may be used to differentiate extreme central pathologies when clonus or trismus is detected.[94]
- *Nerve trunk palpation:* Provocation of symptoms does not necessarily identify the site of nerve tissue injury, because the entire tract can become mechanically sensitive after injury[61,86,95] (e.g. toothache or pain around implants). The mental branch (in the mental foramen on the chin) and the auriculotemporal nerve can be palpated.[62,96] Mandibular branches, including the lingual, interior alveolar, mental and auriculotemporal nerves, are readily palpable. Together with results from the other cranial neural tissue testing, nerve palpation can provide indicators of pain from neurogenic TMD.
- *Neurodynamic testing.* In the temporomandibular region, the ovale foramen of the skull floor, the head of the mandible, the lateral and medial pterygoid muscles are all in direct contact with the mandibular nerve.[93,97] A preliminary study[98] of movement of cranial nerve tissue, using MRI scans, found that the spinomedullar angle changes from 6° to 32° when the cervical spine is moved from neutral to upper cervical flexion, confirming Breig's[108] report that lateral flexion of the head challenges the excursion of the trigeminal nerve. Mouth opening and contralateral laterotrusion load the lingual and inferior alveolar branches.[99,100] Neck flexion and longitudinal movement of the mandible move the auriculotemporal nerve.[101] The proposed examination sequence for the mandibular nerve is a combination of craniocervical flexion, contralateral lateroflexion in about 25 mm mouth opening. It is proposed that this moves the mandibular nerve maximally towards the other side (laterotrusion) without extreme stress on the intra-articular TMJ tissue.[65] Research into this test is in its infancy, but a study using the mandibular neurodynamic test displayed differences in spread and intensity of symptoms and mandibular movement between a whiplash and control group.[65]

At the conclusion of the examination, the clinician is positioned to make a reasoned functional statement from the cardinal signs (pain, noises and range of movement) and additional tests (muscle, joint or neural tests). The results may confirm the sub-classification of pain arising from arthrogenous, myogenic or neurogenic TMD.

MANAGEMENT

During the last decade physiotherapy has become increasingly viable as a treatment option for TMD. There is growing consensus on management strategies between different care-providers who work in the domain of head, neck and orofacial pain.[49]

Persisting head and orofacial pain is a complex entity which can have different sources and multiple contributing/risk factors. This chapter has focused on TMD in persistent head-orofacial pain in full recognition that this is one of many possible pathological sources. The clinician has to decide which temporomandibular, craniofacial, cranioneural and/or craniocervical region(s) are dominant in the patient's pain and functional limitation.

Evidence for Physiotherapy in Temporomandibular Disorders

In the TMD literature, physiotherapy is reputed to relieve musculoskeletal pain and restore normal function, reduce local inflammation and promote regeneration of TMJ tissue. It is usually used as an addition to other treatments.[3] In 2006, two systematic reviews concluded that, despite the criticisms about reliability, validity, outcome measurements and inclusion and exclusion criteria for TMD, exercises, manual therapy, electrotherapy, relaxation training and biofeedback seem to have the best outcomes in TMD treatment.[102,103] Nevertheless contemporary evidence is inconclusive. Two recent randomized controlled trials investigating the long-term effect of physiotherapy on TMD muscle pain and disc displacement without reduction, did not prove the effectiveness of these treatments. In contrast, two studies using a clinical reasoning approach for the treatment of TMD in a chronic cervical headache population determined positive outcomes.[7,8] Patients complaining of chronic cervical headache received orofacial manual therapy in addition to usual care. The patients' symptoms, as well as the temporomandibular and craniocervical physical outcomes, were significantly better at 3 and 6 months in the group receiving therapy including orofacial treatment when compared with the group receiving usual care only. Further randomized controlled trials are required into treatment effectiveness.

A home exercise regimen has been found to be effective in improving the range of mouth opening.[104,105] Importantly, the combination of manual therapy and home exercise individualized to patient's needs has been shown to have superior outcomes.[106] Eight motor control tests are proposed as an option for the basis of an exercise programme, based on impairments found in the individual patient's performance. The tests can be easily transformed into exercises (Fig. 43-3).

Each test is associated with a cue, which may facilitate the movement

- Test 1: Thoracic extension. The thoracic spine follows the person's hand without associated activity of the orofacial and cervical region ('the arrow') (Fig. 43-3A).
- Test 2: Craniocervical extension is performed without increased activity of the mandible, which in turn is controlled by the patient themself with her/ his own hand ('sky viewer') (Fig. 43-3B).
- Test 3: Isolated controlled protrusion of the mandible without associated movement of the facial muscles and the craniocervical region ('rain collector') (Fig. 43-3C).
- Test 4: Protrusion of the tongue. Isolated anterior tongue movement while controlling the hyoid bone without associated activity of the lips and ventral neck muscles ('tongue relaxer') (Fig. 43-3D).
- Test 5: Mouth opening (hinge movement) without shift or sound controlled by the person's own tactical feedback ('breathing fish') (Fig. 43-3E).
- Test 6: Laterotrusion of the mandible. Isolated movement of the mandible without excessive facial and neck activity ('side bite') (Fig. 43-3F).

- Test 7: Controlled protrusion of the mandible with controlled head position ('dog follows boss') (Fig. 43-3G).
- Test 8: Static stabilization test in 20 mm mouth opening in the laterotrusion direction without facial muscle and craniocervical activity. ('stay there') (Fig. 43-3H).

Tests 1 to 4 have a general motor control character; tests 5 to 8 are orientated to mandibular activity. They tend to be more difficult and may be used as a progression. Stoltz et al.[107] found inter-tester reliability (kappa) for these tests ranged from 0.28–0.74. Seven out of eight tests showed substantial reliability ($k > 0.6$). Intra-tester reliability ranged between K 0.48–0.91. Of particular relevance, the tests distinguished chronic from non-chronic TMD (five out of seven tests) but not between a TMD and a control group.

SUMMARY

Non-specific TMD pain may be defined as a separate entity, strongly associated with biomedical, psychosocial and pathophysiological (risk) factors. Screening of these risk factors is part of a systematic examination and the cardinal signs (pain, noises and range of movement) have

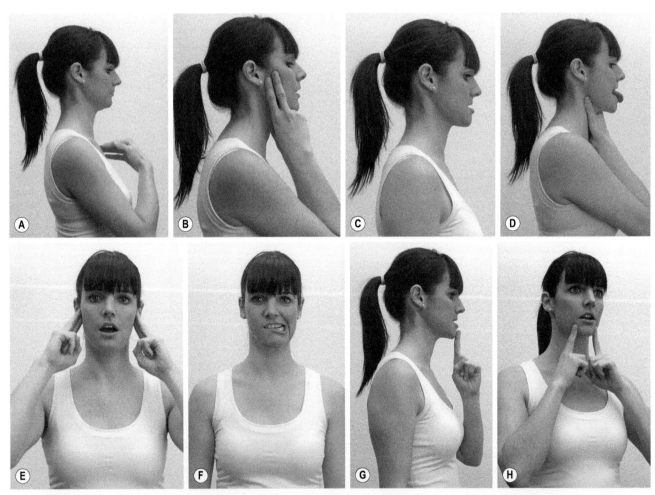

FIGURE 43-3 ■ Motor control tests for the orofacial region. The tests may be used as a basis for further management.

to be proven through clinical tests. These must comply with the principles of MTS. In order to decide on management strategies, trigeminal pain has to be distinguished. Further, the RCD/TMD axis has to be classified before choosing the main neuromusculoskeletal intervention and/or other (pain) management or (facial) rehabilitation modalities.

REFERENCES

1. Ballenberger N, von Piekartz H, Paris-Alemany A, et al. Influence of different upper cervical positions on electromyography activity of the masticatory muscles. J Manipulative Physiol Ther 2012;35:308–18.
2. Nilsson I-M, List T, Drangsholt M. Headache and co-morbid pains associated with TMD pain in adolescents. J Dent Res 2013;92:802–7.
3. De Leeuw R, Klasser G. Orofacial Pain. Guidelines for Assessment, Diagnosis and Management. 5th ed. Quintessence Chicago: The American Academy of Orofacial Pain; 2013.
4. Okeson J. Temporomandibular pains in bells. Orofac Pain 2014;6:329–81.
5. Marklund S, Wänman A. Incidence and prevalence of temporomandibular joint pain and dysfunction. A one-year prospective study of university students. Acta Odontol Scand 2007;65:119–27.
6. Glaros AG, Williams K, Lausten L. Diurnal variation in pain reports in temporomandibular disorder patients and control subjects. J Orofac Pain 2008;22:115–21.
7. Von Piekartz H, Hall T. Orofacial manual therapy improves cervical movement impairment associated with headache and features of temporomandibular dysfunction: a randomized controlled trial. Man Ther 2013;18:345–50.
8. Von Piekartz H, Lüdtke K. Effect of treatment of temporomandibular disorders (TMD) in patients with cervicogenic headache: a single-blind, randomized controlled study. Cranio 2011;29:43–56.
9. Peck C, Goulet JP, Lobbezoo F, et al. Expanding the taxonomy of the diagnostic criteria for temporomandibular disorders. J Oral Rehabil 2014;1:2–23.
10. Schiffman E, Ohrbach R, Truelove EL, et al. The Research Diagnostic Criteria for Temporomandibular Disorders. V: methods used to establish and validate revised Axis I diagnostic algorithms. J Orofac Pain 2010;24:63–78.
11. Schiffman E, Ohrbach R, Truelove E, et al. Diagnostic Criteria for Temporomandibular Disorders (DC/TMD) for Clinical and Research Applications: Recommendations of the International RDC/TMD Consortium Network and Orofacial Pain Special Interest Group. J Oralfac Pain Headache 2014;28:6–27.
12. Benoliel R, Svensson P, Heir GM, et al. Persistent orofacial muscle pain. Oral Dis 2011;17(Suppl. 1):23–41.
13. Wright EF. Referred craniofacial pain patterns in patients with temporomandibular disorders. J Am Dent Assoc 2000;131:1307–15.
14. Schindler H, Svensson P, Türp J, et al. Myosfascial Temporomandibular Disorder Pain. Pathophysiology and Management. The Puzzle of Orofacial Pain. Basel: Karger; 2007.
15. De Boever JA, Carlson GE. Etiology and differential diagnosis. In: Zarb GA, Garlsson GE, Sessle BH, et al., editors. Temporomandibular Joint and Masticatory Muscle Disorders. Munkgaard: Copenhagen; 1994. p. 171–87.
16. Türp J, Greene C, Strub J. Dental occlusion: a critical reflection on past, present and future concepts. J Oral Rehabil 2008;35:446–53.
17. McCarroll R, Naeije M, Kim Y, et al. Short-term effect of a stabilization splint on the asymmetry of submaximal masticatory muscle activity. J Oral Rehabil 1989;16:171–6.
18. Michelotti A, Farella M, Gallo L, et al. Effect of occlusal interference on habitual activity of human masseter. J Dent Res 2005;84:644–8.
19. LeResche L, Saunders K, Von Korff M, et al. Use of exogenous hormones and risk of temporomandibular disorder pain. Pain 1997;69:153–60.
20. Svensson P, Cairns B, Wang K, et al. Injection of nerve growth factor into human masseter muscle evokes long-lasting mechanical allodynia and hyperalgesia. Pain 2003;104:241–7.
21. Cairns B, Svensson P, Wang K, et al. Ketamine attenuates glutamate-induced mechanical sensitization of the masseter muscle in human males. Exp Brain Res 2006;169:467–72.
22. Zubieta JK, Heitzeg MM, Smith Y, et al. COMT val158met genotype affects mu-opioid neurotransmitter responses to a pain stressor. Science (New York, NY) 2003;299:1240–3.
23. Lobbezoo F, Lavigne G. Do bruxism and temporomandibular disorders have a cause-and-effect relationship? J Orofac Pain 1997;11:15–23.
24. Svensson P, List T, Hector G. Analysis of stimulus-evoked pain in patients with myofascial temporomandibular pain disorders. Pain 2001;92:399–409.
25. Glaros AG, Owais Z, Lausten L. Reduction in parafunctional activity: a potential mechanism for the effectiveness of splint therapy. J Oral Rehabil 2007;34:97–104.
26. Mense S, Schiltenwolf M. Fatigue and pain; what is the connection? Pain 2010;148:177–8.
27. Lobbezoo F, Ahlberg J, Glaros A. Bruxism defined and graded: an international consensus. J Oral Rehabil 2013;40:2–4.
28. Von Piekartz H. Management of parafunctional activities and Bruxism. In: Selvararnam P, Nier K, Zuluaga M, editors. Headache, Orofacial Pain and Bruxism. Churchill Livingstone; 2009. p. 261–77.
29. Manfredini D, Cocilovo F, Favero C, et al. Surface electromyography of jaw muscles and kinesiographic recordings: diagnostic accuracy for myofascial pain. J Oral Rehabil 2011;38:791–9.
30. Castroflorio T, Falla D, Wang K, et al. Effect of experimental jaw-muscle pain on the spatial distribution of surface EMG activity of the human masseter muscle during tooth clenching. J Oral Rehabil 2012;39:81–92.
31. McPartland J, Simons D. Myofascial Trigger Points: translating molecular theory into Manual Therapy. In: Dommerholt J, Huijbregts P, editors. Myopfascial Trigger Points. Pathophysiology and Evidence Informed Diagnosis and Management. Boston: Jones and Bartlett Publishers; 2011.
32. Stegenga B, de Bont L, Boering G, et al. Tissue responses to degenerative changes in the temporomandibular joint: a review. J Oral Maxillofac Surg 1991;49:1079–88.
33. Nitzan D. Friction and adhesive forces. Possible underlying causes for temporomandibular joint internal derangement. Cells Tissues Organs 2003;174(1-2):6–16.
34. Delcanho R. Temporomandibular joint arthroscopy. Aust Dent J 2000;45:143.
35. Minakuchi H, Kuboki T, Matsuka Y, et al. Randomized controlled evaluation of non-surgical treatments for temporomandibular joint anterior disk displacement without reduction. J Dent Res 2001;80:924–8.
36. Balasubramaniam R, Ram S. Orofacial movement disorders. Oral Maxillofac Surg Clin North Am 2008;20:273–85.
37. Greene C, Laskin D. Long-term status of TMJ clicking in patients with myofascial pain and dysfunction. J Am Dent Assoc 1988;117:461–5.
38. Larheim T. Role of magnetic resonance imaging in the clinical diagnosis of the temporomandibular joint. Cells Tissues Organs 2005;180:6–21.
39. Schiffman E, Anderson G, Fricton J, et al. The relationship between level of mandibular pain and dysfunction and stage of temporomandibular joint internal derangement. J Dent Res 1992;71:1812–15.
40. Luder H, Bobst P, Schroeder H. Histometric study of synovial cavity dimensions of human temporomandibular joints with normal and anterior disc position. J Oral Rehabil 1993;7:263–74.
41. Westesson P, Bronstein S, Liedberg J. Internal derangement of the temporomandibular joint: morphologic description with correlation to joint function. Oral Surg Oral Med Oral Pathol 1985;59:323–31.
42. Davant T, Greene C, Perry H, et al. A quantitative computer-assisted analysis of disc displacement in patients with internal derangement using sagittal view magnetic resonance imaging. J Oral Maxillofac Surg 1993;51:974–9, discussion 979–81.
43. Santos K, Dutra M, Warmling L, et al. Correlation among the changes observed in temporomandibular joint internal

derangements assessed by magnetic resonance in symptomatic patients. J Oral Maxillofac Surg 2013;71:1504–12.

44. De Leeuw J, Ros WJ, Steenks MH, et al. Multidimensional evaluation of craniomandibular dysfunction. II: pain assessment. J Oral Rehabil 1994;21:515–32.

45. Kavuncu V, Sahin S, Kamanli A, et al. The role of systemic hypermobility and condylar hypermobility in temporomandibular joint dysfunction syndrome. Rheumatol Int 2006;26:257–60.

46. Huddleston Slater J, Lobbezoo F, Onland-Moret N, et al. Anterior disc displacement with reduction and symptomatic hypermobility in the human temporomandibular joint: prevalence rates and risk factors in children and teenagers. J Orofac Pain 2007;21:55–62.

47. De Leeuw R. Post MVA TMD patients endorse more general symptoms than nontrauma TMD patients. J Evid Based Dent Pract 2008;8:246–8.

48. Faralli M, Calenti C, Ibba M, et al. Correlations between posturographic findings and symptoms in subjects with fractures of the condylar head of the mandible. Eur Arch Otorhinolaryngol 2009;266:565–70.

49. Steenks M, Hugger A, De Wijer A. Painful Arthrogenous Temporomandibular Disorders. Pathophysiology, diagnosis, management and prognosis. In: Türp J, Sommer C, Hugger A, editors. The Puzzle of Orofacial Pain. Basel: Karger; 2007. p. 124–53.

50. Rocabado Seaton M, Iglarsh ZA. Musculoskeletal evaluation of the maxillofacial region. In: Musculoskeletal Approach to Maxillofacial Pain. New York: Lippincott Company; 1991. p. 11–117.

51. Haanpää M, Attal N, Backonja M, et al. New PSIG guidelines on neuropathic pain assessment. Pain 2011;152:14–27.

52. Asbury A, Fields H. Pain due to peripheral nerve damage: a hypothesis. Neurology 1984;34:1587–90.

53. Hromada J. Current concepts on the spinal nerves with reference to their function and reparative processes. Acta Chir Orthop Traumatol Cech 1963;30:14–23.

54. Gadient P, Smith J. The neuralgias: diagnosis and management. Curr Neurol Neurosci Rep 2014;14:459–65.

55. Janetta P. Microsurgical approach to the trigeminal nerve for tic douloureux. In: Krayenbühl HP, Maspes E, Sweet W, editors. Progress in Neurological Surgery, vol. 7. Basel: Karger; 1976. p. 180.

56. Yuguang L, Chengyuan W, Meng L, et al. Neuroendoscopic anatomy and surgery of the cerebellopontine angle. J Clin Neurosci 2005;12:256–60.

57. Barba D, Alksne JF. Success of microvascular decompression with and without prior surgical therapy for trigeminal neuralgia. J Neurosurg 1984;60:104.

58. Jannetta P, Bissonette D. Management of failed patient with trigeminal neuralgia. Clin Neurosurg 1985;32:334–47.

59. Renton T, Dawood A, Shah A, et al. Post-implant neuropathy of the trigeminal nerve. A case series. Br Dent J 2012;212:E17.

60. Pedullà E, Meli GA, Garufi A. Neuropathic pain in temporomandibular joint disorders: case-control analysis by MR imaging. Am J Neuroradiol 2009;30:1414–18.

61. Hall T, Elvey R. Nerve trunk pain: physical diagnosis and treatment. Man Ther 1999;4:63–73.

62. Murayama R, Stuginski-Barbosa J, Moraes N, et al. Toothache referred from auriculotemporal neuralgia: case report. Int Endod J 2009;42:845–51.

63. Cavicchi O, Caliceti U, Fernandez I, et al. Laryngeal neuromonitoring and neurostimulation versus neurostimulation alone in thyroid surgery: a randomized clinical trial. Head Neck 2012;34:141–5.

64. Fingleton C, Dempsey L, Smart K, et al. Intraexaminer and interexaminer reliability of manual palpation and pressure algometry of the lower limb nerves in asymptomatic subjects. J Manipulative Physiol Ther 2014;37:97–104.

65. Von Piekartz H. Guidelines for Assessment of Craniomandibular and Craniofacial Region in Craniofacial Pain, Neuromusculoskeletal Assessment, Treatment and Management. Butterworth-Heinemann, Elsevier; 2007. p. 59–83.

66. Dworkin S, Sherman J, Mancl L, et al. Reliability, validity, and clinical utility of the research diagnostic criteria for Temporomandibular Disorders Axis II Scales: depression, non-specific physical symptoms, and graded chronic pain. J Orofac Pain 2002;16:207–20.

67. Langendoen J. Management of craniomandibular disorders. In: Hengeveld E, Banks K, editors. Maitland's Peripheral Manipulation, 5th ed. Management of neuromusculoskeletal disorders, vol. 2. Churchill Livingston; 2013. p. 88–142.

68. Armijo Olivo S, Magee D, Parfitt M. The association between the cervical spine, the stomatognathic system, and craniofacial pain: a critical review. J Orofac Pain 2006;20:271–87.

69. Manfredini D, Castroflorio T, Perinetti G, et al. Dental occlusion, body posture and temporomandibular disorders: where we are now and where we are heading for. J Oral Rehabil 2012;39:463–71.

70. La Touche R, París-Alemany A, von Piekartz H, et al. The influence of cranio-cervical posture on maximal mouth opening and pressure pain threshold in patients with myofascial temporomandibular pain disorders. Clin J Pain 2011;27:48–55.

71. Van Niekerk SM, Louw Q, Vaughan N, et al. Photographic measurement of upper body sitting posture of high school students: a reliability and validity study. BMC Musculoskelet Disord 2008;9:113–19.

72. Watson DH, Trott PH. Cervical headache: an investigation of natural head posture and upper cervical flexor muscle performance. Cephalalgia 1993;13:272–84.

73. Raine S, Twomey L. Head and shoulder posture variation in 160 asymptomatic women and men. Arch Phys Med Rehabil 1997;78:1215–23.

74. Visscher C, Boer W, Lobbezoo F, et al. Is there a relationship between head posture and craniomandibular pain? J Oral Rehabil 2002;29:1030–6.

75. Fernández-de-Las-Peñas C, Coppieters M, Cuadrado M, et al. Patients with chronic tension-type headache demonstrate increased mechano-sensitivity of the supra-orbital nerve. Headache 2008;48:570–7.

76. Archer S, Vig P. Effects of head position on intraoral pressures in Class I and Class II adults. Am J Orthod 1985;87:311–18.

77. Armijo-Olivo S, Rappoport K, Fuentes J. Head and cervical posture in patients with temporomandibular disorders. J Orofac Pain 2011;25:199–209.

78. Lorenz P, von Piekartz H. Profile head measurement of patients with a TMJ in comparison with a control group. Is there a difference? Manuelle Therapie, Thieme (in press).

79. Haas M. Interexaminer reliability for multiple diagnostic test regimens. J Manipulative Physiol Ther 1991;14:95–103.

80. Hesse J, Naeije M, Hansson T. Craniomandibular stiffness in myogenic and arthrogenous CMD patients and control subjects: a clinical and experimental investigation. J Oral Rehabil 1996;23:379–85.

81. Okeson J, Leeuw R. Differential diagnosis of temporomandibular disorders and other orofacial pain disorders. Dent Clin North Am 2011;55:105–20.

82. Anderson G, John MT, Ohrbach R, et al. Influence of headache frequency on clinical signs and symptoms of TMD in subjects with temple headache and TMD pain. Pain 2011;152:765–71.

83. Alonso-Blanco C, Fernández-de-las-Peñas C, de-la-Llave-Rincón A, et al. Characteristics of referred muscle pain to the head from active trigger points in women with myofascial temporomandibular pain and fibromyalgia syndrome. J Headache Pain 2012;13:625–37.

84. Von Piekartz H, Mohr G. Reduction of head and face pain by challenging lateralization and basic emotions: a proposal for future assessment and rehabilitation strategies. J Man Manip Ther 2014;22:25–35.

85. Türp J, Kowalski C, Stohler C. Pain descriptors characteristic of persistent facial pain. J Orofac Pain 1997;11:285–90.

86. Fernández-Pérez A, Villaverde-Gutiérrez C, Mora-Sánchez A, et al. Muscle trigger points, pressure pain threshold, and cervical range of motion in patients with high level of disability related to acute whiplash injury. J Orthop Sports Phys Ther 2012;42:634–41.

87. Hansson P, Backonja M, Bouhassira D. Usefulness and limitations of quantitative sensory testing: clinical and research application in neuropathic pain states. Pain 2007;129:256–9.

88. Fernández-de-Las-Peñas C, Arendt-Nielsen L, Svensson P. Trigeminal and extra-trigeminal hypersensitivity in orofacial pain patients: what are the consequences for further assessment and treatment? In: von Piekartz H, editor. Craniofacial Assessment and Treatment. Stuttgart: Thieme; 2014 [Chapter 5] (in press).

89. Butler D. The Sensitive Nervous System. Adelaide, Australia: Noigroup Publications; 2000.

90. Eliav E, Gracely RH, Nahlieli O, et al. Quantitative sensory testing in trigeminal nerve damage assessment. J Orofac Pain 2004;18:339–44.

91. List T, Leijon G, Svensson P. Somatosensory abnormalities in atypical odontalgia: a case-control study. Pain 2008;139: 333–41.

92. Baad-Hansen L, Pigg M, Ivanovic S. Intraoral somatosensory abnormalities in patients with atypical odontalgia: a controlled multicentre qualitative sensory testing study. Pain 2013;154: 1287–94.

93. Johansson A, Isberg A, Isacsson GA. Radiographic and histologic study of the topographic relations in the temporomandibular joint region: implications for a nerve entrapment mechanism. J Oral Maxillofac Surg 1990;48:953–61, discussion 96.

94. Minami I, Akhter R, Luraschi J, et al. Jaw-movement smoothness during empty chewing and gum chewing. Eur J Oral Sci 2012;120:195–200.

95. Novak C, Mackinnon S. Evaluation of nerve injury and nerve compression in the upper quadrant. J Hand Surg 2005;18: 230–40.

96. Shankland W. Atypical trigeminal neuralgia of the mental nerve: a case study. Cranio 2009;27:19–23.

97. Isberg A, Isacsson G, Williams W, et al. Lingual numbness and speech articulation deviation associated with temporomandibular joint disk displacement. Oral Surgery Oral Medicine Oral Pathology 1987;64:9–14.

98. Doursounian L, Alfonso JM, Iba-Zizen M, et al. Dynamics of the junction between the medulla and the cervical spinal cord: an in vivo study in the sagittal plane by magnetic resonance imaging. Surg Radiol Anat 1989;11:313–22.

99. Benninger B, Kloenne J, Horn J. Clinical anatomy of the lingual nerve and identification with ultrasonography. Br J Oral Maxillofac Surg 2013;51:541–4.

100. Kumar Potu B, Jagadeesan S, Bhat K, et al. Retromolar foramen and canal: a comprehensive review on its anatomy and clinical applications. Morphologie: Bulletin de l'Ass des Anat 2013;97: 31–7.

101. Schroër M, von Piekartz H, Stark W. Movement behaviour of the auriculotemporal nerve during physiological movements of the mandible and cervical spine pilot study using sonographic diagnosis. Man Ther 2012;16:181–90.

102. Medlicott MS, Harris SR. A systematic review of the effectiveness of exercise, manual therapy, electrotherapy, relaxation training, and biofeedback in the management of temporomandibular disorders. Phys Ther 2006;86:955–73.

103. McNeely ML, Armijo Olivo S, Magee D. A systematic review of the effectiveness of physical therapy interventions for temporomandibular disorders. J Phys Ther 2006;86:710–25.

104. Michelotti A, de Wijer A, Steenks M, et al. Home-exercise regimes for the management of non-specific temporomandibular disorders. J Oral Rehabil 2005;32:779–85.

105. Zeno E, Griffin J, Boyd C, et al. The effects of a home exercise program on pain and perceived dysfunction in a woman with TMD: a case study. Cranio 2001;19:279–88.

106. Tuncer AB, Ergun N, Tuncer AH, et al. Effectiveness of manual therapy and home physical therapy in patients with temporomandibular disorders: a randomized controlled trial. J Bodyw Mov Ther 2013;17:302–8.

107. Stotz E, Ballenberger N, von Piekartz H. The reliability of orofacial motor function exercises in TMD versus no TMD. Is there a difference? 2014 (manuscript in preparation).

108. Breig A. Pathologic biomechanics of the cord. In: Breig A, editor. Biomechanics of the Central Nervous System. Stockholm: Almqvist & Wiksell; 1960. p. 120–6.

THORACIC SPINE: MODELS OF ASSESSMENT AND MANAGEMENT

CHAPTER OUTLINE

EDITOR'S INTRODUCTION

The thoracic region is a complex region consisting of five sets of joints for most thoracic segments. It is uniquely encased by ribs, and their attachment to the sternum makes it a stable structure. It can project its influence regionally, for example in breathing or in the way its postural angle influences cervical posture. The research into thoracic spine musculoskeletal disorders is scant in comparison with that undertaken into low back and neck pain disorders. This probably reflects the lower incidence of thoracic pain when compared to the two other regions but this paucity of research should not lessen the importance or impact of thoracic pain disorders on the individual. The volume of research into management methods for thoracic spine disorders is likewise limited. Nevertheless clinicians and researchers are working in the field. In this chapter, authors have been asked to present an overview of two quite different approaches to management of thoracic spine disorders that highlight the diversity which exists in this field. This chapter also brings into discussion the interest and research, particularly over the last decade, into the relationship between the thoracic spine from the musculoskeletal perspective and respiratory function. The diversity in scope within this chapter provides directions for future enquiry.

CHAPTER 44.1 ■ CLINICAL EXAMINATION AND TARGETED MANAGEMENT OF THORACIC MUSCULOSKELETAL PAIN

Quentin Scott

Thoracic spine and chest wall pain (TSP) requires accurate diagnosis for safe and effective management. The clinician must diagnose the presence of a mechanical musculoskeletal movement disorder and exclude other possible causes including disorders of the heart, lungs, pleura and thoracic aorta that can mimic musculoskeletal pain conditions. Thoracic spine function has a significant influence on cervical, lumbar and extremity disorders. Thoracic musculoskeletal pain is common across all age groups[1] and requires thorough and precise clinical examination to ensure accurate diagnosis. This will provide a framework for targeted management addressing specific impairments.

ANATOMICAL AND BIOMECHANICAL CONSIDERATIONS

The thoracic spine can be divided into discrete regions based upon vertebral body dimension,[2,3] zygapophyseal joint orientation or rib joint articulations.[4] The thoracic spine is commonly divided into upper, middle and lower regions based upon anatomy and differences in range of movement and coupled movement patterns.[5] Assessment of thoracic spine movement requires knowledge of zygapophyseal joint orientation and biomechanics and the corresponding rib articulations with their influence on thoracic movement patterns.

An in-depth understanding of the normal range of movement and biomechanics throughout the thorax will allow the clinician to identify faulty movement patterns. The dominant movement of the thoracic spine is axial rotation that mostly occurs in the upper and middle regions.[5-7] Movement studies show greater flexion/extension range of movement and reduced axial rotation in the lower thoracic spine.[5,6]

ASSESSMENT AND DIAGNOSIS OF TSP

Subjective Examination

Area of Symptoms

A detailed description of the area of pain and associated symptoms is the first step in identifying potential sources of nociception. Thoracic pain is commonly referred from the cervical spine and both the abdominal and thoracic viscera.[8,9] In addition, the thoracic spine can refer to the posterior shoulder region, rib cage, anterolateral abdominal wall and iliac crest region.[10,11]

Behaviour of Symptoms

The behaviour of symptoms will further differentiate potential sources of pain, help determine whether the symptoms are mechanical in origin and identify driving mechanisms. Identification of aggravating and easing factors will allow the clinician to explore the relationship between movement behaviour and symptomatology.

Aggravating factors for thoracic spine disorders often encompass one or a combination of the following activities:
- thoracic movement, especially rotation and extension
- upper limb movements, especially into elevation or sustained upper limb activity
- sustained postural load, usually sitting
- cervical motion
- respiration
- repetitive lower limb activities.

Further exploration of aggravating activities may be required to understand the mechanisms involved in the presenting disorder, for example:
- thoracic rotation on pelvis due to computer placement in workplace
- habitual leg crossing driving asymmetrical weight bearing and spinal side bent position
- stroke versus bow side rowing
- dominant arm with overhead sporting activities.

History

A detailed history of the presenting complaint is important to substantiate the mechanisms involved in the onset of pain and progression of symptoms. TSP is often associated with concurrent musculoskeletal symptoms.[1,12,13] Information regarding other musculoskeletal pain assists the clinician to identify contributing factors, for example, chronic low back pain with altered trunk muscle activation patterns leading to reduced thoracic spine mobility and TSP. The history should include details of any treatment of the presenting complaint as this will determine possible future assessment, modes of treatment and the appropriateness of continued management.

Specific Spinal Pathologies

The clinician needs to be aware of specific pathologies that can influence posture and movement, for example:
- Scheuermann's disease
- Ankylosing spondylitis
- deformity due to osteoporotic vertebral compression fracture (Fig. 44-1)
- scoliosis.

The presence of these and other conditions will play a role in the differential diagnosis of TSP disorders.

Red Flags

Red flags are indicators of serious pathology requiring medical referral or further investigations. Inquiries regarding the patient's general health and specific screening questions (such as smoking, history of heart disease, unexplained weight loss) may be necessary to exclude non-musculoskeletal pathology. Questioning for red flags, information regarding behaviour of symptoms (such as consistency and severity) and knowledge of potential sources of thoracic spine and chest wall pain is required to assist identification of presentations that are not mechanical musculoskeletal in origin, for example, the thoracic spine is a common region for metastatic disease. Detailed discussion regarding red flag recognition and presentations is beyond the scope of this section and the reader is directed elsewhere.[14]

Yellow Flags

Yellow flags are indicators of psychosocial factors associated with poor recovery from injury. Psychosocial risk

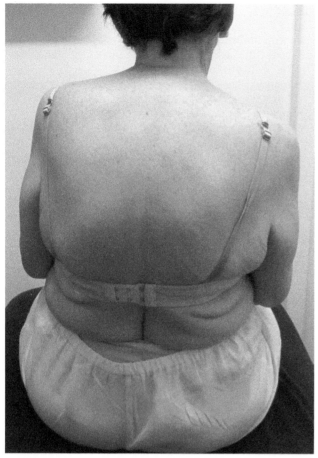

FIGURE 44-1 ■ Increased thoracic kyphosis due to osteoporotic vertebral compression fracture.

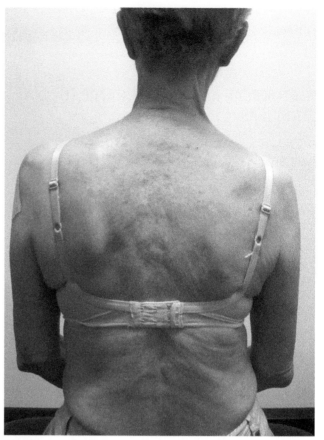

FIGURE 44-2 ■ Increased thoracolumbar extension with poor mid-thoracic, scapula and low lumbar correction in sitting.

factors have been reported in TSP[15] and therefore therapists should be able to identify the presence of yellow flags that will influence management strategies and prognosis.

Physical Examination

Information gained in the subjective examination on the behaviour of symptoms will guide physical examination. The clinician should conduct specific postural, functional, movement and muscle activation assessment to determine faulty movement patterns and motor control strategies.

Posture

Altered thoracic spine posture has been linked to painful movement impairments,[16] reduced shoulder elevation,[17,18] altered scapula kinematics,[17] altered rib cage motion[19,20] and altered chest wall shape.[19]

Assessment of thoracic spine posture focuses on sagittal plane orientation (increased kyphosis vs lordosis), transverse plane orientation (thoracic rotation) and coronal plane orientation (scoliosis). Assessment of the adopted resting posture and how the patient attempts to correct this posture will provide information regarding proprioceptive deficits and possible faulty movement patterns. A common postural correction fault is increased

thoracolumbar junction extension with poor mid-thoracic and scapula correction (Fig. 44-2).

Altered thoracic postures are usually linked to postural faults in other spinal regions, for example, in sitting, increased thoracic kyphosis is often associated with forward head posture and protracted scapulae while decreased kyphosis or flat thoracic spine is seen with increased lumbar flexion (Fig. 44-3). A thoracic posture assessment should also include observation of scapula position and cervical and lumbopelvic regions. Therapist-assisted correction of posture and reassessment of symptomatology will allow further analysis of postural involvement.

An understanding of the effects of age and specific pathologies on the thoracic spine anatomy and resultant thoracic curvature will assist in determining the reversibility of the adopted posture and related movement patterns.

Motion Assessment

Thoracic spine active movement assessment will concentrate on the range and symmetry of thoracic rotation and the range of sagittal plane movement. Careful analysis of movement patterns is required throughout the cervical, thoracic and lumbar spines and more specifically between the regions of the thoracic spine.

When assessing thoracic spine rotation, it is important to observe the pattern of movement, where the movement is occurring and the relationship to pain. It is

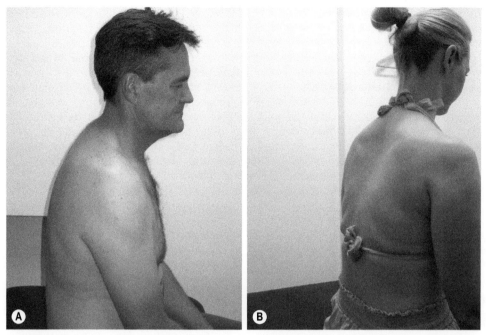

FIGURE 44-3 ■ **(A)** Increased thoracic kyphosis with forward head posture and protracted scapulae. **(B)** Flat thoracic spine with increased lumbar flexion.

possible that restriction in one region of the thorax can lead to increased strain through another region. Thoracic extension can be assessed with bilateral shoulder flexion. The range and pattern of thoracic extension will be linked to postural findings. Increased thoracic kyphosis results in reduced thoracic extension range and possible compensatory patterns in the regions above and below.

Altered thoracic posture can influence the range and pattern of movement coupling.[21] Correction of faulty postural and movement patterns and reassessment of symptomatology and movement behaviour assist identification of driving mechanisms. A common example is reassessment of thoracic rotation following correction of the thoracolumbar position.

Muscle System Assessment

TSP disorders can occur as a result of sub-optimal muscular control of movement leading to increased tissue strain.[16] Assessment of muscle function related to the thoracic spine will involve analysis of posture, functional movement, specific movement tests and specific muscle activation and length tests.

Assessment of the trunk, hip and axioscapula muscle system (which potentially influence the thoracic spine and rib cage) will be determined by the behaviour of symptoms and observation of altered movement patterns. Axioscapula muscle control should be assessed when the behaviour of thoracic symptoms involves upper limb or postural activities. Hip muscle control will be important to assess when the patient reports symptoms with functional activities involving standing and repetitive lower limb movement.

Assessment of breathing patterns will assist in identifying the adopted motor strategy in many TSP disorders. Reduced rib cage mobility has been shown in a low back pain population.[22] This is argued to be the result of the

> **BOX 44-1** | **Diagnosis and Classification of TSP Disorders**
>
> Pathobiological processes
>   Source of nociception
>   Pain mechanisms
>   Patho-anatomical processes
> Exclusion of non-mechanical thoracic pain or serious musculoskeletal pathology
> Presence of structural pathology
> Understanding of faulty thoracic movement and postural patterns
> Muscle system impairment
> Psychosocial involvement

altered relationship between the abdominal muscles, diaphragm and rib cage. Asymmetry in the length and recruitment of the trunk muscles will influence movement of the thoracic spine and rib cage.[16] Different thoracolumbar postures can influence trunk muscle recruitment across the three regions of the spine.[23,24] This has the potential to influence thoracic movement patterns.

Manual Examination

Manual examination of the thoracic spine, rib cage, cervical spine and scapula play an important role in assessment of relative motion and provocation of symptoms in TSP disorders.

Diagnosis

Diagnosis and classification of TSP disorders (Box 44-1) should encompass the possible source of nociception and more importantly the underlying mechanisms to direct the clinician on specific management.

MANAGEMENT OF THORACIC MUSCULOSKELETAL PAIN DISORDERS

Specific management of thoracic musculoskeletal pain disorders is dependent upon accurate diagnostics allowing a targeted approach. The emphasis in the management will depend on the outcome of the physical examination. Thoracic musculoskeletal pain can result from other mechanisms rather than movement restriction. Thoracic musculoskeletal pain disorders make up a heterogeneous group that requires specific treatment approaches to address the presenting impairments.

The main aspects of management will involve a combination of the following.

Postural Correction

Correction of the thoracic spine and other regional postural and proprioceptive impairments is an important starting point in management. Correction of thoracic spine posture should occur in conjunction with cervical spine, scapula, lumbar spine and hip correction, for example, correction of the lumbar spine into neutral posture will be essential before correction of the thoracic spine is possible.

Correction of postural asymmetry in the coronal and transverse planes to ensure no spinal/thoracic rotation or shifting is required in conjunction with correction of sagittal plane postures (Fig. 44-4).

Improve Thoracic Spine Mobility

Optimal thoracic spine function requires the restoration of symmetrical and adequate rotation and appropriate thoracic spine sagittal plane motion. This may be dependent upon factors such as age, degree of thoracic kyphosis and reversibility of the thoracic posture.

Manual therapy directed at both the zygapophyseal joint and rib joint articulations may be required to restore normal movement in cases of restricted segmental motion. Improving movement at one region of the thoracic spine will often reduce stress at another region, for example, specific mobilization of mid-thoracic rotation can improve the overall rotation pattern of movement and reduce lower thoracic strain.

Improving thoracic spine range of motion is also important in the management of cervical spine, lumbar spine and upper limb disorders. Movement dissociation between the different spinal regions will be linked to proprioceptive deficits and the retraining of these aspects will go hand in hand. Restoring improved thoracic spine range and pattern of movement may not occur unless postural deficits in other regions are addressed in conjunction.

Optimize Muscle Function

Goals should be focused on:
• Facilitation of improved thoracic erector spinae endurance and strength. This is indicated in cases of increased thoracic spine kyphosis.
• Facilitation of improved thoracic spine motion control. Improved control may be required either into thoracic rotation, flexion or extension.

Facilitation of motion control may be specific to a region of the thoracic spine and not to the entire thoracic spine. Addressing impairments in thoracic motion control cannot be achieved without first observing the movement patterns of the regions above and below the thoracic spine. Often addressing lumbar spine, cervical spine and scapula muscle function greatly improves thoracic spine muscle impairments.

Address Contributing Impairments

1. Restore normal lumbopelvic and cervical postural and movement patterns. This will assist normalization of trunk musculature that will potentially affect thoracic spine and rib cage mobility.
2. Breathing control to address the relationship between the abdominal muscles, diaphragm and rib cage. This will involve:
   • facilitation of improved abdominal muscle activation and control
   • retraining normal breathing patterns
   • improving lateral rib cage mobility.
3. Axioscapula muscle control. Facilitation of improved axioscapula motor control should occur

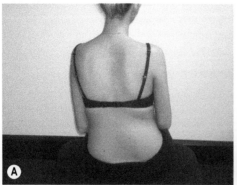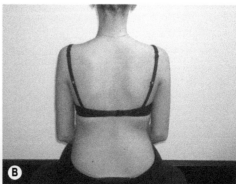

FIGURE 44-4 ■ Correction of right thoracic rotation in conjunction with sagittal plane postural correction.

together with thoracic spine postural and movement retraining.

4. Hip muscle control. Facilitation of optimal hip extensor and abduction strength and endurance in weight-bearing activities is essential to allow appropriate trunk muscle activation strategies during function. This works to prevent adverse effects on thoracic movement and loading patterns.

Precise examination of the thoracic spine will allow the clinician to differentiate thoracic mechanical musculoskeletal from non-mechanical sources. Knowledge of thoracic anatomy, biomechanics, normal range of motion, postures and other regional influences, enables identification of the thoracic movement disorder and underlying mechanisms. This results in a more targeted approach to management.

REFERENCES

1. Briggs AM, Smith AJ, Straker LM, et al. Thoracic spine pain in the general population: prevalence, incidence and associated factors in children, adolescents and adults. A systematic review. BMC Musculoskelet Disord 2009;10:77.
2. Edmondston SJ. Clinical biomechanics of the thoracic spine including the rib cage. In: Boyling JD, Jull GA, editors. Grieve's Modern Manual Therapy The Vertebral Column. 3rd ed. Edinburgh: Churchill Livingstone; 2004.
3. Panjabi MM, Takata K, Goel V, et al. Thoracic human vertebrae. Quantitative three-dimensional anatomy. Spine 1991;16(8):888–901.
4. Lee D. The Thorax: An Integrated Approach. Britsih Columbia: Diane G. Lee Physiotherapist Corporation; 2003.
5. Willems JM, Jull GA, Ng JKF. An in vivo study of the primary and coupled rotations of the thoracic spine. Clin Biomech (Bristol, Avon) 1996;11(6):311–16.
6. White A. Analysis of the mechanics of the thoracic spine in man: an experimental study of autopsy specimens. Acta Orthop Scand 1969;127(Suppl.):1–105.
7. Edmondston SJ, Singer KP. Thoracic spine: anatomical and biomechanical considerations for manual therapy. Man Ther 1997;2(3):132–43.
8. Dwyer A, Aprill C, Bogduk N. Cervical zygapophyseal joint pain patterns. I: a study in normal volunteers. Spine 1990;15(6):453–7.
9. Goodman CC, Snyder TK. Differential Diagnosis for Physical Therapists: Screening for Referral. 5th ed. United States: Elsevier; 2012.
10. Fukui S, Ohseto K, Shiotani M. Patterns of pain induced by distending the thoracic zygapophyseal joints. Reg Anesth 1997;22(4):332–6.
11. Feinstein B, Langton JN, Jameson RM, et al. Experiments on pain referred from deep somatic tissues. J Bone Joint Surg Am 1954;36-A(5):981–97.
12. Murphy S, Buckle P, Stubbs D. A cross-sectional study of self-reported back and neck pain among English schoolchildren and associated physical and psychological risk factors. Appl Ergon 2007;38(6):797–804.
13. Wedderkopp N, Leboeuf-Yde C, Andersen LB, et al. Back pain reporting pattern in a Danish population-based sample of children and adolescents. Spine 2001;26(17):1879–83.
14. Giles IGF, Singer KP, editors. Clinical Anatomy and Management of Thoracic Spine Pain. Oxford: Butterworth Heinemann; 2000.
15. Briggs AM, Bragge P, Smith AJ, et al. Prevalence and associated factors for thoracic spine pain in the adult working population: a literature review. J Occup Health 2009;51(3):177–92.
16. Spitznagle T, Ivens R. Movement system syndromes of the thoracic spine. In: Sahrmann SA, editor. Movement System Impairment Syndromes of the Extremities, Cervical and Thoracic Spines. St Louis: Elsevier Mosby; 2011.
17. Kebaetse M, McClure P, Pratt NA. Thoracic position effect on shoulder range of motion, strength, and three-dimensional scapular kinematics. Arch Phys Med Rehabil 1999;80(8):945–50.
18. Crawford HJ, Jull G. the influence of thoracic posture and movement on range of arm elevation. Physiother Theory Pract 1993; 9:143–8.
19. Lee LJ, Chang AT, Coppieters MW, et al. Changes in sitting posture induce multiplanar changes in chest wall shape and motion with breathing. Respir Physiol Neurobiol 2010;170(3):236–44.
20. Culham EG, Jimenez HA, King CE. Thoracic kyphosis, rib mobility, and lung volumes in normal women and women with osteoporosis. Spine 1994;19(11):1250–5.
21. Edmondston SJ, Aggerholm M, Elfving S, et al. Influence of posture on the range of axial rotation and coupled lateral flexion of the thoracic spine. J Manipulative Physiol Ther 2007;30(3):193–9.
22. Scott QJ, Deeg T, Richardson CA, editors. The Effect of Low Back Pain on Lateral Rib Cage Mobility. Brisbane: MPA Conference; 2005.
23. Caneiro JP, O'Sullivan P, Burnett A, et al. The influence of different sitting postures on head/neck posture and muscle activity. Man Ther 2010;15(1):54–60.
24. O'Sullivan PB, Dankaerts W, Burnett AF, et al. Effect of different upright sitting postures on spinal-pelvic curvature and trunk muscle activation in a pain-free population. Spine 2006;31(19):E707–12.

CHAPTER 44.2 ■ THE THORACIC RING APPROACH™ – A WHOLE PERSON FRAMEWORK TO ASSESS AND TREAT THE THORACIC SPINE AND RIBCAGE

Linda-Joy Lee

Clinicians have long recognized that the thoracic spine can be the silent but underlying cause, or 'driver', for problems elsewhere in the body. Most commonly, the hypothesis is that a stiff thorax creates excessive forces and pain in adjacent areas such as the lumbar spine, neck and shoulder girdle.[1–3]

A challenge for clinicians is how to determine when treatment to the thorax will resolve symptoms either locally or distally. Research on the benefits of thoracic spine treatment is limited and provides conflicting insight into when treatment will improve outcomes; while some subjects show improvements, others report aggravation of symptoms.[1,2] Clinical experiences can be similarly ambiguous. Furthermore, treatment to the thorax may cause adverse experiences such as nausea and sympathetic nervous system symptoms.

To make wise clinical decisions regarding when and how to treat the thorax, the thoracic spine needs to be viewed with a broader lens. Firstly, the thoracic spine needs to be assessed and treated within the context of the three-dimensional 'thoracic ring'.[4-8] Secondly, the thorax needs to be assessed within the context of the whole person and whole body function. That is, in order to determine whether or not treatment to the thorax will positively impact a patient's problem, it is necessary to understand and assess the connections between the thorax and the rest of the body. Thirdly, treatment to the thorax needs to expand beyond techniques that aim to increase mobility, to incorporate training optimal neuromuscular control and muscle balance for optimal movement, load transfer and respiration.

CONNECTING THE THORACIC SPINE AND RIBCAGE AS A SERIES OF 'THORACIC RINGS'

In both research and clinical realms the thoracic spine is commonly considered in isolation from the ribs and ribcage, with separate assessment and treatment techniques for each.[9-12] However, anatomical[13] and recent biomechanical data[14,15] support that where there are anterior attachments, the true functional spinal unit of the thorax is the 'thoracic ring'.[4,8] For example, the fifth thoracic ring is comprised of the right and left fifth ribs, their anterior attachments to the sternum, the T4–T5 thoracic vertebrae and the T4–T5 intervertebral disc.[4-8,10] Therefore there is a need for manual assessment and treatment techniques for the entire thoracic ring.

Thoracic Ring Approach™[16,17] techniques employ palpation points and forces applied around the anterior, lateral and posterior ribcage to assess and treat the three-dimensional thoracic rings.[4-7,16-18] Due to the strong anatomical connections between the ribs and thoracic spine, motion detected at the lateral ribs reflects vertebral motion, and forces applied to the side of the ring impact the vertebral segment as well as the ribs (i.e. the entire ring).[19] Thoracic 'ring palpation'[4-7,17] is applied farthest from the axis of rotation of the thoracic segment and where there is greater amplitude of motion to detect compared to palpation points centrally at the vertebra. Thoracic ring techniques facilitate assessment of inter-ring (segmental) motion and control during functional tasks, as well as analysis of multiple rings and inter-regional relationships simultaneously (Fig. 44-5). Furthermore, thoracic ring palpation and 'thoracic ring correction' techniques[4,5,6,16,17] provide a method to evaluate the connections between a dysfunctional thoracic ring and whole body function.[5,6,17,20]

CONNECTING THE THORAX TO WHOLE BODY FUNCTION: DETERMINING IF THE THORACIC RINGS ARE THE 'DRIVER' FOR THE PATIENT'S PROBLEM

Understanding the role of the thorax in whole body function facilitates more effective clinical reasoning to decide

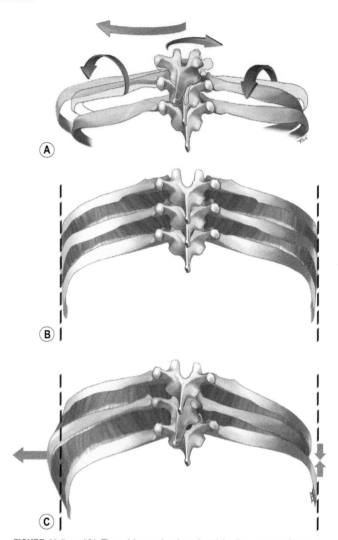

FIGURE 44-5 ■ **(A)** Two 'thoracic rings', with the upper thoracic ring depicting the osteokinematics that occur with right rotation. During right rotation, the vertebra rotates right, the right rib posteriorly rotates and the left rib anteriorly rotates,[10] and there is a left (contralateral) translation of the thoracic ring that can be palpated at the lateral aspect of the ring.[4,5] **(B)** 'Stacked' thoracic rings – when neuromuscular forces are balanced around and between the thoracic rings, optimal alignment is supported and provides a base from which to initiate movement. There is sufficient space between the thoracic rings. Although not all muscles are depicted here, optimal alignment of the thoracic rings is supported by balance between the deep and superficial muscles attaching to the rings. Note that the top vertebra is missing from the superior thoracic ring. If this figure depicts rings 3, 4 and 5, the related vertebral segments include T2–T5. Less muscle bulk over the sides of the rings compared to the posterior aspect of the ring facilitates more accurate analysis of ring motion during functional tasks. **(C)** 'Unstacked' thoracic rings – when force vectors around the thoracic rings are unbalanced, there are multiple patterns of thoracic ring dysfunction that can occur. This figure depicts one potential pattern of non-optimal inter-ring relationships. Compression between the upper and lower rings on the right creates left translation of the middle ring, which is coupled with right rotation. Compression of the rings also creates side bending, which is coupled with rotation. These inter-ring relationships can be assessed simultaneously using thoracic ring palpation techniques. Findings from manual assessment of the posterior joints of the thoracic spine and ribcage need to be interpreted in reference to the position and behaviour of the related thoracic ring. (Reproduced with permission from Linda-Joy Lee Physiotherapist Corp.)

when treatment to the thoracic rings will result in best outcomes. The ultimate goal of treatment is to change the way that patients experience their bodies and to create more optimal strategies for posture, movement and performance. Therefore, when considering any area of the body, the relationship of regional dysfunction to whole body function needs to be assessed and determined.

There are multiple mechanisms by which dysfunction of the thoracic rings, whether painful or not, can drive distal problems as diverse as incontinence, groin pain, Achilles tendinopathy and shoulder impingement. It is not possible to describe these mechanisms in depth here, but based on evidence from anatomy, neurophysiology,

biomechanics and other first principles, several biologically plausible mechanisms have been proposed[6,16,17] (Table 44-1).

Thus, a patient with a dysfunctional thorax can present with a wide variety of symptoms and functional problems. Location of pain or tissue changes does not always correlate to the primary underlying cause of the problem. 'Meaningful Task Analysis (MTA)' was initially proposed as a whole body assessment framework to determine whether or not dysfunction in the thorax was the underlying cause, or 'driver', of the patient's problem.[20] MTA incorporates not only the biomechanical features of a task, but also the emotional, cognitive, social and

TABLE 44-1 Connections Between the Thorax and the Rest of the Body – Examples of Biologically Plausible Mechanisms as to how the Thoracic Rings can Drive Distal Pain and Problems

Anatomical Connections/Role of the Thorax	Possible Mechanisms by Which Dysfunction of the Thoracic Rings can Drive Distal Problems
Direct muscular/myofascial connections between thoracic rings and other regions	Hypertonicity of specific fascicles related to a thoracic ring alters forces at specific segments in the lumbar spine, cervical spine, pelvis and bones of the shoulder girdle
Provides a foundation for shoulder girdle and head/neck function	Rotation/side-bending dysfunction of any thoracic rings creates an asymmetrical foundation for muscle function and load transfer, poor control of thoracic rings results in loss of a stable base for the shoulder girdle, neck and head
Centre of trunk rotation	Altered rotational control of the thorax creates altered forces/loads at other rotational centres in the body (e.g. atlanto-axial joint, hips, subtalar joints)
Closely related to the brachial plexus and subclavian vessels	Twists anywhere in the thorax can create compensatory rotations of the first ring and clavicle, reducing space in the thoracic outlet
Fascial and neural connections to the visceral system	Connect the thoracic rings internally to the neck, cranium, abdominal cavity – for example the pleura of the lungs has connections into the deep cervical fascia; innervation of many viscera comes from thoracic segments → altered neural drive creates gastrointestinal symptoms such as bloating, 'irritable bowel syndrome'
Diaphragm – costal attachments (lower two ribs and lowest four rings)	Altered alignment of multiple thoracic rings changes tension through the muscle fibres and fascia of the diaphragm → alters breathing patterns and can change the shape of apertures for oesophagus, aorta, inferior vena cava → changes blood flow to lower extremity, contributes to oesophageal reflux
Sympathetic trunks run anterior to the heads of the ribs	Tensioning of the sympathetic trunk can occur across multiple levels due to multiple 'unstacked' rings and contribute to sensitization of the sympathetic system and symptoms such as hyperhidrosis, flushing and agitation
Innervation of all abdominal muscles from T7–L1/2 nerve roots, thoracic rings provide attachment/origin for abdominal muscles	'Unstacked' thoracic rings create asymmetrical abdominal muscle recruitment due to altered neural drive, altered position of muscle attachments, or as a compensatory strategy for non-optimal rotational control in the upper thoracic rings → impacts lumbopelvic control, indirect effect on pelvic floor muscle and lumbar paraspinal muscle function
Relationship between intrathoracic and intra-abdominal pressure (IAP)	Excessive superficial muscle activity in the thorax increases IAP → 'pressure belly' creates excessive loads on pelvic floor fascia (contributes to pelvic organ prolapse), or creates sustained increases in pelvic floor muscle activity (contributes to incontinence/pain). Thoracic drivers commonly create asymmetrical patterns of pressure and altered pelvic floor activity due to rotational role
Contributes to control of postural equilibrium, especially in the coronal and transverse planes, because thoracic rings can segmentally and multisegmentally move into lateral translation and rotation to provide control of the centre of mass over the base of support	Poorly controlled thoracic rings, or rings held in one movement pattern create altered loading of lower-extremity structures, especially medial–lateral forces, changes left–right leg weight bearing → alters activation of lower extremity muscles → hip impingement and osteoarthritis, Achilles tendinopathy, metatarsal stress fractures, increased risk for knee ligament injuries[21]
'Stacked' thoracic rings provide a shock-absorbing 'spring' for the trunk	Loss of space between thoracic rings decreases ability to dissipate loads in the trunk → increased loads to the low back on heel strike

contextual features related to a specific problematic or goal-related movement. Meaningful tasks are determined from the patient's story and direct the choice of tasks analysed in the objective assessment.

The clinical decision as to whether or not the thorax should be treated, and which specific thoracic rings to treat, is determined by assessing and manually modifying thoracic ring behaviour during screening tasks related to the patient's meaningful task. For example, for a runner who experiences lateral foot pain on the push-off phase of gait, a relevant screening task is a step forward (Fig. 44-6). If non-optimal alignment, biomechanics or control of any thoracic rings occurs during the task, a 'thoracic ring correction' is performed, whereby optimal thoracic ring alignment, movement and control is provided through gentle but specific manual facilitation at the specific ring level.[4,5,16,17,20] If this 'thoracic ring correction' positively changes (a) ease of task performance, (b)

meaningful complaint/ symptoms and (c) optimizes transfer of loads through other areas of the body, then there is support for the hypothesis of a thoracic ring driver. To further strengthen the hypothesis, manual corrections are also applied to other areas of the body and the impact compared to the thoracic ring correction. In the case of a thoracic ring driver, corrections to other areas either have a negative effect or not as positive an effect as the thoracic ring correction.[4,5,16,17,20] This clinical reasoning framework is a key feature of the Thoracic Ring Approach™[16,17] and the Integrated Systems Model for Pain and Disability.[22]

Therefore the indication to treat the thorax, and specific levels of the thorax, is that the thorax is shown to be a 'driver' in MTA. This provides a clinical rationale to support that treatment to the thoracic rings will result in positive clinical outcomes for whole body function.

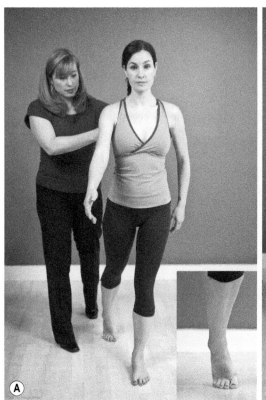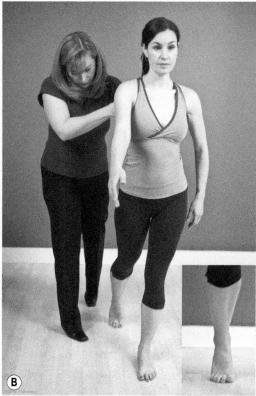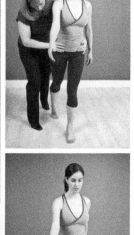

FIGURE 44-6 ■ Meaningful Task Analysis (MTA).[20] To find the driver for the patient's foot pain related to push-off during running, a step forward task is used as a screening task. Multiple areas of non-optimal alignment, biomechanics and/or control (non-optimal load transfer [NOLT]) are identified during the task. **(A)** During left step forward, the right foot demonstrates lateral weight bearing on push-off, with valgus forces at the ankle. At initiation of the step forward, the fourth thoracic ring is felt to translate left, creating a segmental right rotation. Optimally the upper thorax should rotate left, and therefore the movement of the fourth thoracic ring is non-optimal. The resultant left shift of the thorax over the base of support requires the compensatory valgus at the ankle to neutralize the centre of mass over the base of support. Inset: a close-up of the impact of the early left translation of the fourth thoracic ring on the right foot. **(B)** Correction of the fourth thoracic ring during the left step forward task results in optimal weight bearing through the right ankle and foot during push-off, and reduction of the patient's symptoms. Commonly, the starting position of the thoracic rings needs to be corrected by 'stacking' them into optimal inter-ring relationships, then optimal movement and control is manually facilitated during the task. The thorax can drive distal problems in the hip, knee, ankle and foot because of rotational mechanisms and the effect that lateral translation of the thorax has on the centre of mass relative to the base of support. Inset: a close-up of the right foot in push-off in response to the fourth thoracic ring correction. Note the significantly improved position. Application of thoracic ring correction techniques during functional movement analysis allows evaluation of the potential impact that treating specific levels of the thorax will have on symptoms, task performance, and other problematic areas in the kinetic chain. **(C)** The impact of corrections to other areas of NOLT (upper panel: pelvis, and lower panel: foot) is assessed and compared to the impact of the thoracic ring correction. The thoracic ring correction resulted in the best change in task performance, the most positive change on all areas of NOLT, and optimized load transfer through the right foot (area of symptoms). (Reproduced with permission from Linda-Joy Lee Physiotherapist Corp.)

TREATMENT OF THE THORACIC RING DRIVER

Effective treatment will address the underlying impairments of the thoracic rings. Although it is widely held that the most common impairment in the thorax is stiffness, due to the presence of the ribcage,[3,23,24] minimal data support this belief. The intact thorax is mobile in all planes, and in contrast to the limited rotation of the lumbar segments, the primary motion of the thorax is rotation, followed by lateral bending.[25–27] Taken as a whole, the evidence supports that the thorax is inherently flexible in nature.[8]

The capacity for movement within and between the segments of the thorax, along with the requirements for control of upright posture and respiration, requires complex coordination of muscle activity by the central nervous system to meet the demands of stability and movement. Differential control of the deep and superficial thoracic paraspinal muscles occurs in the transverse plane, where the thorax has the greatest movement, for control of opposite rotational perturbations.[28–30]

Clinically, multiple patterns of non-optimal sequencing, force modulation, and synergy between the muscles around the thoracic ring, between the ten thoracic rings and between the rings and other regions of the body have been observed.[4,6,16,17] These non-optimal neuromuscular forces create the appearance of 'stiffness' that is not related to true articular restriction. This proposal is consistent with studies that demonstrate that mobilization and manipulation techniques effect change via neurophysiological mechanisms that alter muscle tone and activity.[31]

Therefore an essential aim of treatment is to create more optimal patterns of muscle recruitment and function related to the thoracic rings. This is addressed through a multimodal treatment program, ensuring that any cognitive and/or emotional components are addressed along with physical impairments. An effective treatment program includes concurrent:

1. addressing impairments such as hypertonic muscles creating non-optimal force vectors on the thoracic rings (remove the old strategy) and
2. training new patterns of neuromuscular activity, balancing muscular synergies and building capacity (strength, endurance) for more optimal control of the thorax. Specific thoracic ring taping supports the exercise process.

Non-optimal force vectors on thoracic rings can arise from multiple structures attaching externally or internally anywhere around the three-dimensional ring. Most common are neuromuscular vectors, but impairments related to the visceral system, myofascial system and articular system are also possible. 'Thoracic ring vector analysis'[32] assesses the location and type of system vectors. The driving rings (usually two sequential thoracic rings) are corrected and 'stacked' into optimal alignment and the location and quality of the resistance to the correction are evaluated. Specific treatment to the structures identified as creating the resistance can then be applied. Tools such as specific myofascial and neuromuscular release, dry needling, muscle energy, mobilization and manipulation can be successful in addressing these impairments. However, often multiple vectors are present. A novel treatment technique, 'thoracic ring stack and breathe',[32] simultaneously releases multiple vectors around and between the thoracic rings, and can be progressed to dynamic contexts to combine release and neuromuscular training (Fig. 44-7).

Notably, it is common to find strong vectors from hypertonicity of muscles positioned laterally and anteriorly around the thoracic rings (e.g. intercostals, serratus anterior, pectoralis minor, oblique abdominals, diaphragm). In these cases, if treatment techniques are focused only posteriorly (e.g. to the erector spinae or posterior articular structures), there is potential to increase imbalances around the thoracic ring and create more dysfunction, even if those levels are the underlying driver. When intercostal hypertonicity is present, assessment and treatment of the two related sequential thoracic rings is essential. If treatment is focused to just one of the thoracic rings, there is potential to make the other ring more dysfunctional. This highlights the importance of assessing force vectors around the entire thoracic ring.

Evaluation of neuromuscular strategies for the thorax needs to include: segmental control (intra-ring and inter-ring), inter-regional control and control of postural equilibrium.[8,33] Exercise prescription is based on control impairments found on assessment. Based on anatomical attachments and research from other areas of the spine, it has been proposed that the deep segmental muscles such as thoracic multifidus and intercostals are architecturally suited to control intra-ring and inter-ring motion.[18] Imagery, visualization and sensory cues combined with specific thoracic ring taping are used to recruit the deep ring control muscles, and this skill is integrated with more complex movement patterns to train synergistic patterns with superficial, multisegmental muscles connecting the thoracic rings to other regions.[4,7,16–18,20]

If dysfunction has been present for any significant period of time, alterations in strength and synergies of muscles between the driving thoracic rings and connected regions will be present. For example, if the upper thoracic rings have functioned in left translation/right rotation, muscles on both sides of the shoulder girdle will have adapted. As old non-optimal patterns are removed, weakness in specific shoulder girdle muscles will become evident and need to be addressed. Exercises that train maintenance of thoracic ring control with shoulder girdle dissociation, both in open and closed chain progressions, provide an intermediate step to more complex movements. Discussion of specific thoracic ring exercise progressions and program design is beyond the scope of this section; however, a brief outline is provided in Table 44-2.

SUMMARY

Shifting from the paradigm that the thorax is stiff and requiring mobilization to one where the thorax is flexible and requiring optimal neuromuscular control provides greater insight into why the thorax can drive distal problems. This moves away from conceptualizing the thorax as a static, stiff box to being a dynamic stack of ten rings,

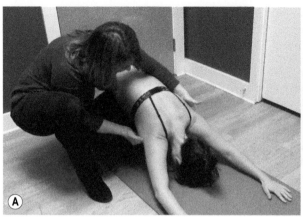
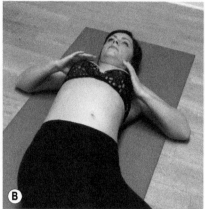
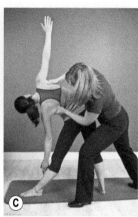

FIGURE 44-7 ■ 'Thoracic ring stack and breathe'.[32] This technique can be performed by the therapist in combination with specific muscle releases (such as the serratus anterior), or taught to patients as a self-release technique. The driving thoracic rings are corrected and manually controlled while different breathing patterns and movements of the trunk and extremities are used to tension different vectors acting on the rings. Over multiple cycles of deep breaths and through movement, the relevant vectors are released, creating a platform to train new muscle recruitment patterns. (**A**) Thoracic ring stack and breathe of rings 3/4 while moving through child's pose to release vectors between the shoulder girdle/arms and the driving thoracic rings. (**B**) Self-stack and breathe of rings 3/4 – the patient self-corrects two sequential thoracic rings on opposite sides, and over several breath cycles moves the pelvis/hips into rotation to release vectors between the driving thoracic rings and the lumbopelvic–hip region. (**C**) Dynamic thoracic ring stack and breathe – the driving thoracic rings are corrected while the patient moves into a functional task and breathes in different patterns. The therapist can modify this to become a training exercise for thoracic ring control by modulating the degree of support and correction provided, giving primarily sensory input and less manual correction support so that the patient actively controls the thoracic rings during movement. (Reproduced with permission from Linda-Joy Lee Physiotherapist Corp.)

TABLE 44-2   **Categories to Consider for Thoracic Ring Exercise Progressions and Program Design**

Segmental control	Intra-ring and inter-ring	Deep muscles; optimal recruitment evidenced by change in ring position and control in response to verbal cues and without superficial muscle activity
Inter-regional control	Thoracic rings – head Thoracic rings – shoulder girdle Include open and closed chain Inversion postures are key to train vertical loading capacity in thorax (e.g. downward dog modified with knees bent → wall handstands → handstand push-ups on wall) Thoracic rings – lumbopelvic/hip (trunk control)	Maintain neutral thoracic ring stacking and dissociate from head movement, shoulder girdle movement (e.g. head rotation, supine horizontal shoulder abduction) Maintain neutral trunk position → during lower extremity challenges (e.g. squats, split squats) → during upper extremity challenges (e.g. wall push-ups, bench push-ups) → combined upper/lower extremity challenges (e.g. front medicine ball throws) Dissociate thoracic ring control in rotation/side-bending patterns – both congruent and incongruent from other regions (e.g. bow and arrow with pulley, lateral medicine ball throws, walking lunges with contralateral trunk rotation)
Postural equilibrium	Thoracic rings – feet (base of support)	Use challenges to postural equilibrium and trunk control in coronal plane (lateral perturbations) while ensuring optimal thoracic ring alignment and control (e.g. deep lateral lunges, star lunges, lateral hops)
Thoracic spring	Ensure thoracic ring control while maintaining vertical space and without bracing or rigidity	Jump squats, lateral hops, skipping

much like a 'slinky' or a shock-absorbing spring. When there is loss of optimal sequencing, force modulation, and synergy between the muscles around the thoracic ring, between the ten thoracic rings and between the rings and other regions of the body, there are many possible consequences throughout the whole body.

The Thoracic Ring Approach™[16,17] incorporates current research on the thorax and provides innovative clinical assessment and treatment skills for the thorax, as well as a clinical reasoning framework that considers the multiple connections between the thorax and other regions of the body. Patients present with non-optimal strategies for their meaningful task that are linked to non-optimal experiences of their body. In thorax-driven cases, treating the thoracic ring(s) in the context of a biopsychosocial model provides the pathway to change these non-optimal strategies and create a positive experience of movement, reconceptualize pain and support optimal strategies for function and performance for the whole person.

REFERENCES

1. Bergman GJD, Winters JC, van der Heijden GJMG, et al. Groningen Manipulation Study. The effect of manipulation of the structures of the shoulder girdle as additional treatment for symptom relief and for prevention of chronicity or recurrence of shoulder symptoms. Design of a randomized controlled trial within a comprehensive prognostic cohort study. J Manipulative Physiol Ther 2002;25(9):543–9.
2. Cleland JA, Glynn P, Whitman JM, et al. Short-term effects of thrust versus nonthrust mobilization/manipulation directed at the thoracic spine in patients with neck pain: a randomized clinical trial. Phys Ther 2007;87(4):431–40.
3. McConnell J. The use of taping for pain relief in the management of spinal pain. In: Boyling JD, Jull GA, et al., editors. Grieve's Modern Manual Therapy: The Vertebral Column. 3rd ed. Edinburgh: Elsevier Churchill Livingstone; 2005. p. 433–42.
4. Lee LJ. Thoracic Stabilization & the Functional Upper Limb: Restoring Stability with Mobility. Vancouver, BC: Course Notes; 2003.
5. Lee LJ. A clinical test for failed load transfer in the upper quadrant: how to direct treatment decisions for the thoracic spine, cervical spine, and shoulder complex. Proceedings of the 2005 Orthopaedic Symposium of the Canadian Physiotherapy Association. London, Ontario, Canada: 2005.
6. Lee LJ. The Role of the Thorax in Pelvic Girdle Pain. Presented at the 6th Interdisciplinary World Congress on Low Back and Pelvic Pain. Barcelona, Spain: 2007 November 7–10.
7. Lee LJ, Lee DG. An integrated multimodal approach to the thoracic spine and ribs. In: Magee DJ, et al., editors. Pathology and Intervention in Musculoskeletal Intervention. Elsevier; 2008.
8. Lee LJ. Motor Control and Kinematics of the Thorax in Pain-Free Function. Australia: University of Queensland; 2013.
9. Giles LGF, Singer KP. The Clinical Anatomy and Management of Thoracic Spine Pain, the Clinical Anatomy and Management of Back Pain Series. Oxford: Butterworth-Heinemann; 2000.
10. Lee DG. Manual Therapy for the Thorax. 1st ed. DOPC, British Columbia: Diane G. Lee Physiotherapist Corp.; 1994.
11. Maitland GD. Vertebral Manipulation. London: Butterworths; 1964.
12. Mitchell FL, Mitchell PKG. The Muscle Energy Manual – Evaluation and Treatment of the Thoracic Spine, Lumbar Spine & Rib Cage. 2nd ed. East Lansing, Michigan: MET press; 2002.
13. Standring S. Gray's Anatomy: The Anatomical Basis of Clinical Practice. 40th ed. Edinburgh: Churchill Livingstone; 2008.
14. Molnar S, Mano S, Kiss L, et al. Ex vivo and in vitro determination of the axial rotational axis of the human thoracic spine. Spine (Phila Pa 1976) 2006;31(26):E984–91.
15. Lee L-J, Chang AT, Coppieters MW, et al. Changes in sitting posture induce multiplanar changes in chest wall shape and motion with breathing. Respir Physiol Neurobiol 2010;170(3):236–44.
16. Lee LJ. Discover the Role of the Thorax in Total Body Function: Introduction to the Thorax 'Ring Approach'. Bergen, Norway: Course Notes; 2011.
17. Lee LJ. The Essential Role of the Thorax in Whole Body Function and the 'Thoracic Ring Approach', Assessment & Treatment Videos. Linda-Joy Lee Physiotherapist Corp; 2012 <www.ljlee.ca>.
18. Lee LJ. Chapter 7: Restoring force closure/motor control of the thorax. In: Lee DG, editor. The Thorax An Integrated Approach. White Rock, BC: Diane G. Lee Physiotherapist Corporation; 2003b.
19. Keene C. Some experiments on the mechanical rotation of the normal spine. J Bone Joint Surg 1906;s2–4(1):69–79.
20. Lee LJ. The essential role of the thorax in restoring optimal function. Keynote presentation at the 2008 Orthopaedic Symposium of the Canadian Physiotherapy Association. Montreal, Canada: 2008.
21. Zazulak BT, Hewett TE, Reeves NP, et al. Deficits in neuromuscular control of the trunk predict knee injury risk: a prospective biomechanical-epidemiologic study. Am J Sports Med 2007;35(7):1123–30.
22. Lee LJ, Lee DG. Chapter 7: Clinical practice – the reality for clinicians. In: Lee DG, editor. The Pelvic Girdle. Elsevier; 2011. p. 255–82.
23. Geelhoed MA, McGaugh J, Brewer PA, et al. A new model to facilitate palpation of the level of the transverse processes of the thoracic spine. J Orthop Sports Phys Ther 2006;36(11):876–81.
24. Takeuchi T, Abumi K, Shono Y, et al. Biomechanical role of the intervertebral disc and costovertebral joint in stability of the thoracic spine. A canine model study. Spine (Phila Pa 1976) 1999;24(14):1414–20.
25. Gregersen GG, Lucas DB. An in vivo study of the axial rotation of the human thoracolumbar spine. J Bone Joint Surg Am 1967;49(2):247–62.
26. Lovett R. The mechanism of the normal spine and its relation to scoliosis. Boston Med Surg J 1905;153:349–58.
27. Watkins R 4th, Watkins R 3rd, Williams L, et al. Stability provided by the sternum and rib cage in the thoracic spine. Spine (Phila Pa 1976) 2005;30(11):1283–6.
28. Lee L-J, Coppieters MW, Hodges PW. Differential activation of the thoracic multifidus and longissimus thoracis during trunk rotation. Spine 2005;30:870–6.
29. Lee L-J, Coppieters MW, Hodges PW. Anticipatory postural adjustments to arm movement reveal complex control of paraspinal muscles in the thorax. J Electromyogr Kinesiol 2009;19(1):46–54.
30. Lee L-J, Coppieters MW, Hodges PW. En bloc control of deep and superficial thoracic muscles in sagittal loading and unloading of the trunk. Gait Posture 2011;33(4):588–93.
31. Bialosky JE, Bishop MD, Price DD, et al. The mechanisms of manual therapy in the treatment of musculoskeletal pain: a comprehensive model. Man Ther 2009;14(5):531–8.
32. Lee LJ. Discover the Thorax – Level 1: Inter-ring Rotational Control for Optimal Trunk Function. Vancouver, BC: Course Notes; 2009.
33. Hodges PW. Neuromechanical control of the spine. Department of Neuroscience. Stockholm, Sweden: Karolinska Institutet; 2003.

CHAPTER 44.3 ■ MANAGEMENT OF THE THORACIC SPINE IN PATIENTS WITH COPD

Nicola Heneghan

Chronic obstructive pulmonary disease (COPD) is a common progressive, preventable and treatable disease, characterized by persistent airflow limitation and associated with an enhanced chronic inflammatory response. Primarily a disease of the lungs, the impact on other body systems, including the musculoskeletal system, is now widely reported, contributing to functional impairments and increased mortality.[1–3]

It is conceivable that some of these co-morbidities may themselves adversely affect pulmonary function, when viewing the respiratory system as a 'whole' (i.e. lungs and related musculoskeletal structures). Collagen degradation or vertebral fractures, which are prevalent in COPD, are likely detrimental to pulmonary function due to pain and thoracic cage restriction.[4] Likewise hyperinflation, a common feature of COPD, results in the ribs adopting a more horizontal orientation, which in turn may contribute to chest wall rigidity and impair inspiratory muscle action.[5]

Evidence-based non-pharmacological management of stable COPD is currently limited to smoking cessation and pulmonary rehabilitation.[3] Pulmonary rehabilitation combines education, psychosocial support and physical exercise, with the latter of these being thought to afford the greatest benefit.[3,6] Generally, physical exercise in pulmonary rehabilitation aims to develop physiological capacity through activities such as stair climbing or walking, rather than promote 'flexibility'. A number of authors have postulated that interventions aimed at increasing chest wall flexibility through 'active therapeutic exercise' or 'passive hands-on manual therapy' may be beneficial to reduce the work of breathing.[7-11]

ANATOMY AND BIOMECHANICS

There are over 112 muscles with attachments directly or indirectly to the thoracic rib cage and through their anatomical relations, likely have a role in supporting respiratory function under normal or abnormal conditions. Grazzini et al.[12] propose an overall shift in the relative contribution that respiratory muscles make to pulmonary function with advancing COPD and a greater involvement of the rib cage; a consequence of physiological and structural diaphragmatic insufficiency. Activation of the accessory respiratory muscles may result in clinically observed postural changes, including a forward head posture and protracted and elevated shoulder girdles.[5,13] While secondary or beneficial for ventilation in the short term, these musculoskeletal adaptations may alter cervicothoracic biomechanics, resulting in musculoskeletal pathologies and pain.[5] It is therefore conceivable that these changes may themselves adversely affect respiratory function.

The thoracic spine provides support posteriorly, and an anchorage for the ribs, thus facilitating respiration in healthy subjects. With the ribs being inextricably linked to the thoracic spine via the costovertebral and costotransverse joints, it is conceivable that abnormalities in spinal motion or posture may exert some influence on pulmonary function. Although in theory it appears reasonable to suppose that changes to musculoskeletal structures such as bones, joints, posture and muscles in the thoracic region have the potential to influence pulmonary function through mechanical alterations, little attention has been given to evaluating this.

RELATIONSHIP BETWEEN THE MUSCULOSKELETAL SYSTEM AND PULMONARY FUNCTION

Most of what is known of this relationship has emerged from research demonstrating reduced pulmonary function in idiopathic spinal scoliosis[14] and osteoporosis.[15] Leong et al.[14] investigated spinal stiffness and compared chest cage motion in young healthy individuals compared to those with scoliosis during a deep breath. They concluded that spinal stiffness contributes to pulmonary dysfunction, with structural abnormalities leading to reduced lung volume, impaired rib movement and altered respiratory muscle mechanics. Harrison et al.[15] concluded from a systematic review of four case-control studies that osteoporosis-related kyphosis was associated with impairment of pulmonary function. Furthermore, the observed pulmonary dysfunction appeared related to the number of vertebral fractures and kyphosis with one study reporting a moderately strong negative association between kyphosis angle and FEV_1.

Altered respiratory biomechanics and pulmonary dysfunction is also evident in older adults. While multifactorial in nature, musculoskeletal changes are highly prevalent and include costal cartilage calcification, costovertebral joint degeneration and decrease in intervertebral space with disc degeneration and respiratory muscle fibre changes.[16-18] Collectively these changes may restrict lung expansion and/or partly explain the observed reduction in total lung capacity seen in older adults.[19] This 'restrictive' pulmonary disorder is in contrast to the airflow obstruction found in COPD, where reduced airflow is secondary to inflammation in the airways.

SYMPTOMATIC FEATURES OF COPD

While dyspnoea is the main symptomatic feature of COPD, cervicothoracic pain has also been recently reported in this patient population,[20] perhaps as a consequence of musculoskeletal structural changes and dysfunction. Recent work by Bentsen et al.[21] reported that prevalence of pain (predominantly neck, shoulders and chest), a common feature of musculoskeletal conditions, was notably higher in patients with COPD (45%) compared to the general population (34%). This is unsurprising given the observed use of accessory respiratory muscles in COPD relating to dyspnoea[20,21] and the adoption of a forward neck posture to open the airways.[5] Interestingly though, Bentsen et al.[21] reported that many COPD subjects had used transcutaneous electrical nerve stimulation/acupuncture to assist in pain management as opposed to other forms of physiotherapy, such as manual therapy or therapeutic exercise.

MANAGEMENT OF COPD TO IMPROVE FLEXIBILITY

Manual Therapy: Passive Interventions

There are a number of studies describing the use of manual therapy techniques for the management of COPD, mainly from the osteopathic and chiropractic literature.[7,8,22-25] Advocates of manual therapy propose that passive techniques, aimed at increasing thoracic mobility, may work to reduce the work of breathing through enhanced oxygen transport and lymphatic return.[7-11] While this theory has not been systematically investigated in COPD, a myofascial release technique did affect heart rate variability (a measure of autonomic activity) in healthy subjects.[26] Henley et al.[26] propose that manual therapy induces autonomic activity resulting in vasodilation, smooth muscle relaxation and increased blood flow. It is proposed that these neurophysiological effects may then facilitate muscle length gains, decrease in pain perception and/or change in tissue tension.

A systematic review of the evidence for the effects of passive manual therapy interventions on pulmonary function in subjects with COPD identified that there is little evidence to currently support or refute the use of manual therapy interventions in the management of COPD.[27] Key problems with the included studies were poor methodological quality of both reporting and conduct of studies; heterogeneity of study type, population, interventions and outcomes; and inadequate statistical analysis and inadequate length of follow-up. Additionally the focus on performance-based measures did not allow for patient-reported measures of well-being such as quality of life or breathlessness to be evaluated. The findings from this review are similar to reviews in asthma, which report that there is insufficient evidence to support or refute use of manipulative therapy in asthma.[9,28]

Exercise: Active Interventions

Respiratory muscle stretch gymnastics (RMSG) is a series of five therapeutic active exercises or 'patterns' of movement (see Box 44-2 and Fig. 44-8) which aims to reduce dyspnoea through increased chest wall flexibility of muscles directly or indirectly related to respiration.[29–31]

BOX 44-2 Respiratory Muscle Stretch Gymnastics

Respiratory Muscle Stretch Gymnastics to be performed in order four times a day[31]
Pattern 1. Elevating and pulling back the shoulders: As you slowly breathe in through your nose, gradually elevate and pull back both shoulders. After taking a deep breath, slowly breathe out through your mouth, relax and lower your shoulders.
Pattern 2. Stretching the upper chest: Place both hands on your upper chest. Pull back your elbows and pull down your chest while lifting your chin and inhaling a deep breath through your nose. Expire slowly through your mouth and relax.
Pattern 3. Stretching the back muscle: Hold your hands in front of your chest. As you slowly breathe in through your nose, move your hands front wards and down, and stretch your back. After deep inspiration, slowly breathe out and resume the original position.
Pattern 4. Stretching the lower chest: Hold the ends of a towel with both hands outstretched at shoulder height. After taking a deep breath, move your arms up while breathing out slowly. After deep expiration, lower your hands and breathe normally.
Pattern 5. Elevating the elbow: Hold one hand behind your head. Take a deep breath through your nose. While slowly exhaling through your mouth, stretch your trunk by raising your elbow as high as is easily possible. Return to the original position while breathing normally. Repeat the process using the alternate hand behind the head.

While RMSG studies used small sample sizes ($n = 12$ for each), these small pre–post[32] and randomized controlled trial[31] studies demonstrate that RMSG may afford some therapeutic benefit in COPD management. Performance-based measures, including the 6-minute walking test, improved significantly with RMSG, with studies reporting a statistically significant increase in distance covered.[31,32] Patient-reported measures of effect also improved with a reduction in dyspnoea at the end of the 6-minute walk[32] and improvements in quality of life were also reported for the RMSG intervention.[32]

Research of exercise to improve pulmonary function in ankylosing spondylitis may provide some support for its inclusion in COPD management.[33,34] Two studies compared usual care with a 3-month home-based programme of spinal flexibility exercises[33,34] and, in the case of Aytekin et al.,[34] they also had a third trial arm that comprised a Global Postural Re-education (GPR®) programme. Both studies found significant improvements in pulmonary function, pain and flexibility in the intervention groups.[33,34] Aytekin et al.[34] reported even more favourable results for the GPR® programme compared with the conventional spinal flexibility programme. GPR® is a physical therapy method developed by Philippe-Emmanuel Souchard (France). The rationale being that fascia exerts an influence on individual muscles that operate concurrently in body regions to facilitate functional movement, also known as 'kinetic chains'. These chains comprise partly of non-contractile tissues and are therefore susceptible to adaptive shortening.[35,36] The aim of GPR® programmes is to stretch the shortened kinetic chains using 15–20-minute stretch holds in one of eight therapeutic postures; it uses the principles of creep, a property of viscoelastic tissue. This is in contrast to a more conventional stretching programme, which targets muscles in isolation, using a timed period counted in seconds. To minimize the development of postural asymmetry, contraction of the antagonist muscles is incorporated into the programme. Evaluation of the content of the GPR® programme would suggest the programme may be suitable for enhancing pulmonary function through the inclusion of specific strengthening and flexibility exercises of 'shortened' muscles, postural muscles, respiratory muscles and trunk muscles.[35] Aside from differences in the programme content and stretch duration, GPR® does share similarities to RMSG. Teodori et al.[36] concluded from a systematic review of the available evidence that GPR® may enhance respiratory muscle strength and chest wall mobility, although no studies of GPR® in patients with respiratory disease or dysfunction have yet been identified.

There are several research reports evaluating the effectiveness of pulmonary rehabilitation in clinically diagnosed restrictive lung disease.[37–39] While results on the whole were favourable and comparable to results of pulmonary rehabilitation in COPD, recruitment was principally based on a restrictive pattern of ventilation from spirometry testing.[38,39] Consequently, there is considerable sample heterogeneity across studies, ranging from interstitial lung disease (pulmonary fibrosis) to non-fibrotic restrictive lung diseases of musculoskeletal origin. This limits the strength of conclusions that can be made

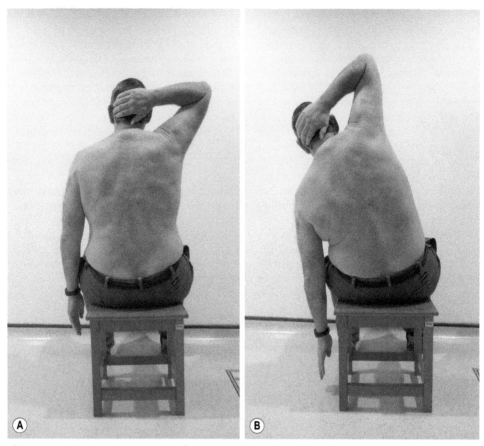

FIGURE 44-8 ■ Respiratory muscle stretch gymnastics. Pattern 5. **(A)** Subject places hand behind head and take a deep breath through the nose. **(B)** While slowly exhaling through the mouth, the subject stretches their trunk by raising the right elbow as high as possible. Subject holds this position and then returns to the original position while breathing normally. This is then repeated for the opposite side.

when discussing restrictive lung diseases of differing aetiology and mechanism. Common across all studies and, in line with other pulmonary rehabilitation studies, the exercise component was focused on developing physiological capacity.[37–39] Justification for rehabilitation being 'solely' focused on developing physiological capacity is questionable given the majority of the sample in one study had restriction of musculoskeletal origin ($n = 20$ from a total sample of 31 had chest wall disease, such as kyphoscoliosis).[39] Naji et al.[37] did, however, differentiate between subjects with interstitial lung disease and skeletal abnormalities, although, with small numbers in each group ($n = 11$, $n = 4$, respectively) and high attrition, they concluded there was much still to be learned, including a question linked to appropriateness of one programme for both groups.

There is a small body of evidence that has sought to evaluate the adjunctive use of a flexibility exercise programme in promoting respiratory biomechanics in the form of RMSG in COPD and GPR® in healthy subjects. While COPD is primarily an obstructive lung disease there appears sufficient evidence to support further research into interventions which promote flexibility of the thoracic cage.

With growing evidence of co-morbid musculoskeletal changes, manual therapy, in the broadest sense may afford some therapeutic benefit to individuals with COPD. Management of such dysfunction, asymptomatic or symptomatic, may complement current approaches to pulmonary rehabilitation where development of physiological capacity is the main focus.

REFERENCES

1. Cooper CB, Dransfield M. The COPD patient in primary care – part 4: understanding the clinical manifestations of a progressive disease. Am J Med 2008;121:S33–44.
2. Barnes PJ, Celli BR. Systemic manifestations and comorbidities of COPD. Eur Respir J 2009;33:1165–85.
3. Global Strategy for the Diagnosis, Management and Prevention of COPD, Global Initiative for Chronic Obstructive Lung Disease (GOLD). 2011 <http://www.goldcopd.org/>; [Accessed 4/1/12].
4. Patel ARC, Hurst JC. Extrapulmonary comorbidities in chronic obstructive pulmonary disease: state of the art. Expert Rev Respir Med 2011;5(5):647–61.
5. Courtney R. The functions of breathing and its dysfunction and their relationship to breathing therapy. Int J Osteopath Med 2009;12:78–85.
6. American Thoracic Society, European Respiratory Society (ATS/ERS) statement on pulmonary rehabilitation. Am J Respir Crit Care Med 2006;173:1390–413.
7. Miller WD. Treatment of visceral disorders by manipulative therapy. In: Goldstein M, editor. The Research Status of Spinal Manipulative Therapy. Bethesda: Dept. HEW; 1975. p. 295–301.
8. Masarsky CS, Weber M. The influence of vertebral manipulation in the management of patients with COPD. JMPT 1988;11:505–10.
9. Hondras MA, Linde K, Jones AP. Manual Therapy for Asthma (Review) 2008. The Cochrane Collaboration. Issue 3 <http://www.cochrane.org/>; [Accessed 4/5/2011].

10. Putt MT, Watson M, Seale H, et al. Muscle stretching technique increases vital capacity and range of motion in patients with chronic obstructive pulmonary disease. Arch Phys Med Rehabil 2008;89(6):1103–7.

11. Noll DR, Johnson JC, Baer RW, et al. The immediate effect of individual manipulation techniques on pulmonary function measures in persons with COPD. Osteopath Med Prim Care 2009;3(9):1–12.

12. Grazzini M, Stendardi L, Gigliotti F, et al. Pathophysiology of exercise dyspnoea in healthy subjects and in patients with chronic obstructive pulmonary disease (COPD). Respir Med 2005;99:1403–12.

13. Chaitow L, Gilbert C, Bradley D. Multidisciplinary Approaches to Breathing Pattern Disorders. Churchill Livingstone; 2002.

14. Leong JCY, Lu WW, Luk KDK, et al. Kinematics of the chest cage and spine during breathing in healthy individuals and in patients with adolescent idiopathic scoliosis. Spine 1999;24(13):1310–15.

15. Harrison RA, Siminoski K, Vethanayagam D, et al. Osteoporosis-related kyphosis and impairments in pulmonary function: a systematic review. J Bone Miner Res 2007;22(3):447–57.

16. Nathan H, Weinberg G, Robin GC, et al. The costovertebral joints, anatomical – clinical observations in arthritis. Arthritis Rheum 1964;7:228–40.

17. Edmondston SJ, Singer KP. Thoracic spine: anatomical and biomechanical considerations for manual therapy. Man Ther 1997;2(3):132–43.

18. Britto RR, Zampa CC, de Oliveira TA, et al. (2007) Effects of the aging process on respiratory function. Gerontology 1997;55:505–10.

19. Scarlata S, Costanzo L, Giua R, et al. Diagnosis and prognostic value of restrictive ventilatory disorders in the elderly: a systematic review of the literature. Exp Gerontol 2012;47:281–9.

20. Lohne V, Heer HC, Andersen M, et al. Qualitative study of pain of patients with chronic obstructive pulmonary disease. Heart Lung 2010;39(3):226–34.

21. Bentsen SB, Rustøen T, Miaskowski C. Prevalence and characteristics of pain in patients with chronic obstructive pulmonary disease compared to the Norwegian general population. J Pain 2011;12(5):539–45.

22. Howell RK, Allen TW, Kappler RE. The influence of osteopathic manipulative therapy in the management of patients with chronic obstructive lung disease. JAOA 1975;74(8):757–60.

23. Witt PL, MacKinnon J. Trager psychophysical integration (TPI); A method to improve chest mobility of patients with chronic lung disease. Phys Ther 1986;66(2):214–17.

24. Noll DR, Degenhardt BF, Johnson JC, et al. Immediate effects of osteopathic manipulative treatment in elderly patients with chronic obstructive pulmonary disease. JAOA 2008;108(5):251–9.

25. Dougherty PE, Engel RM, Vemulpad S, et al. Spinal manipulative therapy for elderly patients with chronic obstructive pulmonary disease: a case series. J Manipulative Physiol Ther 2011;34(6):413–17.

26. Henley CE, Ivins D, Mills M. Osteopathic manipulative treatment and its relationship to autonomic nervous system activity as demonstrated by heart rate variability; a repeated measures study. Osteopath Med Prim Care 2008;2(7):1–8.

27. Heneghan NR, Balanos GM, Adab P, et al. Manual therapy for chronic obstructive airways disease: a systematic review of current evidence. Man Ther 2012;17(6):507–18.

28. Ernst E. Spinal manipulation for asthma: a systematic review of randomised clinical trials. Respir Med 2009;103(12):1791–5.

29. Ito M, Kakizaki F, Tsuzura Y, et al. Immediate effect of respiratory muscle stretch gymnastics and diaphragmatic breathing on respiratory pattern. Respiratory Muscle Conditioning Group. Intern Med 1999;38(2):126–32.

30. Kakizaki F, Shibuya M, Yamazaki T, et al. Preliminary report on the effects of respiratory muscle stretch gymnastics on chest wall mobility in patients with chronic obstructive pulmonary disease. Respir Care 1999;44:409–14.

31. Minoguchi H, Shibuya M, Miyagawa T, et al. Cross-over comparison between respiratory muscle stretch gymnastics and inspiratory muscle training. Intern Med 2002;41:805–12.

32. Yamada M, Kakizaki F, Sibuya M, et al. Clinical effects of four weeks of respiratory muscle stretch gymnastics in patients with chronic obstructive pulmonary disease. Nihon Kyobu Shikkan Gakkai Zasshi 1996;34(6):646–52.

33. Durmuş D, Alayli G, Uzun O, et al. Effects of two exercise interventions on pulmonary functions in the patients with ankylosing spondylitis. Joint Bone Spine 2009;76(2):150–5.

34. Aytekin E, Caglar NS, Ozgonenel L, et al. Home-based exercise therapy in patients with ankylosing spondylitis: effects on pain, mobility, disease activity, quality of life, and respiratory functions. Clin Rheumatol 2012;31(1):91–7.

35. Global Postural Re-education/ Rééducation Posturale Globale® (RPG®). 2012 <https://sites.google.com/site/rpguk123/home>; [Accessed 20/08/12].

36. Teodori RM, Negri JR, Cruz MC, et al. Global postural re-education: a literature review. Rev Bras Fisioter 2011;15(3):185–9.

37. Naji NA, Connor MC, Donnelly SC, et al. Effectiveness of pulmonary rehabilitation in restrictive lung disease. J Cardiopulm Rehabil 2006;26(4):237–43.

38. Kagaya H, Takahashi H, Sugawara K, et al. Effective home-based pulmonary rehabilitation in patients with restrictive lung diseases. Tohoku J Exp Med 2009;218(3):215–19.

39. Salhi B, Troosters T, Behaegel M, et al. Effects of pulmonary rehabilitation in patients with restrictive lung diseases. Chest 2010;137(2):273–9.

CHAPTER 45

LUMBAR SPINE

EDITOR'S INTRODUCTION

The topic of low back pain is enormous and numerous books have been written discussing assessment and a wide range of management approaches. The contemporary issue that has been chosen for discussion in this text recognizes the field of clinical research addressing the problem of heterogeneity in the presentation of patients with musculoskeletal disorders. Subgrouping of patients has been advocated as a method to address this heterogeneity. In theory and practice, patients who share similarities in presentation are grouped by predetermined criteria. The aim of this grouping is to better inform and direct specific therapeutic approaches deemed suitable for this group. Most development and research into subgrouping has occurred in relation to low back pain patients. This chapter on low back pain presents four subgrouping approaches to guide conservative management that have all been developed by physiotherapists from different areas of the world. However, from the perspective of the clinician they present four different and relatively distinct subgrouping approaches whose development has been based on differing criteria. Despite the differences, the research base for each subgrouping approach is growing, which suggests that all have some merit. The physiotherapists who have developed or who are international leaders in these approaches were invited to provide a chapter section that offers a brief overview of the respective subgrouping approach. This allows the reader to better understand, appraise and appreciate the differences and synergies in the approaches and look to current and future research proving the distinct benefit of subgrouping to low back pain patients and their outcomes. Another contemporary issue is training impairments in sensorimotor control that may accompany low back pain and how this is approached. Thus a chapter section explores current thinking and evidence about the role of motor control training in relation to low back pain.

CHAPTER 45.1   ■   THE McKENZIE METHOD OF MECHANICAL DIAGNOSIS AND THERAPY – AN OVERVIEW
Stephen May • Helen Clare

INTRODUCTION

The McKenzie method of mechanical diagnosis and therapy is a unique system of assessment and management, which can be used in the assessment of extremity and spinal musculoskeletal problems. Robin McKenzie first described the method for lumbar spine problems,[1] and then to address cervical and thoracic problems.[2] The original texts have recently been updated and augmented, with the addition of a book introducing the application of the method to patients with extremity musculoskeletal problems.[3–5]

The method uses repeated movements while symptomatic and mechanical responses are being monitored as the key source of information in the physical examination, and then uses these responses to classify patients into mechanical subgroups. The subgroups determine the management strategy, and are classified as derangement, dysfunction or postural syndrome. Patients not meeting the operational definitions for these syndromes can generally be classified in one of the 'other' syndromes. These concepts will be explored more fully below, and then the evidence for their use as a mechanism for determining management strategy will be discussed.

ASSESSMENT

It is important to emphasize that mechanical diagnosis and therapy is not just a system of management, it is primarily a system of assessment and classification. The history component of the assessment follows the usual format including questions about the patient, their problem, its site, whether symptoms are constant or intermittent, the history of the problem, what makes symptoms better or worse, any previous problems or treatments, medication history and questions about Red Flags, perhaps indicating serious spinal pathology that is not suitable for mechanical therapy.

For lumbar spine problems, the physical examination commences with observing posture, and in particular, noting the effect of posture correction on symptoms. If appropriate a neurological examination would be done as part of the baseline assessment. Single movements of flexion, extension and side-gliding are assessed and any pain noted. Side-gliding is assessed as this focuses movement on the lower lumbar spine. The baseline measures from the history and the physical examination are reassessed by the therapist to judge response to management.

The key part of the physical examination is the use of repeated movements. A number of repeated movements could be selected: flexion in standing or lying, extension in standing or lying and side-gliding in standing. However, all of these movements would not be tested in one session; the therapist's clinical decision making determines which movements are examined. In general it will be sagittal movements first as the majority of responses occur in this plane, especially extension. The exception to this is a patient who presents with an acute-onset lateral deformity, which would be addressed first. Sets of about ten repeated movements can be repeated four or five times to determine the response, before another movement might be examined. Operational definitions are provided in Box 45-1.

Repeated Movements

Before the repeated movements are commenced the state of the patient's symptoms are recorded, especially the most distal. After each set of repeated movements, patient's symptoms are monitored again. A series of terms

---

BOX 45-1	Operational Definitions for Mechanical Syndromes and 'Other'[4,5]

DERANGEMENT

- Centralization or progressive abolition of distal pain in response to therapeutic loading
- Each progressive abolition retained over time until all symptoms are abolished
- Back pain is also abolished
- Changes in pain remain better
- Accompanied by changes in mechanical presentation, such as increase in range of movement

ARTICULAR DYSFUNCTION

- Local pain only
- Intermittent pain only
- At least one movement is restricted and restricted movement consistently produces concordant pain at end-range
- No rapid reduction or abolition of symptoms
- No lasting production or peripheralization of symptoms.

CONTRACTILE DYSFUNCTION

- Intermittent pain only
- Concordant pain reproduced with resisted movement
- Active movements may also be painful

POSTURAL SYNDROME

- Local pain only
- Intermittent pain only
- Concordant pain with static loading
- Abolition of pain with postural correction
- No pain with repeated movements
- No loss of range of movement
- No pain during movement

OPERATIONAL DEFINITIONS FOR 'OTHER'

Spinal Stenosis

- Leg symptoms when walking, eased in flexion
- Minimal extension
- Sustained extension provokes leg symptoms

ISTHMIC SPONDYLOLISTHESIS

- Sports-related injury in adolescence
- Worse with static loading

HIP

- Pain on walking, eased with sitting
- Specific pain pattern
- Positive hip tests

SACROILIAC JOINT

- Three or more positive sacroiliac joint pain provocation tests

MECHANICALLY INCONCLUSIVE

- Inconsistent response to loading strategies
- No obstruction to movement

CHRONIC PAIN

- Persistent widespread pain
- Aggravation with all activity
- Exaggerated pain behaviour
- Inappropriate beliefs and attitudes about pain

are used during and after the movements to describe the symptom response; the emphasis and decision making is based on the latter.

The mechanical diagnosis and therapy assessment is initially based on patient exercises only, but both the assessment and the management process allow for *force progressions*, which happen in the following order: patient forces early through to end-range, patient forces end-range with patient overpressure, patient forces with therapist overpressure, and therapist mobilization. As indicated above the overpressures are only used if initial patient-generated forces have been inadequate to generate a clear response. The therapist might choose to test patient overpressures over a 24–48-hour assessment period prior to progressing forces. The initial mechanical diagnosis and therapy assessment is usually conducted in standing, but *force alternatives* include repeated movements in lying, and frontal plane movements, with side-gliding or rotation.

Evidence About the Assessment Process

A systematic review of 48 reliability studies on physical examination procedures for non-specific low back pain conducted on patient populations revealed that most procedures had limited reliability.[6] With an upper threshold of kappa/intra-class correlation coefficient of 0.85, most procedures demonstrated either conflicting evidence or moderate to strong evidence of low reliability. When a lower threshold was used (i.e. a kappa/intra-class correlation coefficient of 0.70), which is still regarded as good, only the procedure of pain response to repeated movements demonstrated moderate evidence for high reliability.

Pain responses to repeated movements, as used when testing for directional preference and centralization, demonstrated reasonably good levels of reliability, and therefore constitute a valid method of determining management strategies. Four studies examined the reliability of the McKenzie classification system itself; three reported kappa values of 0.7 or greater, one reported poor kappa values, but the therapists involved had limited knowledge of the classification system.[6] There is thus reasonable evidence for the reliability of the system among therapists trained in the method.

Several surveys involving over 1500 patients have been conducted with McKenzie-trained therapists to determine the proportions of patients classified in the different mechanical syndromes.[7–9] For lumbar spinal patients the most common classifications were derangement, range 67–75%; dysfunction, 4–6%; postural syndrome, 0–1%; and other, 8–18%. In the derangement category extension (70%), flexion (6%) and lateral movements (24%) centralized, decreased or abolished symptoms, respectively. The findings were very similar for the 111 cervical spine patients where 81% were classified with derangement, 1% as irreducible derangement, 8% with dysfunction, 3% with postural syndrome and 7% with other. Treatment directions for the derangements were also similar: extension (72%), flexion (9%) and lateral movements (19%).[8]

These data were gathered with very diverse methods and from various geographical sites, yet they showed a remarkable consistency. Some 80% or more of these spinal patients were classified into one of the mechanical syndromes of derangement, dysfunction or postural syndrome, with by far the largest group being those with derangement. It is to this classification subgroup that there is the wealth of evidence regarding the prognostic value of centralization and directional preference (see next section). Thus the largest mechanical syndrome subgroup has the most evidence supporting its use in assessment and management.

Evidence Regarding Prognosis

Distal or leg pain can come or go during the natural history of a back pain episode. This is not the same as centralization or directional preference, which must be demonstrated during repeated movements. Directional preference includes centralization but also a decrease in symptoms and/or an increase in a restricted movement in response to therapeutic loading. The distinction between natural history and something which is clinically induced is important as the positive evidence about these clinical phenomena has been derived from their clinically driven nature.

Within physiotherapy examination procedures, no other finding has the prognostic power of centralization, which is defined as the abolition of distal pain *in response to therapeutic loading*. A systematic review of 22 articles assessed the prognostic value of examination procedures. The only evidence for an examination procedure to inform management was for changes in pain location and/or intensity with repeated spinal movements.[10]

A recent systematic review located 54 articles regarding centralization and eight for directional preference.[11] Centralization had a prevalence rate of 44% in 4745 patients, with a higher rate in acute (74%) than subacute or chronic back pain (42%). The prevalence rate of directional preference was 70% in 2368 patients. In other words, these phenomena are commonly encountered clinically. Of 23 studies investigating the prognostic validity of centralization, 21 demonstrated a positive effect in those patients who demonstrated centralization, compared to those who did not. For both centralization and directional preference, seven out of eight studies provided evidence that they are useful treatment effect modifiers. This means that these assessment procedures are evidence-based ways of assessing appropriate management strategies based on these responses.

MANAGEMENT

The classification determines the management. For derangement, the patient performs exercises every 2 to 3 hours that centralize, decrease or abolish their symptoms. At the same time they avoid any sustained provocative positions. For instance, an extension responder might be advised to interrupt sitting every hour by standing and stretching backwards. For dysfunction, the patient performs exercises every 2 to 3 hours that reproduce their symptoms, but leaves them no worse afterwards. Clear advice needs to be given about the reason for doing the exercises (i.e. to remodel 'scar' tissue, the expected response, the need not to be worse after exercising and the need to continue the exercise for many weeks to see an improvement). For a postural syndrome, the patient is advised that it is their sustained, usually sitting posture that is the cause of their symptoms, and that they must interrupt this on a regular basis and should, when sitting, maintain a neutral lumbar posture.

Management is closely linked to the assessment process; the patient is given one exercise to perform on a regular basis, with clear reasoning about why they need to do that exercise or make that adjustment to their posture; and management is very patient-centred. The therapist plays the role of an assessor and advisor, the patient is the main player in their recovery. The therapist equips them with an appropriate exercise, the mechanical therapy component, and also clear reasoning for the exercise, the educational component.

Evidence Regarding Management

When evaluating treatment efficacy the ideal study design is the randomized controlled trial, with systematic reviews being used to analytically summarize this evidence. A number of systematic reviews are relevant in this context (Table 45-1). All are largely supportive of the McKenzie approach or classification-based approaches, though effect sizes are relatively small.

THE 'OTHER' SYNDROMES

As alluded to already, it is recognized that not every patient can be classified into one of the mechanical syndromes, and the ability to classify patients is also a reflection of a therapist's experience and training in the method. Box 45-1 presents a list of what is included in an 'other' category. As can be seen they tend to be more specific classifications. In one survey of 607 patients, 101 (17%) were classified as 'other' in the following ways: mechanically inconclusive 6%, chronic pain state <4%, post-surgery <2%, and Red Flags, stenosis, sacroiliac joint, trauma and spondylolisthesis all around 1% each.[7]

APPLICATION OF MECHANICAL DIAGNOSIS AND THERAPY IN THE CERVICAL SPINE

The principles outlined above apply in exactly the same way with patients with cervical and thoracic problems. As in the lumbar spine, baseline measures of range of movement and neurological status, if appropriate, are taken prior to repeated movements. Again repeated movements tend to start with sagittal plane movements, especially extension, with the key distinction being the importance

---

TABLE 45-1   Conclusions from Systematic Reviews Regarding Evidence for the McKenzie Method and Classification Systems

Reference	Number of RCTs	Remit	Conclusions
Clare et al. 2004[12]	6	Use of McKenzie principles Meta-analysis of data	Short term 8.6% greater reduction in pain, 5.4% greater reduction in disability than controls
Cook et al. 2005[13]	5, high quality (PEDro)	Therapeutic exercises with patients classified using symptom responses	Four out of five significantly better than control group
Machado et al. 2006[14]	11, mostly high quality	McKenzie method Meta-analysis of data	Short term 4.2% greater reduction in pain, 5.2% greater reduction in disability than controls
Slade and Keating 2007[15]	6, high quality	Unloaded exercises; four out of six McKenzie exercises	Short term mean difference favoured McKenzie for pain 0.36–0.63 and for function 0.45–0.47
Fersum et al. 2010[16]	5	Sub-classification systems and matched interventions for manual therapy and exercise	Sub-classification systems significantly better reduction in pain ($p = 0.004$) and disability ($p = 0.0005$) short term, long term for pain ($p = 0.001$)
Kent et al. 2010[17]	4, high quality	Targeted manual therapy or exercise therapy	One study showed McKenzie method had significantly better effects short term
Slater et al. 2012[18]	7, grade quality of evidence low	Sub-classification systems and matched intervention for manual therapy	Significant treatment effects favoured the classification-based treatment compared to controls in pain and disability short and medium term
Surkitt et al. 2012[19]	6–5, high quality (GRADE)	Management using directional preference (DP)	Moderate evidence that DP significantly more effective than controls at short and long term

RCT, Randomized controlled trial.

of retraction and protraction. Retraction involves end-range upper cervical flexion and lower cervical extension,[20] and therefore is regarded as an essential precursor to regaining extension in the cervical spine. Protraction involves end-range upper cervical extension and lower cervical flexion. As this tends to be the common posture assumed during slouched sitting, it is often a symptom provocative position. Repeated movement testing for the cervical spine is most commonly done in sitting in an upright sitting posture. In acute or very severe cases, repeated movements might need to be conducted in lying. In patients failing to regain extension, manual traction in lying might also be used. Home exercises are conducted in sitting or lying position, depending on the physical examination findings.

Regarding frontal plane movements in the cervical spine; two movements are considered: lateral flexion and rotation. The latter is theoretically more associated with upper cervical problems, and lateral flexion with lower cervical problems. In essence both movements are considered with all problems especially if it has been decided lateral rather than sagittal plane forces are needed.

There is much less relevant literature for the cervical spine compared to the lumbar spine. However, it has been noted already that derangement and centralization are commonly found in the cervical spine.[8,21]

CONCLUSIONS

The assessment process of mechanical diagnosis and therapy is indicated for all patients with musculoskeletal symptoms, many of whom will have mechanical syndromes and can be managed with the exercises described in the system. Patients with serious spinal pathology are screened and referred for specialist consultation. Patients with other syndromes are assessed and if they do not meet the criteria of the mechanical syndromes, they will require another evidence-based approach.

The research base for mechanical diagnosis and therapy is substantial and continues to grow. For a fuller reference list go to www.mckenziemdt.org.

REFERENCES

1. McKenzie RA. The Lumbar Spine Mechanical Diagnosis and Therapy. New Zealand: Spinal Publications; 1981.
2. McKenzie RA. The Cervical and Thoracic Spine Mechanical Diagnosis and Therapy. New Zealand: Spinal Publications; 1990.
3. McKenzie RA, May S. The Human Extremities Mechanical Diagnosis and Therapy. New Zealand: Spinal Publications; 2000.
4. McKenzie RA, May S. The Lumbar Spine Mechanical Diagnosis and Therapy. New Zealand: Spinal Publications; 2003.
5. McKenzie RA, May S. The Cervical and Thoracic Spine Mechanical Diagnosis and Therapy. New Zealand: Spinal Publications; 2006.
6. May S. Classification by McKenzie mechanical syndromes: a survey of McKenzie-trained faculty. J Manipulative Physiol Ther 2006;29:637–42.
7. May S, Littlewood C, Bishop A. Reliability of procedures used in the physical examination of non-specific low back pain: a systematic review. Aust J Physiother 2006;52:91–102.
8. Hefford C. McKenzie classification of mechanical spinal pain: profile of syndromes and directions of preference. Man Ther 2007;13:75–81.
9. Werneke MW, Hart D, Oliver D, et al. Prevalence of classification methods for patients with lumbar impairments using the McKenzie syndromes, pain pattern, manipulation and stabilization clinical prediction rules. J Man Manip Ther 2010;18:197–210.
10. Chorti AG, Chortis AG, Strimpakos N, et al. The prognostic value of symptom responses in the conservative management of spinal pain. A systematic review. Spine 2009;34:2686–99.
11. May S, Aina A. Centralization and directional preference: a systematic review. Man Ther 2012;17:497–506.
12. Clare HA, Adams R, Maher CG. A systematic review of efficacy of McKenzie therapy for spinal pain. Aust J Physiother 2004;50:209–16.
13. Cook C, Hegedus EJ, Ramey K. Physical therapy exercise intervention based on classification using the patient response method: a systematic review of the literature. J Man Manip Ther 2005;13:152–62.
14. Machado LAC, de Souza MvS, Ferreira PH, et al. The McKenzie Method for low back pain. A systematic review of the literature with a meta-analysis approach. Spine 2006;31:E254–62.
15. Slade SC, Keating J. Unloaded movement facilitation exercise compared to no exercise or alternative therapy on outcomes for people with non-specific chronic low back pain: a systematic review. J Manipulative Physiol Ther 2007;30:301–11.
16. Fersum KV, Dankaets W, O'Sullivan PB. Integration of sub-classification strategies in RCTs evaluating manual therapy treatment and exercise therapy for non-specific chronic low back pain: a systematic review. Br J Sports Med 2010;44:1054–62.
17. Kent P, Mjosund HL, Petersen DHD. Does targeting manual therapy and/or exercise improve patient outcomes in nonspecific low back pain? A systematic review. BMC Med 2010;8:22.
18. Slater SL, Ford JJ, Richards MC, et al. The effectiveness of subgroup specific manual therapy for low back pain: a systematic review. Man Ther 2012;17:201–12.
19. Surkitt LD, Ford JJ, Hahne AJ, et al. Efficacy of directional preference management for low back pain: a systematic review. Phys Ther 2012;92:652–65.
20. Ordway NR, Seymour RJ, Donelson RG, et al. Cervical flexion, extension, protrusion, and retraction. A radiographic segmental analysis. Spine 1999;24:240–7.
21. Werneke M, Hart DL, Cook D. A descriptive study of the centralisation phenomenon. A prospective analysis. Spine 1999;24:676–83.

CHAPTER 45.2 ■ MULTIDIMENSIONAL APPROACH FOR THE TARGETED MANAGEMENT OF LOW BACK PAIN

Peter O'Sullivan • Wim Dankaerts • Kieran O'Sullivan • Kjartan Fersum

THE FAILURE OF CURRENT PRACTICE

The biomedical approaches to managing low back pain (LBP) have led to an exponential increase in health-care costs, with a concurrent increase in disability and chronicity.[1,2] It has been proposed that this is due in part to the lack of person-centred management based on a validated approach to deal with heterogeneity in the LBP population, and the failure to adopt a biopsychosocial framework based on contemporary evidence.[3]

MULTIDIMENSIONAL CLINICAL REASONING FRAMEWORK FOR LBP

While many classification systems have been advocated in order to deal with the heterogeneity of LBP and enhance treatment matching, few have been validated and tested in randomized trials.[4] Most classification systems are criticized for being unidimensional and failing to reflect the biopsychosocial and heterogenous nature of LBP, thereby limiting the individualization of care.[5] In response to these limitations, a clinical reasoning framework (CRF) has been developed[6] that includes patient triage and incorporates a contemporary biopsychosocial understanding of LBP in order to identify modifiable and non-modifiable factors associated with a person's disorder, to target person-centred care. The CRF has evolved over time from the O'Sullivan classification system which initially focused more on movement control mechanisms,[7] to the CRF which incorporates a biopsychosocial clinical examination combined with screening questionnaires for prognostic risk factors[8,9] and review of radiological and medical investigations where appropriate. A strong therapeutic alliance underpins this process.[10] The different dimensions of the CRF have been published in detail previously,[11] including a detailed appendix in the randomized trial publication.[12] An outline of the different dimensions within the CRF is provided (Fig. 45-1).

Triage: On initial assessment, triage of patho-anatomical factors is required to identify the minority (1–2%) of people with LBP related to serious or systemic Red Flag pathology.[13] For another 5–10%, their LBP is associated with specific pathology with or without radicular features.[14] The remaining 85–90% of people with LBP demonstrate no specific pathology (non-specific LBP), and present with their own unique contributing factors across cognitive, psychosocial, physical and lifestyle domains.[15-19] While patho-anatomical factors such as advanced disc degeneration are associated with an increased risk of LBP,[20] they have a high prevalence in pain-free populations, are not strongly predictive of future LBP and correlate poorly with levels of pain and disability.[21-23] The adverse effects of early magnetic resonance imaging for LBP highlight the risk of iatrogenic disability if spinal imaging is not used sparingly and communicated carefully.[24-26] In the presence of specific pathologies, consideration of all other relevant biopsychosocial domains should also be part of the examination and management process.

Time course of the disorder: Differentiating acute LBP where there is a clear mechanism of injury and inflammatory component, from LBP related to other biopsychosocial factors causing tissue sensitization is important for targeted management (see Fig. 45-1). Frequently, LBP represents a recurrent disorder. Persistent LBP (PLBP) occurs when pain lasts beyond natural healing time (8–12 weeks), where pathology (for a small group), peripheral and central pain mechanisms and maladaptive cognitions, psychosocial factors and behaviours may perpetuate the pain state.

Neurophysiological factors: Pain characteristics reported by patients can range from *mechanically* to *non-mechanically provoked pain* and may reflect different underlying pain mechanisms, providing important directions for targeted rehabilitation and in some cases pharmacology.[27] There is growing evidence that both peripheral (bottom up) and central (top down) pain mechanisms are associated with LBP.[28,29] For example LBP that is localized, mechanically provoked and linked to maladaptive functional and lifestyle behaviours, resulting in abnormal tissue loading, may be associated with nociceptive and inflammatory pain features such as localized heat and pressure hyperalgesia.[30,31] In contrast, 'insidious' pain flares or PLBP linked to other pain and health co-morbidities and high levels of psychosocial and lifestyle stresses, is often widespread and non-mechanical in nature. This may present with either an absence of clinical signs or be associated with exaggerated pain responses to minor mechanical triggers with localized allodynia and/or widespread cold hyperalgesia.[30,32,33] While for some their pain characteristics appear clearly defined, LBP for many presents as a mixed picture reflecting a combination of both peripheral and central pain mechanisms (see Fig. 45-1).[6]

PLBP has also been associated with brain changes such as a loss of grey matter, increased resting brain state, changes in the sensorimotor cortex (i.e. body schema alterations) and loss of endogenous pain inhibition.[34] These factors may contribute to tissue sensitization, as well as altered motor output and movement disturbances, highlighting the important role of the central nervous

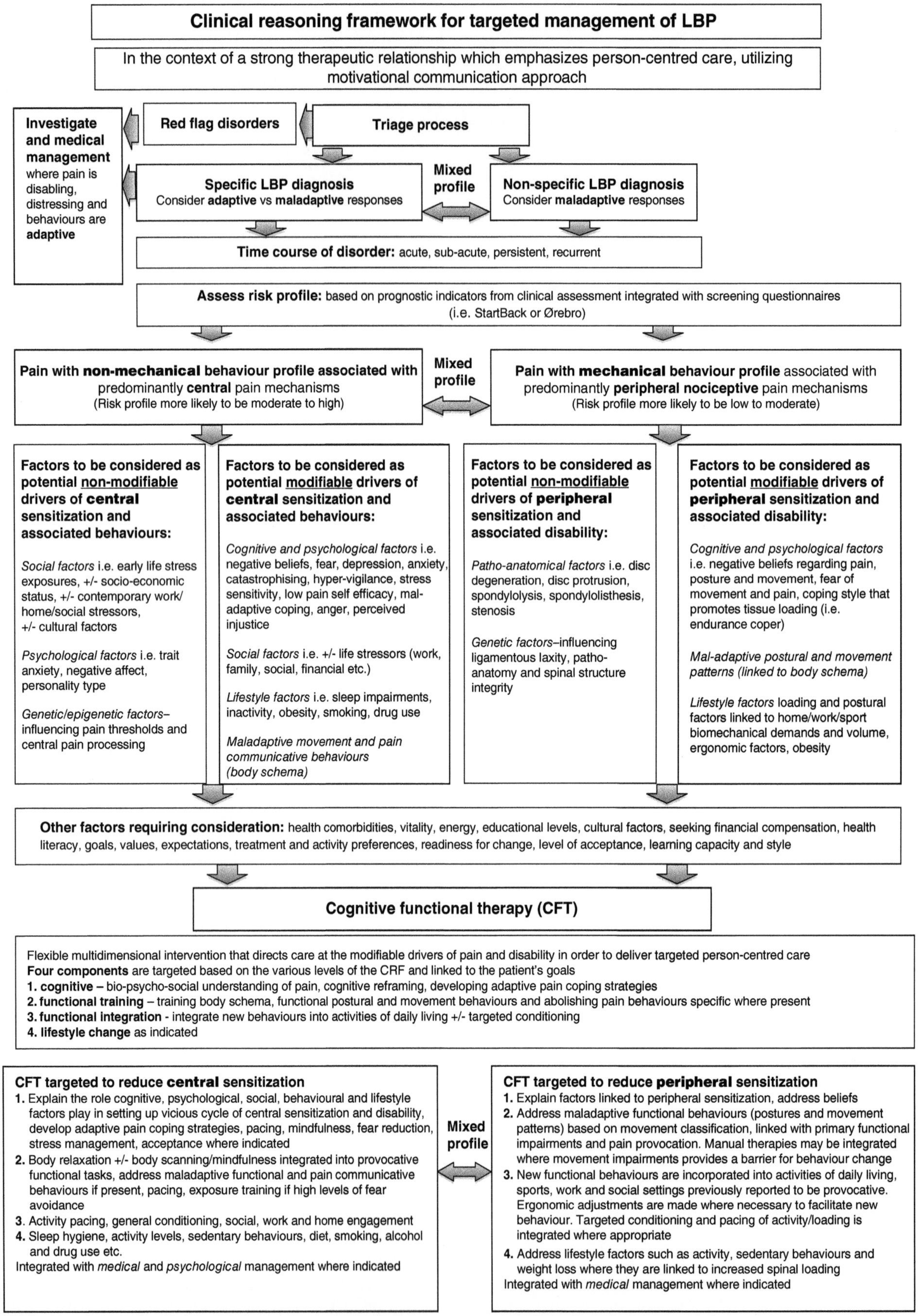

FIGURE 45-1 ■ Clinical reasoning framework for assessment and targeted management of low back pain (LBP). This framework provides an understanding of the clinical reasoning process which directs management towards the modifiable factors linked to the disorder based on prognostic risk factors and underlying pain mechanisms while taking into consideration non-modifiable factors and individual patient characteristics.

system in PLBP.[34,35] For health-care practitioners, gaining insight into pain mechanisms can be achieved through careful clinical examination, quantitative sensory testing and validated questionnaires.[27,36]

Cognitive factors such as negative LBP beliefs, catastrophizing and fear of movement are predictive of disability and are linked to PLBP.[37–40] Many of these negative beliefs gain their origins from health-care practitioners and can have a devastating impact on LBP trajectories.[24,41] **Psychological factors** such as anxiety and depressed mood are also commonly comorbid with PLBP.[42] These factors may act to reinforce maladaptive movement and lifestyle behaviours, enhancing sensitization and disability levels.[43] They may also lead to dysregulation of the hypothalamic–pituitary–adrenal axis, altering central pain processing and immune and neuroendocrine function, promoting central sensitization.[44,45] Screening for, and addressing, these factors is essential for targeted management.[8,9]

Social and cultural factors, although often non-modifiable, may have an influence on pain beliefs, coping and stress load and must be considered in the management of LBP.[43] **Work-related factors** should be investigated where a person is seeking compensation for pain or where work absenteeism or presenteeism are associated with the disorder.[46] Numerous **lifestyle factors** are modifiable and may contribute to both peripheral (via mechanical loading) and central pain mechanisms.[47] There is also evidence of the importance of **health and pain co-morbidities** with LBP and their role in influencing disability levels, general health status and chronicity, as well as providing barriers to management that require special consideration.[15,48,49] **Individual factors** such as the patient goals, preferences, health literacy, levels of acceptance, expectations and readiness for change are important when providing person-centred care in the assessment, management and prognosis of people with LBP.[39,43,50–53]

LBP disorders are frequently associated with pain-related functional behaviours such as altered postures and movement patterns linked to impairments of control, movement and loading.[17] Growing evidence suggests that these behaviours are often maladaptive and provocative in PLBP.[17,30] This is like a 'limp' for a sprained ankle that may be *adaptive* in the acute phase of a traumatic injury; however, when it persists past natural tissue healing time it becomes *maladaptive* and provocative. These behaviours are commonly associated with high levels of trunk muscle co-contraction (excessive 'stability'), are not stereotypical[17,30] and are linked with proprioceptive deficits[54,55] and altered body schema.[56–58] There is growing evidence that they can be characterized based on the presence of functional impairments and directional pain sensitization, providing an opportunity for targeted interventions.[36,59] **Deconditioning** may also occur secondary to activity avoidance, sedentary lifestyles and habitual postures, and may act to reinforce maladaptive movement behaviours associated with the disorder.[37,60] In contrast, endurance copers may present as over-conditioned through 'over activity'.[61] **Pain communicative behaviours** (overt facial and body expressions of pain) are also considered maladaptive in the context of PLBP (in the absence of pathology) and in some cases non-traumatic acute LBP.[62] They correlate with pain catastrophizing, providing opportunities for targeted behavioural management.[63]

There is also growing evidence to support the role genetic factors have on patho-anatomical (i.e. disc degeneration and prolapse) and pain vulnerability in specific populations.[64] While genetic testing is not currently available, family history should be considered in the CRF examination process.

CLINICAL REASONING FRAMEWORK FOR TARGETED MANAGEMENT OF LOW BACK PAIN

Rather than representing a rigid subgrouping system, the CRF provides a flexible framework, providing direction for person-centred clinical assessment and management as outlined in Figure 45-1. Indeed, many of these factors coexist, are not mutually exclusive and have the potential to both peripherally and centrally sensitize spinal structures, reinforcing disability behaviours in the presence or absence of spinal pathology. Some of these factors are modifiable while others are not. Consideration of the relative contribution of the different factors is important for targeted management (in some cases multidisciplinary) as well as realistic prognosis and goal setting.

COGNITIVE FUNCTIONAL THERAPY FOR THE TARGETED MANAGEMENT OF LOW BACK PAIN DISORDERS

Cognitive functional therapy (CFT) was specifically developed as an approach for targeting treatment in patients with LBP where (based on the CRF) maladaptive and modifiable cognitive, psychosocial, functional and lifestyle behaviours are considered provocative of their disorder (Fig. 45-1). The implementation of CFT is adapted to the risk and clinical profile of the patient in order to target both peripheral and central pain drivers of the disorder and associated disability. The primary aims of CFT are to provide a person-centred, biopsychosocial understanding of pain, enhance pain-coping strategies through cognitive restructuring, stress and threat reduction, pain control via targeted functional training and lifestyle change. The functional training is based on the movement classification and discouraging pain behaviours if present, in order to promote pain self-efficacy and confidence by normalizing movements and resuming activities previously avoided or reported as provocative. These are integrated into activities of daily living with physical activation (based on patient preference) in a graduated manner while addressing lifestyle and social factors (such as work) considered to contribute to the disorder. CFT can be integrated with medical management where pain levels dominate and/or psychological management where comorbid mental health disorders are a significant barrier to behavioural change.

Underpinning research has assessed the inter-tester reliability of different aspects of the CRF and shown substantial agreement between trained health-care professionals.[36,59] The efficacy of CFT in patients with PLBP, has been compared with physiotherapy-led exercise and manual therapy in a randomized trial, in primary care, demonstrating long-term benefits.[12] Further research is underway to assess CFT in different care and geographical settings.

The potential mechanisms underlying the therapeutic effect of CFT are likely to be multidimensional. Mediation analyses of the data from a randomized trial[12] show that reductions in pain intensity, improvements in mood and reductions in fear of work were associated with decreased disability. Qualitative data support these findings with people undergoing CFT reporting a changed mind set towards a biopsychosocial understanding of pain, pain controllability and enhanced self-efficacy to achieve lifestyle goals.[65] It is likely that both specific and non-specific treatment effects underpin this process.

SKILLS REQUIRED TO IMPLEMENT THE MULTIDIMENSIONAL APPROACH FOR INDIVIDUALIZED CARE

While the CRF lends itself to any health-care professional managing patients with LBP, CFT requires specific skills across a number of domains. The utilization of motivational interviewing techniques allows for the development of a strong therapeutic alliance within a biopsychosocial framework while identifying and targeting barriers for behavioural change. Diagnostic, observational and interpretive skills are required to triage patients and analyse functional and pain behaviours in order to determine adaptive from maladaptive behaviours. Targeted management requires clinicians to communicate effectively,[66] teach body relaxation strategies,[67] normalize functional movement patterns and discourage pain behaviours,[68] utilizing mindfulness[69] and motivational[70] principles for behavioural change. Feedback (visual, sensory and verbal)[71,72] and activity pacing[73] are components of this process. The biggest obstacle of adopting this approach is often casting off strongly held views that LBP reflects a purely structural problem of the spine, while confidently confronting pain behaviours in patients with pain. In the randomized trial an average of 100 hours of training including patient assessments and management was reported for experienced physiotherapists to reliably implement this approach.[12] Supporting publications, clinical workshops with patients and web-based resources (www.pain-ed.com) are available to assist this process.

SUMMARY

The CRF provides a multidimensional framework in order to diagnose LBP disorders to better target care. The strengths of the CRF, and CFT intervention, approach are that it provides a multidimensional, behaviourally orientated approach to targeted care for patients with LBP, shifting the focus away from treating the symptom of pain to providing clear targets for behavioural change, enhancing pain coping and positive adaptation. It utilizes screening questionnaires and therefore permits integration with other stratification approaches and can be combined with other treatments where indicated. Further research is required, and is ongoing, to further test the validity and clinical utility of this approach.

REFERENCES

1. Deyo RA, Mirza SK, Turner JA, et al. Overtreating chronic back pain: time to back off? J Am Board Fam Med 2009;22:62–8.
2. Dagenais S, Caro J, Haldeman S. A systematic review of low back pain cost of illness studies in the United States and internationally. Spine J 2008;8:8–20.
3. Borkan J, Van Tulder M, Reis S, et al. Advances in the field of low back pain in primary care: a report from the fourth international forum. Spine 2002;27:E128–32.
4. Foster NE, Hill JC, Hay EM. Subgrouping patients with low back pain in primary care: are we getting any better at it? Man Ther 2011;16:3–8.
5. Karayannis NV, Jull GA, Hodges PW. Physiotherapy movement based classification approaches to low back pain: comparison of subgroups through review and developer/expert survey. BMC Musculoskelet Disord 2012;13(1):24.
6. O'Sullivan P. It's time for change with the management of non-specific chronic low back pain. Br J Sports Med 2012;46:224–7.
7. O'Sullivan P. Lumbar segmental instability: clinical presentation and specific stabilizing exercise management. Man Ther 2000;5:2–12.
8. Hill JC, Dunn KM, Lewis M, et al. A primary care back pain screening tool: identifying patient subgroups for initial treatment. Arthritis Care Res 2008;59:632–41.
9. Hockings RL, McAuley JH, Maher CG. A systematic review of the predictive ability of the Orebro Musculoskeletal Pain Questionnaire. Spine 2008;33:E494–500.
10. Hall AM, Ferreira PH, Maher CG, et al. The influence of the therapist-patient relationship on treatment outcome in physical rehabilitation: a systematic review. Phys Ther 2010;90:1099–110.
11. O'Sullivan P. A classification based cognitive functional approach to managing nonspecific chronic low back pain. J Orthop Sports Phys Ther 2012;24:A17–21.
12. Vibe Fersum K, O'Sullivan P, Skouen J, et al. Efficacy of classification based cognitive functional therapy in patients with non-specific chronic low back pain – A randomized controlled trial. Eur J Pain 2013;17:916–28.
13. Henschke N, Maher CG, Refshauge KM, et al. Prevalence of and screening for serious spinal pathology in patients presenting to primary care settings with acute low back pain. Arthritis Rheum 2009;60:3072–80.
14. Koes BW, van Tulder M, Lin CW, et al. An updated overview of clinical guidelines for the management of non-specific low back pain in primary care. Eur Spine J 2010;19:2075–94.
15. Tschudi-Madsen H, Kjeldsberg M, Natvig B, et al. A strong association between non-musculoskeletal symptoms and musculoskeletal pain symptoms: results from a population study. BMC Musculoskelet Disord 2011;12:285.
16. Carroll LJ, Cassidy JD, Côté P. Depression as a risk factor for onset of an episode of troublesome neck and low back pain. Pain 2004;107:134–9.
17. Dankaerts W, O'Sullivan P, Burnett A, et al. Discriminating healthy controls and two clinical subgroups of nonspecific chronic low back pain patients using trunk muscle activation and lumbosacral kinematics of postures and movements: a statistical classification model. Spine 2009;34:1610–18.
18. Hayes C, Naylor R, Egger G. Understanding chronic pain in a lifestyle context the emergence of a whole-person approach. Am J Lifestyle Med 2012;6:421–8.

19. Crombez G, Vlaeyen JWS, Heuts PHTG, et al. Pain-related fear is more disabling than pain itself: evidence on the role of pain-related fear in chronic back pain disability. Pain 1999;80: 329–39.

20. Cheung KM, Karppinen J, Chan D, et al. Prevalence and pattern of lumbar magnetic resonance imaging changes in a population study of one thousand forty-three individuals. Spine 2009;34: 934–40.

21. Carragee EJ, Alamin TF, Miller JL, et al. Discographic, MRI and psychosocial determinants of low back pain disability and remission: a prospective study in subjects with benign persistent back pain. Spine J 2005;5:24–35.

22. Chou R, Fu R, Carrino JA, et al. Imaging strategies for low-back pain: systematic review and meta-analysis. Lancet 2009;373: 463–72.

23. Jarvik JG, Hollingworth W, Heagerty PJ, et al. Three-year incidence of low back pain in an initially asymptomatic cohort: clinical and imaging risk factors. Spine 2005;30:1541–8.

24. Lin IB, O'Sullivan PB, Coffin JA, et al. Disabling chronic low back pain as an iatrogenic disorder: a qualitative study in Aboriginal Australians. BMJ Open 2013;3(4), doi:10.1136/bmjopen-2013-002654.

25. Webster BS, Cifuentes M. Relationship of early magnetic resonance imaging for work-related acute low back pain with disability and medical utilization outcomes. J Occup Environ Med 2010;52: 900–7.

26. Sloan TJ, Walsh DA. Explanatory and diagnostic labels and perceived prognosis in chronic low back pain. Spine 2010;35:E1120–5.

27. Smart KM, Blake C, Staines A, et al. The discriminative validity of "nociceptive," "peripheral neuropathic," and "central sensitization" as mechanisms-based classifications of musculoskeletal pain. Clin J Pain 2011;27:655–63.

28. Üçeyler N, Zeller D, Kahn A-K, et al. Small fibre pathology in patients with fibromyalgia syndrome. Brain 2013;136:1857–67.

29. Woolf CJ. Central sensitization: Implications for the diagnosis and treatment of pain. Pain 2010;152:S2–15.

30. O'Sullivan P. Diagnosis and classification of chronic low back pain disorders: maladaptive movement and motor control impairments as underlying mechanism. Man Ther 2005;10:242–55.

31. Smart KM, Blake C, Staines A, et al. Mechanisms-based classifications of musculoskeletal pain: part 3 of 3: symptoms and signs of nociceptive pain in patients with low back (+/−leg) pain. Man Ther 2012;17:352–7.

32. O'Sullivan P, Waller R, Wright A, et al. Sensory Characteristics of Chronic Non-Specific Low Back Pain: A Subgroup Investigation. Austalian Physiotherapy Association Conference; October 17–20; Melbourne 2013.

33. Smart KM, Blake C, Staines A, et al. Mechanisms-based classifications of musculoskeletal pain: part 1 of 3: symptoms and signs of central sensitisation in patients with low back (±leg) pain. Man Ther 2012;17:336–44.

34. Wand B, Parkitny L, O'Connell N, et al. Cortical changes in chronic low back pain: current state of the art and implications for clinical practice. Man Ther 2011;16:15–20.

35. Moseley GL. Pain, brain imaging and physiotherapy–opportunity is knocking. Man Ther 2008;13:475–7.

36. Vibe Fersum K, O'Sullivan P, Kvåle A, et al. Inter-examiner reliability of a classification system for patients with non-specific low back pain. Man Ther 2009;14:555–61.

37. Vlaeyen J, Linton S. Fear-avoidance model of chronic musculoskeletal pain: 12 years on. Pain 2012;153:1144–7.

38. Sullivan M, Thibault P, Andrikonyte J, et al. Psychological influences on repetition-induced summation of activity-related pain in patients with chronic low back pain. Pain 2009;141:70–8.

39. Briggs AM, Jordan JE, Buchbinder R, et al. Health literacy and beliefs among a community cohort with and without chronic low back pain. Pain 2010;150:275–83.

40. Woby SR, Urmston M, Watson PJ. Self-efficacy mediates the relation between pain-related fear and outcome in chronic low back pain patients. Eur J Pain 2007;11:711–18.

41. Darlow B, Fullen BM, Dean S, et al. The association between health care professional attitudes and beliefs and the attitudes and beliefs, clinical management, and outcomes of patients with low back pain: a systematic review. Eur J Pain 2012;16:3–17.

42. Reichborn-Kjennerud T, Stoltenberg C, Tambs K, et al. Back–neck pain and symptoms of anxiety and depression: a population-based twin study. Psychol Med 2002;32:1009–20.

43. Gatchel RJ, Peng YB, Peters ML, et al. The biopsychosocial approach to chronic pain: scientific advances and future directions. Psychol Bull 2007;133:581–624.

44. Campbell CM, Edwards RR. Mind-body interactions in pain: the neurophysiology of anxious and catastrophic pain-related thoughts. Transl Res 2009;153:97–101.

45. Ren K, Dubner R. Interactions between the immune and nervous systems in pain. Nat Med 2010;16:1267–76.

46. Shaw WS, Van der Windt DA, Main CJ, et al. Early patient screening and intervention to address individual-level occupational factors ("blue flags") in back disability. J Occup Rehabil 2009;19:64–80.

47. Bjorck-van Dijken C, Fjellman-Wiklund A, Hildingsson C. Low back pain, lifestyle factors and physical activity: a population-based study. J Rehabil Med 2008;40:864–9.

48. Hestbaek L, Leboeuf-Yde C, Manniche C. Is low back pain part of a general health pattern or is it a separate and distinctive entity? A critical literature review of comorbidity with low back pain. J Manipulative Physiol Ther 2003;26:243–52.

49. Schneider S, Mohnen SM, Schiltenwolf M, et al. Comorbidity of low back pain: representative outcomes of a national health study in the Federal Republic of Germany. Eur J Pain 2007;11:387–97.

50. Hayes C, Hodson FJ. A whole-person model of care for persistent pain: from conceptual framework to practical application. Pain Med 2011;12:1738–49.

51. Iles RA, Davidson M, Taylor NF, et al. Systematic review of the ability of recovery expectations to predict outcomes in non-chronic non-specific low back pain. J Occup Rehabil 2009;19:25–40.

52. Strand EB, Kerns RD, Christie A, et al. Higher levels of pain readiness to change and more positive affect reduce pain reports–a weekly assessment study on arthritis patients. Pain 2007;127:204–13.

53. Kalauokalani D, Cherkin DC, Sherman KJ, et al. Lessons from a trial of acupuncture and massage for low back pain: patient expectations and treatment effects. Spine 2001;26:1418–24.

54. Sheeran L, Sparkes V, Caterson B, et al. Spinal position sense and trunk muscle activity during sitting and standing in non-specific chronic low back pain: classification analysis. Spine 2012;37:E486–95.

55. O'Sullivan K, Verschueren S, Van Hoof W, et al. Lumbar repositioning error in sitting: healthy controls versus people with sitting-related non-specific chronic low back pain (flexion pattern). Man Ther 2013;18:526–32.

56. Luomajoki H, Moseley G. Tactile acuity and lumbopelvic motor control in patients with back pain and healthy controls. Br J Sports Med 2011;45:437–40.

57. Bray H, Moseley GL. Disrupted working body schema of the trunk in people with back pain. Br J Sports Med 2011;45:168–73.

58. Moseley GL, Gallagher L, Gallace A. Neglect-like tactile dysfunction in chronic back pain. Neurology 2012;79:327–32.

59. Dankaerts W, O'Sullivan P, Straker L, et al. The inter-examiner reliability of a classification method for non-specific chronic low back pain patients with motor control impairment. Man Ther 2006;11:28–39.

60. Smeets RJ, Wittink H, Hidding A, et al. Do patients with chronic low back pain have a lower level of aerobic fitness than healthy controls?: are pain, disability, fear of injury, working status, or level of leisure time activity associated with the difference in aerobic fitness level? Spine 2006;31:90–7.

61. Hasenbring MI, Hallner D, Rusu AC. Fear-avoidance and endurance-related responses to pain: development and validation of the Avoidance-Endurance Questionnaire (AEQ). Eur J Pain 2009;13:620–8.

62. Koho P, Aho S, Watson P, et al. Assessment of chronic pain behaviour: reliability of the method and its relationship with perceived disability, physical impairment and function. J Rehabil Med 2001; 33:128–32.

63. Martel M, Thibault P, Sullivan M. The persistence of pain behaviors in patients with chronic back pain is independent of pain and psychological factors. Pain 2010;151:330–6.

64. Battié MC, Videman T, Parent E. Lumbar disc degeneration: epidemiology and genetic influences. Spine 2004;29:2679–90.

65. Bunzli S, McEvoy S, O'Sullivan P, et al. A Qualitative Investigation of Pathways through Cognitive Functional Therapy for Chronic Low Back Pain. Australian Physiotherapy Association Conference; October 17–20; Melbourne 2013.

66. Darlow B, Dowell A, Baxter GD, et al. The enduring impact of what clinicians say to people with low back pain. Ann Fam Med 2013;11:527–34.

67. Hoffman BM, Papas RK, Chatkoff DK, et al. Meta-analysis of psychological interventions for chronic low back pain. Health Psychol 2007;26:1–9.

68. Dankaerts W, O'Sullivan P, Burnett A, et al. The use of a mechanism-based classification system to evaluate and direct management of a patient with non-specific chronic low back pain and motor control impairment – A case report. Man Ther 2007;12:181–91.

69. Chiesa A, Serretti A. Mindfulness-based interventions for chronic pain: a systematic review of the evidence. J Altern Complement Med 2011;17:83–93.

70. Jones KD, Burckhardt CS, Bennett JA. Motivational interviewing may encourage exercise in persons with fibromyalgia by enhancing self efficacy. Arthritis Care Res 2004;51:864–7.

71. Wand B, Tulloch V, George P, et al. Seeing it helps: movement-related back pain is reduced by visualization of the back during movement. Clin J Pain 2012;28:602–8.

72. Van Hoof W, Volkaerts K, O'Sullivan K, et al. Comparing lower lumbar kinematics in cyclists with low back pain (flexion pattern) versus asymptomatic controls–field study using a wireless posture monitoring system. Man Ther 2012;17:312–17.

73. Macedo LG, Smeets RJEM, Maher CG, et al. Graded activity and graded exposure for persistent nonspecific low back pain: a systematic review. Phys Ther 2010;90:860–79.

CHAPTER 45.3 ■ TREATMENT-BASED CLASSIFICATION SYSTEM

Julie Fritz

What has come to be known as the treatment-based classification (TBC) system was originally disseminated in a publication in 1995 authored by Delitto and colleagues.[1] The timing of this original publication is relevant to its structure and purpose. The mid-1990s corresponded to an overall emphasis on evidence-based practice across all dimensions of health care, and the burgeoning of a body of literature and randomized trials specific to physical therapy treatments for patients with low back pain (LBP).[2,3] The situation then was much as it is today – several treatments commonly used by physical therapists for patients with LBP seem to show some effects, perhaps superior to doing nothing, but overall effect sizes tend to be modest at best.[4,5] A key consideration in interpreting this literature both then and now was the concern that study designs were essentially taking a 'magic bullet' approach to LBP treatment.[6] In other words, a presumption underlying the design of most randomized trials was that a treatment would either 'succeed' or 'fail' for nearly anyone with LBP regardless of clinical presentation. This presumption contradicted the experience of expert clinicians working with patients with LBP who described patterns of clinical findings that were presumed to define subgroups of patients with LBP who would preferentially respond to a particular type of treatment. Many such expert-based symptoms had been described by physical therapists by the mid-1990s, but none had been translated into an ongoing research agenda.[7-12] Questions about optimal strategies for subgrouping patients with LBP and improving patient-centred outcomes remain to this day,[13] but it is certain that the TBC system has contributed significantly to this conversation in the years since its introduction.

The TBC system in its original description was intended for patients with acute or an acute exacerbation of LBP causing substantial pain and limitations in daily activities. The relevance of considering chronicity in the application of the TBC system has been highlighted by subsequent research documenting worse treatment outcomes and increased difficulty classifying patients whose symptoms are chronic.[14,15] After screening patients for any medical Red Flags, the system proposed using the information gathered from the history and physical examination to place a patient into one of four basic classification categories: manipulation, specific exercise (flexion, extension and lateral shift patterns), stabilization and traction. The signs and symptoms originally proposed as the criteria for placing a patient into one of these categories are listed in Table 45-2, and the intervention procedures originally proposed for each category are listed in Table 45-3. The system was based on clinical experience evidence available at the time of its development. Since that time additional research has resulted in various modifications. The original principles guiding the development of the TBC continued to inform ongoing research including the necessity of creating a decision-making system that can be adapted into clinical practice as broadly as possible and the focus on the ultimate goal of improving patient-centred outcomes.

OVERVIEW OF THE TREATMENT-BASED CLASSIFICATION CATEGORIES

Manipulation Classification

Spinal manipulation remains one of the most common treatments used for patients with LBP. The TBC system originally proposed to identify patients likely to benefit from manipulation based on clinical characteristics grounded in the predominant, biomechanically orientated paradigms most popular in the mid-1990s. A great deal of research since that time has raised questions about the validity of these theories explaining the mechanisms of spinal manipulation,[16] and it is therefore not surprising that subsequent research has questioned traditional ways of determining which patients with LBP are most likely to respond to spinal manipulation. The manipulation classification of the TBC system was the first to be evaluated from a more probabilistic research approach that sought to identify clusters of findings that predicted response to spinal manipulation regardless of the alignment of the findings with expert-based paradigms and clinical dogma.[17] The goal of the prediction rule resulting

TABLE 45-2 Signs and Symptoms Originally Proposed as the Criteria for Placing a Patient into a Particular Classification and Revised Criteria Based on Updated Evidence

Manipulation	Asymmetrical lateral flexion range of motion (i.e. capsular pattern of motion restriction) Unilateral low back pain without symptoms into the lower extremities Asymmetrical bony landmarks of the pelvis Positive sacroiliac dysfunction tests (i.e. supine-long sit test, prone knee bend test, standing flexion test)	No symptoms distal to the knee Recent onset of symptoms (<16 days) Low levels of fear-avoidance beliefs (FABQW <19) Hypomobility of the lumbar spine Hip internal rotation range of motion (ROM) (>35° for at least one hip)
Stabilization	Frequent recurrent episodes of LBP with minimal perturbation Hypermobility of the lumbar spine Previous history of lateral shift deformity with alternating sides Frequent prior use of manipulation with dramatic but short-term results Trauma, pregnancy or use of oral contraceptives Relief with immobilization (e.g. bracing)	Younger age (<40 years) Greater general flexibility (post-partum, average SLR ROM >91°) 'Instability catch' or aberrant movements during lumbar flexion/extension ROM Positive findings for the prone instability test For patients who are post-partum: Positive posterior pelvic pain provocation (P4), active straight leg raise (ALSR) and modified Trendelenburg tests Pain provocation with palpation of the long dorsal sacroiliac ligament or pubic symphysis
Specific exercise		
Extension	Symptoms centralize with lumbar extension Symptoms peripheralize with lumbar flexion	Symptoms distal to the buttock Symptoms centralize with lumbar extension Symptoms peripheralize with lumbar flexion Directional preference for extension
Flexion	Symptoms centralize with lumbar flexion Symptoms peripheralize with lumbar extension Diagnosis of lumbar spinal stenosis	Older age (>50 years old) Directional preference for flexion Imaging evidence of lumbar spinal stenosis
Lateral shift	Visible frontal plane deviation of the shoulders relative to the pelvis Asymmetrical side-bending active ROM Painful and restricted extension active ROM	Visible frontal plane deviation of the shoulders relative to the pelvis Directional preference for lateral translation movements of the pelvis
Traction	Signs and symptoms of nerve root compression No movements centralize symptoms	Signs and symptoms of nerve root compression No movements centralize symptoms

TABLE 45-3 Intervention Procedures Originally Proposed for Each Classification and Revised Interventions Based on Updated Evidence

Classification	Original Treatments Proposed by TBC	Updated Treatment Considerations
Manipulation	Manipulation or mobilization techniques targeted to the sacroiliac or lumbar region Active range of motion (ROM) exercises	Manipulation of the lumbopelvic region Active ROM exercises
Stabilization	Trunk strengthening and stabilization exercises Advice to avoid end-range movements and positions Bracing for more severe cases	Promoting isolated contraction and co-contraction of the deep stabilizing muscles (multifidus, transversus abdominus) Strengthening of large spinal stabilizing muscles (erector spinae, oblique abdominals)
Specific exercise		
Extension	End-range extension exercises Avoidance of flexion activities	End-range extension exercises Mobilization to promote extension Avoidance of flexion activities
Flexion	End-range flexion exercises Mechanical traction performed in flexion Avoidance of extension activities	Mobilization or manipulation of the spine and/or lower extremities Exercise to address impairments of strength or flexibility Body-weight-supported treadmill ambulation
Lateral shift	Exercises to correct lateral shift Mechanical or autotraction	Exercises to correct lateral shift Mechanical traction

from this research was to identify patients who were likely to receive rapid, pronounced benefit from spinal manipulation, not to exclude the potential that other patients could not also benefit from the treatment.[17,18] The results, supported by a multi-site randomized trial,[19] indicate that manipulation may be most specifically beneficial for patients between the ages of 18–60 years with no contraindications and an acute onset or exacerbation (about 2 weeks or less) whose symptoms do not extend distal to the knee. The pragmatism and simplicity of this prediction rule are appealing not just within physical therapy practice, but as an opportunity to communicate with physicians about the optimal patients to send rapidly to physical therapy.[20]

Another important lesson learned about the manipulation TBC category relates to generalizability of specific manipulation techniques. Biomechanically focused paradigms for identifying patients likely to benefit from manipulation traditionally placed great emphasis on the specificity of the manipulation technique. Recent research suggests the choice of a specific manipulation technique may not be as relevant as previously thought as long as a thrust manipulation procedure is used.[21,22] Attempts to extend the prediction rule for manipulation to non-thrust mobilization procedures have not been successful.[21,23] The need to consider thrust manipulation and non-thrust mobilization as separate treatment modalities is highlighted by this research and is consistent with more recent theories on the mechanisms of spinal manipulation.[16]

Stabilization Classification

The idea of a subgroup of patients with LBP related to spinal instability has been described for decades, but was initially described as a mechanical condition related to excessive movement between adjacent vertebrae that likely required immobilization or surgical stabilization.[24,25] The original TBC system reflected this perspective, labelling this subgroup 'immobilization' and recommending examination criteria and interventions designed to manage patients who were presumed to have excessive segmental movement (see Tables 45-2 and 45-3). Subsequent research has provided a different perspective by emphasizing the importance of spinal muscles in maintaining and restoring spinal stability, shifting the focus of rehabilitation from 'immobilization' to 'stabilization' or 'motor control'.[26]

The original classification criteria for a stabilization subgroup focused on identifying patients presumed to have excessive segmental movements of the spine (see Table 45-2) such as recurrent LBP episodes, frequent manipulation or self-manipulation with short-term relief, trauma, pregnancy, oral contraceptive use, and positive response to immobilization of the spine. Shifting paradigms on spinal 'instability' and research that employed probabilistic designs to identify patients with LBP likely to respond to exercises designed to improve trunk strength and motor control have resulted in rather different criteria to define this subgroup. The two most important clinical findings appear to be aberrant movement suggestive of poor motor control during active

trunk movement in the sagittal plane and the prone instability test.[27,28] Other findings specific to pregnancy-related LBP have also been proposed.[29]

A persistent challenge with the stabilization subgroup of patients is the optimal treatment strategy. Various motor control exercise programmes have been evaluated, but effect sizes continue to be modest, even among patients believed to fit the stabilization subgroup.[26,28,30,31] Additional research to better understand the needs of patients in this subgroup is needed.

Specific Exercise Classification

The existence of subgroups of patients who preferentially respond to repeated, end-range movements was popularized by McKenzie in the decades preceding the original TBC system description.[12] Consistent with principles of McKenzie, the TBC system identified that the presence of the centralization phenomenon was the primary examination criterion for inclusion in a specific exercise classification, and the movement producing centralization determined the specific direction of exercise required for the patient. Centralization, defined as a situation in which spinal movement or positioning results in movement of symptoms from a distal to a more proximal/midline location, has continued to be shown as an important prognostic factor for patients with LBP.[32,33] A related but distinct finding or directional preference, which occurs when symptoms are diminished, abolished or centralized,[34] may also be useful for identifying the subgroup of patients likely to respond to directional exercises.

There are some studies that lend support to the hypothesis that patients who demonstrate centralization and/or directional preference will preferentially respond to repeated, directional exercises;[35,36] however, a randomized trial that directly addresses this treatment matching hypothesis by evaluating the interaction between directional exercise treatment and these particular examination findings with long-term outcomes has not been conducted. An interesting finding that has emerged from recent investigations is a degree of overlap between patients who fit both the manipulation and specific exercise criteria for extension-orientated treatment.[37] Optimal treatment strategies and sequencing for these patients has not been evaluated.

Traction Classification

Although there was no evidence to support the contention at the time, the original TBC system hypothesized that a subset of patients with LBP existed who were likely to benefit from mechanical traction. The examination criteria defining this subgroup was proposed to be the presence of lower-extremity symptoms and signs of nerve root compression and the absence of centralization with movement testing. Systematic reviews have universally rejected mechanical traction as a potentially beneficial treatment for patients with LBP,[38,39] despite support for the treatment by at least some physical therapists.[40] The research studies used heterogeneous samples of patients with LBP, often with no leg symptoms whatsoever as the basis for the recommendation against using mechanical traction.[41–43] The original TBC system acknowledged that if a traction subgroup did exist, it would include a relatively small proportion of patients with LBP. The mismatch between the TBC system conceptualization of a traction subgroup and existing research prompted a randomized trial to evaluate specific subgrouping factors that may define a traction subgroup.[44] The results suggested that patients with LBP and leg symptoms who fail to centralize with the physical examination and demonstrate a crossed straight leg raise sign may preferentially benefit from mechanical traction.[44] Additional research is needed to further evaluate the validity of these criteria and if appropriate define optimal treatment parameters for mechanical traction.

CONCLUSION

If any classification system is to be useful for clinical practice it must lead to the identification of specific subgroups of patients from data that can be collected during the initial history and physical examination which in turn guided the selection of optimal intervention strategies. The ultimate determination of the value of a classification system is whether or not it improves patient-centred outcomes. Evidence that has emerged since the original description of the TBC system indicates that it may be able to accomplish these objectives for at least some patients with LBP.[14,19,45,46] As with any scientific endeavour, the process of developing and refining a classification system is a dynamic and iterative process that should result in continuous adjustments and improvements.

REFERENCES

1. Delitto A, Erhard RE, Bowling RW. A treatment-based classification approach to low back syndrome: identifying and staging patients for conservative management. Phys Ther 1995;75: 470–89.
2. Sackett DL. A primer on the precision and accuracy of the clinical examination. JAMA 1992;267:2638–44.
3. Sackett DL, Richardson WS, Rosenberg W, et al. Evidence-Based Medicine: How to Practice and Teach EBM. New York: Churchill Livingstone; 2000.
4. Chou R, Atlas SJ, Stanos SP, et al. Nonsurgical interventional therapies for low back pain: a review of the evidence for an american pain society clinical practice guideline. Spine 2009;34:1078–93.
5. Chou R, Huffman LH. Nonpharmacologic therapies for acute and chronic low back pain: a review of the evidence for an American Pain Society/American College of Physicians clinical practice guideline. Ann Intern Med 2007;147:492–504.
6. Delitto A. Research in low back pain: time to stop seeking the elusive "magic bullet". Phys Ther 2005;85:206–8.
7. Atlas SJ, Deyo RA, Patrick DL, et al. The Quebec Task Force classification for Spinal Disorders and the severity, treatment, and outcomes of sciatica and lumbar spinal stenosis. Spine 1996; 21:2885–92.
8. Binkley J, Finch E, Hall J, et al. Diagnostic classification of patients with low back pain: report on a survey of physical therapy experts. Phys Ther 1993;73:138–50.
9. Buchbinder R, Goel V, Bombardier C, et al. Classification systems of soft tissue disorders of the neck and upper limb: do they satisfy methodological guidelines? J Clin Epidemiol 1996;49:141–9.
10. Riddle DL. Classification and low back pain: a review of the literature and critical analysis of selected systems. Phys Ther 1998;78: 708–37.
11. Van Dillen LR, Sahrmann SA, Norton BJ, et al. Reliability of physical examination items used for classification of patients with low back pain. Phys Ther 1998;78:979–88.
12. McKenzie RA. The Lumbar Spine: Mechanical Diagnosis and Therapy. Waikanae, NZ: Spinal Publications New Zealand Ltd.; 1981.
13. Henschke N, Maher CG, Refschauge KM, et al. Low back pain research priorities: a survey of primary care practitioners. BMC Fam Pract 2007;8:40.
14. Apeldoorn AT, Ostelo RW, van Helvoirt H, et al. A randomized controlled trial on the effectiveness of a classification-based system for sub-acute and chronic low back pain. Spine 2012;[Epub ahead of print].
15. Stanton TR, Hancock MJ, Apeldoorn AT, et al. What characterizes people who have an unclear classification using a treatment-based classification algorithm for low back pain? A cross-sectional study. Phys Ther 2013;93:345–55.
16. Bialosky JA, Bishop MD, Price DD, et al. The mechanisms of manual therapy in the treatment of musculoskeletal pain: a comprehensive model. Man Ther 2009;14:531–8.
17. Flynn T, Fritz J, Whitman J, et al. A clinical prediction rule for classifying patients with low back pain who demonstrate short term improvement with spinal manipulation. Spine 2002;27: 2835–43.
18. Fritz JM, Childs JD, Flynn TW. Pragmatic application of a clinical prediction rule in primary care to identify patients with low back pain likely to respond quickly to spinal manipulation. BMC Fam Pract 2005;6:29.
19. Childs JD, Fritz JM, Flynn TW, et al. Validation of a clinical prediction rule to identify patients with low back pain likely to benefit from spinal manipulation. Ann Intern Med 2004;141:920–8.
20. Kramer CD, Koch WH, Fritz JM. Development and outcomes of a program to translate the evidence for spinal manipulation into physical therapy practice. J Man Manip Ther 2013;21:177–86.
21. Cleland JA, Fritz JM, Kulig K, et al. Comparison of the effectiveness of three manual physical therapy techniques in a subgroup of patients with low back pain who satisfy a clinical prediction rule: a randomized clinical trial. Spine 2009;34:2720–9.
22. Sutlive TG, Mabry LM, Easterling EJ, et al. Comparison of short-term responses to two manipulation techniques for patients with low back pain in a military benficiary population. Mil Med 2009;174:750–6.
23. Hancock MJ, Maher CG, Latimer J, et al. Independent evaluation of a clinical prediction rule for spinal manipulative therapy: a randomised controlled trial. Eur Spine J 2008;17:936–43.
24. Fryberg O. Lumbar instability: a dynamic approach by traction-compression radiography. Spine 1987;12:119–29.
25. Kirkaldy-Willis WH, Farfan HF. Instability of the lumbar spine. Clin Orthop 1982;165:110–23.
26. Macedo LG, Maher CG, Latimer J, et al. Motor control exercise for persistent, nonspecific low back pain: a systematic review. Phys Ther 2009;89:9–25.
27. Hicks GE, Fritz JM, Delitto A, et al. Preliminary development of a clinical prediction rule for determining which patients with low back pain will respond to a stabilization exercise program. Arch Phys Med Rehabil 2005;86:1753–62.
28. Rabin A, Shashua A, Pizem K, et al. A clinical prediction rule to identify patients with low back pain who are likely to experience short-term success following lumbar stabilization exercises: a randomized controlled validation study. J Orthop Sports Phys Ther 2014;44:6–13.
29. Stuge B, Laerum E, Kirkesola G, et al. The efficacy of a treatment program focusing on specific stabilizing exercises for pelvic girdle pain after pregnancy: a randomized controlled trial. Spine 2004;29:351–9.
30. Costa LOP, Maher CG, Latimer J, et al. Motor control exercise for chronic low back pain: a randomized placebo-controlled trial. Phys Ther 2009;789:1275–86.
31. Ferreira ML, Ferreira PH, Latimer J, et al. Comparison of general exercise, motor control exercise and spinal manipulative therapy for chronic low back pain: a randomized trial. Pain 2007;131: 31–7.
32. Skytte L, May S, Petersen P. Centralization: its prognostic value in patients with referred symptoms and sciatica. Spine 2005;30: E293–9.

33. Werneke MW, Hart DL, Resnik L, et al. Centralization: prevalence and effect on treatment outcomes using a standardized operational definition and measurement method. J Orthop Sports Phys Ther 2008;38:116–25.

34. Werneke MW, Hart DL, Cuttrone G, et al. Association between directional preference and centralization in patients with low back pain. J Orthop Sports Phys Ther 2011;41:22–31.

35. Browder DA, Childs JD, Cleland JA, et al. Effectiveness of an extension oriented treatment approach in a subgroup of patients with low back pain: a randomized clinical trial. Phys Ther 2007;87:1608–18.

36. Long AL, Donelson R. Does it matter which exercise? A randomized trial of exercise for low back pain. Spine 2004;29:2593–602.

37. Stanton TR, Fritz JM, Hancock MJ, et al. Evaluation of a treatment-based classification algorithm for low back pain: a cross-sectional study. Phys Ther 2011;91:496–509.

38. Gay RE, Brault JS. Evidence-based management of chronic low back pain with traction therapy. Spine J 2008;8:234–42.

39. Harte AA, Baxter GD, Gracey JH. The efficacy of traction for back pain: a systematic review of randomized controlled trials. Arch Phys Med Rehabil 2003;84:1542–53.

40. Harte AA, Gracey JH, Baxter GD. Current use of lumbar traction in the management of low back pain: results of a survey of physio-therapists in the United Kingdom. Arch Phys Med Rehabil 2005;86:1164–9.

41. Schimmel JJ, de Kleuver M, Horsting PP, et al. No effect of traction in patients with low back pain: a single centre, single blind, randomized controlled trial of Intervertebral Differential Dynamics Therapy. Eur Spine J 2009.

42. van der Heijden GJ, Beurskens AJ, Dirx MJ, et al. Efficacy of lumbar traction: A randomised clinical trial. Physiother 1995;81:29–35.

43. Werners R, Pynsent PB, Bulstrode CJK. Randomized trial comparing interferential therapy with motorized lumbar traction and massage in the management of low back pain in a primary care setting. Spine 1999;24:1579–84.

44. Fritz JM, Lindsay W, Matheson JW, et al. Is there a subgroup of patients with low back pain likely to benefit from mechanical traction? Results of a randomized clinical trial and subgrouping analysis. Spine 2007;32:E793–800.

45. Brennan GP, Fritz JM, Hunter SJ, et al. Identifying sub-groups of patients with "non-specific" low back pain: results of a randomized clinical trial. Spine 2006;31:623–31.

46. Fritz JM, Delitto A, Erhard RE. Comparison of a classification-based approach to physical therapy and therapy based on clinical practice guidelines for patients with acute low back pain: a randomized clinical trial. Spine 2003;28:1363–72.

CHAPTER 45.4 ■ MOVEMENT SYSTEM IMPAIRMENT SYNDROMES OF THE LOW BACK

Shirley Sahrmann • Linda Van Dillen

MOVEMENT SYSTEM: INCLUSION NOT EXCLUSION

Classification of patients with low back pain (LBP) has been a major focus of researchers for more than 15 years.[1–9] Classification immediately highlights the issue of diagnosis and labels used by physical therapists and the overall context for these diagnoses. Clearly the name of the profession, which implies treatment by physical means, does not provide a context or an identity for expertise in an anatomical or physiological system of the body[10] as with other health professions. To provide such a context, in June 2013, the American Physical Therapy Association adopted a guiding principle that states 'the identity of physical therapy is the *Movement System* which is the core of physical therapy education, practice, and research.'[11–13]

MOVEMENT SYSTEM IMPAIRMENT SYNDROMES VERSUS MOVEMENT SYSTEM SYNDROMES

The preceding information was provided to clarify why movement system impairment (MSI) syndromes of the lumbar spine are not intended to imply exclusive use of the label movement system. All diagnoses made by physical therapists should be of the movement system (Fig. 45-2). This chapter contains just one approach. The theory of MSI[14,15] is that multiple impairments combine to alter the precise movement of a joint that eventually causes tissue irritation, pain and tissue damage. Another tenet is that 'because movement in the joint occurs too readily and is imprecise, it hurts'. The factors contributing to the painful movement need to be identified to guide treatment. The movement causing the pain is attributed to accessory motion hypermobility in both the range and frequency of occurrence. Accessory arthrokinematic motion is defined as motions between articular surfaces of roll, glide and spin.[16] The premise for the underlying problem of hypermobility is consistent with the characteristics of degenerative disc disease process.[17,18] Similarly, the osteoarthritic process is attributed to small imprecise motions that cause osteophytes that eventually results in hypomobility. The examination is to assess as rigorously as possible the passive and active forces that are causing a deviation in the precision of joint motion. The examination requires attention to manual palpation about the joint segment of interest during passive and active motion. For example, in the lumbar spine, a recommended palpation is on either side of the lumbar spinous processes as the patient rocks backwards in the quadruped position. Often in the rotation syndrome, a small unilateral motion of flexion–rotation can be detected as the patient rocks backwards. The proposed tissue adaptations contributing to the development of the accessory motion hypermobility are illustrated in the kinesiopathological model (Fig. 45-3).

THE KINESIOPATHOLOGICAL MODEL

MSIs are believed to be induced by repeated movements and prolonged alignments of daily activities because these

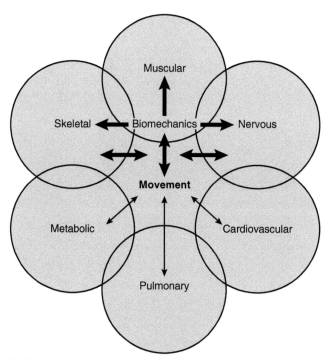

FIGURE 45-2 ■ The human movement system. The musculoskeletal and nervous systems are the primary effectors of movement. Impairments in any effector systems such as muscle weakness, relative stiffness problems, altered activation patterns and pain will affect movement. The other systems are support systems for the effectors, but are also affected by movement and the lack of movement. The examination is designed to detect impairments in the contributing systems and to make a movement system diagnosis. Treatment is based on movement in all forms, from manipulation to mobilization to well-designed exercise programmes and instruction in correct performance of functional and fitness activities. (From: Sahrmann SA. Movement System Impairment Syndromes of the Extremities, Cervical and Thoracic Spines. Elsevier 2010.)

behaviours induce changes in the effector systems that can be considered impairments. Impairment is defined as an abnormality in an anatomical, physiological or psychological system.[19] An impairment can be a non-optimal but also a non-pathological change in the structure and/or function of components of the movement system. The theory is that a pattern of impairments develops that result in a principal impairment that does eventually induce pathological changes in tissues. The multiple impairments comprise the syndrome and in combination contribute to the principal impairment, the diagnosis. The kinesiopathological model depicts these relationships (see Fig. 45-3). The primary mechanism underlying the changes is that the 'body takes the path of least resistance for movement'. Thus the changes in tissues associated with the repeated movements and prolonged alignments shape the path. Daily activities tend to be repetitious with some tissues stretched more than others and some muscles about the joint more active than others. As a consequence a pattern develops because of these tissue adaptations. These adaptations are considered as impairments and are indicative of a loss of optimal balance of tissues about a joint or sometimes even the anterior and posterior musculature of the trunk.

Tissue Adaptations Associated with Repeated Movements and Prolonged Alignment

Relative Flexibility

Flexibility refers to the intrinsic mobility of the motion segment. The term relative is used because the readiness to move becomes more pronounced in a specific direction(s) than in other directions as a result of the repeated movements and prolonged postures of daily activities. For example, in younger individuals lumbar flexion motion often occurs more readily than lumbar extension motions, while in older individuals, movement into extension occurs more readily than movement into flexion.

Relative Stiffness

Relative stiffness refers to the passive tension of muscle and connective tissue that is present during elongation. Stiffness is the resistance to deformation.[20] Stiffness can be defined as the change in tension per unit change in length. In muscle, the connective tissue proteins such as titin and the extracellular matrix with its collagen, are the tissues primarily responsible for stiffness.[21] Hypertrophy of muscle has been shown to increase its stiffness.[22] Just as activities of daily living affect the flexibility of the motion segment, hypertrophy and stiffness are also affected by these activities. The result is that one muscle group crossing the joint can be stiffer than the antagonistic muscle crossing the same joint. As depicted in Figure 45-4, in the prone position when the knee is flexed, the pelvis anteriorly tilts and/or rotates causing lumbar extension and/or rotation. The mechanisms for these motions are that (a) flexibility of the lumbar spine into extension–rotation and (b) the stiffness of tensor fascia lata and/or rectus femoris muscles is greater than the stiffness of the abdominal muscles (which should help to maintain a constant position of the pelvis). The evidence for this readiness of the spine to move during knee flexion will be discussed in the research section of this chapter. Thus movements of the lumbopelvic region are not caused by muscle shortness, but because of the increased spinal flexibility (readiness to move) primarily and relative muscle stiffness secondarily. Therefore stretching the stiff muscles will not stop the spinal motion.[23] Direct efforts have to be made to stop spinal motion and increase the stiffness of the muscle groups that lengthened too readily. In the example given above, the patient needs to stop the spinal motion by contracting the abdominal muscles as part of a programme to hypertrophy those muscles and increase their stiffness. The MSI syndromes are named for the movement direction or alignment that most consistently causes symptoms and is impaired (non-optimal movement), and when corrected the symptoms decrease or are eliminated. The overall strategy for treatment is to prevent the motion and to ensure that the patient is moving in the joints where the movement should be taking place and not moving in joints that should remain relatively still.

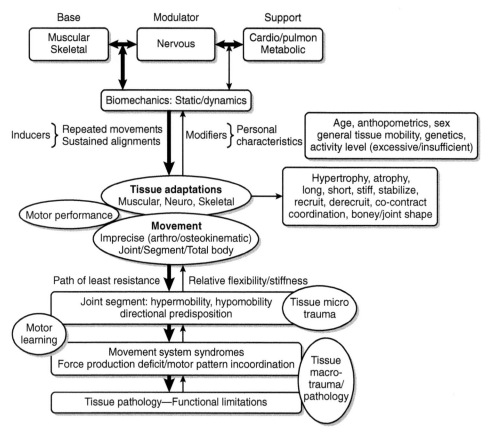

FIGURE 45-3 ■ The kinesiopathologic model. The model is intended to emphasize the general scheme for the development of movement system impairment syndromes. Biomechanics act as an interface between the effector systems and play an important role in the adaptations induced by repeated movements and sustained alignments of daily activities. Personal characteristics are also important modifiers of the types of adaptations that are induced by activity. At the early stage repeated movements can be considered to be characteristic of motor performance but over time and with repetition, the more permanent form of motor learning takes place. The tissue adaptations induce impairments in the movement, which is believed to be in the accessory motion of a joint. This impairment is the result of changes in the relative flexibility of the joint and the relative stiffness of the muscular and connective tissues about the joint. The impaired movement causes tissue microtrauma that becomes macrotrauma. The movement system impairment syndrome is the result of this series of events. In some ways the syndromes can be generally subclassified as to whether the primary deficit is in force production or in motor pattern coordination. Force production deficits require strengthening exercises in addition to ensuring optimal activation patterns while motor pattern coordination deficits require primarily training of activation patterns. (From: Sahrmann SA. Movement System Impairment Syndromes of the Extremities, Cervical and Thoracic Spines. Elsevier, 2010.)

Neuromuscular Activation Patterns

Over time and with repeated use, muscles adapt in response to (a) load; (b) the intensity and frequency of activation; and (c) the duration and magnitude of imposed length changes. The neuromuscular pattern of activation also leads to adaptation that reflects the characteristics of use. This is the basis of the progression from motor performance that is temporary, to motor learning that is permanent.[24] The pattern of neuromuscular activation needs to be assessed, identified and corrected to optimize the treatment programme.

MOVEMENT SYSTEM IMPAIRMENT SYNDROMES OF THE LUMBAR SPINE

The MSI syndromes are lumbar flexion, extension,[25] rotation, flexion–rotation[26] and extension–rotation.[27] The diagnosis of the syndrome is based on the results of an examination that identifies the movement direction and/or alignment that (a) most consistently causes symptoms;

(b) is not performed correctly; and (c) when the performance is corrected the symptoms are eliminated or decrease. The examination consists of tests in standing, supine, side-lying, prone, quadruped and sitting. The tests involve movements of the spine and of the extremities as well as performance of basic functional activities. For the active tests in these positions the patient performs the movement in the preferred or natural way while the therapist observes the pattern of motion. Spinal motion is also observed during basic functional activities. The majority of functional activities involve greater degrees of movement at joints such as the hips and minimal or no movement of the lumbar spine.

General Pattern and Distribution of Syndromes

Lumbar flexion syndromes are more common in younger individuals. The characteristic flexibility of muscles and connective tissue predispose the spine to flexion. Spinal rotation also occurs more readily in the flexed as compared to the extended alignment. Most often those over

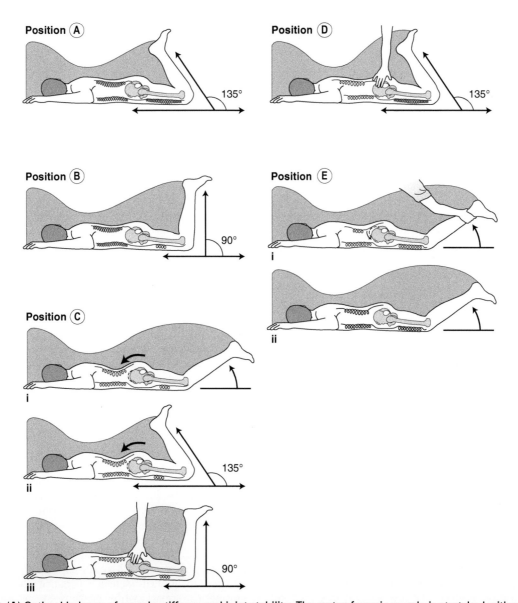

FIGURE 45-4 ■ **(A)** Optimal balance of muscle stiffness and joint stability. The rectus femoris muscle is stretched without compensatory lumbopelvic motion. Therefore the stiffness of the anterior supporting structures of the spine and the passive stiffness of the abdominal muscles are greater than or equal to the stiffness of the rectus femoris muscle. **(B)** Shortness of rectus femoris muscle with counterbalancing stiffness of spinal structures and abdominal muscles. Because the knee flexes to only 90°, the rectus femoris muscle is short and the muscle excursion does not reach the expected standard. However, lumbopelvic compensatory motion is not evident even though the rectus femoris muscle is short. It is not stiffer than the anterior supporting structures of the lumbar spine and the passive extensibility of the abdominal muscles. **(C)** Shortness of rectus femoris muscle with compensatory lumbopelvic motion (position Ci). With knee flexion, compensatory anterior pelvic tilt and lumbar extension occurs, even before the muscle reaches the limit of its excursion. The pelvic tilt increases as the knee flexion range increases (position Cii). When the pelvis is stabilized, which prevents anterior pelvic tilt, the knee flexion is limited to 90° (position Ciii). In contrast to the situation in position B, the shortness of the rectus femoris muscle is associated with compensatory anterior pelvic tilt. Thus not only is the rectus femoris shortened, but its stiffness is also greater than the stiffness of the anterior supporting structures of the lumbar spine and the abdominal muscles. An important implication is that when the rectus femoris muscle is stretched to improve its overall length, the through-the-range stiffness remains. Therefore knee flexion elicits anterior pelvic tilt as long as the rectus femoris muscle is relatively stiffer than the structures preventing the anterior pelvic tilt or the lumbar extension. This phenomenon occurs even though the rectus femoris muscle is able to fully elongate. Correcting the faulty, compensatory pattern requires increasing the stiffness of the abdominal muscles and anterior supporting structures of the spine, in addition to stretching the rectus femoris muscle. It is possible that the compensatory motion occurs only when the rectus femoris muscle reaches the end of its excursion. At this point the resistance is particularly high and thus causes the compensatory motion of the pelvis. In this condition, increasing the length of the rectus femoris muscle eliminates the motion of the pelvis. This condition is not common. **(D)** Compensatory motion without muscle shortness. The knee flexes to 135° (position D), but early in the range there is an associated anterior pelvic tilt and lumbar extension. When the pelvis is stabilized, the knee still flexes to 135°. Clearly the compensatory motion is not associated with a short muscle. The most reasonable explanation is that the anterior supporting structures of the spine and the abdominal muscles are not as stiff as the rectus femoris muscle that has normal length. The relative degree of through-the-range stiffness of the rectus femoris versus the anterior trunk muscles and the anterior supporting structures of the spine is the key factor in determining the movement pattern and in creating the compensatory motion. The compensatory motion occurred long before the muscle reached the end of its range. Correction requires increasing the stiffness of the anterior trunk muscles. **(E)** Compensatory motion with passive flexion controlled by active muscle contraction. When the knee is passively flexed, the stiffness of the rectus femoris muscle is greater than the stiffness of the anterior supporting structures of the spine and the abdominal muscles, which causes compensatory anterior pelvic tilt and lumbar extension (position Ei). When the hamstring muscles actively contract to flex the knee, the compensatory motion is eliminated (position Eii). Possible explanations are that the posterior pelvic tilt elicited by hamstring contraction is sufficient to counteract the stiffness of the rectus femoris. Another explanation is that the abdominal muscles contract enough to counterbalance the anterior pelvic tilt and lumbar extension. (From Sahrmann, S. Diagnosis and Treatment of Movement Impairment Syndromes. Mosby, 2002.)

50 years of age will develop extension or extension-rotation problems. This is consistent with the anatomical changes in the spine of disc degeneration, spondylosis or spondylolysis, spondylolisthesis and spinal stenosis. Rotation motions include those of a specific motion about a vertical axis of the trunk, side-bending and those imposed by lumbopelvic rotation often associated with hip motions. Rotation can cover a wider spectrum of conditions than pure flexion or extension problems and is the most common syndrome component. In summary, the syndromes have a relationship to spinal patho-anatomical changes. These generalizations are intended as a guide and are not meant to imply that these general patterns have 100% application.

Though the labels of flexion, flexion–rotation, extension, extension–rotation or rotation are used, that does not infer that the contributing factors are the same for a given syndrome. There are wide variations in factors that contribute to a given syndrome. The variation in contributing factors is greater for extension, extension–rotation and rotation syndromes than for flexion syndromes. Therefore these labels are not meant to imply that the treatment programme is the same for all individuals with a given label, but the commonality is that the pain-provoking motion is to be avoided. Thus the purposes of the examination are not only to make a diagnosis, but to also identify the contributing factors so that the treatment programme is patient-specific.

Movement System Impairment Examination

The examination is designed to provide the diagnosis, the principal impairment and the contributing factors. An important aspect is that the patient first performs the test motion in the natural or preferred manner (primary test) while the therapist observes the precision of motion and notes the effect on symptoms. Then the therapist instructs the patient in correcting the movement (the secondary test) and notes the effect on symptoms. A major emphasis of the examination is to identify the motions of the spine and extremities that cause pain and teach the patient how to move to eliminate or minimize the symptoms. This modification is necessary not only during specific exercises, but also during all basic functional activities. The belief is that tissues are healing if there are no symptoms. One of the values of the exam is that the patient is also learning what movements cause pain and how to decrease or eliminate the symptoms. Another advantage is that the test items that the patient fails to perform correctly become the exercise. Though the exercises are considered useful, the prevailing belief is that correcting the performance of functional activities is essential to correction of the problem. The basics of the examination are given in Table 45-4. Each test is designed to assess the effect on symptoms associated with a given movement direction and if the movement is impaired. Thus if symptoms increase with forward bending and the lumbar flexion range of motion is excessive, the test is positive for flexion. If the forward bending is corrected and the symptoms decrease that supports the diagnosis of lumbar flexion. The movement direction(s) eliciting symptoms

most frequently is designated as the syndrome or the diagnosis. The examination also provides information about specific muscle performance, such as length, strength, stiffness and activation patterns. Thus the therapist has useful guidelines for developing the exercise programme addressing neuromuscular function.

Treatment

In many ways, when a patient fails a test, that test becomes one of the exercises. Identification of the offending movement direction also provides guidelines for correction of functional activities. As part of the examination, the patient is also learning what movements cause pain and how to correct the movement. Correcting functional activities, which is also a form of therapeutic exercise, is essential. Functional activities include everything from how to roll, sleeping position, how to go from supine to sitting, from sit-to-stand and reverse, how to walk, and how to go up and down stairs. Sitting position and types of chairs need to be assessed as well as any fitness programmes or sports in which the patient participates.

RESEARCH

Clinical and laboratory-based studies of people with chronic LBP who were not in an acute flare-up were used to assess the validity of the classifications and examine elements of the kinesiopathologic model. The steps for these studies were (a) defining a clinical examination;[28] (b) assessing the reliability of examiners to perform the test items;[28-30] (c) determining the examiners' reliability to classify participants;[29,31,32] and (d) assessing the validity of the classifications.[33] Motion-capture instrumentation was used to quantify select aspects of clinical tests, to examine the relationship of those tests for different patient classifications and to examine features of the kinesiopathologic model.

Therapists were reliable in determining the effect on symptoms of specific movement tests and in identifying impaired movement. The classification accuracy was about 70–80%.[31,32,34] The premise that symptoms are related to lumbar spine movement during both direct spinal motion and movement of the extremities was supported by the finding that correction and prevention of spinal motion imposed by extremity movements during examination tests decreased or eliminated symptoms.[35-37] Examples of imposed spinal movement are lumbar flexion–rotation during knee extension in sitting and lumbopelvic rotation during hip rotation in prone position.[35-37] Based on the findings of examination tests associated with direction-specific lumbar motions, validity was demonstrated for extension, extension–rotation and rotation.[33] The underlying premise, that a few degrees of spinal motion that occurs too readily is present in patients with LBP, was supported by motion-capture studies. Among the tests used to assess spinal readiness to move were knee flexion and hip rotation in prone position. For both tests participants with LBP demonstrated earlier and more lumbopelvic rotation than back-healthy participants.[38] The onset of motion in participants with

TABLE 45-4 Movement System Impairment Examination for Low Back Pain

Name_____ M F Hgt_____ Weight _____ Age _____ Date _____
Occupation _____ Fitness Activity _____
Structural characteristics _____
Pain Location: _____ Severity _____

Position	Test	Segment	Impairment	Ext	Rot	Flex
Standing		Spine	Pain			
	Alignment	Thoracic	Kyphosis	E		
			Flat			F
			Swayback	E		
			Asymmetry R L		R	
		Lumbar	Lordosis	E		
			Flat/flex			F
			Asymmetry R L		R	
		Pelvis	Anterior tilt	E		
			Posterior tilt			F
			Lateral tilt		R	
	Forward bend (Fb)	Spine	Pain			F
	Corrected Fb		Pain Y N <			F
	Return Fb		Pain	E		
			Lumbar ext	E		
	Corrected return		Pain Y N <	<E		
	Side-bending		Pain		R	
			Asymmetry		R	
	Rotation		Pain		R	
			Asymmetry		R	
	Single-leg stand		Spine rotation		X	
			Hip drop		X	

Total
Comments:

Position	Test	Segment	Impairment	Ext	Rot	Flex
Supine	Hip flexor length compensation	Lumbopelvic	Anterior tilt	E		
			TFL short/stiff		R	
			Flex short/stiff	E		
			R L asymmetrical		R	
	Position	LE extended	Pain < = >	>E		<F
		LE flexed	Pain < = >	<E		>F
		Support L-spine	Pain < = >	>E		<F
	Hip–knee flexion	Lumbopelvic	pain	E	R	
			Pelvic rotation		R	
	Hip abductor/lateral rot	Lumbopelvic	Pain		R	
			Pelvic rotation		R	
	Abdominal muscles	Pelvis	<2/5	E		
			>2/5			
Side-lying	Position	L-spine	Pain		R	
	Support at waist	L-spine	Pain < = >		R	
	Hip lateral rotation	Lumbopelvic	Pain		R	
			Pelvic rotation		R	
	Hip abductor MMT	Lumbopelvic	Pain		R	
			Weak/long			
	Hip abductor/adductor active	Lumbopelvic	Lateral pelvic tilt		R	

Total
Comments:

Position	Test	Segment	Impairment	Ext	Rot	Flex
Prone	Position	Lumbopelvic	Pain	E		
	Support under abdomen		Pain < = >	<E		>F
	Knee flexion	Lumbopelvic	Pain	E		
	Hip lateral rotation	Lumbopelvic	Pain		R	
			Pelvic rotation		R	
	Hip medial rotation	Lumbopelvic	Pain		R	
			Pelvic rotation		R	

Continued on following page

TABLE 45-4 **Movement System Impairment Examination for Low Back Pain** (Continued)

Position	Test	Segment	Impairment	Ext	Rot	Flex
Quadruped	Position	Lumbopelvic	Pain			
		Alignment	Lumbar flexion			F
			Lumbar rotation		R	
			Thoracic flexion	E		
			Thoracic rotation		R	
	Rocking backwards	Lumbar	Pain			F
			Flexion			F
			Rotation		R	
			Extension	E		
	Shoulder flexion	Lumbar	Pain		R	
			Rotation		R	
Sitting	Flexed	Lumbar	Pain			F
	Flat		Pain			F
	Extended		Pain	E		
	Knee extension	Lumbopelvic	Pain			F
			Flexion-rotation		R	F
Standing	Resting L-spine on wall	Lumbopelvic	Pain < = >	<E		>F
	Shoulder flexion		Pain < = >	>E		
Gait	gait	Lumbopelvic	Pain		R	
			Pelvic rotation		R	
			Hip drop		R	
			L-spine extension	E		

Total
Comments:

Movement System Impairment Diagnosis:
Flexion; extension; rotation; rotation-extension; rotation-flexion

Contributing Factors:

Functional Activities Needing Modification
Walking
Standing
Sitting
Recumbent
  Position
  Rolling
Work arrangement
Recreational/fitness activities

Symptom Modification Activities
Contract abdominals
Back against wall
Sitting
Quadruped
Recumbent: supine prone

Key Exercises

LBP was only a few seconds earlier and less than 5 degrees more than onset of motion in back-healthy participants, supporting the concept that such readiness for lumbar motion is problematic.[38] The lumbopelvic rotation during hip rotation in prone position was also found to elicit symptoms in 60% of the men with LBP but only about 30% of the women.[39-43] Lumbopelvic rotation also occurred earlier, and the early motion was a greater percentage of total lumbopelvic motion in men than in women.[39-42]

Findings from the hip lateral rotation test also demonstrated differences between two of the LBP classifications.[44] The onset of lumboplevic rotation was elicited by the same degree of hip lateral rotation of both the right and left lower extremities in the rotation syndrome, but the onset varied with hip lateral rotation of the right versus the left lower extremity in the extension–rotation syndrome. This finding supports a key concept of relative flexibility, which is that the lumbar spine moves too readily in a specific direction, and that this behaviour varies according to the classification. The finding of symmetrical onset of lumbopelvic rotation in the rotation syndrome and asymmetrical onset in the extension–rotation syndrome was also the same in the test of trunk lateral bending.[45-47] Motion-capture quantification of the early lumbar motion demonstrated symmetrical motion to the right and left in the rotation syndrome and asymmetrical motion in the extension-rotation syndrome. We believe that our research studies are consistent with the belief that early and frequent repetition of small degrees of lumbar motion in specific directions is a contributing factor to tissue microtrauma that becomes macrotrauma. Our studies also support the premise that findings from a clinical examination can reliably and validly classify patients with LBP according to the symptom-producing motions, and on the readiness of the spine to move in a specific direction. Furthermore, because our research has demonstrated that correcting or stopping the spinal motion can decrease or eliminate the symptoms, the most important treatment strategy is that of preventing the offending motion and lumbar stabilization should be emphasized during functional activities and exercises. One study indicated that patients with LBP had more difficulty preventing the lumbopelvic rotation during hip lateral rotation compared to back-healthy participants.[48–50] This finding suggests that specific instruction and training is necessary to achieve optimal results from a stabilization programme.

CONCLUSIONS

The MSI syndrome approach was derived from systematic examination and treatment of patients with LBP. Use of a standard examination indicated that movements of the spine in specific directions consistently elicited symptoms. Correction of the movement or prevention of spinal motion during extremity motions either decreased or eliminated symptoms. A derived kinesiopathologic model proposes that the impaired, painful movements are present before the development of symptoms, thus there are signs before symptoms, and that the impairments (specifically altered activation patterns) are induced by adaptations of the musculoskeletal and nervous system. Key features of the model are that the intrinsic relative (directional) flexibility of the joint and relative stiffness of muscular and connective tissues contribute to a readiness to move. This becomes problematic because the body takes the path of least resistance for movement. The readiness to move in a specific direction is the basis of syndrome classification. Clinical and laboratory studies have assessed the examination, the validity of the classifications and elements of the model. Future research is assessing the effectiveness of classification-specific treatment, the factors inducing the readiness to move and the underlying pathological tissue changes.

REFERENCES

1. Ford JJ, Hahne AJ. Pathoanatomy and classification of low back disorders. Man Ther 2013;18:165–8.
2. Foster NE, Hill JC, Hay EM. Subgrouping patients with low back pain in primary care. are we getting any better at it? Man Ther 2011;16:3–8.
3. McKenzie R. The Lumbar Spine: Mechanical Diagnosis and Therapy. Waikanae: Spinal Publication; 1981.
4. O'Sullivan P. Diagnosis and classification of chronic low back pain disorders: maladaptive movement and motor control impairments as underlying mechanism. Man Ther 2005;10:242–55.
5. Van Dillen L, Sahrmann S, Norton B, et al. Movement system impairment-based categories for low back pain: stage 1 validation. J Orthop Sports Phys Ther 2003;33:126–42.
6. Weiner B. Spine update: the biopsychosocial model and spine care. Spine 2008b;33:219–23.
7. Delitto A, Erhard R, Bowling R. A treatment-based classification approach to low back syndrome: identifying and staging patients for conservative treatment. Phys Ther 1995;75:470–89.
8. Fritz J, Cleland J, Childs J. Subgrouping patients with low back pain: evolution of a classification approach to physical therapy. J Orthop Sports Phys Ther 2007;37:290–302.
9. Kamper SJ, Maher CG, Hancock MJ, et al. Treatment-based subgroups of low back pain. A guide to appraisal of research studies and a summary of current evidence. Best Pract Res Clin Rheumatol 2010;24:181–91.
10. Jull G, Moore A. Physiotherapy's identity. Man Ther 2013;18: 447–8.
11. American Physical Therapy Association. Vision Statement. HOD RC 14-13.
12. American Physical Therapy Association. Guidelines for Vision Statement. HOD RC 15-13.
13. Sahrmann SA. The human movement system – our professional identity. Phys Ther 2014;94(7):1034–42. [Pub online 3/13/2014].
14. Sahrmann SA, editor. Diagnosis and Treatment of Movement Impairment Syndromes. St Louis: Mosby; 2002.
15. Sahrmann SA, editor. Movement System Impairment Syndromes of the Extremities, Cervical and Thoracic Spines. St Louis: Elsevier; 2010.
16. Neumann DA, editor. Kinesiology of the Musculoskeletal System. Foundations of Physical Rehabilitation. St Louis: Mosby; 2002.
17. Onur TS, Wu R, Chu S, et al. Joint instability and cartilage compression in a mouse model of posttraumatic osteoarthritis. J Orthop Res 2014;32:318–23.
18. Wright T. Biomechanical factors in osteoarthritis: the effects of joint instability. HSS J 2012;8:15–17.
19. World Health Organization Definition. <www.who.int/topics/disabilities/en/>.
20. The American Heritage® Dictionary of the English Language, Fourth Edition copyright ©2000 by Houghton Mifflin Company. New York: Houghton Mifflin Company; Updated in 2009.
21. Wang K, McCarters R, Wright J, et al. Regulation of skeletal muscle stiffness and elasticity by titin isoforms: a test of the segmental extension model of resting tension. Proc Natl Acad Sci U S A 1991;88:7101–5.
22. Chleboun G, Howell JN, Conatser RR, et al. The relationship between elbow flexor volume and angular stiffness at the elbow. Clin Biomech 1997;12:383.
23. Moreside JM, McGill SM. Improvements in hip flexibility do not transfer to mobility in functional movement patterns. J Strength Cond Res 2013;27:2635–43.
24. Schmidt R, editor. Motor Control and Learning: A Behavioral Emphasis. 4th ed. Champaign, IL: Human Kinetics; 2005.
25. Harris-Hayes M, Van Dillen LR, Sahrmann SA. Classification, treatment and outcomes of a patient with lumbar extension syndrome. Physiother Theory Pract 2005;21:181–96.
26. Van Dillen LR, Sahrmann SA, Wagner JM. Classification, intervention, and outcomes for a person with lumbar rotation with flexion syndrome. Phys Ther 2005;85:336–51.
27. Maluf KS, Sahrmann SA, Van Dillen LR. Use of a classification system to guide nonsurgical management of a patient with chronic low back pain. Phys Ther 2000;80:1097–111.
28. Van Dillen LR, Sahrmann SA, Norton BJ, et al. Reliability of physical examination items used for classification of patients with low back pain. Phys Ther 1998;78(9):979–88.
29. Harris-Hayes M, Van Dillen LR. The inter-tester reliability of physical therapists classifying low back pain problems based on the movement system impairment classification system. PM R 2009;1:117–26.
30. Luomajoki H, Kool J, de Bruin E, et al. Reliability of movement control tests in the lumbar spine. BMC Musculoskelet Disord 2007;8:90–101.
31. Henry SM, Van Dillen LR, Trombley AR, et al. Reliability of novice raters in using the movement system impairment approach to classify people with low back pain. Man Ther 2013;18:35–40.
32. Norton BJ, Sahrmann SA, Van Dillen FL. Differences in measurements of lumbar curvature related to gender and low back pain. J Orthop Sports Phys Ther 2004;34(9):524–34.
33. Van Dillen LR, Sahrmann SA, Norton BJ, et al. Movement system impairment-based categories for low back pain: stage 1 validation. J Orthop Sports Phys Ther 2003;33:126–42.
34. Trudelle-Jackson E, Sarvaiya-Shah SA, Wang SS. Interrater reliability of a movement impairment-based classification system for

lumbar spine syndromes in patients with chronic low back pain. J Orthop Sports Phys Ther 2008;38:371–6.

35. Van Dillen LR, Sahrmann SA, Norton BJ, et al. Effect of active limb movements on symptoms in patients with low back pain. J Orthop Sports Phys Ther 2001;31(8):402–13.

36. Van Dillen LR, Sahrmann SA, Norton BJ, et al. The effect of modifying patient-preferred spinal movement and alignment during symptom testing in patients with low back pain: a preliminary report. Arch Phys Med Rehabil 2003;84(3):313–22.

37. Van Dillen LR, Maluf KS, Sahrmann SA. Further examination of modifying patient-preferred movement and alignment strategies in patients with low back pain during symptomatic tests. Man Ther 2009;14(1):52–60.

38. Scholtes SA, Gombatto SP, Van Dillen LR. Differences in lumbopelvic motion between people with and people without low back pain during two lower limb movement tests. Clin Biomech 2009;24:7–12.

39. Gombatto SP, Collins DR, Sahrmann SA, et al. Gender differences in pattern of hip and lumbopelvic rotation in people with low back pain. Clin Biomech 2006;21:263–71.

40. Hoffman SL, Johnson MB, Zou D, et al. Sex differences in lumbopelvic movement patterns during hip medial rotation in people with chronic low back pain. Arch Phys Med Rehabil 2011;92: 1053–9.

41. Scholtes SA, Van Dillen LR. Gender-related differences in prevalence of lumbopelvic region movement impairments in people with low back pain. J Orthop Sports Phys Ther 2007;37:744–53.

42. Hoffman SL, Johnson MB, Zou D, et al. Sex differences in lumbopelvic movement patterns during hip medial rotation in people with chronic low back pain. Arch Phys Med Rehabil 2011;92: 1053–9.

43. Hoffman SL, Johnson MB, Zou D, et al. Gender differences in modifying lumbopelvic motion during hip medial rotation in people with low back pain. Rehabil Res Pract 2012;2012:635312.

44. Van Dillen LR, Gombatto SP, Collins DR, et al. Symmetry of timing of hip and lumbopelvic rotation motion in 2 different subgroups of people with low back pain. Arch Phys Med Rehabil 2007;88:351–60.

45. Gombatto SP, Klaesner JW, Norton BJ, et al. Validity and reliability of a system to measure passive tissue characteristics of the lumbar region during trunk lateral bending in people with and people without low back pain. J Rehabil Res Dev 2008;45: 1415–29.

46. Gombatto SP, Norton BJ, Scholtes SA, et al. Differences in symmetry of lumbar region passive tissue characteristics between people with and people without low back pain. Clin Biomech 2008;23:986–95.

47. Gombatto SP, Norton BJ, Sahrmann SA, et al. Factors contributing to lumbar region passive tissue characteristics in people with and people without low back pain. Clin Biomech 2013;28:255–61.

48. Scholtes SA, Norton BJ, Lang CE, et al. The effect of within-session instruction on lumbopelvic motion during a lower limb movement in people with and people without low back pain. Man Ther 2010;15:496–501.

49. Scholtes SA, Norton BJ, Gombatto SP, et al. Variables associated with performance of an active limb movement following within-session instruction in people with and people without low back pain. Biomed Res Int 2013;2013:867–983.

50. Scholtes SA, Norton BJ, Gombatto SP, et al. Variables associated with performance of an active limb movement following within-session instruction in people with and people without low back pain. Biomed Res Int 2013;2013:867–983.

CHAPTER 45.5 ■ THE ROLE OF MOTOR CONTROL TRAINING

Paul Hodges

INTRODUCTION

Rehabilitative and preventative exercise that targets features of sensorimotor control has been applied in the clinical management of low back and pelvic pain for many years. It appears in the clinical literature under many names (e.g. segmental stabilization training,[1] movement impairment syndromes,[2] motor control impairments,[3] motor control training[4]), and is included as a component in many other multimodal approaches.[5] Although exercise approaches that consider sensorimotor changes vary in terms of the features that are prioritized in training, the methods to achieve this and aspects of the underlying philosophy, there are major areas of convergence. Notably, each approach considers that pain, disability and/or recurrence associated with low back pain can be improved by modifying the way in which a person uses their body, and motor learning principles are used to varying degrees to achieve change.[4] Common to these approaches is the proposal that:

- The manner in which a person moves, maintains posture/alignment and/or activates muscle is relevant (in some way) to the presentation of the patient in pain and this may involve peripheral and central elements.
- From the perspective of peripheral nociceptive input, it is assumed that loading on the tissues is relevant and related to the manner in which the

individual uses their body (whether it is related to muscle activity, posture/alignment or movement and too much [e.g. excessive protection] or too little [e.g. poor control of intersegmental motion] control).

- Through careful assessment of the way the person moves and uses their body, the therapist identifies sub-optimal features related to this abnormal loading.
- The therapist identifies a clinical solution to achieve a change in the target feature of sensorimotor control, and this change in muscle activation, posture/alignment and/or movement modifies loading in a manner that affects the patient's symptoms.
- From a central perspective, modification of movement may also have other positive effects (e.g. experience with healthy movement; recovery of body representation). This may impact on pain experience, even in the absence of a contribution of peripheral nociceptive input.

Each element of this proposal requires further consideration to judge the biological plausibility, clinical viability and efficacy of this approach. It is through the systematic investigation of each element that evidence is building, but it is unlikely that this (or any other) approach will be optimal for everyone who presents with low back and pelvic pain. A challenge facing clinical research is to identify the people in pain for whom this approach will be optimal. This chapter overviews the clinical approach and the philosophy underpinning the application of motor control and motor learning principles to low back and pelvic pain.

CLINICAL FRAMEWORK FOR MOTOR CONTROL TRAINING

Basic Principles

Motor control training is an approach that relies on *clinical reasoning* to identify and then modify features of the way a patient uses their body that may be related to their symptoms. This involves careful assessment of posture/alignment, movement and muscle activation; the development of a clinical hypothesis of the relationship between these features and presentation; and relevant clinical techniques to change the target features of sensorimotor control (Fig. 45-5). The basic objective is to optimize motor control. Although early iterations of motor control training assumed that low back and pelvic pain were associated with '*clinical instability*' and the selected treatments aimed to increase control,[6] more recently it has been emphasized that control problems may present across a spectrum of too little, too much, or inaccurate control.[4,7] The former assumption of 'instability' often led to training excessive protection of the spine, which can itself become part of the problem secondary to increased load, reduced movement, etc. Many clinical approaches were developed that aimed to restrict movement with an emphasis on static alignment of spine and pelvis.[8,9] The contemporary view is that motor control should aim to *optimize* control with an emphasis on finding the balance between movement and stiffness. Both movement and stiffness are necessary, and the balance between them depends on the function. *Movement* is critical for shock absorption,[10] load transfer, variation (load sharing), and for the contribution of the trunk and trunk muscles to other functions (e.g. breathing, bladder and bowel function and balance[11]). *Stiffness* is necessary to support load and control excessive displacement.[12] All functions require a different balance across a spectrum; some require greater stiffness, others greater movement. The challenge is to train a patient to function across the spectrum, using the right strategy for the right situation.

Another key aspect is the necessity to consider motor control in the context of the biopsychosocial model of low back pain. Psychosocial issues (e.g. beliefs and attitudes about pain, depression[13,14]) and other biological issues (e.g. inflammatory response[15,16]) influence a patient's response and interact with motor control (e.g. anticipation of pain has a similar effect on motor control as the experience of pain[17,18]).

Contemporary understanding of the adaptations in sensorimotor control to pain and injury forms the foundation of this approach (see Chapter 6).[19] In brief, changes in sensorimotor control that modify the loading on tissue of the spine and pelvis can be characterized by changes in: *muscle morphology and behaviour* associated with enhanced (e.g. increased amplitude, delayed relaxation) or compromised (e.g. delayed/reduced activation, reduced muscle size, decreased fatigue resistance, muscle fibre changes) contribution to lumbopelvic control; *movement* (e.g. reduced movement, reduced acceleration, reduced or increased range, modified

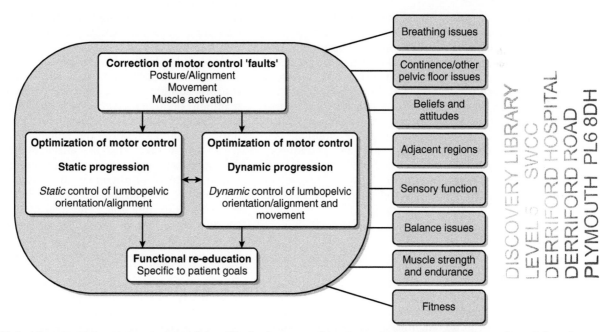

FIGURE 45-5 ■ Clinical framework for motor control training. The basic progression of exercise from identification and retraining of features of sensorimotor control considered to be related to the patient's symptoms, through integration of control of these features in more demanding contexts via static and dynamic progressions and finally into functional training of the tasks the patient has identified as important for them. To the right is an array of features that may present as barriers to recovery of optimal motor control. These should be screened for and included in the intervention as necessary.

sharing of motion between segments [e.g. hip and spine], increased intersegmental translation); *posture* (e.g. sustained position at end of range in any direction, reduced movement in sustained postures, postures associated with increased or decreased muscle activation); and *sensory function*. Although deep muscles of the trunk are commonly compromised, this may not be the critical feature.

A fundamental basis of motor control training is the necessity for the intervention to be individualized to the patient's presentation. It cannot be applied in a uniform manner as exercise needs to be targeted to the individual's unique set of features of muscle activation, posture/alignment and movement that are related to their low back and/or pelvic pain, their unique functional demands, their psychosocial profile and individual differences in learning style. Identifying clinical phenotypes (subgroups) may facilitate the process of selection of priority targets for treatment.

The contemporary approach to motor control training does not come from a single source, but involves an eclectic mix of assessments and treatments. The underlying philosophy has been to combine the most informative (and validated) assessments for muscle activation, posture/alignment and movement, and to draw on a range of approaches to identify optimal methods to achieve a change in motor control and progress the patient to function. A comprehensive review and description of this convergent approach to motor control training has recently been published as the culmination of collaboration between key individuals representing different approaches.[4]

Clinical Application of Motor Control Training

The approach begins with clinical problem solving to identify whether modification of motor control is relevant for the patient, and if so, to optimize posture, movement and muscle activation by addressing the individual patient's presenting features postulated to underpin ongoing symptoms or potential for recurrence. This phase requires careful individual assessment and a test-retest approach to find the optimized behaviour for the individual. Recent developments in subgrouping can facilitate decision making. Subgrouping aids pattern recognition (a feature of practice by skilled clinicians[20]), which provides insight into the likely priority targets (in terms of postures, movements and muscle activation to encourage and/or avoid) for training.

Assessment

Formal assessment compares strategies for muscle activation, posture and movement with a supposed ideal. Assessment of posture involves comparison of alignment in sitting and/or standing against the 'blueprint' ideal spinal and limb alignment, deviations are corrected (e.g. excessive posterior pelvic tilt) and response is evaluated. Muscle activation is analysed in several steps. Firstly, during postural and movement assessment evidence of over/underactivity, atrophy/hypertrophy is

identified. Secondly, formal tests of independent activation of the anterior and posterior deep muscles are conducted to evaluate quality of control of deeper muscles and evidence of overactivity of more superficial muscles. Movement assessment involves comparison of the movement strategy adopted during basic physiological movements (e.g. trunk flexion), standardized functional tasks (e.g. sit-to-stand) and formal movement tests (e.g. hip rotation in prone). The aim is to identify features that deviate from the expected ideal, and to then evaluate the response to correction. The ideal response minimizes pain/discomfort, as well as reduces effort and optimizes other features (e.g. breathing, balance). Figure 45-6 shows some key aspects of assessment.

Correction of Motor Control Faults

The initial phase of training identifies a technique to assist patients to modify target features identified in assessment. Motor learning principles are applied (e.g. segmentation, simplification, feedback, dosage, transfer of training) to modify motor control strategies. Techniques may include cognitive correction with manual guidance, manual cues, instruction and feedback. In the initial phase of skill learning it may be appropriate to target a single aspect of motor control. Ideally, this feature should be one that achieves the greatest change most quickly, either based on relevance for symptoms, potential for correction or patient preference.

Progression of Exercise

Once optimal strategies for correction of each target feature of motor control have been identified and mastered, the next phase progresses exercise through static and dynamic strategies. *Static progression* involves training a patient to optimize control of muscle activation and posture/alignment, and to maintain alignment as load is applied either through movement of limbs or trunk. Although important, the static phase is reasonably straightforward (there is a single goal – to maintain alignment), yet it is critical that patients are also trained to move. *Dynamic progression* involves training a patient to control the spine during movement. This can involve unstable surfaces (relying on the principle that balance cannot be maintained if the spine is stiff), control of alignment and muscle activation as the spine is moved, and control of the spine as a part of whole body function. The final phase involves progression into function. In the *functional re-education* phase the patient is progressed to maintain control of their unique features of posture/alignment, movement and muscle activation that were related to their symptoms in their priority functions. Exercises from a range of different approaches (e.g. pilates, ball exercises, limb-loading tasks, proprioceptive neuromuscular facilitation, Klein-Vogelbach) can be used, sometimes with modification and sometimes according to existing principles. Diversity challenges the individual, maintains motivation and identifies the perfect match for the patient's preferences.

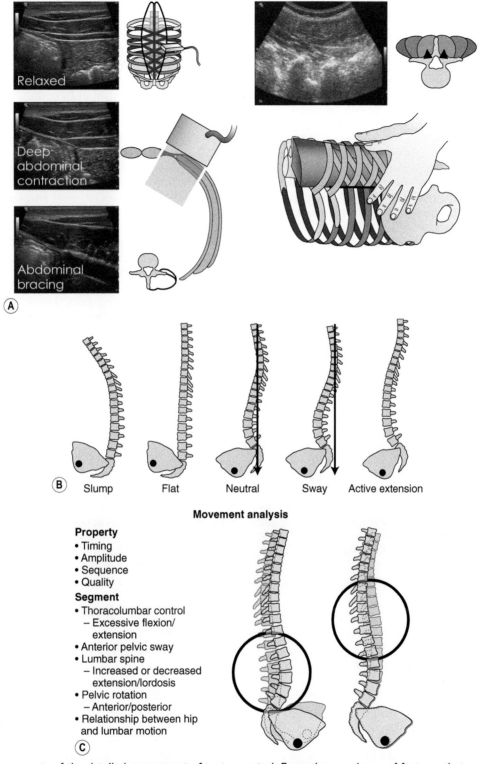

Movement analysis

Property
- Timing
- Amplitude
- Sequence
- Quality

Segment
- Thoracolumbar control
  - Excessive flexion/extension
- Anterior pelvic sway
- Lumbar spine
  - Increased or decreased extension/lordosis
- Pelvic rotation
  - Anterior/posterior
- Relationship between hip and lumbar motion

FIGURE 45-6 ■ Components of the detailed assessment of motor control. Examples are shown of features that can be assessed to build a clinical picture of causes of sub-optimal loading of the spine for an individual patient. (**A**) Muscle activation assessment includes assessment of a patient's ability to activate the deep anterior (left) and posterior (right) trunk muscles to identify deficits in activation and evidence of pattern of over activity. (**B**) Assessment of posture/alignment includes identification of features of posture that deviate from an 'ideal' and then evaluation of the relevance of any identified variation. (**C**) Movement assessment includes analysis of features of movement strategy during basic physiological movements, specific functional tasks, patient-specific functions and formal movement tests. Several key properties of movement are evaluated with specific attention to features of movement that are commonly related to sub-optimal loading.

Potential Barriers to Recovery

It is necessary to consider other features that may present as barriers to recovery for an individual and their relevance for each patient. Such features include aspects of biopsychosocial presentation (e.g. fear/catastrophization, unhealthy pain cognitions) and other physical features that can impact on restoration of optimal motor control. Although not relevant for all patients, individuals may require intervention that targets features such as the contribution of the trunk muscles to continence and breathing disorders (e.g. stress urinary incontinence and chronic airways disease), dysfunction of adjacent joints (e.g. poor foot control, restricted hip mobility), sensory function, balance, strength and endurance, and general physical fitness. Figure 45-5 can be considered a menu from which the necessary interventions can be selected as appropriate for the individual patient.

Common Misconceptions

There are several common misconceptions about motor control training. Firstly, the approach is not focused on a single muscle/muscle group, posture or movement. Several features of motor control may relate to a patient's symptoms and the specific combination to be addressed can only be identified through careful assessment. Secondly, the approach must be tailored to the individual. Subgrouping may aid identification of target features to address, but ultimately each patient needs to be considered as an individual to identify the relevant features of their presentation to influence symptoms. Thirdly, exercise must be progressed to function. Fourthly, the approach is not appropriate for all patients with low back and pelvic pain. Recent work is beginning to identify the patients who will achieve the greatest change with this treatment (see below). Fifthly, the approach does not aim to encourage stiffness. Optimal control involves training a balance between movement and stiffness, and the balance must be trained to match a spectrum of functional demands.

EVIDENCE FOR MOTOR CONTROL TRAINING

How Can Motor Control Training Relieve and Prevent Pain and Disability?

An individual may have ongoing or recurrent pain for several reasons, and motor control training may have different mechanisms. Firstly, pain may involve ongoing nociceptive input from the periphery related to sub-optimal tissue loading and the area may be sensitized. Modification of the loading on the tissues (by changing posture/alignment, movement, or muscle activity) could be expected to reduce symptoms. Tissue loading may be sub-optimal for many reasons. For instance, muscle activation may be too much or too little, movement may be too much or too little, or a posture may load in a direction or duration or involve sub-optimal muscle activation.

Secondly, pain may be centrally maintained by neural processes associated with sensitization. This increased excitability can occur anywhere in the nervous system and is modulated by many factors including cognitive/emotional aspects of pain, and a multitude of synaptic and other neural mechanisms. Optimized motor control could be beneficial: if peripheral nociceptive input maintains some contribution to the pain state;[21] to prevent/manage the development of pain in other body segments secondary to modified motor control; or when experience with healthy movement is beneficial to contribute to resolution of psychosocial and sensitizing mechanisms (e.g. individuals who are fearful of movement/pain/injury).

Thirdly, neuropathic pain is related to nervous system injury. There is often a mechanical aspect, which may be modified by moving more optimally.

Motor control training *could* have an effect across the spectrum of patients in pain. However, for individual cases, better outcomes would be expected if treatments are combined or if treatment is directed at the primary mechanisms which may not be best targeted with motor control training (e.g. fear conditioning).

Is Motor Control Training Effective?

Several systematic reviews confirm the efficacy of motor control training to reduce pain and disability,[22,23] but the results of individual trials vary. Although early trials of individualized intervention targeted to specific subgroups identified large clinical effect sizes,[24–26] the effect has been smaller in recent trials of standardized treatments in patients with non-specific back pain.[27,28] One interpretation of this outcome is that treatment is likely to be most effective if directed in an individualized manner to specific patients. This requires investigation.

Is it Possible to Identify Patients Likely to Respond?

Several recent trials have identified features that appear related to good outcome from this approach. Poor activation of the deep trunk muscles is related to outcome. Patients with poor activation of transversus abdominis at baseline, achieve better improvement in pain.[29,30] Most recently a study has confirmed that patients who score high on a questionnaire of 'lumbar instability' do better with motor control training than graded activity using the principles of cognitive behavioural therapy.[31] On face value, this could suggest patients with instability do better, but the lumbar instability test has never been shown to relate to instability and many elements of the questionnaire could just be indicative of features of nociceptive pain. The questionnaire may simply reflect those who retain a nociceptive component related to sub-optimal tissue loading which may be amenable to motor control training.

Can Motor Control be Changed with Training?

Muscle activation,[32] posture[33] and movement[34] can all be changed with application of motor learning principles. These improvements transfer to function,[32] can be maintained[35] and are related to clinical improvement.[29] Although the evidence is not universal[36] (often because of inadequate methods to assess motor adaptation[37]), there is growing evidence to support the approach.

CONCLUSION

Motor control training is an individualized approach aimed to target features of muscle activation, posture/alignment and movement that contribute to a patient's symptoms. The approach involves an eclectic mix of techniques to restore optimal control via application of motor learning theory. Outcomes are good, but perhaps best when the right patient is targeted with the right treatment. Current research priorities are to address these issues as well as better understand the mechanisms of the approach, with the aim to optimize its application in clinical practice.

REFERENCES

1. Richardson CA, Hodges PW, Hides JA. Therapeutic Exercise for Lumbopelvic Stabilisation: A Motor Control Approach for the Treatment and Prevention of Low Back Pain. Edinburgh: Churchill Livingstone; 2004.
2. Sahrmann S. Diagnosis and Treatment of Movement Impairment Syndromes. St Louis: Mosby Inc; 2002.
3. O'Sullivan P. Diagnosis and classification of chronic low back pain disorders: maladaptive movement and motor control impairments as underlying mechanism. Man Ther 2005;10:242–55.
4. Hodges PW, van Dillen L, McGill S, et al. Integrated clinical approach to motor control interventions in low back and pelvic pain. In: Hodges PW, Cholewicki J, van Dieeneditors J, editors. Spinal Control: The Rehabilitation of Back Pain. Edinburgh: Elsevier; 2013. p. 243–310.
5. Fritz JM, Erhard RE, Hagen BF. Segmental instability of the lumbar spine. Phys Ther 1998;78:889–96.
6. Panjabi MM. The stabilising system of the spine. Part II. Neutral zone and instability hypothesis. J Spinal Disord 1992;5:390–7.
7. Hodges P, Cholewicki J. Functional control of the spine. In: Vleeming A, Mooney V, Stoeckart R, editors. Movement, Stability and Lumbopelvic Pain. Edinburgh: Elsevier; 2007.
8. Chek P. How to Eat, Move and Be Healthy! C.H.E.K Institute; 2004.
9. McGill SM, Karpowicz A. Exercises for spine stabilization: motion/motor patterns, stability progressions, and clinical technique. Arch Phys Med Rehabil 2009;90:118–26.
10. Mok NW, Brauer SG, Hodges PW. Failure to use movement in postural strategies leads to increased spinal displacement in low back pain. Spine 2007;32:E537–43.
11. Hodges P, Gurfinkel VS, Brumagne S, et al. Coexistence of stability and mobility in postural control: evidence from postural compensation for respiration. Exp Brain Res 2002;144:293–302.
12. Cholewicki J, Panjabi MM, Khachatryan A. Stabilizing function of trunk flexor-extensor muscles around a neutral spine posture. Spine 1997;22:2207–12.
13. Leeuw M, Goossens ME, Linton SJ, et al. The fear-avoidance model of musculoskeletal pain: current state of scientific evidence. J Behav Med 2007;30:77–94.
14. Moseley GL. Reconceptualising pain according to its underlying biology. Phys Ther Rev 2007;12:169–78.
15. Wang H, Schiltenwolf M, Buchner M. The role of TNF-alpha in patients with chronic low back pain-a prospective comparative longitudinal study. Clin J Pain 2008;24:273–8.
16. Hodges PW, James G, Blomster L, et al. Can pro-inflammatory cytokine gene expression explain multifidus muscle fiber changes after an intervertebral disc lesion? Spine 2014;39(13):1010–17.
17. Moseley GL, Nicholas MK, Hodges PW. Does anticipation of back pain predispose to back trouble? Brain 2004;127:2339–47.
18. Tucker K, Larsson AK, Oknelid S, et al. Similar alteration of motor unit recruitment strategies during the anticipation and experience of pain. Pain 2012;153:636–43.
19. Hodges PW, Falla D. Interaction between pain and sensorimotor control. In: Jull GA, Moore A, Falla A, et al., editors. Grieve's Modern Musculoskeletal Physiotherapy. 4th ed. UK: Elsevier; 2015; in press.
20. Jones M, Rivett D. Clinical Reasoning for Manual Therapists. Edinburgh: Butterworth Heinemann; 2004.
21. Gracely RH, Lynch SA, Bennett GJ. Painful neuropathy: altered central processing maintained dynamically by peripheral input. Pain 1992;51:175–94.
22. Ferreira PH, Ferreira ML, Maher CG, et al. Specific stabilisation exercise for spinal and pelvic pain: a systematic review. Aust J Physiother 2006;52:79–88.
23. Macedo LG, Maher CG, Latimer J, et al. Motor control exercise for persistent, nonspecific low back pain: a systematic review. Phys Ther 2009;89:9–25.
24. O'Sullivan PB, Twomey LT, Allison GT. Evaluation of specific stabilizing exercise in the treatment of chronic low back pain with radiologic diagnosis of spondylolysis or spondylolisthesis. Spine 1997;22:2959–67.
25. Hides JA, Jull GA, Richardson CA. Long term effects of specific stabilizing exercises for first episode low back pain. Spine 2001;26:243–8.
26. Stuge B, Laerum E, Kirkesola G, et al. The efficacy of a treatment program focusing on specific stabilizing exercises for pelvic girdle pain after pregnancy: a randomized controlled trial. Spine 2004;29:351–9.
27. Goldby LJ, Moore AP, Doust J, et al. A randomized controlled trial investigating the efficiency of musculoskeletal physiotherapy on chronic low back disorder. Spine 2006;31:1083–93.
28. Ferreira ML, Ferreira PH, Latimer J, et al. Comparison of general exercise, motor control exercise and spinal manipulative therapy for chronic low back pain: a randomized trial. Pain 2007;131:31–7.
29. Ferreira PH, Ferreira ML, Maher CG, et al. Changes in recruitment of transversus abdominis correlate with disability in people with chronic low back pain. Br J Sports Med 2010;44:1166–72.
30. Unsgaard-Tondel M, Lund Nilsen TI, Magnussen J, et al. Is activation of transversus abdominis and obliquus internus abdominis associated with long-term changes in chronic low back pain? A prospective study with 1-year follow-up. Br J Sports Med 2012;46:729–34.
31. Macedo LG, Maher CG, Hancock MJ, et al. Predicting response to motor control exercises and graded activity for patients with low back pain: preplanned secondary analysis of a randomized controlled trial. Phys Ther 2014;94(11):1543–54.
32. Tsao H, Hodges PW. Immediate changes in feedforward postural adjustments following voluntary motor training. Exp Brain Res 2007;181:537–45.
33. Falla D, Jull G, Russell T, et al. Effect of neck exercise on sitting posture in patients with chronic neck pain. Phys Ther 2007;87:408–17.
34. Hoffman SL, Johnson MB, Zou D, et al. Effect of classification-specific treatment on lumbopelvic motion during hip rotation in people with low back pain. Man Ther 2011;16:344–50.
35. Tsao H, Hodges PW. Persistence of changes in postural control following training of isolated voluntary contractions in people with recurrent low back pain. J Electromyogr Kinesiol 2008;18:559–67.
36. Wong AY, Parent EC, Funabashi M, et al. Do changes in transversus abdominis and lumbar multifidus during conservative treatment explain changes in clinical outcomes related to nonspecific low back pain? A Systematic Review. J Pain 2014;15:e371–7.
37. Mannion AF, Caporaso F, Pulkovski N, et al. Spine stabilisation exercises in the treatment of chronic low back pain: a good clinical outcome is not associated with improved abdominal muscle function. Eur Spine J 2012;21:1301–10.

THE SACROILIAC JOINT (PELVIC PAIN):

MODELS OF ASSESSMENT AND MANAGEMENT

EDITOR'S INTRODUCTION

Pelvic pain and the joints of the pelvis have fascinated clinicians and researchers from several health disciplines over many decades. The region, not unexpectedly, has attracted interest for women during pregnancy but several studies using anaesthetic blocks have proven that it is a source of pain in the low back region in the general population. Research in the field has increased and knowledge has grown substantially, but it is still a region where there is considerable uncertainly from conservative musculoskeletal perspectives. There is definitive evidence that the pelvic joints can be a source of pain, yet debate continues, for example, about the extent of its capacity for movement. There have been few randomized controlled trials evaluating the conservative treatment approaches for pelvic joint dysfunction. Thus clinical theory and reasoning still play a considerable role in decisions about the aetiology, assessment and management of painful pelvic joint dysfunction. In this chapter, three approaches are presented from internationally renowned clinicians and researchers. They illustrate the synergies and differences that are still present in theory and practice. They were chosen to inform readers of the breadth of current thought and practice.

CHAPTER 46.1 ■ A PERSON-CENTRED BIOPSYCHOSOCIAL APPROACH TO ASSESSMENT AND MANAGEMENT OF PELVIC GIRDLE PAIN

Darren Beales • Peter O'Sullivan

CHALLENGING HEALTH-CARE PRACTITIONER BELIEFS REGARDING THE PELVIS

The pelvis and SIJ (sacroiliac joints), perhaps more than any other joint complex in the body, are shrouded by mystique within the field of manual therapy. Numerous, complex and often confusing theories, assessment procedures and treatment approaches are associated with the pelvis.[1-5] These approaches lack validity and may have a detrimental effect on clinicians' confidence[6] in their manual therapy skills because of a self-perceived inability to 'feel intra-pelvic motion', observe 'displacements' and

- The pelvis and SIJs are designed primarily for load transfer, are inherently stable[7–9] and can safely transfer enormous loads under normal conditions[7]
- The SIJ has very little movement in non-weight-bearing (average 2.5° rotation),[10–14] and even less in weight-bearing (average 0.2° rotation)[15]
- Movement of the SIJs cannot be validly or reliably assessed by manual palpation, particularly in weight-bearing[15–20]
- There is strong evidence that intra-articular displacements within the SIJs do not occur[21] and pelvic manipulation does not alter the position of the pelvic joints[21]
- Asymmetry of the pelvis observed clinically is likely to occur due to changes in the spine and hips secondary to altered pelvic and trunk muscle activity, resulting in directional strain across pain-sensitive structures and not positional changes within the SIJs themselves[21]
- The claim by some health-care practitioners to treat 'non-painful SIJ dysfunction(s)/displacements' for pain in other body locations is not evidence-based
- No study has documented a relationship between ligament laxity of the SIJ and pelvic girdle pain, and relaxin levels are not related to pain or disability during pregnancy[22,23]
- A positive active straight leg raise reflects impaired motor activity of the hip/pelvic region[24,25] associated with sensitized pelvic structures,[26,27] and does not reflect an unstable pelvis
- A clinical diagnosis of SIJ pain can be made by: (a) the finding of pain primarily located to the inferior sulcus of the SIJ, and (b) positive pain provocation stress tests for the SIJ[28]
- The symphysis pubis may be a source of pain, and can be identified through physical examination, though this process has not been validated in the same way as the SIJs. As with the SIJs, there is not a direct relationship between the amount of symphysis movement and pain[29]
- Pelvic girdle pain disorders may be associated with 'excessive' as well as 'insufficient' motor activation of the lumbopelvic and surrounding musculature[25,30–32]
- The strongest predictor of pelvic girdle pain not becoming chronic after pregnancy is the belief that it will not[17]

diagnose complex disorders. Because of this it is important to be clear of the 'facts' regarding the pelvis in the context of current knowledge for both the health-care practitioners (HCPs) and the patient (Box 46-1). Furthermore, transmitting these beliefs to patients can be harmful, contributing to fear, avoidance, hypervigilance and dependency on passive interventions with poor efficacy.

EMBRACING THE BIOPSYCHOSOCIAL MODEL OF PELVIC GIRDLE PAIN

Assessment of pelvic girdle pain (PGP) needs to be considered from a biopsychosocial perspective; screening for Red Flags and specific pathology in the minority, while acknowledging the multifactorial nature of PGP and the importance of identifying both peripheral and/or central mechanism(s) underlying pain and disability in the majority (see Figs 46-1 and 46-2).[33–35] This model is dynamic, flexible and considers both modifiable and non-modifiable factors in order to better target person-centred care (Fig. 46-1).

Neurophysiological Factors

A number of potential factors need to be considered that can result in/modulate both peripheral and central sensitization of pelvic girdle structures (Fig. 46-1). Recent experimental pain research has demonstrated that saline injected into the posterior SIJ ligaments reproduced pain, positive SIJ provocation and active straight leg raise (ASLR) tests similar to the clinical presentation of PGP.[26,36] These findings highlight that sensitization of pelvic ligaments can mimic common clinical presentations in the absence of tissue injury, 'instability' or 'dysfunction'. These findings are mirrored by a parallel study in women with pregnancy-related PGP who demonstrated lower pain pressure thresholds both locally and peripherally, associated with positive clinical tests.[27]

Observed relationships between PGP and central sensitizing factors such as sleep disturbance, depressed mood and anxiety support the concept of top-down sensitizing factors linked to these disorders.[37] These findings suggest that PGP is related to both local and central sensitization affecting the pelvic structures. There is also evidence that factors such as altered body perception are linked to PGP disorders highlighting the potential role of the central nervous system in mediating common patient reports of altered pelvic alignment.[37] Clinical markers of peripheral sensitization are mechanical pain characteristics, local hyperalgesia, positive SIJ provocation tests and ASLR tests, whereas clinical markers of central sensitization are more commonly demonstrated by non-mechanical pain characteristics, widespread pressure and cold sensitization and allodynia.[38,39] Body perception is also important and can be measured with body scanning assessments and the use of body perception questionnaires.[40]

Psychosocial Factors

The vast majority of research investigating psychological features of PGP has been completed in pregnancy-related PGP subjects. However, these factors are also relevant for non-pregnancy-related cases. *Cognitive* factors (thoughts and perceptions) such as fear and negative expectations of recovery impact on pain and disability in PGP patients.[37,41,42] Beliefs such as those related to perceived lumbopelvic weakness are also a potential factor in PGP.[43] It is well known that HCPs' beliefs and communication have an impact on patients' beliefs and management,[44] highlighting the need for HCPs and patients to adopt an evidence-based understanding of the disorder. *Affective* factors (altered mood and emotion) such as depression, stress/emotional distress and catastrophizing have all been shown to be risk factors for ongoing PGP

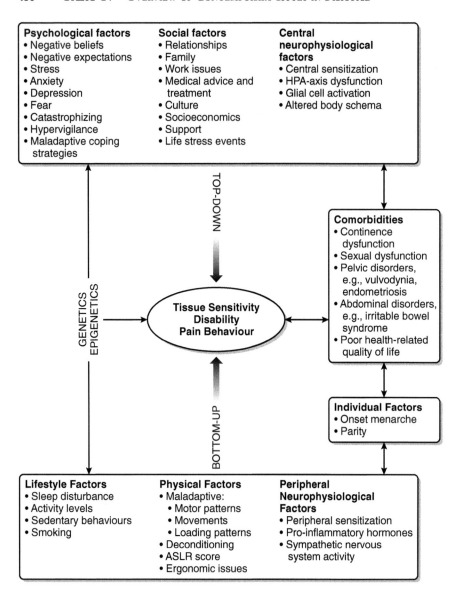

FIGURE 46-1 ■ Biopsychosocial model of pelvic girdle pain. The interaction of contributing factors for an individual result in pain and pain behaviours, which in turn feedback into the system contributing to a vicious pain cycle.

and associated disability.[45–47] *Social* risk factors such as socioeconomic status and work dissatisfaction have been identified as predictors for PGP in numerous studies,[43,48–50] highlighting the potential role of life-stress-related factors in PGP. Clinical screening tools such as the Orebro[51] and STarT Back Screening Tool[52] can be used to identify those people with negative beliefs and high levels of psychological distress, followed up with a careful clinical interview.

Lifestyle Factors

Reduced sleep is associated with chronic PGP.[37] This has previously been shown to influence factors such as pain thresholds and circulating cytokines.[53] Strenuous and more physically demanding employment has also been associated with greater risk of developing PGP,[54,55] highlighting the potential role of peripheral sensitizing factors. Lower general exercise levels have been associated with chronic PGP,[54] while higher exercise levels

prior to pregnancy are associated with lower risk of chronicity.[56] Smoking[48,55] may also contribute to chronicity in PGP. Questioning of lifestyle factors is an important part of the interview process.

Physical Factors – Motor Control Factors

Aberrant motor control strategies have been identified in PGP subjects.[24,25,30,57–59] A significant body of research has investigated motor control patterns related to the ASLR test as high levels of difficulty with an ASLR are predictive of greater levels of disability in PGP.[47,60,61] Evidence suggests increased co-contraction (bracing) of muscles in the presence of persistent PGP.[62–64] We have documented a co-contraction strategy in the abdominal wall of chronic PGP subjects[24,25] linked to bracing of the diaphragm, altered patterns of respiration and generation of increased intra-abdominal pressure, not observed in pain-free subjects.[65] This finding is supported elsewhere.[58] Other research has documented increased activation of the

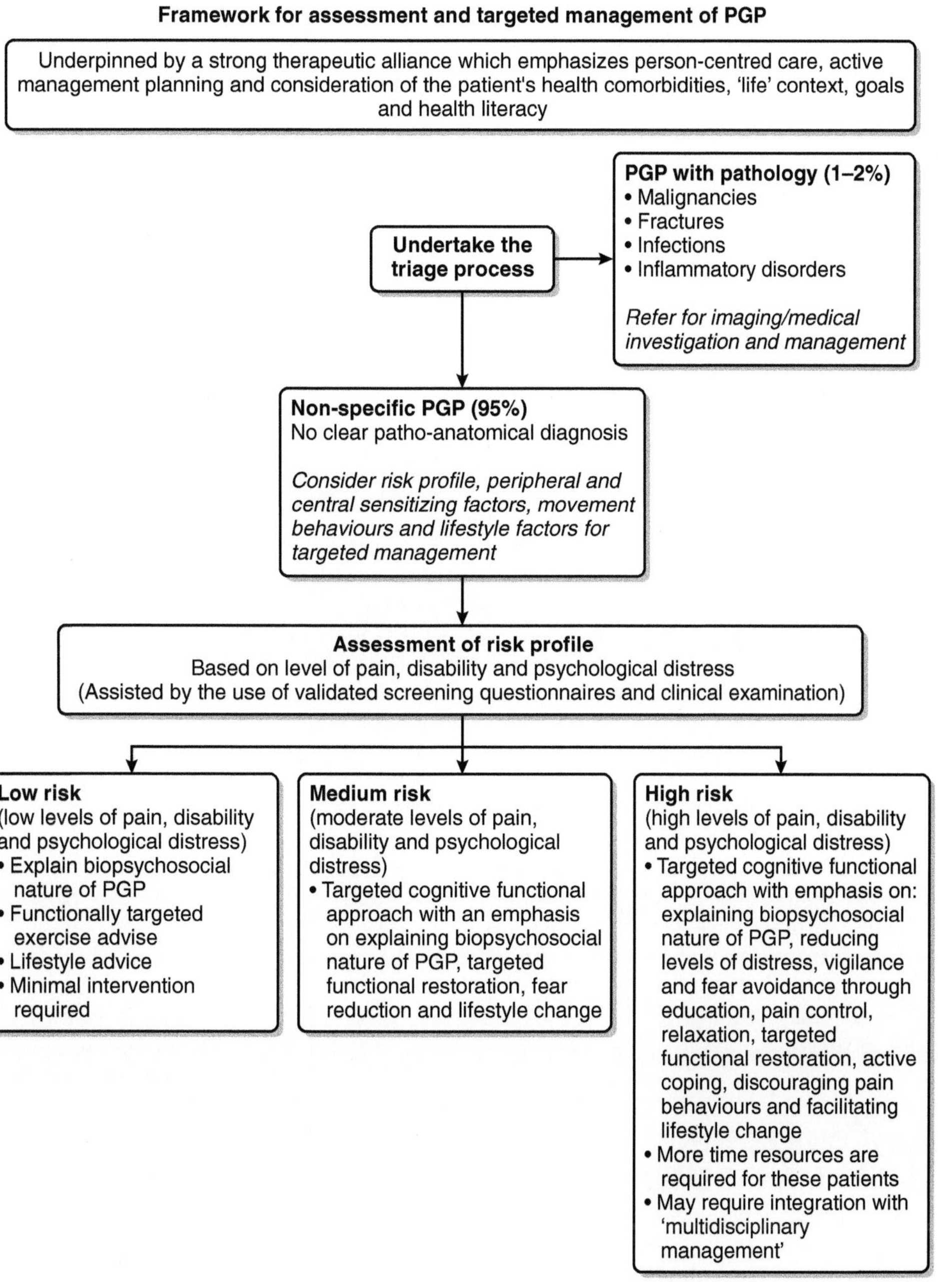

Framework for assessment and targeted management of PGP

Underpinned by a strong therapeutic alliance which emphasizes person-centred care, active management planning and consideration of the patient's health comorbidities, 'life' context, goals and health literacy

Undertake the triage process

PGP with pathology (1–2%)
• Malignancies
• Fractures
• Infections
• Inflammatory disorders

Refer for imaging/medical investigation and management

Non-specific PGP (95%)
No clear patho-anatomical diagnosis

Consider risk profile, peripheral and central sensitizing factors, movement behaviours and lifestyle factors for targeted management

Assessment of risk profile
Based on level of pain, disability and psychological distress
(Assisted by the use of validated screening questionnaires and clinical examination)

Low risk
(low levels of pain, disability and psychological distress)
• Explain biopsychosocial nature of PGP
• Functionally targeted exercise advise
• Lifestyle advice
• Minimal intervention required

Medium risk
(moderate levels of pain, disability and psychological distress)
• Targeted cognitive functional approach with an emphasis on explaining biopsychosocial nature of PGP, targeted functional restoration, fear reduction and lifestyle change

High risk
(high levels of pain, disability and psychological distress)
• Targeted cognitive functional approach with emphasis on: explaining biopsychosocial nature of PGP, reducing levels of distress, vigilance and fear avoidance through education, pain control, relaxation, targeted functional restoration, active coping, discouraging pain behaviours and facilitating lifestyle change
• More time resources are required for these patients
• May require integration with 'multidisciplinary management'

FIGURE 46-2 ■ A clinical framework for pelvic girdle pain (*PGP*) including triage, stratification by risk[51,52] and targeted management of contributing factors.

pelvic floor muscles in PGP patients,[30] consistent with bracing. These 'bracing' motor patterns are commonly observed during the functional analysis of pain provocative postural and movement tasks, challenging the popular belief that PGP is related to a loss of 'core stability'. While these patterns have been described based on group averages, importantly significant individual variations in motor control strategies occur.[24,25,65]

Significant debate exists to the basis of these findings. We propose that in some situations a positive ASLR may represent an adaptive (protective) response to pain across highly sensitized pelvic structures. Attempts to

normalize movement behaviours in this context may be provocative, with the need for the HCP to consider and direct treatment at underlying pain-sensitizing mechanisms prior to or in conjunction with movement training. In many circumstances a positive ASLR appears to represent a maladaptive (provocative) response of the motor system to PGP, by exerting excessive and abnormal load/strain on pain-sensitive structures. Attempts to normalize movement behaviours within a cognitive–functional framework in these cases should result in pain control and increased functional capacity. Identification of individual lumbopelvic motor control strategies during pain-provocative postures and activities is a critical part of the clinical examination in order to determine targets for functional restoration.

Deconditioning of the trunk and lower limbs is common in PGP[66-68] and is likely to be linked to avoidance of movement and activity. This can be assessed with functional movement tests such as squatting, lunging and lifting.

Co-morbidities

Disorders of continence may be comorbid in as many as 50% of women with PGP.[30] Motor dysfunction of the pelvic floor/abdominal cylinder and excessive intra-abdominal pressure generation provides a plausible mechanistic link between these conditions.[30,31,69,70] Various pain disorders both local and peripheral to the pelvis are comorbid with PGP, highlighting the potential role of widespread pain sensitivity linked to abnormal central sensitization.[71]

Genetic and Individual Factors

A familial relationship is known for PGP, with women with PGP more likely to have a mother or sister who also has PGP.[54,72] This may implicate a genetic link,[73] although social and behavioural influences may also mediate this effect. Earlier menarche has been associated with greater risk for developing pregnancy-related PGP,[74] though the exact mechanism for this is unclear. The role of sex and stress hormones on peripheral and central pain mechanisms is well known,[75] although to date there are no definitive studies linking hormones levels to PGP. Additionally increased parity is a risk factor for PGP, although the exact mechanism for this is unknown.[48,54,72,76] Further research is ongoing in this area.

KEY CONSIDERATIONS IN THE BIOPSYCHOSOCIAL MANAGEMENT OF PELVIC GIRDLE PAIN

An expansive, flexible clinical reasoning framework and management system for PGP has been proposed that acknowledges the complex interaction of contributing biopsychosocial factors, while identifying both the mediators as well as the moderators of the disorder in order to target care.[33-35] This cognitive–functional approach has not been fully tested in PGP subjects, but encouraging results have been reported in persistent low back pain subjects.[31,77] Figure 46-2 provides a framework for this approach.

Communication and Language

HCP beliefs have a powerful effect on patient beliefs. Communication and language is an intermediary pathway. Table 46-1 provides examples of HCP messages that have been reported by patients as harmful versus those that have the potential to empower patients to better manage their PGP. Critical to this process is a clear explanation (verbal and written) regarding the interaction of the contributing biopsychosocial factors that underpin the individual's experience of pain sensitization and disability.

Risk Profiling

Growing evidence supports risk profiling of patients with musculoskeletal pain in clinical practice[51,52] to assist with targeting management and resource allocation to those at risk of chronicity This approach can logically be adapted to PGP (Fig. 46-2).

Cognitive–Functional Approach to Management

Consistent with the biopsychosocial nature of 'non-specific' PGP (Fig. 46-1), we propose that management strategies that target modifiable maladaptive cognitive, functional and lifestyle factors that drive pain sensitivity and disability in a person-centred manner should form the basis for care. The importance of a strong therapeutic alliance with empowering communication and language has been emphasized as an over-arching consideration in patient–HCP interactions (Table 46-1). Other specific strategies for cognitive aspects of an individual's presentation include:

- Education regarding patient's contributing factors and vicious cycle of pain from a biopsychosocial perspective.
- Addressing faulty beliefs regarding causes, mechanisms and necessary treatment.
- Address fear, specifically related to the aggravating factors and/or future course.
- Use personally meaningful strategies to reduce stress and anxiety.
- Address pacing issues/avoidance behaviours.
- Address coping strategies (avoidant and endurance).
- Address lifestyle factors such as general physical activity levels, sedentary behaviours, work-related stress and sleep hygiene.
- Utilize realistic, collaborative goal setting.
- Consider patient expectations.

Cognitive considerations support a staged approach to physical restoration aimed at developing pain control and enhancing functional capacity through; body relaxation, normalization of body perception, correcting maladaptive postures and movement patterns, building confidence, conditioning, discouraging pain behaviours and encourage healthy lifestyle changes. Specific functionally based strategies include:

1. Body relaxation techniques – diaphragmatic breathing, body scanning and visual imagery techniques to focus relaxation.
2. Body awareness – isolated lumbopelvic–hip control without excessive co-contraction and breath holding using visual feedback (mirrors and video).
3. Facilitation of normal relaxed postures – lumbopelvic control with relaxed thorax and diaphragmatic breathing.

TABLE 46-1 **Language and Communication is Powerful – It has the Capacity to Harm and Empower**

Messages that Harm	Messages that Heal
Promoting Structural Damage/Dysfunction	**Promote a Biopsychosocial Approach to Pelvic Pain**
'You have an unstable pelvis'	'Pelvic pain means that your pelvic structures are sensitized. Altered postures, muscle tension, lack of sleep, inactivity, stress and worry can sensitize them'
'Your pelvis is out of alignment'	
'Your pelvis goes out of place'	
'Your pelvic pain is because you have a weak core'	'The brain acts as an amplifier – the more you worry about your pain and focus on it the worse it gets'
'Your pelvic ligaments are lax'	'Because you get pain relief with manipulation does **not** mean that your pelvis was out of place. The treatment gives short term pain relief and helps relax the muscles'
'You should use a pelvic belt when you exercise to protect the pelvis'	'Because you get pain relief wearing a pelvic belt does not mean the joints are unstable – it is like putting a brace on a sore knee for support'
Promote a Negative Future Outlook	'When you feel like your pelvis is out of alignment it is usually reflects muscle tension that gives the perception that you are lop-sided'
'Your pelvis will always be unstable'	
'You will always have a weakness now so be careful'	**Promote Trust in the Body**
'You will have to be careful when you get pregnant'	'Your pelvic structures are the strongest structures in the body and can be trusted'
'You won't be able to have a natural birth'	'Pelvis's don't go out of place – they are too strong to do this'
'Having children has wrecked your pelvis – there is nothing you can do now'	'I don't want you to rely on belts and braces, let's teach you ways to be confident in your pelvic structures again'
	'The majority of pelvic girdle pain disorders get better – especially if you have confidence in your body'
Hurt Equals Harm	
'Stop if you feel any pain'	**Encourage Healthy Behaviours**
'Let pain guide you'	'Thinking positively, sleeping well, relaxation and regular exercise will help your pelvic pain'
	'Protecting your pelvis and avoiding movement can make your pain worse – relaxed confident movement helps'
	Encourage Self-Management
	'Let's find a way to give you control over the pain rather than giving short fixes'

These messages are examples given to patients with pelvic girdle pain that resulted in fear and avoidance, and also messages use to empower them to change

4. Retraining normal functional movement patterns (based on patient reports) without breath holding.
5. Discourage pain behaviours such as grimacing, moaning, holding painful body part, limping, avoidance and the persistent use of aids such as braces.
6. Graded integration of movement into previously reported painful, feared and/or avoided tasks, with pain control.
7. Targeted conditioning – lower limbs, trunk and upper limbs as indicated.
8. Lifestyle change – regular physical activity guided by pain levels and patient preference, pacing, sleep hygiene, other general healthy lifestyle considerations (e.g. diet, smoking).

Passive treatments such as manual therapy, massage and acupuncture may be used as an adjunct to a cognitive–functional approach in order to create opportunities for behaviour change. Avoid sole reliance on passive treatments as this may reinforce passive coping strategies. Furthermore it is important that communication related to passive treatment is evidence-based (Box 46-1) and does not contribute to harmful patient beliefs (Table 46-1).

Likely benefits of a cognitive–functional approach include:
• Provides a biopsychosocial understanding of the disorder (Fig. 46-1).
• Facilitates empowerment of the individual for self-management.
• Increased self-confidence and self-efficacy.
• Pain control and reduced disability.

CONCLUSION

We believe that clinicians need to abandon simplistic biomechanical approaches to PGP and adopt an evidence-based approach based on a biopsychosocial understanding of PGP. The challenges of integrating biopsychosocial thinking into health-care education, practice and research are known.[78,79] The model presented here provides a framework for meeting these challenges as well as future research.

REFERENCES

1. Cibulka MT. Understanding sacroiliac joint movement as a guide to the management of a patient with unilateral low back pain. Man Ther 2002;7:215–21.
2. DonTigny RL. Anterior dysfunction of the sacroiliac joint as a major factor in the etiology of idiopathic low back pain syndrome. Phys Ther 1990;70:250–65, discussion 62–5.
3. Kuchera ML. Treatment of gravitational strain pathophysiology. In: Vleeming A, Mooney V, Dorman T, et al., editors. Movement, Stability and Low Back Pain: The Essential Role of the Pelvis. Edinburgh: Churchill Livingstone; 1997. p. 477–99.

4. Oldreive WL. A classification of, and a critical review of the literature on, syndromes of the sacroiliac joint. J Man Manipulative Ther 1998;6:24–30.

5. Sandler SE. The management of low back pain in pregnancy. Man Ther 1996;1:178–85.

6. Nolan D. Column. J Nat Back Exch 2013;25:16–18.

7. Snijders CJ, Vleeming A, Stoeckart R. Transfer of lumbosacral load to iliac bones and legs. Part 1: biomechanics of self-bracing of the sacroiliac joints and its significance for treatment and exercise. Clin Biomech 1993;8:285–94.

8. Vleeming A, Stoeckart R, Volkers AC, et al. Relation between form and function in the sacroiliac joint. Part I: clinical anatomical aspects. Spine 1990;15:130–2.

9. Vleeming A, Volkers AC, Snijders CJ, et al. Relation between form and function in the sacroiliac joint. Part II: biomechanical aspects. Spine 1990;15:133–6.

10. Brunner C, Kissling R, Jacob HA. The effects of morphology and histopathologic findings on the mobility of the sacroiliac joint. Spine 1991;16:1111–17.

11. Jacob HA, Kissling RO. The mobility of the sacroiliac joints in healthy volunteers between 20 and 50 years of age. Clin Biomech 1995;10:352–61.

12. Sturesson B, Selvik G, Uden A. Movements of the sacroiliac joints. A roentgen stereophotogrammetric analysis. Spine 1989;14:162–5.

13. Vleeming A, Buyruk HM, Stoeckart R, et al. An integrated therapy for peripartum pelvic instability: a study of the biomechanical effects of pelvic belts. Am J Obstet Gynecol 1992;166:1243–7.

14. Vleeming A, Van Wingerden JP, Dijkstra PF, et al. Mobility in the sacroiliac joints in the elderly: a kinematic and radiological study. Clin Biomech 1992;7:170–6.

15. Sturesson B, Uden A, Vleeming A. A radiostereometric analysis of movements of the sacroiliac joints during the standing hip flexion test. Spine 2000;25:364–8.

16. Freburger JK, Riddle DL. Using published evidence to guide the examination of the sacroiliac joint region. Phys Ther 2001;81:1135–43.

17. Holmgren U, Waling K. Inter-examiner reliability of four static palpation tests used for assessing pelvic dysfunction. Man Ther 2008;13(1):50–6.

18. Robinson HS, Brox JI, Robinson R, et al. The reliability of selected motion- and pain provocation tests for the sacroiliac joint. Man Ther 2007;12:72–9.

19. van der Wurff P, Hagmeijer RH, Meyne W. Clinical tests of the sacroiliac joint. A systemic methodological review. Part 1: reliability. Man Ther 2000;5:30–6.

20. van der Wurff P, Meyne W, Hagmeijer RH. Clinical tests of the sacroiliac joint. A systematic methodological review. Part 2: validity. Man Ther 2000;5:89–96.

21. Tullberg T, Blomberg S, Branth B, et al. Manipulation does not alter the position of the sacroiliac joint. A roentgen stereophotogrammetric analysis. Spine 1998;23:1124–8, discussion 9.

22. Aldabe D, Ribeiro DC, Milosavljevic S, et al. Pregnancy-related pelvic girdle pain and its relationship with relaxin levels during pregnancy: a systematic review. Eur Spine J 2012;21:1769–76.

23. Vollestad NK, Torjesen PA, Robinson HS. Association between the serum levels of relaxin and responses to the active straight leg raise test in pregnancy. Man Ther 2012;17:225–30.

24. Beales DJ, O'Sullivan PB, Briffa NK. Motor control patterns during an active straight leg raise in chronic pelvic girdle pain subjects. Spine 2009;34:861–70.

25. O'Sullivan PB, Beales DJ, Beetham JA, et al. Altered motor control strategies in subjects with sacroiliac joint pain during the active straight-leg-raise test. Spine 2002;27:E1–8.

26. Palsson TS, Graven-Nielsen T. Experimental pelvic pain facilitates pain provocation tests and causes regional hyperalgesia. Pain 2012;153:2233–40.

27. Palsson TS, Beales D, Slater H, et al. Pregnancy is characterised by widespread deep-tissue hypersensitivity independent of lumbopelvic pain intensity, a facilitated response to manual orthopedic tests and poorer self-reported health. J Pain 2015;In Press. doi:10.1016/j.jpain.2014.12.002.

28. Laslett M, Aprill CN, McDonald B, et al. Diagnosis of sacroiliac joint pain: validity of individual provocation tests and composites of tests. Man Ther 2005;10:207–18.

29. Bjorklund K, Nordstrom ML, Bergstrom S. Sonographic assessment of symphyseal joint distention during pregnancy and post partum with special reference to pelvic pain. Acta Obstet Gynecol Scand 1999;78:125–30.

30. Pool-Goudzwaard AL, Slieker Ten Hove MC, Vierhout ME, et al. Relations between pregnancy-related low back pain, pelvic floor activity and pelvic floor dysfunction. Int Urogynecol J Pelvic Floor Dysfunct 2005;16:468–74.

31. O'Sullivan PB, Beales DJ. Changes in pelvic floor and diaphragm kinematics and respiratory patterns in subjects with sacroiliac joint pain following a motor learning intervention: a case series. Man Ther 2007;12:209–18.

32. Hungerford BA, Gilleard W, Hodges P. Evidence of altered lumbopelvic muscle recruitment in the presence of sacroiliac joint pain. Spine 2003;28:1593–600.

33. O'Sullivan PB, Beales DJ. Diagnosis and classification of pelvic girdle pain disorders, Part 1: a mechanism based approach within a biopsychosocial framework. Man Ther 2007;12:86–97.

34. O'Sullivan PB, Beales DJ. Diagnosis and classification of pelvic girdle pain disorders, Part 2: illustration of the utility of a classification system via case studies. Man Ther 2007;12:e1–12.

35. Beales D, O'Sullivan P. A biopsychosocial model for pelvic girdle pain: a contemporary evidence based perspective. physioscience 2011;7:63–71.

36. Palsson TS, Hirata RP, Graven-Nielsen T. Experimental pelvic pain impairs the performance during the active straight leg raise test and causes excessive muscle stabilization. Clin J Pain 2015;In Press. doi:10.1097/AJP.0000000000000139.

37. Beales DJ, Lutz A, Thompson J, et al. Sleep, kinesiophobia and disturbed body schema are related to disability in chronic pregnancy-related lumbopelvic pain. Australian Physiotherapy Association Conference Week 2013. Melbourne, Australia 2013 31 October-2 November.

38. O'Sullivan P, Waller R, Wright A, et al. Sensory characteristics of chronic non-specific low back pain: a subgroup investigation. Man Ther 2014;19:311–18.

39. Smart KM, Blake C, Staines A, et al. The Discriminative validity of "nociceptive," "peripheral neuropathic," and "central sensitization" as mechanisms-based classifications of musculoskeletal pain. Clin J Pain 2011;27:655–63.

40. Wand BM, James M, Abbaszadeh S, et al. Assessing self-perception in patients with chronic low back pain: development of a back-specific body-perception questionnaire. J Back Musculoskelet Rehabil 2014;27:463–73.

41. Vollestad NK, Stuge B. Prognostic factors for recovery from post-partum pelvic girdle pain. Eur Spine J 2009;18:718–26.

42. Gutke A, Lundberg M, Ostgaard HC, et al. Impact of postpartum lumbopelvic pain on disability, pain intensity, health-related quality of life, activity level, kinesiophobia, and depressive symptoms. Eur Spine J 2011;20:440–8.

43. Ostgaard HC, Andersson GB, Karlsson K. Prevalence of back pain in pregnancy. Spine 1991;16:549–52.

44. Darlow B, Fullen BM, Dean S, et al. The association between health care professional attitudes and beliefs and the attitudes and beliefs, clinical management, and outcomes of patients with low back pain: a systematic review. Eur J Pain 2012;16:3–17.

45. Bjelland EK, Stuge B, Engdahl B, et al. The effect of emotional distress on persistent pelvic girdle pain after delivery: a longitudinal population study. BJOG 2013;120:32–40.

46. Gutke A, Josefsson A, Oberg B. Pelvic girdle pain and lumbar pain in relation to postpartum depressive symptoms. Spine 2007;32:1430–6.

47. Olsson CB, Grooten WJ, Nilsson-Wikmar L, et al. Catastrophizing during and after pregnancy: associations with lumbopelvic pain and postpartum physical ability. Phys Ther 2012;92:49–57.

48. Albert HB, Godskesen M, Korsholm L, et al. Risk factors in developing pregnancy-related pelvic girdle pain. Acta Obstet Gynecol Scand 2006;85:539–44.

49. Berg G, Hammar M, Moller-Nielsen J, et al. Low back pain during pregnancy. Obstet Gynecol 1988;71:71–5.

50. Albert HB, Godskesen M, Westergaard J. Prognosis in four syndromes of pregnancy-related pelvic pain. Acta Obstet Gynecol Scand 2001;80:505–10.

51. Linton SJ, Hallden K. Can we screen for problematic back pain? A screening questionnaire for predicting outcome in acute and subacute back pain. Clinical Journal of Pain 1998;14:209–15.

52. Hill JC, Dunn KM, Lewis M, et al. A primary care back pain screening tool: identifying patient subgroups for initial treatment. Arthritis Rheum 2008;59:632–41.
53. Menefee LA, Cohen MJ, Anderson WR, et al. Sleep disturbance and nonmalignant chronic pain: a comprehensive review of the literature. Pain Med 2000;1:156–72.
54. Larsen EC, Wilken-Jensen C, Hansen A, et al. Symptom-giving pelvic girdle relaxation in pregnancy. I: prevalence and risk factors. Acta Obstet Gynecol Scand 1999;78:105–10.
55. Wu WH, Meijer OG, Uegaki K, et al. Pregnancy-related pelvic girdle pain (PPP), I: terminology, clinical presentation, and prevalence. Eur Spine J 2004;13:575–89.
56. Mogren IM. Previous physical activity decreases the risk of low back pain and pelvic pain during pregnancy. Scand J Public Health 2005;33:300–6.
57. Beales DJ, O'Sullivan PB, Briffa NK. The effects of manual pelvic compression on trunk motor control during an active straight leg raise in chronic pelvic girdle pain subjects. Man Ther 2010;15:190–9.
58. de Groot M, Pool-Goudzwaard AL, Spoor CW, et al. The active straight leg raising test (ASLR) in pregnant women: differences in muscle activity and force between patients and healthy subjects. Man Ther 2008;13:68–74.
59. Hu H, Meijer OG, van Dieen JH, et al. Muscle activity during the active straight leg raise (ASLR), and the effects of a pelvic belt on the ASLR and on treadmill walking. J Biomech 2010;43:532–9.
60. Mens JM, Vleeming A, Snijders CJ, et al. Validity of the active straight leg raise test for measuring disease severity in patients with posterior pelvic pain after pregnancy. Spine 2002;27:196–200.
61. Mukkannavar P, Desai BR, Mohanty U, et al. Pelvic girdle pain in Indian postpartum women: a cross-sectional study. Physiother Theory Pract 2014;30:123–30.
62. Cote JN, Bement MK. Update on the relation between pain and movement: consequences for clinical practice. Clin J Pain 2010;26:754–62.
63. Dankaerts W, O'Sullivan P, Burnett A, et al. Altered patterns of superficial trunk muscle activation during sitting in nonspecific chronic low back pain patients: importance of subclassification. Spine 2006;31:2017–23.
64. Schinkel-Ivy A, Nairn BC, Drake JD. Investigation of trunk muscle co-contraction and its association with low back pain development during prolonged sitting. J Electromyogr Kinesiol 2013;23:778–86.
65. Beales DJ, O'Sullivan PB, Briffa NK. Motor control patterns during an active straight leg raise in pain-free subjects. Spine 2009;34:E1–8.
66. Sjodahl J, Gutke A, Oberg B. Predictors for long-term disability in women with persistent postpartum pelvic girdle pain. Eur Spine J 2013;22:1665–73.
67. Gutke A, Ostgaard HC, Oberg B. Association between muscle function and low back pain in relation to pregnancy. J Rehabil Med 2008;40:304–11.
68. Mens JM, Vleeming A, Snijders CJ, et al. Reliability and validity of hip adduction strength to measure disease severity in posterior pelvic pain since pregnancy. Spine 2002;27:1674–9.
69. Beales DJ, O'Sullivan PB, Briffa NK. Motor control patterns during an active straight leg raise in chronic pelvic girdle pain subjects. Spine 2009;34:861–70.
70. O'Sullivan PB, Beales DJ, Beetham JA, et al. Altered motor control strategies in subjects with sacroiliac joint pain during the active straight-leg-raise test. Spine 2002;27:E1–8.
71. Woolf CJ. Central sensitization: implications for the diagnosis and treatment of pain. Pain 2011;152:S2–15.
72. Mogren IM, Pohjanen AI. Low back pain and pelvic pain during pregnancy: prevalence and risk factors. Spine 2005;30:983–91.
73. Fillingim RB, Wallace MR, Herbstman DM, et al. Genetic contributions to pain: a review of findings in humans. Oral Dis 2008;14:673–82.
74. Bjelland EK, Eberhard-Gran M, Nielsen CS, et al. Age at menarche and pelvic girdle syndrome in pregnancy: a population study of 74973 women. BJOG 2011;118:1646–52.
75. Fillingim RB, Ness TJ. Sex-related hormonal influences on pain and analgesic responses. Neurosci Biobehav Rev 2000;24:485–501.
76. Bjelland EK, Eskild A, Johansen R, et al. Pelvic girdle pain in pregnancy: the impact of parity. Am J Obstet Gynecol 2010;203(146):e1–6.
77. Vibe Fersum K, O'Sullivan P, Skouen JS, et al. Efficacy of classification-based cognitive functional therapy in patients with non-specific chronic low back pain: a randomized controlled trial. Eur J Pain 2012;17:916–28.
78. Foster NE, Delitto A. Embedding psychosocial perspectives within clinical management of low back pain: integration of psychosocially informed management principles into physical therapist practice–challenges and opportunities. Phys Ther 2011;91:790–803.
79. Pincus T, Kent P, Bronfort G, et al. Twenty-five years with the biopsychosocial model of low back pain-is it time to celebrate? A report from the twelfth international forum for primary care research on low back pain. Spine 2013;38:2118–23.

CHAPTER 46.2 ■ THE PELVIC GIRDLE: A LOOK AT HOW TIME, EXPERIENCE AND EVIDENCE CHANGE PARADIGMS

Diane Lee

Scientific research suggests that optimal function of the pelvis is essential for all tasks,[1] and yet agreement is lacking for:

1. What optimal function of the pelvis requires. When should the sacroiliac joint (SIJ) move and when should it not? The biomechanics of the SIJ and pubic symphysis are poorly understood for many tasks that aggravate people with pelvic girdle pain (PGP).
2. Best ways to evaluate the functional status of the pelvis. Even if agreement could be reached on whether the SIJ should move, it has not been established on how to reliably assess it.
3. Best ways to restore optimal function of the pelvis. When, and how, should the SIJ be mobilized or stabilized?

In clinical practice, it is common to see complex patients with a combination of PGP, urinary incontinence, pelvic organ prolapse and/or diastasis rectus abdominis.[2,3] A thorough evaluation often reveals many past injuries, thoughts/beliefs and emotional states that have collectively led to changes in strategies for posture, movement, continence and pelvic organ support. Does the presence of pain, incontinence or prolapse mean the pelvis requires treatment? If not, how should a clinician determine where to intervene to effect the greatest improvement in function and reduction in symptoms? There is little scientific evidence to guide clinicians for these complex, yet common, patients.[4] Clinical reasoning remains the recommended approach for determining the best treatment for the individual patient.[5]

THE INTEGRATED SYSTEMS MODEL FOR DISABILITY AND PAIN

The *Integrated Systems Model for Disability and Pain* (ISM)[6] is a framework to help clinicians organize knowledge and develop clinical reasoning to facilitate wise decisions for treatment. A key feature of this approach is *finding the primary driver*. In short, this involves understanding the relationships between, and within, multiple regions of the body and how impairments in one region can impact the other. Specific tests are used to determine sites of non-optimal alignment, biomechanics and control (defined as *failed load transfer* [FLT]) during analysis of a task. Subsequently, the timing of FLT, as well as the impact of correcting one site on another, is noted. Clinical reasoning of the various results determines the site of the primary driver, or the primary region of the body, that if corrected will have a significant impact on the function of the whole body/person.

Further tests of specific systems (e.g. articular, neural, myofascial, visceral) then determine the underlying impairment causing the non-optimal alignment, biomechanics and/or control of the primary driver for the specific task being assessed. Once the impaired system has been determined, specific techniques and training for release, alignment, control and integration into movement, strength and conditioning can be implemented to improve the function of the primary driver and thus impact the function of the whole body/person.

The ISM approach requires that a clinician is able to reliably perceive (visually and/or kinaesthetically) and interpret joint motion, or lack thereof, during analysis of multiple screening tasks.

The One Leg Standing (OLS) Test

Standing on one leg and flexing the contralateral hip is a task often used to evaluate both mobility and control of the pelvis. Jacob and Kissling determined that 0.4–4.3° of rotation is possible in the non-weight-bearing SIJ in healthy, non-painful subjects.[7] Sturesson and colleagues found no statistical differences in the available range of SIJ motion in subjects with PGP and impairment during OLS.[8-10] These findings suggest that although mobility may vary between subjects, PGP is not predictive of more or less motion at the SIJ.

Hungerford et al. (2004) found that the amplitude of SIJ motion was symmetric in healthy/pain-free subjects and asymmetric in those with PGP.[11] However, Dreyfuss and colleagues found that 20% of healthy/pain-free subjects had movement asymmetries of the SIJ and, again, there appears to be no correlation between PGP and asymmetric SIJ motion.[12] So the question remains as to when noted movement asymmetries of the SIJ are relevant to the clinical picture.

Asymmetric motion of the SIJs during left and right OLS is a sign of FLT (non-optimal alignment and biomechanics) and a key feature of the ISM approach and requires that clinicians can reliably perceive these differences. Unfortunately, inter-tester reliability is lacking for SIJ mobility analysis during this test (Table 46-2). Following a systematic review of commonly used mobility tests for the SIJ, Van der Wurff and colleagues,[13,14] concluded:

> 'Therefore, at this time, it is questionable whether any SIJ tests are of any value for clinical practice[14] [and that] ... There are no indications that 'upgrading' of the methodological quality would have improved the final conclusion[13]'.

When the methods of these studies are considered, several questions arise. How did the testers perceive the information – visually (look at the posterior superior iliac

TABLE 46-2 The Inter-Tester Reliability of Commonly Used Tests for Mobility of the Sacroiliac Joint

Study	Palpation Points	Tactile vs Visual	Finding
Potter and Rothstein (1985)[15]	S2 and inferior PSIS	No comment on tactile versus visual	Unreliable
Carmichael (1987)[16]	Several palpation points	Both visual and tactile	Unreliable
Herzog et al. (1989)[17]	S2 and inferior PSIS	No comment on tactile versus visual	Reliable
Dreyfuss et al. (1994)[12]	S2 and inferior PSIS	No comment on tactile vs. visual	Unreliable
Meijne et al. (1999)[18]	Several palpation points	Both visual and tactile	Unreliable
Van der Wurff et al (2000)[13,14]			Systematic review of all mobility and pain provocation tests of the SIJ and confirm lack of reliability and validity of all mobility tests

spine (PSIS) move relative to the sacrum), kinaesthetically (feel the PSIS move relative to the sacrum), or visually and kinaesthetically and does this matter? Some clinicians appear to have better visual accuracy than kinaesthetic, others have better kinaesthetic sense and a few are good at both. When the clinician is instructed to rely on their predetermined best sense (visual or kinaesthetic), their inter-tester reliability appears to improve, when tested informally during course instruction. Multiple mechanisms may drive this difference; however, those who are less reliable when using vision often have unilateral mobility restrictions of their upper neck. Were the testers in the reliability studies (Table 46-2) screened for asymmetric mobility of their upper neck?

Hungerford et al.[11] also investigated control of SIJ motion on the weight-bearing side during OLS. In the pain-free subjects the innominate remained posteriorly rotated relative to the sacrum, whereas in the PGP population the innominate rotated anteriorly; a movement clinicians can reliably palpate.[19] This research suggests that when assessing control of the SIJ, the key thing to note is any anterior rotation of the innominate relative to the sacrum, a sign of FLT when the pelvis is loaded.

Standing on one leg is a whole body task and a key component of many more complex functional tasks. While the pelvis plays an essential role for standing on one leg, the task requires more than optimal function of the pelvis. When the pelvis fails to transfer load optimally (loses control or fails to move when it should) it is important to consider the impact of the rest of the body on the pelvis and not just assume that the primary problem is within the pelvis.

Multiple studies on subjects with low back and pelvic pain show that motor control changes in the trunk are variable, individual and task-specific. Some muscles are compromised (timing of activation is delayed or absent) while others are augmented (early and increased activation). The common link between tasks and individuals is that the strategy chosen is non-optimal and there are often multiple sites of FLT.

The following brief case report highlights the ISM approach and how clinical experience, and the research evidence, has changed paradigms for understanding what a 'non-moving PSIS relative to the sacrum' during OLS may mean and one possible clinical relevance of a noted movement asymmetry of the SIJ in a subject with multiple sites of FLT and chronic PGP.

CASE REPORT

Jill was a triathlete with a primary complaint of chronic right PGP aggravated by running, her meaningful task. The OLS task is a useful screening test in that it pertains to her meaningful task. During left OLS (Fig. 46-3) her pelvis laterally tilted (abducted) at the left hip (extrinsic pelvic motion) and minimal motion of the right SIJ occurred compared to the left SIJ during right OLS (Fig. 46-4) (i.e. asymmetric intrinsic pelvic motion was present). In addition, her seventh thoracic ring translated to the left and rotated to the right (Fig. 46-5). While these are optimal biomechanics for rotation of a thoracic

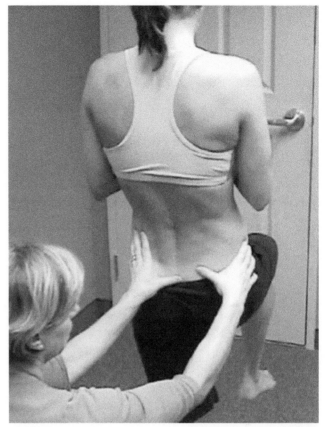

FIGURE 46-3 ■ Active mobility of the right sacroiliac joint during the one leg standing task in this subject reveals only extrinsic motion of the pelvis on the left hip joint (hip joint abduction). No intra-pelvic motion was palpable at the right sacroiliac joint. (Reproduced with permission from Diane G. Lee Physiotherapist Corporation©.)

ring,[20] rotation should not occur during this task and was, therefore, non-optimal (FLT). Increased tone in a specific fascicle of the right iliocostalis lumborum pars thoracis (ILPT) extending from the iliac crest to the right seventh rib (Figs. 46-6) was present.

During right OLS, her right SIJ lost control (the right innominate anteriorly rotated relative to the sacrum) (Fig. 46-7). This motion was intrinsic to, or within, the pelvis. Her seventh thoracic ring continued to translate to the left/rotate to the right and persistent increased tone was noted again in the right ILPT.

There were two sites of FLT for both of these tasks, the seventh thoracic ring and the right SIJ. To determine the primary driver (best region to begin to treat), the timing of FLT was noted during both tasks. The seventh thoracic ring was translated laterally to the left/rotated to the right prior to initiation of weight transfer and this translation/rotation increased before the right SIJ failed to move during left OLS and before the right SIJ lost control during right OLS. This suggested that the seventh thoracic ring was the primary driver. Confirmation of this hypothesis required consideration of the impact of a correction of the pelvis on the seventh thoracic ring alignment, biomechanics and control and then the impact of a pelvic ring correction on the seventh thoracic ring alignment, biomechanics and control during

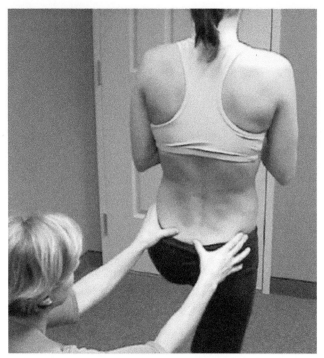

FIGURE 46-4 ■ Active mobility of the left sacroiliac joint in the same subject as Figure 46-3 reveals palpable intra-pelvic motion (i.e. motion between the innominate and the sacrum at the left sacroiliac joint). (Reproduced with permission from Diane G. Lee Physiotherapist Corporation©.)

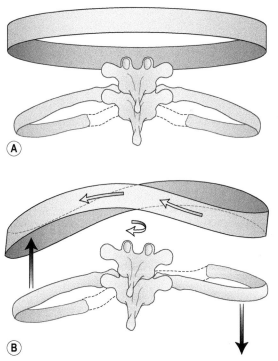

FIGURE 46-5 ■ A thoracic ring has been defined[21] as two adjacent thoracic vertebrae, the left and right ribs that articulate with these vertebrae, the sternum/manubrium and all the associated joints connecting these bones. **(B)** The biomechanics of right rotation of a typical thoracic ring.[20] Left lateral translation occurs in conjunction with right rotation of the thoracic ring. The right rib posteriorly rotates, the left rib anteriorly rotates and at the end of the available range the thoracic spinal segment rotates and side flexes to the right. (Reproduced with permission from Diane G. Lee Physiotherapist Corporation©.)

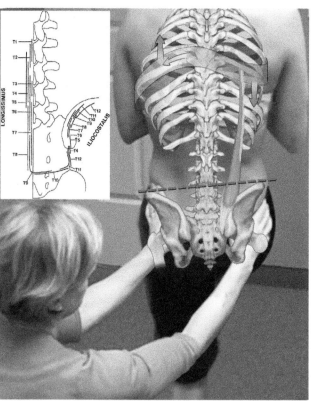

FIGURE 46-6 ■ When a fascicle of the right iliocostalis lumborum pars thoracis (ILPT) extending from the iliac crest to the seventh rib fails to eccentrically lengthen during left one leg standing, posterior rotation of the right innominate can be restricted and posterior rotation of the right seventh rib (inducing a left lateral translation/right rotation of the entire thoracic ring) is facilitated. Inset: Note the specific point of insertion on the iliac crest of the fascicle of the ILPT according to MacIntosh and Bogduk (1991).[22] (Reproduced with permission from Diane G. Lee Physiotherapist Corporation©. This figure is reproduced with permission from the authors and the Spine journal.)

both tasks. Correcting the seventh thoracic ring alignment and control[23] restored the mobility of the right SIJ during left OLS and control of the right SIJ during right OLS, correcting (alignment and control) the pelvis had no impact on the seventh thoracic ring, therefore the seventh thoracic ring was considered to be the driver.

Specific system tests (articular, neural, myofascial and visceral) pertaining to the seventh thoracic ring confirmed that the specific hypertonic fascicle noted in the right ILPT was, in part, responsible for the non-optimal alignment and biomechanics of both the seventh thoracic ring and the pelvic ring. This muscle was one of several trunk muscle dys-synergies, the discussion of which is outside the scope of this chapter. Since much of the neural drive for the abdominal wall and lumbopelvic musculature comes from the lower thorax, it is plausible that low thoracic ring impairments can lead to some muscles being compromised and others augmented, as the evidence has clearly shown. However, what is not known from these studies is the best way to restore synergy and optimal recruitment strategies. According to the ISM approach,[24] treatment was directed to restoring optimal function of the primary driver, the seventh thoracic ring, following which symmetric SIJ mobility and

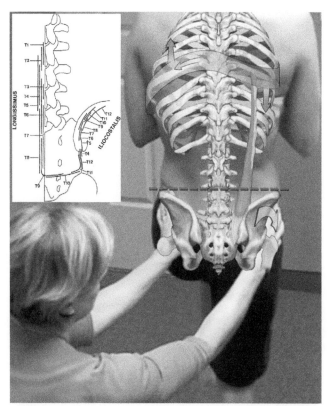

FIGURE 46-7 ■ Two sites of failed load transfer were noted during right one leg standing in this subject, the right SIJ (horizontal arrow on the pelvis) and the seventh thoracic ring (horizontal arrow on the seventh thoracic ring). Inset: Note the specific point of insertion on the iliac crest of the fascicle of the ILPT according to MacIntosh and Bogduk (1991).[22] (This figure is reproduced with permission from the authors and the Spine Journal.)

control was restored without direct intervention to her pelvis.

In this case, the asymmetric mobility of the SIJs was primarily secondary to a hypertonic iliocostalis lumborum pars thoracis (ILPT) and not directly related to a stiff or 'stuck' right SIJ therefore no manual therapy intervention was indicated for her right SIJ. The right SIJ was noted to be not moving when it should (left OLS) and moving when it should not (right OLS); however, the reason was extrinsic to the pelvis. In clinical practice there are many different drivers for pelvic girdle pain; Jill was a thorax-driven PGP case.

CONCLUSION

Clearly, the pelvis can no longer be considered as an individual entity in either assessment or treatment. It is part of a functional whole and tests are required that reflect the essential role it plays in the function, or lack thereof, of multiple systems (posture/equilibrium, musculoskeletal, urogynaecological, respiratory, digestive) and its relationship to multiple regions of the body. When to treat the pelvis and when to look elsewhere for the primary driver requires the skill to not only interpret a finding but to find it reliably. For clinicians, visual and

kinaesthetic senses are foundational tools for assessing the human form in function. Understanding our individual strengths, weaknesses, accuracies and misperceptions enhances our reliability and skills necessary to find a finding. While clinical reasoning can be taught through texts and online media, there will always be a need for hands-on practical courses; this is the art and skill of physiotherapy that is so difficult to measure with science.

The Integrated Systems Model for Disability and Pain is a clinical reasoning approach and 'the advantages of a clinical reasoning approach is that it is responsive to new knowledge and evidence, is flexible and allows for change and growth'.[5] The four editions of *The Pelvic Girdle*[25–28] have evolved over 32 years of clinical practice and clearly reflect how time, experience and evidence challenge paradigms for assessment and treatment of the SIJ. Clinical expertise, a component of evidence-based practice, means having the skill to determine whether or not the SIJ is moving and the clinical reasoning ability to interpret the relevance of the finding for wise treatment decisions. As our clinical expertise for evaluating mobility and control of the SIJ improves, perhaps our ability to demonstrate this scientifically will be confirmed in time for the fifth edition of this text.

REFERENCES

1. Vleeming A, Schuenke MD, Masi AT, et al. The sacroiliac joint: an overview of its anatomy, function and potential clinical implications. J Anat 2012;221(6):537–67.
2. Smith MD, Russell A, Hodges PW. Is there a relationship between parity, pregnancy, back pain and incontinence? Int Urogynecol J 2008;19(2):205–11.
3. Spitznagle TM, Leong FC, Van Dillen LR. Prevalence of diastasis recti abdominis in a urogynecological patient population. Int Urogynecol J Pelvic Floor Dysfunct 2007;18(3):321–8.
4. Vleeming A, Albert HB, Ostgaard HC, et al. European guidelines for the diagnosis and treatment of pelvic girdle pain. Eur Spine J 2008;17:794–819.
5. Jull G. Management of cervical spine disorders: where to now? IFOMPT Quebec City, Canada. 30 September–5 October; 2012.
6. Lee L-J, Lee D. Clinical Practice – The Reality for Clinicians. In: Chapter 7 In The Pelvic Girdle. 4th ed. Edinburgh: Elsevier; 2011.
7. Jacob HAC, Kissling RO. The mobility of the sacroiliac joints in healthy volunteers between 20 and 50 years of age. Clinical Biomechanics 1995;10(7):352–61.
8. Sturesson B. Load and movement of the sacroiliac joint. PhD thesis. Lund University, Sweden 1999.
9. Sturesson B, Selvik G, Uden A. Movements of the sacroiliac joints: a Roentgen stereophotogrammetric analysis. Spine 1989;14(2):162–5.
10. Sturesson B, Uden A, Vleeming A. A radiosteriometric analysis of movements of the sacroiliac joints during the standing hip flexion test. Spine 2000;25(3):364.
11. Hungerford B, Gilleard W, Lee D. Alteration of pelvic bone motion determined in subjects with posterior pelvic pain using skin markers. Clinical Biomechanics 2004;19:456.
12. Dreyfuss P, Dryer S, Griffin J, et al. Positive sacroiliac screening tests in asymptomatic adults. Spine 1994;19(10):1138–43.
13. Van der Wurff P, Hagmeijer R, Meyne W. Clinical tests of the sacroiliac joint. A systematic methodological review: part 1: reliability. Man Ther 2000;5(1):30–6.
14. Van der Wurff P, Meyne W, Hagneijer RHM. Clinical tests of the sacroiliac joint. A systematic methodological review. Part 2: validity. Man Ther 2000;5(2):89–96.
15. Potter NA, Rothstein J. Intertester reliability for selected clinical tests of the sacroiliac joint. Phys Ther 1985;65(11):1671–5.
16. Carmichael JP. Inter- and intra-examiner reliability of palpation for sacroiliac joint dysfunction. J Manipulative Phys Ther 1987;10(4):164–71.

17. Herzog W, Read L, Conway PJW, et al. Reliability of motion palpation procedures to detect sacroiliac joint fixations. J Manipulative Phys Ther 1989;12(2):86–92.
18. Meijne W, van Neerbos K, Aufdemkampe G, et al. Intraexaminer and interexaminer reliability of the Gillet test. J Manipulative Physiol Ther 1999;22(1):4–9.
19. Hungerford B, Gilleard W, Moran M, et al. Evaluation of the reliability of therapists to palpate intra-pelvic motion using the stork test on the support side. J Phys Therapy 2007;87(7):879.
20. Lee D. Biomechanics of the thorax: a clinical model of in vivo function. J Man Manipulative Ther 1993;1:13.
21. Lee D. Manual Therapy for the Thorax. www.dianelee.ca; 1994.
22. MacIntosh JE, Bogduk N. The attachments of the lumbar erector spinae. Spine 1991;16(7):783–92.
23. Lee L-J. Thoracic stabilization & the functional upper limb: restoring stability with mobility, Course Notes. Vancouver, BC. 2003.

24. Lee D, Lee L-J. Clinical Reasoning, Treatment Planning and Case Reports. In: Chapter 9 in: Lee D 2011, The Pelvic Girdle. 4th ed. Edinburgh: Elsevier; 2011.
25. Lee D. The Pelvic Girdle. In: An approach to the Examination and Treatment of the Lumbo-pelvic-hip Region. Edinburgh: Churchill Livingstone; 1989.
26. Lee D. The Pelvic Girdle. In: An Approach to the Examination and Treatment of the Lumbo-pelvic-hip Region. 2nd ed. Edinburgh: Churchill Livingstone; 1999.
27. Lee D. The Pelvic Girdle. In: An Approach to the Examination and Treatment of the Lumbo-pelvic-hip Region. 3rd ed. Edinburgh: Churchill Livingstone; 2004.
28. Lee D. The Pelvic Girdle. In: An Integration of Clinical Expertise and Research. Edinburgh: Churchill Livingstone, Elsevier; 2011.

CHAPTER 46.3 ■ A CRITICAL VIEWPOINT ON MODELS, TESTING AND TREATMENT OF PATIENTS WITH LUMBOPELVIC PAIN

Annelies Pool-Goudzwaard

INTRODUCTION

The lumbopelvic region is a fascinating area considering its evolutionary adaptation to bipedalism and its development through life.[1] Several models have been developed to support clinicians' clinical reasoning in patients with lumbopelvic pain (LPP). This chapter will critically appraise two theoretical models and discuss the abilities and flaws of the diagnostic process. In addition an adapted classification system from O'Sullivan and Beales[2] will be proposed focusing on different motor-strategy patterns of LPP patients,[3–7] describing per group how to intervene.

THEORETICAL MODELS

Models are introduced to simplify and clarify. Two important models are leading in the diagnosis and intervention of LPP: the model of form and force closure[1,8–13] and the debated model of local and global muscles in spinal control.[3,6,7,14]

A. The model of form and force closure is based on the contribution of the sacroiliac joint (SIJ) form and additional compressive forces to create stiffness, ensuring integrity of the pelvic ring during loading.[1,8–11,13] Additional muscle slings or 'cross-bracing structures' are described for optimal force closure.[1,10,13] All muscles with work-lines perpendicular to the SIJs, like transversus abdominus (TrA) and pelvic floor (PF) muscles will be able to increase compressive forces,[8,15] as confirmed by in vitro and in vivo studies,[16–18] although one in vitro study proved the contrary, mimicking solely TrA.[19] Often the form–force closure model is considered scientifically substantiated. However, evidence is lacking that optimal form and force closure is jeopardized in all patients with LPP. Likewise, evidence for the model of myofascial slings, compressing the SIJs via tension in the thoracolumbar fascia is also lacking.[13,20] The model, based on in vitro studies,[1,12,20] is not validated and is questioned for its stiffening effect on the SIJ.[21] Therefore we cannot confirm that non-optimal muscle recruitment of trunk/pelvis/hip muscles will lead to loss of force closure, despite plausible force-transfer via all connected myofascial structures throughout the body.[22]

B. The model of muscular spinal control has developed from static into also including dynamic muscular control.[6,7] Considering the primary model of global and local muscles,[14] recent research points out that the demonstrated separation and simplification of local muscle functioning prior[16,23–25] and separately from global muscles seems too simple to encompass real life.[5,7,26] Anticipatory postural adjustments and preparatory trunk movements are reported in both local and global muscles during activities, for example in walking.[27–31] Recent studies have demonstrated that the most important key factor in spinal control is the ability to respond to challenges either statically or dynamically with variability.[32–34] Healthy subjects tend to use different patterns of contraction of local and global muscles when carrying out the same task.[28,35–37] To enable this, feedback control is plausible.[35] With this knowledge in mind it seems not logical to train all patients in TrA-activation prior to global muscles during all activities. This will introduce 'learned motor control behaviour' and diminish the ability of variability to choose different motor control strategies during activities. Some patients contract their TrA continuously since they understand that otherwise their lumbar spine and/or pelvis will not be (optimally) stabilized.

THE DIAGNOSTIC PROCESS

As clinicians we can diagnose SIJ pain according to evidence-based standards (reliability and validity), by using the multi-test regimen of pain provocation tests.[36–40] But do we have the ability to feel differences in the neutral zone, joint play or end-feel or how the SIJs are positioned? Consider one's palpation ability and interpretation in light of the following facts: (a) anatomical intra- and inter-individual differences in the SIJ's form and position are large;[1,41–43] (b) degrees of motion reported in vivo are very small (mean of 1.2° and maximum 2°);[44] and (c) deformation is present within the innominates during movement.[44] If we are honest we cannot diagnose SIJ mobility and position. Mobility tests do not reach sufficient reliability or validity,[45,46] e.g. palpation of pelvic torque by posterior superior iliac spine and anterior superior iliac spine only reaches a moderate kappa on inter-tester reliability ($\kappa = 0.55$).[46] The same holds for intra-tester reliability ($\kappa = 0.46$) during the standing flexion test.[47] The inter-tester reliability is worse ($\kappa = 0.052$)[47] and a multi-test regimen does not reach sufficient reliability.[44] The Standing Stork test, scoring moderate to good on inter- and intra-tester reliability lacks validity.[47,48] The suspected reduction of movement in the SIJ on the standing side does not occur. In contrast, a displacement of 0.2° occurs in *both* SIJs.[48] Actually, the movement we palpate of the PSIS during the Standing Stork which transcends the 0.2°, may be influenced by the presence of deformation within the innominates.[42]

We can conclude that a level of diagnostic confusion is present which increases the likelihood of inappropriate treatment.[46] Still, clinicians tell patients that their pelvic joints are blocked, twisted, not optimally aligned or unstable. In addition they indicate that pain can be derived from these diagnosed patterns, although tests lack sufficient reliability and validity. By explaining these models as truths to patients we alter their belief system (either positively or negatively). So, how can we diagnose and treat LPP patients if we skip the non-reliable and valid tests?

CLASSIFICATION OF LOW BACK PAIN PATIENTS

Within the algorithm of diagnosing LPP, clinical reasoning should not focus on the possible underlying constructs of pain. By restraining from drawing conclusions if not in accordance with evidence-based standards, the focus can shift to what we can alter to optimize a patient's functioning. This is possible by focusing on motor strategies visible in LPP patients during functional tasks. O'Sullivan and Beales (2007) introduced a classification system describing altered adaptive or maladaptive motor strategies as excessive force closure and reduced force closure, and elicited the importance of central pain processes.[2] Since information is lacking on quantifying differences in force closure, this author suggests an adaptation of the classification model (see Fig. 46-8) by introducing the term 'activity' and adding the motor control loop.[3–7]

Visible differences in patients' motor control can be adaptive and/or compensatory to very different drivers. As clinicians we will never be able to identify what the main driver is. Different sensoric input (Fig. 46-8A) by

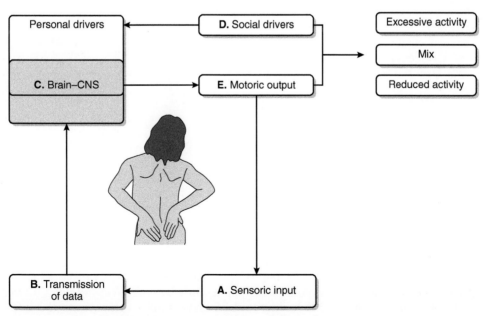

FIGURE 46-8 ■ The adapted classification scheme from O'Sullivan & Beales,[2] incorporating the optimal motor control loop.

altered proprioceptive feedback from joints, ligamentous tissues, tendons and muscle spindles[34,49–51] as well as loss of speed and quality of information transmission can interfere with motor control in LPP patients[52–55] (Fig. 46-8B). The brain (Fig. 46-8C) adapts. Changes are visible within the senso-motoric cortex of the brain.[56–59] Also personal drivers are present (Fig. 46-8C). The intensity of the pain can be influenced by negative emotions,[60,61] fear of pain or damage, directly altering motor control.[62–64] Even more, by observing another's painful action one's own motor control immediately alters during execution of the same action (Pool-Goudzwaard et al., unpublished data). Also, multiple other personal, biological, social and cultural factors (as food involvement)[65] interfere with someone's pain intensity, feelings, behaviour and motor control[67–70] (Fig. 46-8D). The extensive input to and processes within the brain influence the output to the motor system differently in all LPP patients (Fig. 46-8E). We will still see differences in strategies and classify them accordingly.

The proposed classification scheme consists of three groups:

The first group are patients with *excessive* muscle activity during tasks. Signs of this pattern are increased activity in muscles surrounding the abdominal cavity, including the PF, abdominal muscles and the diaphragm (holding breath), leading to an increase of intra-abdominal pressure and stiffening of the spine.[2,18,68–72] Other signs of excessive activity are a decrease of variability, an increase in rigidity, loss of precision in motoric tasks and an inability to relax after muscle activity (Fig. 46-9).[51,52,73] This muscle usage can have negative side effects since higher activity levels within the PF muscles are associated with PF dysfunction such as stress urinary incontinence (OR 4.2) and dyspareunia (OR 42).[18]

The second group within the classification scheme demonstrate *reduced* muscle activity during tasks. A lack of muscle activity can be visible in abdominal and PF muscles.[2] Often the abdomen and the pelvic floor are pushed outwards (Fig. 46-10). This strategy might also increase intra-abdominal pressure when patients hold their breath and provide stretch to the facial sheets surrounding the abdominal cavity, stiffening the spine.[72] These patients may also report PF dysfunctions, for example stress urinary incontinence.[67]

From clinical experience a group of patients demonstrate a *mixed behaviour* with some muscles being very active and others showing reduced activity, for example contracting all abdominal muscles meanwhile pushing the PF downwards.

Differences in strategies can be observed during all kind of activities while focusing on static and dynamic response to increasing difficult tasks.[3,6,74,75] As a start the active straight leg raise (ASLR) test can be used as a suitable low-load task to distinguish between the groups. The ASLR is advocated as a test for load transfer over the pelvis and can be used to diagnose pelvic pain.[67,76–78] Mens et al. (2012) demonstrated high sensitivity and specificity for diagnosing LPP.[78] Some patients score negative on the ASLR,[79] although simultaneous increase of PF activity is demonstrated.[79] During ASLR healthy subjects are able to move the complete pelvis as one,

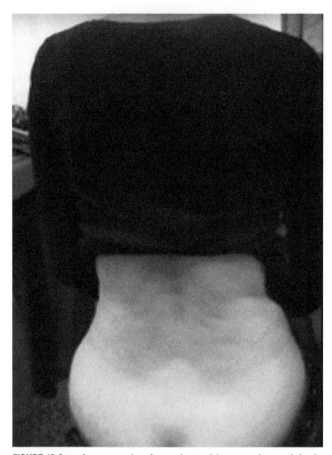

FIGURE 46-9 ■ An example of a patient with excessive activity in muscles. She is not able to relax and sit in a slump position and is continuously contracting her abdominal wall as well as her paraspinal muscles.

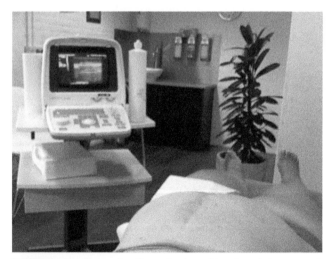

FIGURE 46-10 ■ Example of a patient pushing her abdomen outwards while trying to lift her left leg during an active straight leg raise.

controlling the effect of hip-flexors with contralateral hamstring activity.[80,81] In LPP patients the innominate is pulled forwards on the lifting side, visible during X-ray.[76] LPP patients can demonstrate the different strategies described above[68,80–82]

INTERVENTIONS

Interventions can focus on the restoration of function, with a different emphasis depending on classification-subgroup. As a clinician you can have an impact on the motor loop at several points (Fig. 46-8):

a. Input to the system can be altered by passively moving the lumbopelvic–hip complex,[83] to enlarge input from mechano-sensors. For this proprioceptive firing, a large range of motion is necessary to stimulate as many sensors as possible in the pelvic region. This indicates that we do not mobilize painful SIJs at the end of range, but only increase firing from the mechano-sensors at this end-range. Instead, we want to move the complete lumbopelvic–hip complex in a large range of motion, including either nutation or counter-nutation of the SIJ. The emphasis during these passive movements can be to the non-painful side regarding the importance of pain inhibition on motor control.[84]

b. Although it is not possible to train proprioception located in one single joint or to differentiate between velocity and movement, you can train the patient by drawing attention to positioning. Video recording a patient trying to feel where to stop or move allows instant play back, to make patients aware of what they are doing.

c. It is important to train the brain. Studies have demonstrated that by attention to tasks the changes in the senso-motoric cortex can be normalized.[57,85] Furthermore clinicians have a large influence on a patient's personal belief system since it is driven by what they experience,[86] anticipate,[62,64,86,87] see[65] and hear.[88]

d. Patients should be aware of the influence of the social environment on their pain and behaviour. We as clinicians are part of this social environment and have a direct influence on the patient. In case of fear, giving information that no damage can be done and that movement is necessary to give input to the human body is crucial. Extensive literature is available on the effect of behavioural techniques.[66]

e. One can alter the output to the motoric system; depending into what subgroup you classify the patient. In the subgroup 'excessive activity' the emphasis can be placed on relaxation, breathing freely, decrease in muscle tension and awareness of high muscle activity during tasks. No emphasis needs to be placed on a single muscle group as the TrA.[7] Perhaps the most important effect of training TrA and multifidus lies in optimal reengagement of the senso-motoric cortex instead of a 'stabilizing' effect.[84] When PF dysfunctions are present do not start with TrA training, since TrA and PF muscles co-contract. This might be counterproductive.[89,90] In the subgroup 'reduced activity', the emphasis can be placed on increasing muscle tone and awareness of how muscles can be used during activities. In the mixed group you can train awareness of over- and under-active muscles during activities combining relaxation with training.

For all LPP patients it is crucial to encourage patients to adopt variability in static and dynamic motor control and make them aware of these strategies in daily life.

REFERENCES

1. Vleeming A, Schuenke MD, Masi AT, et al. The sacroiliac joint: an overview of its anatomy, function and potential clinical implications. J Anat 2012;221:537–67.
2. O'Sullivan PB, Beales DJ. Diagnosis and classification of pelvic girdle pain disorders–part 1: a mechanism based approach within a biopsychosocial framework. Man Ther 2007;12:86–97.
3. Reeves NP, Narendra KS, Cholewicki J. Spine stability: lessons from balancing a stick. Clin Biomech 2011;26:325–30.
4. Reeves NP, Narendra KS, Cholewicki J. Spine stability: the six blind men and the elephant. Clin Biomech 2007;22:266–74.
5. Hodges PW, Coppieters MW, MacDonald D, et al. New insight into motor adaptation to pain revealed by a combination of modelling and empirical approaches. Eur J Pain 2013;17:1138–46.
6. Reeves NP, Cholewicki J. Spine system science; a primer on the systems approach. In: Hodges PW, Cholewicky J, van Dieen J, editors. Spinal Control: The Rehabilitation of Back Pain. Edinburgh: Elsevier; 2013.
7. Hodges PW, McGill S, Hides JA. Motor control of the spine and changes in pain: Debate about extrapolation from research observations of motor control strategies to effective treatments for back pain. In: Hodges PW, Cholewicki J, van Dieen J, editors. Spinal Control: The Rehabilitation of Back Pain. Edinburgh: Elsevier; 2013.
8. Snijders CJ, Vleeming A, Stoeckart R. Transfer of lumbosacral load to iliac bones and legs: part 1: biomechanics of self-bracing of the sacroiliac joints and its significance for treatment and exercise. Clin Biomech 1993;8:285–94. [Accessed 12/24/2013 9:44:53 AM].
9. Vleeming A, Stoeckart R, Volkers AC, et al. Relation between form and function in the sacroiliac joint. part I: clinical anatomical aspects. Spine 1990;15:130–2.
10. Vleeming A, Volkers AC, Snijders CJ, et al. Relation between form and function in the sacroiliac joint. part II: biomechanical aspects. Spine 1990;15:133–6.
11. Pool-Goudzwaard AL, Vleeming A, Stoeckart R, et al. Insufficient lumbopelvic stability: a clinical, anatomical and biomechanical approach to 'a-specific' low back pain. Man Ther 1998;3: 12–20.
12. Vleeming A, Pool-Goudzwaard AL, Stoeckart R, et al. The posterior layer of the thoracolumbar fascia. its function in load transfer from spine to legs. Spine (Phila Pa 1976) 1995;20:753–8.
13. Lee D. The Pelvic Girdle: An Integration of Clinical Expertise and Reserach. Edinburgh: Elsevier; 2011.
14. Bergmark A. Stability of the lumbar spine: a study in mechanical engineering. Acta Orthop 1989;60:1–54.
15. Pel JJ, Spoor CW, Goossens RH, et al. Biomechanical model study of pelvic belt influence on muscle and ligament forces. J Biomech 2008;41:1878–84. [Accessed 12/27/2013 5:11:07 AM].
16. Richardson CA, Hides JA, Wilson S, et al. Lumbo-pelvic joint protection against antigravity forces: motor control and segmental stiffness assessed with magnetic resonance imaging. J Gravit Physiol 2004;11:119–22.
17. Richardson CA, Snijders CJ, Hides JA, et al. The relation between the transversus abdominis muscles, sacroiliac joint mechanics, and low back pain. Spine (Phila Pa 1976) 2002;27:399–405.
18. Pool-Goudzwaard A, van Dijke GH, van Gurp M, et al. Contribution of pelvic floor muscles to stiffness of the pelvic ring. Clin Biomech (Bristol, Avon) 2004;19:564–71.
19. Gnat R, Spoor K, Pool-Goudzwaard A. Simulated transversus abdominis muscle force does not increase stiffness of the pubic symphysis and innominate bone: an in vitro study. Clin Biomech 2013;28:262–7.
20. Willard FH, Vleeming A, Schuenke MD, et al. The thoracolumbar fascia: anatomy, function and clinical considerations. J Anat 2012;221:507–36.
21. Bogduk N. Clinical Anatomy of the Lumbar Spine and Sacrum. 3rd ed. Philadelphia, Pa: Churchill Livingstone.; 1997. p. 128
22. Brown SH, McGill SM. Transmission of muscularly generated force and stiffness between layers of the rat abdominal wall. Spine 2009;34:E70–5.

23. Hodges P, Cresswell A, Thorstensson A. Preparatory trunk motion accompanies rapid upper limb movement. Exp Brain Res 1999;124:69–79.

24. Hodges P, Richardson C, Jull G. Evaluation of the relationship between laboratory and clinical tests of transversus abdominis function. Physiother Res Int 1996;1:30–40.

25. Hodges PW, Richardson CA. Altered trunk muscle recruitment in people with low back pain with upper limb movement at different speeds. Arch Phys Med Rehabil 1999;80:1005–12.

26. Allison GT, Morris SL. Transversus abdominis and core stability: has the pendulum swung? Br J Sports Med 2008;42:930–1.

27. Morris SL, Lay B, Allison GT. Corset hypothesis rebutted–transversus abdominis does not co-contract in unison prior to rapid arm movements. Clin Biomech 2012;27:249–54.

28. Morris SL, Lay B, Allison GT. Transversus abdominis is part of a global not local muscle synergy during arm movement. Hum Mov Sci 2013;32:1176–85.

29. Lee L, Coppieters MW, Hodges PW. Anticipatory postural adjustments to arm movement reveal complex control of paraspinal muscles in the thorax. J Electromyogr Kinesiol 2009;19:46–54.

30. Lee L, Coppieters MW, Hodges PW. Differential activation of the thoracic multifidus and longissimus thoracis during trunk rotation. Spine 2005;30:870–6.

31. Saunders SW, Schache A, Rath D, et al. Changes in three dimensional lumbo-pelvic kinematics and trunk muscle activity with speed and mode of locomotion. Clin Biomech 2005;20:784–93.

32. Dupeyron A, Rispens SM, Demattei C, et al. Precision of estimates of local stability of repetitive trunk movements. Eur Spine J 2013;22:2678–85.

33. Willigenburg NW, Kingma I, van Dieen JH. Center of pressure trajectories, trunk kinematics and trunk muscle activation during unstable sitting in low back pain patients. Gait Posture 2013;38:625–30.

34. Willigenburg NW, Kingma I, Hoozemans MJ, et al. Precision control of trunk movement in low back pain patients. Hum Mov Sci 2013;32:228–39.

35. Goodworth AD, Peterka RJ. Contribution of sensorimotor integration to spinal stabilization in humans. J Neurophysiol 2009;102:496–512.

36. Laslett M. Evidence-based diagnosis and treatment of the painful sacroiliac joint. J Man Manipulative Ther 2008;16:142.

37. Van der Wurff P, Hagmeijer R, Meyne W. Clinical tests of the sacroiliac joint: a systematic methodological review. part 1: reliability. Man Ther 2000;5:30–6.

38. van der Wurff P, Meyne W, Hagmeijer RH. Clinical tests of the sacroiliac joint: a systematic methodological review. part 2: validity. Man Ther 2000;5:89–96.

39. van der Wurff P. Clinical diagnostic tests for the sacroiliac joint: motion and palpation tests. Aust J Physiother 2006;52:308.

40. Szadek KM, van der Wurff P, van Tulder MW, et al. Diagnostic validity of criteria for sacroiliac joint pain: a systematic review. J Pain 2009;10:354–68.

41. Bakland O, Hansen JH. The "axial sacroiliac joint". Anat Clin 1984;6:29–36.

42. Pool-Goudzwaard A, Gnat R, Spoor K. Deformation of the innominate bone and mobility of the pubic symphysis during asymmetric moment application to the pelvis. Man Ther 2012;17:66–70.

43. Vleeming A, Van Wingerden J, Dijkstra P, et al. Mobility in the sacroiliac joints in the elderly: a kinematic and radiological study. Clin Biomech 1992;7:170–6.

44. Sturesson B, Uden A, Vleeming A. A radiostereometric analysis of the movements of the sacroiliac joints in the reciprocal straddle position. Spine 2000;25:214–17.

45. van Kessel-Cobelens AM, Verhagen AP, Mens JM, et al. Pregnancy-related pelvic girdle pain: intertester reliability of 3 tests to determine asymmetric mobility of the sacroiliac joints. J Manipulative Physiol Ther 2008;31:130–6.

46. Albert H, Godskesen M, Westergaard J. Evaluation of clinical tests used in classification procedures in pregnancy-related pelvic joint pain. Eur Spine J 2000;9:161–6.

47. Sturesson B, Uden A, Vleeming A. A radiostereometric analysis of movements of the sacroiliac joints during the standing hip flexion test. Spine 2000;25:364–8.

48. Hungerford BA, Gilleard W, Moran M, et al. Evaluation of the ability of physical therapists to palpate intrapelvic motion with the stork test on the support side. Phys Ther 2007;87:879–87.

49. Brumagne S, Cordo P, Lysens R, et al. The role of paraspinal muscle spindles in lumbosacral position sense in individuals with and without low back pain. Spine 2000;25:989–94.

50. Brumagne S, Cordo P, Verschueren S. Proprioceptive weighting changes in persons with low back pain and elderly persons during upright standing. Neurosci Lett 2004;366:63–6.

51. Brumagne S, Janssens L, Janssens E, et al. Altered postural control in anticipation of postural instability in persons with recurrent low back pain. Gait Posture 2008;28:657–62.

52. Claeys K, Brumagne S, Dankaerts W, et al. Decreased variability in postural control strategies in young people with non-specific low back pain is associated with altered proprioceptive reweighting. Eur J Appl Physiol 2011;111:115–23.

53. Radebold A, Cholewicki J, Panjabi MM, et al. Muscle response pattern to sudden trunk loading in healthy individuals and in patients with chronic low back pain. Spine (Phila Pa 1976) 2000;25:947–54.

54. Radebold A, Cholewicki J, Polzhofer GK, et al. Impaired postural control of the lumbar spine is associated with delayed muscle response times in patients with chronic idiopathic low back pain. Spine 2001;26:724–30.

55. Cholewicki J, Silfies SP, Shah RA, et al. Delayed trunk muscle reflex responses increase the risk of low back injuries. Spine 2005;30:2614–20.

56. Tsao H, Galea M, Hodges P. Reorganization of the motor cortex is associated with postural control deficits in recurrent low back pain. Brain 2008;131:2161–71.

57. Tsao H, Tucker K, Hodges P. Changes in excitability of corticomotor inputs to the trunk muscles during experimentally-induced acute low back pain. Neuroscience 2011;181:127–33.

58. Tsao H, Danneels LA, Hodges PW. ISSLS prize winner: smudging the motor brain in young adults with recurrent low back pain. Spine 2011;36:1721–7.

59. Tsao H, Druitt TR, Schollum TM, et al. Motor training of the lumbar paraspinal muscles induces immediate changes in motor coordination in patients with recurrent low back pain. J Pain 2010;11:1120–8.

60. Bruehl S, Liu X, Burns JW, et al. Associations between daily chronic pain intensity, daily anger expression, and trait anger expressiveness: an ecological momentary assessment study. Pain 2012;153:2352–8.

61. Burns JW. Arousal of negative emotions and symptom-specific reactivity in chronic low back pain patients. Emotion 2006;6:309–19.

62. Moseley GL, Nicholas MK, Hodges PW. Does anticipation of back pain predispose to back trouble? Brain 2004;127:2339–46.

63. Moseley GL, Hodges PW. Are the changes in postural control associated with low back pain caused by pain interference? Clin J Pain 2005;21:323–9.

64. Tucker K, Larsson AK, Oknelid S, et al. Similar alteration of motor unit recruitment strategies during the anticipation and experience of pain. Pain 2012;153:636–43.

65. Bell R, Marshall DW. The construct of food involvement in behavioral research: scale development and validation. Appetite 2003;40:235–44.

66. Sarafino EP. Health Psychology: Biopsychosocial Interactions. John Wiley & Sons Inc; 1998.

67. O'Sullivan PB, Beales DJ. Changes in pelvic floor and diaphragm kinematics and respiratory patterns in subjects with sacroiliac joint pain following a motor learning intervention: a case series. Man Ther 2007;12:209–18.

68. Beales DJ, O'Sullivan PB, Briffa NK. Motor control patterns during an active straight leg raise in chronic pelvic girdle pain subjects. Spine 2009;34:861–70.

69. Beales DJ, O'Sullivan PB, Briffa NK. The effects of manual pelvic compression on trunk motor control during an active straight leg raise in chronic pelvic girdle pain subjects. Man Ther 2010;15:190–9.

70. Healey EL, Fowler NE, Burden AM, et al. The influence of different unloading positions upon stature recovery and paraspinal muscle activity. Clin Biomech 2005;20:365–71.

71. Mens J, Hoek van Dijke G, Pool-Goudzwaard A, et al. Possible harmful effects of high intra-abdominal pressure on the pelvic girdle. J Biomech 2006;39:627–35.

72. Hodges PW, Gandevia SC. Changes in intra-abdominal pressure during postural and respiratory activation of the human diaphragm. J Appl Physiol 2000;89:967–76.

73. Brumagne S, Janssens L, Knapen S, et al. Persons with recurrent low back pain exhibit a rigid postural control strategy. Eur Spine J 2008;17:1177–84.

74. Lee AS, Cholewicki J, Reeves NP, et al. Comparison of trunk proprioception between patients with low back pain and healthy controls. Arch Phys Med Rehabil 2010;91:1327–31.

75. Xu Y, Choi J, Reeves NP, et al. Optimal control of the spine system. J Biomech Eng 2010;132:051004.

76. Mens J, Vleeming A, Snijders CJ, et al. The active straight leg raising test and mobility of the pelvic joints. Eur Spine J 1999;8:468–73.

77. Mens JM, Damen L, Snijders CJ, et al. The mechanical effect of a pelvic belt in patients with pregnancy-related pelvic pain. Clin Biomech 2006;21:122–7.

78. Mens JM, Huis In 't Veld YH, Pool-Goudzwaard A. The active straight leg raise test in lumbopelvic pain during pregnancy. Man Ther 2012;17:364–8.

79. Pool-Goudzwaard AL, Slieker TH, Vierhout ME, et al. Relations between pregnancy-related low back pain, pelvic floor activity and pelvic floor dysfunction. Int Urogynecol J Pelvic Floor Dysfunct 2005.

80. Hu H, Meijer OG, van Dieen JH, et al. Muscle activity during the active straight leg raise (ASLR), and the effects of a pelvic belt on the ASLR and on treadmill walking. J Biomech 2010;43:532–9.

81. Hu H, Meijer OG, Hodges PW, et al. Understanding the active straight leg raise (ASLR): an electromyographic study in healthy subjects. Man Ther 2012;17:531–7.

82. de Groot M, Pool-Goudzwaard AL, Spoor CW, et al. The active straight leg raising test (ASLR) in pregnant women: differences in muscle activity and force between patients and healthy subjects. Man Ther 2008;13:68–74.

83. Schleip R, Muller DG. Training principles for fascial connective tissues: scientific foundation and suggested practical applications. J Bodyw Mov Ther 2013;17:103–15.

84. Nijs J, Daenen L, Cras P, et al. Nociception affects motor output: a review on sensory-motor interaction with focus on clinical implications. Clin J Pain 2012;28:175–81.

85. Tsao H, Danneels L, Hodges PW. Individual fascicles of the paraspinal muscles are activated by discrete cortical networks in humans. Clin Neurophysiol 2011;122:1580–7.

86. Moseley GL, Nicholas M, Hodges PW. Pain differs from non-painful attention-demanding or stressful tasks in its effect on postural control patterns of trunk muscles. Exp Brain Res 2004;156:64–71.

87. Moseley GL, Brhyn L, Ilowiecki M, et al. The threat of predictable and unpredictable pain: differential effects on central nervous system processing? Aust J Physiother 2003;49:263–7.

88. Crombez G, Viane I, Eccleston C, et al. Attention to pain and fear of pain in patients with chronic pain. J Behav Med 2013;36:371–8.

89. Sapsford RR, Hodges PW, Richardson CA, et al. Co-activation of the abdominal and pelvic floor muscles during voluntary exercises. Neurourol Urodyn 2001;20:31–42.

90. Bo K, Sherburn M, Allen T. Transabdominal ultrasound measurement of pelvic floor muscle activity when activated directly or via a transversus abdominis muscle contraction. Neurourol Urodyn 2003;22:582–8.

CHAPTER 47

HIP-RELATED PAIN

Kay Crossley • Alison Grimaldi • Joanne Kemp

ARTICULAR AND MUSCLE CONTROL OF THE HIP

Articular and neuromuscular control of the hip is provided by three components working synergistically: (a) bony morphology; (b) passive joint structures such as the acetabular labrum, hip joint capsule and hip ligaments; and (c) hip musculature.

Bony Morphology

The hip joint (femoroacetabular joint) is a synovial joint formed by the head of femur inferiorly and the acetabulum superiorly. The acetabulum sits within the bony pelvis and faces inferiorly, laterally and is normally anteverted (forward facing) by approximately 23°.[1] The femoral head faces superiorly, medially and is anteverted between 10–15° in adults. The anteversion of the acetabulum and head of femur reduces the bony stability in the anterior hip joint. This morphological structure enables the three degrees of movement (i.e. flexion and extension, adduction and abduction, and external and internal rotation).

Passive Joint Structures

Acetabular Labrum

The acetabular labrum extends around the rim of the acetabulum, from the posterior to the anterior aspect of the transverse acetabular ligament.[2] It is considered vital to maintain joint fluid pressure, limiting extravasation of articular cartilage fluid and distributing force to maintain healthy chondral surfaces.[3] The labrum deepens the acetabulum by 21%[4] and absorbs up to 28% of hip joint forces.[4] The acetabular labrum is thinnest and most vulnerable in its anterior aspect. The blood supply enters though the adjacent joint capsule with only the outer third of the labrum vascularized, whereas the inner two-thirds are avascular.[5] Nociceptive free nerve endings are distributed throughout the labrum[6] while the damaged labral tissue contains cytokines,[7] suggesting a nociceptive-producing capacity.

Ligaments of the Hip

The transverse acetabular ligament traverses the acetabular notch, connecting the anterior and posterior labral edges. The collagen fibres forming the deepest layer of labral tissue blend into this ligament. During weight bearing, the head of the femur relocates in the acetabulum, widening the acetabular notch and placing the transverse acetabular ligament under a tensile load.[8]

The ligamentum teres is an intra-articular ligament arising from the fovea of the head of the femur, becoming triangular in shape and inserting into the anterior and posterior aspect of the transverse acetabular ligament.[9] It also communicates with the synovium within the hip.[10] The ligamentum teres has a rich supply of mechanoreceptors and due to its attachment to the transverse acetabular ligament, becomes taut in weight bearing. This suggests a proprioceptive role, especially in weight-bearing activities.[10]

The iliofemoral ligament and pubofemoral ligament reinforce the anterior capsule and limit extremes of extension and abduction. The ischiofemoral ligament has fibres that run in a spiral pattern and limit hyperextension.

Hip Musculature

Dynamic stability is thought to be provided by a synergistic interplay between various hip muscles. Hip muscles may be considered to be stabilizers, prime movers or play a dual role. The stabilization role of each muscle is based on its line of action in relation to the joint axis, its primary action and the ratio between its physiological cross-sectional area (PCSA) relative to muscle fibre length (MFL).[11–13] Muscles with a smaller PCSA to MFL ratio (PCSA cm^2:MFL cm <1.0) are considered to be 'prime movers' of a joint, whereas those muscles with a larger PCSA relative to muscle fibre length (PCSA cm^2:MFL cm >1.0) are considered to be 'joint stabilizers'. Muscles with an equal PCSA and MFL (PCSA cm^2:MFL cm = 1.0) are considered to have the capacity to generate large forces over a variety of muscle lengths, acting as both stabilizers and prime movers. Primary hip stabilizers are thought to locate the head of femur within the acetabulum via posterior, medial or inferior forces exerted on the femoral head. This may minimize stress on potentially vulnerable structures, such as the anterosuperior acetabular labrum and acetabular rim, while maximizing the neuromotor control of the hip. The primary hip stabilizers, with both a PCSA:MFL ratio ≥1.0 and a posterior–medial–inferior line of action, include iliopsoas, gluteus medius, gluteus maximus, quadratus femoris, obturator internus, inferior and superior gemelli, and adductor brevis and pectineus.

JOINT-RELATED HIP PAIN

Background

Hip pain is common in active young to middle-aged men and women. It accounts for approximately 12% of soccer-related injuries,[14] and is the third most common injury in the Australian Football League.[15] In general populations, estimates of prevalence range from 7% in adolescents[16] to 14% in older adults.[17] Joint-related hip pain refers to a number of intra-articular pathologies, including femoroacetabular impingement (FAI), labral pathology and early degenerative change such as chondropathy.[18,19] It has been suggested that hip pain and associated hip morphology and pathology may form part of a continuum where pain and pathology in young to middle-aged people progresses into hip osteoarthritis (OA).[20]

The following section outlines the hip pathologies commonly seen in clinical practice, assessment of patients with hip pain and rationale for the treatment of hip pain.

Femoroacetabular Impingement

FAI refers to variations in hip joint morphology, where the normal sphericity of the head of femur or acetabulum are altered.[21] Diagnosis of these morphological variants can be made from radiographs,[21,22] computerized tomography[23] or magnetic resonance imaging (MRI).[23,24] Femoroacetabular impingement is considered to be a normal variation in hip morphology,[25–27] with the prevalence of cam FAI ranging from 4% in healthy women[28] to 24% in healthy men.[24] Moreover, elite young male basketball players are ten times more likely to have a cam lesion than their aged-matched controls.[29] However, 23% of people with radiographic FAI complain of hip pain,[30] most likely resulting from overload of the adjacent acetabular labrum and intra-articular chondral surfaces.[25,31–33]

There are three types of FAI typically described. The most prevalent is a cam lesion, seen in 78% of people with FAI,[30] which describes the reduction in femoral head neck offset resulting from additional bony tissue at the anterior, superior or anterosuperior aspect of the head neck junction[21,30] (Fig. 47-1). This lesion may increase the shearing forces acting on the anterior labrum and chondral surfaces.[21] Recently, pre-existing cam-type FAI has been identified as a risk factor for hip OA and total hip arthroplasty.[20,34–36] It is unknown whether other factors may explain why certain individuals with cam lesions progress to hip OA whereas others do not.

Pincer impingement is a morphologic variation in the acetabulum observed in approximately 42% of people with FAI.[30] This either manifests as a deep acetabulum, most commonly anteriorly,[21,37] or as a retroverted acetabulum, which leads to an apparent deeper anterior acetabular wall. Pincer-type FAI may directly compress the acetabular labrum between a deep acetabulum and normal, spherical femoral head,[21] leading to labral lesions and subsequent chondral damage. However, pincer impingement appears to be more benign than cam-type

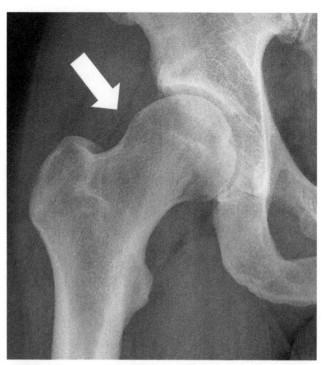

FIGURE 47-1 ■ Cam impingement. The arrow indicates reduced femoral head neck offset.

FAI, resulting in smaller, less-severe chondral lesions.[21] This observation is consistent with a recent report that, in contrast to cam lesions, pincer impingement may protect the hip from OA development.[38] The third type of FAI seen is the mixed presentation where both cam and pincer lesions are seen, which has been reported in 88% of people with FAI.[30]

Acetabular Labral Pathology

Acetabular labral tears can compromise the labral function and therefore directly impact joint health. The prevalence of labral tears is greatest anteriorly,[2,6,39,40] which may be related to the relatively thinner labrum in this region[2,41] or to the presence of cam lesions on the anterosuperior aspect of the femoral head–neck junction.[32] Tears of the acetabular labrum are seen commonly at arthroscopy, with up to 93% of patients undergoing hip arthroscopy having a concomitant labral tear.[40,42] The presence of FAI is associated with labral tears, most likely due to impingement of the labrum between then bony components of the hip.[43–45]

Chondropathy of the Hip

Articular cartilage is a complex structure consisting of chondrocytes and a surrounding extracellular matrix[46] that comprises hydrophilic proteoglycans, including aggrecan, which enable cartilage to withstand very high compressive loads.[46] Articular cartilage is avascular and aneural, relying on the normal distribution of synovial fluid within the joint for nutrition and ongoing optimal health.[47] Factors such as labral tears that impact on the normal function of the synovium and synovial fluid and the distribution of loads imparted to the chondral surfaces have important implications for chondral health. Consequently, chondral lesions of the hip are often seen in conjunction with other hip pathology at hip arthroscopy, especially at the anterior or superior aspect of the acetabular rim and at the chondrolabral junction.[31,42,48] In the knee, meniscal pathology at knee arthroscopy increases the relative risk of knee OA by 3–14 times.[49,50] As such it is possible that factors such as labral pathology[33,51–53] may be associated with an increased the risk of hip chondropathy, and ultimately OA development.[34–36,51,54,55]

Assessment

A comprehensive assessment of the hip joint should include a thorough subjective examination, physical examination and appropriate use of investigations. No single test provides a definitive diagnosis of joint-related hip pain. The most accurate diagnosis of the source of hip pain can only be made when findings from all aspects of assessment are considered.

Key Clinical Diagnostic Features of Joint-Related Hip Pain

While Table 47-1 below describes each pathology as a separate entity, these almost always coexist in clinical practice. The increasing severity of symptoms seen is associated with the progression of degenerative hip disease from FAI to hip OA.

The Role of Imaging: When to and When Not to Image?

Imaging plays an important role in diagnosing the source of hip pain, planning appropriate treatment and establishing a likely prognosis. It should be considered in all patients who have failed to respond to conservative treatment after 6 weeks and prior to undertaking further medical or surgical treatment.

Cam lesions can be assessed with confidence utilizing X-ray. Plain radiographs correlate well with computed tomography and MRI findings and are more accessible for patients and clinicians.[83] An alpha angle >60–65° is considered to indicate a cam lesion.[64,65] The presence of a cam lesion is associated with an increased risk of labral pathology and chondropathy[84] in people with hip pain, and hence its presence may increase clinical suspicion of coexisting lesions. The gold standard imaging for labral pathology is MRI arthrography, which has enhanced accuracy over standard MRI.[67,85] However, whereas standard MRI produces false-positive results (underestimation of labral pathology) with poorer accuracy,[67] newer sequences, including those available with a 3 tesla magnet show promise for the evaluation of labral tears. Similarly, chondropathy can now be assessed using high-resolution MRI, which reveals changes in the chondral matrix.[69] However, these imaging techniques are not yet readily available in clinical practice and arthroscopy remains the gold standard for diagnosis.

Importantly, while imaging may assist with the diagnosis, abnormalities seen on radiographs, computed tomography or MRI provide only part of the picture and should be considered alongside clinical test results.

Red Flags

A number of 'Red Flags' should be considered with any patient presenting with hip pain. These may include rheumatoid and multijoint arthropathies, avascular necrosis of the head of the femur, slipped upper femoral epiphysis, Perthes disease, tumours, synovial chondramatosis, fractured neck of femur and lumbar nerve root compression. If symptoms are not improving as anticipated, a timely referral to the appropriate medical practitioner should be undertaken.

Treatment

First-line treatment of hip joint pain usually comprises conservative management. Medical and surgical management may be included in order to obtain resolution of symptoms if conservative treatment has not succeeded.

Conservative Management

While there is little evidence to guide therapists regarding the most appropriate components of rehabilitation programmes for hip-related pain, commonly reported principles of rehabilitation are hip muscle strengthening, restoration of neuromotor control, addressing remote factors that may alter the kinetic chain function, and unloading the damaged or vulnerable structures.[2,86–90] Conservative therapy generally consists of three components to address these principles: (a) advice; (b) exercise; and (c) manual therapy.

Advice. Advice generally relates to strategies designed to protect and unload vulnerable structures of the hip, based on our understanding of the functional anatomy and biomechanics of the hip. In people with hip pain related to FAI, avoidance of impingement (flexion, internal rotation and adduction or any combination of these activities) as much as possible is advised. Once symptoms have resolved, positions of impingement can be reintroduced in a graduated fashion as long as they remain pain-free. This may involve activity modification on a day-to day basis, such as prolonged sitting in low chairs, as well as during athletic pursuits. For example, footballers may be advised to spend less time changing direction and getting down low to the ball. Gait retraining may also minimize excessive hip extension at the end of stance phase of gait, to decrease the loads on anterior hip joint structures.[91] Since greater body mass index is a feature of those with advancing hip pathology, and will increase hip joint loads, advice regarding weight management is appropriate in this group of patients. General advice relating to the management of hip OA should also be given in those

Table 47-1 Key Clinical Diagnostic Features of Joint-Related Hip Pain

Clinical Diagnostic Features Commonly Seen in All Hip Pathologies
Subjective Examination

Area and nature of pain	Groin, lateral hip, anterior hip, buttock or thigh pain
Aggravating factors	Aggravated by running, kicking, twisting actions, getting in and out of car Deep flexion, prolonged sitting, up and down stairs
Clinical examination	Increased tone and tenderness gluteus medius, piriformis, TFL, iliopsoas, adductor magnus and longus, biceps femoris

Clinical Diagnostic Features Specific to FAI
Subjective Examination

Loading history	Onset of symptoms often after episode of increased loading during sport/activity
Clinical examination	Reduced +/– painful ROM hip flexion,[56] IR@90[56–59] Abduction[60] Pain on FADIR,[56] FABER Reduced strength adduction, ER, flexion, abduction[61] Altered gait in all planes of motion,[62,63] reduced step length
Investigations	X-ray – AP pelvis and lateral Dunn view – Cam lesion: alpha angle >60;[64] >65[65] Pincer lesion: lateral centre edge angle >40[38] CT scan[66]

Clinical Diagnostic Features Specific to Labral Pathology
Subjective Examination

Area and nature of pain	Sometimes ache at rest and night
Aggravating factors	Mechanical symptoms, locking, catching, giving way[2,67]
Loading history	Onset of symptoms possibly after episode of increased loading during sport/activity, but often no cause known
Clinical examination	Reduced ± painful ROM hip flexion, IR@90 Pain on FADIR,[68] FABER Reduced strength[68] Altered gait – reduced step length, reduced hip extension, possibly limp
Investigations	CT scan[66] MRI[69]

Clinical Diagnostic Features Specific to Chondropathy
Subjective Examination

Area and nature of pain	Usually ache at rest and night
Aggravating factors	Mechanical symptoms, locking, catching, giving way Pain on uneven surfaces
Loading history	Sometimes onset following episode of increased load, but often no change in loading pattern reported
Clinical examination	Reduced strength[70] Reduced ROM ±– painful flexion, IR@90[70] ?Increased BMI[71] Painful FADIR, FABER Reduced balance in dynamic tasks[72]
Investigations	dGEMRIC (gadolinium-enhanced) MRI[55,69]

Clinical Diagnostic Features Specific to Hip OA
Subjective Examination

Area and nature of pain	Always ache at rest and night
Aggravating factors	Stiffness, difficulty putting on shoes, getting in and out of car, sitting, sit to stand, prolonged standing, walking, up and down stairs, uneven surfaces
Loading history	Past or current history of high-load occupations and high-intensity sporting activities.[73] Usually no change of load prior to onset
Clinical examination	Reduced ± painful ROM hip flexion ≤115, IR@90 ≤15[74–77] Pain on FADIR, FABER Reduced strength[78,79] Altered gait – reduced step length, reduced hip extension, limp Increased BMI[75,80] Stiffness at end-range ROM tests
Investigations	X-ray – may have joint space narrowing, osteophytes, hypertrophy of subchondral bone, subchondral cysts[81,82]

AP, anteroposterior; *BMI*, Body mass index; *CT*, Computerized tomography; *dGEMRIC*, Delayed gadolinium-enhanced magnetic resonance imaging of cartilage; *ER*, External rotation; *FABER*, Flexion/abduction/external rotation; *FADIR* Flexion/adduction/internal rotation; *FAI*, Femoroacetabular impingement; *IR*, Internal rotation; *MRI*, Magnetic resonance imaging; *ROM*, Range of motion; *TFL*, Tensor fascia lata.

with chondropathy and hip OA, and may include general fitness, lower limb strengthening exercises, chronic disease management, pain management, weight management and coping strategies.

Exercise. Exercise therapies should be individualized for the patient, based on age, gender, personal preference (group-based versus individual exercise programmes, aquatic versus land-based programmes, home versus gym-based programs), desired activity or sporting requirements. While there is no evidence of neuromotor dysfunction in people with hip-related pain, anatomical studies support a theoretical role for their importance in promoting joint stability. Contrasting the lack of evidence for neuromotor control, a number of studies have identified lower muscle strength in people with a variety of hip problems, including FAI,[61] labral tears,[68] post hip arthroscopy[70] and hip OA[78] (see Table 47-1). These impairments are generally observed in all directions, but will be patient-specific.

Conservative management generally includes activity modification and physical therapy including exercise programmes.[92] An exercise programme will usually include specific exercises to strengthen the hip-stabilizing muscle groups, general lower limb strength exercises targeting the gluteal, quadriceps and calf muscles, core and trunk strengthening and adjunctive stretching exercises that do not place the hip into a position of impingement. Strengthening exercises should be progressed from non-weightbearing to weight bearing, to resistance to functional and sports-specific exercises (Figs 47-2 and 47-3).

In recent times a number of studies have suggested optimal exercises to activate the hip abductors[93,94] and hip extensors[94,95] and rotators[96] (see Figs 47-2 and 47-3). Exercises with high activation of these muscles included double leg[95,96] and single leg bridging,[96] side plank with abduction,[94] front plank with extension,[94] single leg squats[94] and resisted band walking.[93] While these studies have been conducted in healthy people without hip pain, they provide a basis for optimal exercises to strengthen hip muscles in people with hip pain.

In addition, exercises to increase fitness and facilitate weight loss should be encouraged in a fashion that does not adversely increase intra-articular loads within the hip joint. Examples of such exercise programmes may include cycling, swimming, walking and modified running programmes tailored to the needs of the individual patient.

Manual Therapy. Manual therapy is commonly used by physiotherapists in the management of hip OA[97] and may include joint mobilizations and soft tissue techniques. Manual therapy aims to increase hip range of motion and reduce stiffness and pain. Hip flexion range is modifiable by physiotherapists and rehabilitation programmes should be targeted to improve this range in patients with hip pain. This may be achieved through the use of manual soft tissue techniques,[98] stretching techniques[98] and hip extension strengthening exercises.[79] Recent studies have shown that manual therapy with patient education results in better outcomes than education alone in people

with hip OA (Fig. 47-4).[99,100] There is minimal evidence to date supporting the use of manual therapy in the management of FAI, labral or chondral pathology, and care should be taken with manual techniques that place a person with painful FAI at end-range impingement. However, contemporary clinical practice suggests that soft tissue and dry-needling techniques aimed at normalizing tone in overactive hip musculature may be beneficial.

Effectiveness of Conservative Therapies

The effectiveness of strengthening interventions in improving physical function outcomes[101,102] and global lower limb strength[101] in people with advanced hip OA has been previously demonstrated. These interventions may improve physical function by altering hip joint loads.[103] However, the efficacy of hip strengthening exercises on pain in people with other hip-related pain is uncertain. Two studies reported a reduction in pain in groups with strength exercise intervention,[101,104] whereas other studies did not see a difference between exercise and education versus education alone.[102,105]

Medical and Surgical Management

With the exception of hip OA, the evidence for the pharmacological management of hip pain is scarce. Recommendations for those with hip OA include paracetamol, oral and topical NSAIDs and intra-articular corticosteroid injections.[106,107] The use of glucosamine and chondroitin-sulphate is not recommended due to lack of supporting evidence in people with hip OA.[106] Intra-articular cortisone injections are sometimes used in contemporary clinical practice in those with FAI, labral pathology and chondropathy prior to surgical management with varied effect. The evidence supporting this practice is minimal, with small case series only indicating a positive effect for up to 12 months.[108] Generally a positive temporary effect is thought to indicate the presence of intra-articular pathology in the hip.

Hip arthroscopy is an orthopaedic surgical procedure that is increasing in popularity, which has contributed to an increased understanding of hip pain and pathology. The primary aims of hip arthroscopy are to reduce pain associated with intra-articular pathology, increase daily and sporting function and possibly reduce the risk of secondary hip OA.[42,109] Hip arthroscopy is considered advantageous over open techniques due to the reduction in risks such as infection and poor wound healing, and a rapid recovery.[42] Outcomes for hip arthroscopy appear positive;[51,110–112] however, to date no studies have compared the efficacy of hip arthroscopy surgery to conservative management in people with hip pain. Moreover, there is little known of the factors that may be associated with outcomes in individuals undergoing hip arthroscopic surgery. Recent studies have reported reduced hip muscle strength and hip joint range of motion[70] exist in people following hip arthroscopy, and altered gait biomechanics pre- and post-operatively.[62,63] It would seem reasonable to include these components in a targeted post-operative rehabilitation programme;

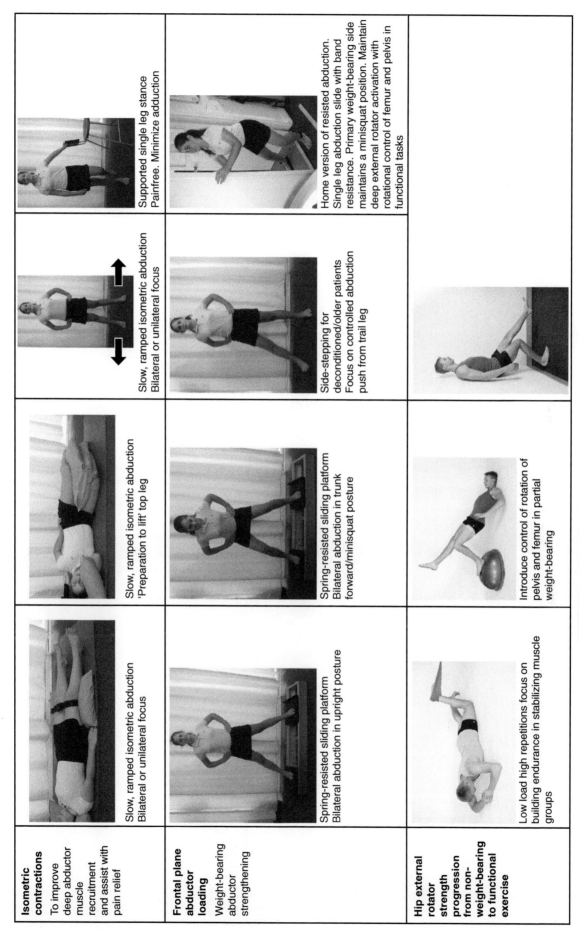

Isometric contractions To improve deep abductor muscle recruitment and assist with pain relief	Slow, ramped isometric abduction Bilateral or unilateral focus	Slow, ramped isometric abduction 'Preparation to lift' top leg	Slow, ramped isometric abduction Bilateral or unilateral focus	Supported single leg stance Painfree. Minimize adduction
Frontal plane abductor loading Weight-bearing abductor strengthening	Spring-resisted sliding platform Bilateral abduction in upright posture	Spring-resisted sliding platform Bilateral abduction in trunk forward/minisquat posture	Side-stepping for deconditioned/older patients Focus on controlled abduction push from trail leg	Home version of resisted abduction. Single leg abduction slide with band resistance. Primary weight-bearing side maintains a minisquat position. Maintain deep external rotator activation with rotational control of femur and pelvis in functional tasks
Hip external rotator strength progression from non-weight-bearing to functional exercise	Low load high repetitions focus on building endurance in stabilizing muscle groups	Introduce control of rotation of pelvis and femur in partial weight-bearing		

FIGURE 47-2 ■ Examples of abductor and external rotator exercises.

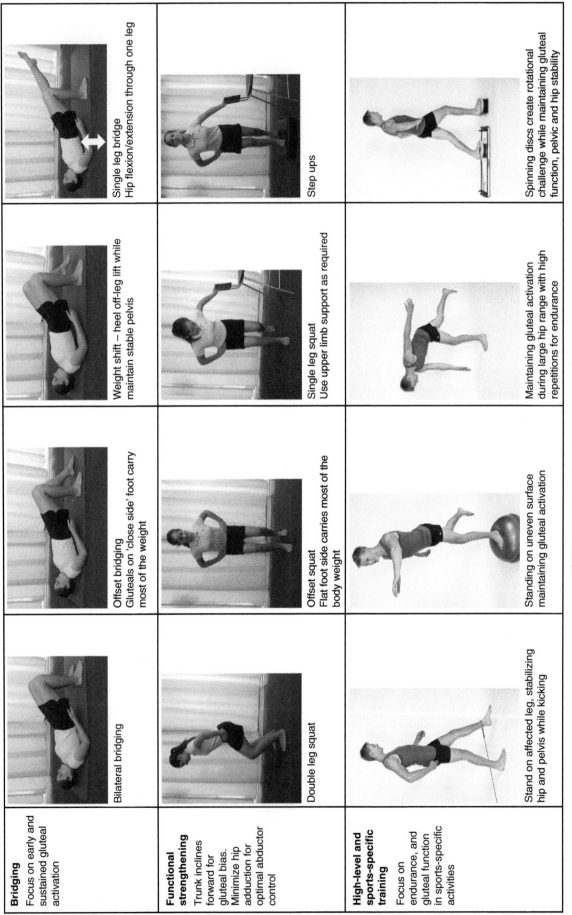

Bridging
Focus on early and sustained gluteal activation

Bilateral bridging

Offset bridging
Gluteals on 'close side' foot carry most of the weight

Weight shift – heel off-leg lift while maintain stable pelvis

Single leg bridge
Hip flexion/extension through one leg

Functional strengthening
Trunk inclines forward for gluteal bias. Minimize hip adduction for optimal abductor control

Double leg squat

Offset squat
Flat foot side carries most of the body weight

Single leg squat
Use upper limb support as required

Step ups

High-level and sports-specific training
Focus on endurance, and gluteal function in sports-specific activities

Stand on affected leg, stabilizing hip and pelvis while kicking

Standing on uneven surface maintaining gluteal activation

Maintaining gluteal activation during large hip range with high repetitions for endurance

Spinning discs create rotational challenge while maintaining gluteal function, pelvic and hip stability

FIGURE 47-3 ■ Examples of extensor exercises.

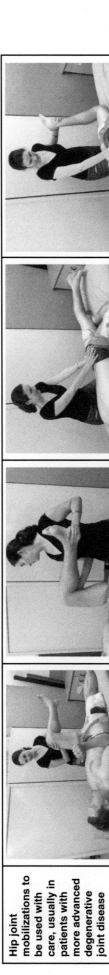

| Hip joint mobilizations to be used with care, usually in patients with more advanced degenerative joint disease | Lateral distraction mobilization with seatbelt | Inferior glide mobilization with seatbelt | Caudal glide mobilization | Rotation mobilization to increase hip rotation range |

FIGURE 47-4 ■ Examples of hip joint mobilization techniques.

however, no studies have tested appropriate rehabilitation programmes.

Controversies, Uncertainties and Future Directions

The concept of FAI as a cause of hip pathology and end-stage hip disease is relatively new, and many uncertainties remain regarding these relationships. Studies have recently indicated a relationship between cam FAI and end-stage hip disease in men[35] and women.[35,36] Cam FAI is more prevalent in men than women in the general population,[24,113] yet the prevalence of end-stage hip disease is roughly equal in men and women.[114] We have a limited understanding of gender-specific risk factors for hip joint-related pain and end-stage hip disease. Factors causing the development of cam FAI are also unclear. The prevalence of cam FAI is greater in young elite male athletes than age-matched controls,[29] and also in people with a family history of FAI.[115] It appears that both genetics and load-related factors play a part in the development of FAI. Moreover, no studies have determined the factors that lead to the development of symptoms in people with FAI. Recently, surgical removal of the cam lesion has become more commonplace with positive reduction of hip symptoms post-operatively.[51] However, it is unclear whether such surgery changes the natural history of the disease in people with cam FAI. Finally, the clinical differential diagnosis of FAI, labral pathology and chondral pathology is difficult, particularly as arthroscopy remains the gold standard for the clinical diagnosis of chondral pathology. However, as the likelihood of these conditions coexisting is high,[71] appropriate conservative management for each of these does not usually vary a great deal. Future studies focusing on each of these issues will greatly increase our understanding of the aetiology and risk factors associated with development of these conditions. This will enable the provision of more appropriate strategies to reduce the likelihood of progression of hip pathology in susceptible individuals.

TENDINOPATHY-RELATED HIP PAIN

Background

Gluteal and proximal hamstring tendinopathies are increasingly recognized sources of pain around the hip and pelvis. Gluteal tendinopathy affects up to 23.5% of women and 8.5% of men between 50–79 years,[116] whereas proximal hamstring tendinopathy may occur or coexist with gluteal tendinopathy in older individuals. However, the prevalence of these conditions is not restricted to older or sedentary populations. Athletes, particularly middle- and long-distance runners, also experience considerable disability and reduced performance secondary to painful gluteal[117–119] or proximal hamstring tendinopathy.[120–123] Despite advances in radiological assessment of pelvic tendinopathies, gold standards in clinical diagnosis and management are yet to be elucidated.

While many general health[124–126] and drug-related factors[127,128] may impact on tendon pain and loadbearing status, mechanical loading has a powerful influence. The homoeostasis within a tendon may be disturbed by a change in type, intensity or frequency of loading stimulus.[129] Load may be applied longitudinally along the tendon fibres (tensile load), or perpendicular to the collagen fibres (compression). Rapid increases in intensity or frequency of tensile loading may result in overload and a net catabolic effect. Similarly, tensile loading of inadequate intensity or frequency (stress deprivation) results in structural degradation and a reduction in the loadbearing capacity of the tendon.[130] Compressive load, commonly encountered at tendon–bone interfaces such as tendon insertion sites, engenders adaptation that increases resistance to compression but weakens the tendon against tensile loading.[131–133] The combination of compression and tensile overload may represent the most noxious environment for a tendon.[134] Using these principles, imposing such forces during assessment and minimizing them during rehabilitation may improve the effectiveness of both.

Assessment

Apart from the cardinal signs of pain experienced directly over the tendon and tenderness on direct palpation, functional and specific tendon-loading tests are key components for the differential diagnosis of tendon-related pain. As confidence in a clinical diagnosis increases with the number of key diagnostic features that are consistent with a particular pathology, considering information gathered from the subjective examination together with results of a battery of clinical tests is recommended.

Key Clinical Diagnostic Features of Tendinopathy-Related Hip Pain

Key diagnostic features and clinical tests described to date in the literature for gluteal[135–141] and proximal hamstring tendinopathy[120,121,135,142] have been outlined in Table 47-2. Note that the diagnostic accuracy of the clinical orthopaedic tests for these tendon pathologies are not well established[143,144] and a comprehensive physical examination of other potential pain sources such as the lumbar spine, peripheral nerves, hip joint and other surrounding soft tissues is also required.

The Role of Imaging: When to and When Not to Image?

Imaging may be required as an adjunct to clinical testing, where there is a history of trauma or marked loss of function (to assess tendon avulsion), or where the clinical diagnosis is unclear and/or there has been a failure to progress with a tendon-focused management plan. Ultrasound or MRI are both useful to assess the tendons and associated bursae at the greater trochanter and ischium.[146–149] MRI has the advantage of providing a wider field of view and may detect other local

Table 47-2   Key Clinical Diagnostic Features of Gluteal and Proximal Hamstring Tendinopathy

Clinical Diagnostic Features Specific to Gluteal Tendinopathy

Subjective Examination

Area of pain	Lateral hip (*GT), extending down the lateral thigh
Aggravating factors	Side lying – pain over GT Walking especially at speed or uphill Stair climbing Stiffness/pain over GT on rising to stand after sitting
Loading history	Onset after change in activity, slip or fall, or may present insidiously A positive test reproduces pain over the greater GT ± the lateral thigh

Physical Examination

Functional loading tasks	Sustained single leg stance[138] Single leg squat, step up, hop[135]
Specific tendon-loading tasks	Passive hip external rotation in 45° F[137] Resisted external derotation test (resisted IR from EOR ER at 90° F, and prone)[138] FABER[136,141] Modified Ober's Test[141]
Palpation	Marked tenderness of the GT[139,140]

Clinical Diagnostic Features Specific to Proximal Hamstring Tendinopathy

Subjective Examination

Area of pain	Ischial pain, extends down the posterior thigh as pain or a feeling of tightness limiting full stride length in running
Aggravating factors	Sitting, particularly on hard surfaces Walking/running particularly with long strides or uphill Forward leaning/forward bending with straight knee Deep lunge or high step up
Loading history	Onset after a change in activity, a slip or fall resulting in a large tensile load (e.g. water skiing or front splits) or a direct compressive blow to the ischium, or may present insidiously A positive test reproduces pain over IT ± the posterior thigh

Physical Examination

Functional loading tasks	Single leg bent knee bridge – Low load Single leg straight-leg bridge (plank) – Moderate load[142] Single leg deadlift – High load[121,135,142]
Specific tendon-loading tasks	Bent Knee Stretch & Modified Bent Knee Stretch Test (Isometric knee F in supine, EOR hip F and knee E)[144,145] Puranen Oravo Test (standing hamstring stretch on bench)[145] Shoe Off Test; Heel Drag Test (isometric load against other foot/floor)[142]
Palpation	Marked tenderness on palpation of the ischial tuberosity, particularly laterally at the semimembranosis origin

E, Extension; *EOR*, End of range; *ER*, External rotation; *F*, Flexion; *FABER*, Flexion/abduction/external rotation; *GMed*, Gluteus medius; *GMin*, Gluteus minimus; *GT*, Greater trochanter; **GT*, the patient should indicate the greater trochanter as the maximal area of pain, or the region from which the pain emanates; *IT*, Ischial tuberosity.

pathologies. Lumbar spine imaging is also often employed for non-responders, to assist in explicating involvement of the spine. Caution is required, however, with the interpretation of imaging abnormalities. Pathology in the lumbar spine, as well as the gluteal and hamstring tendons, is evident in asymptomatic individuals.[146,148,150] Imaging findings must always be considered only alongside clinical test results.

Treatment

Gluteal and proximal hamstring tendinopathy intervention centres on load management. Advice and education regarding minimizing provocative loads is an early priority. A graduated exercise protocol aims to stimulate positive biological changes within the tendon and address any associated aberrant motor patterns. Manual therapy

may be required to help establish and maintain appropriate muscle length and tone, particularly as stretching the affected musculotendinous unit is usually unhelpful due to the accompanying compression–tension load combination.[132]

Gluteal Tendinopathy

For the gluteus medius and minimus tendons the combination of compressive and tensile loads is highest in adduction, when the abductor muscles are working hard at length. For an athlete, a provocative load may be running at speed or hopping, whereas for an older or deconditioned individual, stair climbing or standing on one leg to dress may represent relative overload. Abductor muscle weakness, or a shift in muscle balance or length tension relationship,[151] may result in increased hip adduction.[152] Once symptomatic, compression alone (e.g.

lying on the affected side) or compression with passive adduction will aggravate the condition, particularly if sustained or end-range – sitting with the knees crossed, standing 'hanging on one hip' in adduction, lying on the unaffected side with the affected hip flexed and adducted, hip flexion/adduction stretches. Patients should be educated regarding what constitutes a provocative load and how to avoid or minimize these loads in everyday activities and sport.[153]

The exercise programme aims to reduce pain and improve the efficiency of the hip abductor musculature to minimize the excessive pelvic tilt or shift that increases hip adduction.[154] Early prescription of slowly ramped isometric hip abductor exercises often assists pain relief (see Fig. 47-2), possibly due to the activation of segmental and/or extrasegmental descending pain inhibition mechanisms.[155,156] Weight-bearing functional retraining that aims to minimize hip adduction, progresses from double leg, to offset and then single leg tasks with upper limb support, and ultimately with no support and for athletes more dynamic landing control tasks (see Fig. 47-3). Targeted concentric–eccentric abductor strengthening is often well tolerated quite early if applied without compression. An ideal medium is a sliding platform with spring resistance. Standing on such a platform and actively abducting the hips against resistance allows graduated increases in tensile loading without compression as the hips move from neutral to inner range abduction (see Fig. 47-2).

Proximal Hamstring Tendinopathy

For the proximal hamstring tendons the combination of high compressive and tensile loads occurs in hip flexion, when the tendons wrap around the ischium and the hamstrings are active in this lengthened position.[135,153] The semimembranosis tendon sits deepest and is exposed to greatest compression, which may explain the higher incidence of semimembranosis pathology.[122] Activities and positions utilizing the combination of high compression and active tension should be minimized, for example sustained or loaded trunk forward inclination, walking or running up inclines or high steps, straight-leg deadlifts or similar actions on one leg ('cranes', 'aeroplanes') in the gym. Symptomatic tendons are provoked by compression alone, such as sitting on the ischia, particularly on a hard surface.

The exercise programme provides pain-reducing isometric contractions, and targeted strengthening of the hamstrings and gluteus maximus within the framework of lower quadrant conditioning.[153] Isometric hamstring strengthening is best performed early, in low or no hip flexion to minimize compression (Fig. 47-5). Loading can progress to higher load isometrics and heavy slow loading in the form of hamstring curls, hamstring biased bridge variations and Nordic curls[126] (Fig. 47-5). Achieving good gluteus maximus recruitment is essential during hip extension tasks to avoid relative overload of the hamstring complex. Functional weight-bearing strengthening such as bridging and squatting should be included to re-establish optimal recruitment patterns, commencing at low flexion angles (Fig. 47-3, rows 1 and 2).

Effectiveness of Conservative Therapies

The evidence to date suggests there is no 'magic bullet' solution to tendinopathy, and an exercise-based approach is considered most likely to provide greatest medium- to longer-term results. The challenge for health professionals is to provide improved short- and long-term results. Information on early success of exercise intervention for gluteal tendinopathy is limited to one study reporting a 7% success rate at 1 month,[157] and for proximal hamstring tendinopathy another study reporting a 10% success rate at 3 months.[120] Both studies included a substantial stretching component, the gluteal tendinopathy study included no hip abductor muscle strengthening, and the hamstring study included provocative high compression–high active tension exercises. Patient education and exercise modifications to avoid provocative tendon loads and promote positive adaptation hold great potential for improving outcomes in tendinopathy about the hip.

Controversies, Uncertainties and Future Directions

At this time, one of the greatest controversies with respect to management of tendinopathies is the role of injection therapy – the most common being corticosteroid injections (CSI) and blood-derived products (autologous blood injections and platelet-rich plasma). Although widely used in clinical practice, there is poor evidence regarding their usefulness and unknown effects on local tissue health in the longer term. Despite the short-term pain reduction imparted by CSI in tendinopathic conditions, even a single injection has been shown to delay and reduce outcomes over the medium to longer term.[158,159]

Limited studies have evaluated CSI for gluteal or proximal hamstring tendinopathies. Reduction of lateral hip pain has been reported for 72–75% of patients after 1 month,[157,160] and 41–55% at 3–4 months[157,161,162] following CSI. After 12 months Brinks et al.[161] showed no difference in outcome between groups provided with CSI and 'usual care' (analgesics as required). One retrospective study assessed the effects of CSI on proximal hamstring tendinopathy, describing a 50% success rate at 1 month; however only 24% sustained a positive benefit for more than 6 months.[163]

Injections of biologically active blood products are purported to 'kick start' the healing process by initiating the production of new collagen and stimulating revascularization.[164] No studies to date evaluate the efficacy of autologous blood injections or platelet-rich plasma injections for gluteal or proximal hamstring tendinopathy. From the wider literature a recent review reported inadequate evidence to support platelet-rich plasma injections in tendinopathy management and suggested that 'the use of autologous whole blood should not be recommended'.[165] Much further research is required to clearly establish the efficacy and safety of these and other emerging injectable therapies.

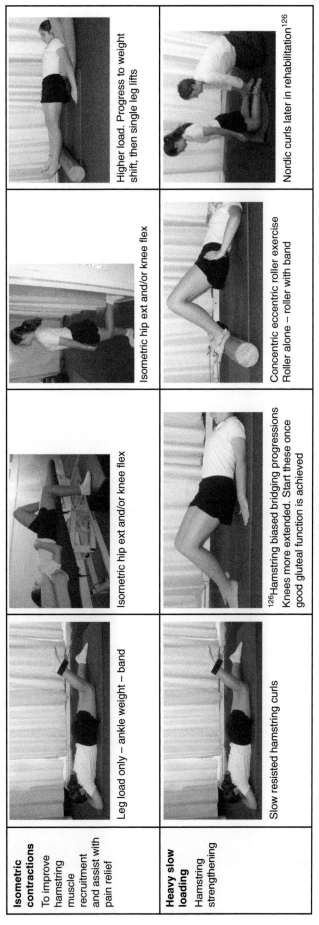

Isometric contractions To improve hamstring muscle recruitment and assist with pain relief			
Leg load only – ankle weight – band	Isometric hip ext and/or knee flex	Isometric hip ext and/or knee flex	Higher load. Progress to weight shift, then single leg lifts
Heavy slow loading Hamstring strengthening			
Slow resisted hamstring curls	[126]Hamstring biased bridging progressions Knees more extended. Start these once good gluteal function is achieved	Concentric eccentric roller exercise Roller alone – roller with band	Nordic curls later in rehabilitation[126]

FIGURE 47-5 ■ Examples of hamstring exercises.

REFERENCES

1. Stem E, O'Connor M, Kransdorf M, et al. Computed tomography analysis of acetabular anteversion and abduction. Skeletal Radiol 2006;35(6):385–9.
2. Lewis CL, Sahrmann SA. Acetabular labral tears. Phys Ther 2006;86(1):110–21.
3. Haemer JM, Carter DR, Giori NJ. The low permeability of healthy meniscus and labrum limit articular cartilage consolidation and maintain fluid load support in the knee and hip. J Biomech 2012;45(8):1450–6.
4. Tan V, Seldes RM, Katz MA, et al. Contribution of acetabular labrum to articulating surface area and femoral head coverage in adult hip joints: an anatomic study in cadavera. Am J Orthop (Belle Mead NJ) 2001;30(11):809–12. [Epub 2002/01/05. eng]; PubMed PMID: 11757858.
5. Petersen W, Petersen F, Tillmann B. Structure and vascularization of the acetabular labrum with regard to the pathogenesis and healing of labral lesions. Arch Orthop Trauma Surg 2003;123(6):283–8.
6. Narvani AA, Tsiridis E, Tai CC, et al. Acetabular labrum and its tears. Br J Sports Med 2003;37(3):207–11. PubMed PMID: 12782544.
7. Dhollander AAM, Lambrecht S, Verdonk PCM, et al. First insights into human acetabular labrum cell metabolism. Osteoarthritis Cartilage 2012;20(7):670–7.
8. Konrath GA, Hamel AJ, Olson SA, et al. The role of the acetabular labrum and the transverse acetabular ligament in load transmission in the hip. J Bone Joint Surg Am 1998;80(12):1781–8.
9. Rao J, Zhou YX, Villar RN. Injury to the ligamentum teres. Mechanism, findings, and results of treatment. Clin Sports Med 2001;20(4):791–9, vii. PubMed PMID: MEDLINE:11675887.
10. Bardakos NV, Villar RN. The ligamentum teres of the adult hip. J Bone Joint Surg Br 2009;91-B(1):8–15.
11. Retchford T, Crossley KM, Grimaldi A, et al. Can local muscles augment stability in the hip? A narrative literature review. J Musculoskelet Neuronal Interact 2013;13(1):1–12.
12. Neumann DA. Kinesiology of the hip: a focus on muscular actions. J Orthop Sports Phys Ther 2010;40(2):82–94.
13. Ward SR, Winters TM, Blemker SS. The architectural design of the gluteal muscle group: implications for movement and rehabilitation. J Orthop Sports Phys Ther 2010;40(2):95–102.
14. Walden M, Hagglund M, Ekstrand J. UEFA Champions League study: a prospective study of injuries in professional football during the 2001–2002 season. Br J Sports Med 2005;39:542–6.
15. Orchard J, Seward H. AFL Injury Report: 2009. Available from: <http://www.afl.com.au/injury%20report/tabid/13706/default.aspx>; 2008.
16. Spahn G, Schiell R, Langlotz A, et al. Hip pain in adolescents: results of a cross-sectional study in German pupils and a review of the literature. Acta Paediatr 2005;94:568–73.
17. Christmas C, Crespo CJ, Franckowiak SC, et al. How common is hip pain among older adults? Results from the Third National Health and Nutrition Examination Survey. J Fam Pract 2002;51(4):345–8. [Epub 2002/04/30. eng]; PubMed PMID: 11978258.
18. Byrd JWT, Jones KS. Prospective analysis of hip arthroscopy with 10-year followup. Clin Orthop Relat Res 2010;468(3):741–6.
19. Clohisy JC, Knaus ER, Hunt DM, et al. Clinical presentation of patients with symptomatic anterior hip impingement. Clin Orthop Relat Res 2009;467(3):638–44, [English].
20. Clohisy JC, Dobson MA, Robison JF, et al. Radiographic structural abnormalities associated with premature, natural hip-joint failure. J Bone Joint Surg Am 2011;93:3–9.
21. Ganz R, Parvizi J, Beck M, et al. Femoroacetabular impingement: a cause for osteoarthritis of the hip. Clin Orthop Relat Res 2003;417:112–20.
22. Tannast M, Kubiak-Langer M, Langlotz F, et al. Noninvasive three-dimensional assessment of femoroacetabular impingement. J Orthop Res 2007;25(1):122–31. PubMed PMID: MEDLINE:17054112.
23. Banerjee P, McLean CR. Femoroacetabular impingement: a review of diagnosis and management. Curr Rev Musculoskelet Med 2011;4(1):23–32. PubMed PMID: MEDLINE:21475562.
24. Reichenbach S, Jüni P, Werlen S, et al. Prevalence of cam-type deformity on hip magnetic resonance imaging in young males: a cross-sectional study. Arthritis Care Res (Hoboken) 2010;62(9):1319–27. PubMed PMID: 20853471.
25. Bardakos NV, Vasconcelos JC, Villar RN. Early outcome of hip arthroscopy for femoroacetabular impingement: the role of femoral osteoplasty in symptomatic improvement. J Bone Joint Surg Br 2008;90(12):1570–5.
26. Byrd JWT, Jones KS. Arthroscopic Femoroplasty in the management of cam-type Femoroacetabular impingement. Clin Orthop Relat Res 2009;467(3):739–46.
27. Pollard TCB, Villar RN, Norton MR, et al. Femoroacetabular impingement and classification of the cam deformity: the reference interval in normal hips. Acta Orthop 2010;81(1):134–41.
28. Gosvig KK, Jacobsen S, Sonne-Holm S, et al. The prevalence of cam-type deformity of the hip joint: a survey of 4151 subjects of the Copenhagen Osteoarthritis Study. Acta Radiol 2008;49(4):436–41. PubMed PMID: 18415788.
29. Siebenrock K, Ferner F, Noble P, et al. The cam-type deformity of the proximal femur arises in childhood in response to vigorous sporting activity. Clin Orthop Relat Res 2011;469:3229–40.
30. Allen D, Beaulé PE, Ramadan O, et al. Prevalence of associated deformities and hip pain in patients with cam-type femoroacetabular impingement. J Bone Joint Surg Br 2009;91(5):589–94.
31. Singh PJ, O'Donnell JM. The outcome of hip arthroscopy in Australian football league players: a review of 27 hips. Arthroscopy: The Journal of Arthroscopic & Related Surgery. 2010;26(6):743–9.
32. Philippon MJ, Weiss DR, Kuppersmith DA, et al. Arthroscopic labral repair and treatment of femoroacetabular impingement in professional hockey players. Am J Sports Med 2010;38(1):99–104.
33. Byrd JWT, Jones KS. Hip Arthroscopy in athletes: 10-year follow-up. Am J Sports Med 2009;37(11):2140–3.
34. Agricola R, Heijboer M, Bierma-Zeinstra S, et al. Cam-type deformities strongly predict total hip replacement within 5 years in those with early symptomatic OA: a prospective cohort study (check). Osteoarthritis Cartilage 2012;20(Suppl. 1):S203.
35. Agricola R, Heijboer MP, Bierma-Zeinstra SMA, et al. Cam impingement causes osteoarthritis of the hip: a nationwide prospective cohort study (CHECK). Ann Rheum Dis 2012.
36. Nicholls AS, Kiran A, Pollard TCB, et al. The association between hip morphology parameters and nineteen-year risk of end-stage osteoarthritis of the hip a nested case-control study. Arthritis Rheum 2011;63(11):3392–400.
37. Siebenrock KA, Schoeniger R, Ganz R. Anterior femoroacetabular impingement due to acetabular retroversion. Treatment with periacetabular osteotomy. J Bone Joint Surg Am 2003;85(2):278–86.
38. Agricola R, Heijboer MP, Roze RH, et al. Pincer deformity does not lead to osteoarthritis of the hip whereas acetabular dysplasia does: acetabular coverage and development of osteoarthritis in a nationwide prospective cohort study (CHECK). Osteoarthritis Cartilage 2013;21(10):1514–21.
39. Farjo LA, Glick JM, Sampson TG. Hip arthroscopy for acetabular labral tears. Arthroscopy 1999;15(2):132–7.
40. McCarthy JC, Noble PC, Schuck MR, et al. The role of labral lesions to development of early degenerative hip disease. Clin Orthop Relat Res 2001;393:25–37.
41. Seldes RM, Tan V, Hunt J, et al. Anatomy, histologic features, and vascularity of the adult acetabular labrum. Clin Orthop Relat Res 2001;382:232–40.
42. Clohisy JC, Baca G, Beaulé PE, et al. Descriptive epidemiology of femoroacetabular impingement: a North American cohort of patients undergoing surgery. Am J Sports Med 2013.
43. Ito K, Minka MA II, Leunig M, et al. Femoroacetabular impingement and the cam-effect. A MRI-based quantitative anatomical study of the femoral head-neck offset. J Bone Joint Surg Br 2001;83(2):171–6.
44. Peelle MW, Della Rocca GJ, Maloney WJ, et al. Acetabular and Femoral Radiographic Abnormalities Associated with Labral Tears. Clin Orthop Relat Res 2005;441:327–33.
45. Tanzer M, Noiseux N. Osseous abnormalities and early osteoarthritis: the role of hip impingement. Clin Orthop Relat Res 2004;429:170–7. PubMed PMID: MEDLINE:15577483.

46. Muir H. The chondrocyte, architect of cartilage. Biomechanics, structure, function and molecular biology of cartilage matrix macromolecules. Bioessays 1995;17(12):1039–47.

47. O'Hara BP, Urban JPG, Maroudas A. Influence of cyclic loading on the nutrition of articular cartilage. Ann Rheum Dis 1990; 49:536–9.

48. McCarthy JC, Lee JA. Hip arthroscopy: indications, outcomes, and complications. J Bone Joint Surg Am 2005;87(5):1138–45.

49. Roos H, Laurén M, Adalberth T, et al. Knee osteoarthritis after meniscectomy: prevalence of radiographic changes after twenty-one years, compared with matched controls. Arthritis Rheum 1998;41(4):687–93.

50. Englund M, Lohmander LS. Risk factors for symptomatic knee osteoarthritis fifteen to twenty-two years after meniscectomy. Arthritis Rheum 2004;50(9):2811–19.

51. Kemp JL, Collins NJ, Makdissi M, et al. Hip arthroscopy for intra-articular pathology: a systematic review of outcomes with and without femoral osteoplasty. Br J Sports Med 2012;46(9): 632–43.

52. Byrd JWT, Jones KS. Hip arthroscopy for labral pathology: prospective analysis with 10-year follow-up. Arthroscopy 2009;25(4): 365–8.

53. Tamura S, Nishii T, Takao M, et al. Associations of hip dysplasia and FAI on modes of acetabular labral tears – 3 dimensional analysis by high-resolution CT arthrography. Osteoarthritis Cartilage 2012;20(Suppl. 1):S214–15.

54. Pollard TCB, Batra RN, Judge A, et al. Genetic predisposition to the presence and 5-year clinical progression of hip osteoarthritis. Osteoarthritis Cartilage 2012;20(5):368–75.

55. Pollard TCB, McNally EG, Wilson DC, et al. Localized cartilage assessment with three-dimensional dGEMRIC in asymptomatic hips with normal morphology and cam deformity. J Bone Joint Surg Am 2010;92(15):2557–69.

56. Ratzlaff C, Simatovic J, Wong H, et al. Reliability of hip examination tests for femoroacetabular impingement (FAI). Arthritis Care Res (Hoboken) 2013;65(10):1690–6.

57. Audenaert EA, Peeters I, Vigneron L, et al. Hip morphological characteristics and range of internal rotation in femoroacetabular impingement. Am J Sports Med 2012;40(6):1329–36.

58. Kapron AL, Anderson AE, Peters CL, et al. Hip internal rotation is correlated to radiographic findings of cam femoroacetabular impingement in collegiate football players. Arthroscopy 2012; 28(11):1661–70.

59. Yuan BJ, Bartelt RB, Levy BA, et al. Decreased range of motion is associated with structural hip deformity in asymptomatic adolescent athletes. Am J Sports Med 2013;41(7):1519–25.

60. Nussbaumer S, Leunig M, Glatthorn J, et al. Validity and test-retest reliability of manual goniometers for measuring passive hip range of motion in femoroacetabular impingement patients. BMC Musculoskelet Disord 2010;11:194–204.

61. Casartelli NC, Maffiuletti NA, Item-Glatthorn JF, et al. Hip muscle weakness in patients with symptomatic femoroacetabular impingement. Osteoarthritis Cartilage 2011;19(7):816–21.

62. Brisson N, Lamontagne M, Kennedy MJ, et al. The effects of cam femoroacetabular impingement corrective surgery on lower-extremity gait biomechanics. Gait Posture 2012;37:258–63.

63. Hunt MA, Gunether JR, Gilbart MK. Kinematic and kinetic differences during walking in patients with and without symptomatic femoroacetabular impingement. Clin Biomech (Bristol, Avon) 2013;5:519–23.

64. Agricola R, Waarsing JH, Thomas GE, et al. Cam impingement: defining the presence of a cam deformity by the alpha angle. Data from the CHECK cohort and Chingford cohort. Osteoarthritis Cartilage 2014;22(2):218–25.

65. Beaulé PE, Hynes K, Parker G, et al. Can the alpha angle assessment of cam impingement predict acetabular cartilage delamination? Clin Orthop Relat Res 2012;470:3361–7.

66. Heyworth B, Dolan M, Nguyen J, et al. Preoperative three-dimensional CT predicts intraoperative findings in hip arthroscopy. Clin Orthop Relat Res 2012;470(7):1950–7.

67. Groh MM, Herrera J. A comprehensive review of hip labral tears. Curr Rev Musculoskelet Med 2009;2(2):105–17. PubMed PMID: MEDLINE:19468871.

68. Yazbek PM, Ovanessian V, Martin RL, et al. Nonsurgical treatment of acetabular labrum tears: a case series. J Orthop Sports Phys Ther 2011;41(5):346–53. PubMed PMID: 21335929.

69. Gold SL, Burge AJ, Potter HG. MRI of hip cartilage. Clin Orthop Relat Res 2012;470:3321–31.

70. Kemp JL, Schache AG, Makdissi M, et al. People with chondropathy have greater physical impairments than those without following hip arthroscopy. Osteoarthritis Cartilage 2013;21(Suppl.): S274.

71. Kemp JL, Makdissi M, Schache AG, et al. Hip chondropathy is prevalent at arthroscopy and is associated with co-existing pathology, but not patient reported outcomes. Osteoarthritis Cartilage 2013;21(Suppl.):S138.

72. Hatton AL, Kemp JL, Brauer SG, et al. Dynamic single-leg balance performance is impaired in individuals with hip chondropathy. Arthritis Care Res (Hoboken) 2013;66(5):709–16.

73. Bierma-Zeinstra S, Koes B. Risk factors and pronostic factors of hip and knee osteoarthritis. Nat Clin Pract Rheumatol 2007;3(2): 78–85.

74. Holla JF, van der Leeden M, Roorda LD, et al. Diagnostic accuracy of range of motion measurements in early symptomatic hip and/or knee osteoarthritis. Arthritis Care Res (Hoboken) 2012;64(1):59–65. [Epub 2011/09/29. eng]; PubMed PMID: 21954179.

75. Holla JFM, Steultjens MPM, van der Leeden M, et al. Determinants of range of joint motion in patients with early symptomatic osteoarthritis of the hip and/or knee: an exploratory study in the CHECK cohort. Osteoarthritis Cartilage 2011;19: 411–19.

76. Arokoski MH, Haara M, Helminen HJ, et al. Physical function in men with and without hip osteoarthritis. Arch Phys Med Rehabil 2004;85(4):574–81. PubMed PMID: 15083432.

77. Altman R, Alarcon G, Appelrouth D, et al. The American College of Rheumatology criteria for the classification and reporting of osteoarthritis of the hip. Arthritis Rheum 1991;34(5):505–14.

78. Arokoski MH, et al. Hip muscle strength and cross sectional area in men with and without hip osteoarthritis. J Rheumatol 2002; 29(10):2185–95.

79. Pua YH, Wrigley TV, Cowan SM, et al. Hip flexion range of motion and physical function in hip osteoarthritis: mediating effects of hip extensor strength and pain. Arthritis Care Res 2009; 61(5):633–40.

80. Lievense AM, Bierma-Zeinstra SMA, Verhagen AP, et al. Influence of obesity on the development of osteoarthritis of the hip: a systematic review. Rheumatology 2002;41(10):1155–62.

81. Altman RD, Gold GE. Atlas of individual radiographic features in osteoarthritis, revised. Osteoarthritis Cartilage 2007;15(Suppl. 1): A1–56.

82. Xu L, Hayashi D, Guermazi A, et al. The diagnostic performance of radiography for detection of osteoarthritis-associated features compared with MRI in hip joints with chronic pain. Skeletal Radiol 2013;42(10):1421–8, [English].

83. Nepple JJ, Kim YJ, Clohisy J. Do plain radiographs correlate with CT for imaging of cam-type femoroacetabular impingement? Clin Orthop Relat Res 2012;470:3313–20.

84. Reichenbach S, Leunig M, Werlen S, et al. Association between cam-type deformities and magnetic resonance imaging–detected structural hip damage: a cross-sectional study in young men. Arthritis Rheum 2011;63(12):4023–30.

85. Zlatkin MB, Pevsner D, Sanders TG, et al. Acetabular labral tears and cartilage lesions of the hip: indirect MR arthrographic correlation with arthroscopy–a preliminary study. AJR Am J Roentgenol 2010;194(3):709–14.

86. Tyler TF, Slattery AA. Rehabilitation of the hip following sports injury. Clin Sports Med 2010;29(1):107–26.

87. Shindle MK, Domb BG, Kelly BT. Hip and pelvic problems in athletes. Oper Tech Sports Med 2007;15(4):195–203.

88. Enseki KR, Martin R, Kelly BT. Rehabilitation after arthroscopic decompression for femoroacetabular impingement. Clin Sports Med 2010;29(2):247–55. PubMed PMID: 20226317.

89. Philippon MJ, Christensen JC, Wahoff MS. Rehabilitation after arthroscopic repair of intra-articular disorders of the hip in a professional football athlete. J Sport Rehabil 2009;18(1): 118–34.

90. Stalzer S, Wahoff M, Scanlan M. Rehabilitation following hip arthroscopy. Clin Sports Med 2006;25(2):337–57.

91. Lewis CL, Sahrmann SA, Moran DW. Effect of hip angle on anterior hip joint force during gait. Gait Posture 2010;32(4): 603–7.

92. Wall PDH, Fernandez M, Griffin DR, et al. Nonoperative treatment for femoroacetabular impingement: a systematic review of the literature. PM R 2013;5(5):418–26.

93. Cambridge EDJ, Sidorkewicz N, Ikeda DM, et al. Progressive hip rehabilitation: the effects of resistance band placement on gluteal activation during two common exercises. Clin Biomech (Bristol, Avon) 2012;27(7):719–24.

94. Boren K, Conrey C, Le Coguic J, et al. Electromyographic analysis of gluteus medius and gluteus maximus during rehabilitation exercises. Int J Sports Phys Ther 2011;6(3):206–23.

95. Fisher BE, Lee Y, Pitsch EA, et al. Method for assessing brain changes associated with gluteus maximus activation. J Orthop Sports Phys Ther 2013;43(4):214–21.

96. Giphart E, Stull J, LaPrade R, et al. Recruitment and activity of the pectineus and piriformis muscles during hip rehabilitation exercises. Am J Sports Med 2012;40(7):1654–63.

97. Cowan SM, Blackburn MS, McMahon K, et al. Current Australian physiotherapy management of hip osteoarthritis. Physiotherapy 2010;96(4):289–95. PubMed PMID: 21056163.

98. Godges JJ, Macrae H, Longdon C, et al. The effects of two stretching procedures on hip range of motion and gait economy. J Orthop Sports Phys Ther 1989;10(9):350–7. [Epub 1989/01/01. eng]; PubMed PMID: 18791317.

99. Bennell K. Physiotherapy management of hip osteoarthritis. J Physiother 2013;59(3):145–57.

100. Poulsen E, Hartvigsen J, Christensen HW, et al. Patient education with or without manual therapy compared to a control group in patients with osteoarthritis of the hip. A proof-of-principle three-arm parallel group randomized clinical trial. Osteoarthritis Cartilage 2013;21(10):1494–503.

101. Rooks DS, Huang J, Bierbaum BE, et al. Effect of preoperative exercise on measures of functional status in men and women undergoing total hip and knee arthroplasty. Arthritis Care Res (Hoboken) 2006;55(5):700–8.

102. Fernandes L, Storheim K, Sandvik L, et al. Efficacy of patient education and supervised exercise vs patient education alone in patients with hip osteoarthritis: a single blind randomized clinical trial. Osteoarthritis Cartilage 2010;18(10):1237–43.

103. Lewis CL, Sahrmann SA, Moran DW. Anterior hip joint force increases with hip extension, decreased gluteal force, or decreased iliopsoas force. J Biomech 2007;40(16):3725–31.

104. French HP, Brennan A, White B, et al. Manual therapy for osteoarthritis of the hip or knee – A systematic review. Man Ther 2011;16(2):109–17.

105. Abbott JH, Robertson MC, Chapple C, et al. Manual therapy, exercise therapy, or both, in addition to usual care, for osteoarthritis of the hip or knee: a randomized controlled trial. 1: clinical effectiveness. Osteoarthritis Cartilage 2013;21(4):525–34.

106. Hochberg MC, Altman RD, April KT, et al. American College of Rheumatology 2012 recommendations for the use of nonpharmacologic and pharmacologic therapies in osteoarthritis of the hand, hip, and knee. Arthritis Care Res (Hoboken) 2012;64(4):465–74.

107. Zhang W, Doherty M, Arden N, et al. Eular evidence based recommendations for the management of hip osteoarthritis: report of a task force of the EULAR Standing Committee for International Clincal Studies Including Therapeutics (ESCISIT). Ann Rheum Dis 2005;64:669–81.

108. Hauser RA, Orlofsky A. Regenerative Injection Therapy (Prolotherapy) for hip labrum lesions: rationale and retrospective study. Open Rehabi J 2013;6:59–68.

109. Ellis HB, Briggs KK, Philippon MJ. Innovation in hip arthroscopy: is hip arthritis preventable in the athlete? Br J Sports Med 2011;45(4):253–8. [Epub 2011 Feb]; PubMed PMID: MEDLINE: 21304160.

110. Clohisy JC, Beaulé PE, O'Malley A, et al. Hip disease in the young adult: current concepts of etiology and surgical treatment. J Bone Joint Surg Am 2008;90(10):2267–81.

111. Robertson WJ, Kadrmas WR, Kelly BT. Arthroscopic management of labral tears in the hip: a systematic review. Clin Orthop Relat Res 2007;455:88–92.

112. Ng VY, Arora N, Best TM, et al. Efficacy of surgery for femoroacetabular impingement: a systematic review. Am J Sports Med 2010;38(11):2337–45.

113. Leunig M, Jüni P, Werlen S, et al. Prevalence of cam and pincer-type deformities on hip MRI in an asymptomatic young Swiss female population: a cross-sectional study. Osteoarthritis Cartilage 2013;21(4):544–50.

114. Dagenais S, Garbedian S, Wai E. Systematic review of the prevalence of radiographic hip osteoarthritis. Clin Orthop Relat Res 2009;467:623–37.

115. Pollard TCB, Villar RN, Norton MR, et al. Genetic influences in the aetiology of femoroacetabular impingement: a sibling study. J Bone Joint Surg Br 2010;92-B(2):209–16.

116. Segal NA, Felson DT, Torner JC, et al. Greater trochanteric pain syndrome: epidemiology and associated factors. Arch Phys Med Rehabil 2007;88(8):988–92. PubMed PMID: 17678660. Pubmed Central PMCID: 2907104.

117. Del Buono A, Papalia R, Khanduja V, et al. Management of the greater trochanteric pain syndrome: a systematic review. Br Med Bull 2012;102:115–31. PubMed PMID: 21893483.

118. Grumet RC, Frank RM, Slabaugh MA, et al. Lateral hip pain in an athletic population: differential diagnosis and treatment options. Sports Health 2010;2(3):191–6. PubMed PMID: 23015937. Pubmed Central PMCID: 3445102.

119. Spiker AM, Dixit S, Cosgarea AJ. Triathlon: running injuries. Sports Med Arthrosc 2012;20(4):206–13. PubMed PMID: 23147090.

120. Cacchio A, Rompe JD, Furia JP, et al. Shockwave therapy for the treatment of chronic proximal hamstring tendinopathy in professional athletes. Am J Sports Med 2011;39(1):146–53. PubMed PMID: 20855554.

121. Fredericson M, Moore W, Guillet M, et al. High hamstring tendinopathy in runners: meeting the challenges of diagnosis, treatment, and rehabilitation. Phys Sportsmed 2005;33(5):32–43. PubMed PMID: 20086362.

122. Lempainen L, Sarimo J, Mattila K, et al. Proximal hamstring tendinopathy: results of surgical management and histopathologic findings. Am J Sports Med 2009;37(4):727–34. PubMed PMID: 19218559.

123. White KE. High hamstring tendinopathy in 3 female long distance runners. J Chiropr Med 2011;10(2):93–9. PubMed PMID: 22014863. Pubmed Central PMCID: 3110412.

124. Del Buono A, Battery L, Denaro V, et al. Tendinopathy and inflammation: some truths. Int J Immunopathol Pharmacol 2011;24(1 Suppl. 2):45–50. PubMed PMID: 21669137.

125. Gaida JE, Ashe MC, Bass SL, et al. Is adiposity an under-recognized risk factor for tendinopathy? A systematic review. Arthritis Rheum 2009;61(6):840–9. PubMed PMID: 19479698.

126. Petersen J, Thorborg K, Nielsen MB, et al. Preventive effect of eccentric training on acute hamstring injuries in men's soccer: a cluster-randomized controlled trial. Am J Sports Med 2011;39(11):2296–303. PubMed PMID: 21825112.

127. de Oliveira LP, Vieira CP, Da Re Guerra F, et al. Statins induce biochemical changes in the Achilles tendon after chronic treatment. Toxicology 2013;311(3):162–8. PubMed PMID: 23831763.

128. Wise BL, Peloquin C, Choi H, et al. Impact of age, sex, obesity, and steroid use on quinolone-associated tendon disorders. Am J Med 2012;125(12):1228.e23–8. PubMed PMID: 23026288. Pubmed Central PMCID: 3502655.

129. Magnusson SP, Langberg H, Kjaer M. The pathogenesis of tendinopathy: balancing the response to loading. Nat Rev Rheumatol 2010;6(5):262–8. PubMed PMID: 20308995.

130. Thornton GM, Shao X, Chung M, et al. Changes in mechanical loading lead to tendonspecific alterations in MMP and TIMP expression: influence of stress deprivation and intermittent cyclic hydrostatic compression on rat supraspinatus and Achilles tendons. Br J Sports Med 2010;44(10):698–703. PubMed PMID: 18801769.

131. Almekinders LC, Weinhold PS, Maffulli N. Compression etiology in tendinopathy. Clin Sports Med 2003;22(4):703–10. PubMed PMID: 14560542.

132. Cook JL, Purdam C. Is compressive load a factor in the development of tendinopathy? Br J Sports Med 2012;46(3):163–8. PubMed PMID: 22113234.

133. Vogel KG, Ordog A, Pogany G, et al. Proteoglycans in the compressed region of human tibialis posterior tendon and in ligaments. J Orthop Res 1993;11(1):68–77. PubMed PMID: 8423522.

134. Soslowsky LJ, Thomopoulos S, Esmail A, et al. Rotator cuff tendinosis in an animal model: role of extrinsic and overuse factors. Ann Biomed Eng 2002;30(8):1057–63. PubMed PMID: 12449766.

135. Cook JL, Purdam CR. The challenge of managing tendinopathy in competing athletes. Br J Sports Med 2014;48(7):506–9. PubMed PMID: 23666020.

136. Fearon AM, Scarvell JM, Neeman T, et al. Greater trochanteric pain syndrome: defining the clinical syndrome. Br J Sports Med 2013;47(10):649–53.

137. Bird PA, Oakley SP, Shnier R, et al. Prospective evaluation of magnetic resonance imaging and physical examination findings in patients with greater trochanteric pain syndrome. Arthritis Rheum 2001;44(9):2138–45.

138. Lequesne M, Mathieu P, Vuillemin-Bodaghi V, et al. Gluteal tendinopathy in refractory greater trochanter pain syndrome: diagnostic value of two clinical tests. Arthritis Rheum 2008;59(2):241–6.

139. Tortolani P, Carbone JJ, Quartararo LG. Greater trochanteric pain syndrome in patients referred to orthopedic spine specialists. Spine J 2002;2(4):251–4.

140. Williams BS, Cohen SP. Greater trochanteric pain syndrome: a review of anatomy, diagnosis and treatment. Anesthesia and analgesia. Anesth Analg 2009;108(5):1662–70.

141. Woodley SJ, Nicholson HD, Livingstone V, et al. Lateral hip pain: findings from magnetic resonance imaging and clinical examination. J Orthop Sports Phys Ther 2008;38(6):313–28.

142. Bowman KFJ, Cohen SB, Bradley JP. Operative management of partial-thickness tears of the proximal hamstring muscles in athletes. Am J Sports Med 2013;41(6):1363–71.

143. Reiman MP, Goode AP, Hegedus EJ, et al. Diagnostic accuracy of clinical tests of the hip: a systematic review with meta-analysis. Br J Sports Med 2013;47(14):893–902. PubMed PMID: 22773321.

144. Reiman MP, Loudon JK, Goode AP. Diagnostic accuracy of clinical tests for assessment of hamstring injury: a systematic review. J Orthop Sports Phys Ther 2013;43(4):223–31. PubMed PMID: 23321899.

145. Cacchio A, Borra F, Severini G, et al. Reliability and validity of three pain provocation tests used for the diagnosis of chronic proximal hamstring tendinopathy. Br J Sports Med 2012;46(12):883–7. PubMed PMID: 22219215.

146. Blankenbaker DG, Ullrick SR, Davis KW, et al. Correlation of MRI findings with clinical findings of trochanteric pain syndrome. Skeletal Radiol 2008;37(10):903–9. PubMed PMID: 18566811.

147. Connell DA, Bass C, Sykes CA, et al. Sonographic evaluation of gluteus medius and minimus tendinopathy. Eur Radiol 2003;13(6):1339–47. PubMed PMID: 12764651.

148. De Smet AA, Blankenbaker DG, Alsheik NH, et al. MRI appearance of the proximal hamstring tendons in patients with and without symptomatic proximal hamstring tendinopathy. AJR Am J Roentgenol 2012;198(2):418–22. PubMed PMID: 22268187.

149. Petchprapa CN, Bencardino JT. Tendon injuries of the hip. Magn Reson Imaging Clin N Am 2013;21(1):75–96. PubMed PMID: 23168184.

150. Jensen MC, Brant-Zawadzki MN, Obuchowski N, et al. Magnetic resonance imaging of the lumbar spine in people without back pain. N Engl J Med 1994;331(2):69–73. PubMed PMID: 8208267.

151. Grimaldi A. Assessing lateral stability of the hip and pelvis. Man Ther 2011;16(1):26–32. PubMed PMID: 20888285.

152. Birnbaum K, Siebert CH, Pandorf T, et al. Anatomical and biomechanical investigations of the iliotibial tract. Surg Radiol Anat 2004;26(6):433–46. PubMed PMID: 15378277.

153. Grimaldi A. Lateral Hip Pain with Dr Alison Grimaldi. Physioedge Podcasts 2012.

154. Grimaldi A, Mellor R, Bennell K, et al. Gluteal tendinopathy: a proposed pathoaetiological mechanism-based management approach. Submitted. 2014.

155. Kosek E, Ekholm J. Modulation of pressure pain thresholds during and following isometric contraction. Pain 1995;61(3):481–6. PubMed PMID: 7478692.

156. Kosek E, Lundberg L. Segmental and plurisegmental modulation of pressure pain thresholds during static muscle contractions in healthy individuals. Eur J Pain 2003;7(3):251–8. PubMed PMID: 12725848.

157. Rompe JD, Segal NA, Cacchio A, et al. Home training, local corticosteroid injection, or radial shock wave therapy for greater trochanter pain syndrome. Am J Sports Med 2009;37(10):1981–90. PubMed PMID: 19439758.

158. Coombes BK, Bisset L, Vicenzino B. Efficacy and safety of corticosteroid injections and other injections for management of tendinopathy: a systematic review of randomised controlled trials. Lancet 2010;376(9754):1751–67. PubMed PMID: 20970844.

159. Scott A, Khan KM. Corticosteroids: short-term gain for long-term pain? Lancet 2010;376(9754):1714–15. PubMed PMID: 20970846.

160. Labrosse JM, Cardinal E, Leduc BE, et al. Effectiveness of ultrasound-guided corticosteroid injection for the treatment of gluteus medius tendinopathy. AJR Am J Roentgenol 2010;194(1):202–6. PubMed PMID: 20028924.

161. Brinks A, van Rijn RM, Willemsen SP, et al. Corticosteroid injections for greater trochanteric pain syndrome: a randomized controlled trial in primary care. Ann Fam Med 2011;9(3):226–34. PubMed PMID: 21555750. Pubmed Central PMCID: 3090431.

162. Cohen SP, Strassels SA, Foster L, et al. Comparison of fluoroscopically guided and blind corticosteroid injections for greater trochanteric pain syndrome: multicentre randomised controlled trial. BMJ 2009;338:b1088. PubMed PMID: 19366755. Pubmed Central PMCID: 2669115.

163. Zissen MH, Wallace G, Stevens KJ, et al. High hamstring tendinopathy: MRI and ultrasound imaging and therapeutic efficacy of percutaneous corticosteroid injection. AJR Am J Roentgenol 2010;195(4):993–8. PubMed PMID: 20858830.

164. Marx RE. Platelet-rich plasma (PRP): what is PRP and what is not PRP? Implant Dent 2001;10(4):225–8. PubMed PMID: 11813662.

165. de Vos RJ, van Veldhoven PL, Moen MH, et al. Autologous growth factor injections in chronic tendinopathy: a systematic review. Br Med Bull 2010;95:63–77. PubMed PMID: 20197290.

CHAPTER 48

THE KNEE: INTRODUCTION

CHAPTER OUTLINE

CHAPTER 48.1 ■ ACUTE KNEE INJURIES

Lee Herrington

INTRODUCTION

If external or internal forces directed at the knee are of sufficient magnitude and duration, they will result in structural disruption of one or more of the anatomical structures in and around the joint. Tissue failure will result if stress is applied too quickly, exceeds the tissue's tolerance limits or if it is applied repetitively without sufficient time for recovery. This type of failure has been termed dynamic overload. Dynamic overload of the tissue may be a result of an acceleration or deceleration injury. An acceleration injury occurs when the body or body parts are stationary or moving slower than the applied force. The injury producing force accelerates the body or body part beyond the tissue's ability to withstand or resist that force, such as when a footballer is being tackled and the force of contact by the opposing player's foot against the lateral aspect of the leg exceeds the ability of the medial collateral ligament to resist the force, potentially resulting in damage. In the case of deceleration injury, the body or body parts are rapidly decelerated. Examples include landing from a jump or attempting to stop and quickly change direction (cutting). If the body is not able to oppose these forces the resulting movement would apply a substantial valgus force on the knee, which is the classic mechanism for anterior cruciate ligament injury.

Acceleration injuries are typically related to contact injuries, whereas deceleration injuries usually involve no contact with external loads or forces (i.e. other players) as the forces are generated internally. While prevention of contact injuries may be difficult, if not impossible, it would appear that if dynamic overload of the tissues could be prevented during the deceleration phase, then the risk of injury is reduced and potentially removed. In order to achieve this, the loads involved in sporting and functional activities need to be understood. Appreciation of the loads involved in dynamic overload is important in preventing deceleration injuries, because when rehabilitating an individual post injury (or surgical repair of that injury), the goal is to restore pain-free function and prevent the injury reoccurring. This is essentially the same as attempting to prevent the injury happening in the first instance, and the person involved requires rehabilitation in a manner that has the end goal of developing the intrinsic ability (strength and neuromuscular control) to match the loads involved, thereby preventing tissue stress and injury from occurring.

COMMON ACUTE KNEE INJURIES

Injury to the anterior cruciate ligament (ACL) would appear to be by far the most debilitating acute knee injury, followed by injury to the menisci, collateral ligaments then posterior cruciate ligament. Definitive statistics are unavailable. However, acute knee injury may account for 14–40% of all acute musculoskeletal injuries.[1,2] Meniscal injury may be responsible for 9% of all acute musculoskeletal trauma, with collateral ligaments 7% and anterior cruciate ligament 4%.[3] Meniscal injuries have been reported to occur at a rate of 0.3–0.6 per 1000 (training) hours,[4] rising to 3–13 per 1000 (training) hours in a military population.[5] ACL injury rates are around 0.1–0.4 per 1000 (training) hours;[4] however, injury rate may be as high as 1 in 20 females who play soccer and basketball at a competitive level.[6]

NATURE OF LOADS

Non-contact deceleration injuries typically involve a failure to control multidirectional forces. One of the most common movement patterns associated with knee injury is that of dynamic valgus collapse (Fig. 48-1), which has been associated with injury to the ACL, medial collateral ligament, medial and lateral meniscus and articular joint surfaces.[7] Dynamic valgus collapse involves the sudden deceleration of the knee, with the limb if uncontrolled, moving into a position of hip adduction and internal rotation, knee abduction and tibial external rotation and with the knee often slightly flexed during either landing or cutting. All of these factors contribute to generating substantial knee external abduction and flexor moments, along with a rapid increase in vertical ground reaction force (compressive loading to the joint).

Increased knee abduction and flexor moments have been associated with ACL injury[6] and patellofemoral joint pain.[8] Elevated vertical ground reaction forces (VGRF) have been associated with joint irritation and degeneration,[7] increased meniscal loading and damage,[9] increased tibiofemoral joint anterior shear loads[10] and raised patellofemoral joint reaction force.[11] Typical VGRF values associated with common tasks would be 1.5–2.5 times body weight when running, 2.5–3 times body weight (when landing from a forward hop) and rapidly changing direction (cutting) and 1.5–3 times body weight landing from a 30 cm box. Knee abduction moments typically range from 0.6 Newton metre per kilogram body weight (Nm/kg) during running, to 0.4–0.9 Nm/kg during cutting (depending on angle) and

0.5–1 Nm/kg during single leg landing from a 30–40 cm box. These forces increase considerably once the scenario is 'more real', for example dribbling a basketball or holding a lacrosse stick and cutting increases the load by greater than 0.3 Nm/kg.[12,13] The levels of loads described here are substantial for those working towards full rehabilitation of the knee following injury and preventing injury (or re-injury) as they represent the minimum level of force the body is required to generate to control these potentially deleterious forces. The ability to absorb these forces during dynamic tasks may alter the internal or external forces acting on the joint and potentially decrease the loading placed on the passive joint structures.[10] The hip abductor external rotator muscle group has to be able to generate a minimum force equivalent to 60% of body weight for multiple repetitions in order to counter the forces pushing the knee into valgus (external knee abduction moment) during a variety of functional tasks, as described above. Likewise, to counter the VGRF, the combined closed chain lower limb extensor muscle strength must be equal to or greater than twice body weight, to match the typical loads applied to the body.

The key components in dealing with these forces in order to prevent injury or re-injury will be the development of sufficient strength to counteract the loads applied and appropriate neuromuscular control strategies to apply the strength in an appropriate manner.

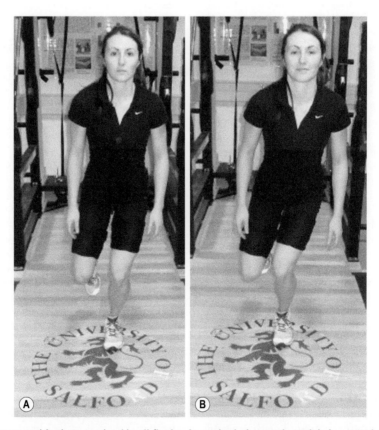

FIGURE 48-1 ■ (A) Good alignment, hip, knee and ankle all flexing in sagittal plane only, pelvis in neutral position, trunk aligned over pelvis. (B) Poor movement showing valgus collapse, involves foot pronation, knee abduction, hip adduction and internal rotation, tilting of the pelvis and leaning of the trunk.

STRENGTHENING

The immediate post-injury (or post-surgery) period is often characterized by significant reduction in function due to pain, joint effusion and decreased muscle activation. If these issues are not addressed they are likely to substantially impact on long-term functional performance.[6]

Muscle Inhibition

Quadriceps muscle weakness is a common consequence of knee injury. The decrement in quadriceps function has been termed arthrogenic muscle inhibition (AMI).[14] AMI is a neurological decline in muscle activation resulting from both pain and joint effusion.[15] AMI hinders rehabilitation by preventing strength gains in the quadriceps. AMI becomes problematic if it is not reversed and muscle function restored, as this can lead to decreased functional ability and biomechanical deficits,[16] re-injury and the development of osteoarthritis.[17] The management of AMI requires a multifacet approach involving the use of a number of treatment modalities, directed at sensory control and aimed at altering the motor drive, increasing the stimulus to the muscle.[17]

One approach to preventing AMI is to incorporate means to block or modify the sensory signals that are generating the inhibitory stimulus. Fundamentally this will involve reducing pain and knee effusion. The use of cryotherapy appears to be beneficial in reducing AMI developed in the presence of knee effusion,[18,19] as does transcutaneous electrical stimulation (TENS).[18] Both these modalities block sensory pain signalling. There appears to be little evidence other than anecdotal for the use of either compression or elevation to control effusion, though they may be considered.[16] To improve motor stimulus, muscle stimulation appears beneficial in reducing AMI[20] either when used in conjunction with an exercise programme[21,22] or to provide a superimposed twitch (involuntary muscle contraction) alongside a volitional isometric quadriceps contraction.[23] High-load resistance training may also prove useful.[24] Electromyographic biofeedback may be beneficial in overcoming AMI, although this is supported by a single case study.[25]

Strength, Power and Work Capacity Development

Once normal activation patterns for quadriceps have been established, progressive strengthening is then required. Quadriceps strength deficits following ACL reconstruction have been related to restricted knee motion during gait[26] and poorer self-reported function.[27] This quadriceps weakness is associated with decreased knee flexion on landing[26,28] with consequential increase in joint loading[29] and the potential for secondary joint injury. When considering the mode of training, Risberg et al.[30] reported that closed chain activities (e.g. squatting and step ups) in isolation were associated with a 20% deficit in quadriceps strength compared with training involving a combination of open (knee extension) and closed kinetic chain exercises. This indicates the need to incorporate both joint isolation (open kinetic chain)

exercises and closed chain exercises to optimize strength recovery. Alongside sufficient strength, the ability to generate force rapidly (power) will substantially impact on functional performance, especially the performance of sport-specific speed- and agility-based tasks.[31] Both Angelozzi et al.[32] and Myer et al.[33] reported significant deficits in the rate of force development in patients post ACL reconstruction surgery despite successfully returning to sport, this may predispose the athlete to increased risk of secondary injury.[34,35]

Decreased gluteal muscle activity has been associated with increased knee valgus angles and abduction moments during a variety of functional tasks,[9] with improvements in hip abduction-lateral rotation strength and activation leading to superior neuromuscular control and alignment of the lower limb.[8,36] Hollman et al.[37] reported that strength and recruitment of gluteal muscles were significant factors in maintaining limb alignment upon landing. Consequently, training should target both isolated strength and coordinated activation within patterns of movement. Homan et al.[38] demonstrated that individuals with poor gluteal strength used a greater proportion of their maximal isometric voluntary contraction during landing tasks, so work capacity (endurance) will also be a factor to consider when training these individuals. The single-leg squat was the best exercise for recruitment of the gluteus medius and maximus activation in combination, so might provide the most appropriate intervention[39] (Fig. 48-2).

DEVELOPMENT OF NEUROMUSCULAR CONTROL

When landing or cutting the impact with the ground creates forces and moments of force that not only accelerate flexion of the hip, knee and ankle dorsiflexion, but in resolving the forces involved, create multdirectional loads on the knee joint. It has been proposed[10] that the greater the energy absorption by muscle during these tasks, the greater the potential decrease in the amount of energy transferred to the capsule-ligamentous and articular tissues of the knee. In order to undertake this role successfully, the muscular system must not only acquire sufficient strength to match the forces involved, but also must be suitably trained to coordinate the application of this muscular force. This coordination involves appropriate timing of muscle force, as well as the appropriate degree and direction of force. Essentially, the sole aim of neuromuscular training is to educate the neuromuscular system to react in an appropriate and timely manner to reduce the loads on the passive joint structures of the knee.

Neuromuscular rehabilitation requires the regaining of symmetrical motion and appropriate movement strategies in order to limit deleterious loads and motion, to reduce risk of re-injury and improve function.[14] Simple verbal and visual feedback given in isolation can positively influence both landing and running biomechanics. Feedback is a fundamental tool to enhance learning and performance of motor skills and may be the quickest and simplest form of training available. Feedback has

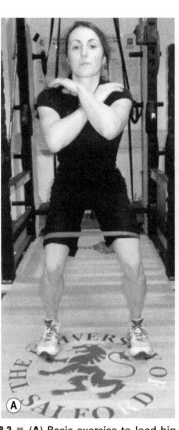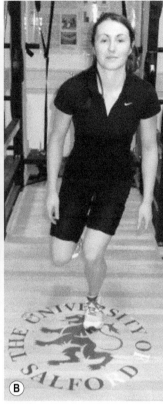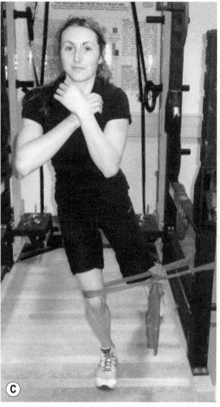

FIGURE 48-2 ■ **(A)** Basic exercise to load hip abductor and external rotators during squatting task, they squat pushing out against band. **(B)** Progression onto single-leg squat which increased load on hip abductor external rotator muscles. **(C)** Progression of load onto hip abductor external rotator muscles, then squat while pushing out against band.

been shown to be a vital part of motor skill learning associated with optimizing lower limb movements, decreasing VGRF, knee valgus angles and moments.[40,41] Neuromuscular training therefore needs to incorporate appropriate verbal and visual feedback to optimize (re-) learning the skill.

Neuromuscular rehabilitation often relies on closed skill activities carried out in a set order,[42] which typically involves repeated practices of the closed skill (identical movement tasks in stable predictable environments most often carried out at a pace defined by the participant). To more appropriately reflect the motor skill requirements of sports and dynamic functional movements in everyday life, the programmes require progressively increasing the complexity where more open skill (non-planned skills/ tasks) elements become incorporated in a more random fashion, once the closed skill tasks have been mastered.[43] This involves activities that are initially controlled and self-paced, allowing the participant to understand and master the specifics of the appropriate movement patterns in environments that are predictable and static and allow the individual to plan their movements in advance (closed skill practice).[44] The activities then progress to incorporate more random elements, where the environment is unpredictable and changing and the participant needs to adapt their movements in response (open skill practice).[44]

A progressive structured neuromuscular training programme that develops the participant's movement and landing skills through progressively more challenging tasks is depicted in Figures 48-3 and 48-4. The programme evolves progressively through an initial phase involving discrete closed movements in a block practice format, an intermediate phase, which incorporates a combination of some closed and some controlled open skill elements, and finally, practice elements that involve open movements in a random practice format.[44]

Limb loading is performed using a closed kinetic chain. Initially, activities are introduced to improve movement skills and control during limb loading tasks prior to undertaking load acceptance (landing) tasks.[32] This is followed by introducing loads and reducing stability, as demonstrated in a single-leg squat (Fig. 48-2). A qualitative assessment scoring system during both unilateral limb load and load acceptance activities has been described and discussed elsewhere.[32,45] Structured verbal plus video input significantly reduces both VRGF and knee valgus angles on landing[34] and should be incorporated in the rehabilitation programme.

Progression within the closed skill training element and the open skill element are described within Figures 48-3 and 48-4, respectively. Jump landing training significantly reduces knee abduction moments and angles and VGRF[46] improve performance[47] and reduce the risk of ACL injury.[6]

CONCLUSION

Rehabilitation of a deceleration dynamic overload injury to the knee requires an appreciation of the nature of the

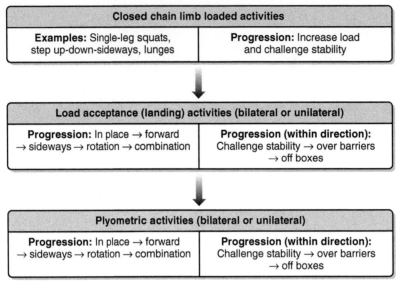

Key: → = indication of progression from one to the next

FIGURE 48-3 ■ Progression of unilateral loading and load acceptance tasks during closed skill practice.

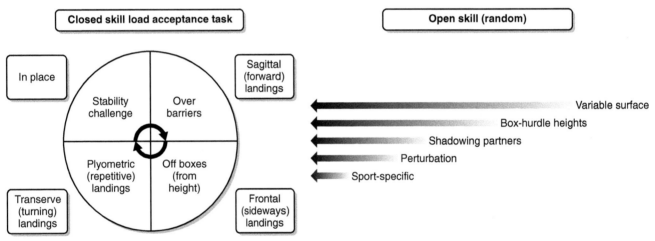

FIGURE 48-4 ■ Progression of unilateral load acceptance tasks during open skill practice.

forces involved in both the injury itself and during the tasks set that are specific to the injured individual and the overall demands of the sport. Once understood, controlling these forces becomes the paramount goal of rehabilitation to prevent further overload of the tissues. Control of these forces initially requires sufficient strength within the muscular system and then, appropriate neuromuscular control strategies to coordinate the application of the muscular force at the appropriate time and with the appropriate degree and direction of force. In order to attain the first goal, appropriate progressive resistance training principles must be applied to regain the proper levels of strength and force development. To successfully achieve the second rehabilitation goal, a motor skill learning programme needs be undertaken where the patient is able to apply appropriate movement strategies, to minimize injury risk, in an open randomly changing environment.

REFERENCES

1. Button K, Iqbal A, Letchford R, et al. Clinical effectiveness of knee rehabilitation techniques and implications for a self-care model. Physiotherapy 2012;98:288–300.
2. Van Middelkoop M, van Linschoten C, Berger M, et al. Knee complaints seen in general practice: active sport participants versus non-sport participants. BMC Musculoskelet Disord 2008;19: 9–36.
3. Schappert S, Burt C. Ambulatory care visits to physician offices, hospital outpatient departments and emergency departments: United states, 2001–2002. Vital Health Stat 2006;13: 1–66.
4. Wasserstein D, Khoshbin A, Dwyer T, et al. Risk factors for recurrent anterior cruciate ligament reconstruction: a population study in Ontario, Canada. Am J Sports Med 2013;41:2099–107.
5. Jones J, Burks R, Owens B, et al. Incidence and risk factors associated with meniscal injuries among active service US military service members. J Athl Train 2012;47:67–73.
6. Hewett T, Di Stasi S, Myer G. Current concepts for injury prevention in athletes after anterior cruciate ligament reconstruction. Am J Sports Med 2013;41:216–24.

7. Logerstedt D, Snyder-Mackler L, Ritter R, et al. Knee pain and mobility impairments: meniscal and articular cartilage lesions. J Orthop Sports Phys Ther 2010;40:A1–35.

8. Khayambashi K, Mohammadkhani Z, Ghaznavi K, et al. The effects of isolated hip abductor and external rotator muscle strengthening on pain, health status, and hip strength in females with patellofemoral pain: a randomized controlled trial. J Orthop Sports Phys Ther 2012;42:22–9.

9. Zazulak B, Hewett T, Reeves N, et al. Deficits in neuromuscular control of the trunk predict knee injury risk: a prospective biomechanical-epidemiological study. Am J Sports Med 2007;35:1123–30.

10. Norcross M, Blackburn T, Goerger B, et al. The association between lower extremity energy absorption and biomechanical factors related to anterior cruciate ligament injury. Clin Biomech 2010;25:1031–6.

11. Grabiner M, Feuerbach J, Lundin T, et al. Visual guidance to force plates does not influence ground reaction variability. J Biomech 1999;28:1115–17.

12. Chaudhari A, Andriacchi T. The mechanical consequences of dynamic frontal plane limb alignment for non-contact ACL injury. J Biomech 2006;39:330–8.

13. Fedie R, Caristedt K, Willson J, et al. Effect of attending to a ball during a side cut maneuver on lower extremity biomechanics in male and female athletes. Sports Biomech 2010;9:165–77.

14. Hurley M. The effects of joint damage on muscle function, proprioception and rehabilitation. Man Ther 1997;2:11–17.

15. Palmieri-Smith R, Villwock M, Downie B, et al. Pain and effusion and quadriceps activation and strength. J Athl Train 2013;48:186–91.

16. Palmieri-Smith R, Thomas A, Woitys E. Maximising quadriceps strength after ACL reconstruction. Clin Sports Med 2009;27:405–24.

17. Hart J, Ingersoll C. Quadriceps EMG frequency content following isometric lumbar extension. J Electromyogr Kinesiol 2010;20:840–4.

18. Hopkins J, Ingersoll C, Edwards J, et al. Cryotherapy and transcutaneous electric neuromuscular stimulation decrease arthrogenic muscle inhibition of vastus medialis after knee joint effusion. J Athl Train 2002;37:25–31.

19. Rice D, McNair P, Dalbeth N. Effects of cryotherapy on arthrogenic muscle inhibition using an experimental model of knee swelling. Arthritis Rheum 2009;61:78–83.

20. Jubeau M, Gondin J, Martin A, et al. Differences in twitch potentiation between voluntary and stimulated quadriceps contractions of equal intensity Scand. Sand J Med Sci Sports 2009;30:1–7.

21. Fitzgerald G, Piva S, Irrgang J. A modified neuromuscular electrical stimulation protocol for quadriceps strength training following anterior cruciate ligament reconstruction. J Orthop Sports Phys Ther 2003;33:492–501.

22. Hasegawa S, Kobayashi M, Arai T, et al. Effect of early implementation of electrical muscle stimulation to prevent muscle atrophy and weakness in patients after anterior cruciate ligament reconstruction. J Electromyogr Kinesiol 2011;21:622–30.

23. Ediz L, Ceylan M, Turktas U, et al. A randomised controlled trial of electrostimulation effects on effusion, swelling and pain recovery after anterior cruciate reconstruction: a pilot study. Clin Rehabil 2011;26:413–22.

24. Aagaard P, Simonsen E, Andersen J, et al. Neural inhibition during maximal eccentric and concentric quadriceps contractions: effect of resistance. J Appl Physiol 2000;89:2249–57.

25. Maitland M, Ajemain S, Suter E. Quadriceps femoris and hamstring muscle function in a person with an unstable knee. Phys Ther 1999;79:66–75.

26. Lewek M, Rudolph K, Axe M, et al. The effect of insufficient quadriceps strength on gait after anterior cruciate ligament reconstruction. Clin Biomech 2002;17:56–63.

27. Schmitt L, Paterno M, Hewett T. The impact of quadriceps femoris strength asymmetry on functional performance at return to sport following anterior cruciate ligament reconstruction. J Orthop Sports Phys Ther 2012;42:750–9.

28. Morrissey M, Hooper D, Drechsler W, et al. Relationship of leg muscle strength and knee function in the early period after anterior cruciate ligament reconstruction. Scand J Med Sci Sports 2004;14:360–6.

29. Becker R, Berth A, Nehring M, et al. Neuromuscular quadriceps dysfunction prior to osteoarthritis of the knee. J Orthop Res 2004;22:768–73.

30. Risberg M, Holm I, Myklebust G, et al. Neuromuscular training versus strength training during the first 6 months after anterior cruciate ligament reconstruction: a randomised clinical trial. Phys Ther 2007;87:1–14.

31. Herrington L, Myer G, Horsley I. Task based rehabilitation protocol for elite athletes following anterior cruciate ligament reconstruction: a clinical commentary. Phys Ther Sport 2013;14:188–98.

32. Angelozzi M, Madaama M, Corsica C, et al. Rate of force development as an adjunctive outcome measure for return to sport decisions after anterior cruciate ligament reconstruction. J Orthop Sports Phys Ther 2012;42:772–80.

33. Myer G, Martin L, Ford K, et al. No association from time from surgery with functional deficits in athletes after anterior cruciate ligament reconstruction. Am J Sports Med 2012;40:2256–63.

34. Di Stasi S, Myer G, Hewett T. Neuromuscular training to target deficits associated with second anterior cruciate ligament injury. J Orthop Sports Phys Ther 2013;43:777–92.

35. Comfort P, Allen M, Graham-Smith P. Comparison of peak ground reaction force and rate of force development during variations of the power clean. J Strength Cond Res 2011;25:1235–9.

36. Philippon M, Decker M, Giphart J, et al. Rehabilitation exercise progression for the gluteus medius muscle with consideration for iliopsoas tendinitis: an in-vivo electromyography study. Am J Sports Med 2011;39:1777–85.

37. Hollman J, Hohl J, Kraft J, et al. Modulation of frontal plane kinematics by hip extensor strength and gluteus maximus recruitment during a jump landing task in healthy women. J Sport Rehabil 2013;22:184–90.

38. Homan K, Norcross M, Goerger B, et al. The influence of gluteal activity and lower extremity kinematics. J Electromyogr Kinesiol 2013;23:411–15.

39. Distefano L, Clark M, Padua D. Evidence supporting balance training in healthy individuals: a systematic review. J Strength Cond Res 2009;23:18–31.

40. Cowling E, Steele J, McNair P. Effect of verbal instructions on muscle activity and risk of injury to the anterior cruciate ligament during landing. Br J Sports Med 2003;37:126–30.

41. Milner C, Fairbrother J, Srivatsan A, et al. Simple verbal instruction improves knee biomechanics during landing in female athletes. Knee 2012;19:399–403.

42. McCormick B. Task complexity and jump landings in injury prevention for basketball players. J Strength Cond Res 2012;34:89–92.

43. Verstegen M, Falsone S, Orr R, et al. Suggestions from the field for return to sports participation following anterior cruciate ligament reconstruction: American football. J Orthop Sports Phys Ther 2012;42:337–44.

44. Herrington L, Comfort P. Training for prevention ACL injury: incorporation of progressive landing skill challenges into a program. J Strength Cond Res 2013;35:59–65.

45. Whatman C, Hing W, Hulme P. Physiotherapist agreement when visually rating movement quality during lower extremity functional screening tests. Phys Ther Sport 2012;13:87–96.

46. Munro A, Herrington L. The effect of videotape augmented feedback on drop jump landing strategy: implications for anterior cruciate ligament and patellofemoral joint injury prevention. Knee 2014;21(5):891–5.

47. Herrington L. The effects of 4 weeks of jump training on landing knee valgus and crossover hop performance in female basketball players. J Strength Cond Res 2010;24:3427–32.

CHAPTER 48.2 ■ PATELLOFEMORAL PAIN

Kay Crossley • Sallie Cowan • Bill Vicenzino

ARTICULAR AND MUSCLE CONTROL OF THE PATELLOFEMORAL JOINT

Anatomy and Motor Control of the Patellofemoral Joint and Adjacent Structures

The patellofemoral joint (PFJ) is the articulation between the patella and the femoral trochlea. The patella is a sesamoid bone located within the patellar ligament, with five facets that articulate with the femur. The geometry of these facets varies between individuals and may affect patellar tracking.[1–3] In healthy individuals, aspects of the femoral trochlea including its depth, as well as the shape and height of the lateral trochlea, can affect patellar tracking.[4–8] From 20–30° of knee flexion, the patella is confined within the trochlea and hence, the bony joint components provide inherent stability. However, outside of this range there is little intrinsic bony support for the patella and stability must be provided by other soft tissue structures, both passively and actively.

Lateral passive support is provided by the fibrous superficial and deep lateral retinacula. Fibrous expansions from vastus lateralis[9] and the iliotibial band (ITB) contribute to these retinacula, with additional lateral support provided by two distal components of the ITB.[10,11] Since most of the lateral retinaculum arises from the ITB, excessive lateral tracking may occur if the ITB is tight. Medially, the retinaculum is thinner and is thought to be less significant in influencing patellar tracking. Three ligaments described as joint capsule thickenings, the patellofemoral, patellomeniscal and patellotibial ligaments, lie beneath the retinaculum.[7] Of these, the medial patellofemoral ligament is the primary restraint to lateral patellar translation, with the others thought to be less important.[12–14]

Thus, the PFJ is inherently unstable and relies heavily on active stabilization via the muscular system. The most important muscular support is provided by the quadriceps, in particular vastus medialis and lateralis (VL). The vastus medialis is generally divided into two components – the vastus medialis obliquus (VMO) and the vastus medialis longus. While there is some conjecture as to whether these are separate entities, most authors agree that the two components have differing functions due to their fibre orientation, attachments and thus angle of force on the patella.[15–20] The oblique alignment of VMO provides a mechanical advantage for stabilizing the patella, which counterbalances the larger cross-sectional area and thus force-producing capacity of VL. Indeed, studies indicate that while VMO is unable to extend the knee on its own, it is active throughout knee extension aiding in centralizing the patella within the trochlea and enhancing the efficiency of VL.[16,21,22] In addition, a recent in vivo study demonstrated that improving VMO function also reduces the load imposed on the lateral cartilage of the patellofemoral joint.[23] Electromyographic studies

support this synergistic relationship between the vasti, with studies demonstrating a relatively balanced relationship in terms of magnitude and timing of activation during a wide variety of tasks.[8,24–36]

Anatomy of Remote Structures and Impact on the Patellofemoral Joint

There are a number of other factors that may impact on the PFJ – these include structures both proximal and distal to the joint. Proximally, these factors include femoral internal rotation,[37–40] altered hip motor control,[41,42] increased apparent knee valgus[38,43,44] and inadequate flexibility of hamstrings, ITB and tensor fascia latae.[40,45] Distally, factors include increased tibial rotation, pronated foot type[39] and inadequate flexibility of gastrocnemius.[40]

PATELLOFEMORAL PAIN

Background

Patellofemoral pain (PFP) is the term for PFJ disorders that is preferred over synonyms such as anterior knee pain, patellofemoral pain syndrome and chondromalacia patellae.[46] The prevalence of PFP is high in active populations[39,45,47–51] and PFP frequently accounts for presentations to general medical[52,53] and sports medicine[49,54] practitioners. PFP generally refers to pain in the anterior aspect of the knee (sometimes retro-patellar and occasionally referring symptoms to the posterior aspects of the knee). It is often referred to as a 'diagnosis of exclusion', i.e. made when other potential sources of pain (e.g. meniscal, patellar tendon) are ruled out. Nociception from any or all of the PFJ structures such as synovium, subchondral bone[55,56] or the infrapatellar fat pad[57–59] may result in the individual experiencing pain.

Patellofemoral pain is mostly associated with activities that load the PFJ, such as stair ambulation, squatting, rising from sitting and running. Both extrinsic and intrinsic factors can modulate PFJ load. Extrinsic factors are those that affect the external forces exerted on the body during weight-bearing activities (e.g. body mass, speed of gait, surfaces, footwear, frequency of loading). Factors related to the individual (intrinsic factors) can also influence PFJ alignment and hence, the distribution of the PFJ loads (e.g. the geometry of the femoral trochlea, increased foot pronation, increased femoral and tibial rotation and increased tightness of the ITB, as described above).

Evidence for Impairments in Local Motor Control in Patellofemoral Pain

In people with PFP it is proposed that the normal balanced activation of VMO and VL is disrupted.

Inadequate motor control of VMO may result in a lateral shift of the patellar[60] or an increase in lateral patellofemoral pressure.[61] Indeed, individuals with PFP produce less quadriceps torque than those without pain,[62,63] but there is controversy in the literature regarding an imbalance in the magnitude of vasti activation in PFP.[31-33,64-70] Disrupted vasti motor control may also take the form of delayed activation of VMO relative to VL, and a number of studies have supported this line of thought and demonstrated a delay in both reflex onset time and electromyographic activation of VMO relative to VL.[31,70-76] However, there is also some conflict with a number of authors describing no differences in electromyographic onsets.[32,33,67,70,77,78] These inconsistencies may in part be accounted for by a wide variation in electromyographic methodology[79] and the inherent heterogeneity in the PFP population.

Evidence for Impairments in Remote Contributors to Patellofemoral Pain

Clinically, poor hip and pelvic muscle control are commonly addressed in the treatment of PFP, and evidence to support this association is increasing. Greater femoral internal rotation has been associated with PFP[80] and may contribute to its development.[39] There is also evidence for decreased hip abductor and rotator strength in PFP,[81-86] alteration in gluteus medius motor control,[87-89] decreased sagittal plane balance stability[90] and decreased trunk side flexion strength.[88] However, not all studies have described dysfunction in hip abductor and external rotator strength or motor control in individuals with PFP.[88,91] Distally, excessive subtalar joint pronation[92] has been linked with greater tibial segment[93] and hip joint internal rotation. In addition, restricted ankle dorsiflexion is associated with decreased knee flexion angles during squatting,[93] which may be a risk factor for PFP.[39] However, it appears that the evidence supporting distal impairments in people with PFP is less than for proximal.[80]

Assessment

A comprehensive assessment of the PFJ should include a thorough interview (history, symptom mapping and description), physical examination and appropriate use of investigations. No single test provides a definitive diagnosis of PFP and the findings from all aspects of assessment are considered.

Key Clinical Diagnostic Features of Patellofemoral Pain

Key diagnostic features and clinical tests are described in Table 48-1. Note that the diagnostic accuracy of the clinical tests for PFP are not well established and a comprehensive physical examination of other potential pain sources such as other knee structures, hip joint, lumbar spine and other surrounding soft tissues is also required. In addition, all patients presenting with anterior knee pain should be assessed for other conditions (e.g. osteochondritis dissecans, slipped capital femoral epiphysis,

Perthes or other hip conditions, tumours, stress fractures, apophysitis, tendinopathies).

The Role of Imaging

Imaging is rarely needed in the assessment of PFP. Radiographs and computerized tomography provide information on the morphology of the joint and presence of osteoarthritis, in addition to screening for serious pathology if suspected. Magnetic resonance imaging provides greater information on the soft tissue structures and some of the newer sequences (T2 relaxation times and T1ρ) hold promise to evaluate the early stages of cartilage damage.[94,95] Interpretation of imaging abnormalities must always be considered alongside clinical test results.

Treatment

Conservative treatments are the cornerstone of PFP management. Effective treatments usually integrate techniques that target the local PFJ factors, in addition to the more remote (distal and proximal) factors. There are many different approaches that can be used to address these factors, including exercise, manual therapy, taping, bracing and foot orthoses. In practice, many or all of these approaches are used, in isolation or in combination, depending on the patient's presentation, clinician's expertise and the preferences of both patient and clinician.

Exercise

Exercise forms a major part of PFP management and generally includes: (a) vasti retraining; (b) hip muscle retraining; (c) strengthening/endurance building for lower limb and trunk muscles; (d) coordination and balance training; and (e) retraining of functional activities (including sports- or work-related).

1. Vasti retraining is recommended to restore the motor control of the medial and lateral vasti. Retraining focuses on increasing the patient's ability to activate their VMO, ideally with little VL activity or lateral hamstring co-contraction. We can use the principals of motor retraining, applied within three phases: (a) formal motor skill training; (b) integration of skill into low-load tasks; and (c) progression to higher load tasks.

   Participants are taught to activate their VMO in different positions (e.g. sitting, lying, standing) or different degrees of knee flexion, hip abduction or knee rotation. Many patients need a variety of strategies to assist VMO activation, including imagery or visual cues, facilitation techniques (e.g. palpation, taping, dry needles/acupuncture, feedback [e.g. surface EMG, real-time ultrasound, tactile or visual]), or inhibitory techniques to reduce overactivity in the VL or lateral hamstrings (e.g. inhibitory taping, feedback).

   After mastering the ability to achieve and maintain a VMO contraction, the patient is progressed through tasks, based on their ability to maintain control and the absence of significant pain. The absence of significant pain can be measured with

---

TABLE 48-1   Key Clinical Diagnostic Features of Patellofemoral Pain

Clinical Diagnostic Features Specific to Patellofemoral Pain

Interview

Area of pain	Usually anterior, but might be medial, lateral or infrapatellar. Pain is frequently vague or not specific to a palpable structure
Aggravating factors	Activities that load the PFJ – such as stair climbing, prolonged sitting with knee flexion or rising from sitting, squatting, lunging, running (especially downhill)
Noises/other symptoms	May have clicks, clunks or crepitus May report giving way. Possibly due to subluxation or quadriceps muscle inhibition
Loading history	Often insidious, may occur after change in loading/activity or following acute knee injury

Physical Examination

Observation – standing	VMO wasting may be obvious, might observe alterations in motor control; generalized quadriceps wasting or weakness might be present Altered static alignment/postures may be evident (e.g. femoral internal rotation, knee valgus, foot pronated with lowered medial longitudinal arch)
Observation-functional tasks	Global deficits might be evident during simple tasks (e.g. walking), or only be evident in higher loaded tasks (e.g. running, hopping or single-leg squat). Frequent deficits include: • Loss of knee flexion control during weight acceptance phase • Poor control of trunk and pelvis • Poor control of femoral internal rotation (observed as apparent knee valgus) • Poor control of foot alignment (e.g. excessively pronated)
Functional loading tasks	Activities that load the PFJ (e.g. single-leg squat, hop or stairs) will aggravate pain PFJ taping often decreases pain
Palpation	Tenderness on medial or lateral facets of patella, might be tender in infrapatellar (including fat pad) region or may have no tenderness ITB lateral retinaculum might be tender/tight on palpation Might have effusion, usually small supra- or infrapatellar soft tissue swelling
Knee range of motion	Most commonly normal, occasionally restricted when severe
PFJ movement	Might be malaligned (e.g. laterally tilted and positioned) Movements are often restricted – could be in any direction but commonly on medial glide
Flexibility	May have loss of flexibility – hamstrings and quadriceps, but also ITB, iliopsoas and triceps surae
Strength	Specific loss of control might be evident (e.g. VMO/quadriceps, hip external rotators), but must assess for more global loss of strength (including trunk and hip musles, triceps surae)

ITB, Iliotibial band; *PFJ,* Patellofemoral joint; *VMO,* vastus medialis obliquus.

---

the pain monitoring system[96] (where pain is recorded on a 10-cm visual analogue scale) and pain levels of 0–2 are considered safe. Pain levels up to 5 momentarily during exercise or immediately following exercise are acceptable, but not extending to the following morning. Examples of low-load tasks include lunges, squats and step ups (Fig. 48-5A–D). For these tasks, further progressions can be made from minimal weight bearing (using hand rails or other supports) to full weight bearing (and eventually added loading) and through various knee flexion ranges (Fig. 48-5E–H).

2. Hip muscle retraining may be required to improve motor control of the hip abductors, external rotators and extensors. The principles are the same as for vasti retraining, and the two programmes are easily integrated, such that the gluteal muscles are activated in a coordinated manner with the VMO during tasks such as lunge, squat and step (Fig. 48-5C–H). The hip abductors and external rotators work to maintain a level pelvis and hence, simple instructions may be used during exercises including: 'keep the pelvis level/horizontal' (to control hip adduction) and 'keep the knee centre over the foot centre' (to control femoral internal rotation).

3. Lower limb muscle strengthening/endurance building is likely to be necessary for all patients. Adequate strength and endurance are needed, especially in the quadriceps, hip muscles, trunk muscles and triceps surae. Strengthening programmes may be commenced early (see above for maintaining control and monitoring pain) and progressed according to patient response and American College of Sports Medicine guidelines.[97] For many patients, a generalized strengthening programme alone can result in reduced pain and improved function. However, patients with poor vasti or gluteal coordination may be unable to progress through a strengthening programme without first addressing their motor control deficits.

4. Coordination and balance training is essential to restore lower limb function. This retraining is generally combined with other exercise prescription and will involve a variety of tasks.

5. Retraining of functional activities is usually the final stage of the exercise-based interventions. People with PFP may need to return to high loaded activities, which involve knee flexion during full weight bearing (e.g. stair descent, deep squats), or higher intensity activities such as running. In order to

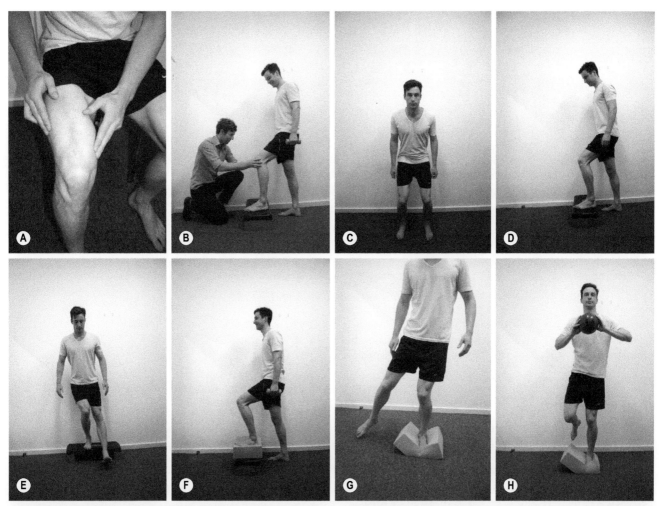

FIGURE 48-5 ■ Vasti retraining. Activation of vastus medialis obliquus in different positions, including low and higher loading activities. **(A)** Retraining focuses on increasing the patient's ability to activate their vastus medialis obliquus, ideally with little vastus lateralis activity or lateral hamstring co-contraction. **(B)** Progressing to low-load activity (e.g. partial weight-bearing lunge), maintaining feedback on activation, as well as position of knee and hip, relative to foot. **(C)** Double-leg squat. **(D)** Step up. **(E)** Single-leg step down. **(F)** Step up with additional loads. **(G)** Single-leg squat/balance. **(H)** Combine gluteal and vasti control with balance and proprioception.

progress to these high PFJ loaded activities, patients need additional training. They need to train their motor control, strength and endurance in the quadriceps and global muscles (e.g. triceps surae, hip and trunk muscles), balance and coordination in these higher loading tasks. The choice of exercise and decisions to progress are based on the patient's needs, their ability to maintain control and the absence of significant pain.

Taping

Patellar taping has been used to manage PFP since it was first described by Jenny McConnell in 1986.[98] While researchers and clinicians agree that patellar tape can effectively reduce a patient's pain, the mechanisms underpinning these taping effects still remain unclear. It is likely that positive benefits are imparted partly due to subtle changes in patellar position and PFJ contact area[99] and partly due to changes in motor control,[100] or cutaneous/proprioceptive input. Regardless of the mechanism, patellar tape provides temporary pain relief that can be used to improve compliance and performance with an exercise programme and enable pain-free activities of daily living (e.g. stairs), work or sports. The commonly used taping techniques (Fig. 48-6A) to reduce pain include: (a) medial glide; (b) medial tilt; (c) fat pad unloading; (d) superior tilt; or (e) rotation. Adverse skin reactions are frequently encountered and are best avoided with the use of adhesive gauze (e.g. Fixomull,™ Smith & Nephew), skin preparation (protective barrier or plastic skin) and advice not to remove the tape too quickly.

An alternative taping technique is to tape the tibia into a relative internal rotation on the femur (or relative external rotation of the femur on the tibia)[101] (Fig. 48-6B). This particular technique is based on the premise that internal rotation of the knee will reduce the Q-angle and lower stresses in the PFJ. As for the patellar taping techniques, test–re-test of a symptom provocative physical task (e.g. stair climbing, squatting) with and without the

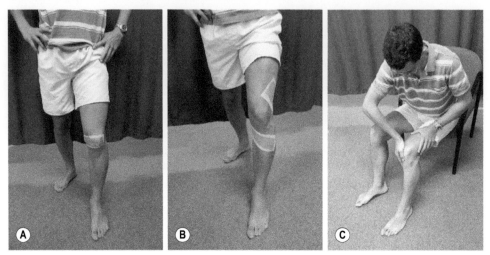

FIGURE 48-6 ■ Taping and manual therapy. **(A)** Patellofemoral taping: medial glide. **(B)** Mulligan tibiofemoral taping. Taping the tibia into relative internal rotation on the femur. **(C)** Self patellofemoral mobilizations. Tilting the medial border of the patella posteriorly (i.e. medial tilt).

tape in situ can be used by clinicians to evaluate the appropriateness of using this technique in any specific individual patient.

Manual Therapy

Manual therapy for PFP involves joint and soft tissue mobilization, manipulation and massage. Joint mobilizations might include manual gliding techniques of the patellofemoral or tibiofemoral joints, whereas soft tissue therapies could involve friction massage of tight lateral retinacula structures and deep tissue massage or myofascial release massage applied to the fascia/muscles of the thigh (predominantly anterolateral). The emphasis is on sustained loading of the soft tissues,[102] usually in a position that lengthens the treated soft tissues (e.g. for lateral retinacula structures: medial tilt of patella, tibiofemoral joint in approximately 30–90° flexion (Fig. 48-6C). Applied passively by either the patient or clinician, these techniques are designed to optimize movement and facilitate the exercise programme. Studies evaluating efficacy of such techniques applied in isolation show a lack of benefit,[103] which supports the common clinical practice that manual therapy is seldom or never done in isolation.

Foot Orthoses

In-shoe foot orthoses have been recommended as a treatment option for PFP. This is based on the premise that these devices reduce the amount of foot pronation and hence, tibial rotation.[104] In so doing, these devices reverse part of the abnormal biomechanics often associated with PFP. Their application in isolation is clinically not uncommon, but evidence indicates that their effect is optimized if delivered as part of a multimodal management care plan.[103]

There is preliminary, low-level evidence indicating that a favourable response to foot orthoses occurs in those with greater peak rear foot eversion[105] or greater

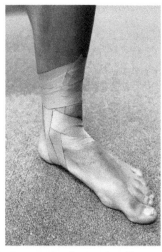

FIGURE 48-7 ■ Anti-pronation foot taping. Symptom modification test–re–test approach of assessing the potential benefit of foot orthoses, in this case using some reverse 6 anti-pronation tape.

difference in mid foot width between weight bearing and non-weight bearing.[106] Currently this evidence is difficult for the clinician to directly apply to an individual patient. To decide if a patient is likely to benefit from a foot orthosis, the clinician might consider using a test–re–test approach of observing a symptom-provocative physical task (e.g. stair climbing, jogging) without and with an anti-pronation foot taping technique (Fig. 48-7) or a temporary orthosis.[107] A substantial improvement in the patient's ability to perform the symptom-provocative task could indicate a potential benefit of foot orthoses. Preliminary evidence also suggests that immediate improvements with foot orthoses predict beneficial effects 12 weeks later.[108]

Effectiveness of Treatments

There is considerable evidence for the efficacy of different treatment approaches for PFP. Systematic reviews and meta-analyses provide level I evidence for the use of multimodal interventions (combination of retraining, strengthening, balance/coordination, functional retraining, taping and manual therapy)[103] and also for individual treatments in isolation.[100,103,109] Recent reviews conclude that tailored patellar taping immediately reduces pain with a large effect, while other techniques have only small (untailored medial patellar taping) or negligible (Kinesio Tape® Tex) effects on pain in the immediate term.[100] There is limited evidence for better short-term outcomes with foot orthoses versus flat inserts,[103,109] versus wait and see[110] and beneficial effects for exercise (versus control), closed chain exercises (versus open chain exercises) and acupuncture (versus control).[108] While there is no level I evidence for the use of hip strengthening for PFP, recent randomized controlled trials (level II evidence) support the use of hip-strengthening programmes to reduce pain and improve function.[111,112] However, there is moderate evidence for no additive effectiveness of knee braces to exercise therapy on pain and conflicting evidence on function.[113]

The evidence suggests that, in implementing evidence-based practice for the conservative management of PFP, clinicians can employ a multimodal treatment, or individual components (except bracing), based on patient preferences and presentations and clinician preferences and expertise.

EMERGING ISSUES AND NEW ADVANCES

Hip muscle dysfunction has long been identified as a feature of PFP[41,42] and there are an increasing number of studies evaluating the effects of hip-strengthening protocols for the treatment of PFP. However, due to the imprecise relationship between hip strength and biomechanics, and evidence that hip biomechanics are better predictors of PFP than hip strength,[114,115] one emerging area of research centres on the retraining of movement patterns. This emerging area of clinically relevant research consists of employing strategies that change lower limb biomechanics, such as using a variety of feedback methods from real-time gait analysis systems[116] to mirrors,[117] changing stride frequency[118] and running barefoot.[119] While such techniques show promise for patients with aberrant lower limb biomechanics, further research is required to test the efficacy of these programmes. Also, as advances are made in low-cost technologies (e.g. Nintendo Wii,® Microsoft Kinect,® ViMove by DorsaVi®) it may be possible to use such devices to provide real-time feedback to retrain movement in the clinic or home.

Another significant paradigm shift in the field of PFP, has been the awareness that the natural history of PFP is not one of spontaneous recovery in a proportion of those with PFP.[120,121] Most notably, there is increasing speculation that PFP may be a prelude to patellofemoral osteoarthritis.[120,122] While no current studies have prospectively studied people with PFP to verify this relationship, a case-control study[123] observed that individuals undergoing an arthroplasty for patellofemoral osteoarthritis were

more likely (odds ratio 2.31, 95% confidence interval 1.37–3.88) to report having had patellofemoral pain as an adolescent than those patients undergoing an arthroplasty for isolated tibiofemoral osteoarthritis. Clearly, more research is required to confirm the link between PFP and patellofemoral osteoarthritis, but recent reports using newer imaging sequences report adverse changes (T1ρ relaxation times) in the patellar cartilage of patients with patellofemoral pain that correlate strongly with the severity of patellar tilt.[94] Also, Farrokhi et al.[124] identified elevated patellofemoral stress in people with PFP as a potential mechanism underpinning a link between PFP and structural joint disease. Until studies identify whether PFP and patellofemoral osteoarthritis exist along a continuum of disease, clinicians who treat patients with persistent PFP should consider the possibility of early degenerative joint changes.

CONTROVERSIES, UNCERTAINTIES AND FUTURE DIRECTIONS

Patellofemoral chondral/cartilage lesions are problematic and fairly common among young adults with PFP. While a number of surgical treatment options are available, including microfracture, autologous or juvenile chondrocyte implantation, osteochondral autograft transfer and osteochondral allograft implantation, there is a paucity of evidence for their effectiveness. Additionally, non-surgical approaches are increasingly being used. These include injections of hyaluronic acid, platelet-rich plasma or other cytokines concentrated from autologous blood[125] and stem cells.

Basic science, pre-clinical and clinical studies suggest a promising role for platelet-rich plasma injections for cartilage injuries and joint pain. However, the specifics of platelet-rich plasma treatment, including the volume of plasma, number of injections and intervening interval, have not yet been optimized. Clinical acceptance of platelet-rich plasma therapies has occurred quickly, probably because of both the safety profile and the relative ease of preparation. However, there is no high-quality evidence that supports its extensive clinical use.[125] Similarly, the clinical evidence for other injection treatments is currently lacking.

There are many new directions in the management of PFP. Perhaps the most relevant area will be the move to develop interventions that are more targeted to the patient.

REFERENCES

1. Ahmed AM, Burke DL, Hyder A. Force analysis of the patellar mechanism. J Orthop Res 1987;5:69–85.
2. van Kampen A, Huiskes R. Three dimensional tracking pattern of the human patella. J Orthop Res 1990;8:372–82.
3. Heegaard J, Leyvraz PF, van Kampen A, et al. Contribution of joint geometry and soft tissue structures on patellar stability. Trans Orthop Res 1994;40:667.
4. Farahmand F, Tahmasbi MN, Amis AA. Lateral force-displacement behaviour of the human patella and its variation with knee flexion – a biomechanical study in vitro. J Biomech 1998;31: 1147–52.
5. Grelsamer RP, Klein JR. The biomechanics of the patellofemoral joint. J Orthop Sports Phys Ther 1998;28(5):286–97.

6. Senavongse W, Tantisatirapong T. Patellofemoral joint instability: a biomechanical study. Int J Appl Biomed Eng 2008;1(1): 61–4.

7. Fulkerson JP, Shea KP. Current concepts review: disorder of patellofemoral alignment. J Bone Joint Surg Am 1990;72A:1424–9.

8. Reynolds L, Levin T, Medeiros J, et al. EMG activity of vastus medialis obliquus and vastus lateralis and there role in patella alignment. Am J Phys Med 1983;62:61.

9. Reider B, Marshall JL, Koslin D, et al. The anterior aspect of the knee joint. J Bone Joint Surg Am 1981;63A:351–6.

10. Terry GC, Hughston JC, Norwood LA. The anatomy of the iliopatellar band and iliotibial tract. Am J Sports Med 1986;14:39–45.

11. Williams PL, Warwick R. Grays Anatomy. 36th ed. Edinburgh: Churchill Livingstone; 1980.

12. Conlan T, Garth WP, Lemons JE. Evaluation of the medial soft-tissue restraints of the extensor mechanism of the knee. J Bone Joint Surg Am 1993;75A:682–93.

13. Desio SM, Burks RT, Bachus KN. Soft tissue restraints to lateral patellar translation in the human knee. Am J Sports Med 1998;26(1):59–65.

14. Hautamaa PV, Fithian DC, Kaufman KR, et al. Medial soft tissue restraints in lateral patellar instability and repair. Clin Orthop Relat Res 1998;349:174–82.

15. Bose K, Kanagasuntherum R, Osman M. Vastus medialis oblique: an anatomical and physiological study. Orthopaedics 1980;3: 880–90.

16. Lieb FJ, Perry J. Quadriceps function. J Bone Joint Surg Am 1968;50-A:1535–48.

17. Raimondo RA, Ahmad CS, Blankevoort L, et al. Patellar stabilization – a quantitative evaluation of the vastus medialis obliquus muscle. Orthopedics 1998;21(7):791–5.

18. Scharf W, Weinstable R, Othrner E. Anatomical separation and clinical importance of two different parts of the vastus medialis muscle. Acta Anat 1985;123:108–11.

19. Thiranagama R. Nerve supply of the human vastus medialis muscle. J Anat 1990;170:193–8.

20. Amis AA, Senavongse W, Bull AM. Patellofemoral kinematics during knee flexion–extension: an in vitro study. J Orthop Res 2006;24:2201–11.

21. Bull AMJ, Senavongse WW, Taylor AR, et al., editors. The Effect of the Oblique Portions of the Vastus Medialis and Lateralis on Patellar Tracking. 11th Conference of the ESB; 1998; Toulouse, France.

22. Goh JCH, Lee PYC, Bose K. A cadaver study of the function of the oblique part of vastus medialis. J Bone Joint Surg Am 1995;2: 225–31.

23. Elias JJ, Kilambi S, Goerke DR, et al. Improving vastus medialis obliquus function reduces pressure applied to lateral patellofemoral cartilage. J Orthop Res 2009;27:578–83.

24. Spairani L, Barbero M, Cescon C, et al. An electromyographic study of the vastii muscles during open and closed kinetic chain submaximal isometric exercises. Int J Sports Phys Ther 2012; 7(6):617–26.

25. Duffell LD, Dharni H, Strutton PH, et al. Electromyographic activity of the quadriceps components during the final degrees of knee extension. J Back Musculoskeletal Rehabil 2011;24(4): 215–23.

26. Brownstein BA, Lamb RL, Mangine RE. Quadriceps torque and integrated eletromyography. J Orthop Sports Phys Ther 1985;6:309–14.

27. Gryzlo SM, Patek RM, Pink M, et al. Electromyographic analysis of knee rehabilitation exercises. J Orthop Sports Phys Ther 1994;20:36–43.

28. Isear JA, Erickson JC, Worrell TW. EMG analysis of lower extremity muscle recruitment patterns during an unloaded squat. Med Sci Sports Exerc 1997;29(4):532–9.

29. Karst GM, Willett GM. Reflex response times of vastus medialis oblique and vastus lateralis in normal subjects and in subjects with patellofemoral pain – letter of response. J Orthop Sports Phys Ther 1997;26(2):108–9.

30. Lange GW, Hintermeister RA, Schlegel T, et al. Electromyographic and kinematic analysis of graded treadmill walking and the implications for knee rehabilitation. J Orthop Sports Phys Ther 1996;23(5):294–301.

31. Mariano P, Caruso I. An electromyographic investigation of subluxation of the patella. J Bone Joint Surg Am 1979;61:169–71.

32. Morrish GM, Woledge RC. A comparison of the activation of muscles moving the patella in normal subjects and in patients with chronic patellofemoral problems. Scand J Rehabil Med 1997;29(1): 43–8.

33. Powers CM, Landel RF, Perry J. Timing and intensity of vastus muscle activity during functional activities in subjects with and without patellofemoral pain. Phys Ther 1996;76:946–55.

34. Signorile JF, Kacsik D, Perry A, et al. The effect of knee and foot position on the electromyographical activity of the superficial quadriceps. J Orthop Sports Phys Ther 1995;22(1):2–9.

35. Smith GP, Howe TE, Oldham JA, et al. Assessing quadriceps muscles recruitment order using rectified averaged surface EMG in young normals and 'weak' and healthy elderly subjects. Clin Rehabil 1995;9(1):40–6.

36. Wild JJ, Franklin TD, Woods GW. Patellar pain and quadriceps rehabilitation: an EMG study. Am J Sports Med 1982;10:12–15.

37. Noehren B, Pohl MB, Sanchez Z, et al. Proximal and distal kinematics in female runners with patellofemoral pain. Clin Biomech 2012;27(4):366–71. PubMed PMID: 22071426.

38. Barton CJ, Levinger P, Webster KE, et al. Walking kinematics in individuals with patellofemoral pain syndrome: a case control study. Gait Posture 2011;33(2):386–91.

39. Boling M, Padua D, Marshall S, et al. A prospective investigation of biomechanical risk factors for patellofemoral pain syndrome. Am J Sports Med 2009;37(11):2108–16.

40. Grayson TH. Disorders of the Patellofemoral Joint. 2nd ed. Baltimore: Williams and Wilkins; 1990.

41. Powers CM. The influence of altered lower-extremity kinematics on patellofemoral joint dysfunction: a theoretical perspective. J Orthop Sports Phys Ther 2003;33(11):639–46. PubMed PMID: WOS:000186785000002.

42. Prins MR, van der Wurff P. Females with patellofemoral pain syndrome have weak hip muscles: a systematic review. Aust J Physiother 2009;55:9–15.

43. Messier S, Davis S, Curl W, et al. Etiological factors associated with patellofemoral pain in runners. Med Sci Sports Exerc 1991;23(9):1008–15.

44. Callaghan MJ. What does proprioception testing tell us about patellofemoral pain? Man Ther 2011;16(1):46–7. [Epub 2010/08/13. eng]; PubMed PMID: 20702131.

45. Witvrouw E, Lysens R, Bellemans J, et al. Intrinsic risk factors for the development of anterior knee pain in an athletic population. A two-year prospective study. Am J Sports Med 2000;28(4):480–9. PubMed PMID: 10921638.

46. Davis IS, Powers CM. Patellofemoral pain syndrome: proximal, distal, and local factors, an international retreat, April 30-May 2, 2009, Fells Point, Baltimore, MD. J Orthop Sports Phys Ther 2010;40(3):A1–16.

47. Rathleff MS, Roos EM, Olesen JL, et al. Lower mechanical pressure pain thresholds in female adolescents with patellofemoral pain syndrome. J Orthop Sports Phys Ther 2013;43(6):414–21. [Epub 2013/03/20. eng]; PubMed PMID: 23508216.

48. Barber Foss KD, Myer GD, Chen SS, et al. Expected prevalence from the differential diagnosis of anterior knee pain in adolescent female athletes during preparticipation screening. J Athl Train 2012;47(5):519–24. [Epub 2012/10/17. eng]; PubMed PMID: 23068589. Pubmed Central PMCID: 3465032.

49. Taunton JE, Ryan MB, Clement DB, et al. A retrospective case-control analysis of 2002 running injuries. Br J Sports Med 2002;36:95–101.

50. Van Tiggelen D, Cowan S, Coorevits P, et al. Delayed vastus medialis obliquus to vastus lateralis onset timing contributes to the development of patellofemoral pain in previously healthy men. Am J Sports Med 2009;37(6):1099–105.

51. Duvigneaud N, Bernard E, Stevens V, et al. Isokinetic assessment of patellofemoral pain syndrome: a prospective study in female recruits. Isokinet Exerc Sci 2008;16(4):213–19. PubMed PMID: ISI:000262452000002. [English].

52. van Middelkoop M, van Linschoten R, Berger MY, et al. Knee complaints seen in general practice: active sport participants versus non-sport participants. BMC Musculoskelet Disord 2008;9:36. PubMed PMID: ISI:000254554000001.

53. Wood L, Muller S, Peat G. The epidemiology of patellofemoral disorders in adulthood: a review of routine general practice morbidity recording. Prim Health Care Res Dev 2011;12(2): 157–64.

54. Baquie P, Brukner P. Injuries presenting to an Australian sports medicine centre: a 12 month study. Clin J Sport Med 1997;7: 28–31.

55. Insall J, Falvo KA, Wise DW. Chondromalacia Patellae. A prospective study. J Bone Joint Surg Am 1976;58(1):1–8.

56. Fulkerson JP. Diagnosis and treatment of patients with patellofemoral pain. Am J Sports Med 2002;30(3):447–56.

57. Tsirbas A, Paterson RS, Keene GCR. Fat pad impingement: a missed cause of patello femoral pain? Aust J Sci Med Sport 1990;December:24–6.

58. Fulkerson JP. Disorders of the Patellofemoral Joint. 3rd ed. Baltimore: Williams & Wilkins; 1997.

59. Matthews LS, Sonstegard DA, Henke JA. Load bearing characteristics of the patello-femoral joint. Acta Orthop 1977;48(5): 511–16.

60. Sakai N, Lou Z-P, Rand JA, et al. The influence of weakness in the vastus medialis oblique muscle on the patellofemoral joint: an in vitro biomechanical study. Clin Biomech 2000;15:335–9.

61. Neptune RR, Wright IC, van den Bogert AJ. The influence of orthotic devices and vastus medialis strength and timing on patellofemoral loads during running. Clin Biomech 2000;15(8):611–18. [Epub 2000/08/11. eng]; PubMed PMID: 10936434.

62. Powers CM, Perry J, Hsu A, et al. Are patellofemoral pain and quadriceps femoris muscle torque associated with locomotor function? Phys Ther 1997;77(10):1063–75.

63. Thomee R, Renstrom P, Karlsson J, et al. Patellofemoral pain syndrome in young women. II. Muscle function in patients and healthy controls. Scand J Med Sci Sports 1995;5:245–51.

64. Boucher J, King M, Lefebre R, et al. Qudriceps femoris muscle activity in patellofemoral pain syndrome. Am J Sports Med 1992; 20(5):527–32.

65. Petschnig R, Baron R, Engel A, et al. Objectivation of the effects of knee problems on vastus medialis and vastus lateralis with EMG and dynamometry. Phys Med Rehabil 1991;2:50–4.

66. Miller JP. Vastus medialis obliquus and vastus lateralis activity in patients with and without patellofemoral pain syndrome. J Sport Rehabil 1997;6:1–10.

67. Sheehy P, Burdett RC, Irrgang JJ, et al. An electromyographic study of vastus medialis oblique and vastus lateralis activity while ascending and descending steps. J Orthop Sports Phys Ther 1998;27:423–9.

68. Coqueiro K, Bevilaqua-Grossi D, Berzin F, et al. Analysis on the activation of the VMO and VLL muscles during semisquat exercises with and without hip adduction in individuals with patellofemoral pain syndrome. J Electromyogr Kinesiol 2005;15:596–603.

69. Souza DR, Gross M. Comparison of vastus medialis obliquus: vastus lateralis muscle integrated electromyographic ratios between healthy subjects and patients with patellofemoral pain. Phys Ther 1991;71(4):310–20.

70. Cavazzuti L, Merlo A, Orlandi F, et al. Delayed onset of electromyographic activity of vastus medialis obliquus relative to vastus lateralis in subjects with patellofemoral pain syndrome. Gait Posture 2010;32:290–5.

71. Cesarelli M, Bifulco P, Bracale M. Study of the control strategy of the quadriceps in anterior knee pain. IEEE Trans Rehabil Eng 2000;8:330–41.

72. Cowan SM, Bennell KL, Hodges PW, et al. Delayed onset of electromyographic activity of vastus medialis obliquus relative to vastus lateralis in subjects with patellofemoral pain syndrome. Arch Phys Med Rehabil 2001;82(2):183–9. [Epub 2001/03/10. eng]; PubMed PMID: 11239308.

73. Perez PL, Gossman MR, Lechner D, et al., editors. Electromyographic Temporal Characteristics of the Vastus Medialis Oblique and the Vastus Lateralis in Women with and without Patellofemoral Pain. 12th International Congress of the World Confederation for Physical Therapy; 1995; Washington, DC, U.S.A.

74. Witvrouw E, Delvaux K, Lysens R, et al. Reflex response times of vastus medialis oblique and vastus lateralis in normal subjects and in subjects with patellofemoral pain – response. J Orthop Sports Phys Ther 1997;26(2):109–10.

75. Voight M, Weider D. Comparative reflex response times of the vastus medialis and the vastus lateralis in normal subjects and subjects with extensor mechanism dysfunction. Am J Sports Med 1991;10:131–7.

76. Cowan SM, Hodges PW, Bennell KL, et al. Altered vastii recruitment when people with patellofemoral pain syndrome complete a

77. postural task. Arch Phys Med Rehabil 2002;83(7):989–95. PubMed PMID: ISI:000176600700017.

77. Grabiner MD, Koh MA, Von Haefen I. Effect of concomitant hip joint adduction and knee joint extension forces on quadriceps activation. Eur J Exp Musculoskeletal Res 1992;1:155–60.

78. Karst GM, Willett GM. Onset timing of electromyographic activity in the vastus medialis oblique and vastus lateralis muscles in subjects with and without patellofemoral pain syndrome. Phys Ther 1995;75(9):813–23.

79. Chester R, Smith T, Sweeting D, et al. The relative timing of VMO and VL in the aetiology of anterior knee pain: a systematic review and meta-analysis. BMC Musculoskelet Disord 2008;9:64.

80. Barton CJ, Levinger P, Menz HB, et al. Kinematic gait characteristics associated with patellofemoral pain syndrome: a systematic review. Gait Posture 2009;30(4):405–16. PubMed PMID: WOS: 000273040200002.

81. Magalhaes E, Abdalla R, Fukuda T, et al. A comparison of hip strength between sedentary females with and without patellofemoral pain syndrome. J Orthop Sports Phys Ther 2010; 40:641–7.

82. Nakagawa T, Moriya E, Maciel C, et al. Trunk, pelvis, hip, and knee kinematics, hip strength, and gluteal muscle activation during a single-leg squat in males and females with and without patellofemoral pain syndrome. J Orthop Sports Phys Ther 2012;42:491–501.

83. Ireland ML, Willson JD, Ballantyne BT, et al. Hip strength in females with and without patellofemoral pain. J Orthop Sports Phys Ther 2003;33(11):671–6. [Epub 2003/12/13. eng]; PubMed PMID: 14669962.

84. Cichanowski HR, Schmitt JS, Johnson RJ, et al. Hip strength in collegiate female athletes with patellofemoral pain. Med Sci Sports Exerc 2007;39(8):1227–32. PubMed PMID: ISI: 000248581500004.

85. Robinson R, Nee RJ. Analysis of hip strength in females seeking physical therapy treatment for unilateral patellofemoral pain syndrome. J Orthop Sports Phys Ther 2007;37(5):232–8.

86. Bolgla LA, Malone TM, Umberger BR, et al. Hip strength and hip and knee kinematics during stair descent in females with and without patellofemoral pain syndrome. J Orthop Sports Phys Ther 2008;38(1):12–18.

87. Aminaka N, Pietrosimone BG, Armstrong CW, et al. Patellofemoral pain syndrome alters neuromuscular control and kinetics during stair ambulation. J Electromyogr Kinesiol 2011;21:645–51.

88. Cowan SM, Crossley KM, Bennell KL. Altered hip and trunk muscle function in individuals with patellofemoral pain. Br J Sports Med 2009;43(8):584–8. [Epub 2008/10/08. eng]; PubMed PMID: 18838402.

89. Brindle TJ, Mattacola C, McCrory J. Electromyographic changes in the gluteus medius during stair ascent and descent in subjects with anterior knee pain. Knee Surg Sports Traumatol Arthrosc 2003;11(4):244–51. [Epub 2003/04/16. eng]; PubMed PMID: 12695878.

90. Negahban H, Etemadi M, Naghibi S, et al. The effects of muscle fatigue on dynamic standing balance in people with and without patellofemoral pain syndrome. Gait Posture 2013;37(3):336–9.

91. Hollman JH, Galardi CM, Lin I-H, et al. Frontal and transverse plane hip kinematics and gluteus maximus recruitment correlate with frontal plane knee kinematics during single-leg squat tests in women. Clin Biomech 2014;29:468–74.

92. Tiberio D. The effect of excessive subtalar joint pronation on patellofemoral mechanics: a theoretical model. J Orthop Sports Phys Ther 1987;9(4):160–5. [Epub 1987/01/01. eng]; PubMed PMID: 18797010.

93. Macrum E, Bell DR, Boling M, et al. Effect of limiting ankle-dorsiflexion range of motion on lower extremity kinematics and muscle-activation patterns during a squat. J Sport Rehabil 2012;21(2):144–50.

94. Thuillier DU, Souza RB, Wu S, et al. T1r imaging demonstrates early changes in the lateral patella in patients with patellofemoral pain and maltracking. Am J Sports Med 2013;41(8):1813–18.

95. Li X, Benjamin C, Link TM, et al. In vivo T1r and T2 mapping of articular cartilage in osteoarthritis of the knee using 3T MRI. Osteoarthritis Cartilage 2007;15:789–97.

96. Thomee R. A comprehensive treatment approach for patellofemoral pain syndrome in young women. Phys Ther 1997;77(12): 1690–703.

97. Garber CE, Blissmer B, Deschenes MR, et al. Quantity and quality of exercise for developing and maintaining cardiorespiratory, musculoskeletal, and neuromotor fitness in apparently healthy adults: guidance for prescribing exercise. Med Sci Sports Exerc 2011;43(7):1334–59.

98. McConnell J. The management of chondromalacia patellae: a long term solution. Aust J Physiother 1986;32(4):215–23.

99. Crossley KM, Cowan SM, Bennell KL, et al. Patellar taping: is clinical success supported by scientific evidence? Man Ther 2000;5(3):142–50.

100. Barton C, Balachandar V, Lack S, et al. Patellar taping for patellofemoral pain: a systematic review and meta-analysis to evaluate clinical outcomes and biomechanical mechanisms. Br J Sports Med 2013;48(6):417–24.

101. Mulligan B, editor. 'NAGS', 'SNAGS', 'MWMS'. 6th ed. Wellington, New Zealand: Hutcheson Bowman and Stewart Ltd; 2010.

102. McConnell J. Management of patellofemoral problems. Man Ther 1996;1:60–6.

103. Collins NJ, Bisset LM, Crossley KM, et al. Efficacy of nonsurgical interventions for anterior knee pain: systematic review and meta-analysis of randomized trials. Sports Med 2012;42(1):31–48. [Epub 2011/12/14. eng]; PubMed PMID: 22149696.

104. Mills K, Blanch P, Chapman AR, et al. Foot orthoses and gait: a systematic review and meta-analysis of literature pertaining to potential mechanisms. Br J Sports Med 2010;44(14):1035–46.

105. Barton CJ, Menz HB, Levinger P, et al. Greater peak rear foot eversion predicts foot orthoses efficacy in individuals with patellofemoral pain syndrome. Br J Sports Med 2011;45:697–701.

106. Vicenzino B, Collins N, Cleland J, et al. A clinical prediction rule for identifying patients with patellofemoral pain who are likely to benefit from foot orthoses: a preliminary determination. Br J Sports Med 2008;44(12):doi: 10.1136/bjsm.2008.052613.

107. Vicenzino B. Foot orthotics in the treatment of lower limb conditions: a musculoskeletal physiotherapy perspective. Man Ther 2004;9(4):185–96.

108. Barton CJ, Menz HB, Crossley KM. Clinical predictors of foot orthoses efficacy in individuals with patellofemoral pain. Med Sci Sports Exerc 2011;43(9):1603–10. PubMed PMID: WOS: 000293951800001.

109. Barton CJ, Munteanu SE, Menz HB, et al. The efficacy of foot orthoses in the treatment of individuals with patellofemoral pain syndrome: a systematic review. Sports Med 2010;40(5):377–95. [Epub 2010/05/04. eng]; PubMed PMID: 20433211.

110. Mills K, Blanch P, Dev P, et al. A randomised control trial of short term efficacy of in-shoe foot orthoses compared with a wait and see policy for anterior knee pain and the role of foot mobility. Br J Sports Med 2012;46(4):247–52.

111. Fukuda TY, Melo WP, Zaffalon BM, et al. Hip posterolateral musculature strengthening in sedentary women with patellofemoral pain syndrome: a randomized controlled clinical trial with 1-year follow-up. J Orthop Sports Phys Ther 2012;42(10):823–30.

112. Khayambashi K, Mohammadkhani Z, Ghaznavi K, et al. The effects of isolated hip abductor and external rotator muscle strengthening on pain, health status, and hip strength in females with patellofemoral pain: a randomized controlled trial. J Orthop Sports Phys Ther 2012;42(1):22–9.

113. Swart NM, Van Linschoten R, Bierma-Zeinstra SMA, et al. The additional effect of orthotic devices on exercise therapy for patients with patellofemoral pain syndrome: a systematic review. Br J Sports Med 2012;46(8):570–7.

114. Rathleff MS, Rathleff CR, Crossley KM, et al. Hip strength and patellofemoral pain – a systematic review. Br J Sports Med 2014;48(14):1088.

115. Noehren B, Hamill J, Davis I. Prospective evidence for a hip etiology in patellofemoral pain. Med Sci Sports Exerc 2013;45(6): 1120–4.

116. Noehren B, Scholz J, Davis I. The effect of real-time gait retraining on hip kinematics, pain and function in subjects with patellofemoral pain syndrome. Br J Sports Med 2011;45(9):691–6.

117. Willy RW, Scholz JP, Davis IS. Mirror gait retraining for the treatment of patellofemoral pain in female runners. Clin Biomech 2012;27(10):1045–51.

118. Lenhart RL, Thelen DG, Wille CM, et al. Increasing running step rate reduces patellofemoral joint forces. Med Sci Sports Exerc 2014;46(3):557–64.

119. Bonacci J, Vicenzino B, Spratford W, et al. Take your shoes off to reduce patellofemoral joint stress during running. Br J Sports Med 2014;48(6):425–8.

120. Thomas MJ, Wood L, Selfe J, et al. Anterior knee pain in younger adults as a precursor to subsequent patellofemoral osteoarthritis: a systematic review. BMC Musculoskelet Disord 2010;11:201.

121. Collins NJ, Bierma-Zeinstra SMA, Crossley KM, et al. Prognostic factors for patellofemoral pain: a multicentre observational analysis. Br J Sports Med 2013;47:227–33.

122. Crossley KM, Hinman RS. The patellofemoral joint: the forgotten joint in knee osteoarthritis. Osteoarthritis Cartilage 2011; 19(7):765–7. PubMed PMID: WOS:000293323000001.

123. Utting MR, Davies G, Newman JH. Is anterior knee pain a predisposing factor to patellofemoral osteoarthritis? Knee 2005;12: 362–5.

124. Farrokhi S, Keyak JH, Powers CM. Individuals with patellofemoral pain exhibit greater patellofemoral joint stress: a finite element analysis study. Osteoarthritis Cartilage 2011;19(3):287–94.

125. Andia I, Maffulli N. Platelet-rich plasma for managing pain and inflammation in osteoarthritis. Nat Rev Rheumatol 2013;9(12): 721–30.

CHAPTER 48.3 ■ KNEE OSTEOARTHRITIS

Kim Bennell • Rana Hinman • Melanie Holden • George Peat

IMPACT ON INDIVIDUALS AND SOCIETY

Individuals with knee osteoarthritis (OA) frequently experience chronic pain, functional limitations, psychological problems and reduced quality of life.[1–6] Rates of co-morbidity are high, with many people reporting additional conditions, including cardiac diseases, type 2 diabetes, obesity and other joint pain.[7] Several recent studies have reported higher all-cause mortality in individuals with knee OA compared with the general population,[8–10] possibly due to co-morbidities[8] or presence of low-grade chronic systemic inflammation.[10]

The reported prevalence of knee OA varies greatly, from 6.3–70.8%, depending on the sample and whether OA is defined by radiographs, symptoms or self-reported diagnosis.[11] The prevalence will continue to rise as the population ages[12] and as levels of obesity, a risk factor, continue to grow.[13] The cost implications of knee OA are considerable, with costs related to lost productivity, community and social services for OA, and from a range of treatments, particularly knee joint replacement surgery.[14] Given the considerable individual and societal burden of knee OA, treatments that reduce symptoms and slow functional decline are needed[15] while efforts to discover structural disease-modifying interventions continue.

CONCEPTS OF OSTEOARTHRITIS

Osteoarthritis, often erroneously referred to as 'wear-and-tear' or 'degenerative joint disease', has been traditionally viewed as a disease primarily involving progressive destruction of articular cartilage that causes joint dysfunction and pain.[16] However, inconsistent correlation between clinical symptoms and radiographic OA challenge the view that pain is simply a result of cartilage damage. Plain radiographs offer a relatively limited, late view of OA pathology and an increasing body of literature is now based on magnetic resonance imaging (MRI). Studies using this more sensitive imaging modality have also only found weak associations between knee pain and cartilage volume and thickness.[17] Thus articular cartilage, normally aneural and avascular, seems unlikely to be a major direct contributor to symptoms.[18,19]

Pathologically, OA is now known to involve all joint tissues, including cartilage, bone, synovium/capsule, ligaments and muscle, and there is increased cell activity and new tissue formation within all of the joint, including remodelling of bone adjacent to synovial joints, and new bone formation (osteophyte) at the joint margins.[20] This paints a rather different picture from that of 'wear-and-tear', to one of 'wear-and-repair' in which osteoarthritis is conceptualized as a repair process that is generally slow, but efficient.[20] Longitudinal studies with up to 14 years of follow-up show that the course of OA varies between individuals and is not always progressive.[21,22]

Inflammation, previously believed to be irrelevant to knee OA,[16] is now believed to be an important factor directly linked to clinical symptoms and cartilage degradation.[23,24] In both the early and late phases of OA, inflammation of the synovial membrane (synovitis) is common.[24,25] Why the synovium becomes inflamed in OA remains controversial. The most accepted hypothesis is that once degraded, cartilage fragments contact the synovium, which reacts by producing excess inflammatory mediators (enzymes) that are responsible for cartilage degeneration. These enzymes cause further breakdown of cartilage that in turn increases synovial inflammation,[23] and a vicious cycle is formed.

Although pathological changes go some way to explaining the pain mechanisms involved in OA, MRI features suggestive of OA (including cartilage damage, osteophytes and bone marrow lesions) are also commonly found in individuals with no knee pain.[18] Other factors must play a part:[26] OA may be best conceptualized within a biopsychosocial framework in which pain results from a complex interaction between structural changes, social and psychological factors.[19,27,28] Clear evidence now exists showing that psychological and social factors, including helplessness, anxiety, depression, self-efficacy and participation restriction, are associated with knee pain and OA.[6,29,30] Variability in pain over time has been linked to fluctuations in psychological factors;[6] however, the causal direction of this relationship is difficult to determine and questions remain about whether psychological factors influence pain or vice versa.[6,26]

RISK FACTORS FOR DEVELOPMENT AND PROGRESSION

The development of knee OA results from both local joint-specific factors and systemic factors (Fig. 48-8).[31] Women are not only more likely to have OA than men, but they also have more severe OA.[32] Other systemic risk factors include race/ethnicity, genetics and diet.[31,33] Obesity and being overweight are well-established local risk factors for knee OA,[34] as are knee injury[35] and occupation, particularly jobs requiring both carrying and kneeling or squatting.[36] There is mixed evidence on the effects of physical activity, exercise and sport on knee OA, with some studies suggesting an increased risk of OA in those who exercise more regularly or intensely,[37] but others showing no association between recreational activity, running, or generally high activity levels and knee OA.[31,38] Other local risk factors for knee OA include joint biomechanics, knee alignment and joint laxity.[33]

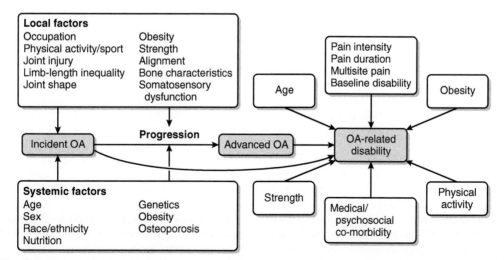

FIGURE 48-8 ■ Risk factors for osteoarthritis (*OA*) and related disability. (Reprinted from PM & R. Suri P, Morgenroth DC, Hunter DJ. Epidemiology of osteoarthritis and associated comorbidities, S10–19. © 2012, with permission from Elsevier.)

Comparatively few studies have examined risk factors for structural progression of knee OA. For many potential risk factors there is still only limited or conflicting evidence on their relationship to disease progression[39] and challenges in the design and interpretation of these studies may be a contributory factor.[33,40] However, there is fairly consistent evidence linking older age, varus knee alignment, presence of OA in multiple joints, radiographic severity at baseline, and higher body mass index to higher risk of future progression of knee OA.[39] A number of studies have also evaluated the course of functional status over time in individuals with knee OA. Increasing age, greater pain and functional limitations, obesity, poor general health and concurrent co-morbidities are all predictors of poor functional outcome in knee OA. However, lower levels of mental health symptoms including anxiety and depression, greater self-efficacy and social support, and regular physical activity appear to protect against functional decline.[31]

THE ROLE OF BIOMECHANICS AND NEUROMUSCULAR FACTORS

Joint loading, acting within the context of systemic and local joint-specific susceptibility, plays a role in the aetiology of knee OA.[41] Since direct measurement of joint loads in vivo is generally not feasible in humans, three-dimensional gait analysis is typically used to infer compressive joint loads during walking. For knee OA, the most relevant and widely studied load parameter is the external knee adduction moment (KAM) in the frontal plane, generated because the ground reaction force vector passes medial to the joint centre. This moment forces the knee into varus, compressing the medial joint compartment and stretching lateral structures. As such, the KAM has been used as an indicator of medial joint load.[42,43] Of importance, longitudinal studies have found that higher KAM indices are associated with an increased risk of structural progression in people with knee OA.[44,45] Given this, physical therapy interventions that reduce the KAM may slow disease progression.

Impairments in the local mechanical environment and neuromotor control systems, such as malalignment, varus thrust and altered muscle-activation patterns, exist and can influence knee load and thereby structural progression. Malalignment, particularly varus malalignment in those with medial compartment OA, often arises or worsens as a consequence of the osteoarthritic process due to cartilage loss, bony attrition and meniscal damage. The presence of malalignment is a clinical marker of the likelihood of both structural deterioration[46] and decreases in function.[47]

Failure to dynamically control frontal plane motion at the knee joint can manifest as a visually observed varus thrust with dynamic worsening or abrupt onset of varus alignment in the early part of stance phase.[48] Varus thrust is associated with higher knee load during walking,[49,50] faster disease progression[49] and greater pain during weight-bearing activities.[51] Another consequence of lack of dynamic control may be symptomatic knee instability reported by the patient as buckling, slipping or giving

way of the knee during weight-bearing activities.[52] This has been identified as a problem in a substantial proportion of individuals with knee OA affecting their ability to function.[52,53] The causes of varus thrust and self-reported instability are likely to be multifactorial, resulting from factors such as passive joint laxity, structural damage, muscle weakness, pain and altered neuromuscular control. A better understanding of the underlying causes is needed to help design appropriate interventions to stabilize the knee and reduce these phenomena.

Neuromuscular function is important to balance external moments applied to the knee joint[54,55] and improve the dynamic stability of the joint during walking. However, alterations in neuromuscular function may increase knee load.[56] Muscle weakness is consistently found in people with knee OA.[57] Recent interest in the patterns of muscle activation associated with knee OA suggests that some patients adopt a co-contraction strategy involving activation of many muscles in a less specific fashion.[58-60] While these neuromuscular alterations most likely represent coping strategies and thus may have short-term benefits, they may have long-term negative consequences by altering the distribution and increasing the magnitude of load and potentially speeding structural disease progression. This has led to the recommendation that novel exercise approaches designed to reduce levels of co-contraction should be developed to address these neuromuscular changes.[58,60] However, if co-contraction is an adaptive response, then removing this strategy without addressing more appropriate means to control joint stability may be detrimental. The most effective form of physical therapy to address these impairments is currently not known.

DIAGNOSIS AND ASSESSMENT

Diagnosis

In the absence of any agreed 'gold standard', the diagnosis of knee OA may be made on clinical grounds without normally requiring imaging or laboratory investigations.[33] After excluding important differential diagnoses,[61] a working diagnosis of OA may be applied to patients aged 45 years and over, reporting persistent joint pain that is worse with use, and morning stiffness lasting no more than half an hour.[20] The presence of known risk factors and classical symptoms and signs may help strengthen clinical suspicion (Box 48-1), serving mainly to identify the more advanced cases.[63-66] However, it should be noted that many clinical signs may not have the level of reliability or diagnostic validity one might wish for clinical decision making.[33,67-69]

Under a working diagnosis of OA, practitioners will confront a spectrum of clinical and pathological severity ranging from intermittent symptoms to constant aches with severe, acute exacerbations[70-72] and from early structural changes visible only on MRI[3,73] to complete loss of joint space.[74] While many patients clearly value having a diagnosis,[75] the benefits of this cannot be assumed[76,77] and time and care must be taken over its explanation to patients. Emerging with a new or reinforced belief that

BOX 48-1	Risk Factors, Symptoms and Signs that Should Be Associated with Increased Clinical Suspicion of Knee Osteoarthritis

Older age
Higher body mass index
Family history of osteoarthritis
History of previous ligament/cartilage injury to knee
History of repetitive, cumulative, or heavy loading (for example, as part of occupation)
Persistent knee pain*
Reduced function*
Limited duration knee stiffness (<30 minutes)*
Coarse crepitus*
Restricted knee flexion range of motion*
Bony enlargement*
Fixed flexion deformity
Modest effusion

*Key criteria from EULAR Task Force recommendations[62]

'it's my age', 'it's wear-and-tear, and therefore inevitably progressive and activity/exercise are contra-indicated', or 'nothing can be done' should be taken as a strong indicator of a failed consultation.

Beyond Diagnosis

Assessment serves many purposes other than diagnosis. Careful evaluation of pain and functional limitation is integral to many of these purposes, but cannot be adequately understood within a strict biomedical framework (Fig. 48-8). Pain experience and function are influenced by a wider set of determinants, some potentially modifiable, whose identification requires a more holistic assessment (e.g. Table 48-2).

A myriad patient-reported outcome measures are available to the clinician and there are many excellent published reviews of these instruments to guide selection.[78] Further attempts to streamline and simplify the administration of patient-reported outcome measures for routine clinical practice are underway.[79–81] Simple, easily interpretable measures already exist, such as a standardized 0–10 numerical rating scale for pain intensity. The use of physical performance tests is recommended to complement the picture gained from patient-reported outcome measures with an evaluation of what the patient can do[82,83] (Table 48-3).

TREATMENT STRATEGIES

Management of knee OA has traditionally focused on treatment of pain and disability associated with established disease. However, there is interest in treatment that can also slow or prevent structural progression to advanced disease. Regardless of the management goals, treatment for knee OA should be individualized based on assessment findings and be patient-centred involving shared decision making between the patient and clinician. The optimal management of knee OA requires a combination of non-pharmacological and

pharmacological treatment strategies[85] with surgery reserved for end-stage disease that is unresponsive to other interventions. Education, exercise and if appropriate, weight loss, are the core recommended treatments for knee OA.

Given the chronicity of the disease, treatments that encourage patient self-management are particularly important. Furthermore, treatments need to address both the physical and psychosocial issues identified on assessment and referral to other appropriate health professionals may be required. A more patient-focused communication style that involves reassurance, encouragement, support, empathy, asking questions and listening is associated with greater therapeutic alliance between the clinician and patient and improves patient outcomes.[86,87] Adherence is greater when clinicians are perceived as supportive rather than paternalistic,[88] and clinicians need to ensure that their communication style promotes, rather than hinders, patient self-management.

Education

Patient education is an integral component of knee OA treatment and should cover a range of topics including pain management, exercise, diet, activity–rest cycling, goal-setting and problem solving. Educational strategies that improve the patient's understanding of the neurophysiology and neurobiology of pain can have a positive effect on chronic musculoskeletal pain.[2,89] Key messages for patients with knee OA have been identified through a consensus exercise involving over 50 international experts and patients.[90]

Exercise

Exercise is universally recommended by clinical guidelines for the management of all patients with knee OA.[91–93] Systematic reviews and meta-analyses consistently support the short-term benefit of exercise for improving pain and physical function in people with knee OA,[94–96] even those with severe disease awaiting total joint replacement.[97] For those who are overweight/obese, the combination of exercise and dietary weight loss is more effective for symptoms than either treatment alone.[98] Although the magnitude of benefits may be considered small-to-moderate, this is comparable to reported estimates for simple analgesics and oral non-steroidal anti-inflammatory drugs for OA pain.[99] Importantly, exercise is associated with relatively few side effects compared to drug treatments. In contrast to symptomatic benefit from exercise, evidence from a limited number of studies to date does not show any effects of exercise in reducing knee load[100–102] or in slowing structural disease progression in people with knee OA.[103]

Clinical guidelines for managing OA[92] strongly recommend that people with knee OA participate in cardiovascular and/or resistance land-based exercise, as well as aquatic exercise. In particular, aquatic exercise may be useful for those who are overweight/obese or who have severe disease. Results of a recent systematic review support a combination of strengthening, flexibility and

TABLE 48-2 Holistic Assessment

Holistic Assessment

Assess the effect of osteoarthritis on the person's function, quality of life, occupation, mood, relationships and leisure activities. Below are example topics

The patient's existing thoughts	The patient's support network	The patient's mood	Pain assessment	Effect of osteoarthritis on:	Other musculoskeletal pain	Co-morbidities
• What concerns do they have? • What are their expectations? • What do they know about osteoarthritis?	• Is the patient isolated or do they have a carer? • How is the main support giver coping? • What are their ideas, concerns and expectations?	• Screen for depression • Are there any other stresses in their life? **The patient's attitude to exercise** • Previous exercise experience • Beliefs about exercise • Potential barriers and facilitators to exercise	Assess: • Self-help strategies the patient is using • Current drugs being used, including their doses, frequency, timing and any possible side effects • Evidence of pain catastrophizing • Self-efficacy around pain managements	• Activities of daily living • Family duties • Hobbies • Lifestyle expectations • Quality of sleep • Energy levels • Their occupation, including short- and long-term ability to perform their job (are any adjustments to home or workplace required?)	• Is there evidence of a chronic pain syndrome? • Are there other treatable sources of pain (for example, peri-articular pain or bursitis)?	• If two or more morbidities, consider any interaction • Is the patient fit for surgery? • Assess the most appropriate therapy • Is the patient prone to falls?

(Adapted from[20])

TABLE 48-3 **Description of the Minimum Core Set of Physical Performance Measures for Hip and Knee Osteoarthritis* as Recommended by the Osteoarthritis Research Society International[83]**

Test	Equipment Needed	Description
30-second chair stand test	• Timer/stop watch • Straight back chair with a 44 cm (17 inch) seat height, preferably without arms	Maximum number of chair stand repetitions possible in 30 seconds
40 m fast-paced walk test	• Timer/stop watch • 10 m marked walkway with space to safely turn around at each end • 2 cones placed approximately 2 m beyond each end of the walkway • Calculator to convert time to speed	A fast-paced walking test that is timed over 4 × 10 m for a total of 40 m performed in comfortable footwear
Stair climb test	• Timer/stop watch • Set of stairs	Time in seconds it takes to ascend and descend a flight of stairs. The number of stairs will depend on individual availability

*There are currently no consensus recommendations for performance tests in younger patients at high risk of osteoarthritis, although Kroman et al.[84] provide a review of the evidence on these.

aerobic exercise for improving function.[94] Neither the type[96] nor intensity[104,105] of the strengthening exercise appears to influence outcome. More recently, neuromuscular exercise typically performed in functional weight-bearing positions and emphasizing quality and efficiency of movement, as well as alignment of the trunk and lower limb joints, has been promoted for knee OA.[106] In addition to structured exercise, encouraging and supporting patients to increase overall physical activity levels is also important.[107] Effect sizes for individual supervised exercise treatments are greater than those for class-based programmes and home exercise.[95] Furthermore, 12 or more directly supervised exercise sessions with a health professional significantly improve pain and function to a greater extent when compared with less than 12 supervised exercise sessions.[95] While this may be the case, there is still unwillingness in many healthcare settings to fund this level of intervention as a core component of knee OA care.

While effective in the short term, the benefits of exercise decline over the longer term due to lack of adherence.[108] A dose–response relationship has been demonstrated between adherence rates and exercise effects.[109] A complex array of factors can influence adherence. These include attitude towards exercise, perceived severity of knee symptoms (those with more severe symptoms are most likely to adhere), ideas about the cause of arthritis (those thinking arthritis is due to age or 'wear-and-tear' are less adherent) and the perceived effectiveness of the intervention. Numerous strategies have been suggested to help improve adherence to exercise in people with OA,[110] including individualizing the exercise programme, educating about the disease process and benefits of exercise, regular monitoring from the therapist, integrating behavioural graded activity principles, use of 'booster sessions', self-monitoring, reinforcement by other individuals, telephone and/or mail contact as well as participating in exercise with a spouse or other family member.[111]

An important common misperception is that pain during exercise in patients with knee OA indicates joint damage. Although experiences of pain when exercising may assist decisions about exercise dosage, patients should be advised that it is normal to feel some discomfort or pain during exercise. Practical exercise prescription tips for physiotherapists are shown in Box 48-2.

Manual Therapy

Manual therapy is often used in the management of knee OA,[112] generally in combination with other interventions such as exercise. There are a limited number of clinical trials of manual therapy with relatively recent systematic reviews reporting fair evidence for short-term benefits and limited evidence for long-term benefits of manual therapy, although the studies had a high risk of bias.[113,114] Another systematic review and meta-analysis suggested that the addition of manual therapy to exercise may be more effective than exercise alone.[115] However, none of the studies included in this review directly compared the treatments as was done in a more recent randomized controlled trial involving 206 people with hip or knee OA.[116] In this high-quality study, manual physiotherapy provided significant benefits for pain and disability over usual care that were sustained to 1 year. However, there was no added benefit from the combination of manual physiotherapy and exercise and indeed the combination was generally less effective or at best no more effective than either intervention alone. The authors reasoned that, given a fixed clinic visit time, combining manual therapy and exercise therapy necessitates reducing the dose of both, compared with a clinic visit focusing on one or the other and that this may have explained the results. Nonetheless, the results show the benefits of manual therapy for people with knee OA.

Braces

Neoprene or elastic sleeves are the simplest and cheapest type of knee braces available. Although they offer little joint support, they provide compression and warmth and have been shown to significantly improve quality of life and function.[117] Unloader braces are semi-rigid knee

---

BOX 48-2	Practical Exercise Prescription for Patients with Knee Osteoarthritis

- As similar reductions in pain and improvements in function can be gained with various types of exercise, the patient should chose the type of exercise they prefer
- An exercise programme to improve muscle strength, aerobic capacity and flexibility is recommended
- Strengthening exercises should target major lower limb muscles such as the quadriceps, hip abductors and extensors, hamstrings and gastrocnemius
- Aerobic exercise such as walking can also assist in weight loss/prevention of weight gain and in improving mood and anxiety
- Aquatic exercise may be beneficial for those who are overweight/obese or those with more severe disease
- Tai chi may be a useful exercise option for some
- Balance exercises should be included if assessment reveals balance impairments or if the patient has a history of falls
- Increasing overall general physical activity levels during everyday life is important in addition to structured exercise
- Treatment benefits in terms of reduced pain and improved function can be gained from individual, class-based and home-based programmes
- Although individual treatments show the greatest treatment benefits for pain and function, superiority of one delivery mode over the other remains unclear
- Group exercise and home exercise are similarly effective and patient preference should be considered in the decision-making process of preferred delivery mode
- Home-based programmes can be supplemented with supervised programmes (class or individual) to maximize the cost-effective benefits
- Discomfort or pain during exercise is to be expected. However, severe or intense pain during exercise, pain that does not subside to usual levels within a few hours after exercise, increased night pain following exercise, or swelling or increased swelling in the hours following exercise or the next morning indicate that the type or dosage of exercise need to be modified

braces designed for people with predominant medial or lateral tibiofemoral joint OA and varus or valgus malalignment. They apply an external three-point corrective force that improves symptoms[118] and reduces biomechanical load on the affected compartment[119,120] as well as muscle activation and co-contraction levels.[121] Thus, valgus bracing offers great potential for slowing disease progression in medial knee OA if load reduction can be sustained. Long-term studies are now required to evaluate the effects of bracing on joint structure.

For patients with patellofemoral joint (PFJ) OA or whose predominant symptoms arise from the PFJ, a patellofemoral brace may be useful. These aim to unload the lateral compartment of the PFJ by applying a force to the patella in a medial direction.[122] However, the symptomatic benefits are unclear. No significant effects on pain were noted in a cross-over trial comparing patellofemoral bracing to a control bracing condition in people with lateral PFJ OA and anterior knee pain

symptoms. In contrast, a recent parallel-group RCT showed that 6-week use of a patellofemoral brace (compared to no brace) resulted in significant reductions in knee pain, and in the volume of bone marrow lesions (lesions seen in the subchondral bone on MRI and a marker of disease progression) in the PFJ.[123] These promising results are the first evidence that bracing may be able to influence underlying joint structure in knee OA.

Footwear and Orthoses

Given that knee OA is mechanically driven,[124] and footwear and shoe insoles can influence the centre of pressure at the foot (and thus knee load via the knee lever arm),[125,126] these strategies may assist in the management of patients with knee OA, and may, in fact, have the ability to slow disease progression.

Most research has focused on lateral wedge insoles. A recent systematic review, which evaluated the effect of lateral wedges on the external KAM,[127] demonstrated that these insoles reduced the peak KAM. Unfortunately, the load-reducing effects of lateral wedges have not translated into clinically meaningful reductions in pain[128] nor slowing of structural disease progression (cartilage volume on MRI) when compared to neutral insoles.[129] In contrast, the limited literature available evaluating medial wedges for lateral tibiofemoral OA suggests that these insoles can reduce pain in women with bilateral valgus malalignment.[130] Given the dearth of studies evaluating the clinical effects of other shoe orthoses in knee OA such as shock-absorbing insoles[131] and medial arch supports, the usefulness of these is not yet known.

Clinical guidelines recommend every patient with knee OA receive advice concerning appropriate footwear.[85,91] Compared to barefoot walking regular off-the-shelf shoes increase medial knee load by 7–14%, depending on shoe type.[127] Shoe types that are more likely to increase medial knee load include high-heeled shoes and shoes that promote foot stability rather than mobility.[132–138] Biomechanical evidence suggests lightweight, flat and flexible footwear may be optimal for knee OA. Recently, novel innovative footwear has been developed specifically to reduce knee loads in people with knee OA. Shoes with 'variable stiffness' soles (where the lateral sole is stiffer compared to medial) can reduce the KAM compared to shoes with a uniformly stiff sole,[139,140] but do not appear to significantly reduce knee pain. 'Mobility' shoes incorporate a flexible grooved sole (and engineered to mimic barefoot walking) and can also reduce the peak KAM by 8% compared to self-selected walking shoes;[141] however, the efficacy of these shoes in treating symptoms of knee OA has not been evaluated. Unstable rocker-soled shoes (Masai Barefoot Technology®) have been proposed as an option for knee OA given their potential to improve gait stability and reduce joint load.[142] These shoes reduce peak KAM by up to 13% in overweight males (who are at risk of developing knee OA);[143] however, a 12-week randomized controlled trial comparing unstable shoes to normal walking shoes showed no symptomatic effects in a sample with symptomatic knee OA.[142] Thus, at present, it is not clear what role innovative shoe designs may play, if any, in managing symptoms associated with knee OA.

Gait Aids and Gait Retraining

Emerging research suggests that gait retraining can reduce the KAM during walking, and thus may have potential as a structure-modifying treatment strategy. A systematic review of gait modification strategies identified 14 different strategies that have been evaluated for their effects on the KAM.[144]

Use of a walking cane is conditionally recommended in clinical guidelines for knee OA.[92] Biomechanical evidence shows that using a cane in the contralateral hand can reduce the KAM by 6–17%.[145] Greatest offloading of the knee occurs when greater amounts of body weight are placed through the cane, when body weight is placed through the cane earlier (rather than later) during stance phase of gait, and when the cane is placed at a greater lateral distance away from the affected limb. Thus, it is important that clinicians train patients with knee OA to use walking canes appropriately in order to ensure maximum benefit. There has been one RCT evaluating the efficacy of walking canes in people with knee OA,[146] reporting that 60 days of cane use significantly reduced pain, improved physical function and reduced analgesic use. Further research is now required to determine whether long-term use of a cane can have disease-modifying effects.

Acupuncture

Meta-analyses show that acupuncture is effective for the treatment of chronic pain, including OA.[147] One recent systematic review concluded that acupuncture can be considered one of the more effective physical treatments for alleviating knee OA pain in the short term.[148] The addition of acupuncture to exercise delivered by physiotherapists was also cost-effective.[149] The benefits of acupuncture may result from factors over and above the specific effects of needling such as positive expectation of treatment benefit.[147]

CONCLUSION

Treatment of knee OA requires a biopsychosocial approach with an emphasis on assisting the patient to self-manage their condition. Education, exercise and, if appropriate, weight loss, are key treatments recommended by all clinical guidelines. Attention to adherence strategies is important to ensure longer-term benefits. To date, there are no established structural disease-modifying treatments. However, given the link between higher knee load and disease progression, treatments that reduce knee load such as braces, modified footwear, gait aids and gait retraining have potential.

REFERENCES

1. Neame R, Doherty M. Osteoarthritis update. Clin Med 2005;5:207–10.
2. Hurley MV. Muscle dysfunction and effective rehabilitation of knee osteoarthritis: what we know and what we need to find out. Arthritis Rheum 2003;49:444–52.
3. Hunter DJ, Zhang W, Conaghan PG, et al. Systematic review of the concurrent and predictive validity of MRI biomarkers in OA. Osteoarthritis Cartilage 2011;19:557–88.
4. Jordan KM, Arden NK, Doherty M, et al. EULAR Recommendations 2003: an evidence based approach to the management of knee osteoarthritis: report of a Task Force of the Standing Committee for International Clinical Studies Including Therapeutic Trials (ESCISIT). Ann Rheum Dis 2003;62:1145–55.
5. Murphy SL, Lyden AK, Phillips K, et al. Subgroups of older adults with osteoarthritis based upon differing comorbid symptom presentations and potential underlying pain mechanisms. Arthritis Res Ther 2011;13:R135.
6. Wise BL, Niu J, Zhang Y, et al. Psychological factors and their relation to osteoarthritis pain. Osteoarthritis Cartilage 2010;18:883–7.
7. de Rooij M, Steultjens MPM, Avezaat E, et al. Restrictions and contraindications for exercise therapy in patients with hip and knee osteoarthritis and co-morbidity. Phys Ther Rev 2013;18:101–11.
8. Betancourt MCC, Dehghan A, Campos N, et al. Osteoarthritis and mortality: meta-analysis of two prospective cohorts. Osteoarthritis Cartilage 2013;21:s151.
9. Hunter DJ. Osteoarthritis. Best Pract Res Clin Rheumatol 2011;25:801–14.
10. Nuesch E, Dieppe P, Reichenbach S, et al. All cause and disease specific mortality in patients with knee or hip osteoarthritis: population based cohort study. BMJ 2011;342:d1165.
11. Pereira D, Peleteiro B, Araujo J, et al. The effect of osteoarthritis definition on prevalence and incidence estimates: a systematic review. Osteoarthritis Cartilage 2011;19:1270–85.
12. Wilmoth JR. Demography of longevity: past, present, and future trends. Exp Gerontol 2000;35:1111–29.
13. James WP. The epidemiology of obesity: the size of the problem. J Intern Med 2008;263:336–52.
14. OECD. 2011. Health at a Glance 2011: OECD Indicators, OECD Publishing. <http://dx.doi.org/10.1787/health_glance-2011-en>.
15. Bennell K. Physiotherapy management of hip osteoarthritis. J Physiother 2013;59:145–57.
16. Jordan JM, Gracely RH. A special osteoarthritis and cartilage issue on pain in osteoarthritis. Osteoarthritis Cartilage 2013;21:1143–4.
17. Hunter DJ, Arden N, Conaghan PG, et al. Definition of osteoarthritis on MRI: results of a Delphi exercise. Osteoarthritis Cartilage 2011;19:963–9.
18. Guermazi A, Niu J, Hayashi D, et al. Prevalence of abnormalities in knees detected by MRI in adults without knee osteoarthritis: population based observational study (Framingham Osteoarthritis Study). BMJ 2012;345:e5339.
19. Hunter DJ, Guermazi A, Roemer F, et al. Structural correlates of pain in joints with osteoarthritis. Osteoarthritis Cartilage 2013;21:1170–8.
20. NICE. Osteoarthritis: National Clinical Guideline for Care and Management in Adults. Guideline. London: National Institute for Health and Clinical Excellence, UK; 2008 Report No: CG59 Contract No: CG59.
21. Leyland KM, Hart D, Javaid MK, et al. The natural history of radiographic knee osteoarthritis: a fourteen year population-based cohort study. Arthritis Rheum 2012;64(7):2243–51. doi:10.1002/art.34415.
22. Soni A, Kiran A, Hart DJ, et al. Prevalence of reported knee pain over twelve years in a community-based cohort. Arthritis Rheum 2012;64:1145–52.
23. Berenbaum F. Osteoarthritis as an inflammatory disease (osteoarthritis is not osteoarthrosis! Osteoarthritis Cartilage 2013;21:16–21.
24. Sellam J, Berenbaum F. The role of synovitis in pathophysiology and clinical symptoms of osteoarthritis. Nat Rev Rheumatol 2010;6:625–35.
25. Ayral X, Pickering EH, Woodworth TG, et al. Synovitis: a potential predictive factor of structural progression of medial tibiofemoral knee osteoarthritis – results of a 1 year longitudinal arthroscopic study in 422 patients. Osteoarthritis Cartilage 2005;13:361–7.
26. Neogi T. The epidemiology and impact of pain in osteoarthritis. Osteoarthritis Cartilage 2013;21:1145–53.

27. Dieppe PA, Lohmander LS. Pathogenesis and management of pain in osteoarthritis. Lancet 2005;365:965–73.

28. Hunter DJ, McDougall JJ, Keefe FJ. The symptoms of osteoarthritis and the genesis of pain. Rheum Dis Clin North Am 2008;34:623–43.

29. Schneider S, Junghaenel DU, Keefe FJ, et al. Individual differences in the day-to-day variability of pain, fatigue, and well-being in patients with rheumatic disease: associations with psychological variables. Pain 2012;153:813–22.

30. Wilkie R, Peat G, Thomas E, et al. Factors associated with restricted mobility outside the home in community-dwelling adults ages fifty years and older with knee pain: an example of use of the International Classification of Functioning to investigate participation restriction. Arthritis Rheum 2007;57:1381–9.

31. Suri P, Morgenroth DC, Hunter DJ. Epidemiology of osteoarthritis and associated comorbidities. PM R 2012;4:S10–19.

32. Srikanth VK, Fryer JL, Zhai G, et al. A meta-analysis of sex differences prevalence, incidence and severity of osteoarthritis. Osteoarthritis Cartilage 2005;13:769–81.

33. Zhang Y, Jordan JM. Epidemiology of osteoarthritis. Clin Geriatr Med 2010;26:355–69.

34. Felson D, Lawrence R, Dieppe P, et al. Osteoarthritis: new insights: part 1: the disease and its risk factors. Ann Intern Med 2000;133:635–46.

35. Lohmander LS, Englund PM, Dahl LL, et al. The long-term consequence of anterior cruciate ligament and meniscus injuries: osteoarthritis. Am J Sports Med 2007;35:1756–69.

36. Felson DT, Hannan MT, Naimark A, et al. Occupational physical demands, knee bending, and knee osteoarthritis: results from the Framingham Study. J Rheumatol 1991;18:1587–92.

37. Blagojevic M, Jinks C, Jeffery A, et al. Risk factors for onset of osteoarthritis of the knee in older adults: a systematic review and meta-analysis. Osteoarthritis Cartilage 2010;18:24–33.

38. Felson DT, Niu J, Clancy M, et al. Effect of recreational physical activities on the development of knee osteoarthritis in older adults of different weights: the Framingham Study. Arthritis Rheum 2007;57:6–12.

39. Chapple CM, Nicholson H, Baxter GD, et al. Patient characteristics that predict progression of knee osteoarthritis: a systematic review of prognostic studies. Arthritis Care Res 2011;63:1115–25.

40. Zhu Y. Bias introduced by conditioning on an intermediate variable: comment on the article by Zhang et al. Arthritis Care Res 2011;63:784.

41. Brandt KD, Dieppe P, Radin E. Etiopathogenesis of osteoarthritis. Med Clin North Am 2009;93:1–24, xv.

42. Zhao D, Banks SA, Mitchell KH, et al. Correlation between the knee adduction torque and medial contact force for a variety of gait patterns. J Orthop Res 2007;25:789–97.

43. Schipplein OD, Andriacchi TP. Interaction between active and passive knee stabilizers during level walking. J Orthop Res 1991;9:113–19.

44. Miyazaki T, Wada M, Kawahara H, et al. Dynamic load at baseline can predict radiographic disease progression in medial compartment knee osteoarthritis. Ann Rheum Dis 2002;61:617–22.

45. Bennell KL, Bowles KA, Wang Y, et al. Higher dynamic medial knee load predicts greater cartilage loss over 12 months in medial knee osteoarthritis. Ann Rheum Dis 2011;70:1770–4.

46. Sharma L, Song J, Dunlop D, et al. Varus and valgus alignment and incident and progressive knee osteoarthritis. Ann Rheum Dis 2010;69:1940–5.

47. Sharma L, Song J, Felson DT, et al. The role of knee alignment in disease progression and functional decline in knee osteoarthritis. JAMA 2001;286:188–95.

48. Chang AH, Chmiel JS, Moisio KC, et al. Varus thrust and knee frontal plane dynamic motion in persons with knee osteoarthritis. Osteoarthritis Cartilage 2013;21:1668–73.

49. Chang A, Hayes K, Dunlop D, et al. Thrust during ambulation and the progression of knee osteoarthritis. Arthritis Rheum 2004;50:3897–903.

50. Kuroyanagi Y, Nagura T, Kiriyama Y, et al. A quantitative assessment of varus thrust in patients with medial knee osteoarthritis. Knee 2012;19:130–4.

51. Lo GH, Harvey WF, McAlindon TE. Associations of varus thrust and alignment with pain in knee osteoarthritis. Arthritis Rheum 2012;64:2252–9.

52. Felson DT, Niu J, McClennan C, et al. Knee buckling: prevalence, risk factors, and associated limitations in function. Ann Intern Med 2007;147:534–40.

53. Fitzgerald GK, Piva SR, Irrgang JJ. Reports of joint instability in knee osteoarthritis: its prevalence and relationship to physical function. Arthritis Rheum 2004;51:941–6.

54. Shelburne KB, Torry MR, Pandy MG. Contributions of muscles, ligaments, and the ground-reaction force to tibiofemoral joint loading during normal gait. J Orthop Res 2006;24:1983–90.

55. Sritharan P, Lin YC, Pandy MG. Muscles that do not cross the knee contribute to the knee adduction moment and tibiofemoral compartment loading during gait. J Orthop Res 2012;30:1586–95.

56. Winby CR, Lloyd DG, Besier TF, et al. Muscle and external load contribution to knee joint contact loads during normal gait. J Biomech 2009;42:2294–300.

57. Bennell KL, Wrigley TV, Hunt MA, et al. Update on the role of muscle in the genesis and management of knee osteoarthritis. Rheum Dis Clin North Am 2013;39:145–76.

58. Childs JD, Sparto PJ, Fitzgerald GK, et al. Alterations in lower extremity movement and muscle activation patterns in individuals with knee osteoarthritis. Clin Biomech 2004;19:44–9.

59. Heiden TL, Lloyd DG, Ackland TR. Knee joint kinematics, kinetics and muscle co-contraction in knee osteoarthritis patient gait. Clin Biomech 2009;24:833–41.

60. Hortobagyi T, Westerkamp L, Beam S, et al. Altered hamstring-quadriceps muscle balance in patients with knee osteoarthritis. Clin Biomech (Bristol, Avon) 2005;20:97–104.

61. Porcheret M, Healey E, Dziedzic K, et al. Osteoarthritis: a modern approach to diagnosis and management. Arthritis Res UK 2011;6:1–9.

62. Zhang W, Doherty M, Peat G, et al. EULAR evidence-based recommendations for the diagnosis of knee osteoarthritis. Ann Rheum Dis 2010;69:483–9.

63. Schouten JS, Valkenburg HA. Classification criteria: methodological considerations and results from a 12 year following study in the general population. J Rheumatol Suppl 1995;43:44–5.

64. Peat G, Duncan RC, Wood LR, et al. Clinical features of symptomatic patellofemoral joint osteoarthritis. Arthritis Res Ther 2012;14:R63.

65. Peat G, Thomas E, Duncan R, et al. Clinical classification criteria for knee osteoarthritis: performance in the general population and primary care. Ann Rheum Dis 2006;65:1363–7.

66. Peat G, Thomas E, Duncan R, et al. Estimating the probability of radiographic osteoarthritis in the older patient with knee pain. Arthritis Rheum 2007;57:794–802.

67. Cibere J, Bellamy N, Thorne A, et al. Reliability of the knee examination in osteoarthritis: effect of standardization. Arthritis Rheum 2004;50:458–68.

68. Wood L, Peat G, Wilkie R, et al. A study of the noninstrumented physical examination of the knee found high observer variability. J Clin Epidemiol 2006;59:512–20.

69. Riddle DL. Validity of clinical measures of frontal plane knee alignment: data from the osteoarthritis initiative. Man Ther 2012;17:459–65.

70. Gooberman-Hill R, Woolhead G, Mackichan F, et al. Assessing chronic joint pain: lessons from a focus group study. Arthritis Rheum 2007;57:666–71.

71. Hawker GA, Stewart L, French MR, et al. Understanding the pain experience in hip and knee osteoarthritis – an OARSI/OMERACT initiative. Osteoarthritis Cartilage 2008;16:415–22.

72. Marty M, Hilliquin P, Rozenberg S, et al. Validation of the KOFUS (Knee Osteoarthritis Flare-Ups Score). Joint Bone Spine 2009;76:268–72.

73. Cibere J, Zhang H, Thorne A, et al. Association of clinical findings with pre-radiographic and radiographic knee osteoarthritis in a population-based study. Arthritis Care Res 2010;62:1691–8.

74. Kellgren JH, Lawrence JS. Rheumatism in miners. II. X-ray study. Br J Ind Med 1952;9:197–207.

75. Arthritis and Musculoskeletal Alliance. Standards of Care for People with Osteoarthritis. 2004.

76. Bedson J, McCarney R, Croft P. Labelling chronic illness in primary care: a good or a bad thing? Br J Gen Pract 2004;54:932–8.

77. Moynihan R, Doust J, Henry D. Preventing overdiagnosis: how to stop harming the healthy. BMJ 2012;344:e3502.

78. Collins NJ, Misra D, Felson DT, et al. Measures of knee function: International Knee Documentation Committee (IKDC)

Subjective Knee Evaluation Form, Knee Injury and Osteoarthritis Outcome Score (KOOS), Knee Injury and Osteoarthritis Outcome Score Physical Function Short Form (KOOS-PS), Knee Outcome Survey Activities of Daily Living Scale (KOS-ADL), Lysholm Knee Scoring Scale, Oxford Knee Score (OKS), Western Ontario and McMaster Universities Osteoarthritis Index (WOMAC), Activity Rating Scale (ARS), and Tegner Activity Score (TAS). Arthritis Care Res 2011;63:S208–28.

79. Fries JF, Cella D, Rose M, et al. Progress in assessing physical function in arthritis: PROMIS short forms and computerized adaptive testing. J Rheumatol 2009;36:2061–6.

80. Broderick JE, Schneider S, Junghaenel DU, et al. Validity and reliability of patient-reported outcomes measurement information system instruments in osteoarthritis. Arthritis Care Res 2013;65: 1625–33.

81. Arthritis Res UK & Chartered Society of Physiotherapy. The Musculoskeletal Patient-Reported Outcome Measure (M-PROM). 2013.

82. Stratford PW, Kennedy DM. Performance measures were necessary to obtain a complete picture of osteoarthritic patients. J Clin Epidemiol 2006;59:160–7.

83. Dobson F, Hinman RS, Roos EM, et al. OARSI recommended performance-based tests to assess physical function in people diagnosed with hip or knee osteoarthritis. Osteoarthritis Cartilage 2013;21:1042–52.

84. Kroman SL, Roos EM, Bennell KL, et al. Measurement properties of performance-based outcome measures to assess physical function in young and middle-aged people known to be at high risk of hip and/or knee osteoarthritis: a systematic review. Osteoarthritis Cartilage 2014;22(1):26–39.

85. Zhang W, Moskowitz RW, Nuki G, et al. OARSI recommendations for the management of hip and knee osteoarthritis, part II: OARSI evidence-based, expert consensus guidelines. Osteoarthritis Cartilage 2008;16:137–62.

86. Pinto RZ, Ferreira ML, Oliveira VC, et al. Patient-centred communication is associated with positive therapeutic alliance: a systematic review. J Physiother 2012;58:77–87.

87. Hall AM, Ferreira PH, Maher CG, et al. The influence of the therapist-patient relationship on treatment outcome in physical rehabilitation: a systematic review. Phys Ther 2010;90:1099–110.

88. Chan DK, Lonsdale C, Ho PY, et al. Patient motivation and adherence to postsurgery rehabilitation exercise recommendations: the influence of physiotherapists' autonomy-supportive behaviors. Arch Phys Med Rehabil 2009;90:1977–82.

89. Louw A, Diener I, Butler DS, et al. The effect of neuroscience education on pain, disability, anxiety, and stress in chronic musculoskeletal pain. Arch Phys Med Rehabil 2011;92:2041–56.

90. Nicholson P, French S, Hodges P, et al., editors. Key patient messages. OARSI Scientific Congress; 2014; Paris: Osteoarthr Cartilage.

91. Fernandes L, Hagen KB, Bijlsma JW, et al. EULAR recommendations for the non-pharmacological core management of hip and knee osteoarthritis. Ann Rheum Dis 2013;72:1125–35.

92. Hochberg MC, Altman RD, Toupin April K, et al. American College of Rheumatology 2012 recommendations for the use of nonpharmacologic and pharmacologic therapies in osteoarthritis of the hand, hip, and knee. Arthritis Care Res 2012;64:465–74.

93. Conaghan PG, Dickson J, Grant RL. Care and management of osteoarthritis in adults: summary of NICE guidance. BMJ 2008;336:502–3.

94. Uthman OA, van der Windt DA, Jordan JL, et al. Exercise for lower limb osteoarthritis: systematic review incorporating trial sequential analysis and network meta-analysis. BMJ 2013;347: f5555.

95. Fransen M, McConnell S. Exercise for osteoarthritis of the knee. Cochrane Database Syst Rev 2008;(4):CD004376.

96. Pelland L, Brosseau L, Wells G, et al. Efficacy of strengthening exercises for osteoarthritis (part I): a meta-analysis. Phys Ther Rev 2004;9:77–108.

97. Wallis JA, Taylor NF. Pre-operative interventions (non-surgical and non-pharmacological) for patients with hip or knee osteoarthritis awaiting joint replacement surgery – a systematic review and meta-analysis. Osteoarthritis Cartilage 2011;19:1381–95.

98. Messier SP, Mihalko SL, Legault C, et al. Effects of intensive diet and exercise on knee joint loads, inflammation, and clinical outcomes among overweight and obese adults with knee osteoarthritis: the IDEA randomized clinical trial. JAMA 2013;310: 1263–73.

99. Zhang W, Nuki G, Moskowitz RW, et al. OARSI recommendations for the management of hip and knee osteoarthritis: part III: changes in evidence following systematic cumulative update of research published through 2009. Osteoarthritis Cartilage 2010;18:476–99.

100. Bennell KL, Hunt MA, Wrigley TV, et al. Hip strengthening reduces symptoms but not knee load in people with medial knee osteoarthritis and varus malalignment: a randomised controlled trial. Osteoarthritis Cartilage 2010;18:621–8.

101. Foroughi N, Smith RM, Lange AK, et al. Lower limb muscle strengthening does not change frontal plane moments in women with knee osteoarthritis: a randomized controlled trial. Clin Biomech 2011;26:167–74.

102. Lim BW, Hinman RS, Wrigley TV, et al. Does knee malalignment mediate the effects of quadriceps strengthening on knee adduction moment, pain, and function in medial knee osteoarthritis? A randomized controlled trial. Arthritis Rheum 2008;59:943–51.

103. Mikesky AE, Mazzuca SA, Brandt KD, et al. Effects of strength training on the incidence and progression of knee osteoarthritis. Arthritis Rheum 2006;55:690–9.

104. Tanaka R, Ozawa J, Kito N, et al. Efficacy of strengthening or aerobic exercise on pain relief in people with knee osteoarthritis: a systematic review and meta-analysis of randomized controlled trials. Clin Rehabil 2013;27:1059–71.

105. Jan M, Lin C, Lin Y, et al. Effects of weight-bearing versus nonweight-bearing exercise on function, walking speed, and position sense in participants with knee osteoarthritis: a randomized controlled trial. Arch Phys Med Rehabil 2009;90:897–904.

106. Ageberg E, Link A, Roos EM. Feasibility of neuromuscular training in patients with severe hip or knee OA: the individualized goal-based NEMEX-TJR training program. BMC Musculoskelet Disord 2010;11:126.

107. Dunlop DD, Song J, Semanik PA, et al. Objective physical activity measurement in the osteoarthritis initiative: are guidelines being met? Arthritis Rheum 2011;63(11):3372–82.

108. Pisters MF, Veenhof C, van Meeteren NL, et al. Long-term effectiveness of exercise therapy in patients with osteoarthritis of the hip or knee: a systematic review. Arthritis Rheum 2007;57:1245–53.

109. Ettinger WH Jr, Burns R, Messier SP, et al. A randomized trial comparing aerobic exercise and resistance exercise with a health education program in older adults with knee osteoarthritis. The Fitness Arthritis and Seniors Trial (FAST). JAMA 1997;277:25–31.

110. Jordan JL, Holden MA, Mason EE, et al. Interventions to improve adherence to exercise for chronic musculoskeletal pain in adults. Cochrane Database Syst Rev 2010;(20):CD005956.

111. Marks R. Knee osteoarthritis and exercise adherence: a review. Curr Aging Sci 2012;5:72–83.

112. Walsh NE, Hurley MV. Evidence based guidelines and current practice for physiotherapy management of knee osteoarthritis. Musculoskeletal Care 2009;7:45–56.

113. Brantingham JW, Bonnefin D, Perle SM, et al. Manipulative therapy for lower extremity conditions: update of a literature review. J Manipulative Physiol Ther 2012;35:127–66.

114. French HP, Brennan A, White B, et al. Manual therapy for osteoarthritis of the hip or knee – a systematic review. Man Ther 2011;16:109–17.

115. Jansen MJ, Viechtbauer W, Lenssen AF, et al. Strength training alone, exercise therapy alone, and exercise therapy with passive manual mobilisation each reduce pain and disability in people with knee osteoarthritis: a systematic review. J Physiother 2011;57 :11–20.

116. Abbott JH, Robertson MC, Chapple C, et al. Manual therapy, exercise therapy, or both, in addition to usual care, for osteoarthritis of the hip or knee: a randomized controlled trial. 1: clinical effectiveness. Osteoarthritis Cartilage 2013;21(4):525–34.

117. Kirkley A, Webster-Bogaert S, Litchfield R, et al. The effect of bracing on varus gonarthrosis. J Bone Joint Surg Am 1999;81: 539–48.

118. Brouwer R, Jakma T, Verhagen A, et al. Braces and orthoses for treating osteoarthritis of the knee. Cochrane Lib 2005;(1): CD004020.

119. Lindenfeld TN, Hewett TE, Andriacchi TP. Joint loading with valgus bracing in patients with varus gonarthrosis. Clin Orthop Relat Res 1997;344:290–7.

120. Pollo FE, Otis JC, Backus SI, et al. Reduction of medial compartment loads with valgus bracing of the osteoarthritic knee. Am J Sports Med 2002;30:414–21.

121. Fantini Pagani CH, Willwacher S, Kleis B, et al. Influence of a valgus knee brace on muscle activation and co-contraction in patients with medial knee osteoarthritis. J Electromyogr Kinesiol 2013;23:490–500.

122. McWalter EJ, Hunter DJ, Harvey WF, et al. The effect of a patellar brace on three-dimensional patellar kinematics in patients with lateral patellofemoral osteoarthritis. Osteoarthritis Cartilage 2011;19:801–8.

123. Felson D, Parkes M, Gait A, et al. A Randomised Trial Of A Brace For Patellofemoral Osteoarthritis Targeting Knee Pain and Bone Marrow Lesions. ACR Annual Meeting, San Diego, USA. 2013.

124. Andriacchi TP, Mundermann A. The role of ambulatory mechanics in the initiation and progression of knee osteoarthritis. Curr Opin Rheumatol 2006;18:514–18.

125. Kean CO, Bennell KL, Wrigley TV, et al. Modified walking shoes for knee osteoarthritis: mechanisms for reductions in the knee adduction moment. J Biomech 2013;46:2060–6.

126. Hinman RS, Bowles KA, Metcalf BB, et al. Lateral wedge insoles for medial knee osteoarthritis: effects on lower limb frontal plane biomechanics. Clin Biomech 2012;27:27–33.

127. Radzimski AO, Mundermann A, Sole G. Effect of footwear on the external knee adduction moment – a systematic review. Knee 2012;19:163–75.

128. Parkes MJ, Maricar N, Lunt M, et al. Lateral wedge insoles as a conservative treatment for pain in patients with medial knee osteoarthritis: a meta-analysis. JAMA 2013;310:722–30.

129. Bennell K, Bowles K, Payne C, et al. Lateral wedge shoe insoles for medial knee osteoarthritis: 12 month randomised controlled trial. BMJ 2011;342:2912.

130. Rodrigues P, Ferreira A, Pereira R, et al. Effectiveness of medial-wedge insole treatment for valgus knee osteoarthritis. Arthritis Care Res 2008;59:603–8.

131. Turpin KM, De Vincenzo A, Apps AM, et al. Biomechanical and clinical outcomes with shock-absorbing insoles in patients with knee osteoarthritis: immediate effects and changes after 1 month of wear. Arch Phys Med Rehabil 2012;93:503–8.

132. Kerrigan D, Johansson J, Bryant M, et al. Moderate-heeled shoes and knee joint torques relevant to the development and progression of knee osteoarthritis. Arch Phys Med Rehabil 2005;86:871–5.

133. Kerrigan D, Karvosky M, Lelas J, et al. Men's shoes and knee joint torques relevant to the development and progression of knee osteoarthritis. J Rheumatol 2003;30:529–33.

134. Kerrigan D, Lelas J, Karvosky M. Women's shoes and knee osteoarthritis. Lancet 2001;357:1097–8.

135. Kerrigan DC, Todd MK, Riley PO. Knee osteoarthritis and high-heeled shoes. Lancet 1998;351:1399–401.

136. Shakoor N, Sengupta M, Foucher KC, et al. Effects of common footwear on joint loading in osteoarthritis of the knee. Arthritis Care Res 2010;62:917–23.

137. Sacco IC, Trombini-Souza F, Butugan MK, et al. Joint loading decreased by inexpensive and minimalist footwear in elderly women with knee osteoarthritis during stair descent. Arthritis Care Res 2012;64:368–74.

138. Trombini-Souza F, Kimura A, Ribeiro AP, et al. Inexpensive footwear decreases joint loading in elderly women with knee osteoarthritis. Gait Posture 2011;34:126–30.

139. Erhart JC, Dyrby CO, D'Lima DD, et al. Changes in in vivo knee loading with a variable-stiffness intervention shoe correlate with changes in the knee adduction moment. J Orthop Res 2010;28:1548–53.

140. Erhart JC, Mundermann A, Elspas B, et al. A variable-stiffness shoe lowers the knee adduction moment in subjects with symptoms of medial compartment knee osteoarthritis. J Biomech 2008;41:2720–5.

141. Shakoor N, Lidtke RH, Sengupta M, et al. Effects of specialized footwear on joint loads in osteoarthritis of the knee. Arthritis Rheum 2008;59:1214–20.

142. Nigg B, Emery C, Hiemstra L. Unstable shoe construction and reduction of pain in osteoarthritis patients. Med Sci Sports Exerc 2006;38:1701–8.

143. Buchecker M, Wagner H, Pfusterschmied J, et al. Lower extremity joint loading during level walking with Masai barefoot technology shoes in overweight males. Scand J Med Sci Sports 2012;22:372–80.

144. Simic M, Hinman RS, Wrigley TV, et al. Gait modification strategies for altering medial knee joint load: a systematic review. Arthritis Care Res 2011;63(3):405–26.

145. Simic M, Bennell KL, Hunt MA, et al. Contralateral cane use and knee joint load in people with medial knee osteoarthritis: the effect of varying body weight support. Osteoarthritis Cartilage 2011;19:1330–7.

146. Jones A, Silva PG, Silva AC, et al. Impact of cane use on pain, function, general health and energy expenditure during gait in patients with knee osteoarthritis: a randomised controlled trial. Ann Rheum Dis 2012;71:172–9.

147. Vickers AJ, Cronin AM, Maschino AC, et al. Acupuncture for chronic pain: individual patient data meta-analysis. Arch Intern Med 2012;172:1444–53.

148. Corbett MS, Rice SJ, Madurasinghe V, et al. Acupuncture and other physical treatments for the relief of pain due to osteoarthritis of the knee: network meta-analysis. Osteoarthritis Cartilage 2013;21:1290–8.

149. Whitehurst DG, Bryan S, Hay EM, et al. Cost-effectiveness of acupuncture care as an adjunct to exercise-based physical therapy for osteoarthritis of the knee. Phys Ther 2011;91:630–41.

CHAPTER 49

ANKLE INJURY

Claire Hiller • Kathryn Refshauge

Ankle injuries are among the most common injuries in both sporting and non-sporting populations.[1-5] The most common ankle injuries presenting to the clinic are ankle sprains and ankle fractures. It is not the intent of this chapter to discuss detailed assessment and management of these conditions, but rather to highlight the recent issues and advances in the area of ankle sprain and the related syndesmosis injury and chronic ankle instability, and fracture.

EPIDEMIOLOGY

Acute ankle sprains are among the most common sporting injuries[4] and are responsible for a high proportion of attendances at emergency centres.[2] A recent meta-analysis found that the incidence of ankle sprains was higher in female athletes, the young, and athletes of indoor and court sports. However, the pooled prevalence across subgroups was similar, being approximately 11% of all injuries.[3] The incidence of lateral sprains (0.93 per 1000 athlete exposures) was almost three times higher than syndesmosis sprains (0.38) and nine times higher than medial sprains (0.06).[3] The majority of studies on incidence of ankle injuries have focused primarily on lateral ankle sprain; however, the incidence of syndesmosis injury appears to be increasing.

Syndesmosis sprain, also known as a 'high' ankle sprain, is a sprain of the soft tissues of the inferior tibiofibular joint. Originally, only the interosseous membrane was considered to constitute the syndesmosis. Recent evidence suggests that an injury of any of the following anatomic structures is considered a syndesmosis sprain: the ankle interosseous membrane, the interosseous ligament, the anterior tibiofibular ligament and the posterior inferior tibiofibular ligament with its transverse ligament.[6] The inferior tibiofibular joint is a very stable joint due to both bony congruence and ligamentous restraints.[6] The inferior tibiofibular joint is so strong it is reported that the syndesmosis and ankle mortise only widen 1 mm during normal gait.[7] An increase in this widening by as little as 1 mm decreases the contact area of the tibiofibular joint by 42%.[8]

The reported incidence of ankle syndesmosis injury varies between 1%[9] and 25%[10] of all ankle sprains. This wide range may be due to a real increase in incidence, or may be due to improved diagnosis of syndesmosis injury. While ankle sprains are easily recognized, diagnosis of syndesmosis injuries has proved more elusive. However, recent evidence has improved diagnostic accuracy of syndesmosis injury using simple tests available in any setting.

Chronic ankle instability (CAI) is the most commonly used term to describe ongoing problems following an ankle sprain.[11] Reported problems include recurrent sprain, the ankle feeling unstable or giving way, altered range of motion (either increased laxity or stiffness) and pain.[12] These problems may exist in isolation or combination.[13] CAI can result in disability, decreased physical activity or job participation,[14-17] and the development of ankle osteoarthritis.[18]

CAI appears to be highly prevalent. A systematic review found that between 15% and 64% of people had not recovered 3 years after their ankle sprain.[19] It has been reported that 8% of people in the general population have ongoing problems after ankle sprain, and for the majority these problems had persisted for more than 10 years.[15] Despite research increasing exponentially in the past few years, much remains unknown about CAI.

PROGNOSIS

The typical clinical course after a lateral ankle sprain is a marked decrease in pain and increase in function within 2 weeks.[19] Whereas most people recover, up to 18% still have problems years later.[15] While it appears intuitive that the severity of a lateral ankle sprain would be related to recovery time or likelihood of residual problems, evidence for this is lacking.[20] Currently it is unknown who will develop ongoing problems after an ankle sprain, unless the injury involves the joint.

It has frequently been reported that recovery from an ankle syndesmosis injury takes longer than recovery from a lateral ankle sprain.[9,21-23] The reported delayed recovery varies widely, ranging from 2 to 20 times that of lateral ankle sprain. To increase precision, and overcome some of the methodological flaws of previous studies, a recent prospective study used magnetic resonance imaging (MRI) to determine recovery times for syndesmosis injury. This study found that it took four times longer to return to sport or activity after syndesmosis injury than after ankle sprain (62 versus 15 days mean recovery time).[24] The same study found that any person with a lateral ankle sprain or syndesmosis injury who had not recovered within 2 weeks of injury, was likely to have prolonged recovery if the vertical jump height was reduced or the score on the Fear Avoidance Beliefs Questionnaire Sport subscale was high.[24] In addition, a positive squeeze test or an increased tenderness on palpation of the anterior interosseous membrane has been found to be strongly related to time to return to sport.[25-27]

There has been no investigation of prognosis for people who have developed CAI, except for an acknowledgement that some injuries ultimately progress to post-traumatic ankle osteoarthritis.[18]

RISK FACTORS

Many risk factors for ankle injuries have been proposed with few definitive findings. The risk of an ankle injury was found to be increased in people with greater postural sway, lower postural stability, decreased eccentric inversion strength at slow speeds of isokinetic testing, and higher concentric plantarflexion strength at high speeds of isokinetic testing.[28] However, no risk factors have been substantiated for an initial ankle sprain. Systematic reviews of studies which investigated mixed groups of participants (i.e. those with and those without a previous history of sprain) have suggested that females of younger age,[3] with poor postural control,[29,30] and limited dorsiflexion[29] are at higher risk of future ankle sprain.

There are no confirmed risk factors for syndesmosis injury, and unlike other ankle sprains a previous ankle sprain or high ankle sprain does not appear to increase the likelihood of re-injury.[31] One study noted that there is a higher risk of syndesmosis injury among American football players who play on artificial surfaces compared with natural grass.[10]

The only confirmed predictor for CAI is a history of previous ankle sprain.[20] A recent systematic review of prospective studies that followed people after their first sprain to identify those who developed CAI, found only four studies. The score on the Cumberland Ankle Instability Tool (a questionnaire to measure ankle instability with excellent psychometric properties)[32] and number of foot lifts in 30 seconds with the eyes closed[33] did not predict re-sprain. One study found that severity of the index sprain predicted re-sprain but methodological issues suggest that the findings should be interpreted with caution.[20]

DIAGNOSIS

It is now clear that early, accurate diagnosis of the specific ankle injury is critical to ensure effective treatment that is specific to the injury. The diagnoses that are most commonly missed are fracture, syndesmosis injury, talar dome lesion or occasionally the less common injuries and abnormalities such as subtalar sprain or tarsal coalition.[34]

Imaging is often used to confirm differential diagnosis of ankle injury. X-rays are mainly used for identifying bony injury (e.g. fractures or a tibiofibular diastasis associated with a syndesmosis injury).[35] The use of stress X-rays for lateral ligament[36] or syndesmosis injury[37] does not have high diagnostic accuracy. MRI has the best diagnostic accuracy for ligament and syndesmosis injury[36,38,39] but is relatively expensive to be considered for routine use. Ultrasound imaging is cheap and quick but reliability and accuracy of diagnosis are strongly operator-dependent. Most research in the area of ultrasound diagnosis has used expert radiographers rather than trained clinicians, and demonstrated that ultrasound has a high degree of accuracy for diagnosis of acute[36] and chronic ATFL injury[40,41] and anterior tibiofibular ligament injury.[42] One recent study compared bedside ultrasound in the emergency department, utilized by clinicians with 6 hours of training, with MRI to identify ATFL injury. The results of bedside ultrasound were comparable to MRI indicating that the use of real-time ultrasound in the clinic has promise for initial triaging and decisions for further investigations.[43]

Fracture

One of the important differential diagnoses at initial presentation is the possible presence of an ankle fracture. It is not uncommon for a lateral sprain to be accompanied by an avulsion fracture, particularly in children. Ankle syndesmosis injuries are usually incomplete, but may be accompanied by an ankle fracture or less commonly by a fracture of the proximal fibula.[44]

The Ottawa Ankle Rules (OAR) should be utilized to rule out fractures or the need for X-rays.[45] X-rays should only be ordered if there is pain in either malleolar zone and any of: bone tenderness at either malleolar tip, or along the distal 6 cm of the posterior edge of the tibia or fibular, or inability to bear weight for four steps both immediately after injury and in the clinician's rooms. The likelihood of an acute injury being an ankle fracture when the OAR is negative is around 1.4%.[46]

A modification of the OAR has been developed for paediatric use to further decrease exposure to X-rays.[47] On clinical examination, if the only findings are tenderness and swelling over the distal fibula or adjacent lateral ligaments distal to the tibial anterior joint line, an X-ray is not required. These injuries have been deemed low-risk ankle injuries that can be managed conservatively. Such low-risk injuries include lateral ankle sprains, non-displaced Salter–Harris types I and II fractures of the distal fibula and avulsion fractures of the distal fibula or lateral talus.[47] Although all investigations of the OAR have been conducted in emergency departments, it is highly likely that the decision rules would generalize to most clinicians in any setting.

Ankle Sprain

Inversion Sprain

The mechanism of injury for an inversion sprain has long been believed to be inversion of the plantar flexed ankle.[48] However, recent case reports using three-dimensional biomechanical analysis of real-time ankle sprain incidents, report that inversion with internal rotation may be a more important mechanism.[49]

The primary clinical diagnostic tests for inversion sprain are the anterior drawer and talar tilt tests. Despite their common use there is little evidence of their diagnostic accuracy.[50] It may be that the anterior drawer test carried out 4–5 days post injury, together with the presence of pain on palpation of the ligament, and evidence of bruising, may be more accurate diagnostic indicators of a ligament sprain.[51]

There are a number of systems used to grade the severity of an ankle sprain injury[52] with no system having evidence for high reliability or validity, and none is universally accepted. For the clinician it is more important to ensure identification of severe pathologies and any associated injuries to ensure implementation of the most appropriate treatment and timely referral if required.

Syndesmosis Injury

During the history, a high index of suspicion should be raised that the injury has disrupted the ankle syndesmosis if the mechanism of injury involved external rotation of the foot. Other physical findings consistent with syndesmotic injuries include palpatory tenderness over the syndesmotic ligaments and swelling proximal to the ankle joint line.[53]

Many diagnostic clinical tests have been proposed but until recently there has been little evidence to support their use. A recent systematic review of diagnostic tests for syndesmosis injury found only two studies that examined the validity of some tests.[54] Diagnostic validity of the anterior drawer, cotton, dorsiflexion, external rotation and fibula translation tests was poor. Results for validity of the squeeze test were conflicting (LR −1.50 to +1.50), and reliability of other diagnostic tests was variable. Intra-rater reliability was high in terms of percentage close agreement (PCA) for the squeeze, cotton, external rotation and dorsiflexion tests (PCA >83%). Inter-rater reliability was good (intraclass correlation coefficient >0.70) for the external rotation stress test, and fair to poor for the squeeze, dorsiflexion, cotton, anterior drawer and fibular translation tests (intraclass correlation coefficient <0.46).[54]

More recently, diagnostic accuracy of the clinical examination for syndesmosis injury was determined by comparing test findings with findings on MRI.[55] Eight symptoms and five physical signs were investigated. Symptoms included mechanism of injury (dorsiflexion and external rotation of the foot), inability to continue to play or walk, pain or dysfunction out of proportion to injury, pain in the shank or knee during injury, swelling above the ankle, inability to hop, pain during lunge with external rotation of the foot, and presence of a posterior impingement. Five diagnostic tests were investigated: palpation of syndesmosis ligaments; palpation of deltoid ligament; squeeze test; dorsiflexion lunge with compression; and dorsiflexion with external rotation stress test. The dorsiflexion with external rotation test was found to have the highest sensitivity (71%) and the squeeze test the highest specificity (88%). A combination of the two tests did not further improve sensitivity or specificity. Of all investigated symptoms, the only one to reach the predetermined level of 70% sensitivity was the inability to hop, and for specificity were pain out of proportion to the injury (whether too much or too little in relation to the mechanism) and pain in the shank or knee.

Taken together, these findings suggest the key questions in the history include: mechanism of injury (dorsiflexion or external rotation); inability to walk; or inability to perform a single leg hop. If any of the syndesmosis ligaments are painful to palpation and the dorsiflexion and rotation test is positive, then the squeeze test should be performed to confirm the injury. If the squeeze test is positive then it is very likely to be a syndesmosis injury and MRI is recommended (Table 49-1).

TABLE 49-1 **Summary of Recommended Syndesmosis Clinical Diagnostic Test Protocols**

	Protocol	Positive Findings	Rationale
Syndesmosis ligament palpation ©Amy Sman	Palpation of anterior tibiofibular ligament/ posterior inferior tibiofibular ligament –transverse ligament/ interosseous ligament/ interosseous membrane[25,56,57]	Report of pain during palpation of the ligament/ membrane[25,56,57]	The classic feature of ankle syndesmosis injury is thought to be palpatory tenderness over the anterior and posterior tibiofibular ligaments and between the tibia and fibula.[53,58] Tenderness proximally along the interosseous membrane was indicative of a longer time to recovery[25] and a more severe injury[59]

Continued on following page

TABLE 49-1 **Summary of Recommended Syndesmosis Clinical Diagnostic Test Protocols** (Continued)

	Protocol	Positive Findings	Rationale
Dorsiflexion-external rotation test 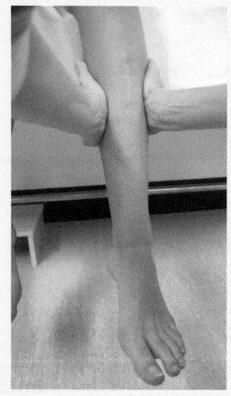©Amy Sman	Leg is stabilized in 90° knee flexion, the ankle in maximal dorsiflexion, and an external rotation stress to the injured foot and ankle is applied[23]	Reproduction of anterolateral pain over the syndesmosis area	The test is thought to reproduce pain over the ankle syndesmosis ligaments by mimicking the commonly described mechanism of injury[23,60–62]
Squeeze test	Patient sitting over side of the bed. Compression of fibula and tibia above the midpoint of the calf[9,61,63,64]	Replication of pain in the area of the ankle syndesmosis[9,61,63,64]	Biomechanical analysis confirmed that the calf compression causes separation at the distal tibiofibular joint.[63] It is thought to increase tension in the remaining ankle syndesmosis ligament fibres, resulting in pain at the ankle[65]

©Amy Sman

Chronic Ankle Instability

Diagnosis of CAI is relatively straightforward. Patients presenting with ongoing problems following an ankle sprain, including; pain, recurrent injury, mechanical ankle instability and functional ankle instability are likely to have CAI. There have been a number of methods developed to measure these different aspects of CAI. The two recommended by the International Ankle Consortium to measure functional (or perceived) instability are the Cumberland Ankle Instability Tool[32] and the Identification of Functional Ankle Instability.[66] A score of ≤27 out of 30 on the Cumberland Ankle Instability Tool is interpreted as indicating presence of functional ankle instability, although a score of ≤24 is recommended for research. A score of ≥10 out of 37 for the Identification of Functional Ankle Instability is also interpreted as presence of functional ankle instability.[12] A paediatric version of the

Cumberland Ankle Instability Tool has been developed for use in people aged 8 years and older.[67] For measuring disability related to CAI the Foot and Ankle Ability measure[68] and Foot and Ankle Outcome Score are recommended.[69]

IMPAIRMENTS

Once diagnosed, it is the impairments that are treated rather than the actual pathology. Typically, physical examination of a peripheral injury involves comparison of test results with the unaffected limb. However, the contralateral limb is likely not a useful comparator for determining impairment or monitoring progress. In addition to the prevalence of bilateral ankle problems, there is evidence that deficits are bilateral even after unilateral injury, e.g. in postural control and various balance tests, following an ankle sprain.[70]

Common impairments following acute ankle sprain are pain, swelling, reduced range of motion and decreased balance. Pain and swelling usually resolve quickly. The volume of swelling is only moderately correlated with injury severity[51] and is not associated with self-assessed function.[71] However, swelling that has not resolved within one month is related to ongoing decreased function and quality of life.[71,72] Reduced ankle range of motion occurs due to pain, swelling or loss of normal accessory joint motion in the ankle or subtalar joints.[73,74] Dorsiflexion is the most commonly impaired motion. Although ankle laxity improves during the first 6 to 12 weeks, it commonly persists for at least one year post injury.[75] The extent of ligament laxity is not associated with level of self-reported function.[76]

Both strength of the ankle muscles and postural control[30,70] are impaired following an ankle sprain. Strength may take up to 4 months post injury to normalize.[77–80]

Chronic ankle instability results in similar impairments to those of acute ankle sprain. Impairments identified from the highest level of evidence (i.e. in systematic reviews) include changes in morphology of the talus,[81] muscle weakness,[81,82] impaired balance or postural stability,[30,70,81,83,84] and decreased proprioceptive ability.[84,85] However, only specific types of muscle contraction or strength ratios are affected[81,82,84] and, similarly, only some aspects of proprioception are impaired.[81,84] Recent findings are indicative of changes in the central organization of movement in people with CAI. Not only are there bilateral postural deficits,[33,86] but also proximal changes in muscle patterns,[87–90] alterations in planned movement patterns[91–95] and changes in cortical[96,97] and peripheral sensory excitability.[98–100] It is currently thought that there may be an association between subgroups of CAI and various deficits;[13,91] however, there is no definitive evidence to support this proposal. It appears that the deficits experienced by people with CAI may be highly individual.[13] Clinicians should therefore take care to examine the presenting patient and not use a routine formula for treatment.

MANAGEMENT

Evidence and guidelines for the treatment of ankle sprains has been summarized and published in several countries over recent years. The reader is directed to these for a more detailed summary of the literature.[101–106] There are no studies of treatment for the conservative management of syndesmosis injuries. Overall, the majority of ankle sprains can be effectively managed using conservative treatments.

Surgery should rarely be considered.[107] Lateral sprains with severe mechanical joint instability, and syndesmosis injuries that also involve fractures or frank diastasis, require surgery. Currently the most common surgical techniques for severe syndesmosis injury are screws or suture buttons.[108] While both have excellent outcomes, suture buttons appear to provide a more accurate method of syndesmosis stabilization.[109]

Ankle Sprain

Conservative treatment in the initial phase after sprain, usually consists of the (P)RICE regimen for acute soft tissue injuries,[106] even though not all individual elements have strong evidence to support their use.[110] Protection in the form of functional support rather than immobilization is effective for most ankle sprains,[107] with the possible exception of severe sprains which may benefit from a rigid form of immobilization for a short (up to 10 days) period.[111] Functional support involves the use of a removable device and it appears that a semi-rigid brace is better than other supports (e.g. an elastic bandage) in terms of functional outcome and total cost.[112] The preferred type of functional support depends on the outcome required. A systematic review comparing the types of functional support (elastic bandage, tape, semi-rigid support and lace-up ankle support) found them to be equally effective for reducing pain, swelling, ankle instability and preventing recurrent sprain.[113] A semi-rigid support appeared more effective for earlier return to sport, and tape resulted in a higher rate of skin complications. A recent comparison of an Aircast ankle brace with an elastic support bandage demonstrated a significant improvement in ankle function at 10 days and 1 month when using the ankle brace.[114] The use of a protective device for a prolonged period for lateral ankle sprain is occasionally used, but has no research evidence to support its use, and is not recommended.

Manual therapy has been applied in a number of ways to treat ankle sprains.[115] In the acute phase both passive anteroposterior glide of the talus[116,117] and osteopathic ankle manipulation[118] reduced pain and increased dorsiflexion range of motion in the short term after lateral ankle sprain. For treatment in the subacute phase mobilization with movement, as described by Mulligan, a chiropractic mortise adjustment technique and an anteroposterior glide of the talus were all shown to improve ankle range of motion, reduce pain and improve function.[115]

Medications of various types have been suggested for ankle sprains. There is strong evidence that the use of non-steroidal anti-inflammatory drugs (NSAIDs) during the first 2 weeks following ankle sprain, administered orally or topically, is more effective than a placebo.[102] Non-steroidal anti-inflammatory drugs (Piroxicam) reduced pain and swelling and improved function in the short term with continued better functional outcomes than placebo for at least 6 months.[119] However, care should be taken to monitor early mobilization levels if choosing this option as the study also noted an increase in ankle instability in the treated group.

Exercise training includes interventions to restore range of motion, strength and sensorimotor function.[102] Various forms of exercise training have been shown to result in more rapid recovery for sprains of any severity,[120-123] although one study with apparently contradictory findings found that supervised rehabilitation was not superior to conventional treatment for recovery in participants in the Netherlands.[124] Both groups improved, potentially because usual care included home exercises in addition to early mobilization and ankle protection.

There is little evidence for the use of electrophysical agents for treatment of acute ankle sprains.[103,104,125] Ultrasound is not effective and should not be used in the treatment of acute ankle sprains.[126,127]

Syndesmosis Injury

No study to date has evaluated treatment for syndesmosis injury, and therefore recommendations must, of necessity, be based on logic and clinical wisdom. For stable injuries that involve the syndesmosis, the most common management is protection in a boot or brace for varying lengths of time[7,21,53,128,129] followed by rehabilitation. Tape has also been suggested when a brace is not suitable, and usually consists of a modified circumferential application placed above the malleoli with or without a modified subtalar sling.[53]

Clinical wisdom and logic would also caution against the use of manual therapy techniques at the ankle in the early stages of syndesmosis injury, as dorsiflexion widens the ankle mortise and places the syndesmotic ligaments under further stress. It is reasonable to assume that end-range dorsiflexion and weight-bearing activities also be avoided in the acute phase due to the potential for widening of the ankle mortise.

During later-stage rehabilitation, care should be taken with return to exercise, and consideration given to delaying activities with plyometrics, and cutting or changing direction manoeuvres. These activities could force the foot into external rotation relative to the tibia, thereby increasing strain of the syndesmosis.

Chronic Ankle Instability

Management of CAI encompasses a range of treatment options, all of which have limited evidence for their efficacy. The most common intervention is exercise, of varying forms, including elements variously described as 'balance', 'neuromuscular', strength and 'functional' training. While there is evidence that some form of exercise programme is more effective than no training for reducing sensorimotor deficits or improving function,[130] the size of the effect is moderate at best.[131] Furthermore, the variety of combinations of training modes, frequency and duration of exercise investigated precludes identification of the effective component(s).[131]

Manual therapy for CAI is effective for some outcomes, but not others. Mobilization techniques to improve ankle range of motion were shown to be mostly effective.[132-135] The techniques improved sports-related activities,[132] pain and function,[134,136] but did not change dynamic balance or activities of daily living.[132]

Orthotics for treating CAI should be used with caution. While orthotics have been shown to improve proprioceptive and balance abilities[137-140] the effect may not be greater than that of an exercise or rehabilitation intervention alone.[140]

Prevention of Further Ankle Sprain

The use of an external brace or ankle tape has been shown to decrease the recurrence of ankle sprains.[107,141] A recent randomized controlled trial compared an 8-week progressive home-based neuromuscular training programme with wearing an ankle brace for 12 months during sports activities, and a combination of the neuromuscular programme and 8 weeks of wearing the brace.[142] Bracing was more effective than training for reducing ankle sprain recurrence, but not the severity of sprain. While useful for sporting activities, such an intervention does not aid prevention when not wearing the brace during activities of daily living or for those who play a sport where braces are not permitted. Tape has also been shown to be effective although the rate of skin complications is higher and the long-term cost is greater. It would appear that using a brace or tape should be considered a long-term protective strategy for people participating in sports activities. Their use should continue after the rehabilitation training programme has finished.

CONCLUSION

Early accurate diagnosis of ankle injury is essential, in particular the identification of a fracture or syndesmosis injury, to ensure early effective management and to prevent further harm. Early identification of a syndesmosis injury is important as some common treatment techniques should be avoided or modified. While the 'simple sprain' is the most common presenting injury, there is no treatment 'recipe'. Treatment must be individualized according to findings on clinical examination, particularly for people who develop chronic ankle instability after sprain. However, the most effective treatment appears to be an exercise-based programme which involves strength, balance, neuromuscular and functional components.

REFERENCES

1. Boyce SH, Quigley MA. Review of sports injuries presenting to an accident and emergency department. Emerg Med J 2004;21(6):704–6.
2. Bridgman SA, Clement D, Downing A, et al. Population based epidemiology of ankle sprains attending accident and emergency units in the West Midlands of England, and a survey of UK practice for severe ankle sprains. Emerg Med J 2003;20(6):508–10.
3. Doherty C, Delahunt E, Caulfield B, et al. The incidence and prevalence of ankle sprain injury: a systematic review and meta-analysis of prospective epidemiological studies. Sports Med 2014;44(1):123–40.
4. Fong DT, Hong Y, Chan LK, et al. A systematic review on ankle injury and ankle sprain in sports. Sports Med [Review] 2007;37(1):73–94.
5. Marinos G, Giannopoulos A, Vlasis K, et al. Primary care in the management of common orthopaedic problems. Qual Prim Care 2008;16(5):345–9.
6. Lebech M, Andersen O, Christensen NC, et al. Feasibility of neonatal screening for toxoplasma infection in the absence of prenatal treatment. Danish Congenital Toxoplasmosis Study Group. Lancet 1999;353(9167):1834–7.
7. Lin CF, Gross ML, Weinhold P. Ankle syndesmosis injuries: anatomy, biomechanics, mechanism of injury, and clinical guidelines for diagnosis and intervention. J Orthop Sports Phys Ther 2006;36(6):372–84.
8. Hermans JJ, Beumer A, de Jong TA, et al. Anatomy of the distal tibiofibular syndesmosis in adults: a pictorial essay with a multi-modality approach. J Anat 2010;217(6):633–45.
9. Hopkinson WJ, St Pierre P, Ryan JB, et al. Syndesmosis sprains of the ankle. Foot Ankle 1990;10(6):325–30.
10. Hunt KJ, George E, Harris AH, et al. Epidemiology of syndesmosis injuries in intercollegiate football: incidence and risk factors from National Collegiate Athletic Association injury surveillance system data from 2004–2005 to 2008–2009. Clin J Sport Med 2013;23(4):278–82.
11. Delahunt E, Coughlan GF, Caulfield B, et al. Inclusion criteria when investigating insufficiencies in chronic ankle instability. Med Sci Sports Exerc [Review] 2010;42(11):2106–21.
12. Gribble PA, Delahunt E, Bleakley C, et al. Selection criteria for patients with chronic ankle instability in controlled research: a position statement of the international ankle consortium. J Orthop Sports Phys Ther 2013;43(8):585–91.
13. Hiller CE, Kilbreath SL, Refshauge KM. Chronic ankle instability: evolution of the model. J Athl Train [Research Support, Non-U.S. Gov't] 2011;46(2):133–41.
14. Arnold BL, Wright CJ, Ross SE. Functional ankle instability and health-related quality of life. J Athl Train 2011;46(6):634–41.
15. Hiller CE, Nightingale EJ, Raymond J, et al. Prevalence and impact of chronic musculoskeletal ankle disorders in the community. Arch Phys Med Rehabil 2012;93(10):1801–7.
16. Konradsen L, Bech L, Ehrenbjerg M, et al. Seven years follow-up after ankle inversion trauma. Scand J Med Sci Sports 2002;12(3):129–35.
17. Wikstrom EA, Tillman MD, Chmielewski TL, et al. Self-assessed disability and functional performance in individuals with and without ankle instability: a case control study. J Orthop Sports Phys Ther 2009;39(6):458–67.
18. Valderrabano V, Hintermann B, Horisberger M, et al. Ligamentous posttraumatic ankle osteoarthritis. Am J Sports Med 2006;34(4):612–20.
19. van Rijn RM, van Os AG, Bernsen RM, et al. What is the clinical course of acute ankle sprains? A systematic literature review. Am J Med [Review] 2008;121(4):324–31 e6.
20. Pourkazemi F, Hiller CE, Raymond J, et al. Predictors of chronic ankle instability after an index lateral ankle sprain: a systematic review. J Sci Med Sport 2014;17(6):568–73.
21. Osbahr DC, Drakos MC, O'Loughlin PF, et al. Syndesmosis and lateral ankle sprains in the national football league. Orthopedics 2013;36(11):e1378–84.
22. Wright RW, Barile RJ, Surprenant DA, et al. Ankle syndesmosis sprains in national hockey league players. Am J Sports Med 2004;32(8):1941–5.
23. Boytim MJ, Fischer DA, Neumann L. Syndesmotic ankle sprains. Am J Sports Med 1991;19(3):294–8.
24. Sman AD, Hiller CE, Rae K, et al. Prognosis of ankle syndesmosis injury. Med Sci Sports Exerc 2014;46(4):671–7.
25. Nussbaum ED, Hosea TM, Sieler SD, et al. Prospective evaluation of syndesmotic ankle sprains without diastasis. Am J Sports Med 2001;29(1):31–5.
26. Miller BS, Downie BK, Johnson PD, et al. Time to return to play after high ankle sprains in collegiate football players: a prediction model. Sports Health 2012;4(6):504–9.
27. Sikka RS, Fetzer GB, Sugarman E, et al. Correlating MRI findings with disability in syndesmotic sprains of NFL players. Foot Ankle Int 2012;33(5):371–8.
28. Witchalls J, Blanch P, Waddington G, et al. Intrinsic functional deficits associated with increased risk of ankle injuries: a systematic review with meta-analysis. Br J Sports Med [Meta-Analysis Research Support, Non-U.S. Gov't Review] 2012;46(7):515–23.
29. de Noronha M, Refshauge KM, Herbert RD, et al. Do voluntary strength, proprioception, range of motion, or postural sway predict occurrence of lateral ankle sprain? Br J Sports Med 2006;40(10):824–8, discussion 828.
30. McKeon PO, Hertel J. Systematic review of postural control and lateral ankle instability, part I: can deficits be detected with instrumented testing. J Athl Train 2008;43(3):293–304.
31. Sman AD, Hiller CE, Rae K, et al. Predictive factors for ankle syndesmosis injury in football players: a prospective study. J Sci Med Sport 2014;17(6):586–90.
32. Hiller CE, Refshauge KM, Bundy AC, et al. The Cumberland ankle instability tool: a report of validity and reliability testing. Arch Phys Med Rehabil [Research Support, Non-U.S. Gov't] 2006;87(9):1235–41.
33. Hiller CE, Refshauge KM, Herbert RD, et al. Balance and recovery from a perturbation are impaired in people with functional ankle instability. Clin J Sport Med [Comparative Study Research Support, Non-U.S. Gov't] 2007;17(4):269–75.
34. Brukner P, Khan K, Karlsson J. Acute ankle injuries. In: Brukner P, Khan K, editors. Clinical Sports Medicine. 3rd ed. Sydney: McGraw-Hill.; 2006. p. 612–31.
35. Harper MC, Keller TS. A radiographic evaluation of the tibiofibular syndesmosis. Foot Ankle 1989;10(3):156–60.
36. Oae K, Takao M, Uchio Y, et al. Evaluation of anterior talofibular ligament injury with stress radiography, ultrasonography and MR imaging. Skeletal Radiol 2010;39(1):41–7.
37. Pakarinen H, Flinkkila T, Ohtonen P, et al. Intraoperative assessment of the stability of the distal tibiofibular joint in supination-external rotation injuries of the ankle: sensitivity, specificity, and reliability of two clinical tests. J Bone Joint Surg Am 2011;93(22):2057–61.
38. Oae K, Takao M, Naito K, et al. Injury of the tibiofibular syndesmosis: value of MR imaging for diagnosis. Radiology 2003;227(1):155–61.
39. Takao M, Ochi M, Oae K, et al. Diagnosis of a tear of the tibiofibular syndesmosis. The role of arthroscopy of the ankle. J Bone Joint Surg Br 2003;85(3):324–9.
40. Cheng Y, Cai Y, Wang Y. Value of ultrasonography for detecting chronic injury of the lateral ligaments of the ankle joint compared with ultrasonography findings. Br J Radiol 2014;87(1033):20130406.
41. Hua Y, Yang Y, Chen S, et al. Ultrasound examination for the diagnosis of chronic anterior talofibular ligament injury. Acta Radiol 2012;53(10):1142–5.
42. Mei-Dan O, Kots E, Barchilon V, et al. A dynamic ultrasound examination for the diagnosis of ankle syndesmotic injury in professional athletes: a preliminary study. Am J Sports Med 2009;37(5):1009–16.
43. Gun C, Unluer EE, Vandenberk N, et al. Bedside ultrasonography by emergency physicians for anterior talofibular ligament injury. J Emerg Trauma Shock 2013;6(3):195–8.
44. Norkus SA, Floyd RT. The anatomy and mechanisms of syndesmotic ankle sprains. J Athl Train 2001;36(1):68–73.
45. Stiell IG, McKnight RD, Greenberg GH, et al. Implementation of the Ottawa ankle rules. JAMA 1994;271(11):827–32.
46. Bachmann LM, Kolb E, Koller MT, et al. Accuracy of Ottawa ankle rules to exclude fractures of the ankle and mid-foot: systematic review. BMJ [Meta-Analysis Review] 2003;326(7386):417.
47. Boutis K, Grootendorst P, Willan A, et al. Effect of the Low Risk Ankle Rule on the frequency of radiography in children with ankle injuries. CMAJ [Clinical Trial Multicenter Study Research Support, Non-U.S. Gov't] 2013;185(15):E731–8.

48. Koenig MD. Ligament Injuries of the Foot and Ankle in Adult Athletes. In: DeLee JC, Drez D, Miller MD, editors. DeLee and Drez's Orthopaedic Sports Medicine. 3rd ed. Philadelphia: Saunders/Elsevier.; 2010. p. 1912–60.

49. Fong DT, Ha SC, Mok KM, et al. Kinematics analysis of ankle inversion ligamentous sprain injuries in sports: five cases from televised tennis competitions. Am J Sports Med 2012;40(11): 2627–32.

50. Croy T, Koppenhaver S, Saliba S, et al. Anterior talocrural joint laxity: diagnostic accuracy of the anterior drawer test of the ankle. J Orthop Sports Phys Ther 2013;43(12):911–19.

51. van Dijk CN, Mol BW, Lim LS, et al. Diagnosis of ligament rupture of the ankle joint. Physical examination, arthrography, stress radiography and sonography compared in 160 patients after inversion trauma. Acta Orthop Scand [Comparative Study] 1996;67(6):566–70.

52. Fong DT, Chan YY, Mok KM, et al. Understanding acute ankle ligamentous sprain injury in sports. Sports Med Arthrosc Rehabil Ther 2009;1:14.

53. Mulligan EP. Evaluation and management of ankle syndesmosis injuries. Phys Ther Sport 2011;12(2):57–69.

54. Sman AD, Hiller CE, Refshauge KM. Diagnostic accuracy of clinical tests for diagnosis of ankle syndesmosis injury: a systematic review. Br J Sports Med 2013;47(10):620–8.

55. Sman AD, Hiller CE, Rae K, et al. Diagnostic accuracy of clinical tests for ankle syndesmosis injury. Br J Sports Med 2013. doi:10.1136/bjsports-2013-092787 [Epub ahead of print].

56. Taylor DC, Englehardt DL, Bassett Iii FH. Syndesmosis sprains of the ankle. The influence of heterotopic ossification. Am J Sports Med 1992;20(2):146–9.

57. Mullins JF, Sallis JG. Recurrent sprain of the ankle joint with diastasis. J Bone Joint Surg Br 1958;40-B(2):270–3.

58. Williams GN, Jones MH, Amendola A. Syndesmotic ankle sprains in athletes. Am J Sports Med 2007;35(7):1197–207.

59. Alonso A, Khoury L, Adams R. Clinical tests for ankle syndesmosis injury: reliability and prediction of return to function. J Orthop Sports Phys Ther 1998;27(4):276–84.

60. Ogilvie-Harris DJ, Reed SC. Disruption of the ankle syndesmosis: diagnosis and treatment by arthroscopic surgery. Arthroscopy 1994;10(5):561–8.

61. Magee D. Lower Leg, Ankle and Foot. Orthopedic Physical Assessment. 4th ed. Saunders; 2002. p. 765–809.

62. Beumer A, Swierstra BA, Mulder PGH. Clinical diagnosis of syndesmotic ankle instability: evaluation of stress tests behind the curtains. Acta Orthop Scand 2002;73(6):667–9.

63. Teitz CC, Harrington RM. A biomechanical analysis of the squeeze test for sprains of the syndesmotic ligaments of the ankle. Foot Ankle Int 1998;19(7):489–92.

64. Kiter E, Bozkurt M. The crossed-leg test for examination of ankle syndesmosis injuries. Foot Ankle Int 2005;26(2):187–8.

65. Wataru Miyamoto MT. Management of chronic disruption of the distal tibiofibular syndesmosis. World J Orthop 2011;2(1):1–6.

66. Simon J, Donahue M, Docherty C. Development of the Identification of Functional Ankle Instability (IdFAI). Foot Ankle Int 2012;33(9):755–63.

67. Mandarakas M, Hiller CE, Rose KJ, et al. Measuring ankle instability in pediatric Charcot-Marie-Tooth disease. J Child Neurol 2013;28(11):1456–62.

68. Carcia CR, Martin RL, Drouin JM. Validity of the Foot and Ankle Ability Measure in athletes with chronic ankle instability. J Athl Train 2008;43(2):179–83.

69. Roos EM, Brandsson S, Karlsson J. Validation of the foot and ankle outcome score for ankle ligament reconstruction. Foot Ankle Int 2001;22(10):788–94.

70. Wikstrom EA, Naik S, Lodha N, et al. Balance capabilities after lateral ankle trauma and intervention: a meta-analysis. Med Sci Sports Exerc 2009;41(6):1287–95.

71. Aiken AB, Pelland L, Brison R, et al. Short-term natural recovery of ankle sprains following discharge from emergency departments. J Orthop Sports Phys Ther 2008;38(9):566–71.

72. Man IO, Morrissey MC. Relationship between ankle-foot swelling and self-assessed function after ankle sprain. Med Sci Sports Exerc 2005;37(3):360–3.

73. Denegar CR, Hertel J, Fonseca J. The effect of lateral ankle sprain on dorsiflexion range of motion, posterior talar glide, and joint laxity. J Orthop Sports Phys Ther 2002;32(4):166–73.

74. Wolfe MW, Uhl TL, Mattacola CG, et al. Management of ankle sprains. Am Fam Physician 2001;63(1):93–104.

75. Hubbard-Turner T. Relationship between mechanical ankle joint laxity and subjective function. Foot Ankle Int 2012;33(10): 852–6.

76. Croy T, Saliba S, Saliba E, et al. Talofibular interval changes after acute ankle sprain: a stress ultrasonography study of ankle laxity. J Sport Rehabil [Research Support, Non-U.S. Gov't] 2013; 22(4):257–63.

77. Holme E, Magnusson SP, Becher K, et al. The effect of supervised rehabilitation on strength, postural sway, position sense and re-injury risk after acute ankle ligament sprain. Scand J Med Sci Sports 1999;9(2):104–9.

78. Konradsen L, Olesen S, Hansen HM. Ankle sensorimotor control and eversion strength after acute ankle inversion injuries. Am J Sports Med 1998;26(1):72–7.

79. Leanderson J, Bergqvist M, Rolf C, et al. Early influence of an ankle sprain on objective measures of ankle joint function. A prospective randomised study of ankle brace treatment. Knee Surg Sports Traumatol Arthrosc [Clinical Trial Randomized Controlled Trial] 1999;7(1):51–8.

80. Wilkerson GB, Pinerola JJ, Caturano RW. Invertor vs. evertor peak torque and power deficiencies associated with lateral ankle ligament injury. J Orthop Sports Phys Ther 1997;26(2): 78–86.

81. Hiller CE, Nightingale EJ, Lin CW, et al. Characteristics of people with recurrent ankle sprains: a systematic review with meta-analysis. Br J Sports Med [Meta-Analysis Research Support, Non-U.S. Gov't Review] 2011;45(8):660–72.

82. Arnold BL, Linens SW, de la Motte SJ, et al. Concentric evertor strength differences and functional ankle instability: a meta-analysis. J Athl Train 2009;44(6):653–62.

83. Arnold BL, De La Motte S, Linens S, et al. Ankle instability is associated with balance impairments: a meta-analysis. Med Sci Sports Exerc 2009;41(5):1048–62.

84. Munn J, Sullivan SJ, Schneiders AG. Evidence of sensorimotor deficits in functional ankle instability: a systematic review with meta-analysis. J Sci Med Sport 2010;13(1):2–12.

85. Witchalls J, Waddington G, Blanch P, et al. Ankle instability effects on joint position sense when stepping across the active movement extent discrimination apparatus. J Athl Train 2012; 47(6):627–34.

86. Hale SA, Hertel J, Olmsted-Kramer LC. The effect of a 4-week comprehensive rehabilitation program on postural control and lower extremity function in individuals with chronic ankle instability. J Orthop Sports Phys Ther 2007;37(6):303–11.

87. Brown C, Bowser B, Simpson KJ. Movement variability during single leg jump landings in individuals with and without chronic ankle instability. Clin Biomech (Bristol, Avon) 2012;27(1): 52–63.

88. Friel K, McLean N, Myers C, et al. Ipsilateral hip abductor weakness after inversion ankle sprain. J Athl Train 2006;41(1):74–8.

89. Gribble PA, Hertel J, Denegar CR. Chronic ankle instability and fatigue create proximal joint alterations during performance of the Star Excursion Balance Test. Int J Sports Med 2007;28(3): 236–42.

90. Sedory EJ, McVey ED, Cross KM, et al. Arthrogenic muscle response of the quadriceps and hamstrings with chronic ankle instability. J Athl Train 2007;42(3):355–60.

91. Brown C, Padua D, Marshall SW, et al. Individuals with mechanical ankle instability exhibit different motion patterns than those with functional ankle instability and ankle sprain copers. Clin Biomech (Bristol, Avon) 2008;23(6):822–31.

92. Delahunt E, Monaghan K, Caulfield B. Altered neuromuscular control and ankle joint kinematics during walking in subjects with functional instability of the ankle joint. Am J Sports Med 2006; 34(12):1970–6.

93. Fu SN, Hui-Chan CW. Modulation of prelanding lower-limb muscle responses in athletes with multiple ankle sprains. Med Sci Sports Exerc 2007;39(10):1774–83.

94. Wikstrom EA, Bishop MD, Inamdar AD, et al. Gait termination control strategies are altered in chronic ankle instability subjects. Med Sci Sports Exerc 2010;42(1):197–205.

95. Hass CJ, Bishop MD, Doidge D, et al. Chronic ankle instability alters central organization of movement. Am J Sports Med 2010; 38(4):829–34.

96. Needle AR, Palmer JA, Kesar TM, et al. Brain regulation of muscle tone in healthy and functionally unstable ankles. J Sport Rehabil 2013;22(3):202–11.
97. Pietrosimone BG, Gribble PA. Chronic ankle instability and corticomotor excitability of the fibularis longus muscle. J Athl Train 2012;47(6):621–6.
98. Needle AR, Charles BBS, Farquhar WB, et al. Muscle spindle traffic in functionally unstable ankles during ligamentous stress. J Athl Train 2013;48(2):192–202.
99. Hoch MC, McKeon PO, Andreatta RD. Plantar vibrotactile detection deficits in adults with chronic ankle instability. Med Sci Sports Exerc 2012;44(4):666–72.
100. Powell MR, Powden CJ, Houston MN, et al. Plantar cutaneous sensitivity and balance in individuals with and without chronic ankle instability. Clin J Sport Med 2014;24(6):490–6.
101. McKay G, Cook J. Evidence-Based Clinical Statement: Physiotherapy Management of Annkle Injuries in Sport. Victoria: Australian Physiotherapy Association; 2006.
102. Kaminski TW, Hertel J, Amendola N, et al. National Athletic Trainers' Association position statement: conservative management and prevention of ankle sprains in athletes. J Athl Train [Practice Guideline Review] 2013;48(4):528–45.
103. Kerkhoffs GM, van den Bekerom M, Elders LA, et al. Diagnosis, treatment and prevention of ankle sprains: an evidence-based clinical guideline. Br J Sports Med 2012;46(12):854–60.
104. Martin RL, Davenport TE, Paulseth S, et al. Ankle stability and movement coordination impairments: ankle ligament sprains. J Orthop Sports Phys Ther 2013;43(9):A1–40.
105. Seah R, Mani-Babu S. Managing ankle sprains in primary care: what is best practice? A systematic review of the last 10 years of evidence. Br Med Bull 2011;97:105–35.
106. Polzer H, Kanz KG, Prall WC, et al. Diagnosis and treatment of acute ankle injuries: development of an evidence-based algorithm. Orthop Rev (Pavia) 2012;4(1):e5.
107. Petersen W, Rembitzki IV, Koppenburg AG, et al. Treatment of acute ankle ligament injuries: a systematic review. Arch Orthop Trauma Surg 2013;133(8):1129–41.
108. Hunt KJ. Syndesmosis injuries. Curr Rev Musculoskelet Med 2013;6(4):304–12.
109. Naqvi GA, Cunningham P, Lynch B, et al. Fixation of ankle syndesmotic injuries: comparison of tightrope fixation and syndesmotic screw fixation for accuracy of syndesmotic reduction. Am J Sports Med 2012;40(12):2828–35.
110. van den Bekerom MP, Struijs PA, Blankevoort L, et al. What is the evidence for rest, ice, compression, and elevation therapy in the treatment of ankle sprains in adults? J Athl Train 2012;47(4):435–43.
111. Lamb SE, Marsh JL, Hutton JL, et al. Mechanical supports for acute, severe ankle sprain: a pragmatic, multicentre, randomised controlled trial. Lancet 2009;373(9663):575–81.
112. Kemler E, van de Port I, Backx F, et al. A systematic review on the treatment of acute ankle sprain: brace versus other functional treatment types. Sports Med 2011;41(3):185–97.
113. Kerkhoffs GMMJ, Struijs PAA, Marti RK, et al. Different functional treatment strategies for acute lateral ankle ligament injuries in adults. Cochrane Database Syst Rev 2002;(3):CD002938.
114. Boyce SH, Quigley MA, Campbell S. Management of ankle sprains: a randomised controlled trial of the treatment of inversion injuries using an elastic support bandage or an Aircast ankle brace. Br J Sports Med [Clinical Trial Comparative Study Multicenter Study Randomized Controlled Trial] 2005;39(2):91–6.
115. Loudon JK, Reiman MP, Sylvain J. The efficacy of manual joint mobilisation/manipulation in treatment of lateral ankle sprains: a systematic review. Br J Sports Med 2014;48(5):365–70.
116. Cosby NL, Koroch M, Grindstaff TL, et al. Immediate effects of anterior to posterior talocrural joint mobilizations following acute lateral ankle sprain. J Man Manip Ther 2011;19(2):76–83.
117. Green T, Refshauge K, Crosbie J, et al. A randomized controlled trial of a passive accessory joint mobilization on acute ankle inversion sprains. Phys Ther 2001;81(4):984–94.
118. Eisenhart AW, Gaeta TJ, Yens DP. Osteopathic manipulative treatment in the emergency department for patients with acute ankle injuries. J Am Osteopath Assoc 2003;103(9):417–21.
119. Slatyer MA, Hensley MJ, Lopert R. A randomized controlled trial of piroxicam in the management of acute ankle sprain in

Australian Regular Army recruits. The Kapooka Ankle Sprain Study. Am J Sports Med 1997;25(4):544–53.
120. van Rijn RM, van Ochten J, Luijsterburg PA, et al. Effectiveness of additional supervised exercises compared with conventional treatment alone in patients with acute lateral ankle sprains: systematic review. BMJ [Comparative Study Evaluation Studies Research Support, Non-U.S. Gov't Review] 2010;341:c5688.
121. van Rijn RM, van Heest JA, van der Wees P, et al. Some benefit from physiotherapy intervention in the subgroup of patients with severe ankle sprain as determined by the ankle function score: a randomised trial. Aust J Physiother [Randomized Controlled Trial Research Support, Non-U.S. Gov't] 2009;55(2):107–13.
122. Bleakley CM, O'Connor SR, Tully MA, et al. Effect of accelerated rehabilitation on function after ankle sprain: randomised controlled trial. BMJ 2010;340:c1964.
123. van Os AG, Bierma-Zeinstra SM, Verhagen AP, et al. Comparison of conventional treatment and supervised rehabilitation for treatment of acute lateral ankle sprains: a systematic review of the literature. J Orthop Sports Phys Ther 2005;35(2):95–105.
124. van Rijn RM, van Os AG, Kleinrensink GJ, et al. Supervised exercises for adults with acute lateral ankle sprain: a randomised controlled trial. Br J Gen Pract [Multicenter Study Randomized Controlled Trial Research Support, Non-U.S. Gov't] 2007;57(543):793–800.
125. Lin CW, Hiller CE, de Bie RA. Evidence-based treatment for ankle injuries: a clinical perspective. J Man Manip Ther 2010;18(1):22–8.
126. van den Bekerom MP, van der Windt DA, Ter Riet G, et al. Therapeutic ultrasound for acute ankle sprains. Cochrane Database Syst Rev 2011;(6):CD001249.
127. Verhagen EA. What does therapeutic ultrasound add to recovery from acute ankle sprain? A review. Clin J Sport Med [Comment Research Support, Non-U.S. Gov't] 2013;23(1):84–5.
128. Clanton TO, Paul P. Syndesmosis injuries in athletes. Foot Ankle Clin 2002;7(3):529–49.
129. Miller TL, Skalak T. Evaluation and treatment recommendations for acute injuries to the ankle syndesmosis without associated fracture. Sports Med 2014;44(2):179–88.
130. de Vries JS, Krips R, Sierevelt IN, et al. Interventions for treating chronic ankle instability. Cochrane Database Syst Rev 2011;(8):CD004124.
131. O'Driscoll J, Delahunt E. Neuromuscular training to enhance sensorimotor and functional deficits in subjects with chronic ankle instability: a systematic review and best evidence synthesis. Sports Med Arthrosc Rehabil Ther Technol 2011;3:19.
132. Gilbreath JP, Gaven SL, Van Lunen BL, et al. The effects of Mobilization with Movement on dorsiflexion range of motion, dynamic balance, and self-reported function in individuals with chronic ankle instability. Man Ther 2014;19(2):152–7.
133. Reid A, Birmingham TB, Alcock GK. Efficacy of mobilization with movement for patients with limited dorsiflexion after ankle sprain: a crossover trial. Physiotherapy Canada 2007;59(3):166–72.
134. Pellow JE, Brantingham JW. The efficacy of adjusting the ankle in the treatment of subacute and chronic grade I and grade II ankle inversion sprains. J Manipulative Physiol Ther 2001;24(1):17–24.
135. Hoch MC, McKeon PO. Joint mobilization improves spatiotemporal postural control and range of motion in those with chronic ankle instability. J Orthop Res 2011;29(3):326–32.
136. Hoch MC, Andreatta RD, Mullineaux DR, et al. Two-week joint mobilization intervention improves self-reported function, range of motion, and dynamic balance in those with chronic ankle instability. J Orthop Res 2012;30(11):1798–804.
137. Sesma AR, Mattacola CG, Uhl TL, et al. Effect of foot orthotics on single- and double-limb dynamic balance tasks in patients with chronic ankle instability. Foot Ankle Spec [Research Support, Non-U.S. Gov't] 2008;1(6):330–7.
138. Gabriner ML, Braun BA, Houston MN, et al. The effectiveness of foot orthotics on improving postural control in individuals with chronic ankle instability: a critically appraised topic. J Sport Rehabil 2013;[Epub ahead of print].
139. Hadadi M, Mousavi ME, Fardipour S, et al. Effect of soft and semirigid ankle orthoses on Star Excursion Balance Test performance in patients with functional ankle instability. J Sci Med Sport 2013;17(4):430–3.

140. Lee HJ, Lim KB, Jung TH, et al. Changes in balancing ability of athletes with chronic ankle instability after foot orthotics application and rehabilitation exercises. Ann Rehabil Med 2013;37(4): 523–33.

141. Dizon JM, Reyes JJ. A systematic review on the effectiveness of external ankle supports in the prevention of inversion ankle sprains among elite and recreational players. J Sci Med Sport 2010;13(3):309–17.

142. Janssen KW, van Mechelen W, Verhagen EA. Bracing superior to neuromuscular training for the prevention of self-reported recurrent ankle sprains: a three-arm randomised controlled trial. Br J Sports Med 2014;48(16):1235–9.

THE SHOULDER

CHAPTER 50.1 ■ SHOULDER ASSESSMENT

Eric Hegedus • Jeremy Lewis

INTRODUCTION

Musculoskeletal problems involving the shoulder are common, with a reported lifetime prevalence as high as 67%.[1] Complaints increase with age and are common in the fifth to seventh decades.[2-4] Of concern is the fact that 40–54% of people with shoulder problems report continued symptoms up to 3 years after initial onset.[3,5,6] These symptoms are frequently associated with substantial morbidity.

The main role of the shoulder is to position the hand to permit the upper limb to perform activities ranging from the performance of high-powered, explosive activities, such as serving in tennis, to placing the hand within the visual field to perform highly skilled prehensile tasks such as writing. The shoulder also places the upper limb and hand to facilitate weight bearing through the upper extremity in activities such as gymnastics. Pain, loss of movement, instability, muscle imbalance and loss of strength and endurance may have a detrimental impact on shoulder function.

The complexity of the shoulder and its wide spectrum of function create challenges in assessment and diagnosis. The principal aims of shoulder assessment are to collect meaningful information that informs clinical decision making, aids in diagnosis and directs efficient and effective management of shoulder dysfunction. This chapter will address the first two aims.

ASSESSMENT OVERVIEW AND CLINICAL DECISION MAKING

There are several models of clinical decision making that explain how a clinician uses the information gathered in an assessment. In cases where the examiner is a new learner or when an experienced examiner is confronted with an unfamiliar set of signs and symptoms, hypothetical–deductive reasoning is typified by the gathering of data in a step-wise fashion, from general to specific, to confirm or refute a working hypothesis. The process described in this chapter is such an approach. This chapter will progress systematically from the patient interview, to screening, to motion testing and, finally, to orthopaedic tests where the issue of diagnostic accuracy will be discussed.

Knowledge of epidemiological data provides valuable information when examining the shoulder. This will be discussed briefly in the following section.

The Importance of Epidemiology Data in Shoulder Assessment and Diagnosis

Certain pathologies and diagnoses have a greater chance of existing in defined patient populations. In other words, pre-test or pre-assessment probability is higher for certain pathologies in specific populations. For example, without a history of trauma, a rotator cuff tear would be uncommon in the average 15-year-old but rotator cuff tendinopathy may occur in a young elite swimmer. For a person aged between 40 and 60 years there is roughly a 25% chance of a rotator cuff tear which rises to approximately 50% in people in their 80s.[7,8] Two of the stronger diagnostic test clusters for rotator cuff tear incorporate an age-over-60 component.[9,10] Another example pertains to patients with a first-time traumatic dislocation. The dislocation is almost certain to recur if the individual is under the age of 20 years and almost certain not to happen again if over the age of 40 years.[11-13] Importantly for diagnosis, individuals over the age of 40 years who have had a dislocation are likely to have a rotator cuff tear in addition to instability and, regardless of age, clinicians should be aware of the possibility of a bony lesion like a Hill–Sachs or Bankart. As a final example, degenerative changes in the acromioclavicular joint are not likely in the young but for those aged 61–88 years, the likelihood is 90%.[14] Knowing the baseline probability helps the systematic assessment, outlined hereafter, to be more accurate.

THE PATIENT INTERVIEW, FLAGS AND ESTABLISHING A BASELINE FOR OUTCOMES

A systematic examination begins with a review of all relevant medical records and reports and a patient interview. At this stage it is important for the clinician to screen for Red and Yellow Flags, gain an understanding of how the shoulder dysfunction is affecting the patient as a whole, and to determine the patient's short- and long-term needs. Red Flags are serious conditions that require referral. Common Red Flags are reports of trauma, fever or chills, unremitting night pain, bilateral symptoms and unintentional, substantial weight loss. An affirmative response to a single Red Flag question may not be a reason for an immediate referral but a cluster typically would be.[15,16] It is essential to continuously monitor changes in the individual's health status for changes to Red Flag status.

The presence of Yellow Flags such as negative coping mechanisms, anxiety, depression and kinesiophobia are associated with a negative outcome.[17,18] Prognostic factors associated with a negative outcome in patients with shoulder pain include concurrent neck pain, high pain intensity and symptoms greater than 3 months' duration.[3,19,20] Factors correlated with a positive outcome are lower disability at baseline and less pain-catastrophizing behaviour.[21] Psychosocial factors may be more important predictors in those with chronic shoulder pain.[21]

Self-report outcome measures further enhance patient history by detailing the effects of the injury or illness on the patient's quality of life including function. They may be categorized as generic, disease-specific, site- and region-specific, and dimension-specific. A review of all self-report measures is beyond the scope of this chapter, but we will touch on a few here. Generic measures for people with musculoskeletal shoulder conditions may include; the single assessment numeric evaluation (SANE),[22] the P4 pain scale,[23] and the patient-specific functional scale (PSFS).[24] Shoulder- and region-specific outcome measures that should be considered to inform assessment and outcome include the nine-item quick disabilities of the arm, shoulder or the *Quick*-DASH-9,[25] the full DASH,[26] and the Shoulder Pain and Disability Index (SPADI).[27] In a throwing athlete with shoulder pain, the Kerlan–Jobe Orthopaedic Clinic Shoulder and Elbow Score (KJOC-SES)[28] should be considered.

Physical performance measures should be included at baseline and are thought to capture a different component of function than self-report measures.[29] Physical performance measures may be less affected by pain and psychosocial variables than are self-report measures.[30] Currently, physical performance measures are not well

supported by research confirming their validity, reliability and responsiveness. Table 50-1 presents a short list of physical performance measures for the shoulder, a brief description of how to perform them and the population in which they have been studied.

PHYSICAL EXAMINATION

Observation

The patient interview helps direct and is followed by a physical examination. The initial steps of the examination include an assessment of posture and identification of any deviations of posture from an expected norm, as well as gathering clinical clues that may later support a diagnosis (e.g. swelling, ecchymosis, muscle atrophy and scapular dyskinesis). It is important to acknowledge that although postural assessment is considered to be an integral part of the shoulder examination, definitive research evidence providing guidance on how to perform a postural examination and, importantly, how to interpret findings are currently unavailable. For example, an increase in the thoracic kyphosis may be observed, and a hypothesis that this postural deviation contributes to the patient's shoulder pain has been formulated.[35] However, currently this hypothesis has no definitive support.[36,37] Similar uncertainties surround the concept of scapular dyskinesis and discord exists between clinicians. Some suggest that scapular dyskinesis is an important clinical finding due to its correlation with pathology,[38,39] whereas others have found no correlation.[40–42] Even when scapular dyskinesis is found, there is little agreement about which components and what magnitude constitute dyskinesis.[43] What is known currently is that scapular dyskinesis is not diagnostic of any particular pathology but it still may be an important impairment to address when treating patients with shoulder pain.[44,45]

The Screening Examination

After observation, the physical examination involves an appropriate screening examination. For example, the upper quarter screen (UQS) is used for patients who report shoulder pain and radiating symptoms down the arm. The UQS aims to determine whether the source of

TABLE 50-1	**Recommended Upper Extremity Physical Performance Measures**		
Test	**Assesses**	**Population**	
FIT-HaNSA[31]	Work-specific tasks	Younger, working	
CKCUEST[32]	Single arm stability	Mostly young, athletic males	
UQYBT[33]	Mobility, stability, endurance	College-aged, military population	
Single Arm Shot Put[34]	Power	Healthy, recreationally active adults	

FIT-HaNSA, Functional impairment test-hand and neck/shoulder/arm; *CKCUEST*, Closed kinetic chain upper extremity stability test; *UQYBT*, Upper quarter Y-balance test.

the pain is in the neck, shoulder, or other region and whether the impairments are of neurologic origin. The UQS combines active cervical spine motions and functional movements of the shoulder and, when relevant, testing of dermatomes, myotomes, reflexes, vibration sense and upper motoneuron testing. An examination of vascular status (see Chapter 35) may also be required. It is necessary to appropriately screen the cervical and thoracic regions to determine if they are involved with the presenting shoulder symptoms.

Active Motion, Passive Motion, Palpation and Muscle Testing

The focused physical examination of the shoulder commences with examination of active shoulder range of motion (ROM), passive ROM (physiological and accessory motions as indicated), palpation and muscle

performance testing. Methods for measuring impairments such as range of movement and strength have been published.[46,47] The known diagnostic accuracies for these components of the shoulder examination can be found in Table 50-2. These procedures are followed by orthopaedic special tests, which are considered to form an integral component of the physical examination.

Orthopaedic Special Tests and Diagnostic Accuracy

Tests have been devised to identify lesions in specific tissues, such as the labrum, the rotator cuff, the acromioclavicular joint, subacromial bursa and the biceps. The diagnostic accuracy of a clinical test is determined by comparing the clinical finding against a 'gold standard' comparator. For the shoulder, the comparator would typically be direct observation during surgery (soft tissue

---

TABLE 50-2 Best Available Evidence of the Diagnostic Accuracy of the Shoulder Examination

Test Name	Pathology	Sensitivity/ Specificity	LR LR+/LR−	Screen (Sc) Diagnose (D) Both (B) Neither (N) Unknown(?)
History	Any	?	?	?
Observation				
Shrug sign (during elevation)[48]	OA	91/57	0.16	Sc
	Adhesive capsulitis	95/50	0.10	
	Rotator cuff tendinopathy	96/53	0.08	
Motion Testing (Active, Passive, Accessory)				
Sulcus sign[49]	Superior labral tear	17/93	2.43	N
Anterior drawer test[50]	Anterior instability	53/85	3.53	N
Palpation				
Supraspinatus[51]	Tendinopathy	92/41	0.19	Sc
Biceps[51]	Tendinopathy	85/48	0.31	N
AC joint[52]	AC pathology	96/10	0.40	N
Muscle Testing				
Infraspinatus test[53]	Impingement	56/87	4.39	N
Empty can[10]	Impingement	44/90	4.20	N
Orthopaedic Special Tests				
Apprehension[54]	Anterior instability	72/96	18.0	D
Relocation[50]	Anterior instability	81/92	10.1/0.1	B
Surprise[55]	Anterior instability	92/89	8.4/0.08	B
Passive distraction[56]	SLAP lesion	53/94	8.3	D
Passive compression[57]	SLAP lesion	82/86	5.7/0.2	B
Dynamic labral shear-modified[58]	Any labral tear	72/98	36	D
Belly-off[59]	Subscapularis tendinopathy	86/91	9.7/0.14	B
Belly press[60]	Subscapularis tendinopathy	40/98	20.0	D
Modified belly press[59]	Subscapularis tendinopathy	80/88	6.7/0.23	B
Bear hug[60]	Subscapularis tendinopathy	60/92	7.23	D
Bony apprehension[61]	Bony instability	94/84	5.9/0.07	B
OMPT[62]	Bony abnormality	84/99	84.0	D
Lateral Jobe[63]	Rotator cuff tear (RCT)	81/89	7.4/0.21	B
ERLS[64]	Full-thickness tear	46/49	7.2	D
AC resisted extension[65]	AC Joint Pathology	72/85	4.8	D

AC, Acromioclavicular; *ERLS*, external rotation lag sign; *LR*, likelihood ratio; *OA*, osteoarthritis; *OMPT*, olecranon manubrium percussion test; *SLAP*, superior labral anterior to posterior.

TABLE 50-3	**Determining the Accuracy of Clinical Tests**		
		'Gold Standard' Reference Test **(Examples Include: MRI, US, Arthroscopic Visualization)**	
		Condition/Disorder Present	**Condition/Disorder Not Present**
Clinical test	**Positive clinical finding** (e.g. pain, weakness, instability)	True positive (A)	False positive (B)
	Negative clinical finding (e.g. no pain, weakness or instability)	False negative (C)	True negative (D)

US, ultrasound; *MRI,* magnetic resonance imaging.
Interpretation:
Sensitivity = A/(A + C) (Ideal 100%)
Specificity = D/(B + D) (Ideal 100%)
Positive likelihood ratio (LR+) = Sensitivity/1 − Specificity >3 = useful, >10 = very useful
Negative likelihood ratio (LR−) = 1 − Sensitivity/Specificity <0.33 = useful, <0.1 = very useful

lesions), a radiograph (bony lesions) or injection (impingement syndrome). The underlying principle is that observed structural failure is the cause or is associated with symptoms. Table 50-3 details how the accuracy of clinical tests is determined.

Sensitivity, specificity and positive and negative likelihood ratios are the most robust metrics in determining diagnostic accuracy. For a clinician to derive confidence that the findings of an orthopaedic test may help rule in or rule out the presence of a condition or specific structural pathology the test must be positive if the condition is present and negative if not present. The sensitivity and specificity of any test must be considered together, not one component in isolation. For example, the Neer sign[66] is a clinical procedure involving scapula stabilization with shoulder flexion and over-pressure. If the patient informs the clinician that the procedure is painful (positive test) then the presence of subacromial impingement may be considered. Alternatively, impingement may be ruled out if no pain (negative test) is reproduced during the procedure. The assumption with this interpretation is that the orthopaedic test findings for every patient may be classified as a true positive or a true negative so that both sensitivity and specificity are 100%. Currently there are no orthopaedic tests with these stellar metrics.

Likelihood ratios (LR) may be more useful. As demonstrated in Table 50-3, both LR+ and LR− combine sensitivity and specificity into one number. A test with a strong LR+ moves the examiner closer to a diagnosis and a test with a strong LR− moves the clinician further away from a diagnosis. At the beginning of this chapter, we discussed baseline probabilities found in epidemiological literature. An LR+ of 5.0 or greater and LR− of 0.20 or less are moderately to highly valuable in modifying the baseline probability to the extent of ruling in or ruling out a pathology, respectively. As either the LR+ or LR− approaches a value of 1.0, the value of the diagnostic test diminishes to the point where it insignificantly modifies the baseline probability.

Clinicians should have knowledge of the sensitivity, specificity and positive and negative LRs of clinical tests. Despite the widespread clinical use of these shoulder orthopaedic tests to inform a diagnosis, there is surprisingly little evidence to support their diagnostic utility.[45,67,68]

The diagnostic accuracy and use of these tests has been challenged,[45,67,68] as there are a substantial number of people without shoulder symptoms who have identifiable structural pathology on imaging.[69] Published reviews have discussed this issue in detail.[45]

Clustering tests and measures together, a standard procedure in physical examination, helps to improve diagnosis. Nevertheless studies examining clustered tests rarely show values better than the most accurate tests, but possibly because the best tests in combination have not been studied.[68] Table 50-2 summarizes the most accurate tests from the highest-quality research studies. It is important to appreciate that the diagnostic accuracy of even the best clinical tests is determined by comparison with observed structural failure (which may be asymptomatic and not the cause of symptoms), and as such, interpretation of clinical findings derived from even these best tests must be made in light of all of the other information gathered from the patient assessment. Determining which structures are involved in the patient's presentation and differentiation between different musculoskeletal shoulder disorders remains difficult.[45,70–72]

SUMMARY

The shoulder is a highly complex, multijoint system that has a wide array of functional demands that require mobility and stability. Assessment to reach a diagnosis and inform clinical decision making needs to be both thorough and systematic. The assessment process (Fig. 50-1) must also incorporate knowledge of epidemiology and baseline probability with best evidence, and an appreciation of patient aspirations, desires and values. Where evidence is unclear, clinicians should rely even more heavily on clinical decision making, which some call the 'art' of physiotherapy. The clinical decision-making model described in this chapter is the hypothetical–deductive model. Although this method progresses more rapidly with experience and is most comprehensive, it is also the slowest. More experienced clinicians take shortcuts by using pattern-recognition or heuristic decision making. In order to minimize false assumptions and misdiagnoses, especially with the

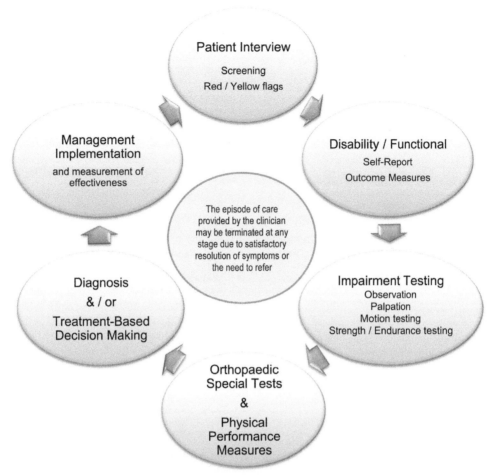

FIGURE 50-1 ■ Components of a systematic, thorough physical examination.

heuristic model, the clinician is obliged to regularly review research databases to update and synthesize knowledge. Also, it is important to realize that the assessment process is an ongoing continuum and as the patient's condition changes, additional assessment is mandatory. Following the process outlined in this chapter and summarized in Figure 50-1 ensures a systematic, thorough and ongoing assessment process.

REFERENCES

1. Meyers OL, Jessop S, Klemp P. The epidemiology of rheumatic disease in a rural and an urban population over the age of 65 years. S Afr Med J 1982;62(12):403–51. [Epub 1982/09/11].
2. Bot SD, van der Waal JM, Terwee CB, et al. Incidence and prevalence of complaints of the neck and upper extremity in general practice. Ann Rheum Dis 2005;64(1):118–23. [Epub 2004/12/21].
3. van der Windt DA, Koes BW, Boeke AJ, et al. Shoulder disorders in general practice: prognostic indicators of outcome. Br J Gen Pract 1996;46(410):519–23. [Epub 1996/09/01].
4. Picavet HS, Schouten JS. Musculoskeletal pain in the Netherlands: prevalences, consequences and risk groups, the DMC(3)-study. Pain 2003;102(1–2):167–78. [Epub 2003/03/07].
5. Macfarlane GJ, Hunt IM, Silman AJ. Predictors of chronic shoulder pain: a population based prospective study. J Rheumatol 1998;25(8):1612–15. [Epub 1998/08/26].
6. Winters JC, Sobel JS, Groenier KH, et al. The long-term course of shoulder complaints: a prospective study in general practice. Rheumatology (Oxford) 1999;38(2):160–3. [Epub 1999/05/26].
7. Yamaguchi K, Ditsios K, Middleton WD, et al. The demographic and morphological features of rotator cuff disease. A comparison of asymptomatic and symptomatic shoulders. J Bone Joint Surg Am 2006;88(8):1699–704. [Epub 2006/08/03].
8. Yamamoto A, Takagishi K, Osawa T, et al. Prevalence and risk factors of a rotator cuff tear in the general population. J Shoulder Elbow Surg 2010;19(1):116–20. [Epub 2009/06/23].
9. Litaker D, Pioro M, El Bilbeisi H, et al. Returning to the bedside: using the history and physical examination to identify rotator cuff tears. J Am Geriatr Soc 2000;48(12):1633–7. [Epub 2000/12/29].
10. Park HB, Yokota A, Gill HS, et al. Diagnostic accuracy of clinical tests for the different degrees of subacromial impingement syndrome. J Bone Joint Surg Am 2005;87(7):1446–55. [Epub 2005/07/05].
11. Marans HJ, Angel KR, Schemitsch EH, et al. The fate of traumatic anterior dislocation of the shoulder in children. J Bone Joint Surg Am 1992;74(8):1242–4. [Epub 1992/09/01].
12. Postacchini F, Gumina S, Cinotti G. Anterior shoulder dislocation in adolescents. J Shoulder Elbow Surg 2000;9(6):470–4. [Epub 2001/01/13].
13. Deitch J, Mehlman CT, Foad SL, et al. Traumatic anterior shoulder dislocation in adolescents. Am J Sports Med 2003;31(5):758–63. [Epub 2003/09/17].
14. Needell SD, Zlatkin MB, Sher JS, et al. MR imaging of the rotator cuff: peritendinous and bone abnormalities in an asymptomatic population. AJR Am J Roentgenol 1996;166(4):863–7. [Epub 1996/04/01].
15. Henschke N, Maher CG, Ostelo RW, et al. Red flags to screen for malignancy in patients with low-back pain. Cochrane Database Syst Rev 2013;(2):CD008686, [Epub 2013/03/02].
16. Ross MD, Boissonnault WG. Red flags: to screen or not to screen? J Orthop Sports Phys Ther 2010;40(11):682–4. [Epub 2010/11/03].
17. Parr JJ, Borsa PA, Fillingim RB, et al. Pain-related fear and catastrophizing predict pain intensity and disability independently

using an induced muscle injury model. J Pain 2012;13(4):370–8. [Epub 2012/03/20].

18. Cho CH, Jung SW, Park JY, et al. Is shoulder pain for three months or longer correlated with depression, anxiety, and sleep disturbance? J Shoulder Elbow Surg 2013;22(2):222–8. [Epub 2012/06/29].

19. Kuijpers T, van der Windt DA, van der Heijden GJ, et al. Systematic review of prognostic cohort studies on shoulder disorders. Pain 2004;109(3):420–31.

20. Kuijpers T, van der Windt DA, Boeke AJ, et al. Clinical prediction rules for the prognosis of shoulder pain in general practice. Pain 2006;120(3):276–85.

21. Reilingh ML, Kuijpers T, Tanja-Harfterkamp AM, et al. Course and prognosis of shoulder symptoms in general practice. Rheumatology (Oxford) 2008;47(5):724–30. [Epub 2008/04/16].

22. Williams GN, Gangel TJ, Arciero RA, et al. Comparison of the Single Assessment Numeric Evaluation method and two shoulder rating scales. Outcomes measures after shoulder surgery. Am J Sports Med 1999;27(2):214–21. [Epub 1999/04/02].

23. Stratford PW, Dogra M, Woodhouse L, et al. Validating self-report measures of pain and function in patients undergoing hip or knee arthroplasty. Physiother Can 2009;61(4):189–94, discussion 95–6. [Epub 2010/09/03].

24. Stratford PW, Gill C, Westaway M, et al. Assessing disability and change on individual patients: a report of a patient specific measure. Physiother Can 1995;47:258–63.

25. Gabel CP, Yelland M, Melloh M, et al. A modified QuickDASH-9 provides a valid outcome instrument for upper limb function. BMC Musculoskelet Disord 2009;10:161. [Epub 2009/12/22].

26. Beaton DE, Katz JN, Fossel AH, et al. Measuring the whole or the parts? Validity, reliability, and responsiveness of the Disabilities of the Arm, Shoulder and Hand outcome measure in different regions of the upper extremity. J Hand Ther 2001;14(2):128–46. [Epub 2001/05/31].

27. Roach KE, Budiman-Mak E, Songsiridej N, et al. Development of a shoulder pain and disability index. Arthritis Care Res 1991;4(4):143–9. [Epub 1991/12/01].

28. Domb BG, Davis JT, Alberta FG, et al. Clinical follow-up of professional baseball players undergoing ulnar collateral ligament reconstruction using the new Kerlan-Jobe Orthopaedic Clinic overhead athlete shoulder and elbow score (KJOC Score). Am J Sports Med 2010;38(8):1558–63. [Epub 2010/03/31].

29. Wright AA, Cook CE, Baxter GD, et al. Relationship between the Western Ontario and McMaster Universities Osteoarthritis Index Physical Function Subscale and physical performance measures in patients with hip osteoarthritis. Arch Phys Med Rehabil 2010;91(10):1558–64. [Epub 2010/09/30].

30. Terwee CB, van der Slikke RM, van Lummel RC, et al. Self-reported physical functioning was more influenced by pain than performance-based physical functioning in knee-osteoarthritis patients. J Clin Epidemiol 2006;59(7):724–31. [Epub 2006/06/13].

31. Kumta P, MacDermid JC, Mehta SP, et al. The FIT-HaNSA demonstrates reliability and convergent validity of functional performance in patients with shoulder disorders. J Orthop Sports Phys Ther 2012;42(5):455–64. [Epub 2012/01/28].

32. Goldbeck T, Davies G. Test-retest reliability of the closed kinetic chain upper extremity stability test: a clinical field test. Sport Rehabil 2000;9(1):35–45.

33. Gorman PP, Butler RJ, Plisky PJ, et al. Upper quarter y balance test: reliability and performance comparison between genders in active adults. J Strength Cond Res 2012;26(11):3043–8. [Epub 2012/01/10].

34. Negrete RJ, Hanney WJ, Kolber MJ, et al. Can upper extremity functional tests predict the softball throw for distance: a predictive validity investigation. Int J Sports Phys Ther 2011;6(2):104–11. [Epub 2011/06/30].

35. Theisen C, van Wagensveld A, Timmesfeld N, et al. Co-occurrence of outlet impingement syndrome of the shoulder and restricted range of motion in the thoracic spine–a prospective study with ultrasound-based motion analysis. BMC Musculoskelet Disord 2010;11:135. [Epub 2010/07/01].

36. Lewis JS, Green A, Wright C. Subacromial impingement syndrome: the role of posture and muscle imbalance. J Shoulder Elbow Surg 2005;14(4):385–92. [Epub 2005/07/15].

37. Lewis JS, Valentine RE. The pectoralis minor length test: a study of the intra-rater reliability and diagnostic accuracy in subjects with and without shoulder symptoms. BMC Musculoskelet Disord 2007;8:64. [Epub 2007/07/11].

38. Ludewig PM, Cook TM. Alterations in shoulder kinematics and associated muscle activity in people with symptoms of shoulder impingement. Phys Ther 2000;80(3):276–91. [Epub 2000/03/01].

39. Kibler WB, Sciascia A, Wilkes T. Scapular dyskinesis and its relation to shoulder injury. J Am Acad Orthop Surg 2012;20(6):364–72. [Epub 2012/06/05].

40. Graichen H, Stammberger T, Bonel H, et al. Three-dimensional analysis of shoulder girdle and supraspinatus motion patterns in patients with impingement syndrome. J Orthop Res 2001;19(6):1192–8. [Epub 2002/01/10].

41. Mell AG, LaScalza S, Guffey P, et al. Effect of rotator cuff pathology on shoulder rhythm. J Shoulder Elbow Surg 2005;14(1 Suppl. S):58S–64S. [Epub 2005/02/24].

42. Ratcliffe E, Pickering S, McLean S, et al. Is there a relationship between Subacromial Impingement Syndrome and scapular orientation?: A systematic review. Br J Sports Med 2013;In Press.

43. Ludewig PM, Reynolds JF. The association of scapular kinematics and glenohumeral joint pathologies. J Orthop Sports Phys Ther 2009;39(2):90–104. [Epub 2009/02/06].

44. Wright AA, Wassinger CA, Frank M, et al. Diagnostic accuracy of scapular physical examination tests for shoulder disorders: a systematic review. Br J Sports Med 2013;47(14):886–92. [Epub 2012/10/20].

45. Lewis JS. Rotator cuff tendinopathy/subacromial impingement syndrome: is it time for a new method of assessment? Br J Sports Med 2009;43(4):259–64. [Epub 2008/10/08].

46. Valentine RE, Lewis JS. Intraobserver reliability of 4 physiologic movements of the shoulder in subjects with and without symptoms. Arch Phys Med Rehabil 2006;87(9):1242–9. [Epub 2006/08/29].

47. Lewis JS, Valentine RE. Intraobserver reliability of angular and linear measurements of scapular position in subjects with and without symptoms. Arch Phys Med Rehabil 2008;89(9):1795–802. [Epub 2008/09/02].

48. Jia X, Ji JH, Petersen SA, et al. Clinical evaluation of the shoulder shrug sign. Clin Orthop Relat Res 2008;466(11):2813–19. [Epub 2008/06/11].

49. Nakagawa S, Yoneda M, Hayashida K, et al. Forced shoulder abduction and elbow flexion test: a new simple clinical test to detect superior labral injury in the throwing shoulder. Arthroscopy 2005;21(11):1290–5. [Epub 2005/12/06].

50. Farber AJ, Castillo R, Clough M, et al. Clinical assessment of three common tests for traumatic anterior shoulder instability. J Bone Joint Surg Am 2006;88(7):1467–74. [Epub 2006/07/05].

51. Toprak U, Ustuner E, Ozer D, et al. Palpation tests versus impingement tests in Neer stage I and II subacromial impingement syndrome. Knee Surg Sports Traumatol Arthrosc 2013;21(2):424–9. [Epub 2012/03/29].

52. Walton J, Mahajan S, Paxinos A, et al. Diagnostic values of tests for acromioclavicular joint pain. J Bone Joint Surg Am 2004;86-A(4):807–12. [Epub 2004/04/08].

53. Michener LA, Walsworth MK, Doukas WC, et al. Reliability and diagnostic accuracy of 5 physical examination tests and combination of tests for subacromial impingement. Arch Phys Med Rehabil 2009;90(11):1898–903. [Epub 2009/11/06].

54. Jia X, Petersen SA, Khosravi AH, et al. Examination of the shoulder: the past, the present, and the future. J Bone Joint Surg Am 2009;91(Suppl. 6):10–18. [Epub 2009/11/26].

55. Gross ML, Distefano MC. Anterior release test. A new test for occult shoulder instability. Clin Orthop Relat Res 1997;339:105–8. [Epub 1997/06/01].

56. Schlechter JA, Summa S, Rubin BD. The passive distraction test: a new diagnostic aid for clinically significant superior labral pathology. Arthroscopy 2009;25(12):1374–9. [Epub 2009/12/08].

57. Kim YS, Kim JM, Ha KY, et al. The passive compression test: a new clinical test for superior labral tears of the shoulder. Am J Sports Med 2007;35(9):1489–94. [Epub 2007/05/05].

58. Ben Kibler W, Sciascia AD, Hester P, et al. Clinical utility of traditional and new tests in the diagnosis of biceps tendon injuries and superior labrum anterior and posterior lesions in the shoulder. Am J Sports Med 2009;37(9):1840–7. [Epub 2009/06/11].

59. Bartsch M, Greiner S, Haas NP, et al. Diagnostic values of clinical tests for subscapularis lesions. Knee Surg Sports Traumatol Arthrosc 2010;18(12):1712–17. [Epub 2010/04/09].

60. Barth JR, Burkhart SS, De Beer JF. The bear-hug test: a new and sensitive test for diagnosing a subscapularis tear. Arthroscopy 2006;22(10):1076–84. [Epub 2006/10/10].
61. Bushnell BD, Creighton RA, Herring MM. The bony apprehension test for instability of the shoulder: a prospective pilot analysis. Arthroscopy 2008;24(9):974–82. [Epub 2008/09/02].
62. Adams SL, Yarnold PR, Mathews JJt. Clinical use of the olecranon-manubrium percussion sign in shoulder trauma. Ann Emerg Med 1988;17(5):484–7. [Epub 1988/05/01].
63. Gillooly JJ, Chidambaram R, Mok D. The lateral Jobe test: a more reliable method of diagnosing rotator cuff tears. Int J Shoulder Surg 2010;4(2):41–3. [Epub 2010/11/13].
64. Miller CA, Forrester GA, Lewis JS. The validity of the lag signs in diagnosing full-thickness tears of the rotator cuff: a preliminary investigation. Arch Phys Med Rehabil 2008;89(6):1162–8. [Epub 2008/05/28].
65. Chronopoulos E, Kim TK, Park HB, et al. Diagnostic value of physical tests for isolated chronic acromioclavicular lesions. Am J Sports Med 2004;32(3):655–61. [Epub 2004/04/20].
66. Neer CS 2nd. Impingement lesions. Clin Orthop Relat Res 1983;173:70–7. [Epub 1983/03/01].
67. Hegedus EJ, Goode A, Campbell S, et al. Physical examination tests of the shoulder: a systematic review with meta-analysis of individual tests. Br J Sports Med 2008;42(2):80–92, discussion. [Epub 2007/08/28].
68. Hegedus EJ, Goode AP, Cook CE, et al. Which physical examination tests provide clinicians with the most value when examining the shoulder? Update of a systematic review with meta-analysis of individual tests. Br J Sports Med 2012;46(14):964–78. [Epub 2012/07/10].
69. Girish G, Lobo LG, Jacobson JA, et al. Ultrasound of the shoulder: asymptomatic findings in men. AJR Am J Roentgenol 2011; 197(4):W713–19. [Epub 2011/09/24].
70. Luime JJ, Verhagen AP, Miedema HS, et al. Does this patient have an instability of the shoulder or a labrum lesion? JAMA 2004;292(16):1989–99. [Epub 2004/10/28].
71. de Winter AF, Jans MP, Scholten RJ, et al. Diagnostic classification of shoulder disorders: interobserver agreement and determinants of disagreement. Ann Rheum Dis 1999;58(5):272–7. [Epub 1999/05/04].
72. Norregaard J, Krogsgaard MR, Lorenzen T, et al. Diagnosing patients with longstanding shoulder joint pain. Ann Rheum Dis 2002;61(7):646–9. [Epub 2002/06/25].

CHAPTER 50.2 ■ ROTATOR CUFF TENDINOPATHY AND SUBACROMIAL PAIN SYNDROME

Jeremy Lewis • Karen Ginn

INTRODUCTION

Of the myriad musculoskeletal conditions affecting the shoulder, subacromial impingement (pain) syndrome (SIS) and rotator cuff (RC) tendinopathy are considered to be the most common. There is uncertainty if SIS represents a primary pathology. The pain, weakness and associated morbidity associated with SIS are hypothesized to be primarily due to dysfunction of the RC and not due to a primary mechanical abrasion from the undersurface of the acromion onto the RC.[1] This clinical presentation is also known as painful arc syndrome, RC syndrome and RC disease.

The RC tendon is composed of the tendons of the supraspinatus, infraspinatus, teres minor and subscapularis that interdigitate and fuse together before inserting onto the humeral tuberosities. This structural arrangement improves resistance to failure when the RC is under load because (a) tension in one muscle may be distributed over a wider area and (b) it reduces stress within the tendon during extremes of movement.[2] The RC tendon is confluent, multilayered and interwoven and the supraspinatus tendon is made up of six to nine structurally independent parallel fascicles separated by endotendon and lubricant that facilitates sliding.[3] To support the wide range of functions demanded of the shoulder, the RC contributes to movement, stability and sensory–motor control of the glenohumeral joint. The large range of movement implies that during end-range activities different parts of the RC will be relatively compressed and stretched. This may lead to internal friction and compression within the tendons (see Chapters 10.1 and 10.2).

Uncertainty exists as to the cause of RC pathology with hypotheses including; extrinsic mechanisms such as subacromial impingement, intrinsic mechanisms such as internal tendon failure, and combinations of the two. These hypotheses have been reviewed in detail.[3,4] Other potential causes include weakness and recruitment and timing abnormalities, which may lead to anomalous humeral head translation during movement.[5,6]

ROTATOR CUFF FUNCTION

All RC muscles produce rotation torque at the shoulder: subscapularis (anterior RC) is an internal rotator and infraspinatus, teres minor and supraspinatus (posterior RC) are external rotators.[7–9] Evidence indicates that supraspinatus does not initiate shoulder abduction.[10,11]

The traditional view of the role of the RC muscles to provide functional shoulder joint stability is that they contribute in equal proportions[12] to compress the humeral head into the glenoid fossa during all shoulder movements to limit humeral head translation.[13] In addition, they function to depress the humeral head to prevent potential superior translation of the humerus due to deltoid activity.[14] Recent evidence that the RC muscles are recruited at significantly different activity levels during shoulder flexion and extension suggests that this explanation of the mechanism whereby the RC provides dynamic shoulder joint stability may require revision.[15,16] Shoulder flexion recruits the posterior RC (infraspinatus and supraspinatus) at significantly higher levels than during extension, whereas the subscapularis (anterior RC) is recruited at significantly higher levels during extension.[15,17] This reciprocal recruitment pattern of the RC during sagittal plane shoulder movement is not load-dependent and occurs at low, medium and high loads.[15] Simultaneous recruitment of all the RC muscles in equal proportions, therefore, does not appear to be an essential requirement to achieve dynamic shoulder joint stability.

The direction-specific recruitment pattern of the RC during sagittal plane shoulder movement was found to be highly synchronous with the muscles producing shoulder flexion and extension.[15] This suggests that the different parts of the RC function to stabilize the shoulder joint by counterbalancing potential anterior–posterior humeral head translation forces generated by the muscles producing flexion and extension, respectively.[15] The RC, therefore, functions to prevent potential superior translation of the humeral head due to deltoid activity as well as potential anterior and posterior translation due to flexor and extensor muscle activity, respectively.

The view that the RC muscles are functioning as stabilizers of the shoulder joint during all shoulder movements may also require revision. Maximal isometric shoulder adduction tasks are associated with minimal to low levels of RC muscle activity,[18] suggesting that either activity in shoulder adductor muscles does not produce translation forces on the humeral head, or that muscles other than the RC are functioning to stabilize the shoulder joint during adduction. More research is required to better understand the role of the RC as stabilizers.

Activation of the RC muscles has implications for axio-scapular muscle function. As the RC muscles take their origin from the scapula, contraction of the RC has the potential to move the scapula away from the midline.[19] Therefore, coordinated contraction of axio-scapular muscles to provide a stable muscular anchor for the scapula is necessary for optimal RC function.[19]

DIAGNOSIS

SIS is most probably a collection of clinical symptoms and not a clinical entity. It is unlikely that the Neer sign and Hawkins test are identifying an actual condition but are more likely to be reproducing symptoms that may include underlying RC pathology. The incidence of RC tendinopathy has been reported to range from 0.3% to 5.5% and the point prevalence from 2.4% to 21% across all age groups.[20] However, many people choose not to report their symptoms, and as outlined in Chapter 50.1, deriving a definitive diagnosis of RC pathology is difficult.[21–24] Therefore interpreting epidemiological data and deriving inferences need to be done with caution.

Studies have demonstrated that many people without symptoms have structural pathology in the region[25,26] and there is no robust way of determining if the presenting symptoms are due to the observed structural failure.[1,24] This has implications for clinical decision making, including recommendations for surgery.[1,24]

In order to derive a clinical diagnosis of RC pathology other potential causes of shoulder pain, for example referral from the cervical spine, glenohumeral joint instability or osteoarthritis, should be excluded.[27] Pain associated with RC tendinopathy may extend over the shoulder and/or lateral and proximal upper arm. It is exacerbated by arm movements, particularly overhead activities, and frequently increases at night.[27] A recent systematic review reported that the most accurate pain provocation test for detecting RC tendinopathy was the painful arc test: pain occurring in mid-range shoulder abduction had the highest LR and no pain during shoulder abduction the lowest LR.[28] As all the RC muscles produce rotation torque at the shoulder, assessment of active and passive rotation ROM and rotation strength will aid in diagnosing RC pathology. It is recommended that, if possible, these tests be performed at 90° abduction[29] where electromyographic studies suggest that RC muscles are more specifically recruited.[16] Limitation of movement that occurs only with active motion suggests impairment of the RC muscles and although associated with diagnostic uncertainty, external and internal rotation lag tests have been identified as the most accurate clinical tests for identifying full-thickness RC tears.[28] Pain and weakness when testing shoulder external rotation strength have been found to be the most accurate test for detecting symptomatic RC disease.[28] However, it is important to reiterate that none of these tests are definitive and other sources of pain and weakness must be considered and excluded.[24]

In a recent investigation of individuals with unilateral RC tendinopathy, Roy et al.[30] used transcranial magnetic stimulation to map both the infraspinatus on the side with symptoms and the asymptomatic side. Their findings suggested that decreased corticospinal excitability was observed on the symptomatic side and that this asymmetry was related to chronicity, but not to intensity of pain. This investigation is the first to observe this type of change associated with RC tendinopathy, and it is extremely relevant for clinicians as it suggests cortical reorganization occurs in the presence of pain and may contribute to explaining the poor correlation between local tendon imaging changes and symptoms.[1,24] Further research is needed to determine if the pain associated with RC tendinopathy is driving the cortical changes or vice versa and whether exercise as therapy and other interventions, such as lifestyle factors (Chapters 11 and 37), influence the cortical changes associated with RC pathology.

TREATMENT

The main intervention for treating SIS and RC tendinopathy is active exercise therapy.[31] The limited data available suggest that implementing a programme of physiotherapist-supervised exercises confers clinical benefit in the short and longer term when compared to no treatment or placebo treatment. In patients with mixed shoulder disorders, including SIS and RC pathology, significantly greater recovery, function and ROM was demonstrated in the group receiving exercise after 1 month compared to those receiving no treatment.[32] People diagnosed with RC disease who received exercise therapy demonstrated significant functional benefit at 2.5 years follow-up compared with a placebo group.[33]

Over the past decade a number of randomized clinical trials have been published which clearly demonstrate that an exercise-based approach should be considered first in the management of RC tendinopathy and SIS.[34,35] Not only do these studies suggest that no additional benefit is conferred from surgical intervention, but an exercise-based approach is also associated with substantial savings for health funding bodies. Haahr et al.[36] reported at 1-year follow-up that there was no difference in outcomes between subacromial decompression and exercise for a group of 90 people diagnosed with SIS. At 4- to 8-year follow-up they again concluded no significant clinical difference in outcome between the groups with more payments for sick leave being required in the surgical group.[37] Ketola et al. concluded that exercise was as effective as surgery at 1-year follow-up[38] and again at 5-year follow-up,[39] arguing that subacromial decompression was not cost-effective and exercise should be given first priority. The average number of physiotherapy treatments ranged from seven to 19 sessions (each lasting 60 minutes), and physiotherapy care pathways should be developed using these data as a minimal acceptable standard. Specific exercise approaches have demonstrated positive outcomes in patients diagnosed with SIS[40] and full-thickness[41] and massive RC tears.[42] Ainsworth et al.[42] demonstrated positive outcomes at 3 and 6 months using a specific exercise approach for people with massive RC tears. There is a paucity of research comparing surgical repair and exercise for partial- and full-thickness tears of the RC. With the exception of those who have sustained traumatic tears of the RC, and due to the poor correlation between structural failure and symptoms, it would appear to be advisable to trial exercise therapy first and if desired outcomes are not being achieved at specific time points then an onward referral for a surgical opinion would be warranted.

Although exercise appears to be the most valuable type of treatment for SIS and RC pathology, many exercise strategies have been proposed and little evidence is available to guide the clinician to the most appropriate and effective exercises. Although it is often advocated that particular exercises target particular shoulder muscles it is clear from many electromyographic studies that most exercises elicit significant levels of activity in a large number of shoulder muscles.[43,44] This is to be expected since movements of the humerus and scapula occur simultaneously to produce full-range movement of the shoulder and because the RC and axio-scapular muscles must also be recruited to prevent muscle forces from destabilizing the humeral head and scapula, respectively.

A thorough examination of shoulder movement quality and muscle function should determine the choice of treatment goals and appropriate exercises.[29] All parameters of muscle function should be considered, including active and passive length; isometric, concentric and eccentric strength; inner, mid and outer range strength; strength balance; and recruitment pattern/rhythm. As RC and axio-scapular muscles perform both mover and

stabilizer roles, exercises should be tailored to address these different functional roles as well as performed in a manner related to the specific functional needs of the patient.

Although different rationale have been proposed to justify exercise strategies to treat SIS and RC pathology,[45,46] a number of common guiding principles emerge. Evidence suggests that shoulder ROM and muscle power may improve when pain is reduced.[4,5] Pain, weakness and loss of normal function are features associated with RC pathology. Pain, which may be irritable and present at night, may be addressed by relative rest and supported by appropriate medication and intra-subacromial bursal injection therapy.[4] Acute or acute on chronic tendon pain may be associated with a proliferation of tendons cells and both glucocorticoids and analgesics (e.g. bupivacaine) have been reported to reduce tenocyte numbers[47,48] with possible equal clinical benefit.[49,50] Injections into the subacromial bursa, as part of an appropriately structured rehabilitation programme, may be beneficial in managing the pain. Weakness may be real or caused by pain inhibition or a combination of both, and may be addressed by pain management and a graduated exercise programme. It may be appropriate to provide advice to avoid painful shoulder activities and initially perform exercises in a pain-free manner to promote normal muscle function and movement patterns as part of the management programme.[51] The restoration of normal movement patterns is a principal aim of exercise programmes whether they are designed to address painful tendons,[4] altered scapular kinematics[29] or abnormal neuromuscular control.[51] Exercise therapy should be performed in a controlled and graduated manner whether the aim is to exercise an under-loaded RC tendon,[4] to improve motor control by gradually increasing the complexity of the exercises[51] or to achieve conscious scapular control before progressing to scapular and RC strengthening exercises.[24,29] Patients should be advised that the exercise programme will need to be done regularly over a number of weeks and months to achieve the ongoing mechanical stimulation to restore and maintain tendon health or to restore normal RC and axio-scapular muscle length, strength and/or motor control patterns.[29,51]

It is important to recognize that people diagnosed with RC pathology who do not respond to exercise therapy and other treatments including medications, injections and surgery may have non-peripherally mediated pain mechanisms, with their experience of pain being due to central sensitization.[52,53]

WHAT ELSE INFLUENCES OUTCOME?

Although exercise therapy is the mainstay of the management for SIS and RC tendinopathy,[4] other interventions may contribute to improving clinical outcomes. The available evidence from randomized controlled trials supports the use of subacromial corticosteroid injection for RC disease, although its effect may be small and short-lived.[54]

The evidence to support the inclusion of manual therapy with exercise for the treatment of SIS and RC pathology varies depending on where the passive mobilization/manipulation techniques are applied. Adding manual therapy applied to the cervicothoracic vertebral region and/or thorax to exercise therapy confers short- to medium-term clinical benefit compared to exercise therapy alone.[55,56] Conversely, the addition of manual therapy applied to the shoulder region joints (glenohumeral, acromioclavicular and sternoclavicular joints) to exercise therapy and advice does not appear to result in additional clinical benefit.[57] The long-term benefit of adding manual therapy to exercise in the treatment of SIS and RC pathology is not known.

The evidence for low-level laser therapy in the management of RC tendinopathy, although not definitive, suggests it may be beneficial.[58] The use of therapeutic ultrasound and extracorporeal shock wave therapy for non-calcific RC tendinosis does not appear to be supported; however, there may be some benefit for calcific tendinosis.[59,60] Taping may also be beneficial in the short term[61] but again more robust research is required.

Cigarette smoking appears to be a risk factor in RC pathology[62] and smoking cessation may be beneficial in the management of this condition. Future research may also establish an improvement in the outcome of RC pathology with dietary management.[63–65]

MEASURING OUTCOME

Measuring the effectiveness of clinical intervention is an essential component of clinical practice to guide treatment progression and evaluate treatment outcome. For interventions targeting the RC, outcome measures would typically include measuring; pain,[38] shoulder range of movement[66] and strength,[67] and may include thoracic[68] and scapular[69] posture. More important than these measurements of impairment, are measurements of function and disability that should be evaluated using validated outcome measures such as; the DASH, Quick-DASH and SPADI.[70–72]

POSTURE AND MUSCLE IMBALANCE

Deviations from an ideal posture and associated muscle imbalances are considered to be mechanisms that result in pain and movement abnormality. Although upper body postural abnormalities are frequently associated with SIS and RC tendon pathology,[73,74] evidence supporting postural abnormalities in the pathogenesis of these shoulder pathologies is lacking.[75] No study has found that treatment directed at improving posture can in fact change posture in the long term in people with shoulder symptoms or that a change in posture is the reason for long-term improvements in function and reductions in pain.[76]

It has been suggested that in the presence of the classic forward head posture, there is an associated increase in the thoracic kyphosis and changes in scapular posture, such that the scapula tilts anteriorly and downwards.[74]

Downward scapular rotation and excessive anterior tilt are frequently attributed to shortening of the pectoralis minor.[77] With the patient supine a distance of greater than 2.5 cm from the treatment couch to the posterior acromion has been attributed to a short pectoralis minor muscle.[77] However, the evidence supporting scapular posture and muscle imbalance in the aetiology of SIS and RC pathology remains at best equivocal. A recent systematic review failed to identify evidence for a consistent alteration in scapular posture across studies that investigated SIS and scapular position.[78] Research on the pectoralis minor length test failed to identify differences in people with and without shoulder pain, with the distance being marginally greater in people with no symptoms.[79] In addition, if poor posture and a concomitant alteration in scapular posture does lead to irritation of the RC, the pathology should occur on the superior (bursal) surface of tendon. A recent narrative review summarizing findings of observational studies reported that the majority of RC tendon pathology was observed to occur on the joint side of the tendon or within the tendon, a finding that largely refutes the acromial abrasion theory.[1] As an alternative to the examination of static posture to inform management, an approach that assesses dynamic changes to posture may be warranted.[24]

CONCLUSIONS

Further research is essential to identify methods of facilitating more accurate diagnosis of RC pathology and exclude other sources of pain experienced in the shoulder. It is important to appreciate that there is a poor correlation between pain, symptoms and imaging findings. The implication is that structural pathology identified by current imaging modalities may not necessarily be the cause of symptoms. The tissue changes, chemicals or changes in motor recruitment responsible for the symptoms remain elusive, and in others the symptoms may result from central sensitization. It is clear that a biopsychosocial approach to assessment and management is essential. There is mounting evidence supporting exercise therapy in the management of RC tendinopathy and the challenge is to identify more effective ways to deliver this type of intervention. Patient education and lifestyle management are also important components that support successful rehabilitation.

REFERENCES

1. Lewis JS. Subacromial impingement syndrome: a musculoskeletal condition or a clinical illusion? Phys Ther Rev 2011;16(5): 388–98.
2. Clark JM, Harryman DT 2nd. Tendons, ligaments, and capsule of the rotator cuff. Gross and microscopic anatomy. J Bone Joint Surg 1992;74(5):713–25.
3. Lewis JS. Rotator cuff tendinopathy. Br J Sports Med 2009;43(4): 236–41. [Epub 2008/09/20].
4. Lewis JS. Rotator cuff tendinopathy: a model for the continuum of pathology and related management. Br J Sports Med 2010;44(13): 918–23.
5. Chester R, Smith TO, Hooper L, et al. The impact of subacromial impingement syndrome on muscle activity patterns of the shoulder

complex: a systematic review of electromyographic studies. BMC Musculoskelet Disord 2010;11:45. [Epub 2010/03/11].

6. Cools A, Witvrouw E, Declercq G, et al. Scapular muscle recruitment patterns: trapezius muscle latency with and without impingement symptoms. Am J Sports Med 2003;31(4):542–9.

7. Boettcher C, Ginn K, Cathers I. What is the optimal exercise for supraspinatus strengthening? Med Sci Sports Exerc 2009;41(11):1979–83.

8. Dark A, Ginn K, Halaki M. The effect of increasing resistance on shoulder muscle activity levels during commonly-used rotator cuff exercises. Phys Ther 2007;87(8):1039–46.

9. Reinold M, Wilk K, Flesig G, et al. Electromyographis analysis of the rotator cuff and deltoid musculature during common shoulder external rotation exercises. J Orthop Sports Phys Ther 2004;34(7):385–94.

10. van Linge B, Mulder JD. Function of the supraspinatus muscle and its relation to the supraspinatus syndrome: an experimental study in man. J Bone Joint Surg 1963;45B(4):750–4.

11. Reed D, Cathers I, Halaki M, et al. Does supraspinatus initiate shoulder abduction? J Electromyogr Kinesiol 2012.

12. Sharkey N, Marder R, Hansen P. The entire rotator cuff contributes to elevation of the arm. J Orthop Res 1994;12:699–708.

13. Lippitt S, Matsen F. Mechanisms of glenohumeral joint stability. Clin Orthop 1993;291:20–8.

14. Sharkey N, Marder R. The rotator cuff opposes superior translation of the humeral head. Am J Sports Med 1995;23(3):270–5.

15. Wattanaprakornkul D, Cathers I, Halaki M, et al. The rotator cuff muscles have a direction specific recruitment pattern during flexion and extension exercises. J Sci Med Sport 2011;14:376–82.

16. Boettcher C, Cathers I, Ginn K. Shoulder muscle recruitment strategies are task specific. J Sci Med Sport 2010;[Epub 10.1016/j.jsams.2010.03.008].

17. Wattanaprakornkul D, Halaki M, Boettcher C, et al. A comprehensive analysis of muscle recruitment patterns during shoulder flexion: an electromyographic study. Clin Anat 2011;24(6):619–26.

18. Reed D, Halaki M, Ginn K. The rotator cuff muscles are activated at low levels during shoulder adduction: an experimantal study. J Physiother 2010;56(4):259–64.

19. Kibler W. The role of the scapula in athletic shoulder function. Am J Sports Med 1998;26(2):325–37.

20. Littlewood C, May S, Walters S. Epidemiology of rotator cuff tendinopathy: a systematic review. Shoulder Elbow 2013;5(4):256–65.

21. Boettcher CA, Ginn KA, Cathers I. The 'empty can' and 'full can' tests do not selectively activate supraspinatus. J Sci Med Sport 2009;12(4):435–9.

22. Lewis JS, Tennent TD. How effective are diagnostic tests for the assessment of rotator cuff disease of the shoulder? In: MacAuley D, Best TM, editors. Evidenced Based Sports Medicine. 2nd ed. London: Blackwell Publishing; 2007.

23. Hegedus EJ, Goode AP, Cook CE, et al. Which physical examination tests provide clinicians with the most value when examining the shoulder? Update of a systematic review with meta-analysis of individual tests. Br J Sports Med 2012;46(14):964–78. [Epub 2012/07/10].

24. Lewis JS. Rotator cuff tendinopathy/subacromial impingement syndrome: is it time for a new method of assessment? Br J Sports Med 2009;43(4):259–64.

25. Frost P, Andersen JH, Lundorf E. Is supraspinatus pathology as defined by magnetic resonance imaging associated with clinical sign of shoulder impingement? J Shoulder Elbow Surg 1999;8(6):565–8.

26. Girish G, Lobo LG, Jacobson JA, et al. Ultrasound of the shoulder: asymptomatic findings in men. AJR Am J Roentgenol 2011;197(4):W713–19. [Epub 2011/09/24].

27. Gomoll A, Katz J, Warner J, et al. Rotator cuff disorders: recognition and management among patients with shoulder pain. Arth Rheum 2004;50(12):3751–61.

28. Hermans J, Luime J, Meuffels D, et al. Does this patient with shoulder pain have rotator cuff disease? the rational clinical examination systematic review. JAMA 2013;310(8):837–47.

29. Ellenbecker T, Cools A. Rehabilitation of shoulder impingement syndrome and rotator cuff injuries: an evidenced-based review. Br J Sports Med 2010;44:319–27.

30. Roy JS, Ngomo S, Mercier C. Is asymmetry in corticospinal excitability of the infraspinatus muscle correlated with shoulder-specific

outcomes following rotator cuff tendinopathy? 12th International Congress on Shoulder and Elbow Surgery and 4th International Congress of Shoulder and Elbow Therapists; Nagoya, Japan. 2013.

31. van der Heijden GJMG. Shoulder disorders: a state-of-the-art review. Ballieres Clin Rheumatol 1999;13(2):287–309.

32. Ginn K, Herbert R, Khouw W, et al. A randomised, controlled clinical trial of a treatment for shoulder pain. Phys Ther 1997;77(8):802–11.

33. Brox J, Gjengedal E, Uppheim G, et al. Arthroscopic surgery versus supervised exercises in patients with rotator cuff disease (stage ii impingement syndrome): a prospective, randomised, controlled study in 125 patients with 2.5 year follow-up. J Shoulder Elbow Surg 1999;8(2):102–11.

34. Coghlan J, Buchbinder R, Green S, et al. Surgery for rotator cuff disease. Cochrane Database Syst Rev 2008;(1):CD005619.

35. Gebremariam L, Hay E, Koes B, et al. Effectiveness of surgical and postsurgical interventions for subacromial impingment syndrome: a systematic review. Arch Phys Med Rehabil 2011;92:1900.

36. Haahr JP, Ostergaard S, Dalsgaard J, et al. Exercises versus arthroscopic decompression in patients with subacromial impingement: a randomised, controlled study in 90 cases with a one year follow up. Ann Rheum Dis 2005;64(5):760–4.

37. Haahr JP, Andersen JH. Exercises may be as efficient as subacromial decompression in patients with subacromial stage II impingement: 4–8-years' follow-up in a prospective, randomized study. Scand J Rheumatol 2006;35(3):224–8.

38. Ketola S, Lehtinen J, Arnala I, et al. Does arthroscopic acromioplasty provide any additional value in the treatment of shoulder impingement syndrome?: a two-year randomised controlled trial. J Bone Joint Surg 2009;91(10):1326–34.

39. Ketola S, Lehtinen J, Rousi T, et al. No evidence of long-term benefits of arthroscopicacromioplasty in the treatment of shoulder impingement syndrome: five-year results of a randomised controlled trial. Bone Joint Res 2013;2(7):132–9. [Epub 2013/07/10].

40. Holmgren T, Hallgren H, Oberg B, et al. Effect of specific exercise staregy on need for surgery in patients with subacromial impingement syndrome: randomised controlled study. BMJ 2012;344:e787.

41. Kuhn J, Dunn W, Sanders R, et al. Effectiveness of physical therapy in treating atraumatic full-thickness rotator cuff tears: a multicenter prospective cohort study. J Shoulder Elbow Surg 2013;22:1371–9.

42. Ainsworth R, Lewis JS, Conboy V. A prospective randomized placebo controlled clinical trial of a rehabilitation programme for patients with a diagnosis of massive rotator cuff tears of the shoulder. Shoulder Elbow 2009;1(1):55–60.

43. Boettcher C, Ginn K, Cathers I. Standard maximum isometric voluntary contraction tests for normalizing shoulder muscle EMG. J Orthop Res 2008;26(12):1591–7.

44. Hintermeister R, Lange G, Schultheis J, et al. Electromagnetic activity and applied load during shoulder rehabilitation exercises using elastic resistance. Am J Sports Med 1998;26(2):210–20.

45. Ben-Yishay A, Zuckermann J, Gallagher M, et al. Pain inhibition of shoulder strength in patients with impingement syndrome. Orthopedics 1994;17:685–8.

46. Brox J, Roe C, Saugen E, et al. Isometric abduction muscle activation in patients with rotator tendinosis of the shoulder. Arch Phys Med Rehabil 1997;78:1260–7.

47. Scutt N, Rolf CG, Scutt A. Glucocorticoids inhibit tenocyte proliferation and Tendon progenitor cell recruitment. J Orthop Res 2006;24(2):173–82. [Epub 2006/01/26].

48. Scherb MB, Han SH, Courneya JP, et al. Effect of bupivacaine on cultured tenocytes. Orthopedics 2009;32(1):26. [Epub 2009/02/20].

49. Alvarez CM, Litchfield R, Jackowski D, et al. A prospective, double-blind, randomized clinical trial comparing subacromial injection of betamethasone and xylocaine to xylocaine alone in chronic rotator cuff tendinosis. Am J Sports Med 2005;33(2):255–62.

50. Ekeberg OM, Bautz-Holter E, Tveita EK, et al. Subacromial ultrasound guided or systemic steroid injection for rotator cuff disease: randomised double blind study. Br Med J 2009;338:a3112.

51. Ginn K, Cohen M. Exercise therapy aimed at restoring neuromuscular control for the treatment of shoulder pain: a randomised comparative clinical trial. J Rehabil Med 2005;37:115–22.

52. Gwilym SE, Oag HC, Tracey I, et al. Evidence that central sensitisation is present in patients with shoulder impingement syndrome

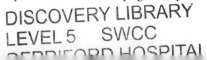

and influences the outcome after surgery. J Bone Joint Surg Br 2011;93(4):498–502. [Epub 2011/04/06].

53. Gifford L. The 'central' mechanisms. In: Gifford L, editor. Topical issues in pain 1. Falmouth: CNS Press; 1998. p. 67–80.

54. Buchbinder R, Green S, Youd J. Corticosteroid injections for shoulder pain. Cochrane Database Syst Rev 2009.

55. Bang M, Deyle G. Comparison of supervised exercise with and without manual physical therapy for patients with shoulder impingement syndrome. J Orthop Sports Phys Ther 2000;30(3):126–37.

56. Bergman G, Winters J, Groenier K, et al. Manipulative therapy in addition to usual care for patients with shoulder dysfunction and pain. Ann Intern Med 2004;141:432–9.

57. Yiasemides R, Halaki M, Cathers I, et al. Does passive joint mobilization of shoulder region joints provide additional benefit over advice and exercise alone for people who have shoulder pain and minimal movement restriction? A randomized controlled trial. Phys Ther 2011;91(2).

58. Tumilty S, Munn J, McDonough S, et al. Low level laser treatment of tendinopathy: a systematic review with meta-analysis. Photomed Laser Surg 2010;28(1):3–16. [Epub 2009/08/28].

59. Green S, Buchbinder R, Hetrick S. Physiotherapy interventions for shoulder pain. Cochrane Database Syst Rev 2003;(2):CD004258.

60. Huisstede B, Gebremariam L, Sande Rvd, et al. Evidence for effectiveness of extracorporal shock-wave therapy (ESWT) to treat calcific and non-calcific rotator cuff tendinosis e A systematic review. Man Ther 2011;16(11):419–33.

61. Teys P, Bisset L, Collins N, et al. One-week time course of the effects of Mulligan's Mobilisation with Movement and taping in painful shoulders. Man Ther 2013;18(5):372–7. [Epub 2013/02/09].

62. Baumgarten KM, Gerlach D, Galatz LM, et al. Cigarette smoking increases the risk for rotator cuff tears. Clin Orthop Relat Res 2010;468(6):1534–41. [Epub 2009/03/14].

63. Radak Z, Takahashi R, Kumiyama A, et al. Effect of aging and late onset dietary restriction on antioxidant enzymes and proteasome activities, and protein carbonylation of rat skeletal muscle and tendon. Exp Gerontol 2002;37(12):1423–30.

64. Fallon K, Purdam C, Cook J, et al. A 'polypill' for acute tendon pain in athletes with tendinopathy? J Sci Med Sport Med Aust 2008;11(3):235–8. [Epub 2007/12/14].

65. Lewis JS, Sandford FM. Rotator cuff tendinopathy: is there a role for polyunsaturated Fatty acids and antioxidants? J Hand Ther 2009;22(1):49–56.

66. Valentine RE, Lewis JS. Intraobserver reliability of 4 physiologic movements of the shoulder in subjects with and without symptoms. Arch Phys Med Rehabil 2006;87(9):1242–9.

67. Dollings H, Sandford F, O'Conaire E, et al. Shoulder strength testing: the intra-and inter-tester reliability of routine clinical tests, using the PowerTrack II Commander. Shoulder Elbow 2012;4(2):131–40.

68. Barrett E, McCreesh K, Lewis J. Reliability and validity of non-radiographic methods of thoracic kyphosis measurement: a systematic review. Man Ther 2014;19(1):10–17.

69. Lewis JS, Valentine RE. Intraobserver reliability of angular and linear measurements of scapular position in subjects with and without symptoms. Arch Phys Med Rehabil 2008;89(9):1795–802.

70. Gabel CP, Yelland M, Melloh M, et al. A modified QuickDASH-9 provides a valid outcome instrument for upper limb function. BMC Musculoskelet Disord 2009;10:161. [Epub 2009/12/22].

71. Beaton DE, Katz JN, Fossel AH, et al. Measuring the whole or the parts? Validity, reliability, and responsiveness of the Disabilities of the Arm, Shoulder and Hand outcome measure in different regions of the upper extremity. J Hand Ther 2001;14(2):128–46. [Epub 2001/05/31].

72. Roach KE, Budiman-Mak E, Songsiridej N, et al. Development of a shoulder pain and disability index. Arthritis Care Res 1991;4(4):143–9.

73. Grimsby O, Gray J. Interrelation of the spine to the shoulder girdle. In: Donatelli R, editor. Physical Therapy of the Shoulder. 3rd ed. New York: Churchill Livingstone; 1997. p. 95–129.

74. Gray J, Grimsby O. Interrelationship of the spine, rib cage, and shoulder. In: Donatelli R, editor. Physical Therapy of the Shoulder. 4th ed. Edinburgh: Churchill Livingston; 2004. p. 133–85.

75. Lewis JS, Green A, Wright C. Subacromial impingement syndrome: the role of posture and muscle imbalance. J Shoulder Elbow Surg 2005;14(4):385–92.

76. McClure PW, Bialker J, Neff N, et al. Shoulder function and 3-dimensional kinematics in people with shoulder impingement syndrome before and after a 6-week exercise program. Phys Ther 2004;84(9):832–48.

77. Sahrmann S. Diagnosis and treatment of movement impairment syndromes. London: Mosby; 2002.

78. Ratcliffe E, Pickering S, McLean S, et al. Is there a relationship between subacromial impingement syndrome and scapular orientation? A systematic review. Br J Sports Med 2013;[Epub 2013/11/01].

79. Lewis JS, Valentine RE. The pectoralis minor length test: a study of the intra-rater reliability and diagnostic accuracy in subjects with and without shoulder symptoms. BMC Musculoskelet Disord 2007;8(1):64.

CHAPTER 50.3 ■ THE UNSTABLE SHOULDER

Lyn Watson • Tania Pizzari • Jane Simmonds • Jeremy Lewis

INTRODUCTION

The glenohumeral joint (GHJ) requires a large range of multi-planar motion to enable the upper limb to perform multiple and complex functional tasks that range from precision activities such as writing to high-powered explosive activities commonplace in sport. Passive and dynamic structures are required to maintain congruence between the humeral head and glenoid fossa in order to stabilize the GHJ during all shoulder movements and activities.[1] Deficits in these structures may lead to GHJ instability and be associated with substantial disability due to loss of normal movement, pain and kinesiophobia, resulting in compromised function and reduced quality of life.[2]

GHJ instability represents a spectrum of disorders with overlapping syndromes that range from complete dislocation of the joint to excessive uncontrolled translation of the humeral head leading to secondary shoulder symptoms.[1,3–7] Although a number of classification systems for shoulder instability have been proposed, none have gained universal acceptance. This creates difficulties not only for diagnosis and inter-professional communication, but also for evaluation and comparisons of treatments across trials.[1,8] The FEDS system, which evaluates the patient perception of frequency, aetiology, direction and severity of the instability, is the only system to date that has been tested for reliability and content validity.[8] However, this system has been criticized for eliminating multidirectional instability and pain in the overhead athlete from the classification, and for failing to address voluntary instability.[9]

Shoulder instability may occur as a result of traumatic injury, repetitive use, or be inherited.[1] In the absence of an accepted classification system, it may be appropriate to use an individual or algorithmic approach to the diagnosis and management of instability.[10] A well-structured clinical examination that systematically documents the factors associated with each individual suffering from instability enables the clinician to determine the direction, severity, functional impact and most appropriate management pathway. In this chapter, instability will be classified according to direction, and will cover unidirectional instabilities (anterior, posterior or inferior) and multidirectional instability.

Anterior shoulder instability is the predominant direction of instability. The incidence of anterior shoulder dislocation is estimated to range from 8.2 to 56.3 dislocations per 100 000 people per year,[11-14] with an estimated prevalence of 1.7%.[8] These data almost certainly underestimate the prevalence of instability as they relate to joint dislocations and not to other forms of instability such as subluxations, which may occur at rates five times higher than dislocations in young athletes.[15]

Although posterior dislocation is less common than anterior, there is a higher rate of associated bone and soft tissue injury.[16] Posterior dislocations are considered to account for only 2–3% of all shoulder instabilities. However, the majority of posterior dislocations are missed on initial examination,[16] and posterior subluxation or translational instability may be easily overlooked and misdiagnosed as 'impingement' pain or tight posterior capsule. Assessment of humeral head translation during flexion and horizontal flexion may help identify excessive posterior translation of the humeral head. Posterior instabilities may be associated with increased joint laxity and with multidirectional instability. Increased retroversion of the glenoid fossa may also be associated with posterior instability.[17]

Multidirectional instability (MDI) may be defined as symptomatic glenohumeral subluxation or dislocation in more than one direction as a result of repetitive microtrauma, muscle incoordination and congenital differences in the joint.[18-21] The quintessential finding of this clinical condition is the presence of symptomatic inferior instability (sulcus sign) in addition to anterior and posterior dislocations or subluxations of the shoulder.[22-24] The literature presents varying opinions on whether two or three directions of instability are required to be classified as MDI, whether the onset is always atraumatic[23,25-29] or whether MDI exists at all.[8]

Following traumatic dislocations, the shoulder joint is more susceptible to recurrent dislocation due to instability. Two-thirds of all anterior dislocations are reported to recur in patients aged less than 20 years old.[30,31] These rates drop slightly (to approximately 40%) in those aged between 20 and 40 years and are further reduced (less than 15%) in people aged over 40 years.[31] With respect to posterior dislocations, an overall recurrence rate of 17.7% has been reported and is highest in younger people.[32]

ASSESSMENT

Interview

The FEDS classification system identifies the patient interview as the most important component of the examination.[8] Many features of the patient's history may alter the clinicians' decision-making process for both the clinical examination and treatment strategies. A history of trauma increases the likelihood of a structural lesion such as a labral tear, and this might place the patient at risk of recurrence and the possible need for surgery. A sudden increase or worsening of symptoms may suggest the onset of a structural lesion associated with repetitive microtrauma in a person who has been classified with atraumatic instability. However, as discussed in Chapter 50.1 (Shoulder Assessment) not all structural lesions are symptomatic.[33,34]

The frequency of instability impacts on treatment planning, and people with recurrent dislocations that substantially affect function are more likely to require surgical stabilization. The direction of instability experienced by the individual is also important to establish, as this will influence rehabilitation strategies. Some individuals are able to clearly define and even demonstrate the direction(s) of their shoulder instability and may even be able to reduce a dislocation of the GHJ independently. Others may sense that the shoulder is unstable but may not be able to accurately describe the direction(s) of the instability.[20,25,35]

Pain patterns may vary[1] although the most likely description is global shoulder pain, ill-defined and rather vague in location, that is often activity- or position-specific.[19,20,25] In patients with an inferior component to their instability pattern, paraesthesia may develop, particularly with use of the arm by the side, such as when carrying or writing.[35]

Physical Examination

In standing, active ranges of movement are performed to ascertain where in the ROM the instability occurs. In particular, abduction, flexion, horizontal flexion (in varying ranges of flexion) and external rotation (through varying ranges of abduction) are observed since these commonly demonstrate through-range subluxations.[24,36-38]

Treatment direction tests involve determining the influence of changing the thoracic kyphosis, scapular position and humeral head position on symptoms, in isolation or combination.[34,39-41] Decreasing the thoracic kyphosis is associated with a concomitant posterior scapular tilt. These procedures may be applied to any movement, posture and orthopaedic test that reproduce the individual's symptoms.[34,40,41]

These types of correction techniques will help determine whether the patient's instability symptoms will respond to rehabilitation and help direct the direction of the rehabilitation protocol. One specific suggestion involves positioning the scapula in a combination of slight (10°) upward rotation, elevation (1–2 cm) and 5° posterior tilt (Fig. 50-2).[40,41]

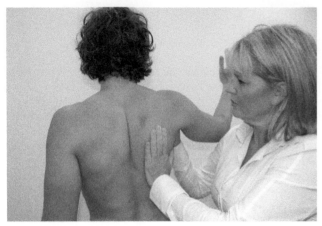

FIGURE 50-2 ■ Scapular positioning in a combination of slight (10°) upward rotation, elevation (1–2 cm) and 5° posterior tilt.

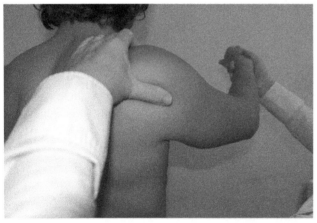

FIGURE 50-3 ■ Manually applied anteriorly directed force on the humeral head.

Humeral head procedures that involve an anteriorly (Fig. 50-3) or posteriorly directed force may be achieved manually,[34,40,41] with seatbelts or neoprene straps. The advantage of a neoprene shoulder fixation belt[34] is that they may be applied with varying force and directions as well as during functional activities such as weight bearing (push up) and throwing and may also be used in treatment (Fig. 50-4).

Orthopaedic Instability Tests

Shoulder assessment including the orthopaedic instability tests has been discussed in Chapter 50.1, and a comprehensive review has been published.[42] There is a possible risk of dislocation when performing the tests designed to assess instability and as such they must be performed cautiously. When performing these tests a positive finding for instability is increased translation associated with reproduction of the patient's symptoms (pain, guarding or apprehension).[20,43,44]

MANAGEMENT

Anterior Dislocation

Following dislocation, management typically involves reduction and immobilization, followed by rehabilitation to strengthen the shoulder.[45] Historically, surgery has been reserved for recurrent dislocations, associated GHJ trauma, or the presence of ongoing symptoms.[46] However, robust evidence supports surgical intervention over conservative management for the prevention of recurrence in young active males following primary anterior dislocation.[26,45,46] Surgery is associated with few complications and has also been shown to produce superior functional outcomes in comparison to conservative management.[45] The high risk of recurrent dislocations in young active males, combined with evidence that recurrence potentially leads to damage of the passive stabilizing structures[47] and that cumulative trauma may result in higher degrees of osteoarthritis,[48] suggests a surgical approach as first-line treatment should be considered.[49,50]

The reluctance to adopt surgical intervention as the primary management approach possibly stems from a lack of confidence in the research evidence and the limited generalizability of the findings to the general population.[50] Variations in the types of surgical interventions and conservative management provision exist in the literature.[45,46,50] It is therefore impossible to conclude that the studies to date have compared 'best practice' surgical intervention with 'best practice' conservative intervention. It should also be considered that some individuals will have success with conservative management, while others may require stabilization. While respecting patient values and understanding their aspirations, identifying those that may benefit from the most appropriate conservative treatment[51] will help avoid unnecessary surgery.[52]

The best surgical technique following anterior dislocation remains a matter of debate.[53] Although arthroscopic surgery is becoming increasingly popular,[54] a recent Cochrane review[55] reported no definitive differences in outcome between arthroscopic and open surgery to anteriorly stabilize the shoulder.

A bony (non-anatomical) procedure (e.g. Latarjet–Bristow) is advocated for patients at high risk of recurrence[56] in preference to a soft tissue, arthroscopic repair. Currently, there is no consensus as to what constitutes best post-surgical rehabilitation.

Following an acute dislocation where no fracture has occurred, immobilization is generally prescribed (typically for 2 weeks) until pain is reduced. The duration and position of immobilization after anterior dislocation have been debated.[57] For people under the age of 30 years there may be no difference in recurrence rates when immobilized in internal rotation for less than 1 week when compared to 3 weeks or even longer periods of immobilization.[58] Additionally, duration of immobilization in internal rotation does not appear to impact on outcome.[51,52,59] Similar recurrence rates are reported following immobilization in external rotation for 0, 3, or 6 weeks.[60] Compliance rates for immobilization in both internal and external rotation are typically low.[61]

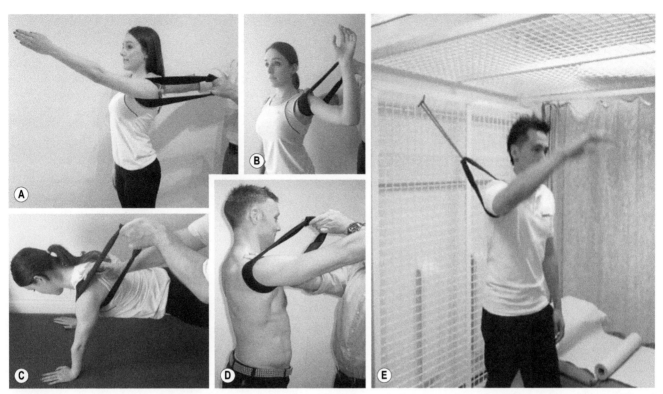

FIGURE 50-4 ■ Humeral head 'positioning' procedures applied with a purpose-built neoprene shoulder fixation strap. Anterior (A) and posterior (P) glides with varying pressures and inclinations may be applied during weight-bearing and non-weight-bearing activities of variable speeds and complexities. Examples shown: **(A)** A–P glide during shoulder flexion; **(B)** A–P superior glide during shoulder abduction-external rotation; **(C)** A–P glide during weight bearing; **(D)** P–A glide during flexion; and **(E)** A–P/superior during shoulder rehabilitation. (Shoulder Fixation Belt: www.LondonShoulderClinic.com)

Immobilization in external rotation has gained attention in the past decade with cadaveric and magnetic resonance studies demonstrating greater approximation of the anterior soft tissue to the glenoid when compared to internal rotation.[62–64] However, subsequent randomized controlled trials comparing immobilization in internal rotation with external rotation have produced equivocal findings.[61,65–67] Appropriately designed research is required to advance knowledge in these areas.

Posterior Dislocation

There is a paucity of research evidence guiding the management of posterior dislocations.[68] Conservative management is recommended for at least 6 months following successful reduction with no substantial fracture, rotator cuff tear or ongoing instability.[16,17]

Anterior or Posterior Subluxation and Multidirectional Instability (MDI)

Anterior and posterior subluxations occur when the humeral head translates excessively but does not dislocate. This may result from structural lesions (such as labral tears or capsule and ligament attenuation) or as a result of weakened or decreased muscular control.[1] Exercise therapy is commonly recommended as the initial treatment strategy for these instabilities.[18–20,69] This is based on the rationale that strengthening the scapular

and rotator cuff muscles compensates for the lack of passive stability and assists in active control of the shoulder.[20,70] Poor muscle patterning is uncoordinated muscle activation strategies that result in aberrant scapulo-humeral movement patterns that compromise humeral head control and may increase the risk of GHJ subluxation. Muscle patterning is recognized as a contributing factor in MDI[71] and rehabilitation is considered the primary treatment option. Despite this recommendation, the evidence for exercise-based management of MDI remains uncertain due to studies of low quality and a high risk of bias.[72] When conservative treatment is unsuccessful, surgery, usually to tighten the inferior capsule, may be considered.[19,20] Studies that have compared surgical intervention with conservative treatment for MDI have demonstrated improvements in favour of surgery for impairment outcomes and improvements in favour of conservative management for patient-focused outcomes.[73–76] Definitive conclusions are not available due to a lack of appropriately designed research.[72]

Conservative Rehabilitation Principles

Currently there are no randomized controlled trials that compare conservative management to control or sham treatment. A number of protocols have been published[77] and these are based on physiological and biological evidence of shoulder joint stability. Table 50-4 outlines conservative management, including the acute phase where

TABLE 50-4 Management Guidelines Post Reconstruction Surgery or Dislocation

Stage of Rehabilitation	Acute Management Immediately Post-Surgery or Dislocation	Acute Management Approximately 2–6 Weeks	Stage 1: Scapula Setting Phase	Stage 2: Coronal Plane 0–45° Abduction	Stage 3: Posterior Musculature 0–45° Abduction	Stage 4: Flexion	Stage 5: Coronal/ Sagittal Plane 45–90°	Stage 6: Isolated Strength Drills	Stage 7: Overhead/ Functional
Components	Shoulder immobilization Pain relief Elbow/wrist exercises	Passive and active assisted range of motion Isometric scapula muscle strength	Upward rotation shrug	Standing ER with light band resistance (0° abduction) Standing IR with band resistance (0° abduction)	Shrugs Side lie ER Standing ER with heavier band Standing row (0° abduction progress to 45° abduction)	Forward punch in scapula plane	ER and IR at 90° abduction Flexion at 90° Horizontal flexion/ extension	Posterior deltoid Anterior deltoid Middle deltoid (short lever abduction)	Deltoid >90° IR >90° ER >90° Flexion >90° Sport-specific part drills
Dosage	Continual immobilization for approximately 2 weeks post-surgery, immobilization time may vary by surgeon	Scapula setting: 20 repetitions 3 × per day	Goal: 0.5 kg–1 kg × 20 reps in standing	Goal: ER/IR: full arc 3 × 20 reps against medium resistance	Goal: Shrugs 3 × 20 reps with 2 kg Side lie ER with 1 kg moderate to heavy resistance ER 3 × 20 moderate to heavy resistance Row: 45° abduction, heavy band 3 × 20 reps	Goal: × 20 reps up to 45° with light to moderate band resistance as able to control	Goal: ER/IR: full arc × 20 reps against medium resistance × 20 reps up to 90° with moderate band resistance HF/HE × 20 reps pain-free light resistance	Goal: All exs: 3–4 kg at arc of motion required for function	Control of drill × 20 reps Strength drills × 12 (increased load) Low load high reps for endurance, high load high reps for strength
Progression		Commence passive movement when pain allows or according to surgeon protocol	Commence upward rotation shrug when able to control setting drill	Start with no weight in standing, if unable to perform complete shrugs in side lying	Commence ER approximately 1 week prior to IR If unable to complete standing ER with control perform standing shoulder extension initially	Regress to stage 3 if poor control, pain or posterior subluxation during exercise	Higher-level resistance bands/ weights can be prescribed if required for sport or function and can be controlled	Commence post. deltoid first, progress from standing rows to bent over Then introduce mid. deltoid (standing punch to flexion 90°) Then commence ant. deltoid	Progress to strength drills as required and whole practice of sports-specific drills
Precautions	Avoid positions of risk Anterior instability: abduction combined with external rotation Posterior instability: flexion with horizontal flexion +/− internal rotation	If predisposed, individuals may experience an increase in neck pain performing the shrug. Deep neck flexor exercises may be required, or supine/ side-lying shrugs initially	Continue upward rotation shrug, only progress stage when individual has good scapular and humeral head control Exercises should not elicit symptoms			Care must be taken in flexion for patients with posterior instability	Ensure humeral head is articulating in a central position in abduction/ external rotation positions at 90°		

ant. deltoid, anterior deltoid; ER, external rotation; ex, exercises; IR, internal rotation; mid. deltoid, middle deltoid; post. deltoid, posterior deltoid...

an individual is post-surgery or post-dislocation, followed by the stages of rehabilitation for individuals with MDI or subluxing instabilities or for individuals following the acute phase post injury or surgery.

GENERALIZED JOINT HYPERMOBILITY, JOINT HYPERMOBILITY SYNDROME AND SHOULDER INSTABILITY

Generalized joint hypermobility (GJH) is a unifying feature of Ehlers–Danlos syndrome (EDS), Marfan syndrome and osteogenesis imperfecta which are all heritable disorders of connective tissue (HDCT) that affect the connective tissue matrix proteins.[78] In recent decades joint hypermobility syndrome (JHS), a more common connective tissue disorder with a mixed phenotype of the heritable disorders of connective tissues, has been identified. JHS is considered to be an atypical HDCT, sharing overlapping features with EDS, Marfan syndrome and osteogenesis imperfecta.[78] Many authorities now consider JHS to be indistinguishable from EDS (hypermobility type).[79] The term JHS is used in this section to describe these inseparable entities.

The reported point prevalence of GJH and JHS in the adult general population is 10 to 30% and 0.75% respectively.[78,80] The point prevalence of JHS reported in musculoskeletal rheumatology and physiotherapy outpatient settings ranges from 30–60%.[81–83]

Currently there is no biomedical test to diagnose JHS and therefore the diagnosis is based on clinical examination. The Brighton Criteria (Box 50-1) may be used to reach a diagnosis in both adults and children.[84] Symptoms of JHS frequently commence in early childhood, are amplified during adolescence and may continue into adult life.[84,85] The predominant presenting complaints are musculoskeletal dysfunction and pain. Numerous extra-articular manifestations are also reported.[78,85,86]

Individuals with GJH and JHS may present with a wide range of shoulder pathologies. Pain is often more profound in those with JHS. Muscular weakness, fatigue, altered scapular position,[87] scapular dyskinesia, poor proprioception, maladaptive postural changes and subsequent chronic pain states are common[88,89] and may cascade towards regional chronic pain states.

Although individuals with GJH and JHS are susceptible to traumatic instability,[90,91] they also commonly present with multidirectional and unidirectional instability unrelated to trauma.[88] Very minor events may create recurring episodes of shoulder displacement and ongoing pain, resulting in increasing disability. Correct and early recognition and classification of the instability in this patient population will lead to appropriate management and avoid unnecessary surgery, which in some cases may exacerbate symptoms and disability.[88]

Management requires a multifaceted approach due to the nature of the condition. Initial rehabilitation should focus on education, joint protection and training the motor control system.[92] Closed kinetic chain exercises, using biofeedback to enhance proprioception from mirrors, tape, exercise balls and hands-on facilitation may be helpful in the early stages.[92] Later, hydrotherapy/

| **BOX 50-1** | **Brighton Criteria** |

MAJOR CRITERIA

- A Beighton score of 4/9 or greater (either currently or historically)
- Arthralgia for longer than 3 months in four or more joints

MINOR CRITERIA

- A Beighton score of 1, 2, or 3/9 (0, 1, 2 or 3 if aged 50+)
- Arthralgia (for 3 months or longer) in one to three joints or back pain for (for 3 months or longer), spondylosis, spondylolysis/spondylolisthesis
- Dislocation/subluxation in more than one joint, or in one joint on more than one occasion. Soft tissue rheumatism: three or more lesions (e.g. epicondylitis, tenosynovitis, bursitis)
- Marfanoid habitus (tall, slim, span/height ration 1.03 upper: lower segment ration less than 0.89, arachnodactyly (positive Steinberg/wrist signs)
- Abnormal skin striae, hyperextensibility, thin skin, papery scarring
- Eye signs: drooping eyelids or myopia or antimongoloid slant
- Varicose veins or hernia or uterine/rectal prolapse

A diagnosis is made on the basis of:

- Two major criteria
- One major plus two minor criteria
- Four minor criteria
- Two minor criteria and unequivocally affected first-degree relative in family history
- JHS is excluded by the presence of Marfan or Ehlers–Danlos syndromes other than the EDS hypermobility type (formerly EDS III).

NB: Criteria Major 1 and Minor 1 are mutually exclusive, as are Major 2 and Minor 2.

(Grahame et al.[84])
EDS, Ehlers–Danlos syndrome; *JHS*, joint hypermobility syndrome.

---

aquatic rehabilitation and a graduated strength, endurance and plyometric functional rehabilitation programme may be implemented. More challenging cases often require additional pain management and input from a multidisciplinary team.

REFERENCES

1. Lewis A, Kitamura T, Bayley JIL. (ii) The classification of shoulder instability: new light through old windows! Curr Orthop 2004;18(2):97–108.
2. Gartsman GM, Brinker MR, Khan M, et al. Self-assessment of general health status in patients with five common shoulder conditions. J Shoulder Elbow Surg 1998;7(3):228–37.
3. Garth WP Jr, Allman FL Jr, Armstrong WS. Occult anterior subluxations of the shoulder in noncontact sports. Am J Sports Med 1987;15(6):579–85.
4. Jobe CM, Iannotti JP. Limits imposed on glenohumeral motion by joint geometry. J Shoulder Elbow Surg 1995;4(4):281–5.
5. Salomonsson B, Sforza G, Revay S, et al. Atraumatic shoulder instability. Discussion of classification and results after capsular imbrication. Scand J Med Sci Sports 1998;8(6):398–404.
6. Walch G, Boileau P, Noel E, et al. Impingement of the deep surface of the supraspinatus tendon on the posterosuperior glenoid rim: an arthroscopic study. J Shoulder Elbow Surg 1992;1(5):238–45.
7. Yamaguchi K, Flatow EL. Management of multidirectional instability. Clin Sports Med 1995;14(4):885–902.

8. Kuhn JE. A new classification system for shoulder instability. Br J Sports Med 2010;44(5):341–6.

9. Shea KP. ISAKOS Consensus shoulder instability classification system. Shoudler Concepts 2013: Consensus and Concerns ISAKOS Upper Extremity Committees 2009–2013. Springer; 2013.

10. Murray IR, Ahmed I, White NJ, et al. Traumatic anterior shoulder instability in the athlete. Scand J Med Sci Sports 2013;23(4): 387–405.

11. Liavaag S, Svenningsen S, Reikeras O, et al. The epidemiology of shoulder dislocations in Oslo. Scand J Med Sci Sports 2011; 21(6):e334–40.

12. Nordqvist A, Petersson CJ. Incidence and causes of shoulder girdle injuries in an urban population. J Shoulder Elbow Surg 1995;4(2):107–12.

13. Simonet WT, Melton LJ 3rd, Cofield RH, et al. Incidence of anterior shoulder dislocation in Olmsted County, Minnesota. Clin Orthop Relat Res 1984;186:186–91.

14. Kroner K, Lind T, Jensen J. The epidemiology of shoulder dislocations. Arch Orthop Trauma Surg 1989;108(5):288–90.

15. Owens BD, Duffey ML, Nelson BJ, et al. The incidence and characteristics of shoulder instability at the United States Military Academy. Am J Sports Med 2007;35(7):1168–73.

16. Rouleau DM, Hebert-Davies J. Incidence of associated injury in posterior shoulder dislocation: systematic review of the literature. J Orthop Trauma 2012;26(4):246–50.

17. Tannenbaum E, Sekiya JK. Evaluation and management of posterior shoulder instability. Sports Health 2011;3(3):253–63.

18. An YH, Friedman RJ. Multidirectional instability of the glenohumeral joint. Orthop Clin North Am 2000;31(2):275–85.

19. Bahu MJ, Trentacosta N, Vorys GC, et al. Multidirectional instability: evaluation and treatment options. Clin Sports Med 2008; 27(4):671–89.

20. Guerrero P, Busconi B, Deangelis N, et al. Congenital instability of the shoulder joint: assessment and treatment options. J Orthop Sports Phys Ther 2009;39(2):124–34.

21. Mallon WJ, Speer KP. Multidirectional instability: current concepts. J Shoulder Elbow Surg 1995;4(1 Pt 1):54–64.

22. Ide J, Maeda S, Yamaga M, et al. Shoulder-strengthening exercise with an orthosis for multidirectional shoulder instability: quantitative evaluation of rotational shoulder strength before and after the exercise program. J Shoulder Elbow Surg 2003;12(4):342–5.

23. McFarland EG, Kim TK, Park HB, et al. The effect of variation in definition on the diagnosis of multidirectional instability of the shoulder. J Bone Joint Surg Am 2003;85-A(11):2138–44.

24. Neer CS 2nd, Foster CR. Inferior capsular shift for involuntary inferior and multidirectional instability of the shoulder. A preliminary report. J Bone Joint Surg Am 1980;62(6):897–908.

25. Fischer SP. Arthroscopic treatment of multidirectional instability. Sports Med Arthrosc 2004;12(2):127–34.

26. Chahal J, Marks PH, Macdonald PB, et al. Anatomic Bankart repair compared with nonoperative treatment and/or arthroscopic lavage for first-time traumatic shoulder dislocation. Arthroscopy 2012;28(4):565–75.

27. Gerber C, Nyffeler RW. Classification of glenohumeral joint instability. Clin Orthop Relat Res 2002;400:65–76.

28. Joseph TA, Williams JS Jr, Brems JJ. Laser capsulorrhaphy for multidirectional instability of the shoulder. An outcomes study and proposed classification system. Am J Sports Med 2003;31(1): 26–35.

29. Throckmorton TW, Dunn W, Holmes T, et al. Intraobserver and interobserver agreement of International Classification of Diseases, Ninth Revision codes in classifying shoulder instability. J Shoulder Elbow Surg 2009;18(2):199–203.

30. Hovelius L, Augustini BG, Fredin H, et al. Primary anterior dislocation of the shoulder in young patients. A ten-year prospective study. J Bone Joint Surg Am 1996;78(11):1677–84.

31. Simonet WT, Cofield RH. Prognosis in anterior shoulder dislocation. Am J Sports Med 1984;12(1):19–24.

32. Robinson CM, Seah M, Akhtar MA. The epidemiology, risk of recurrence, and functional outcome after an acute traumatic posterior dislocation of the shoulder. J Bone Joint Surg Am 2011; 93(17):1605–13.

33. Miniaci A, Mascia AT, Salonen DC, et al. Magnetic resonance imaging of the shoulder in asymptomatic professional baseball pitchers. Am J Sports Med 2002;30(1):66–73.

34. Lewis JS. Rotator cuff tendinopathy/subacromial impingement syndrome: is it time for a new method of assessment? Br J Sports Med 2009;43(4):259–64.

35. VandenBerghe G, Hoenecke HR, Fronek J. Glenohumeral joint instability: the orthopedic approach. Semin Musculoskelet Radiol 2005;9(1):34–43.

36. Ozaki J. Glenohumeral movements of the involuntary inferior and multidirectional instability. Clin Orthop Relat Res 1989;238: 107–11.

37. Inui H, Sugamoto K, Miyamoto T, et al. Three-dimensional relationship of the glenohumeral joint in the elevated position in shoulders with multidirectional instability. J Shoulder Elbow Surg 2002;11(5):510–15.

38. Jobe FW, Kvitne RS, Giangarra CE. Shoulder pain in the overhand or throwing athlete. The relationship of anterior instability and rotator cuff impingement. Orthop Rev 1989;18(9):963–75.

39. Magarey ME, Jones MA. Specific evaluation of the function of force couples relevant for stabilization of the glenohumeral joint. Man Ther 2003;8(4):247–53.

40. Watson LA, Pizzari T, Balster S. Thoracic outlet syndrome part 1: clinical manifestations, differentiation and treatment pathways. Man Ther 2009;14(6):586–95.

41. Watson LA, Pizzari T, Balster S. Thoracic outlet syndrome part 2: conservative management of thoracic outlet. Man Ther 2010; 15(4):305–14.

42. Hegedus EJ, Goode AP, Cook CE, et al. Which physical examination tests provide clinicians with the most value when examining the shoulder? Update of a systematic review with meta-analysis of individual tests. Br J Sports Med 2012;46(14):964–78.

43. Kuhn JE, Helmer TT, Dunn WR, et al. Development and reliability testing of the frequency, etiology, direction, and severity (FEDS) system for classifying glenohumeral instability. J Shoulder Elbow Surg 2011;20(4):548–56.

44. Tennent TD, Beach WR, Meyers JF. A review of the special tests associated with shoulder examination. Part II: laxity, instability, and superior labral anterior and posterior (SLAP) lesions. Am J Sports Med 2003;31(2):301–7.

45. Godin J, Sekiya JK. Systematic review of rehabilitation versus operative stabilization for the treatment of first-time anterior shoulder dislocations. Sports Health 2010;2(2):156–65.

46. Handoll HH, Almaiyah MA, Rangan A. Surgical versus nonsurgical treatment for acute anterior shoulder dislocation. Cochrane Database Syst Rev 2004;(1):CD004325.

47. Habermeyer P, Gleyze P, Rickert M. Evolution of lesions of the labrum-ligament complex in posttraumatic anterior shoulder instability: a prospective study. J Shoulder Elbow Surg 1999;8(1): 66–74.

48. Ogawa K, Yoshida A, Ikegami H. Osteoarthritis in shoulders with traumatic anterior instability: preoperative survey using radiography and computed tomography. J Shoulder Elbow Surg 2006; 15(1):23–9.

49. Boone JL, Arciero RA. First-time anterior shoulder dislocations: has the standard changed? Br J Sports Med 2010;44(5):355–60.

50. Monk AP, Garfjeld Roberts P, Logishetty K, et al. Evidence in managing traumatic anterior shoulder instability: a scoping review. Br J Sports Med 2013 Aug 21;doi:10.1136/bjsports-2013-092296; [Epub ahead of print].

51. Van Tongel A, Rosa F, Heffernan G, et al. Long-term result after traumatic anterior shoulder dislocation: what works best? Musculoskelet Surg 2011;95(Suppl. 1):S65–70.

52. Hovelius L, Olofsson A, Sandstrom B, et al. Nonoperative treatment of primary anterior shoulder dislocation in patients forty years of age and younger. a prospective twenty-five-year follow-up. J Bone Joint Surg Am 2008;90(5):945–52.

53. Randelli P, Taverna E. Primary anterior shoulder dislocation in young athletes: fix them! Knee Surg Sports Traumatol Arthrosc 2009;17(12):1404–5.

54. Malhotra A, Freudmann MS, Hay SM. Management of traumatic anterior shoulder dislocation in the 17- to 25-year age group: a dramatic evolution of practice. J Shoulder Elbow Surg 2012;21(4): 545–53.

55. Pulavarti RS, Symes TH, Rangan A. Surgical interventions for anterior shoulder instability in adults. Cochrane Database Syst Rev 2009;(4):CD005077.

56. Balg F, Boileau P. The instability severity index score. A simple pre-operative score to select patients for arthroscopic or open

shoulder stabilisation. J Bone Joint Surg Br 2007;89(11): 1470–7.

57. Cutts S, Prempeh M, Drew S. Anterior shoulder dislocation. Ann R Coll Surg Engl 2009;91(1):2–7.

58. Paterson WH, Throckmorton TW, Koester M, et al. Position and duration of immobilization after primary anterior shoulder dislocation: a systematic review and meta-analysis of the literature. J Bone Joint Surg Am 2010;92(18):2924–33.

59. Scheibel M, Kuke A, Nikulka C, et al. How long should acute anterior dislocations of the shoulder be immobilized in external rotation? Am J Sports Med 2009;37(7):1309–16.

60. Itoi E, Hatakeyama Y, Itoigawa Y, et al. Is protecting the healing ligament beneficial after immobilization in external rotation for an initial shoulder dislocation? Am J Sports Med 2013;41(5): 1126–32.

61. Liavaag S, Brox JI, Pripp AH, et al. Immobilization in external rotation after primary shoulder dislocation did not reduce the risk of recurrence: a randomized controlled trial. J Bone Joint Surg Am 2011;93(10):897–904.

62. Liavaag S, Stiris MG, Lindland ES, et al. Do Bankart lesions heal better in shoulders immobilized in external rotation? Acta Orthop 2009;80(5):579–84.

63. Miller BS, Sonnabend DH, Hatrick C, et al. Should acute anterior dislocations of the shoulder be immobilized in external rotation? A cadaveric study. J Shoulder Elbow Surg 2004;13(6):589–92.

64. Itoi E, Sashi R, Minagawa H, et al. Position of immobilization after dislocation of the glenohumeral joint. A study with use of magnetic resonance imaging. J Bone Joint Surg Am 2001;83-A(5):661–7.

65. Itoi E, Hatakeyama Y, Kido T, et al. A new method of immobilization after traumatic anterior dislocation of the shoulder: a preliminary study. J Shoulder Elbow Surg 2003;12(5):413–15.

66. Itoi E, Hatakeyama Y, Sato T, et al. Immobilization in external rotation after shoulder dislocation reduces the risk of recurrence. A randomized controlled trial. J Bone Joint Surg Am 2007; 89(10):2124–31.

67. Finestone A, Milgrom C, Radeva-Petrova DR, et al. Bracing in external rotation for traumatic anterior dislocation of the shoulder. J Bone Joint Surg Br 2009;91(7):918–21.

68. Paul J, Buchmann S, Beitzel K, et al. Posterior shoulder dislocation: systematic review and treatment algorithm. Arthroscopy 2011; 27(11):1562–72.

69. Burkhead WZ Jr, Rockwood CA Jr. Treatment of instability of the shoulder with an exercise program. J Bone Joint Surg Am 1992;74(6):890–6.

70. Beasley L, Faryniarz DA, Hannafin JA. Multidirectional instability of the shoulder in the female athlete. Clin Sports Med 2000; 19(2):331–49.

71. Jaggi A, Lambert S. Rehabilitation for shoulder instability. Br J Sports Med 2010;44(5):333–40.

72. Warby SA, Pizzari T, Ford JJ, et al. The effect of exercise-based management for multidirectional instability of the glenohumeral joint: a systematic review. J Shoulder Elbow Surg 2014;23(1): 128–42.

73. Illyes A, Kiss J, Kiss RM. Electromyographic analysis during pull, forward punch, elevation and overhead throw after conservative treatment or capsular shift at patient with multidirectional shoulder joint instability. J Electromyogr Kinesiol 2009;19(6):e438–47.

74. Kiss J, Damrel D, Mackie A, et al. Non-operative treatment of multidirectional shoulder instability. Int Orthop 2001;24(6): 354–7.

75. Kiss RM, Illyes A, Kiss J. Physiotherapy vs. capsular shift and physiotherapy in multidirectional shoulder joint instability. J Electromyogr Kinesiol 2010;20(3):489–501.

76. Tillander B, Lysholm M, Norlin R. Multidirectional hyperlaxity of the shoulder: results of treatment. Scand J Med Sci Sports 1998;8(6):421–5.

77. Gibson K, Growse A, Korda L, et al. The effectiveness of rehabilitation for nonoperative management of shoulder instability: a systematic review. J Hand Ther 2004;17(2):229–42.

78. Hakim A, Grahame R. Joint hypermobility. Best Pract Res Clin Rheumatol 2003;17(6):989–1004.

79. Tinkle BT, Bird HA, Grahame R, et al. The lack of clinical distinction between the hypermobility type of Ehlers-Danlos syndrome and the joint hypermobility syndrome (a.k.a. hypermobility syndrome). Am J Med Genet A 2009;149A(11):2368–70.

80. Klemp P, Williams SM, Stansfield SA. Articular mobility in Maori and European New Zealanders. Rheumatology 2002;41(5):554–7.

81. Clark CJ, Simmonds JV. An exploration of the prevalence of hypermobility and joint hypermobility syndrome in Omani women attending a hospital physiotherapy service. Musculoskeletal Care 2011;9(1):1–10.

82. Connelly E. The prevalence of joint hypermobility and joint hypermobility syndrome (JHS) in patients presenting to a London neuromusculoskeletal triage clinic and the impact of JHS on quality of life. UK: Master of Science: University of Herfordshire; 2013.

83. Grahame R, Hakim A. High prevalence of joint hypermobility syndrome in clinic referrals to a north London community hospital. Rheumatology 2004;43(3 Suppl. 1):198.

84. Grahame R, Bird HA, Child A. The revised (Brighton 1998) criteria for the diagnosis of benign joint hypermobility syndrome (BJHS). J Rheumatol 2000;27(7):1777–9.

85. Murray KJ. Hypermobility disorders in children and adolescents. Best Pract Res Clin Rheumatol 2006;20(2):329–50.

86. Engelbert RHH, Scheper MC. Joint hypermobility with and without musculoskeletal complaints: a physiotherapeutic approach. Int Musculoskelet Med 2011;33(4):146–50.

87. Moghadam AN, Salimee MM. A comparative study on scapular static position between females with and without generalized joint hyper mobility. Med J Islam Repub Iran 2012;26(3):97–102.

88. Jaggi A, Lambert S. Regional complications in joint hypermobility syndrome: the shoulder joint. In: Hakim A, Keer R, Grahame R, editors. Hypermobility, fibromyalgia, and chronic pain. Edinburgh: Churchill Livingstone/Elsevier; 2010. p. 197–205.

89. Simmonds JV, Keer RJ. Hypermobility and the hypermobility syndrome. Man Ther 2007;12(4):298–309.

90. Cameron KL, Duffey ML, DeBerardino TM, et al. Association of generalized joint hypermobility with a history of glenohumeral joint instability. J Athl Train 2010;45(3):253–8.

91. Muhammad AA, Jenkins P, Ashton F, et al. Hypermobility a risk factor for recurrent shoulder dislocations. Br J Sports Med 2013;47(10):e3.

92. Keer R, Simmonds J. Joint protection and physical rehabilitation of the adult with hypermobility syndrome. Curr Opin Rheumatol 2011;23(2):131–6.

CHAPTER 50.4 ■ POSTERIOR SHOULDER TIGHTNESS

John Borstad • **Jeremy Lewis**

OVERVIEW

Posterior shoulder tightness is suspected when glenohumeral internal rotation and/or horizontal adduction ROM are decreased. This reduction of normal movement may result from decreased extensibility of the posterior glenohumeral joint capsule, the posterior shoulder muscles, or a combination of both. Increased humeral retroversion may also contribute to a decrease in ROM, but is distinct from posterior shoulder tightness.[1] The first published account of posterior shoulder tightness was described in association with shoulder ROM alterations in baseball pitchers.[2] Posterior shoulder tightness occurs frequently in throwing athletes but may also occur in the general population.[3] Many uncertainties exist regarding posterior shoulder tightness, including whether or not it is even a real phenomenon related to soft tissue structure or mechanics.

MECHANISMS

In throwing athletes, it is proposed that posterior shoulder tightness is caused by reduced posterior capsule extensibility.[4] During the deceleration phase of throwing, the posterior shoulder muscles contract eccentrically to absorb energy created during the acceleration phase. However, muscle function may decline with fatigue, such that the posterior capsule shares deceleration loads. Over time, cyclic capsule loading leads to contracture and fibrosis, decreased capsule extensibility and altered motion.[5] It is hypothesized that tensile loading triggers cellular and metabolic processes that synthesize tissue in an effort to protect the capsule against further loading.[4]

Increased muscle stiffness, a short-term consequence of fatiguing eccentric contractions, may also contribute to posterior shoulder tightness in throwing athletes.[6] However, this mechanism remains speculative because long-term eccentric exercise results in increased ROM and protection against further muscle adaptations.[7] Adhesions between the posterior capsule and shoulder external rotators have also been described and may contribute to motion loss.[5]

Other hypotheses for the development of posterior shoulder tightness include adaptations resulting from ageing or activity. Changes associated with ageing such as increased collagen cross-links, variations in collagen expression and reduced elasticity may reduce capsular extensibility.[8] Osteoarthritis involving the posterior glenoid fossa may result in local tissue changes.[9] Labourers may develop tightness through work demands that repetitively load the posterior cuff and capsule complex.[10] For muscle, increased cross-bridge engagement or stiffness of the parallel or series elastic components may cause tightness.[11] Importantly, all these proposed mechanisms remain hypothetical.

EVIDENCE

Evidence of posterior shoulder tightness is based primarily on clinical observation. Characteristic motion loss patterns are consistently noted in throwing athletes, and interventions to increase posterior shoulder extensibility often reverse these patterns.[12-16] Similarly, increased internal rotation ROM is reported after cutting the posterior capsule in cadaver experiments[17] and releasing the capsule arthroscopically in vivo.[7] Likewise, experimental shortening of cadaver posterior capsules results in motion losses similar to those exhibited by throwing athletes,[18,19] but it is not known if shortening is equivalent to contracture and fibrosis in vivo. The characteristic motion losses are associated with thickened posterior shoulder structures[20,21] including the capsule,[22] but no studies have correlated motion loss with muscle extensibility. Arthroscopic evaluation identified visible posterior capsule contracture and fibrosis, but quantification or comparison to asymptomatic shoulders was not performed. While these associations provide validity to posterior shoulder tightness as an impairment, direct evidence that verifies the existence of posterior shoulder tightness is lacking.

DIAGNOSIS

Posterior shoulder tightness is currently assessed by quantifying glenohumeral joint internal rotation and/or horizontal adduction ROM. Intra- and inter-rater reliability of each method is reported as good to excellent,[23-25] yet construct validity has not been established. Both measurements produced lower strain on the posterior capsule of cadavers than a position of 60° flexion and passive internal rotation.[18] This measurement also accurately identifies capsule tightness in throwers and has high intra-rater reliability. Motion must be compared to the contralateral shoulder motion to determine if tightness exists. A concern with all posterior shoulder tightness measurements is their inability to distinguish between capsule tightness, muscle tightness and humeral retroversion. In addition, the influence of scapula position on these measurements may affect their interpretation and this has not been examined.

MANAGEMENT

Alleviating posterior shoulder tightness appears possible through stretching and/or manual therapy. Two stretch positions are commonly used and both are effective.[14] The 'sleeper stretch' is performed by passively internally rotating the shoulder when side lying on the affected side with the arm flexed to near 90°. The cross-body stretch is performed by elevating the arm to 90° and passively adducting the humerus towards the chest. Both stretches can be administered by the clinician or the patient. The cross-body stretch may be more effective than the sleeper stretch, while both improved tightness more than a non-stretch control group.[14] Contract–relax techniques may also reduce posterior shoulder tightness.[15]

Several studies have demonstrated that manual interventions focused on increasing posterior capsule extensibility, when added to stretching and strengthening exercises, may decrease tightness.[13,16,26] Manual therapy may be more effective if initially applied in the open position of the glenohumeral joint and progressed to more flexed and internally rotated positions.[27]

RECOMMENDATIONS

Despite evidence that posterior shoulder tightness is associated with shoulder injury in throwing athletes, the relative importance of the impairment remains unknown. Specifically, prevalence rates in symptomatic non-throwers, the degree of tightness that is clinically meaningful and the risk of developing shoulder pain when posterior shoulder tightness is present are key unknown factors. Longitudinal studies that verify the development of posterior shoulder tightness are warranted, as are studies that establish the mechanisms by which capsule or muscle tightness occur. The optimum posterior shoulder measurements must be determined, with an emphasis on discerning capsule from muscle, controlling for the influence of humeral retroversion and establishing validity. Finally, the most effective interventions for reversing posterior shoulder tightness, including treatment dose, still need to be determined.

REFERENCES

1. Crockett HC, Gross LB, Wilk KE, et al. Osseous adaptation and range of motion at the glenohumeral joint in professional baseball pitchers. Am J Sports Med 2002;30(1):20–6.
2. Pappas AM, Zawacki RM, McCarthy CF. Rehabilitation of the pitching shoulder. Am J Sports Med 1985;13(4):223–35.
3. Ticker JB, Beim GM, Warner JJ. Recognition and treatment of refractory posterior capsular contracture of the shoulder. Arthroscopy 2000;16(1):27–34.
4. Burkhart SS, Morgan CD, Kibler WB. The disabled throwing shoulder: spectrum of pathology Part I: pathoanatomy and biomechanics. Arthroscopy 2003;19(4):404–20.
5. Yoneda M, Nakagawa S, Mizuno N, et al. Arthroscopic capsular release for painful throwing shoulder with posterior capsular tightness. Arthroscopy 2006;22(7):801.e1–e5, –.
6. Oyama S, Myers JB, Blackburn JT, et al. Changes in infraspinatus cross-sectional area and shoulder range of motion with repetitive eccentric external rotator contraction. Clin Biomech (Bristol, Avon) 2011;26(2):130–5.
7. Potier TG, Alexander CM, Seynnes OR. Effects of eccentric strength training on biceps femoris muscle architecture and knee joint range of movement. Eur J Appl Physiol 2009;105(6):939–44.
8. Freemont AJ, Hoyland JA. Morphology, mechanisms and pathology of musculoskeletal ageing. J Pathol 2007;211(2):252–9.
9. Madry H, Luyten FP, Facchini A. Biological aspects of early osteoarthritis. Knee Surg Sports Traumatol Arthrosc 2012;20(3): 407–22.
10. Kim SG, Akaike T, Sasagaw T, et al. Gene expression of type I and type III collagen by mechanical stretch in anterior cruciate ligament cells. Cell Struct Funct 2002;27(3):139–44.
11. Kragstrup TW, Kjaer M, Mackey AL. Structural, biochemical, cellular, and functional changes in skeletal muscle extracellular matrix with aging. Scand J Med Sci Sports 2011;21(6):749–57.
12. Laudner KG, Sipes RC, Wilson JT. The acute effects of sleeper stretches on shoulder range of motion. J Athl Train 2008;43(4): 359–63.
13. Manske RC, Meschke M, Porter A, et al. A randomized controlled single-blinded comparison of stretching versus stretching and joint mobilization for posterior shoulder tightness measured by internal rotation motion loss. Sports Health 2010;2(2):94–100.
14. McClure P, Balaicuis J, Heiland D, et al. A randomized controlled comparison of stretching procedures for posterior shoulder tightness. J Orthop Sports Phys Ther 2007;37(3):108–14.
15. Moore SD, Laudner KG, McLoda TA, et al. The immediate effects of muscle energy technique on posterior shoulder tightness: a randomized controlled trial. J Orthop Sports Phys Ther 2011; 41(6):400–7.
16. Tyler TF, Nicholas SJ, Lee SJ, et al. Correction of posterior shoulder tightness is associated with symptom resolution in patients with internal impingement. Am J Sports Med 2010;38(1):114–19.
17. Moskal MJ, Harryman DT 2nd, Romeo AA, et al. Glenohumeral motion after complete capsular release. Arthroscopy 1999; 15(4):408–16.
18. Borstad JD, Dashottar A. Quantifying strain on posterior shoulder tissues during 5 simulated clinical tests: a cadaver study. J Orthop Sports Phys Ther 2011;41(2):90–9.
19. Grossman MG, Tibone JE, McGarry MH, et al. A cadaveric model of the throwing shoulder: a possible etiology of superior labrum anterior-to-posterior lesions. J Bone Joint Surg Am 2005; 87(4):824–31.
20. Tehranzadeh AD, Fronek J, Resnick D. Posterior capsular fibrosis in professional baseball pitchers: case series of MR arthrographic findings in six patients with glenohumeral internal rotational deficit. Clin Imaging 2007;31(5):343–8.
21. Tuite MJ, Petersen BD, Wise SM, et al. Shoulder MR arthrography of the posterior labrocapsular complex in overhead throwers with pathologic internal impingement and internal rotation deficit. Skeletal Radiol 2007;36(6):495–502.
22. Thomas SJ, Swanik CB, Higginson JS, et al. A bilateral comparison of posterior capsule thickness and its correlation with glenohumeral range of motion and scapular upward rotation in collegiate baseball players. J Shoulder Elbow Surg 2011;20(5):708–16.
23. Laudner KG, Stanek JM, Meister K. Assessing posterior shoulder contracture: the reliability and validity of measuring glenohumeral joint horizontal adduction. J Athl Train 2006;41(4):375–80.
24. Myers JB, Oyama S, Wassinger CA, et al. Reliability, precision, accuracy, and validity of posterior shoulder tightness assessment in overhead athletes. Am J Sports Med 2007;35(11):1922–30.
25. Tyler TF, Nicholas SJ, Roy T, et al. Quantification of posterior capsule tightness and motion loss in patients with shoulder impingement. Am J Sports Med 2000;28(5):668–73.
26. Tate AR, McClure PW, Young IA, et al. Comprehensive impairment-based exercise and manual therapy intervention for patients with subacromial impingement syndrome: a case series. J Orthop Sports Phys Ther 2010;40(8):474–93.
27. Cools AM, Declercq G, Cagnie B, et al. Internal impingement in the tennis player: rehabilitation guidelines. Br J Sports Med 2008;42(3):165–71.

CHAPTER 50.5 ■ FROZEN SHOULDER CONTRACTION SYNDROME

Jeremy Lewis

INTRODUCTION

The term frozen shoulder was introduced by Codman in 1934[1] describing it as a condition of unknown aetiology, being difficult to treat but certain to resolve. In 1945, Neviaser,[2] based on a case series of ten patients, suggested the term adhesive capsulitis better described the pathology, due to the observations of inflammation, fibrosis and adhesions within the axillary fold and to the anatomic neck of the humerus. However, more recent evidence supports thickening and contracture of the inferior GHJ capsule, without adhesions to the humerus.[3] As such, the term adhesive capsulitis may not appropriately describe the condition. Terminology has evolved to include primary frozen shoulder, which is used when the cause of the condition is of idiopathic origin, and secondary frozen shoulder when it is deemed to have occurred following a specific event such as trauma, following surgery or associated with an underlying condition such as calcific tendinosis. Zuckerman and Rokito[4] have further classified secondary frozen shoulder into systemic, extrinsic and intrinsic categories. In Japan and China the term 'the 50-year-old shoulder' is used reflecting the mean age of onset. Yang et al.[5] used the term frozen shoulder syndrome and Bunker[6] advocated use of the term 'contraction of the shoulder' arguing this best encompasses the clinical and histological presentation. The myriad terminology reflects poor understanding of the patho-aetiology and lack of clinical consensus. The term frozen shoulder has been described as a 'waste-can diagnosis'[7] as it is often applied to any stiff and painful presentation of the shoulder. Additionally, current use of the term frozen shoulder may be ambiguous and lead to complacency as it suggests the shoulder will 'thaw' and return to normal with or without treatment. This may be incorrect as research suggests recovery may not be complete even after 11 years post onset.[8] The suggestion by Bunker[6] for the term 'contracture of the shoulder' may be more suitable, but this does not take into account the often severe pain associated with the condition. As such, the term frozen shoulder contraction syndrome (FSCS) may be more appropriate.

EPIDEMIOLOGY

Uncertainty remains as to the lifetime prevalence and annual incidence of FSCS. Nevasier and Hannifan[9] presented epidemiological data from published studies that suggested FSCS occurs in 2–5% of the population, with women more commonly affected than men, with the non-dominant hand more frequently involved, and that 20–30% will develop the condition bilaterally. Although these data have been cited in publications for many decades, considerable uncertainty persists as to the accuracy of these statistics. Issues such as diagnosis and inclusion criteria in the original studies may have possibly resulted in over-reporting and misinterpretation of the epidemiology. Bunker[6] has described that the condition is equally distributed between men and women and the incidence is 0.75%. This may be comparable with an estimated annual incidence of 0.24% reported in general practice in the Netherlands.[10] Diabetes, hypothyroidism, lower body mass index and a family history of frozen shoulder may be risk factors for idiopathic frozen shoulder.[11] Smith et al.[12] identified diabetes and a sibling with frozen shoulder as risk factors for developing FSCS in those undergoing arthroscopic capsular release. Others have also identified a genetic predisposition[13,14] and ethnicity may also be involved, as people born in the British Isles or having parents/grandparents born in the British Isles, may be at greater risk of suffering from the condition.[11]

NATURAL HISTORY

FSCS is typically described as progressing through three phases: freezing, frozen and thawing. In most cases FSCS is characterized by the onset of pain that generally becomes severe and disabling, and is often described as excruciating when the shoulder moves suddenly. Pain is present at night and is usually severe and disrupts sleep. In association with the pain, the shoulder becomes progressively stiff and movement substantially reduced. Clinically, the severity of pain will vary as will the degree of stiffness between individuals. Codman[1] described that recovery will occur and should be expected. Reeves[15] reported that the average duration of the condition is 30.1 months (range 1 to 3.5 years), observing that the longer the second or stiff/frozen stage, the longer the third or thawing/recovery phase. Other studies suggest substantially longer duration of symptoms. Shaffer et al.[8] reported that 50% of people diagnosed with idiopathic frozen shoulder had ongoing shoulder pain and/or shoulder stiffness at an average 7-year follow-up. In contrast, Miller et al.[16] reported in a retrospective analysis that all patients achieved pain-free shoulder movement during activities of daily living. These conflicting data suggest that the natural history of frozen shoulder may be variable. They may also reflect different diagnostic criteria, variation in outcome measurements and procedures, bias and the possibility of concomitant shoulder presentations. Routinely informing people diagnosed with FSCS that the condition always resolves with or without treatment, may be inaccurate and misleading. The natural history may follow the shape of a bell curve with the majority of people taking 2 to 3 years for the symptoms to resolve and a percentage on either side of the peak experiencing symptoms for considerably shorter or longer durations. Although the pain may settle and the function may return, this does not necessarily mean full range of movement is always restored. Kanbe et al.[17] described adhesions of the long head of biceps to the rotator interval, which may contribute to ongoing movement restriction.

DIAGNOSIS

There is no definitive diagnostic test for FSCS, and diagnosis is based on physical examination and the absence of radiographic abnormalities. Cyriax and Cyriax[18] described FSCS as being a capsular restriction of the shoulder involving some limitation of internal rotation, with a greater limitation of passive abduction, with the greatest limitation of passive external rotation. Zuckerman and Rokito[4] published a consensus document describing frozen shoulder as a restriction of both active and passive shoulder motion with shoulder radiographs being essentially normal except for the possible presence of osteopenia or calcific tendinosis. They further described primary frozen shoulder as idiopathic in origin and secondary when the underlying aetiology was identifiable. Intrinsic secondary frozen shoulder occurred in the presence of rotator cuff and biceps tendinopathy and calcific tendinosis, and extrinsic secondary frozen shoulder being associated with pathology remote from the shoulder such as ipsilateral breast surgery, cervical radiculopathy, chest wall tumour, cerebrovascular accident and humeral or clavicular fracture. Systemic secondary frozen shoulder occurred in the presence of conditions such as diabetes and thyroid abnormalities. However, a definitive relationship between many of these conditions and frozen shoulder remains uncertain.

The importance of a radiograph cannot be underestimated as many conditions affecting the shoulder manifest with pain and stiffness.[6,19] Locked glenohumeral dislocations, substantial glenohumeral degenerative changes, avascular necrosis of the humeral head, fractures, osteosarcomas and calcific tendinosis are examples of conditions that would usually be associated with reduced joint movement and pain. In these conditions, the radiological presentation would demonstrate pathology. Bunker[6] argued that a diagnosis of frozen shoulder should be considered if clinically there is an equal restriction of active and passive shoulder external rotation range and that radiologically the shoulder radiograph is reported as normal. This remains the simplest diagnostic procedure and research is required to fully validate this method. It may be necessary to test external rotation range in a number of positions to ensure that there are no compensatory movements for lost glenohumeral external rotation.[20] Clinic assessment for FSCS may need to be tested over time as the condition may not have declared itself in the initial clinical visit. Additionally, the presence of pain, for reasons other than FSCS, may lead to the individual rigidly fixing the shoulder, possibly due to fear of increased pain on movement and this may be misdiagnosed as a FSCS.

MANAGEMENT

FSCS is difficult to treat and there is little consensus as to what constitutes optimal evidence-based treatment and as mentioned FSCS is frequently described in three stages: (a) frozen or pain; (b) freezing or stiffness; and (c) thawing or recovery phase.[15] Others have described it as a four-stage process.[7] Once diagnosis has been confirmed, an alternative approach used by the author is to divide the condition into two phases: (a) more pain than stiff and (b) more stiff than pain.

People suffering with FSCS require education detailing what is known about the natural history and expected outcomes, as well as being made aware of treatment alternatives and outcomes of each in an unbiased and patient-focused manner. It is incumbent upon the clinician to be aware of the research evidence, its generalizability, as well as its quality. People with FSCS are frequently informed that the condition will get better with or without treatment and supervised neglect is preferable to physiotherapy. This was the conclusion reported in a non-randomized investigation employing a quasi-experimental design with a high risk of bias,[21] and as such these recommendations must be interpreted cautiously. In addition, the treatment offered in the 'supervised neglect' group should also be considered as physiotherapy.

Data from 2370 people diagnosed with frozen shoulder suggested that therapeutic benefit may be achieved with procedures such as joint mobilization and exercise, and poorer outcomes may be associated with ultrasound and massage.[22] A limitation of these data is that inclusion

and assessment criteria for FSCS were not specified other than patient's being classified with the ICD-9 code 726.0. Mobilization therapy may be beneficial in the management of FSCS. A randomized comparison of high- (Maitland grade III-IV) and low-(grade II) grade glenohumeral inferior, anterior and posterior mobilization procedures in 100 people with frozen shoulder for an average of 20 treatments over 12 weeks suggested that significant improvements occurred in both groups over 12 months. A trend for greater clinical improvement (movement and pain) was observed in the high-grade mobilization group.[23] In a study of 28 people with frozen shoulder, both end-range mobilizations and mobilization with movement demonstrated greater clinical effectiveness than mid-range mobilizations over a 12-week period.[5] A control group was not included in either study and as such, without a 'no treatment' control group it is not clear if improvement was due to natural recovery.

In a small pilot randomized clinical study ($n = 27$) no significant difference in pain and functional ability as measured by the SPADI was identified between an osteopathic (Neil-Asher) deep soft tissue technique and a group given manual therapy and exercise, and another (termed placebo) comprised of breathing exercise, pain-free range of movement exercises and effleurage. Gains in shoulder abduction range were greatest in the deep soft tissue group. This study only reported short-term results (12 weeks) post-intervention and the number and details of interventions were not described.[24] The SPADI involves five questions concerning pain and eight pertaining to functional movement. As no difference in outcome was detected in SPADI between the groups, the importance of an increase in abduction range must be interpreted cautiously and more research is required.

In a small, short-term follow-up randomized clinical trial, deep heating (12 sessions over 4 weeks) involving short-wave diathermy followed by stretching appeared to produce favourable results in people diagnosed with frozen shoulder.[25] There may also be some short-term benefit with 12 laser treatments administered over 12 weeks combined with home exercises.[26]

Acupuncture is commonly used to treat FSCS; however, the quality of the evidence supporting its effectiveness is generally poor. Maund et al.[27] concluded that there is insufficient evidence to make definitive recommendations regarding the use of acupuncture in the treatment of frozen shoulder. However, on the basis of one randomized controlled trial deemed to be of high quality,[28] two systematic reviews[29,30] concluded that acupuncture combined with exercise may confer moderate benefit in the short term.

Although popular, there is a paucity of definitive evidence for the use of corticosteroid (CS) injections in the management of FSCS. A synthesis of the evidence suggests that CS injections may reduce pain and improve function in the short term,[27,31,32] and that the benefit may be enhanced in both the short term and medium term when guided intra-articular CS injections are combined with physiotherapy.[27,32] Carette et al.[32] reported best outcomes in a group randomized to receive image-guided injections up to 1 year post onset and physiotherapy, which involved twelve, 1-hour sessions over 4 weeks.

TABLE 50-5	Frozen Shoulder Contraction Syndrome: Injection Therapy and Physiotherapy Care Pathway	
Assessment	**Stage I to Early Stage II (Pain > Stiffness) Corticosteroid Injection and Physiotherapy**	**Late Stage II to Stage III: (Stiffness > Pain) Hydro-Distension and Physiotherapy**
• Sexes are affected equally with approximate peak onset of 52 years for men and 55 for women • Full patient interview and physical examination. Screen for Yellow and Red Flags and monitor during treatment • Equal restriction of active and passive external rotation • Radiographs normal • Organize blood tests to screen for diabetes and other related health conditions • Outcome measures Consider: ROM, Pain, Function, SPADI, DASH, Quick-DASH, EQ-5D-5L, PGIC, Patient Satisfaction • Fully inform patient. Determine care pathway based on evidence and patient's values. Consider following as possible pathway	• Screen for contraindications and special precautions for an intra-articular small-volume corticosteroid and lidocaine injection • If no CIs/SPs, explain risks and benefits, gain consent, proceed with ultrasound-guided small-volume corticosteroid and lidocaine injection (strong evidence short term and moderate evidence medium term) • Perform the injection as an ultrasound-guided procedure (or use another imaging guidance). No radiation associated with ultrasound • RCTs have not demonstrated a difference between location, dosage and volume of injection • During the first week gentle self-assisted and active movements • Second to fourth weeks, mobilization, soft tissue massage, passive movements, self-assisted movements, exercises as tolerated • Consider re-injecting at 4/52 if pain not under control. No more than three times in 1 year and at least 1 month between injections • Injection procedures may overlap across the stages and be performed concomitantly. If unable to inject consider: [need to screen for CIs] • Laser, mobilization, soft tissue massage, passive movements, acupuncture, exercise, short-wave diathermy • Oral steroid and suprascapular nerve blocks are also procedures associated with clinical benefit Main references: Maund et al.,[27] Favejee et al.[30]	• Screen for CI and SP to image guided GHJ intra-articular lidocaine and large-volume NaCl injection (i.e. hydro-distension) • Consider USGI as no radiation associated with ultrasound • If no CIs/SPs, explain risks and benefits, gain consent, proceed with hydro-distension procedure if: • ROM not restored from CS and lidocaine injection, or • First presentation to clinic when in stiffness > pain stage (moderate evidence; NNT-pain 2, NNT-ROM/function: 3) • Immediately following the procedure: Passive movements and PNF • Instruct home programme involving regular (hourly if possible) active movements, self-assisted active movements and stretching on day of procedure and regularly on following days • In clinic: mobilization, PNF, progress home programme • If required repeat hydro-distension at one week • Injection procedures may overlap across the stages and be performed concomitantly Main references: Favejee et al.,[30] Buchbinder et al.[35] Notes: • Monitor outcome measures • Ensure adequate physiotherapy is embedded within care pathway • For physiotherapists not currently providing ultrasound-guided injections, develop care pathways with orthopaedic and radiology colleagues • In refractory cases and if improvement not as expected, consider orthopaedic referral for opinion on capsular release

CI, contraindication; *CS*, corticosteroid; *DASH*, Disability of the Arm Shoulder and Hand; *GHJ*, glenohumeral joint; *NNT*, numbers needed to treat for benefit; *PGIC*, patient global impression of change; *PNF*, proprioceptive neuromuscular facilitation; *Quick-DASH*, Quick Disability of the Arm Shoulder and Hand; *ROM*, range of movement; *SP*, special precaution; *SPADI*, Shoulder Pain and Disability Index; *USGI*, ultrasound-guided injection. Adapted from www.LondonShoulderClinic.com (01/2014).

Physiotherapy treatments varied according to the stage of the frozen shoulder and included active and assisted range of movement exercises, ultrasound, mobilization, ice and strengthening. In an attempt to elucidate the optimal dose of ultrasound-guided intra-articular CS to treat FSCS (freezing or stiff stage) Yoon et al.[33] reported significant improvement in the CS groups when compared to the placebo group (analgesic only) but no difference between the CS groups using the SPADI, shoulder pain and shoulder range of movement as outcome measures, and recommended the use of low-dose CS.

Arthrographic hydro-distension is a technique that involves injecting large volumes of sodium chloride into the glenohumeral joint under imaging guidance. The aim of the procedure is to distend the contracted joint capsule. It is a procedure that is now performed by

appropriately skilled physiotherapists in the United Kingdom.[34] A systematic review[35] concluded that the procedure was associated with a numbers needed to treat for benefit of 2 for pain reduction, and a numbers needed to treat of 3 for improvement in function in patients diagnosed with FSCS. Range of shoulder movement (but not pain and function) is enhanced when physiotherapy (manual therapy and exercise) is provided after the hydro-distension procedure.[36]

Manipulation under anaesthetic involves scapular stabilization with shoulder flexion, abduction and adduction, followed by maximal shoulder internal and external rotation (with the elbow flexed). Tearing of the contracted capsule may be felt or heard. The evidence supporting manipulation under anaesthetic is poor. Kivimaki et al.[37] randomized 127 people with frozen shoulder to manipulation under anaesthetic and physiotherapy-directed exercises and to physiotherapy exercises alone. They did not detect any difference at 6, 12, 26 and 52 weeks. Of concern, in a study of 30 people undergoing manipulation under anaesthetic, arthroscopy revealed haemarthrosis in all patients following the procedure, and in addition to other iatrogenic intra-articular damage; four people (13%) were observed to have suffered SLAP (superior labral anterior to posterior) lesions, partial tears of the subscapularis were detected in three people, and anterior labral detachment were detected in four people, with an associated osteochondral lesion detected in one person.[38]

Arthroscopic capsular release of the shoulder involves combinations of glenohumeral joint distension, capsular debridement, ligament splitting, loosening of adhesions, shoulder movement, shoulder manipulation and post-surgical physiotherapy. Usually following surgery there is a need to take a week or longer off work. The procedure is not supported by robust research and conclusions from published case series are therefore at high risk of bias.[39,40] Grant et al.[41] concluded that the quality of evidence available is low and the current available data demonstrate little benefit for a capsular release instead of, or in addition to, a manipulation under anaesthetic.

Health funding bodies are appropriately demanding ways of reducing the cost of health-care delivery while maintaining and improving outcomes. Chapter 40 (Advanced roles in musculoskeletal physiotherapy) discusses a physiotherapy-led initiative for the management of FSCS. The pathway comprises assessment, imaging, ultrasound-guided CS injection and hydro-distension procedures, embedded within a physiotherapy rehabilitation programme, entirely led and performed by physiotherapists.[34] This treatment package is provided at a fraction of the cost of the surgical procedures used to treat FSCS. It would be beneficial to appropriately compare the physiotherapy-led programme and capsular release procedure for clinical outcomes, adverse events, economic analysis and patient satisfaction. Additionally, hydro-distension is performed in a clinic and the patient is free to go home soon after the procedure and is not associated with additional time off work.

CONCLUSION

FSCS may be less common than suggested in the literature; however, when present it is associated with substantial pain, movement restriction and morbidity. The literature is beset with studies that are frequently small and have high levels of bias, from which conclusions to underpin clinical practice are difficult to extract with confidence. There is a paucity of literature supporting physiotherapy interventions for FSCS, but it is potentially incorrect to state that supervised neglect is preferential to physiotherapy. Manipulation under anaesthetic appears to be no more effective than physiotherapy and is associated with possible joint damage. Capsular release is not supported by robust scientific evidence and has not been comprehensively compared

to physiotherapist-led care pathways for FSCS that include ultrasound-guided CS injections and hydro-distension procedures embedded within physiotherapy exercise and mobilization treatment (Table 50-5). Much is still to be learnt about frozen shoulder and a better name for this disorder may be FSCS.

REFERENCES

1. Codman E. The Shoulder: rupture of the supraspinatus tendon and other lesions in or about the subacromial bursa. Boston: Thomas Todd Company; 1934.
2. Neviaser J. Adhesive capsulitis of the shoulder. A study of the pathological findings in periarthritis of the shoulder. J Bone Joint Surg (Am) 1945;27(2):211–22.
3. Wiley AM. Arthroscopic appearance of frozen shoulder. Arthroscopy 1991;7(2):138–43. [Epub 1991/01/01].
4. Zuckerman JD, Rokito A. Frozen shoulder: a consensus definition. J Shoulder Elbow Surg 2011;20(2):322–5. [Epub 2010/11/06].
5. Yang JL, Chang CW, Chen SY, et al. Mobilization techniques in subjects with frozen shoulder syndrome: randomized multiple-treatment trial. Phys Ther 2007;87(10):1307–15. [Epub 2007/08/09].
6. Bunker T. Time for a new name for frozen shoulder-contracture of the shoulder. Shoulder Elbow 2009;1:4–9.
7. Neviaser RJ, Neviaser TJ. The frozen shoulder. Diagnosis and management. Clin Orthop Relat Res 1987;223:59–64. [Epub 1987/10/01].
8. Shaffer B, Tibone JE, Kerlan RK. Frozen shoulder. A long-term follow-up. J Bone Joint Surg 1992;74(5):738–46.
9. Neviaser AS, Hannafin JA. Adhesive capsulitis: a review of current treatment. Am J Sports Med 2010;38(11):2346–56. [Epub 2010/01/30].
10. van der Windt DA, Koes BW, Deville W, et al. Effectiveness of corticosteroid injections versus physiotherapy for treatment of painful stiff shoulder in primary care: randomised trial. BMJ 1998;317(7168):1292–6. [Epub 1998/11/07].
11. Wang K, Ho V, Hunter-Smith DJ, et al. Risk factors in idiopathic adhesive capsulitis: a case control study. J Shoulder Elbow Surg 2013;22(7):e24–9. [Epub 2013/01/29].
12. Smith CD, White WJ, Bunker TD. The associations of frozen shoulder in patients requiring arthroscopic release. Shoulder Elbow 2012;4(2):87–9.
13. Hakim AJ, Cherkas LF, Spector TD, et al. Genetic associations between frozen shoulder and tennis elbow: a female twin study. Rheumatology 2003;42(6):739–42. [Epub 2003/05/06].
14. Hirschhorn P, Schmidt JM. Frozen shoulder in identical twins. Joint Bone Spine 2000;67(1):75–6. [Epub 2000/04/25].
15. Reeves B. The natural history of the frozen shoulder syndrome. Scand J Rheumatol 1975;4(4):193–6. [Epub 1975/01/01].
16. Miller MD, Wirth MA, Rockwood CA Jr. Thawing the frozen shoulder: the 'patient' patient. Orthopedics 1996;19(10):849–53. [Epub 1996/10/01].
17. Kanbe K, Inoue K, Inoue Y. Dynamic movement of the long head of the biceps tendon in frozen shoulders. J Orthop Surg (Hong Kong) 2008;16(3):295–9. [Epub 2009/01/08].
18. Cyriax J, Cyriax P. Cyriax's Illustrated Manual of Orthopaedic Medicine. 2nd ed. Oxford: Butterworth Heinemann; 1993.
19. Sano H, Hatori M, Mineta M, et al. Tumors masked as frozen shoulders: a retrospective analysis. J Shoulder Elbow Surg 2010;19(2):262–6. [Epub 2009/07/04].
20. Valentine RE, Lewis JS. Intraobserver reliability of 4 physiologic movements of the shoulder in subjects with and without symptoms. Arch Phys Med Rehabil 2006;87(9):1242–9.
21. Diercks RL, Stevens M. Gentle thawing of the frozen shoulder: a prospective study of supervised neglect versus intensive physical therapy in seventy-seven patients with frozen shoulder syndrome followed up for two years. J Shoulder Elbow Surg 2004;13(5):499–502.
22. Jewell DV, Riddle DL, Thacker LR. Interventions associated with an increased or decreased likelihood of pain reduction and improved function in patients with adhesive capsulitis: a retrospective cohort study. Phys Ther 2009;89(5):419–29. [Epub 2009/03/10].

23. Vermeulen HM, Rozing PM, Obermann WR, et al. Comparison of high-grade and low-grade mobilization techniques in the management of adhesive capsulitis of the shoulder: randomized controlled trial. Phys Ther 2006;86(3):355–68.

24. Greenhalgh S, Self J. Red flags: A guide to identifying serious pathology of the spine. Edinburgh: Churchill Livingstone Elsevier; 2006.

25. Leung MS, Cheing GL. Effects of deep and superficial heating in the management of frozen shoulder. J Rehabil Med 2008;40(2):145–50. [Epub 2008/05/30].

26. Stergioulas A. Low-power laser treatment in patients with frozen shoulder: preliminary results. Photomed Laser Surg 2008;26(2):99–105. [Epub 2008/03/18].

27. Maund E, Craig D, Suekarran S, et al. Management of frozen shoulder: a systematic review and cost-effectiveness analysis. Health Technol Assess 2012;16(11):1–264. [Epub 2012/03/13].

28. Sun KO, Chan KC, Lo SL, et al. Acupuncture for frozen shoulder. Hong Kong Med J 2001;7(4):381–91. [Epub 2002/01/05].

29. Jain TK, Sharma NK. The effectiveness of physiotherapeutic interventions in treatment of frozen shoulder/adhesive capsulitis: a systematic review. J Back Musculoskeletal Rehabil 2013;27(3):247–73.

30. Favejee MM, Huisstede BM, Koes BW. Frozen shoulder: the effectiveness of conservative and surgical interventions–systematic review. Br J Sports Med 2011;45(1):49–56. [Epub 2010/07/22].

31. Blanchard V, Barr S, Cerisola FL. The effectiveness of corticosteroid injections compared with physiotherapeutic interventions for adhesive capsulitis: a systematic review. Physiotherapy 2010; 96(2):95–107. [Epub 2010/04/28].

32. Carette S, Moffet H, Tardif J, et al. Intraarticular corticosteroids, supervised physiotherapy, or a combination of the two in the treatment of adhesive capsulitis of the shoulder: a placebo-controlled trial. Arthritis Rheum 2003;48(3):829–38.

33. Yoon SH, Lee HY, Lee HJ, et al. Optimal dose of intra-articular corticosteroids for adhesive capsulitis: a randomized, triple-blind, placebo-controlled trial. Am J Sports Med 2013;41(5):1133–9. [Epub 2013/03/20].

34. O'Connaire E, Lewis JS. Arthrographic hydrodistension for frozen shoulder. A physiotherapy-led initiative in primary care. Available from: <http://www.health.org.uk/media_manager/public /75/programme_library_docs/Central%20London%20-%20 Frozen%20Shoulder.pdf>; 2011.

35. Buchbinder R, Green S, Youd JM, et al. Arthrographic distension for adhesive capsulitis (frozen shoulder). Cochrane Database Syst Rev 2008;(1):CD007005, [Epub 2008/02/07].

36. Buchbinder R, Youd JM, Green S, et al. Efficacy and cost-effectiveness of physiotherapy following glenohumeral joint distension for adhesive capsulitis: a randomized trial. Arthritis Rheum 2007;57(6):1027–37. [Epub 2007/08/01].

37. Kivimaki J, Pohjolainen T, Malmivaara A, et al. Manipulation under anesthesia with home exercises versus home exercises alone in the treatment of frozen shoulder: a randomized, controlled trial with 125 patients. J Shoulder Elbow Surg 2007;16(6):722–6. [Epub 2007/10/13].

38. Loew M, Heichel TO, Lehner B. Intraarticular lesions in primary frozen shoulder after manipulation under general anesthesia. J Shoulder Elbow Surg 2005;14(1):16–21. [Epub 2005/02/22].

39. Fernandes MR. Arthroscopic capsular release for refractory shoulder stiffness. Rev Assoc Med Bras 2013;59(4):347–53. [Epub 2013/07/16].

40. Dattani R, Ramasamy V, Parker R, et al. Improvement in quality of life after arthroscopic capsular release for contracture of the shoulder. Bone Joint J 2013;95-B(7):942–6. [Epub 2013/07/03].

41. Grant JA, Schroeder N, Miller BS, et al. Comparison of manipulation and arthroscopic capsular release for adhesive capsulitis: a systematic review. J Shoulder Elbow Surg 2013;22(8):1135–45. [Epub 2013/03/21].

CHAPTER 51

ELBOW

Brooke Coombes • Leanne Bisset • Bill Vicenzino

INTRODUCTION

Anatomically, the elbow is a complex joint with a large range of motion, many musculotendinous attachments and several traversing neurovascular structures. Its elaborate design allows this joint to position the hand in space and act as a stabilizer for lifting, carrying, pushing, pulling and throwing. The complex anatomy and biomechanics of the elbow, combined with a large spectrum of pathology, presents a challenge for the treating clinician. This chapter presents an overview of contemporary issues in examination and differential diagnosis, along with the conservative rehabilitation programmes for various elbow injuries, synthesizing the current evidence with clinical reasoning.

CLINICAL INTERVIEW

History

Establishing the mechanism of injury is important following traumatic injuries to gain an understanding of the original injury, any concomitant injuries and timeframes for healing. For the post-surgical patient, additional information should be gained from the surgeon to understand the surgical procedure, and any limitations in range of motion due to joint stability or fixation. For non-traumatic injuries, it is equally important to question the nature, duration and evolution of symptoms, including exposure to repetitive occupational or sporting risks. A combination of physical exertion and repetitive elbow and wrist movements is a strong risk factor for epicondylalgia and other non-specific elbow disorders in working populations.[1] Lateral epicondylalgia is more common in racket sports,[2] whereas overhead throwing athletes are predisposed to medial elbow injury. It is important to ascertain if the condition has occurred before or if there is a history of other upper extremity injury or surgery.

Symptoms

Thorough questioning of the location, quality, intensity and behaviour of pain is insightful. Snapping or clicking during supination/extension with associated pain over the posterolateral elbow region may implicate posterolateral rotatory instability. Other symptoms of instability, including clumsiness, heaviness, fatigue or loss of control, are important to clarify, particularly in the throwing athlete. The presence and location of any numbness or paraesthesia may help determine potential sites of compression or irritation of nerves around the elbow. Given most sites around the elbow involve dynamic structures, their temporal nature and relationship to throwing or occupational tasks provides important information.[3] Patterns of symptoms or behaviours that indicate an urgent medical or psychological problem should be highlighted during the clinical interview. For example, symptoms of sudden swelling may indicate infection, inflammation or compartment syndrome, while malignancy may be considered if severe progressive pain is unrelated to activity.

Functional Demands

It is essential to determine if any limitations on daily activities, work, sport or hobbies exist. For the throwing athlete, specific information should be obtained about symptoms while throwing, including what phase, after how many throws, and the presence of paraesthesia or symptoms of instability. Questioning should extend to details of work status and timing for return to work. Failure to gain information about the functional demands placed on the elbow may limit diagnosis and effective treatment planning.

Co-morbidity

There is strong evidence that musculoskeletal co-morbidity has an adverse impact on the overall prognosis of musculoskeletal problems[4,5] and may influence treatment planning. For these reasons, examination of the spine, shoulder, wrist and hand is also essential. Concomitant pathology may exist, for example trauma-associated fractures or soft tissue injuries at the wrist, or pain secondary to the use of substitution patterns when elbow range of motion (ROM) or strength is insufficient.

Outcome Measures

There is a need for greater consensus and standardization of outcomes concerning the elbow to allow comparison between trials and clinical practice. Patient-reported outcomes are advocated over observer-based scoring systems for examination of elbow pain and function because of lack of agreement and heterogeneous weighting of outcomes.[6–8] Patient-rated instruments vary in specificity or focus, some are joint-specific (e.g. Oxford Elbow Score), or condition-specific (e.g. the Patient-Rated Tennis Elbow Evaluation), while others are applicable to the whole upper limb (e.g. Disability of Arm Shoulder or Hand). An advantage of using a specific outcome measure that is focused on the condition (or anatomical site), is it is likely to be the most responsive to change in that condition. However, kinesiological theory suggests that the upper extremity operates as a single functional unit and the latter may be more relevant for examining conditions that tend to affect more than one joint or are associated with many co-morbidities. A recent systematic review of the validity, reliability and responsiveness of elbow-specific clinical rating systems found the Oxford Elbow Score was the only outcome with good or excellent quality methods based on the COSMIN checklist.[9] Research into the use of rating scales in patients following traumatic elbow injury is currently lacking.[10]

PHYSICAL EXAMINATION OF THE ELBOW

Many elbow conditions and associated investigations and tests used to differentiate between conditions have yet to be evaluated for their accuracy (i.e. the sensitivity and specificity). In the following paragraphs, we provide a description of key physical tests for examination of the elbow, highlighting the diagnostic and prognostic relevance of findings.

Range of Motion

Goniometry is useful, especially for monitoring the effectiveness of treatments to improve ROM. The measurement error for this instrument is estimated to be 5° for elbow flexion–extension and 9° for forearm rotation.[11] The patterns of loss of elbow motion and passive examination, including assessment of the end feel and accessory movements, are also informative and may direct the clinician to the structures limiting motion. For example, motion deficits secondary to capsular joint stiffness should be differentiated from that secondary to two-joint muscle length, such as the biceps, triceps or forearm muscles. When assessing forearm rotation it is essential to examine accessory movements at both proximal and distal radio-ulnar joints, as both may contribute to limited pronation and supination.[12]

Elbow Stability

Elbow instability can be viewed on a continuum from mild laxity to severe and recurrent dislocation that progresses from the lateral to the medial side of the elbow and may involve soft tissue and/or bone.[13] Elbow instability can be classified according to the following:[13]
- articulations involved (radial head, elbow)
- direction of displacement (valgus, varus, anterior, posterolateral rotatory)
- degree of displacement (subluxation, dislocation)
- timing (acute, chronic, recurrent)
- presence or absence of fractures.

Diagnosis of elbow instability is usually made with a combination of history, physical examination, imaging and arthroscopic examination. Several clinical tests to elucidate symptoms of instability are described in Table 51-1. However, it is important to recognize that findings on physical examination are commonly subtle and examination of instability may need to be performed with the patient under sedation or with stress radiography.[13,14]

Lateral Instability

Under acute axial loading (e.g. a fall on an outstretched hand), there is progressive involvement of soft and bony structures about the elbow. Initially, the lateral ulnar rotates posterolaterally, injuring the lateral collateral and lateral ulnar collateral ligaments, while the integrity of the anterior band of the medial collateral ligament (MCL) remains intact.[13] This injury results in valgus and posterolateral rotatory instability (PLRI, stage 1). PLRI is rarely seen as an overuse injury, but rather as a consequence of acute trauma[20] and may be combined with secondary radio-capitellar joint compression and posteromedial impingement in people with long-standing instability. PLRI is diagnosed through the patient history and through the lateral pivot-shift manoeuvre of the elbow (see Table 51-1). Patients may complain of recurrent snapping or clicking during supination/extension with associated pain over the posterolateral elbow region. The patient may report difficulty or a feeling of instability while performing activities such as pushing up from a chair or attempting a push up with forearm supination. When demonstrating these tasks, the patient will be reluctant to fully extend the elbow in weight bearing. In addition, they may also report painful catching, clicking or a feeling of instability during elbow flexion/extension, particularly around 40° of elbow flexion with forearm supination. Posterolateral subluxation usually reduces in pronation, which is thought to be due to greater contact at the radio-humeral joint and therefore greater transmission of axial forces across the radio-humeral joint in pronation compared with supination,[21] particularly in the presence of an intact MCL.

Stage 2 instability involves incomplete elbow dislocation that results in tearing of the lateral collateral ligament (LCL) complex as well as anterior and posterior soft tissue disruption. Lastly, stage 3 involves a full elbow dislocation that may involve rupture to some or all of the MCL as well as fractures of the radial head and/or coronoid process.[13] The terrible triad injury of the elbow involves a combination of coronoid process and radial head fractures, and elbow dislocation. It often results in recurrent instability, development of degenerative changes and persistent long-term disability.[13,22–24] Often a trauma seen in younger people, long-term complications include persistent instability, non-union, malunion and radio-ulnar fusion.[13]

Medial Instability

Medial instability may also be approached on a spectrum, from micro tears of the MCL in response to repetitive overload that eventually leads to partial or full ligament tears.[25,26] The chronic valgus overload that leads to valgus

TABLE 51-1   Clinical Tests for Elbow Instability

Indication	Test	Description	Positive Result
Ulnar collateral ligament injury[15]	Abduction stress test	Patient's elbow in 90° flexion Examiner applies valgus force while palpating the medial joint line	Pain Medial joint space opening of 2 mm greater than the uninjured elbow
	Moving valgus stress test	Patient's shoulder in 90° abduction and external rotation Examiner applies valgus stress to flexed elbow, then extends the elbow while maintaining the valgus elbow/external shoulder rotation force	Pain between 120° and 70° of elbow flexion Sensitivity 100%, specificity 75%[16]
	Modified milking manoeuvre	Patient's shoulder in adduction and maximum external rotation and elbow flexed to 70° Examiner applies valgus stress by pulling down on patient's thumb and palpating the medial joint line with their other hand	Pain Medial joint space opening
Posterolateral rotatory instability (PLRI)[17]	Lateral pivot shift[18]	Patient supine with shoulder flexed and externally rotated and forearm supinated Examiner flexes the elbow while applying valgus, supination and axial compression	Skin dimple or prominent radial head Apprehension/pain at 40° flexion Clunk or relief with further flexion (joint reduced)
	Posterolateral rotary drawer test[14]	Examiner pulls the proximal lateral forearm posteriorly	Skin dimple Apprehension
	Table top relocation test[19]	Patient standing in front of a table with affected hand on the lateral edge of the table (a) Patient performs a press-up with the elbow pointing laterally (forearm supinated) (b) Above repeated while the examiner prevents posterior subluxation of the radial head (c) Removal of examiner support	 (a) Apprehension/pain at approximately 40° flexion (b & c) Relief and recurrence of symptoms, respectively

instability is most common in throwing athletes. The late cocking and early acceleration phases of throwing, when the elbow is in flexion, create excessive repetitive valgus forces generated by high angular velocities.[27-29] There are significant negative consequences associated with chronic valgus instability, including compression stress in the radio-humeral joint, traction stress in the medial compartment (flexor-pronator muscles, medial epicondyle epiphysis, ulnar nerve) and posteromedial impingement, all of which can lead to chronic pain and be career-ending for an athlete.[20] In contrast, an acute injury to the MCL may be associated with a compression fracture of the radial neck, and ligament injury should be suspected if a radial head fracture is identified radiographically.

Muscle–Tendon Function

Physical evaluation of musculotendinous function is useful for determining the presence and extent of both acute, traumatic injuries and chronic degenerative conditions, including tendinopathy. Patients with lateral epicondylalgia present with lateral elbow pain with resisted wrist extension test (Cozens test), resisted middle finger extension test and/or the Mills test, in which the examiner passively pronates the forearm, flexes the wrist and extends the elbow. Patients with medial epicondylalgia have pain with resisted wrist flexion when the elbow is extended fully, while resisted elbow flexion and supination is used to test for distal biceps tendinopathy.

Palpation

Systematic palpation of local elbow structures may be useful in the differential diagnosis of the source of localized pain in some elbow conditions. For example, tenderness of the lateral epicondyle and/or common extensor tendon origin is typical of lateral epicondylalgia, whereas pain over the posterolateral elbow, particularly in the younger patient, may implicate involvement of the synovial plica. Patients with medial epicondylalgia experience pain that is localized just anterior and distal to the common flexor muscle origin, whereas patients with ulnar collateral ligament injury typically have point tenderness approximately 2 cm distal to the medial epicondyle. However, forearm tenderness is found in lateral epicondylalgia, fibromyalgia and cervical referred pain, reducing the specificity of palpation as a stand-alone diagnostic test.

Nerve Function

Examination of nerve function associated with elbow injury is multifaceted and should proceed in a systematic fashion based on clinical interview. Table 51-2 presents a

TABLE 51-2   **Clinical Tests for Provocation of Peripheral Nerves at the Elbow**

Indication	Test	Description	Positive Result
Ulnar neuropathy	Tinel's test[33]	Examiner taps lightly at the ulnar nerve at medial epicondylar groove	Tingling radiating to fourth or fifth digits
	Flexion compression test[33]	Patient's elbow maximally flexed with wrist in neutral, sustained for 60 seconds while the examiner applies compression proximal to the cubital tunnel	Tingling in the ulnar nerve distribution within 60 seconds
	Elbow flexion test[34]	Maximal elbow flexion combined with maximal wrist extension, sustained for 5 seconds	Reproduction of paraesthesia or pain Sensitivity 25%, specificity 100%
	Shoulder internal rotation elbow flexion test[34]	Patient positioned in 90° abduction, 10° flexion and maximal internal rotation of the shoulder, maximal supination, wrist and finger extension sustained for 5 seconds	Reproduction of symptoms within the ulnar nerve distribution Sensitivity 87%, specificity 98%
Radial tunnel syndrome	Resisted supination	Resisted supination with elbow extended	Pain distal to lateral epicondyle

selection of nerve provocation tests. In the general population, the presence of pain about the elbow and sensory loss or associated paraesthesias is often the first diagnostic clue to a nerve problem, whereas motor weakness is a much later finding.[3] In throwing athletes, the first symptoms can be fatigue and loss of velocity or control. Several neural provocation tests of the upper extremity have been described, in which a series of positions are sequentially applied to increase or decrease stress on nerve branches at the elbow.[30,31] The reader is referred to other texts or chapters for description of these tests.[32] There is considerable debate regarding the diagnostic validity of neural provocation tests, and results should be combined with findings from the interview, imaging and other physical tests.[32] Others have shown that provocative tests provide marginal value over routine clinical examination for diagnosing ulnar neuropathy at the elbow.[33]

The ulnar nerve is the most commonly affected nerve around the elbow and the second most common neuropathy in the upper limb, after carpal tunnel syndrome.[35] Ulnar neuropathy at the elbow may occur after traumatic rupture of the MCL or secondary to chronic medial elbow instability, as seen in throwing athletes. Symptoms are commonly related to repetitive or prolonged elbow flexion, resulting in neural traction rather than dynamic compression in the cubital tunnel.[34] Subluxation of the ulnar nerve is reported in 11% of healthy individuals and may not be related to a higher incidence of ulnar neuropathy at the elbow.[36] Subluxation of the ulnar nerve may be examined by palpating the nerve as the elbow is flexed.

Nerve compression may occur anywhere within the radial tunnel.[37,38] However, the posterior interosseus nerve (PIN), a motor branch of the common radial nerve, is most commonly compressed as it passes between two portions of the superior border of supinator at the arcade of Froshe. Motor weakness of the finger and thumb extensors and abductor pollicis longus has traditionally been considered the primary clinical feature of PIN involvement.[38,39] An alternative, sometimes disputed syndrome associated with PIN dysfunction is radial tunnel syndrome. The features of radial tunnel syndrome are similar to lateral epicondylalgia, with patients reporting pain over the proximal dorsal aspect of the forearm that is aggravated by repetitive or resisted forearm supination/pronation and middle finger extension, localized tenderness on palpation over the lateral epicondyle, with a history of repetitive manual activity.[38-41] The difficulty in differentiating radial tunnel syndrome from lateral epicondylalgia is reflected in the low level of accuracy (37–52%) using history and physical tests in the diagnosis of radial tunnel syndrome.[42,43]

Strength

Clinically useful measures of elbow and grip strength may be obtained using hand-held isometric devices and compared to either the contralateral arm, or in cases of bilateral involvement, to normative values.[44] The dominant arm is reported to be 6–8% stronger than the nondominant arm for gripping and forearm rotation and 4% stronger for elbow flexion and extension strength.[44] A standardized test position of 90° of elbow flexion and neutral forearm position is recommended[45] for testing of elbow strength, because reduced ROM in some conditions precludes positioning in full pronation or supination.[44]

Maximal grip strength has been found to be of limited use in clinical populations, such as lateral epicondylalgia or arthritic disease, where pain interferes with maximal voluntary effort.[46,47] The pain-free grip test, which measures the amount of force that the patient generates to the onset of pain, is commonly performed in patients with lateral epicondylalgia and correlates more strongly with pain and disability and perceived improvement than maximal strength in this population.[48,49] Most protocols recommend testing with the elbow in relaxed extension and forearm pronation, three times with 1-minute intervals, using the average of these repetitions to compare between affected and unaffected sides.[50] An alternative testing position with the elbow flexed 90° and forearm in neutral forearm rotation is also used.

Diagnostic Imaging

Radiographs remain the initial imaging choice following traumatic elbow injuries to establish the initial injury, any associated fractures or displacement, as well as to evaluate post-reduction alignment and bony healing. The elbow extension test[51] has been proposed as a simple test to effectively rule out the need for radiography. Patients with a recent elbow injury who cannot fully extend their elbow after injury should be referred for radiography, as they have a nearly 50% chance of fracture. For those able to fully extend their elbow, radiography can be deferred but the patients should return if symptoms have not resolved within 7–10 days. Caution should be used in children and in patients with suspected olecranon fracture.

Magnetic resonance imaging (MRI) has been reported to be highly specific (100% specificity, 57% sensitivity) for detecting ulnar collateral ligament tears.[52] Complete or large tears on MRI respond more poorly to rehabilitation than partial tears, indicating MRI plays a role in both diagnosis and predicting outcomes.[53] Computed tomography and MRI arthrography have been shown to be very sensitive for the detection of full or partial articular cartilage lesions of the elbow.[54]

Reports on the accuracy of ultrasound for diagnosis of lateral epicondylalgia are variable. Some studies have found relatively high sensitivity but low specificity in the detection of symptomatic lateral epicondylalgia,[55] whereas others have found high specificity using a combination of grey-scale changes and power Doppler examination of neovascularity.[56] The latter study concluded that ultrasound can be used to conclusively rule out lateral epicondylalgia as a diagnosis and should prompt the clinician to consider other causes for lateral elbow pain. If the patient complains of clicking or locking, MRI and computed tomography or magnetic resonance arthrography may be used to detect other pathologies, such as loose bodies, instability, annular ligament injury or elbow synovial fold syndrome.[57,58] Clarke et al.[59] found large tears of the common extensor tendon and tears of the lateral collateral ligament were significantly correlated with poorer response to conservative treatment. The presence of neovascularity demonstrated no correlation with change in pain or disability suggesting it may be a poor indicator of prognosis.

Ultrasound may also be useful in diagnosing nerve compression (Fig. 51-1) by detecting swelling and hypoechogenicity of the nerve or identifying secondary causes such as cysts.[59–62] Follow-up of patients with ulnar neuropathy at the elbow after a median of 14 months found pronounced ulnar nerve thickening at the time of the diagnosis was associated with poor outcome, especially in conservatively treated cases, indicating that sonography provides prognostic as well as diagnostic information.[63]

Electrophysiological testing is reported to be beneficial in evaluating ulnar neuropathy and PIN syndrome, while is difficult to perform and rarely helpful for examining the median nerve at the elbow or radial tunnel syndrome.[3] Throwing-related nerve injuries are typically exertional, so electrodiagnostic testing immediately after throwing may be helpful.[3]

CONSERVATIVE MANAGEMENT OF THE ELBOW

The elbow must have mobility, stability and strength and be pain-free to allow independent function in daily activities including the physical demands of work and recreation. Optimal outcome after elbow injury requires the therapist to address all aspects of elbow function. In order to effectively treat a patient with an acute traumatic injury, an understanding of tissue healing, potential stresses to tissues and treatment techniques to protect the injured structures is essential. Early and continued communication with the surgeon regarding the injured structures, specifics about any surgical intervention, stability of fracture fixation and joint stability may be required. For non-traumatic injuries, an understanding of the onset of pathology as well as the individual's premorbid functional level are important. The following paragraphs and Table 51-3 describe the current evidence for conservative rehabilitation of acute traumatic and non-traumatic injuries of the elbow.

Acute Traumatic Injuries of Bone and Ligaments

While several systematic reviews are available for treating acute traumatic injuries of the elbow, few offer guidance

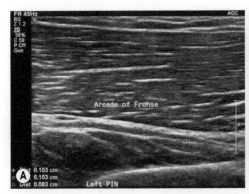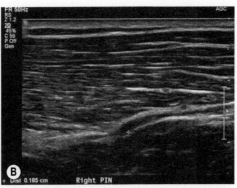

FIGURE 51-1 ■ Posterior interosseus nerve impingement at the arcade of Froshe. (From Qld XRay Pty Ltd, Australia.)

TABLE 51-3 Elbow Conditions and Treatments

Injury/Condition	Timing	Treatment	Precautions and Indications
Simple acute dislocation	First 3–5 days 6–8 weeks	Closed reduction, rest in an elbow splint, followed by active ROM in pronation to avoid subluxing positions Rehabilitation when both MCL and LCL are injured should use active motion with the humerus in either the horizontal or vertical orientations, irrespective of forearm rotation, to minimize valgus and varus loads[64]	Forearm supination facilitates radial head subluxation posterolaterally, therefore pronation may protect against PLRI.[65] Careful monitoring of the patient's progress is necessary, and presence of subluxation or dislocation during the rehabilitation phase (particularly in the first 3 weeks following reduction) may indicate the need for an elbow brace that limits supination and varus/valgus forces[13] Passive motion should be avoided in early rehabilitation phases as it may cause alterations in varus–valgus angulation and internal–external rotation of the ulna relative to the humerus[64]
Stable injury either post-reduction or post-surgery	Immediately	Active ROM of all unaffected joints, including shoulder, wrist and hand, and the unaffected arm	Safe limits to ROM should be determined at surgery or post-reduction of dislocation, to avoid stress to healing MCL and LCL[66], particularly end-of-range extension[66]
	Begin as early as pain and inflammation allow, on average 1–5 days post-surgery or relocation[12,22,90–92]	Commence active ROM through the safe (stable) zone, in a gravity-assisted position for elbow flexion/extension Early triceps activation included to minimize possible scarring of the posterior capsule[67] Progress to anti-gravity as tolerated	
	4–6 weeks, with good fracture healing and joint stability[12]	Elbow passive ROM: gentle 20-second sustained holds end of range, repeated four to five times to avoid the stretch reflex[67] Passive force should be directed through the distal radius and ulna and not the wrist or hand, to avoid stressing the passive restraints of the wrist[12] Progressive resistance exercises: for elbow flexors and extensors, strengthening should begin in pain-free arcs of motion with light resistance with hand or cuff weights or resistive bands with progression of ROM and resistance as tolerated. Strengthening in pronation and supination begins with the elbow in 90° of flexion using a weighted bar Strengthening of muscles at uninvolved joints may be started within the first week as tolerated Once good ROM and strength of the upper extremity are achieved, work- and sport-specific conditioning may begin as necessary to allow the patient to safely and confidently return to activity. Suggested exercises for rehabilitation of elbow injuries and principles guiding prescription can be found elsewhere[68]	Painful stretching should be avoided as it elicits guarding and spasm and limits progression When there is significant elbow or forearm instability, strengthening may be delayed until 6–8 weeks. The ability of the scapular musculature to form a stable base for the upper extremity is important to regain ROM and strength at the elbow, forearm and wrist. Correct form should be emphasized to prevent stresses to healing ligaments or fractures. For example, a patient may compensate for limited supination by shoulder adduction and external rotation, which causes a valgus stress on the elbow
	Once adequate fracture and soft tissue healing is achieved and the joint is considered stable	Manual therapy techniques (e.g. passive accessory glides if capsular tightness is limiting motion) Grade I or II mobilizations to decrease pain and oedema, grade III or IV mobilizations carefully applied to increase motion Simple distraction may be more helpful than accessory glides, as intra-articular translation during normal elbow flexion and extension is minimal[69]	Passive joint mobilizations are never used on an unstable elbow Manual force should be specifically applied to each structure identified as being involved, recognizing that joints outside the elbow may contribute to limited elbow motion. For example, both anterior mobilization of the radial head and posterior mobilization of the distal radius on the ulnar may be applied to improve supination, whereas the reverse is appropriate for pronation[69]

TABLE 51-3   Elbow Conditions and Treatments (Continued)

Injury/Condition	Timing	Treatment	Precautions and Indications
Acute medial collateral ligament mid-substance tear	0–6 weeks	Following surgical repair, patient is in protective bracing for 6 weeks[70]	
Subacute or chronic isolated ulnar collateral ligament injury		It is recommended that throwing be avoided for the first 2–3 months, during which night splitting and ROM exercises for the elbow flexors and forearm pronators is commenced.[93] Strengthening of the elbow extensors should be avoided because of potential valgus stress. Once pain-free, a progressive strengthening programme for all muscle groups about the elbow and shoulder can be commenced. Active flexion/extension motion in supination stabilizes the MCL-deficient elbow[71,72]	Throwing athletes with complete tears found on MRI are less likely to be rehabilitated successfully and surgical intervention might be considered earlier in these patients[15]
Posterolateral rotatory instability		Active flexion/extension motion in pronation stabilizes the LCL-deficient elbow, even in the presence of disruption to the common extensor origin[64,73–76] Biceps, triceps and forearm muscles should be strengthened Medial elbow musculature promotes elbow stability in forearm supination and the lateral musculature in pronation[77] Anconeus activation should be included as a stabilizer for the posterolateral corner[14]	
Ulnar neuropathy		Active rest, in which gentle physical therapy, icing and anti-inflammatories are given. Immobilization is used only for severe cases and is very brief, only until acute symptoms subside. After approximately 4 weeks, a graduated throwing programme is started[3]	Avoid prolonged movements or positions that provoke symptoms Night splinting and nerve gliding exercises did not produce additional improvement[78]
Radial neuropathy		Throwing athletes: activity modification, ice, anti-inflammatories and splinting to support both the elbow and the wrist[3]	Throwing athletes often do strenuous wrist extensor exercises, and these should be reduced during the recovery phase to diminish the irritation of the radial nerve and its branches[3]
Lateral epicondylalgia	At diagnosis	Mobilization with movement, manual therapy in combination with pain-free grip, isometric, concentric[68,79,80] or eccentric wrist extension, and supination/pronation[81] Cervical spine manual and exercise therapy techniques, particularly in patients reporting cold hyperalgesia, severe pain and disability[82] Global upper limb strength and conditioning Retraining sensorimotor function, including attention to re-establishing optimal wrist posture during gripping tasks, as well as proximal strength conditioning[83,84]	

LCL, lateral collateral ligament; MCL, medial collateral ligament; PLRI, posterolateral rotatory instability; ROM, range of motion.

on conservative management options. Two Cochrane systematic reviews of treatments for elbow fractures[85,86] did not identify any randomized controlled trial (RCT) of conservative treatments, while systematic review of treatments for elbow dislocation[87] identified only two, small underpowered RCTs. One trial[88] found no significant differences between early mobilization of the elbow versus 3 weeks of cast immobilization, while the other trial[89] found no significant differences between surgical repair of torn ligaments versus 2 weeks of cast immobilization.

For a stable fracture and/or a stable reduction post-dislocation, early active ROM has been shown to result in better outcomes versus prolonged immobilization.[12,22,90–92] Acute fracture dislocations require open reduction internal fixation, which involves stabilizing the fracture sites and repair of ligaments to facilitate early active ROM (Table 51-3).[13] Information obtained from the surgeon regarding healing status will determine if it is appropriate. Simple dislocations, in the absence of associated fractures, have a good long-term prognosis. Specific exercises for rehabilitation of elbow injuries and principles guiding prescription can be found elsewhere.[68]

Elbow Instability

Management of PLRI requires surgical repair, as they are unlikely to correct in the long term, once established. Avulsion of the MCL from the medial epicondyle may be managed through direct surgical reattachment. It is important to note the importance of the radial head as a secondary stabilizer against valgus forces in the elbow, and saving the radial head after dislocation should be considered to maintain valgus stability.[13,70]

There is no published literature comparing surgical and conservative management of ulnar collateral ligament injury. Generally, localized injury to the ulnar collateral ligament is initially treated non-surgically. However, throwing athletes with complete tears found on MRI are less likely to be rehabilitated successfully and surgical intervention might be considered earlier in these patients.[15] In their study of the outcome of conservative management of athletes with ulnar collateral ligament injury, Rettig et al.[93] found 42% were able to return to pre-injury level of competition after a minimum of 3 months rest and rehabilitation exercises, an average of 24.5 weeks after diagnosis (Table 51-3).

Much less is known about the role of conservative management of PLRI. If injury to the lateral collateral ligament complex is present, patients should avoid placing the arm in an abducted or internally rotated position to prevent varus opening of the elbow, which may impair ligament healing. Exercises in prone lying with external rotation of the shoulder should be avoided for the same reason. Study of the role of muscle contributions to elbow stability, indicates that biceps, triceps and the forearm muscles contribute to dynamic elbow stability by producing joint compression forces. Recent findings[77] suggest the medial elbow musculature mostly affects elbow stability with the arm in supination and

the lateral musculature in pronation, where the passive tension in the respective muscles is increased. Anconeus, which originates near the lateral epicondyle and inserts broadly onto the ulnar in a fan shape, seems designed to serve its major function as a dynamic stabilizer, particularly in the prevention of lateral or posterolateral instability.[14]

Lateral Epicondylalgia

Several high-quality RCTs have evaluated the efficacy of a multimodal programme of elbow mobilization with movement and exercise for lateral epicondylalgia, finding evidence of short-term benefit on pain and function.[46,94] No difference was found in the long term compared to either wait-and-see or placebo injection, in which approximately 93–100% of individuals enrolled in the trials reported complete recovery or much improvement at 1 year.

Systematic review of the effectiveness of manipulative therapy in treating lateral epicondylalgia[95] found the use of Mulligan's mobilization with movement effective in providing immediate, short-term and long-term benefits. A comprehensive description of techniques can be found in the following review papers, along with discussion of potential physiological rationales for immediate improvements in pain-free grip.[96,97] Immediate benefits have also been demonstrated using manipulative therapy directed at the cervical spine compared to placebo or control conditions,[95] while its addition to local elbow treatments was found to improve pain and disability at 6 weeks and 6 months compared to local elbow treatment alone.[95,98] A cross-sectional study of individuals with lateral epicondylalgia but without significant neck pain identified impairment on manual examination at C4–C5, C5–C6 and C6–C7 segmental levels in comparison to healthy controls.[99]

Several systematic reviews can be found evaluating exercise interventions for lateral epicondylalgia.[100–102] While they are in agreement that resistance exercise results in substantial improvement in pain and grip strength, optimal mode and dosing remains undefined. Eccentric exercise has been the most studied; however, there is no conclusive evidence of its superiority over other protocols.[102] A protocol of progressive resistance exercises is recommended as a part of a multimodal therapy programme and described in detail elsewhere.[68,79,80] The rationale for progressive loading is to improve local muscular strength and endurance as well as stimulating tendon remodelling.[103] It is recommended that loading commence in a pain-free capacity. This may be particularly important for individuals with severe pain and disability, who demonstrate widespread mechanical hyperalgesia and bilateral cold hyperalgesia.[82] Evidence of bilateral sensorimotor impairments and global upper limb weakness can be found in unilateral lateral epicondylalgia.[83,84,104,105] Based on these findings, a comprehensive exercise programme should incorporate retraining of wrist positioning during gripping, as well as address proximal strength deficits and scapulothoracic conditioning.

Posterolateral Impingement

Posterolateral impingement can be clinically confused with lateral epicondylalgia, potentially resulting in mismanagement and failure to respond to treatment. In contrast to lateral epicondylalgia, posterolateral impingement is more common in young adult athletes. The symptoms are non-specific, with pain located posterolaterally to the elbow, not directly over the lateral epicondyle or common extensor origin or muscle/tendon tissue, with or without symptoms of clicking or locking. If the patient does complain of clicking or locking, then other pathologies must be ruled out (e.g. loose bodies, instability or annular ligament injury).[57,58] MRI and computed tomography or magnetic resonance arthrography may be useful in the diagnosis of elbow synovial fold syndrome. Late diagnosis may result in mechanical degeneration of articular cartilage.[106,107] While several case reports describe successful outcomes following surgical removal of an inflamed or hypertrophied synovial fold,[106,107] few discuss conservative treatment options or prognosis. Anti-inflammatory medication, manual therapy and avoidance of aggravating activities, such as tennis or throwing, followed by a graduated return to these tasks are recommended. As in rehabilitation of epicondylalgia, exercise programmes should emphasize scapulothoracic posture and shoulder strength.

Medial Epicondylalgia

In the systematic review of manual therapy and exercise interventions by Hoogvliet et al.,[108] no study of medial epicondylalgia was found. Exercise prescription is currently based on that of lateral epicondylalgia, with emphasis on the wrist flexors and pronators rather than extensors. If present, concomitant ligament laxity or ulnar nerve irritation should be addressed.

Ulnar Neuropathy

The ulnar nerve is the most commonly affected nerve around the elbow and the second most common compression neuropathy in the upper limb, after carpal tunnel syndrome.[35] Compression of the nerve resulting in neuropraxia or neuropathic signs and symptoms is commonly related to repetitive or prolonged elbow flexion. Ulnar nerve involvement may occur secondary to medial elbow instability, after traumatic rupture of the MCL or chronic laxity as seen in throwing athletes.

Cochrane systematic review of treatments for ulnar neuropathy[109] found only one randomized trial of conservative treatment. This trial found that information on avoiding prolonged movements or positions that provoke symptoms was effective in improving subjective discomfort[78] (Table 51-3). None of the conservative treatments improved muscle strength. In another prospective study of patients with ulnar neuropathy, Beekman[52] found only 16% of affected arms were in complete remission, 28% had improved, 34% were stable and 22% were progressive after a median follow-up of 14 months. While not designed to investigate the most optimal treatment for patients with ulnar neuropathy at the elbow, they found that patients undergoing surgery more frequently reported a remission or improvement (61%) than those treated conservatively (35%).

Keefe and Lintner[3] provide guidelines for conservative treatment of early ulnar neuropathy in the throwing athlete. If symptoms recur despite an adequate period of conservative care, then surgery should be considered. They advise that the chance for success with conservative measures is smaller in individuals with multiple recurrences, and thus advocate decompression and ulnar nerve transposition sooner rather than later for the throwing athlete with multiple recurrences or chronic symptoms. Treatment of ulnar nerve injuries should start with consideration of the status of the ulnar collateral ligament as even minor laxity has been shown to contribute to ulnar nerve injuries in throwing athletes, and must be addressed to prevent recurrence.[3]

Radial Nerve Entrapment

In radial tunnel syndrome, the patient complains of pain that is deep and characterized as an ache. The pain is worse at night or after throwing, and is located just distal to the lateral epicondyle in the extensor muscle mass. There are rarely sensory or motor changes. In contrast to radial tunnel syndrome, PIN entrapment often occurs after a long history of lateral forearm or elbow pain followed by notable loss of PIN-supplied muscles, causing weak wrist extension with radial deviation. The differentiating feature between radial tunnel syndrome and PIN syndrome is the presence or absence of motor weakness. Given that motor weakness may be more a function of the severity rather than the location of compression, these two syndromes may be considered to be variants on the same pathology.[38]

Neurogenically mediated lateral elbow/forearm pain may be defined as a vague, diffuse, aching pain in the extensor muscles of the proximal forearm, possibly radiating into the dorsal aspect of the hand, or as a sharp shooting pain along the dorsal aspect of the forearm.[37] Pain is increased by resisted supination of the extended elbow. Tenderness can be elicited by palpation over the supinator muscle, approximately 4–5 cm distal to the lateral epicondyle. Electrophysiological tests are often inconclusive;[37] however, compression of the nerve as it passes through the supinator bundle may be confirmed through skilled ultrasound imaging (Fig. 51-1). A recent systematic review[110] found no RCTs concerning radial tunnel syndrome. As PIN entrapment may lead to permanent injury, the threshold for surgical release of the nerve is reported to be lower for this disorder than radial tunnel syndrome.[3] Non-operative treatment has been described for the throwing athlete (Table 51-3).[3] If there is no improvement after 3 months of conservative management, then surgical release can be undertaken.

CONCLUSION

Given the expanding knowledge base of the unique biomechanics of the elbow complex and the physiological changes that occur with both acute and chronic injuries, a review in this area is timely. This chapter identifies a need for more RCTs comparing different conservative approaches using standardized outcomes to optimise rehabilitation after elbow injury.

Acknowledgement

Dr Sanjay Dhupelia and Qld XRay (Australia) for provision of Figure 51-1 and technical advice on ultrasound imaging.

REFERENCES

1. Herquelot E, Bodin J, Roquelaure Y, et al. Work-related risk factors for lateral epicondylitis and other cause of elbow pain in the working population. Am J Ind Med 2013;56:400–9.
2. Hsu S, Moen T, Levine W, et al. Physical examination of the athlete's elbow. Am J Sport Med 2012;40:699–708.
3. Keefe DT, Lintner DM. Nerve injuries in the throwing elbow. Clin Sports Med 2004;23:723–42.
4. Mallen CD, Peat G, Thomas E, et al. Prognostic factors for musculoskeletal pain in primary care: a systematic review. Br J Gen Pract 2007;57:655–61.
5. Smidt N, Lewis M, Van Der Windt D, et al. Lateral epicondylitis in general practice: course and prognostic indicators of outcome. J Rheumatol 2006;33:2053–9.
6. MacDermid JC, Michlovitz SL. Examination of the elbow: linking diagnosis, prognosis, and outcomes as a framework for maximizing therapy interventions. J Hand Ther 2006;19:82–97.
7. Riedel K, Beaton DE. Update on the state of outcome measurement in total elbow arthroplasty research: identifying a need for consensus. J Bone Joint Surg Am 2013;95:e97 91–8.
8. Turchin DC, Beaton DE, Richards RR. Validity of observer-based aggregate scoring systems as descriptors of elbow pain, function, and disability. J Bone Joint Surg Am 1998;80:154–62.
9. The B, Reininga IH, El Moumni M, et al. Elbow-specific clinical rating systems: extent of established validity, reliability, and responsiveness. J Shoulder Elbow Surg 2013;22:1380–94.
10. Dowrick AS, Gabbe BJ, Williamson OD, et al. Outcome instruments for the assessment of the upper extremity following trauma: a review. Injury 2005;36:468–76.
11. Armstrong AD, MacDermid JC, Chinchalkar S, et al. Reliability of range-of-motion measurement in the elbow and forearm. J Shoulder Elbow Surg 1998;7:573–80.
12. Bano KY, Kahlon RS. Radial head fractures – advanced techniques in surgical management and rehabilitation. J Hand Ther 2006;19:114–35.
13. O'Driscoll S, Jupiter J, King G, et al. The unstable elbow. J Bone Joint Surg Am 2000;82:724–38.
14. O'Driscoll SW. Classification and evaluation of recurrent instability of the elbow. Clin Orthop Relat Res 2000:34–43.
15. Freehill MT, Safran MR. Diagnosis and management of ulnar collateral ligament injuries in throwers. Curr Sports Med Rep 2011;10:271–8.
16. O'Driscoll SWM, Lawton RL, Smith AM. The 'moving valgus stress test' for medial collateral ligament tears of the elbow. Am J Sport Med 2005;33:231–9.
17. Anakwenze OA, Kancherla VK, Iyengar J, et al. Posterolateral rotatory instability of the elbow. Am J Sport Med 2014;42:485–91.
18. O'Driscoll SW, Horii E, Carmichael SW, et al. The cubital tunnel and ulnar neuropathy. J Bone Joint Surg Br 1991;73:613–17.
19. Arvind CH, Hargreaves DG. Table top relocation test – New clinical test for posterolateral rotatory instability of the elbow. J Shoulder Elbow Surg 2006;15:500–1.
20. Cain E, Dugas J, Wolf R, et al. Elbow injuries in throwing athletes: a current concepts review. Am J Sport Med 2003;31:621–35.
21. Morrey B, An K, Stormont T. Force transmission through the radial head. J Bone Joint Surg 1988;70–A:250–256.
22. Broberg M, Morrey B. Results of treatment of fracture-dislocations of the elbow. Clin Orthop 1987;216:109–19.
23. Hotchkiss R. Fractures and Dislocations of the Elbow. Philadelphia USA: Lippincott-Raven; 1996.
24. Ring D, Jupiter J. Current concepts review. Fracture-dislocation of the elbow. J Bone Joint Surg Am 1998;80:566–80.
25. Azar F, Andrews J, Wilk K, et al. Operative treatment of ulnar collateral ligament injuries of the elbow in athletes. Am J Sport Med 2000;28:16–23.
26. Jobe F, Stark H, Lombardo S. Reconstruction of the ulnar collateral ligament in athletes. J Bone Joint Surg Am 1986;68:1158–63.
27. Feltner M. Three-dimensional interactions in a two-segment kinetic chain. Part II: application to the throwing arm in baseball pitching. Int J Sport Biomech 1989;5:420–50.
28. Fleisig G, Andrews J, Dillman C, et al. Kinetics of baseball pitching with implications about injury mechanisms. Am J Sport Med 1995;23:233–9.
29. Werner SL, Fleisig GS, Dillman CJ, et al. Biomechanics of the elbow during baseball pitching. J Orthop Sports Phys Ther 1993;17:274–8.
30. Butler D. Mobilisation of the Nervous System. Melbourne: Churchill Livingstone; 1991.
31. Elvey RL. Physical evaluation of the peripheral nervous system in disorders of pain and dysfunction. J Hand Ther 1997;10:122–9.
32. Nee RJ, Jull G, Vicenzino B, et al. The validity of upper-limb neurodynamic tests for detecting peripheral neuropathic pain. J Orthop Sports Phys Ther 2012;42:413–24.
33. Beekman R, Schreuder AH, Rozeman CA, et al. The diagnostic value of provocative clinical tests in ulnar neuropathy at the elbow is marginal. J Neurol Neurosurg Psychiatry 2009;80:1369–74.
34. Ochi K, Horiuchi Y, Tanabe A, et al. Shoulder internal rotation elbow flexion test for diagnosing cubital tunnel syndrome. J Shoulder Elbow Surg [AM] 2012;21:777–81.
35. Bonzentka D. Cubital tunnel syndrome pathophysiology. Clin Orthop Relat Res 1998;351:90–4.
36. Van Den Berg PJ, Pompe SM, Beekman R, et al. Sonographic incidence of ulnar nerve (sub)luxation and its associated clinical and electrodiagnostic characteristics. Muscle Nerve 2013;47:849–55.
37. Kotnis NA, Chiavaras MM, Harish S. Lateral epicondylitis and beyond: imaging of lateral elbow pain with clinical-radiologic correlation. Skeletal Radiol 2012;41:369–86.
38. Tennent T, Woodgate A. Posterior interosseous nerve dysfunction in the radial tunnel. Curr Orthop 2008;22:226–32.
39. Vrieling C, Robinson P, Geertzen J. Posterior interosseous nerve syndrome: literature review and report of 14 cases. Eur J Plast Surg 1998;21:196–202.
40. Lawrence T, Mobbs P, Fortems Y, et al. Radial tunnel syndrome. A retrospective review of 30 decompressions of the radial nerve. J Hand Surg B 1995;20:454–9.
41. Lister G, Belsole R, Kleinert H. The radial tunnel syndrome. J Hand Surg [Am] 1979;4:52–9.
42. Ferdinand B, Rosenberg Z, Schweitzer M, et al. MR imaging features of radial tunnel syndrome: initial experience. Radiology 2006;240:161–8.
43. Ritts G, Wood M, Linscheid R. Radial tunnel syndrome. A ten-year surgical experience. Clin Orthop Relat Res 1987;219:201–5.
44. Askew LJ, An KN, Morrey BF, et al. Isometric elbow strength in normal individuals. Clin Orthop Relat Res 1987;261–6.
45. Fess E. Grip strength. In: Casanova J, editor. Clinical Assessment Recommendations. Chicago: American Society of Hand Therapists; 1992. p. 41–5.
46. Bisset L, Beller E, Jull G, et al. Mobilisation with movement and exercise, corticosteroid injection, or wait and see for tennis elbow: randomised trial. Br Med J 2006a;333:939–41.
47. Helliwell PS, Howe A, Wright V. An evaluation of the dynamic qualities of isometric grip strength. Ann Rheum Dis 1988;47:934–9.
48. Smidt N, van der Windt DAWM, Assendelft WJ, et al. Interobserver reproducibility of the assessment of severity of complaints, grip strength, and pressure pain threshold in patients with lateral epicondylitis. Arch Phys Med Rehabil 2002;83:1145–50.
49. Stratford P, Levy D. Assessing valid change over time in patients with lateral epicondylitis at the elbow. Clin J Sport Med 1994;4:88–91.
50. Lim EC. Pain free grip strength test. J Physiother 2013;59:59.
51. Appelboam A, Reuben AD, Benger JR, et al. Elbow extension test to rule out elbow fracture: multicentre, prospective validation and

observational study of diagnostic accuracy in adults and children. BMJ 2008;337:a2428.

52. Timmerman LA, Schwartz ML, Andrews JR. Preoperative evaluation of the ulnar collateral ligament by magnetic resonance imaging and computed tomography arthrography. Evaluation in 25 baseball players with surgical confirmation. Am J Sport Med 1994;22:26–32.

53. Kim NR, Moon SG, Ko SM, et al. MR imaging of ulnar collateral ligament injury in baseball players: value for predicting rehabilitation outcome. Eur J Radiol 2011;80:e422–6.

54. Waldt S, Bruegel M, Ganter K, et al. Comparison of multislice CT arthrography and MR arthrography for the detection of articular cartilage lesions of the elbow. Eur Radiol 2005;15:784–91.

55. Levin D, Nazarian LN, Miller TT, et al. Lateral epicondylitis of the elbow: US findings. Radiology 2005;237:230–4.

56. du Toit C, Stieler M, Saunders R, et al. Diagnostic accuracy of power Doppler ultrasound in patients with chronic tennis elbow. Br J Sports Med 2008;42:572–6.

57. Cerezal L, Rodriguez-Sammartino M, Canga A, et al. Elbow synovial fold syndrome. Am J Roentgenol 2013;201:W88–96.

58. Huang G, Lee C, Lee H, et al. MRI, arthroscopy, and histologic observations of an annular ligament causing painful snapping of the elbow joint. Am J Roentgenol 2005;185:397–9.

59. Clarke A, Ahmad M, Curtis M, et al. Lateral elbow tendinopathy. Correlation of ultrasound findings with pain and functional disability. Am J Sport Med 2010;38:1209–14.

60. Beekman R, Schoemaker M, van der Plas J, et al. Diagnostic value of high-resolution sonography in ulnar neuropathy at the elbow. Neurology 2004;62:767–73.

61. Konin G, Nazarian L, Walz D. US of the elbow: indications, technique, normal anatomy, and pathologic conditions. Radiographics 2013;33:E125–47.

62. Yoon J, Hong S-J, Kim B-J, et al. Ulnar nerve and cubital tunnel ultrasound in ulnar neuropathy at the elbow. Arch Phys Med Rehabil 2008;89:887–9.

63. Beekman R, Wokke JH, Schoemaker MC, et al. Ulnar neuropathy at the elbow: follow-up and prognostic factors determining outcome. Neurology 2004;63:1675–80.

64. Alolabi B, Gray A, Ferreira LM, et al. Rehabilitation of the medial- and lateral collateral ligament-deficient elbow: an in vitro biomechanical study. J Hand Ther 2012;25:363–72.

65. Dodds S, Fishler T. Terrible triad of the elbow. Orthop Clin North Am 2013;44:47–58.

66. King G, Morrey B, An K. Stabilizers of the elbow. J Shoulder Elbow Surg 1993;2:165–74.

67. Davila SA, Johnston-Jones K. Managing the stiff elbow: operative, nonoperative, and postoperative techniques. J Hand Ther 2006;19:268–81.

68. Vicenzino B, Hing W, Rivett D, et al., editors. Mobilisation with Movement: The Art and the Science. Chatswood NSW: Elsevier; 2011.

69. Lockard M. Clinical biomechanics of the elbow. J Hand Ther 2006;19:72–80.

70. Morrey B. Instructional course lectures: complex instability of the elbow. J Bone Joint Surg 1997;79-A:460–9.

71. Armstrong A, Dunning C, Faber K, et al. Rehabilitation of the medial collateral ligamentdeficient elbow: an in vitro biomechanical study. J Hand Surg [Am] 2000;25:1051–7.

72. Pichora J, Fraser G, Ferreira L, et al. The effect of medial collateral ligament repair tension on elbow joint kinematics and stability. J Hand Surg [Am] 2007;32:1210–17.

73. Dunning C, Zarzour Z, Patterson S, et al. Muscle forces and pronation stabilize the lateral ligament deficient elbow. Clin Orthop Relat Res 2001;388:118–24.

74. Fraser G, Pichora J, Ferreira L, et al. Lateral collateral ligament repair restores the initial varus stability of the elbow: an in vitro biomechanical study. J Orthop Trauma 2008;22:615–23.

75. McKee M, Schemitsch E, Sala M, et al. The pathoanatomy of lateral ligamentous disruption in complex elbow instability. J Shoulder Elbow Surg 2003;12:391–6.

76. O'Driscoll S, Morrey B, Korinek S, et al. Elbow subluxation and dislocation. A spectrum of instability. Clin Orthop 1992; 280:186–97.

77. Seiber K, Gupta R, McGarry MH, et al. The role of the elbow musculature, forearm rotation, and elbow flexion in elbow stability: an in vitro study. J Shoulder Elbow Surg 2009;18:260–8.

78. Svernlov B, Larsson M, Rehn K, et al. Conservative treatment of the cubital tunnel syndrome. J Hand Surg Eur Vol 2009;34:201–7.

79. Coombes B, Bisset L, Connelly L, et al. Optimising corticosteroid injection for lateral epicondylalgia with the addition of physiotherapy: a protocol for a randomised control trial with placebo comparison. BMC Musculoskelet Disord 2009;10:doi:10.1186/1471-2474-1110-1176.

80. Pienimaki TT, Tarvainen TK, Siira PT, et al. Progressive strengthening and stretching exercises and ultrasound for chronic lateral epicondylitis. Physiotherapy 1996;82:522–30.

81. Navsaria R, Ryder D, Lewis J, et al. The Elbow-EpiTrainer: a method of delivering graded resistance to the extensor carpi radialis brevis. Effectiveness of a prototype device in a healthy population. Br J Sports Med 2013.

82. Coombes B, Bisset L, Vicenzino B. Thermal hyperalgesia distinguishes those with severe pain and disability in unilateral lateral epicondylalgia. Clin J Pain 2012;28:595–601.

83. Alizadehkhaiyat O, Fisher AC, Kemp GJ, et al. Upper limb muscle imbalance in tennis elbow: a functional and electromyographic assessment. J Orthop Res 2007;25:1651–7.

84. Bisset LM, Russell T, Bradley S, et al. Bilateral sensorimotor abnormalities in unilateral lateral epicondylalgia. Arch Phys Med Rehabil 2006;87:490–5.

85. Gao Y, Zhang W, Duan X, et al. Surgical interventions for treating radial head fractures in adults. Cochrane Database Syst Rev 2013. doi:10.1002/14651858.CD008987.pub2.

86. Wang Y, Zhuo Q, Tang P, et al. Surgical interventions for treating distal humeral fractures in adults. Cochrane Database Syst Rev 2013;doi:10.1002/14651858.CD009890.pub2.

87. Taylor F, Sims M, Theis J-C, et al. Interventions for treating acute elbow dislocations in adults. Cochrane Database Syst Rev 2012;doi:10.1002/14651858.CD007908.pub2.

88. Rafai M, Largab A, Cohen D, et al. Pure posterior luxation of the elbow in adults: immobilization or early mobilization. A randomized prospective study of 50 cases. Chir Main 1999;18:272–8.

89. Josefsson PO, Gentz CF, Johnell O, et al. Surgical versus nonsurgical treatment of ligamentous injuries following dislocation of the elbow joint. A prospective randomized study. J Bone Joint Surg Am 1987;69:605–8.

90. Kuntz DG Jr, Baratz ME. Fractures of the elbow. Orthop Clin North Am 1999;30:37–61.

91. Liow RY, Cregan A, Nanda R, et al. Early mobilisation for minimally displaced radial head fractures is desirable. A prospective randomised study of two protocols. Injury 2002;33:801–6.

92. Saati AZ, McKee MD. Fracture-dislocation of the elbow: diagnosis, treatment, and prognosis. Hand Clin 2004;20:405–14.

93. Rettig AC, Sherrill C, Snead DS, et al. Nonoperative treatment of ulnar collateral ligament injuries in throwing athletes. Am J Sport Med 2001;29:15–17.

94. Coombes BK, Bisset L, Brooks P, et al. Effect of corticosteroid injection, physiotherapy, or both on clinical outcomes in patients with unilateral lateral epicondylalgia: a randomized controlled trial. J Am Med Assoc 2013;309:461–9.

95. Herd C, Meserve B. A systematic review of the effectiveness of manipulative therapy in treating lateral epicondylalgia. J Man Manip Ther 2008;16:225–37.

96. Vicenzino B. Lateral epicondylalgia: a musculoskeletal physiotherapy perspective. Man Ther 2003;8:66–79.

97. Vicenzino B, Cleland JA, Bisset L. Joint manipulation in the management of lateral epicondylalgia: a clinical commentary. J Man Manip Ther 2007;15:50–6.

98. Cleland JA, Flynn TW, Palmer JA. Incorporation of manual therapy directed at the cervicothoracic spine in patients with lateral epicondylalgia: a pilot clinical trial. J Man Manip Ther 2005;13:143–51.

99. Coombes BK, Bisset L, Vicenzino B. Bilateral cervical dysfunction in patients with unilateral lateral epicondylalgia without concomitant cervical or upper limb symptoms: a cross-sectional case-control study. J Manipulative Physiol Ther 2014;37:79–86.

100. Cullinane FL, Boocock MG, Trevelyan FC. Is eccentric exercise an effective treatment for lateral epicondylitis? A systematic review. Clin Rehabil 2014;28:3–19.

101. Raman J, MacDermid JC, Grewal R. Effectiveness of different methods of resistance exercises in lateral epicondylosis – a systematic review. J Hand Ther 2012;25:5–25.

102. Woodley BL, Newsham-West RJ, Baxter GD. Chronic tendinopathy: effectiveness of eccentric exercise. Br J Sports Med 2007;41:188–99.

103. Coombes BK, Bisset L, Vicenzino B. A new integrative model of lateral epicondylalgia. Br J Sports Med 2009b;43:252–8.

104. Bisset LM, Coppieters MW, Vicenzino BT. Sensorimotor deficits remain at 12 months despite conservative treatment in patients with tennis elbow. Arch Phys Med Rehabil 2009;90:1–8.

105. Coombes B, Bisset L, Vicenzino B. Elbow flexor and extensor muscle weakness in lateral epicondylalgia. Br J Sports Med 2012a;46:449–53.

106. Antuna S, O'Driscoll S. Snapping plicae associated with radiocapitellar chondromalacia. Arthroscopy 2001;17:491–5.

107. Steinert A, Goebel S, Rucker A, et al. Snapping elbow caused by hypertrophic synovial plica in the radiohumeral joint: a report of three cases and review of literature. Arch Orthop Trauma Surg 2010;130:347–51.

108. Hoogvliet P, Randsdorp MS, Dingemanse R, et al. Does effectiveness of exercise therapy and mobilisation techniques offer guidance for the treatment of lateral and medial epicondylitis? A systematic review. Br J Sports Med 2013;47:1112–19.

109. Caliandro P, La Torre G, Padua R, et al. Treatment for ulnar neuropathy at the elbow. Cochrane Database Syst Rev 2011;CD006839.

110. Rinkel WD, Schreuders TA, Koes BW, et al. Current evidence for effectiveness of interventions for cubital tunnel syndrome, radial tunnel syndrome, instability, or bursitis of the elbow: a systematic review. Clin J Pain 2013;29:1087–96.

CHAPTER 52

WRIST/HAND

Anne Wajon

Achieving the best possible functional outcome following hand injury requires careful understanding of anatomy and pathology, together with a team approach involving the patient, therapist and surgeon. This chapter will integrate clinical reasoning into the assessment, diagnosis and management of a variety of common hand and wrist conditions. Emerging issues and new advances in the care of the hand-injured patient, providing directions that reflect advances in practice, will also be discussed.

While some hand conditions require immobilization for adequate tissue healing, many others will suffer from persistent stiffness if the hand is not permitted to move during the healing period.

PRINCIPLES OF ASSESSMENT

History

When assessing a patient with a hand or wrist complaint, it is essential to take a detailed history. This will enable the clinician to develop 'hypotheses about the probable location and type of pathology, the clinical symptoms to be treated, possible strategies to manage the problem, contraindications or precautions to examination and treatment procedures' (p 117).[1]

Mechanism of Injury

Identifying the mechanism of injury will help to establish the general direction and force applied to the hand during an injury, and identify the potential structures involved. Other patients will not be able to identify a mechanism of injury and may describe an insidious onset of symptoms. Careful questioning might reveal a contributing factor in their activities of daily living, such as a sudden increase in computer use or caring for a new child. Identification of these contributing factors will provide guidance for patient education in the long-term relief of symptoms.

Previous Injuries

It is also important to identify whether the patient has any underlying pathology or had suffered previous injuries to the affected hand. A history of waking with tingling in the fingers at night, joint stiffness following previous fracture, or pre-existing pain condition (or arthritis) will need to be taken into consideration when planning treatment goals and functional outcomes. The treatment strategy will need to consider all pathologies affecting the hand, particularly ensuring that any newly prescribed exercise programme will not aggravate a previous condition.

Clinical Context

Considering the importance of the hand in everyday life, particularly in relation to the patient's hand dominance, knowledge of their occupation, hobbies and sports is essential.

Does the individual have any special requirements that will help determine appropriate management? For example, will a young mother presenting with de Quervains syndrome be able to modify her postures and handholds when managing the baby to allow the condition to resolve?

Examination

It is essential to have a thorough understanding of the anatomical structures likely to be involved. It is beyond the scope of this text to review all structures involved; however, they will be discussed where relevant to the pathology being presented.

Inspection

Observing the hand at rest and during use will provide an invaluable insight. Considering that there is very little muscle or fat coverage on the hand and wrist, any local pathology can be identified by areas of discoloration (bruising/redness) and swelling. Further, inspecting for wasting of intrinsic muscles, presence of wounds and scars, and general bony alignment will be important.

Sensation

It is important to determine the location of any paraesthesia or numbness, as location of areas of altered sensation may be helpful in assessing for involvement of peripheral nerves. Further, it is possible to map recovery of sensation following peripheral nerve injury by using sensibility and manual muscle tests.[2]

Range of Motion

It is helpful to develop a routine sequence of movements in assessing the hand and wrist. This sequence may be altered if the patient complains of any exacerbation of symptoms. A finger goniometer is particularly useful in measuring the small joints of the hand.

The fingers should be measured for gross range of extension and flexion. However, if there is local pathology at the proximal interphalangeal joint of one digit, it might be appropriate to measure both gross and isolated range of motion. For isolated proximal interphalangeal joint measurements, measure proximal interphalangeal joint flexion with the metacarpophalangeal joint extended, and conversely, measure proximal interphalangeal extension with the metacarpophalangeal joint flexed. This will help eliminate involvement of the long forearm extensors and flexors in restricting joint range of motion.

Measurements of the thumb are more complicated because of the flexibility afforded by the carpometacarpal joint. The interphalangeal and metacarpophalangeal joints should be measured for extension and flexion, and the carpometacarpal joint measured for palmar and radial abduction, retropulsion (ability to lift thumb off the table) and opposition (ability to touch tip of little finger and slide down to distal palmar crease of little finger).

Measurements of the wrist include extension, flexion, radial and ulnar deviation. It is helpful to allow the fingers to curl while measuring wrist extension, and for the fingers to straighten when measuring wrist flexion, otherwise the long finger flexors and extensors will limit range of wrist motion. Additionally, measures of forearm rotation, pronation and supination, should be taken with the elbow positioned next to the waist. Either an inclinometer or regular small joint goniometer may be used.

Assessment of range of motion will contribute to determining whether the restriction is due to joint stiffness and muscle tightness, and additionally whether any of these movements reproduce the patient's pain.

Strength

Muscles are tested for isometric strength. The hand-held dynamometer is a reliable way to measure isometric forearm strength,[3] however it does not necessarily relate to overall hand function and task performance.[4] Standard assessment of grip strength involves the patient being seated with the arms by their side, the elbow flexed at 90°, and the forearm and wrist in neutral.[5] Traditionally, a hydraulic hand dynamometer is used, and the mean of three trials recorded. However a study comparing the reliability of one versus three grip strength trials found that one maximal trial is 'as reliable as, and less painful than, either the best of, or mean of, three trials' (p. 318).[6]

Pinch strength may be tested in three positions: tip pinch (two point), chuck pinch (three point) and lateral pinch. Results will vary according to the patient's age, sex, occupation and hand dominance. The dominant hand is usually stronger than the non-dominant hand, and it would be expected that patient's strength would improve as they progress through their rehabilitation.

Specific manual muscle testing can be performed to determine whether there is peripheral nerve involvement. A simple test for radial nerve function involves resistance of the extensor carpi radialis and extensor carpi ulnaris; for the median nerve abductor pollicis brevis, and for the ulnar nerve abductor digiti minimi.

Additional individual muscle tests may be indicated following a peripheral nerve laceration, in the presence of suspected nerve compression, or in the presence of limited range of motion in the hand. It may be appropriate to perform a full manual muscle test of the upper limb in certain conditions. Comprehensive texts are available which detail how this may be performed.[7]

Palpation and Provocative Tests

Palpation provides information regarding temperature, swelling, bony involvement, soft tissue thickening and pain, and will be useful in determining which structure(s) might be contributing to the patient's symptoms. This will further assist in determining which provocative tests are appropriate.

A number of provocative tests have been described to assist in the diagnosis of specific pathological conditions in the hand, wrist and elbow. To determine the usefulness of these tests, Valdes and LaStayo[8] performed a literature review and determined positive (LR+) and negative (LR–) likelihood ratios. They proposed that provocative tests with a LR+ ≥2.0, or a mean LR– of ≤0.5, from two or more studies that scored ≥8/12 on the MacDermid rating scale[9] would be highly recommended. Tests that met this criteria include Phalen's, Tinel's and modified compression test for carpal tunnel syndrome,[10] the scaphoid shift test for scapholunate instability,[11] and Tinel's and elbow flexion test for cubital tunnel syndrome.[12]

It is important to remember that provocative tests are not used in isolation, but considered in a clinical reasoning framework that incorporates subjective assessment, clinical intuition and experience.

Investigations

Plain radiographs are useful for assessing fractures, dislocations and osteoarthritis. Complex fracture anatomy is more clearly identified with computed tomography, whereas magnetic resonance imaging is indicated when there is a suspected subtle fracture or soft tissue involvement. In particular, magnetic resonance imaging is useful for investigations for scapholunate instability, triangular fibrocartilage complex (TFCC) trauma or occult ganglions. Ultrasound is helpful in the analysis of suspected soft tissue problems such as digital pulley injuries, tendon ruptures, ganglions or tendinopathy. Nevertheless, one should be cautious when interpreting imaging results as there can be a poor correlation between clinical symptoms and radiological findings.[13]

PRINCIPLES OF MANAGEMENT

Hand Therapy

Hand therapists are physical therapists or occupational therapists who incorporate patient education, exercise prescription, custom-made splints and casts, modalities, and attention to ergonomic and postural issues in their treatments. Their goal is to improve patient function and independence with work tasks, sports, hobbies and other activities of daily living.

Immobilization

Prolonged immobilization after finger fractures or joint injuries may result in persistent stiffness, chronic pain and deformity. It is recommended that an early motion programme that avoids re-stressing injured structures, be encouraged to prevent joint contracture and adhesions of the gliding soft tissues of the extensor and flexor tendons.[14]

It is recommended that the hand be supported in the intrinsic plus position, known as the 'position of safe immobilization', during fracture healing. This position involves metacarpophalangeal joint flexion of 60–90°, interphalangeal extension at 0° and the wrist in approximately 30° extension. The thumb should be positioned in mid palmar/radial abduction and the forearm in neutral, unless otherwise indicated. This position minimizes contracture of collateral ligament and joint capsular structures and addresses the 'ultimate functional demands of the hand requiring length and extensibility of the dorsal skin' (p. 6).[15] Not only is it essential that any splinting or casting does not include joints that do not need to be immobilized, but it is important that the fracture is sufficiently stable to allow early motion, otherwise complications of pain and persistent stiffness are likely to arise.[16] As swelling begins to subside it is important to reassess if the applied immobilization is continuing to provide adequate support or needs remoulding to ensure fit and avoid pressure areas.

Oedema Control

A fracture to the hand will injure adjacent and surrounding soft tissues, resulting in oedema that may contribute to persistent swelling and stiffness if not appropriately managed. Cold therapy has been shown to reduce pain at rest and with movement, and reduce functional disability when compared with placebo in a prospective randomized controlled trial of 74 patients with a sports-related soft tissue injury.[17] Additionally, rest, compression, elevation and protected mobilization can help to reduce oedema following acute injury or surgery.

Scar and Wound Care

Massage is performed to reduce adhesion of scars, assist in oedema reduction and reduce hypersensitivity. Patients are instructed to perform massage four to six times per day to the affected area. Additionally, various silicone products can be useful to flatten raised or thickened scars. Silicone gel sheets are available commercially and patients are instructed to wear them if appropriate at night for up to 3 months following surgery.

Exercises

Exercises are designed to regain full range of motion without causing any increase in pain or inflammation. Specific tendon gliding exercises[18] may be useful for maximizing differential tendon glide between flexor digitorum profundus and flexor digitorum superficialis (Fig. 52-1). It is important to educate patients to perform exercises carefully and accurately to avoid inadvertently compensating with unaffected joints.

MANAGING COMMON CONDITIONS

Fractures

Metacarpal and Phalangeal Fractures

Metacarpal and phalangeal fractures are relatively common in sporting injuries, and may result in considerable functional impairments, including pain, stiffness and weakness, if not managed well. It is essential to consider whether the fracture is stable, is in correct anatomical alignment, and whether there are any other associated soft tissue injuries. Mal-alignment of the fracture will result in mal-rotation of the digits, and this may interfere with the ability to return to full function.

Conservative treatment is appropriate if the fracture is stable, in good alignment and only minimally displaced. The hand may be splinted in the position of safe immobilization, supporting the adjacent digit and the joints above and below the fracture site.

Acute swelling may be controlled by cryotherapy, elevation and compression. The patient is instructed to begin pain-free active range of motion exercises immediately, and by 4 weeks, it is likely that a set of buddy straps will replace the splint for light activities. Generally it is advisable that the patient is instructed to continue using the splint for any sporting or at-risk activities until the 6-week time period. At this time, any residual stiffness or weakness should be resolved by specific blocking exercises, appropriate splinting and progression of a resisted strengthening programme.

Blocking exercises attempt to isolate the movement to the involved joint, and involve supporting the phalanx or metacarpal below the stiff joint. For example, holding the proximal interphalangeal joint in extension will facilitate isolated distal interphalangeal joint flexion exercise, alternatively holding the metacarpophalangeal joint flexed will facilitate active proximal interphalangeal joint extension. By 8 to 10 weeks, any persistent joint stiffness may be addressed by applying a dynamic splint that holds the stiff joint at the end of available range, for an extended period of time.[19]

If the fracture is unstable or rotated, or intra-articular at the proximal interphalangeal joint, it is advisable to refer the patient to a hand surgeon to discuss whether internal fixation is required.

Distal Radius Fractures

Distal radius fractures are common in the elderly, although they may occur in any age group. A dorsally displaced fracture is known as a Colles fracture, whereas a volarly displaced fracture is referred to as a Smith's type fracture.[20] Stable fractures in good alignment may be managed in a short arm cast; however, comminuted fractures with intra-articular involvement may require either closed or open reduction with internal fixation.

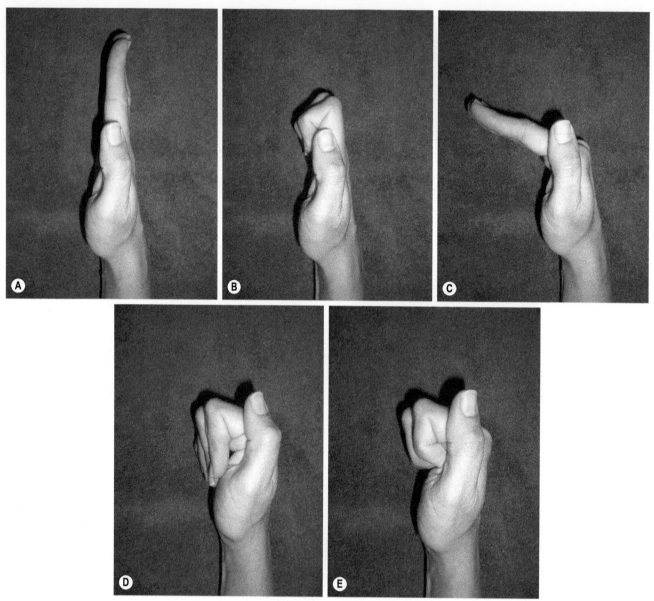

FIGURE 52-1 ■ Tendon gliding exercises.

During the period of immobilization, it is important that the patient exercises the uninvolved digits and is able to move the thumb, fingers and elbow freely within the cast. Once the cast is removed (usually at around 6 weeks post fracture) the patient should be instructed to perform a routine set of exercises, aiming to regain wrist extension and flexion, and forearm pronation and supination. Often the use of heat with stretch can facilitate the early return of motion once the cast is removed, and a graded programme of grip and forearm strengthening is helpful to improve strength and confidence with return to functional tasks.

Scaphoid Fractures

The scaphoid is the most commonly fractured carpal bone, accounting for 60% of carpal fractures and 11% of hand fractures in Norway.[21] Scaphoid fractures should be suspected in any cases where 'trauma involved the hand and/or wrist, particularly falls onto an outstretched hand' (p. 1370).[22] Initial radiographic findings may be reported as normal; however, tenderness in the anatomical snuffbox, accompanying swelling and loss of grip strength are suggestive of a scaphoid fracture and warrant presumptive casting and repeat radiography or a magnetic resonance imaging investigation after 10 to 14 days. Acute stable or incomplete fractures may be treated conservatively[23] by immobilization for 6 to 8 weeks. Subsequent radiographs must confirm fracture union before immobilization is discontinued and the patient started on a programme of exercises for regaining range of motion and strength. Although options for immobilization of scaphoid fractures include a long arm cast, a below-elbow cast or a scaphoid cast including the thumb carpometacarpal and metacarpal joints, current evidence suggests there is no advantage of any one particular cast over another,[24] and no significant difference in the rate of non-union between the various types of cast.[25] Based on the information available to date, it would seem reasonable for surgeons and therapists to continue to follow their casting preference. Alternatively, some patients may consider surgical treatment of non-displaced or minimally displaced fractures to achieve an earlier return to work, even though these short-term benefits may be associated with an increased risk of osteoarthritis.[26]

Unfortunately, the diagnosis of scaphoid fracture may be delayed, and non-union or malunion can result. This may lead to chronic pain, weakness and stiffness, ultimately leading to early osteoarthritis.[27] Internal fixation is appropriate in these individuals, as well as those with displaced scaphoid waist fractures, proximal pole fractures and fractures resulting in loss of carpal alignment.[28]

Tendon Injury

Mallet Injury

The most common injury to the distal interphalangeal joint of the digits is a mallet finger injury. Commonly people will complain that they were struck on the tip of the finger by a ball, or they 'caught' the finger when tucking in the sheets. The traumatic incident may be insignificant. The resultant loss of active extension of the distal interphalangeal joint (Fig. 52-2) is due to either a small avulsion fracture of the insertion of the extensor tendon, or a rupture of the tendon itself.

The mallet finger injury responds well to a period of conservative splinting. In the absence of a fracture, the distal interphalangeal joint is held in constant slight hyperextension for up to 8 weeks. If there is an avulsion fracture, the distal interphalangeal joint is held in neutral extension for 6 weeks. It is essential to remind the patient to continue to exercise the uninvolved proximal interphalangeal joint and to care for the skin. During the 6- to 8-week period of immobilization, the patient must maintain the extension force to the distal interphalangeal joint at all times, even if the splint is removed for skin care. Splinting options include a cylindrical-style thermoplastic splint or a dorsally based static distal interphalangeal

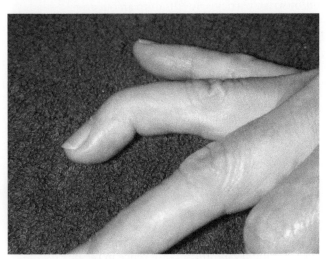

FIGURE 52-2 ■ Mallet finger deformity.

joint extension splint. A recent comparative study between these two different style splints identified an improved extension lag of 5° in the cylindrical group in comparison to the 9° lag after immobilization in a lever-type thermoplastic splint.[29] The amount of oedema, the patient's contribution to skin care and compliance with splint wearing, and the expertise of the therapist will determine which style of splint is appropriate for any given patient.

Boutonniere

A true boutonniere deformity of the finger presents with proximal interphalangeal flexion and distal interphalangeal hyperextension. It occurs following rupture of the central slip (extensor apparatus) on the dorsum of the proximal interphalangeal joint. The distal interphalangeal joint hyperextends as the lateral bands of the extensor mechanism sublux volarly at the proximal interphalangeal joint, and their extension force is transmitted to the distal interphalangeal joint. Acutely, the proximal interphalangeal joint is passively correctable into full extension, but left untreated, will ultimately develop into a flexion contracture with increasing proximal interphalangeal joint flexion. Patients presenting with this condition should be treated conservatively with 4 weeks in a splint that holds their proximal interphalangeal joint in full extension, while allowing the distal interphalangeal joint to flex. Subsequently, they may be managed with a Capener splint[30] that takes the extension load off the proximal interphalangeal joint, and allows the joint to move through a protected range of flexion.

Flexor Tendon – Flexor Digitorum Profundus Avulsion

The flexor digitorum profundus tendon may be avulsed at its insertion to the distal phalanx when a player is grabbing an opponent's jersey during a game of rugby or American football. As the opponent pulls or runs away, the distal interphalangeal joint is forcibly hyperextended, resulting in rupture of the flexor digitorum profundus tendon. The patient will report that they are unable to actively flex the distal interphalangeal joint. Active flexion of the proximal interphalangeal joint should not be affected due to the action of the FDS tendon. Patients presenting with this injury should be immediately referred to a hand surgeon for surgical intervention.

Joint Injury

Volar Plate Injury at the Proximal Interphalangeal Joint

The volar plate is a mobile, thick and fibrocartilaginous structure attached to the anterior margin of the base of the middle phalanx.[31] It is commonly injured when the joint is forced into hyperextension while attempting to catch a ball, and this results in a small avulsion fracture of the volar plate. Trauma to the volar plate may be successfully managed by a dorsal blocking splint to prevent the joint from being fully straightened for the first 3 weeks. Initially, the splint will be moulded to prevent the joint from extending in the last 20 to 30° of range, while the patient is encouraged to actively flex towards the palm. Alternatively, a custom-made thermoplastic figure-of-eight splint may be fitted.[32]

Each week, the splint is remoulded to allow a further 10° extension. By 3 weeks, the patient is encouraged to wear either the straightened dorsal splint or buddy straps for protection during sport and physical activities, until the 6-week time period. It is important that flexion exercises are performed during the early healing phase. By 6 weeks, blocked extension exercises can be added. Unfortunately, some people complain of persistent stiffness and may require dynamic splinting to regain full range of proximal interphalangeal joint extension.

Swan-neck Deformity

Chronic injury to the volar plate may result in a patient presenting with a 'swan-neck' deformity. This deformity of proximal interphalangeal joint hyperextension and distal interphalangeal flexion can lead to considerable functional handicap, making it difficult to flex at the proximal phalangeal joint during grasping activities. It can be managed by the application of a small 'figure-of-eight' splint that prevents the proximal interphalangeal joint from fully extending, while still allowing full flexion range.

Collateral Ligament Injury

The collateral ligaments of the proximal interphalangeal joint protect the joint from lateral force, and become increasingly tense with flexion of the joint.[31] Collateral ligament injuries are common with ball sports, and will result in a swollen, stiff and painful joint. Stress testing of the collateral ligament will reproduce pain and confirm whether there is any joint laxity. It is useful to assess integrity of the collateral ligaments at the proximal interphalangeal joint in full extension and slight flexion to help determine at which angle the joint is least stable. Conservative management includes oedema control with a compressive bandage, tendon gliding exercises and buddy straps to maintain the proximal interphalangeal joint in neutral deviation during motion. Although it may take 12 to 24 months for morning stiffness and residual swelling to resolve, most people will manage with little functional deficit.

Ulnar Collateral Ligament Injury of the Thumb

The metacarpophalangeal joint of the thumb is most commonly injured when a radially directed impact forces the thumb into abduction and hyperextension. The resultant injury to the ulnar collateral ligament is referred to as skier's thumb, as this is a common injury in this sport. Symptoms include local swelling, pain and tenderness to palpation, instability and weakness during pinch. Pain will be reproduced when stressing the ulnar collateral ligament by applying a valgus force to the metacarpophalangeal joint in extension and at 30° of flexion. A complete tear is diagnosed when there is no solid endpoint

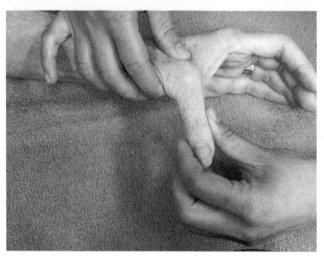

FIGURE 52-3 ■ Stress testing of ulnar collateral ligament injury.

(Fig. 52-3) on stress testing.[33] If it is associated with a Stener lesion, whereby the proximal end of the torn ligament flips out over the adductor aponeurosis, surgical repair will be required.[34] A postero-anterior stress radiograph with a difference of more than 15 degrees should be surgically explored for a Stener lesion.[35]

If there is laxity on stress testing, but a firm and painful end feel, it may be assumed that the patient has suffered a partial tear and can be managed with a custom-made thumb splint which prevents any radial force being transmitted to the metacarpophalangeal joint. It should be worn for up to 6 weeks, depending on the degree of laxity and pain with stress testing. The splint may be removed for gentle pain-free active range of motion and proprioceptive exercises. After the 6-week period of splinting the patient may be instructed to wean out of the splint, and while being careful to avoid any lateral stress to the metacarpophalangeal joint when out of the splint, they could begin pinch and grip strengthening with exercise putty. At this stage, they should be advised to continue with the splint during heavy lifting or gym work, or to use strapping tape to provide an intermediate amount of support while resuming sporting activities, possibly for up to 3 months.

Wrist Instabilities

Patients may present with wrist pain following either acute trauma or with a history of chronic pain related to overuse. The pain may be local or diffuse, and taking a thorough history and performing a careful examination will assist in determining which structures are contributing to their symptoms.

There are various degrees of instability and many structures that may cause pain, but for the purpose of this chapter, only scapholunate and ulnar carpal instabilities will be presented.

Scapholunate Ligament

The scapholunate ligament is commonly injured in a fall on an outstretched hand and will result in central dorsal wrist pain. Patients frequently complain that this pain is aggravated by weight bearing on an extended wrist. The scaphoid shift test[11] is commonly used to test for scapholunate instability. The examiner moves the wrist from ulnar deviation towards radial deviation while maintaining pressure with their thumb on the scaphoid tubercle. This stresses the scapholunate ligament and restricts the normal flexion that occurs during the movement from radial to ulnar deviation.[36]

As the scapholunate interosseous ligament is supplied by mechanoreceptors and ligamentomuscular reflexes, a new approach to rehabilitation for dynamic instability will incorporate proprioceptive retraining, specifically conscious training of muscles that protect the scapholunate joint and unconscious neuromuscular training incorporating joint stability and posture.[37] It has been identified that the dart-throwing motion is a stable and controlled plane of motion that results in less scaphoid and lunate motion than pure wrist flexion–extension,[38] while being a more functional plane of motion for most activities of daily living.

Rehabilitation of patients with a scapholunate ligament injury initially includes splinting for pain relief, and education regarding avoiding aggravating activities. Once the initial pain has begun to settle, it is appropriate to introduce proprioceptive awareness training including joint position sense and kinaesthesia. It is important to avoid any strong resisted gripping at this stage as this is only likely to increase gapping of the scapholunate ligament as the hand is compressed onto the carpus. Progression of proprioceptive and strengthening exercises will include isometric training, eccentric training, isokinetic training and co-activation based on Hagert's principles of conscious neuromuscular rehabilitation.[37] Late-stage rehabilitation should aim to 'restore the neuromuscular reflex patterns that exist in a normal joint' (p. 11) and may include training with a Powerball or slosh pipe (Fig. 52-4). These devices provide an unpredictable and multidirectional stimulus to the wrist, which requires a coordinated unconscious contraction of wrist agonists and antagonists.[37]

Distal Radio-ulnar Joint and Ulnocarpal Complex

Ulnar-sided wrist pain may occur following a sudden twisting injury to the wrist, with or without a fall. Stability of the distal radio-ulnar joint relies on both muscular and ligamentous restraints. Structures include pronator quadratus, extensor carpi ulnaris, interosseous membrane and the triangular fibrocartilage complex.[39]

Aggravating activities may include tennis or golf; however, it is not uncommon to develop ulnar-sided wrist pain following distal radius fracture. Additionally, occupational, degenerative or anatomical factors may contribute to ulnar-sided wrist pain.

Provocative tests for the TFCC include the TFCC stress test and the TFCC stress test with compression.[36] Both tests involve 'placing the wrist in ulnar deviation while applying a shear force across the ulnar complex of the wrist' (p. 249), while the TFCC stress test with compression additionally applies axial compression. However

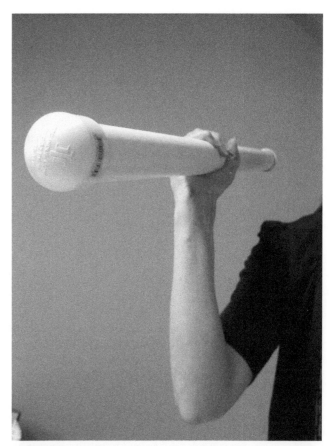

FIGURE 52-4 ■ Slosh pipe for scapholunate ligament instability.

a recent study investigating the accuracy of provocative tests for diagnosing wrist ligament injuries suggests that these tests have limited value,[36] although when combined with magnetic resonance imaging, the proportion of correct diagnoses improved by 13%.

Depending on the severity of symptoms, patients with ulnar-sided wrist pain may be managed with an ulnar carpal support attached to a soft wrist splint, which attempts to pronate the subluxed carpus.[40] Others find a 'WristWidget™' may be sufficient support, especially for those who find that wearing the brace while weight bearing through an extended wrist relieves their pain (http://www.wristwidget.com/protocol.html). For those with more persistent symptoms, it may be necessary to support the wrist and forearm in a thermoplastic wrist splint until symptoms begin to settle.

Patients with ulnar carpal instability should be instructed in the importance of activity modification, specifically to prevent loading the wrist in ulnar deviation, or extension and radial deviation which can place excessive traction on the ulnocarpal ligaments.[41] Exercises should aim to improve dynamic neuromuscular stability of the TFCC.

Considering the natural tendency when making a closed fist is for the carpal bones to supinate, increasing tension at the TFCC, treatment should concentrate on muscles that result in pronation of the carpus. A recent cadaveric study[42] concluded that the extensor carpi ulnaris tendon and its sheath offer dynamic stability for the wrist by providing a pronation effect on the distal carpal row.

Further, extensor carpi ulnaris may be considered the only dynamic stabilizer on the ulnar side of the wrist.[43] Exercises for neuromuscular control may include isokinetic, isometric, eccentric, co-activation and reactive muscle activation exercises.[37]

Osteoarthritis

The development of osteoarthritis may be considered the 'end-stage of a disease that originates in the tissues supporting the joint' (p. 278).[44] These structures include the cartilage, subchondral bone, synovium, ligaments, nerves and peri-articular muscles. Osteoarthritis frequently affects the small joints of the hand, and while most people over the age of 55 will have some radiographic changes consistent with osteoarthritis,[13] the correlation between severity of symptoms and radiographic changes is low.[45]

Thumb Carpometacarpal Joint

Pain at the base of the thumb is particularly common in postmenopausal women in the fifth to seventh decades of life.[46] It is frequently located either at the palmar surface of the trapeziometacarpal joint, or more dorsally, between the base of the first and second metacarpals. The pain is most often aggravated by opening jars, writing, turning taps and sustained grip activities; however, in cases of more advanced arthritis, it can also result in a constant dull aching pain. Radiographs may reveal joint space narrowing, sclerosis, articular debris and joint subluxation.[47] Severe (stage IV) joint degeneration will be associated with scaphotrapezotrapezoidal joint involvement and these patients will often complain of wrist pain along with pain at the base of the thumb. Careful palpation of the scaphotrapezotrapezoidal joint and trapezium, just distal to the scaphoid, will assist in determining the source of symptoms.[48] Further, axial compression and rotation of the first metacarpal on a stabilized trapezium (the grind test) is a recommended manoeuvre[8] for reproducing pain and crepitus at the joint.[48]

A variety of splinting options are available for patients with pain at the base of the thumb; however, there is no evidence to support the superiority of one over another.[49] In general, a more flexible neoprene style splint is appropriate for those with mild symptoms, and the rigid thermoplastic style splint is useful for those with more severe pain that limits most activities of daily living. The long opponens splint will be helpful for those with scaphotrapezotrapezoidal joint involvement as it supports the wrist, while the short opponens splint should suffice if the pain is limited to the carpometacarpal joint. Alternatively, the Colditz 'push' splint[50] or the three-point strap splint[51] may be useful for more specific task performance activities, including writing, stringed instrument playing and crafts.

While there is no evidence to support the superiority of one exercise programme over another, there is a general consensus that exercise may improve function, pain and strength.[49,52] Guidelines for the performance of exercises may be found in a recent narrative review by Valdes and Heyde.[53] They suggest that exercises should be pain-free and not lead to an aggravation of pain for more than 2 hours after the activity. A retrospective review of a dynamic stability approach to the treatment of this common condition reported a reduction in pain and disability scores with a combination of splinting, web space release, mobilizations to provide distraction and to reduce dorsal subluxation, first dorsal interosseous strengthening and taping.[54]

Anatomical studies have recently identified the presence of mechanoreceptors in the dorsal carpometacarpal joint ligaments,[55] supporting their proprioceptive role in enhancing joint stability. This has led the author to develop specific exercises for neuromuscular retraining, particularly concentrating on activities that address instability. These exercises include improving the patient's awareness and control of the alignment of their thumb while tracing along the line of a tennis ball with the tip of the thumb. It may be necessary to wear the small three-point strap splint[51] to prevent hyperextension of the metacarpophalangeal joint if they are unable to control this themselves (Fig. 52-5). Similarly, they may practice tearing sheets of paper while 'maintaining the thumb joints in an ideal arc',[56] incorporate use of chopsticks to improve joint position sense and neuromuscular control, or enhance stability by rotating a credit card in exercise putty.

The specific intervention that is appropriate for any given patient will depend on the severity of the patient's symptoms at the time, and their response to treatment provided. Failure of symptom relief with such conservative interventions may lead the therapist to consider whether graded motor imagery could be useful for chronic pain, as recent research has suggested

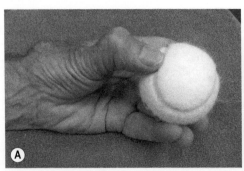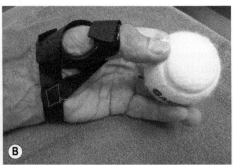

FIGURE 52-5 ■ Trace line on tennis ball for proprioceptive training **(A)**, but consider using three-point splint to control metacarpophalangeal joint alignment if necessary **(B)**.

sensitization mechanisms may contribute to symptoms in this population.[57] Surgery may be an appropriate intervention for ongoing debilitating pain and limitation of function.

Soft Tissue Conditions

Carpal Tunnel Syndrome

Carpal tunnel syndrome is the most common neuropathy,[58] affecting 3.8% of the population. Personal risk factors include being female, increased basal metabolic rate and age, while workplace risk factors included high job strain.[59] Patients usually present with nocturnal pins and needles and numbness in the median nerve distribution. Various tests may be used to assess for carpal tunnel syndrome, including Phalen's test, the hand elevation test, Hoffman-Tinel's sign, the carpal compression test and the tourniquet test.[10] An electrodiagnostic study of the median nerve may be considered the reference standard and is useful to exclude other diagnoses and stage the severity of carpal tunnel syndrome.[60]

Treatment approaches include nocturnal splinting with the wrist in neutral, and while it may be necessary to continue this for 6 weeks, it is likely that night splinting will provide immediate relief. Additionally, nerve and tendon gliding,[61] and median nerve sliding exercises[58] are considered helpful, as is education regarding aggravating postural factors. Constant tingling and numbness in the median nerve distribution, wasting of abductor pollicis brevis or failure of symptom relief with conservative measures will necessitate surgical review for consideration of decompression.

De Quervain's Disease

De Quervain's disease is the result of thickening of the first extensor tendon sheath, and is considered the result of intrinsic degenerative mechanisms.[62] It is common in young mothers and home renovators who perform repeated unaccustomed activities requiring sustained pinch or grasp with radio-ulnar deviation. The diagnosis of de Quervain's disease is made by history and physical examination. Symptoms include pain over the radial styloid, with tenderness and swelling of the first extensor compartment and reproduction of pain with resisted thumb extension or the Finkelstein's manoeuvre.[63] The Finkelstein's manoeuvre will reproduce pain at the radial styloid in affected people and involves the patient making a fist over a flexed thumb, and then moving the wrist into ulnar deviation.

Conservative intervention includes splinting in a custom-made thermoplastic splint, which immobilizes the wrist and thumb but allows interphalangeal joint motion, education regarding avoidance of aggravating activities and postures, and tendon and nerve glides. Gradual improvement in symptoms over a 4- to 6-week period of conservative intervention should be expected, and may lead the therapist to wean the patient into a flexible neoprene thumb and wrist support and progress into a neuromuscular rehabilitation programme. It is essential that activity modifications are maintained to prevent return of symptoms. Referral to a hand surgeon should be considered following failure of conservative intervention over a 6- to 12-week period, or the presence of bilateral symptoms. Other options include a corticosteroid injection or surgical release of the first dorsal compartment for more persistent and severe cases.

Trigger Finger

Trigger finger is more common in women in the fifth to sixth decades of life[64] and most commonly affects the thumb, middle and ring fingers in otherwise healthy individuals. The onset of triggering may be insidious, yet it has also been associated with direct trauma, de Quervain's disease, diabetes mellitus and osteoarthritis.[65]

Patients report a triggering or snapping sensation when they attempt to straighten their fingers from a full fist, but in more severe cases, find they are unable to straighten their finger without assistance from their other hand. Most cases are due to thickening of the digit's annular (A1) pulley, restricting the smooth glide of the flexor tendon through the fibro-osseous tunnel, and resulting in a nodule forming on the tendon sheath. This nodule moves proximally during flexion, but gets caught at the A1 pulley on extension.

Conservative management involves splinting the digit to prevent the friction of the tendon gliding through the A1 pulley. A small metacarpophalangeal joint blocking splint that permits IP joint flexion may be sufficient; however, if this small splint does not prevent clicking or locking with movement, a dorsal finger splint that immobilizes the proximal interphalangeal and distal interphalangeal joints may be required. Failure of a 6-week trial of splinting may indicate the need for a corticosteroid injection, which is considered effective and safe in the management of trigger finger.[66] Those who fail to achieve long-lasting relief with either splinting or a repeat steroid injection may require surgical release.

Complex Regional Pain Syndrome

Complex regional pain syndrome type 1 describes a population of patients who have incapacitating pain and impairment in function without an identifiable peripheral nerve injury. The resulting pain is often disproportionate to the severity of the injury and is associated with abnormal sensory, motor, sudomotor, vasomotor and/or trophic changes.[67] Emerging approaches to treatment include graded motor imagery,[68] incorporating left/right judgements, imagined movements and mirror therapy. Other approaches include sensorimotor retraining,[69] functional active exercises and neuroscience education.[70] A recent systematic review of neuroscience education has found positive effects on pain perception, disability and catastrophization, and may give patients the confidence to move without anxiety about causing further tissue injury.[70]

REFERENCES

1. Refshauge K, Latimer J, Maher C. The History. In: Refshauge K, Gass E, editors. Musculoskeletal Physiotherapy. Clinical Science

and Evidence-Based Practice. 2nd ed. Butterworth Heinemann; 2004. p. 117–63.

2. Skirven T, Osterman AL, Fedorczyk J, et al. Sensibility Assessment for Nerve Lesions-in-Continuity and Nerve Lacerations. 6th ed. Philadelphia, PA: Elsevier Mosby; 2011.

3. Bohannon R. Testing isometric limb muscle strength with dynamometers. Crit Rev Phys Rehabil Med 1990;2:75–86.

4. Herzberg G. Muscle Testing. In: Refshauge K, Gass E, editors. Musculoskeletal Physiotherapy. Clinical Science and Evidence-Based Practice. Butterworth Heinemann; 2004.

5. Fess E. Grip Strength. 2nd ed. Chicago: American Society of Hand Therapists; 1992. p. 41–5.

6. Codham F, Lewis J, Lee H. The reliability of one vs. three grip trials in symptomatic and asymptomatic subjects. J Hand Ther 2006;19(3):318–26.

7. Hislop H, Avers D, Brown M. Daniels and Worthingham's Muscle Testing. Techniques of Manual Examination and Performance Testing. 9th ed. St Louis, Missouri: Elsevier Saunders; 2014.

8. Valdes K, LaStayo P. The value of provocative tests for the wrist and elbow: a literature review. J Hand Ther 2013;26(1):32–42, quiz 43.

9. MacDermid JC, Wessel J. Clinical diagnosis of carpal tunnel syndrome: a systematic review. J Hand Ther 2004;17(2):309–19.

10. Amirfeyz R, Clark D, Parsons B, et al. Clinical tests for carpal tunnel syndrome in contemporary practice. Arch Orthop Trauma Surg 2010;131(4):471–4.

11. Watson H, Ashmead D, Makhlouf V. Examination of the scaphoid. J Hand Surg 1988;13:657–60.

12. Kroonen LT. Cubital tunnel syndrome. Orthop Clin North Am 2012;43(4):475–86.

13. Dahaghin S, Bierma-Zeinstra S, Ginai AZ, et al. Prevalence and pattern of radiographic hand osteoarthritis and association with pain and disability (the Rotterdam study). Ann Rheum Dis 2005;64(5):682–7.

14. Oetgen ME, Dodds SD. Non-operative treatment of common finger injuries. Curr Rev Musculoskelet Med 2007;1(2):97–102.

15. Wilton J. Hand Splinting. Principles of design and fabrication. Bath Press, Avon: WB Saunders Company Ltd; 1997.

16. Putnam M. Posttraumatic stiffness in the hand. Clin Orthop Relat Res 1996;327:182–90.

17. Airaksinen OV, Kyrklund N, Latvala K, et al. Efficacy of cold gel for soft tissue injuries: a prospective randomized double-blinded trial. Am J Sports Med 2003;31(5):680–4.

18. Wehbe MA. Tendon gliding exercises. Am J Occup Ther 1987;41(3):164–7.

19. Glasgow C, Tooth LR, Fleming J, et al. Dynamic splinting for the stiff hand after trauma: predictors of contracture resolution. J Hand Ther 2011;24(3):195–206.

20. Prosser R. The Wrist. In: Prosser R, Conolly WB, editors. Rehabilitation of the Hand and Upper Limb. Butterworth Heinemann; 2003. p. 109–75.

21. Hove L. Epidemiology of scaphoid fractures in Bergen, Norway. Scandinavian. Scand J Plast Reconstr Surg Hand Surg 1999;33(4):423–6.

22. Baldassarre R, Huges T. Investigating suspected scaphoid fracture. Br Med J 2013;346:1370.

23. Geissler W, Adams J, Bindra R, et al. Scaphoid fractures: what's hot, what's not. Instr Course Lect 2012;61:71–84.

24. Alshryda S, Shah A, Odak S, et al. Acute fractures of the scaphoid bone: systematic review and meta-analysis. Surgeon 2012;10(4):218–29.

25. Doornberg J, Buijze G, Ham S, et al. Nonoperative treatment for acute scaphoid fractures: a systematic review and meta-analysis of randomized controlled trials. J Trauma 2011;71(4):1073–81.

26. Buijze G, Doornberg J, Ham S, et al. Surgical compared with conservative treatment for acute nondisplaced or minimally displaced scaphoid fractures. J Bone Joint Surg 2010;92:1534–44.

27. Meyer C, Chang J, Stern P, et al. Complications of distal radial and scphoid fracture treatment. J Bone Joint Surg 2013;95A(16):1518–26.

28. Meermans G, Verstreken F. Influence of screw design, sex, and approach in scaphoid fracture fixation. Clin Orthop Relat Res 2012;470(6):1673–81.

29. Tocco S, Boccolari P, Landi A, et al. Effectiveness of cast immobilization in comparison to the gold-standard self-removal orthotic intervention for closed mallet fingers: a randomized clinical trial. J Hand Ther 2013;26(3):191–201.

30. Pratt A, Burr N, Grobbelaar AO. A prospective review of open central slip laceration repair and rehabilitation. J Hand Surg [Am] 2002;27B(6):530–4.

31. Palastanga N, Field D, Soames R. Anatomy and Human Movement: Structure and Function. 5th ed. Butterworth Heinemann Elsevier; 2006.

32. Laporte J, Berrettoni B, Seitz W, et al. The figure-of-eight splint for prominal interphalangeal joint volar plate injuries. Orthop Rev 1992;21(4):457–62.

33. Ritting A, Baldwin P, Rodner C. Ulnar collateral ligament injury of the thumb metacarpophalangeal joint. Clin J Sport Med 2010;20(2):106–12.

34. Samora J, Harris J, Greiesser M, et al. Outcomes after injury to the thumb ulnar collateral ligament – a systematic review. Clin J Sport Med 2013;23(4):247–54.

35. Fujiwara H, Oda R, Kubo T. Re-evaluation of stress radiographic findings for preoperative diagnosis of Stener lesion. J Hand Surg 2013;38(8):906–7.

36. Prosser R, Harvey L, LaStayo P, et al. Provocative wrist tests and MRI are of limited diagnositc value for suspected wrist ligament injuries: a cross-sectional study. J Physiother 2011;57(4):247–52.

37. Hagert E. Proprioception of the wrist joint: a review of current concepts and possible implications on the rehabilitation of the wrist. J Hand Ther 2010;23:2–17.

38. Moritomo H, Apergis EP, Herzberg G, et al. IFSSH Committee Report of Wrist Biomechanics Committee: biomechanics of the so-called dart-throwing motion of the wrist. J Hand Surg 2007;32(9):1447–52.

39. Hagert E, Chim H, Moran SL. Anatomy of the distal radioulnar joint and ulnocarpal complex. In: Greenberg JA, editor. American Society for Surgery of the Hand. 2013. p. 11–21.

40. Prosser R. Conservative management of ulnar carpal instability. Aust J Physiother 1995;41(1):41–6.

41. Moritomo H, Murase T, Arimitsu S, et al. Change in length of the ulnocarpal ligaments during radiocarpal motion: possible impact on triangular fibrocartilage complex foveal tears. J Hand Surg [Am] 2008;33(8):1278–86.

42. Salva-Coll G, Garcia-Elias M, Leon-Lopez M, et al. Role of the extensor carpi ulnaris and its sheath on dynamic carpal stability. J Hand Surg 2011;37:544–8.

43. Leon-Lopez M, Salva-Coll G, Garcia-Elias M, et al. Role of the extensor carpi ulnaris in the stabilization of the lunotriquetral joint. An experimental study. J Hand Ther 2013;26(4):312–17.

44. Hagert ELJ, Ladd A. Innervation patterns of thumb trapeziometacarpal joint ligaments. J Hand Surg 2012;37A:706–14.

45. Zhang W, Doherty M, Leeb BF, et al. EULAR evidence based recommendations for the management of hand osteoarthritis: Report of a Task Force of the EULAR Standing Committee for International Clinical Studies Including Therapeutics (ESCISIT). Ann Rheum Dis 2007;66(3):377–88.

46. Swigart C, Eaton R, Glickel S, et al. Splinting in the treatment of arthritis of the first carpometacarpal joint. J Hand Surg [Am] 1999;24A:86–91.

47. Eaton R, Glickel S. Trapeziometacarpal osteoarthritis. Staging as a rationale for treatment. Hand Clin 1987;3(4):455–71.

48. Skirven T. Clinical examination of the wrist. J Hand Ther 1996;9(2):96–107.

49. Wajon A, Ada L. No difference between two splint and exercise regimens for people with osteoarthritis of the thumb: a randomised controlled trial. Aust J Physiother 2005;51:245–9.

50. Colditz J. The biomechanics of a thumb carpometacarpal immobilisation splint. J Hand Ther 2000;13(3):228–35.

51. Wajon A. The thumb strap splint for dynamic instability of the trapeziometacarpal joint. J Hand Ther 2000;13(3):236–7.

52. Davenport BJ, Jansen V, Yeandle N. Pilot randomized controlled trial comparing specific dynamic stability exercises with general exercises for thumb carpometacarpal joint osteoarthritis. Hand Therapy 2012;17(3):60–7.

53. Valdes K, Von der Heyde R. An exercise program for carpometacarpal osteoarthritis based on biomechanical principles. J Hand Ther 2012;25:251–63.

54. O'Brien VH, Giveans MR. Effects of a dynamic stability approach in conservative intervention of the carpometacarpal joint of the thumb: a retrospective study. J Hand Ther 2013;26(1):44–52.

55. Hagert E, Mobargha N. The role of proprioception in osteoarthritis of the hand and wrist. Curr Rheumatol Rev 2012;8:278–84.
56. Colditz JC. Dynamic loading posture of the thumb: the Colditz tear test. J Hand Ther 2013;26(4):360–2.
57. Chiarotto A, Fernandez-de-Las-Penas C, Castaldo M, et al. Bilateral pressure pain hypersensitivity over the hand as potential sign of sensitization mechanisms in individuals with thumb carpometacarpal osteoarthritis. Pain Med 2013;14(10):1585–92.
58. Coppieters MW, Alshami AM. Longitudinal excursion and strain in the median nerve during novel nerve gliding exercises for carpal tunnel syndrome. J Orthop Res 2007;25(7):972–80.
59. Harris-Adamson C, Eisen EA, Dale AM, et al. Personal and workplace psychosocial risk factors for carpal tunnel syndrome: a pooled study cohort. Occup Environ Med 2013;70:529–37.
60. Boland RA, Kiernan MC. Assessing the accuracy of a combination of clinical tests for identifying carpal tunnel syndrome. J Clin Neurosci 2009;16(7):929–33.
61. Rozmaryn LM, Dovelle S, Rothman ER, et al. Nerve and tendon gliding exercises and the conservative management of carpal tunnel syndrome. J Hand Ther 1998;11(3):171–9.
62. Clarke M, Lyall H, Grant J, et al. The histopathology of de Quervain's disease. J Hand Surg [Am] 1998;23(6):732–4.
63. Batteson R, Hammond A, Burke F, et al. The de Quervain's screening tool: validity and reliability of a measure to support clinical diagnosis and management. Musculoskeletal Care 2008; 6(3):168–80.
64. Makkouk AH, Oetgen ME, Swigart CR, et al. Trigger finger: etiology, evaluation, and treatment. Curr Rev Musculoskelet Med 2007;1(2):92–6.
65. Nimigan A, Ross D, Gan B. Steroid injections in the management of trigger fingers. Am J Phys Med Rehabil 2006;85(1):36–43.
66. Peters-Veluthamaningal C, van der Windt D, Winters D, et al. Corticosteroid injection for de Quervain's tenosynovitis. Cochrane Database Syst Rev 2009;(3):1–19.
67. Harden RN, Bruehl S, Stanton-Hicks M, et al. Proposed new diagnostic criteria for complex regional pain syndrome. Pain Med 2007;8(4):326–31.
68. Moseley GL. Graded motor imagery is effective for long-standing complex regional pain syndrome: a randomised controlled trial. Pain 2004;108(1–2):192–8.
69. Flor H, Diers M. Sensorimotor training and cortical reorganization. NeuroRehabilitation 2009;25:19–27.
70. Louw A, Diener I, Butler DS, et al. The effect of neuroscience education on pain, disability, anxiety, and stress in chronic musculoskeletal pain. Arch Phys Med Rehabil 2011;92(12): 2041–56.

PART V

FUTURE DIRECTIONS

CHAPTER 53

FUTURE DIRECTIONS IN RESEARCH AND PRACTICE

Gwendolen Jull • Ann Moore • Deborah Falla •
Jeremy Lewis • Christopher McCarthy • Michele Sterling

For much of the 20th century, musculoskeletal conditions were not the pre-eminent concern of Western governments or health-funding bodies nor were they a funding priority area for health-care research. This is understandable as other diseases such as diphtheria, chicken pox, small pox, measles, tuberculosis, pertussis, pneumococcal disease, polio, tetanus, thyroid and others were of far more concern. We now live in a very different world. Vaccines have controlled many of the diseases of the early part of the century. Life expectancy in the United States at the beginning of the 20th century was 47 years and by the end was approaching 78 years. The impact of musculoskeletal disorders grew.

The magnitude of the problem of musculoskeletal conditions was effectively brought to prominence, and the World Health Organization (WHO) established the Bone and Joint Decade 2000–2010 which, notably, has been extended for another decade (Bone and Joint Decade 2010–2020). As one outcome of this worldwide initiative, the Global Burden of Disease study confirmed the immense burden associated with musculoskeletal conditions across all developed and developing countries.[1] Such evidence as well as WHO initiatives has drawn attention to musculoskeletal disorders internationally, generated momentum in research and is changing health attitudes and policies. Musculoskeletal disorders are a major cause of pain, physical disability and attendant distress. Frequently they have a profound and detrimental impact on an individual's quality of life. They are a major reason for health-related work absence and as such, have a substantial detrimental impact on countries' economies, both in terms of lost productivity and the percentage of gross domestic product spent on managing these conditions. Musculoskeletal conditions are rarely a direct cause of death, but as exercise is considered to be essential in the treatment of common illnesses such as obesity, diabetes, cancer, depression, anxiety and stress and cardiorespiratory disease, the lack of mobility associated with musculoskeletal pathology will directly contribute to the morbidity and mortality associated with these diseases. With an ageing and more sedentary population the impact of these problems experienced by the individual will increase exponentially.

Physiotherapists with their body of knowledge, clinical and research expertise are perfectly placed to rise to the challenges and make a significant contribution to enhancing the prevention and management of musculoskeletal disorders. Many have already done so by contributing to high-quality musculoskeletal research that is being used to address these issues and inform health-care policy. The work presented in this text is testament to some of the research currently being undertaken internationally. However, there is still a significant amount of work to be completed across the spectrum of health-care provision (primary, secondary and tertiary rehabilitation) to provide more effective management and treatments for musculoskeletal conditions.

Physiotherapists working with other health-care colleagues need to develop innovative ways to prevent musculoskeletal disease to reduce the burden and detriment of musculoskeletal disease experienced by individuals and society, with primary prevention being the ideal. Physiotherapists in clinical, community, work, sport, education or research environments are well placed to contribute to population health initiatives such as promoting active lifestyles to optimize musculoskeletal health at all stages of life. However, there are still substantial gaps in our knowledge regarding both the optimal and valid methods of physical screening towards primary prevention of injury or overuse syndromes for a range of individuals, from those trying to maintain the desired fitness level and healthy lifestyle to those involved in competitive sport. Likewise conclusive knowledge as to what constitutes the safest and the most effective means of staying active and promoting musculotendinous health across all ages and co-morbidities without detrimentally impacting on these tissues remains elusive.

Physiotherapists have a large stake in secondary prevention of painful musculoskeletal disorders and much laboratory and clinical research has already been undertaken into the neurosciences, pathokinesiology and pathophysiology towards development of optimal management methods. Knowledge has grown enormously and therapeutics have improved. However, the results from randomized controlled trials reveal that the effect sizes of most treatments are, at best, modest for most conditions. The heterogeneity of patient presentations within a diagnostic category (e.g. subacute low back pain, shoulder impingement syndrome) is held to contribute to these poor to modest mean group outcomes when all individuals are managed with the same treatment regimen. It is now well known that the relative contribution of sensory, motor, psychological and social mechanisms in a patient's pain condition will vary considerably between individuals, and different mechanisms will have different weighting at any point in time. This heterogeneity has spurred interest into concepts of subgrouping and, over the last decade, creation of clinical prediction rules to try to best fit the intervention to the patient. The notion that one treatment fits all sizes has been dispelled. However, it could be questioned if we are yet even aware of all of the criteria on which individuals should be characterized towards prescribing a particular intervention. More research is required across the spectrum 'from bench top to bedside'. More knowledge is required about, for example, the role of genetics and an individual's biological make-up with respect to propensity for musculoskeletal disorders and chronic pain; how biological and psychosocial features interrelate and how they might moderate or mediate a painful musculoskeletal disorder. In persistent spinal pain, there has been somewhat of a dismissal of the presence of ongoing peripheral sources of nociception. Yet, for instance, in the case of chronic whiplash-associated disorders, this position is proving to be inaccurate. Nevertheless further research is necessary to understand the role that peripheral sources of nociception play in a patient's pain, disability and psychological distress. This is becoming more feasible with advanced imaging and diagnostic techniques continuing to develop. Physiotherapy management is not the panacea for all musculoskeletal ills and more clarity is required to clearly understand which sensory, movement, neuromuscular and sensorimotor features are able to be modified by physiotherapy management strategies and what features may mitigate against a successful outcome from these treatment approaches.

There has been a tendency to regard each episode of musculoskeletal pain as a new acute episode. What has become clear is that musculoskeletal disorders and especially spinal pain are usually recurrent in nature over several decades of an individual's life, if not a lifetime. Similarly, it is well recognized that when a joint such as the knee is subjected to significant trauma, the arthritic process may be initiated prematurely. Thus it is considered a necessary step to view musculoskeletal disorders as likely recurrent and progressive disorders, not as repetitions of an acute episode, if effective rehabilitation programmes are to be designed. Thus an important focus for future rehabilitation practices and research is the prevention of recurrence or transition to chronicity and, with our ageing population, effective methods to slow disease progression. This opens questions such as what can physical interventions achieve against certain disease markers, what 'dosages' of exercise are required to achieve the required change in neuromuscular control, will the training produce permanent change, or does the brain have to be constantly tuned with a maintenance programme?

Tertiary prevention is a vital area to optimize an individual's quality of life and lower the personal and financial burden of persistent or progressive musculoskeletal disorders in our ageing populations. The areas of education, self-management programmes and maintenance care become important strategies to refine and optimize their effect. More attention needs to be given to patient perspectives through qualitative research. For example, there is a need to ensure that differences in therapists' and patients' perspectives of self-management

are understood, recognized and articulated in order for self-management programmes to be more effectively utilized and tailored to particular needs. There are many 'topics' within education but it still remains to be determined what is the most effective education/advice that individuals require for certain conditions or circumstances and which produce best outcomes, especially in terms of enhanced quality of life. Likewise, there is a range of face-to-face and electronic channels to deliver education at a group or individual basis, but the best ways and the best times to deliver this intervention for education or self-management strategies to have the greatest impact has not yet been established. It is likewise not known which models of care best slow musculoskeletal disease progression, but it is anticipated that it will be a multimodal model, for example, education, exercise, various aides/supports and pharmacological interventions. How delivery affects models of care needs to be questioned. For example, will extended personal contact with patients with chronic musculoskeletal disorders decrease distress and increase their compliance with activity and exercise. Benefits of this low-cost approach to-long-term care have been shown with other chronic diseases, but is yet to be proven with musculoskeletal disorders.

Research may inform new directions in management, but ensuring that the evidence translates to a change in practice is a challenge faced by all professionals. It behoves institutions training future generations of physiotherapists to design and deliver contemporary curricula and ensure that their graduates are intelligent consumers of research and well skilled in communication, educational approaches and research-informed therapeutics. Knowledge is being generated at a rapid pace. As well as research to generate knowledge, research is also required to determine the best methods of delivery of continuing professional development for practicing clinicians to ensure this knowledge is translated into practice, and results in changes in practice behaviour and improved patients outcomes. Continuing professional development for physiotherapists has some unique challenges especially regarding expert physical skill acquisition to implement new assessment or management practices.

This fourth edition of *Grieve's Modern Musculoskeletal Physiotherapy* is evidence of a vibrant research and clinical culture in the field of musculoskeletal disorders internationally. There is no doubt that mechanistic and clinical research have progressed the field substantially in the last decade. The aim for the next decade of research is to build on this knowledge and further refine practices so that the outcome is a notable reduction in the burden of musculoskeletal disease across all developed and developing countries.

REFERENCE

1. Lim SS, Vos T, Flaxman AD, et al. A comparative risk assessment of burden of disease and injury attributable to 67 risk factors and risk factor clusters in 21 regions, 1990–2010: a systematic analysis for the Global Burden of Disease Study 2010. Lancet 2012; 380(9859):2224–60.

Page numbers followed by 'f' indicate
figures, 't' indicate tables, and 'b' indicate
boxes.

611